AF251672

CANCER AND THE HEART

Third Edition

CANCER AND THE HEART

Third Edition

Michael S. Ewer, MD, JD, PhD
Professor, Department of Cardiology
The University of Texas MD Anderson Cancer Center
Houston, Texas

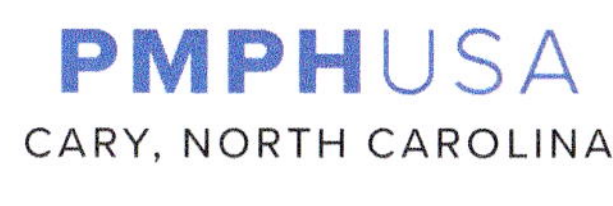

PMPHUSA
CARY, NORTH CAROLINA
2019

PMPH USA, Ltd.

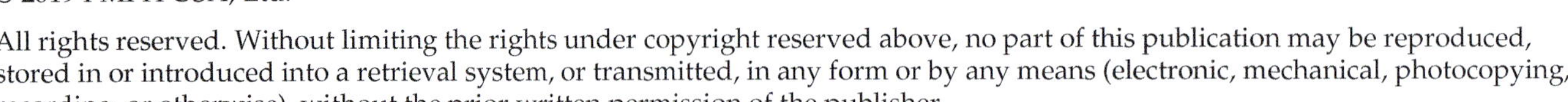

1140 Kildaire Farm Road, Suite 200-5
Cary, NC 27511
Tel: 919-502-4220
Fax: 919-502-7673
E-mail: info@pmph-usa.com

© 2019 PMPH USA, Ltd.

All rights reserved. Without limiting the rights under copyright reserved above, no part of this publication may be reproduced, stored in or introduced into a retrieval system, or transmitted, in any form or by any means (electronic, mechanical, photocopying, recording, or otherwise), without the prior written permission of the publisher.

19 20 21 22/KING/9 8 7 6 5 4 3 2 1

ISBN-13   978-1-60795-297-8
ISBN-10   1-60795-297-1
eISBN-13   978-1-60795-964-9

Printed in the United States of America by King Printing.
Editor: Linda H. Mehta; Copyeditor/Typesetter: diacriTech; Cover designer: Allison Dibble

Library of Congress Cataloging-in-Publication Data

Names: Ewer, Michael S., editor.

Title: Cancer and the heart / [edited by] Michael S. Ewer.

Other titles: Cancer and the heart (Ewer)

Description: Third edition. | Raleigh, North Carolina : PMPH USA, 2019. |
    Includes bibliographical references and index.

Identifiers: LCCN 2019019282 (print) | LCCN 2019020122 (ebook) |
    ISBN 9781607959649 (ebook) | ISBN 9781607952978 (hardcover) | ISBN 1607952971
    (hardcover) | ISBN 9781607959649 (eISBN)

Subjects: | MESH: Heart Diseases—etiology | Heart—drug effects |
    Heart—radiation effects | Neoplasms—complications | Neoplasms—therapy |
    Cardiotoxicity—complications

Classification: LCC RC280.H45 (ebook) | LCC RC280.H45 (print) | NLM WG 210 |
    DDC 616.1/207—dc23

LC record available at https://lccn.loc.gov/2019019282

Sales and Distribution

Canada
Login Canada
300 Saulteaux Cr.
Winnipeg, MB R3J 3T2
Phone: 1.800.665.1148
Fax: 1.800.665.0103
www.lb.ca

Foreign Rights
John Scott & Company
International Publisher's Agency
P.O. Box 878
Kimberton, PA 19442, USA
Tel: 610-827-1640
Fax: 610-827-1671
rights@johnscottco.us

*United Kingdom, Europe, Middle East,
Africa, Singapore, Thailand, Philippines,
Indonesia, Vietnam, Pacific Rim, Korea,*

*Australia, New Zealand, Papua New
Guinea, Fiji, Tonga, Solomon Islands,
Cook Islands, Malaysia*
Eurospan Limited
3, Henrietta Street, Covent Garden
London WC2E 8LU, UK
Tel: Within the UK: 0800 526830
Outside UK: +44 (0)20 7845 0868
http://www.eurospanbookstore.com

*India, Bangladesh, Pakistan, Sri Lanka,
Nepal*
**Jaypee Brothers Medical Publishers
Pvt. Ltd.**
4838, 24 Ansari Road
Darya Ganj
New Delhi- 110002, India
Phone: +91 11 23272143
Fax: +91 11 23276490
www.jaypeebrothers.com

People's Republic of China
People's Medical Publishing House
International Trade Department
No. 19, Pan Jia Yuan Nan Li
Chaoyang District
Beijing 100021, P.R. China
Tel: 8610-67653342
Fax: 8610-67691034
www.pmph.com/en

Notice: The authors and publisher have made every effort to ensure that the patient care recommended herein, including choice of drugs and drug dosages, is in accord with the accepted standard and practice at the time of publication. However, since research and regulation constantly change clinical standards, the reader is urged to check the product information sheet included in the package of each drug, which includes recommended doses, warnings, and contraindications. This is particularly important with new or infrequently used drugs. Any treatment regimen, particularly one involving medication, involves inherent risk that must be weighed on a case-by-case basis against the benefits anticipated. The reader is cautioned that the purpose of this book is to inform and enlighten; the information contained herein is not intended as, and should not be employed as, a substitute for individual diagnosis and treatment.

Dedication

To the many thousands of patients, each of whom helps us as the knowledge base that ultimately gave rise to *Cancer and the Heart* evolves. Their courage and dedication as they face serious disease and the effects of harsh treatments continues to drive our efforts to learn from them.

To our colleagues who provide us with continued support and helpful criticism as we bring new ideas, insights, and concepts to *Cancer and the Heart*.

And to our families and friends who have endured our preoccupation regarding the creation of this new edition of *Cancer and the Heart*. They have stood by us as we searched, researched, wrote, edited, and ultimately will bask in the pride of another edition that culminates this huge effort.

A special thank you for Teresa Diez who worked with exceptional diligence as the various manuscripts and graphics arrived, evolved, and eventually were deemed "finished."

—**Michael S. Ewer, MD, JD, PhD**

Contents

Contributors...*ix*

Foreword ....*xv*

Preface...*xvii*

Chapter 1. Principles of Oncologic Chemotherapy and Immunotherapy *by* Luis E. Fayad, Alison Woo, and Larry W. Kwak 1

Chapter 2. Pharmacology of Cardio-Oncology *by* Emanuela Salvatorelli, Pierantonio Menna, and Giorgio Minotti 11

Chapter 3. Anthracycline Cardiotoxicity: Clinical Aspects, Recognition, Monitoring, Treatment, and Prevention *by* Michael S. Ewer 47

Chapter 4. Trastuzumab-Associated Cardiotoxicity *by* Thomas M. Suter and Michael S. Ewer 79

Chapter 5. Mechanisms of Anti-HER2 Cardiotoxicity: Interference with Neuregulin-1 Cardioprotective Signaling *by* Zarha Vermeulen, Vincent Segers, and Gilles W. De Keulenaer 89

Chapter 6. Checkpoint Inhibitors *by* Lavanya Kondapalli, Rupal O'Quinn, and Joseph R. Carver 103

Chapter 7. Effects of Radiation Therapy on the Cardiovascular System *by* David J. Cutter, Carolyn W. Taylor, Kazem Rahimi, Paul McGale, Vanessa Ferreira, Matthew Burrage, Sindu Vivekanandan, Maria Hawkins, and Sarah C. Darby...119

Chapter 8. Cardiac Amyloidosis *by* Syed Wamique Yusuf.......................................185

Chapter 9. Cardiac Arrhythmias in the Cancer Patient *by* Asif Jafferani, Syed Wamique Yusuf, and Steven M. Ewer 197

Chapter 10. Cardiac Ultrasonography, Doppler Imaging, and Related Techniques for Cancer Patients *by* Jose Banchs and Thomas H. Marwick 219

Chapter 11. Diagnosis of Cardiac Tumors *by* Ali Agha, Purvi Parwani, and Juan C. Lopez-Mattei.......................................237

Chapter 12. Pericardial Disease in the Cancer Patient *by* Steven M. Ewer................................243

Chapter 13. Arterial and Venous Thromboembolic Diseases in Cancer Patients *by* Elie Mouhayar...263

Chapter 14. Cardiac Tumors *by* Daniel Perry, Monika Leja, Scott Schuetze, Shanda H. Blackmon, and Michael J. Reardon 279

Chapter 15. Carcinoid Heart Disease *by* Saamir A. Hassan 309

Chapter 16. Cardiac Monitoring During Clinical Trials *by* Nicolas Palaskas and Michael S. Ewer 315

Chapter 17. Cardiovascular Toxicity of Antiangiogenic Therapy: Mechanisms and Management by Divyanshu Mohananey, Rohit Kumar, and Tochi M. Okwuosa.................................329

Chapter 18. Heart–Lung Interactions in the Cancer Patient *by* Vickie R. Shannon and Saadia A. Faiz.....................................351

Chapter 19. Cardiac Emergencies Among Cancer Patients *by* Carmen P. Escalante and Sai-Ching Jim Yeung.................................423

Chapter 20. Cardiac Considerations for Treating Cancer in Infants and Children *by* Neha Bansal, Rofida Nofal, Sanjeev Aggarwal, Vivian I. Franco, Emma R. Lipshultz, Stephen E. Sallan, and Steven E. Lipshultz...447

Chapter 21. Infectious Endocarditis in Cancer Patients *by* Eduardo Yepez Guevara, Jose Banchs, David J. Tweardy, and Javier Adachi 477

Chapter 22. Magnetic Resonance Imaging and Therapeutic Radiation in Cancer Patients with Implanted Pacemaker or Defibrillator Devices *by* Kaveh Karimzad...491

Chapter 23. Cardiovascular Interventions for Cancer Patients *by* Ezequiel Muñoz, Brian Greet, Konstantinos Marmagkiolis, and Cezar Iliescu...501

Chapter 24. Psychosocial Considerations in Treating the Cancer Patient with Heart Disease *by* Anecita P. Fadol 527

Chapter 25. Preoperative Assessment of the Cancer Patient for Noncardiovascular Surgery *by* Marc A. Rozner, Shital Vachhani, Teresa Moon, and January Y. Tsai......543

Chapter 26. Advanced Heart Failure in Patients with Cancer *by* Sadeer G. Al-Kindi and Guilherme H. Oliveira............................561

Chapter 27. Pregnancy and the Heart in Cancer Patients and Survivors *by* Kara A. Thompson 587

Chapter 28. Exercise in the Cancer Patient: Cardiac Considerations *by* Susan C. Gilchrist 599

Index 607

Contributors

Javier Adachi, MD [21]
Professor
Department of Infectious Diseases, Infection Control,
  and Employee Health
Division of Internal Medicine
The University of Texas MD Anderson Cancer Center
Houston, Texas

Sanjeev Aggarwal, MD [20]
Associate Professor
Wayne State University School of Medicine
Children's Hospital of Michigan
Detroit, Michigan

Ali Agha, MD [11]
Department of Internal Medicine
University of Texas Health Science Center at Houston
Houston, Texas

Sadeer G. Al-Kindi, MD [26]
Advanced Heart Failure and Transplantation Center
  and Onco-Cardiology Program
Harrington Heart & Vascular Institute
University Hospitals Cleveland Medical Center
Case Western Reserve University School of Medicine
Cleveland, Ohio

Jose Banchs, MD [10, 21]
Associate Professor
Department of Cardiology
Division of Internal Medicine
The University of Texas MD Anderson Cancer Center
Houston, Texas

Neha Bansal, MD [20]
Associate Professor
Wayne State University School of Medicine
Children's Hospital of Michigan
Detroit, Michigan

Shanda H. Blackmon, MD, MPH [14]
Department of Thoracic Surgery
Mayo Clinic
Rochester, Minnesota

Matthew Burrage, MBBS, FRACP [7]
Oxford Centre for Clinical Magnetic Resonance
  Research

Division of Cardiovascular Medicine
Radcliffe Department of Medicine
University of Oxford
John Radcliffe Hospital
Oxford, United Kingdom

Joseph R. Carver, MD [6]
Chief of Staff, Abramson Cancer Center
Division of Cardiology, Department of Medicine
Perelman School of Medicine
University of Pennsylvania
Philadelphia, Pennsylvania

David J. Cutter, DPhil, FRCR [7]
Clinical Trial Service Unit
Nuffield Department of Population Health
University of Oxford
Oxford, United Kingdom

Sarah C. Darby, PhD [7]
Clinical Trial Service Unit
Nuffield Department of Population Health
University of Oxford
Oxford, United Kingdom

Gilles W. De Keulenaer, MD, PhD [5]
Laboratory of Physiopharmacology
University of Antwerp
Antwerp, Belgium

Carmen P. Escalante, MD [19]
Professor and Chair
Department of General Internal Medicine, Ambulatory
  Treatment and Emergency Care
Division of Internal Medicine
The University of Texas MD Anderson Cancer Center
Houston, Texas

Michael S. Ewer, MD, JD, PhD [3, 4, 16]
Professor
Department of Cardiology
Division of Internal Medicine
The University of Texas MD Anderson Cancer Center
Houston, Texas

Steven M. Ewer, MD [9, 12]
Associate Professor
Division of Cardiovascular Medicine

University of Wisconsin School of Medicine and Public Health
Madison, Wisconsin

Anecita P. Fadol, MSN, PhD, RN [24]
Associate Professor
Departments of Nursing and Cardiology
The University of Texas MD Anderson Cancer Center
Houston, Texas

Saadia A. Faiz, MD [18]
Associate Professor
Department of Pulmonary Medicine
Division of Internal Medicine
The University of Texas MD Anderson Cancer Center
Houston, Texas

Luis E. Fayad, MD [1]
Associate Professor
Department of Lymphoma/Myeloma
Division of Cancer Medicine
The University of Texas MD Anderson Cancer Center
Houston, Texas

Vanessa Ferreira, MD, FRCP [7]
Department of Cardiovascular Medicine
University of Oxford
Oxford, United Kingdom

Vivian I. Franco, MD, MPH [20]
Wayne State University School of Medicine
Children's Hospital of Michigan
Detroit, Michigan

Susan C. Gilchrist, MD, MS [28]
Associate Professor,
Department of Clinical Cancer Prevention
Division of Cancer Prevention and Population Sciences
The University of Texas MD Anderson Cancer Center
Houston, Texas

Brian Greet, MD [23]
Fellow, Clinical Cardiac Electrophysiology Fellowship
Texas Heart Institute
Baylor College of Medicine
Baylor St. Luke's Medical Center
Houston, Texas

Eduardo Yepez Guevara, MD [21]
Department of Internal Medicine—Infectious Diseases
The University of Texas Health Science Center at Houston
Houston, Texas

Saamir A. Hassan, MD [15]
Associate Professor
Department of Cardiology
Division of Internal Medicine
The University of Texas MD Anderson Cancer Center
Houston, Texas

Maria Hawkins, FRCR [7]
Clinical Trial Service Unit
Nuffield Department of Population Health
University of Oxford
Oxford, United Kingdom

Cesar A. Iliescu, MD, FACC, FSCAI [23]
Professor, Department of Cardiology
Director, Cardiac Catheterization Laboratory
Division of Internal Medicine
The University of Texas MD Anderson Cancer Center
Houston, Texas

Asif Jafferani, MD [9]
Division of Cardiovascular Medicine
University of Wisconsin School of Medicine and Public Health
Madison, Wisconsin

Kaveh Karimzad, MD [22]
Associate Professor
Department of Cardiology
Division of Internal Medicine
The University of Texas MD Anderson Cancer Center
Houston, Texas

Lavanya Kondapalli, MD [6]
Assistant Professor of Cardiology-Medicine
UCHealth Heart and Vascular Center—Anschutz
Aurora, Colorado

Rohit Kumar, MD [17]
Department of Internal Medicine
John H Stroger, Jr. Hospital of Cook County
Chicago, Illinois

Larry W. Kwak, MD, PhD [1]
Vice President and Deputy Director
Comprehensive Cancer Center
Director, Toni Stephenson Lymphoma Center
Dr. Michael Friedman Professor of Translational Medicine
Professor, Department of Hematology and Hematopoietic Stem Cell Transplantation
City of Hope
Duarte, California

Monika Leja, MD [14]
Assistant Professor
Cardiology Clinic | Cardiovascular Center
Michigan Medical
University of Michigan
Ann Arbor, Michigan

Emma R. Lipshultz, BA [20]
Clinical Research Coordinator
Dana-Farber Cancer Institute
Boston, Massachusetts

Steven E. Lipshultz, MD [20]
Department of Pediatrics
Wayne State University School of Medicine
Children's Hospital of Michigan
Detroit, Michigan

Konstantinos Marmagkiolis, MD [23]
Adjunct Associate Professor
Department of Cardiology
Division of Internal Medicine
The University of Texas MD Anderson Cancer Center
Houston, Texas

Juan C. Lopez-Mattei, MD [11]
Assistant Professor
Departments of Cardiology and Diagnostic Imaging
Division of Internal Medicine
The University of Texas MD Anderson Cancer Center
Houston, Texas

Thomas H. Marwick, MBBS, PhD [10]
Director and Chief Executive
Baker Heart and Diabetes Institute Central Australia
Melbourne, Victoria, Australia

Paul McGale, PhD [7]
Clinical Trial Service Unit
Nuffield Department of Population Health
University of Oxford
Oxford, United Kingdom

Pierantonio Menna, PhD [2]
Member, Antimicrobial Stewardship Working Group
Department of Medicine and Unit of Drug Sciences
University Campus Bio-Medico
Rome, Italy

Giorgio Minotti, MD [2]
Dean, Department of Medicine and Surgery
University Campus Bio-Medico
Rome, Italy

Divyanshu Mohananey, MD [17]
Department of Internal Medicine
John H Stroger, Jr. Hospital of Cook County
Chicago, Illinois

Teresa Moon, MD [25]
Associate Professor
Department of Anesthesiology and Perioperative
  Medicine
Division of Anesthesiology and Critical Care
The University of Texas MD Anderson Cancer Center
Houston, Texas

Elie Mouhayar, MD [13]
Professor
Department of Cardiology
Division of Internal Medicine
The University of Texas MD Anderson Cancer Center
Houston, Texas

Ezequiel Muñoz, MD [23]
Internal Medicine Resident
John H. Stroger, Jr. Hospital of Cook County
Chicago, Illinois

Rofida Nofal, MD [20]
Hematology/Oncology Department
University of San Francisco
Benioff Children's Hospital
Oakland, California

Tochi M. Okwuosa, DO [17]
Assistant Professor
Division of Cardiology
Rush University Medical Center
Chicago, Illinois

Guilherme H. Oliveira, MD [26]
Advanced Heart Failure and Transplantation Center
  and Onco-Cardiology Program
Harrington Heart & Vascular Institute
University Hospitals Cleveland Medical Center
Case Western Reserve University School of Medicine
Cleveland, Ohio

Rupal P. O'Quinn, MD [6]
Assistant Professor of Clinical Medicine
Penn Heart and Vascular Center
Perelman Center for Advanced Medicine
Philadelphia, Pennsylvania

Nicolas Palaskas, MD [16]
Department of Cardiology
Division of Internal Medicine

The University of Texas MD Anderson Cancer Center
Houston, Texas

Purvi Parwani, MBBS [11]
Assistant Professor of Medicine
Loma Linda University School of Medicine
Loma Linda, California

Daniel Perry, MD [14]
Resident, Department of Internal Medicine
Michigan Medicine
University of Michigan School of Medicine
Ann Arbor, Michigan

Kazem Rahimi, MD [7]
Department of Cardiology
John Radcliffe Hospital
Oxford Radcliffe Hospitals NHS Trust
Oxford, United Kingdom

Michael J. Reardon, MD [14]
Clinical Professor of Cardiac Surgery
Houston Methodist Hospital
Houston, Texas

Marc A. Rozner, MD [25]
Associate Professor
Department of Anesthesiology and Perioperative
   Medicine
Division of Anethesiology and Critical Care
The University of Texas MD Anderson Cancer Center
Houston, Texas
Deceased

Stephen E. Sallan, MD [20]
Quick Family Chair of Pediatric Oncology
Professor of Pediatrics
Dana-Farber Cancer Institute
Harvard Medical School
Boston, Massachusetts

Emanuela Salvatorelli, PhD [2]
Department of Medicine and Unit of Drug Sciences
University Campus Bio-Medico
Rome, Italy

Scott Schuetze, MD, PhD [14]
Professor of Medical Oncology and Internal Medicine
Michigan Medicine
University of Michigan School of Medicine
Ann Arbor, Michigan

Vincent Segers, PhD [5]
Laboratory of Physiopharmacology
University of Antwerp
Antwerp, Belgium

Vickie R. Shannon, MD [18]
Professor
Department of Pulmonary Medicine
Division of Internal Medicine
The University of Texas MD Anderson Cancer Center
Houston, Texas

Thomas M. Suter, MD [4]
Department of Cardiology
University of Bern
Bern University Hospital
Bern, Switzerland

Carolyn W. Taylor, DPhil [7]
Clinical Trial Service Unit
Nuffield Department of Population Health
University of Oxford
Oxford, United Kingdom

Kara A. Thompson, MD [27]
Assistant Professor
Department of Cardiology
Division of Internal Medicine
The University of Texas MD Anderson Cancer Center
Houston, Texas

January Y. Tsai, MD [25]
Associate Professor
Department of Anesthesiology and Perioperative
   Medicine
Division Head, Division of Internal Medicine
The University of Texas MD Anderson Cancer Center
Houston, Texas

David J. Tweardy, MD [21]
Division Head, Internal Medicine-Clinical
Division of Internal Medicine
The University of Texas MD Anderson Cancer Center
Houston, Texas

Shital Vachhani, MD [25]
Associate Professor
Department of Anesthesiology and Perioperative
   Medicine
Division of Anesthesiology and Critical Care
The University of Texas MD Anderson Cancer Center
Houston, Texas

Zarha Vermeulen, PharmD [5]
Laboratory of Physiopharmacology
University of Antwerp
Antwerp, Belgium

Sindu Vivekanandan, FRCR [7]
Clinical Trial Service Unit
Nuffield Department of Population Health
University of Oxford
Oxford, United Kingdom

Alison Woo, BA, MS [1]
Program Manager
Lymphoma/Myeloma—Research
The University of Texas MD Anderson Cancer Center
Houston, Texas

Sai-Ching Jim Yeung, MD, PhD [19]
Professor
Department of Emergency Medicine
Division of Internal Medicine
The University of Texas MD Anderson Cancer Center
Houston, Texas

Syed Wamique Yusuf, MD [8, 9]
Professor
Department of Cardiology
Division of Internal Medicine
The University of Texas MD Anderson Cancer Center
Houston, Texas

Foreword

Over the last 60 years, the field of cardio-oncology has evolved significantly. Oncologists have long been concerned about cardiac reserves for surgical candidates, the effects of radiation on the heart, and how patients with underlying cardiac conditions might fare when treated for cancer. It wasn't until the discovery that anthracyclines cause heart failure, however, that integrating cardiac evaluations and testing became a part of the oncologic practice.

The University of Texas MD Anderson Cancer Center was among the first cancer hospitals to introduce techniques like cardiac ultrasound along with the now, nearly forgotten, parameters of systolic time intervals, apex-cardiography, and vector electrocardiography. MD Anderson was the first cancer center to have a vigorous heart biopsy program, initially implemented to manage patients receiving anthracyclines, but presently optimized to expand patient care and research involving newer classes of anticancer agents. Our institution also has the first cancer treatment-related cardiac catheterization laboratory.

In December 2017, when I became MD Anderson's fifth president and reflected on the institution's contributions to this field, one of my desires for advancements in years to come was to broaden therapeutic options for patients with cancer, including patients with underlying cardiac conditions. As we continue to advance research and harness genomic and immunologic tools, several new cancer treatment strategies could raise concerns of cardiac dysfunction. Such concerns include those related to new imaging techniques; updated understanding of how cancer drugs affect cardiac structure and function; modern initiatives of cardiac protection for both chemotherapy and radiation therapy patients; and cardiac complications related to checkpoint inhibitors. It is in this context that various authors, from MD Anderson as well as other internationally-recognized authorities, present the third edition of *Cancer and the Heart*.

I hope that you find this material stimulating, interesting and, most importantly, useful. Our collective hope is that the material herein will ultimately serve to help cancer patients in Texas, across the nation and all over the world better tolerate the burdens of their treatment. For those further along in their cancer journey, we hope that this knowledge will help these survivors lead lives more fully, without experiencing potentially avoidable cardiac complications. This work advances us further down the road to our ultimate goal—to end cancer, once and for all.

—Peter WT Pisters, MD
President
The University of Texas MD Anderson Cancer Center

PREFACE

Cancer and heart disease remain the two most common causes of death in developed countries. While these entities may be separate and distinguishable from each other, they are not mutually exclusive; they often coexist in individual patients, and when they occur concurrently or sequentially they constitute a complex group of problems that form the basis of what is now often described as onco-cardiology or cardio-oncology.

From the perspective of public health, societal initiatives to reduce hazardous exposure and positively modify lifestyles have contributed to a safer environment and have made a positive impact in reducing devastation and suffering. Nonetheless, we still expend a huge proportion of our national gross domestic product on the prevention, diagnosis, treatment, and support for patients afflicted with cancer and heart disease. Much has been written about these diseases. Perusal of the available resources reveals huge tomes that delve into these illnesses in considerable detail. Notwithstanding the successes in both fields and the availability of much scientific literature, much remains to be studied, analyzed, and ultimately introduced into research endeavors as well as into the practice patterns of physicians who deal with cancer patients who have cardiac concerns. It is with this in mind that a third edition of *Cancer and the Heart* is offered with the hope that the contents and perspective show insight and relevance.

The material herein focuses on the complex interactions of multiple disease states in patients who have cancer, and who either have or are deemed to be at increased risk of acquiring significant heart disease. It is the integration of this material that is often fragmented in other resources, or is not available in a concise format elsewhere. The distinguished group of contributing authors believe that an up-to-date resource for clinicians and investigators will help to fill this void. Our ultimate goal is to offer assistance in elevating and individualizing medical care in order to improve quality of life for these challenging patients with onco-cardiologic concerns. Additionally, we hope that this book will help researchers who endeavor to translate both basic and clinical research into practical approaches for patient care.

The first chapters of this book address the effects of cancer treatment on the heart. The material in this section concerns anthracyclines, the chemical agents that directly destroy myocytes; these agents were the first that introduced clinicians to the risk of heart disease as an adverse effect of cancer care. The cardiac effects of other anticancer drugs, many of which affect the heart in ways other than direct myocyte destruction, are also included in this section. In employing these anti-cancer drugs, clinicians recognize the deliberate exposure to patients of toxic therapies, and do so with the anticipation that the degree of secondary organ injury can be mitigated. We have, in essence, "picked our poison," while at the same time striving to preserve cardiac function. These agents and their troublesome sequelae, when administered alone or in combination, are, hopefully, placed in clinical perspective. Injury, however, is not limited to chemical agents; radiation effects on the heart are also considered in this section.

The next group of chapters deal with a variety of cardiac imaging techniques spanning the gamut from older "tried and true" modalities to those that are considered more modern and more sophisticated. The discussions here are focused on the specific clinical problems experienced by physicians and their cancer patients who have cardiac disease and require different imaging strategies. Imaging techniques employed with the intent to identify and protect those at risk increased as well as techniques to follow patients both during and long after exposure of their therapy for malignancy so as to identify toxicity outliers are also discussed.

The final chapters examine a number of other related subjects that are vitally important to cancer patients and those who care for them. Specific groups of patients who additionally have other organ or organ system dysfunction are discussed in this section.

In writing and editing this book we have been cognizant of the difficulties in balancing the various concerns that arise when a patient has more than one disease, and where the optimal management strategies of one affects the treatment, management, or progression of the other. We know of no broader or more problematic example than that of the cancer patient with heart disease. We recognize that treating heart disease in cancer patients may not always fit the guidelines and strategies suggested by major organizations such as the American Heart Association or the American College of Cardiology; we understand that treating patients whose disease state affects multiple organ systems requires balances and compromises in order to optimize outcome. Interestingly, guidelines have been defined recently for the treatment and evaluation of cardiac concerns in cancer patients resulting in considerable unity as to the standards of the various aspects of supportive care. As clinicians and researchers interested in cancer and the heart, we recognize that the optimal management of a tumor may not serve as the best possible outcome for a patient who subsequently succumbs to treatment-related cardiotoxicity. Likewise, a compromise in oncologic care with an over-cautious approach to cardioprotection may compromise survival. This book is intended to help clinicians recognize these dilemmas and help them and their patients cope with the uncertainties that undoubtedly will continue to arise.

Finally, the authors recognize that our knowledge is expanding at a very rapid rate. We never stop learning; our education is, to a large extent, at the mercy of our colleagues and our patients. While they are too numerous to mention individually, we take this opportunity to thank our colleagues for their guidance, the education they provide, their mentorship, their collegiality, the criticism they provide us with, their friendship, and, last but not least, their wisdom. Our patients provide the clinical experience upon which we observe, and upon which we continue to learn.

—Michael S. Ewer, MD, JD, PhD
Professor of Medicine

1 Principles of Oncologic Chemotherapy and Immunotherapy

Luis E. Fayad ■ *Alison Woo* ■ *Larry W. Kwak*

INTRODUCTION

The treatment of malignant conditions requires a clear understanding of the principles of neoplastic cell growth kinetics, pharmacokinetic, and pharmacodynamic variability, pharmacologic mechanisms of drug action, mechanisms of drug resistance, and drug interactions. There has been a significant increase in the knowledge of molecular oncology, and with the identification of multiple targets for new agents, there has been an extensive expansion of the oncology drug pipeline. Numerous ongoing trials are studying these new compounds. This chapter will discuss the major classes of chemotherapy and immunotherapy agents currently approved for the treatment of different malignancies.

THE CELL CYCLE AND TUMOR GROWTH PATTERN

The growth pattern of different neoplastic cells can affect the biological behavior of these cells and their responses to different antineoplastic agents. While some cells are not dividing and are terminally differentiated, malignant cells are in a continuous proliferation rate. Others can stay in a nondividing stage, but can eventually be recruited into the cell cycle.

The cell cycle has four distinct phases. The G1 phase consists of cells that recently finished their division and will continue proliferation. After a variable amount of time, these cells will begin to synthesize DNA, and the S phase will start. DNA synthesis will continue during the S phase, and once DNA synthesis is completed, he cell will enter a period of rest called the G2 phase. After this period, the cell will enter the M phase, which is the mitotic period, where chromosome condensation occurs and the cells divide. During the M phase many cells are more sensitive to the antineoplastic activity of a specific group of drugs called cell cycling drugs (vinca alkaloids, alkylating agents, antimetabolites). Finally, resting cells that are not actively dividing are described as being in the G0 phase. The transition between the different cell-cycle phases are regulated by specific signaling proteins. Abnormal signaling can be found in different neoplastic processes.

PHARMACOKINETIC AND PHARMACODYNAMIC VARIABILITY

■ Pharmacokinetics and Pharmacodynamics

The practicing physicians must be aware of drug toxicities and manage drugs with a narrow therapeutic index. Atkinson et al. has defined pharmacokinetics as "the quantitative analysis of the process of drug absorption, distribution, and elimination that determines the time course of drug action." In contrast, pharmacodynamics is directly related to drug-induced clinical outcomes,[1] and links drug dosing and kinetics to clinical drug effects, including toxicities or efficacy. Both pharmokinetic and pharmodynamic factors can complicate the treatment of individual cancer patients, and the practicing oncologist must deal with these situations on a daily basis.

Pharmacokinetics depends on many different factors, primarily bioavailability, volumes of distribution, protein binding, clearance, elimination half-life, and dose proportionality.

The most clinically useful parameter in drug therapy is clearance, which is a reflection of all the body processes that contribute to drug elimination, that is, what the body does to the drug. Clearance is defined as dose/AUC. The definition of clearance is the volume of drug eliminated per unit of time. In cancer treatment, the importance of clearance is enhanced because clearance is the only parameter that correlates with area under the concentration versus time curve (AUC), a useful measure of systemic drug exposure.

Overcoming interindividual variation in clearance is fundamental to the analysis of pharmaco-kinetics.[2] To use the appropriate dosing of chemotherapy agents, one method is to use the drugs according to body surface area (BSA), expressed in mg/m^2, to achieve a uniform AUC in patients with different sizes. Despite the widespread use of BSA to achieve this goal, correlation between clearance and BSA is weak, but remains a common practice.[3,4]

Liver metabolism and renal clearance are the most important mechanisms for drug clearance. Platinum-derived drugs are mostly eliminated by glomerular filtration, and doxorubicin, vincristine, etoposide, and others are metabolized by the liver. Other drugs are metabolized in the liver to their active form, and the metabolites are eliminated in the urine. Guidelines to adjust the doses of different drugs according to the degree of organ dysfunction are available for the practicing oncologist.

Pharmacogenomic Variability

Genetic factors may be involved in the variability in drug action and toxicity. Pharmacogenomics attempts to define the influence of genetic differences on drug dynamic and kinetics.[5] Genetic variations can be found in certain specific-drug metabolizing enzymes, such as CYP2C9 and CYP2D6. The best characterized example in clinical oncology is the inherited deficiency of the enzyme thiopurine methyltransferase (TPMT) that results in an excess in toxicity and poor tolerance to thiopurine.[6] Irinotecan, a drug approved in the treatment of colon cancer, has an active metabolite SN-38. Genetic variations associated with a deficiency in dihydropyrimidine dehydrogenase (DPD) activity, the rate-limiting catabolic enzyme responsible for the clearance of 5-luorouracil (5-FU), have been identified in some patients who had fatal toxicities with standard doses of this drug. Individual variation in the toxicity with irinotecan could be explained by genetic polymorphism in gene encoding the UDP-glucoronosyltransferase (UGT)1A1 enzyme that is involved in clearance of the active metabolite of SN-38.[7] Polymorphisms in the IgG Fc receptor FcgammaRIIIa may correlate with responses to rituximab-based treatments, presumably because of their role in antibody-dependent cellular cytotoxicity. Most recently, IgG Fc receptor FcgammaRIIIa 158 V/F polymorphism correlates with rituximab-induced neutropenia after autologous transplantation in patients with non-Hodgkin lymphoma.[8–10]

The identification of mutations in the epidermal growth factor receptor (EGFR) in non–small-cell lung carcinoma (NSCLC) and their correlation with response of EGFR inhibitors has become an important factor in the field of cancer genomics and therapeutics. Higher responses to erlotinib (Tarceva) and to gefitinib (Iressa) have been found in patients with NSCLC of Asian origin, since they have more frequent mutations in EFGR.[11]

CHEMOTHERAPY AGENTS (CLASSIFIED BY MECHANISM OF ACTION)

Many therapeutic agents are used in oncology, with new drugs being approved every year. We will summarize the most important drugs according to their mechanism of action (Table 1-1).

Alkylating Agents

Alkylating agents are one the most common group of chemotherapy agents used in the treatment of different malignancies. Alkylating agents impair cell function by forming covalent bonds with the amino, carboxyl, sulfhydryl, and phosphate groups of biologically important molecules. The most common and important targets of alkylation are DNA, RNA, and proteins. The nitrogen at the 7 position of guanine in DNA is particularly susceptible to alkylation. Alkylating agents require the cell to be in proliferation mode, but are not cell-cycle dependent. The mechanisms of resistance are by glutathione conjugation or by enhanced DNA repair mechanisms.[12]

Nitrosoureas

The nitrosoureas are distinguished by their high liposolubility and chemical instability. They spontaneously decompose into two highly reactive intermediates, chloroethyl diazohydroxide and isocyanate. The lipophilic nature of the nitrosoureas enables easier passage across the blood-brain barrier, achieving therapeutic CNS concentrations, a reason why they are used to treat brain tumors, including CNS lymphomas and lioblastomas.

Platinum Agents

Cisplatin is an inorganic heavy metal complex that has activity similar to cell-cycle phase-nonspecific alkylating agents. Cisplatins produce intrastrand and interstrand DNA cross-links and form DNA adducts, thus inhibiting the synthesis of DNA, RNA, and proteins preferentially at the nitrogen 7 position in the guanine and adenine residues to form a variety of monofunctional and bifunctional adducts. The exact sequences that lead to cell death after the formation of platinum-DNA adducts have not yet been elucidated. Cells treated with platinum showed evidence of apoptosis. Carboplatin has the same active diamine platinum moiety as cisplatin, but is bonded to a carboxylate group, which gives it better water solubility and slower hydrolysis compared with cisplatin. This alters the toxicity profile, causing more myelosuppression, but less nephrotoxicity, nausea, vomiting, and neuropathy, compared with cisplatin. These two drugs are used in the treatment of lung cancer (often in combination with taxanes, gemcitabine, or vinorelbine), germ cell tumors (where cisplatin is the preferred drug over carboplatin), lymphomas (in combination with other

TABLE 1-1   Chemotherapeutic agents classified by mechanism of action

MAJOR CLASS	SUBCLASS	EXAMPLES
Alkylating agents	Nitrogen mustard	mechlorethamine, chlorambucil, melphalan, estramustine, cyclophosphamide, ifosfamide, bendamustine
	Nitrosoureas	carmustine, lomustine, streptozotocin
	Alkyl sulfonate	busulfan
	Platinum complexes	cisplatin, oxaliplatin, carboplatin
	Aziridine	thiotepa
	Nonclassic alkylators	dacarbazine, procarbazine, temozolomide
Antimetabolites	Folate analogs	methotrexate, pemetrexed, pralatrexate
	Purine analogs	fludarabine, bendamustine (partially), 6-mercaptopurine, clofarabine, thioguanine, nelarabine
	Adenosine analogs	cladribine, pentostatin
	Pyrimidine analogs	cytarabine, gemcitabine, capecitabine, floxuridine, fluorouracil
	Substitute urea	hydroxyurea
Natural products	Enzymes	asparaginase, peg-asparaginase
	Camptothecin analogs	irinotecan, topotecan
	Microtubule agents	paclitaxel, docetaxel, vinblastine, vincristine, vinorelbine, epothilon
	Epipodophyllotoxins	etoposide, teniposide
	Antitumor antibiotics	bleomycin, mitomycin, dactinomycin, daunorubicin, doxorubicin, epirubicin, idarubicin, mitoxantrone, valrubicin
Targeted therapies	Monoclonal antibodies	rituximab, alemtuzumab, denileukin diftitox, ofatumumab, Y^{90} ibritumomab tiuxetan, I^{131} tositumomab, trastuzumab,cetuximab, panitumumab, bevacizumab
	mTOR inhibitors	everolimus, temsirolimus
	HDAC inhibitors	vorinostat, depsipeptide
	Molecular targeted therapies	imatinib, dasatinib, nilotinib, bortezomib, lapatinib, sorafenib, sunitinib
	Other biological agents	interferon-α, interleukin-2

drugs), and some sarcomas. Oxaliplatin, on the other hand, has been approved for the use in GI malignancies, especially in the adjuvant setting of colon cancer. Oxaliplatin also has been used, especially in Europe as part of salvage regimen for non-Hodgkin lymphomas as single agent, or in combination with drugs such as gemcitabine. The main dose-limiting toxicity of oxaliplatin is sensory neuropathy. The mechanism of resistance to platinum-containing regimens can be related to reduced accumulation, inactivation, increased DNA repair, and increased DNA damage tolerance.[13]

■ Antimetabolites

Antimetabolites are structural analogs of the naturally occurring metabolites involved in DNA and RNA synthesis. As more knowledge of those path ways has been obtained, more compounds are being developed. Antimetabolites exert their cytotoxic activity either by competing with a metabolite that is normally incorporated into DNA or RNA, or by competing with normal metabolites for the catalytic or regulatory site of a key enzyme. Because of their mechanism of action, metabolites are often more active when cells are in the S phase and have little or no activity when the cells are in G0 phase. These drugs are therefore more effective against tumors that have a high growth rate. Most antimetabolites have a nonlinear dose response, which means that after a certain dose no additional cells are killed with increased dosing. The antimetabolites can be divided into folate analogs, purine analogs, adenosine analogs, pyrimidine analogs, and substituted urea.[14]

■ Folate Analogs

Methotrexate (MTX) is a tight-binding inhibitor of dihydrofolate reductase (DHFR) a critical enzyme in folate metabolism, since this enzyme keeps the folate pool in its reduced form, tetrahydrofolate. The precise mechanism of MTX remains a subject of continuous debate. The most accepted mechanism is that inhibition of DHFR depletes the pool of tetrahydrofolate, which results in the inhibition of de novo thymidylate and purine biosynthesis as well as inhibition of protein synthesis. Cellular resistance to MTX remains a challenge to its clinical efficacy. There are several mechanisms suspected to be involved in MTX resistance, such as alterations in antifolate transport by either a defect in the reduced folate carrier or folate receptor protein, decreased capacity to polyglutamate MTX by different mechanisms, amplification of the DHFR gene, alterations in the target enzyme DHFR, and other mechanisms that go beyond the scope of this chapter. The drug is used for nonmalignant conditions such

as rheumatoid arthritis at low doses, and high doses are used in certain conditions such as central nervous system lymphomas and osteosarcomas. The drug also has been used intrathecally for patients with leptomeningeal malignancies. When high systemic doses are used, rescue with leucovorin is used to decrease significant toxicities. The most important side effects, which are associated with the dose and method of administration, include mucositis, renal and liver toxicity, cytopenias, and skin rashes. Encephalopathy or pneumonitis is rarely seen.

■ New Antifolates

Pemetrexed (Alimta) is a pyrrolopyrimidine, multitargeted antifolate analog that targets multiple enzymes involved in folate metabolism, including thymidylate synthase (TS), DHFR, glycinamide ribonucleotide formyltransferase, and aminoimidazole carboxamide formyltransferase. The dose-limiting toxicities are mucositis, myelosuppression, and skin rash. The drug is approved for lung cancer as single agent and in combination therapy.

Pralatrexate (PDX, 10-propargyl 10-deaza-aminopterin) is a new chemotherapeutic agent with promising activity in T-cell lymphomas and non–small-cell lung cancer. It has been granted approval by the Food and Drug Administration (FDA) for use in the treatment of relapsed and refractory peripheral T-cell lymphomas (PTCL). Pralatrexate was rationally designed to have high affinity for the one carbon-reduced folate carrier (RFC-1), which leads to better cellular internalization of the drug and a greater antitumor effect than methotrexate. Raltitrexed is another inhibitor of the DHFR that is currently under study, mostly for treating colon cancer.

■ 5-Fluoropyrimidines

The fluoropyrimidine 5-fluorouracil (5FU) is inactive in its parent form and requires intracellular activation to exert its cytotoxic effect. The drug readily enters the cells by the facilitated uracil transport mechanism. This compound is metabolized to its cytotoxic form by different pathways. It is transformed to FUdR by thymidine phosphorylase. Subsequent phosphorylation of FUdR by thymidine kinase results in the active metabolite 5-fluoro-2-deoxyuridine monophosphate (FdUMP). FdUMP forms a stable covalent complex with TS. The inhibition of TS leads to the depletion of deoxythymidine triphosphate (dTTP), interfering with DNA synthesis and repair. This is the main mechanism of action for 5FU. There are other pathways of how 5FU works, but their detailed description is beyond the scope of this chapter. This drug has been used mostly in gastrointestinal malignancies, such as colon cancer, stomach cancer, and pancreatic cancer. The drug is used in other breast cancer protocols. Topical administration has been used for skin cancer. The main toxicity of 5FU is gastrointestinal with mucositis, diarrhea, and myelosuppression.

Capecitabine is a fluoropyrimidine with a bioavailability of 80% by oral administration. Once activated, have a similar mechanism of action than FU. The drug has similar toxicities as 5-FU, with the addition of hand-foot syndrome. The drug is approved for treating colon cancer and breast cancer.

Cytarabine(1β-D-arabinofuranosylcytosine;AraC) is one of several arabinose nucleosides and is one of the main agents for the treatment of acute myelogenous leukemia. The drug is also used in the treatment of other hematologic malignancies, including acute lymphoblastic leukemias and Hodgkin and non-Hodgkin lymphomas.

Ara-C enters the cell by nucleoside transport proteins, and once in the cytoplasm, requires activation for its cytotoxicity. Ara-C is converted to aracytidine monophosphate (Ara-CMP), by the enzyme deoxycytidine kinase (dCK). This enzyme is the rate-limiting step for the anabolism of Ara-C. Other steps finally convert the drug to aracytidine triphosphate (Ara-CTP), which inhibits DNA polymerase, delta DNA-polymerase, and beta DNA-polymerase. By different mechanisms, cytarabine interferes with DNA elongation. Ara-C is more effective in the S phase of the cell cycle. The main toxicities are severe myelosuppression, infections, bleeding, gastrointestinal toxicity with mucositis and diarrhea, and nausea and vomiting. Central nervous system toxicity has been reported specifically in the elderly and when high doses of cytarabine are used.

Gemcitabine is transported by a similar mechanism as cytarabine. The drug, five times more lipophilic than cytarabine, accumulates at higher doses in the cells. The activation of the drug occurs by similar mechanisms as cytarabine. The main drug toxicity is myelosuppression. Gemcitabine is mostly used in pancreatic cancer, lung cancer, breast, and other carcinomas. The drug has activity in non-Hodgkin and Hodgkin lymphomas and has been used in combination with other drugs in the salvage setting.

Fludarabine is a nucleoside analogue, with activity in hematologic malignancies, including chronic lymphocytic leukemias and indolent B-cell lymphomas. The main toxicity is myelosuppression and risk for infections, some of which are opportunistic.

◾ Natural Products

A wide variety of compounds with antitumor activity have been isolated from natural substances, such as algae, plants, fungi, and bacteria. Some of these products are now semisynthetic or synthetically designed based on the parent compound.

◾ Antitumor Antibiotics

Bleomycin, a classic antitumor antibiotic, preferentially intercalates DNA at guanine-cytosine and guanine-thymine sequences, resulting in spontaneous oxidation and formation of free oxygen radicals, causing strand breakage. This drug is given intravenously and the main side effect is pulmonary toxicity, causing pulmonary fibrosis, particularly in individuals with preexisting pulmonary conditions, smokers, or seniors. The drug is used today mostly in combination chemotherapy for germ cell tumors and Hodgkin lymphomas.

◾ Anthracyclines

The anthracycline antibiotics are products of the fungus Streptomyces percetus varcaesius. The anthracyclines have a similar chemical structure, with a basic anthracycline structure containing a glycoside bound to an amino sugar, daunosamine. The anthracyclines have many mechanisms of action. The most important ones are intercalation between DNA base pairs and inhibition of DNA-topoisomerases I and II. The most commonly used anthracyclines are doxorubicin, idarubicin, epirubicin, and daunorubicin. They have wide indications in oncology including breast cancer, leukemias, lymphomas, endometrial cancer, and soft tissue sarcomas. They are administered intravenously and metabolized by the liver, requiring dose adjustments for liver toxicity. Idarubicin and epirubicin are thought to be less cardiotoxic, one of the main cumulative toxicities associated with this group of drugs, which will be discussed extensively in another chapter. Oxygen radical formation from reduced doxorubicin intermediates is thought to be one of the mechanisms of cardiotoxicity. The most important predictor for cardiotoxicity in patients receiving these drugs is history of arterial hypertension. Other important side effects associated with anthracyclines include myelosuppression, alopecia, mucositis, and nausea.

◾ Epipodophyllotoxins

Etoposide is a semisynthetic epipodophyllotoxin extracted from the root of *Podophyllum peltatum* (mandrake plant). The mechanism of action occurs by inhibiting topoisomerase II activity by stabilizing the DNA-topoisomerase II complex; this stabilization results in the inability of the cell to synthesize DNA, and the cell cycle is arrested in G1 phase. This drug can be used orally, but is mostly used intravenously. Because the drug is metabolized by the liver, this requires making adjustments in patients with liver dysfunction. The main side effects include hypotension and myelosuppression. This drug is widely used in different malignancies and is the cornerstone treatment for germ cell tumors in combination with platinum-containing regimens, and for treating small cell carcinoma of the lung, certain sarcomas, leukemias, and lymphomas, in both the frontline and in the recurrent setting (including transplant preparative regimens). Recent reports suggest that etoposide can be useful to replace doxorubicin in the regimen rituximab-CHOP (R-CEOP) in patients with cardiac conditions with contraindication to anthracyclines. The results were similar to those obtained with historical controls receiving standard R-CHOP.

■ Vinca Alkaloids

The vinca alkaloids, derived from the periwinkle plant vinca rosea, are a classic cell cycle-dependent drug. They enter the cell and bind rapidly to tubulin, which occurs in the S phase at a site different from the binding site associated with paclitaxel. Once this binding occurs, the polymerization of the microtubules is blocked, resulting in impaired mitotic spindle formation in the M phase. These drugs are administered intravenously, together with include vincristine, vinblastine, vindesine, and vinorelbine. They are metabolized by the liver, and doses must be adjusted for patients with liver dysfunction. Neurotoxicity and constipation are two of the most common toxicities associated with these agents, especially in patients treated with vincristine. Myelosuppression is another side effect of all except vincristine. The indications of these drugs are for the treatment of patients with lymphomas, lung cancer, and certain sarcomas.

■ Taxanes

Paclitaxel (Taxol) and doxetacel (Taxotere) are semi-synthetic derivatives from extracted precursors from the yew plant. They have a novel 14-member ring, the taxane, which promotes microtubular assembly and stability, blocking the cell cycle during the mitosis. Doxetacel, which is more potent than paclitaxel in enhancing microtubular assembly, also induces apoptosis. The drugs are administered intravenously, and the most common side effects include myelosuppression, neuropathy, and alopecia. Few patients can develop fluid retention and cardiac bradyarrhythmias. Hypersensitivity reactions are rare now that prophylaxis is given. Taxanes are used in the treatment for non–small-cell carcinoma of the lungs, head and neck cancers, breast cancer, ovarian cancer, and Kaposi sarcoma.

■ Camptothecin Analogs

Camptothecin analogs include two drugs, irinotecan (Camptosar) and topotecan (Hycamtin). These semi-synthetic analogs of the alkaloid camptothecin, derived from the Chinese ornamental tree Camptotheca acuminate, are inhibitors of topoisomerase I and interrupt the elongation phase of DNA replication. The most common toxicities of these drugs include myelosuppression, cholinergic syndrome with cramps, flushing, bradycardia, tearing, vomiting, and visual accommodation problems. Diarrhea is also frequent in patients treated with irinotecan, a drug with the main indication for treatment of colon cancer, which also has a substantial activity in small cell carcinoma of the lung. Topotecan is indicated mainly for the treatment of recurrent ovarian cancer and recurrent small cell carcinoma of the lung. Topotecan requires dose adjustments for patients with renal dysfunction, and irinotecan requires dose adjustments for patients with hepatic dysfunction.

IMMUNOTHERAPY

■ Monoclonal Antibodies

Chimeric or humanized monoclonal antibodies have changed the treatment of malignancies. Monoclonal antibodies can be naked or conjugated to toxins or radioisotopes. They also can be bispecific. Rituximab, Ofatumumab,

Y90 Ibritumomab tioxetan, I131 Tositumomab Rituximab was the first monoclonal antibody approved for the treatment of humans. It is a chimeric monoclonal antibody against anti-CD20, a surface marker found on most B-cell lymphomas. The mechanism of action is unclear and can be related to complement activation, cell derived immunity, or induction of apoptosis. The drug is administered intravenously, and the main side effects include administration reactions with fever and hypersensitivity, especially during the first dose. Mild myelosuppression and reactivation of viral infections have also been described. Its use is approved as a single agent in recurrent CD20+ indolent lymphomas. In combination with chemotherapy, rituximab has been found to be superior to chemotherapy alone in diffuse large B-cell lymphomas and in indolent B-cell lymphomas, with improvement in the overall response, complete responses, time to treatment failure, and survival.

New monoclonal antibodies against CD20 are currently under study, including ofatumumab, recently approved for the treatment of recurrent chronic lymphocytic leukemia.[15]

I131 tositumomab (Bexxar) and Y90 ibritumomabtiuxetan (Zevalin) are conjugated murine anti-CD20 monoclonal antibodies to radioisotopes that have activity in lymphomas. The main side effects are infusion reactions and delayed prolonged myelosuppression, with tositumomab causing hypothyroidism in some patients because of the radioactive iodine. These drugs are approved for the treatment of recurrent CD20+ indolent and transformed B-cell lymphomas.

■ Alemtuzumab (Campath)

Alemtuzumab is an anti-CD52 marker expressed in both B- and T-cell lymphocytes. It is a very potent antibody and has been approved for use in treating refractory chronic lymphocytic leukemia. Its side effects include infusion reactions, which occur less often when administered subcutaneously instead intravenously, the more traditional route of administration. Other side effects include cytopenia and infections, in particular, reactivation of cytomegalovirus. The drug is also used in T-cell lymphomas and cutaneous T-cell lymphomas. Cardiac toxicity has been reported in some patients receiving this drug.

■ Bevacizumab (Avastin)

Bevacizumab is a naked monoclonal antibody that binds to vascular endothelial growth factor (VEGF). Bevacizumab binds VEGF and prevents ligand-induced VEGF receptor activation, which blocks the stimulation of endothelial cell growth and inhibits new blood vessel formation, thus preventing further secretion of VEGF. The main side effects are increased incidence of thrombosis, hypertension, and delays in the healing of wounds. The drug is used in metastatic colon cancer, but is also used in renal cancer, glioblastomas, lung cancer, and breast cancer.

■ Trastuzumab (Herceptin)

Trastuzumab is another monoclonal antibody that has shown modest activity as single agent in patients with metastatic breast carcinoma who overexpress HER-2-NEU. It has been proven to increase the activity of chemotherapy in those patients as well. In the adjuvant setting was found to be better than placebo when used in addition to standard chemotherapy. The drug has shown cardiotoxicity, therefore, cardiac monitoring is necessary.

■ Cetuximab (Erbitux) and Panitumumab (Vectibix)

Cetuximab is a monoclonal antibody that binds epidermal growth factor on the surface of the cells, ultimately leading to downregulation of this signaling pathway. The drug has been found to be active in a subset of patients with metastatic colon cancer.[16] The drug also was shown to improve in the outcomes when added to radiation when compared with radiation alone in patients with locally advanced head and neck cancers.[17] The main side effects are rash, acne, and rare infusion reactions.

Panitumumab is another monoclonal antibody targeting EGFR and is approved for use in patients with metastatic colorectal cancer who failed standard chemotherapy.

TARGETED THERAPIES

There are many new targeted therapies, and with increased knowledge of tumor biology, more options are available. We will briefly mention some of the most important ones.

Imatinib Mesylate, Dasatinib, Nilotinib Imatinib mesylate is a classical targeted therapy and inhibits Bcr-Abl tyrosine kinase in patients with Philadelphia-positive (Ph+) chronic myelogenous leukemia (CML). Originally synthesized as an inhibitor of platelet derived growth factor, it is also a potent inhibitor of the c-kit tyrosine kinase. Its use has changed the management of patients of Ph+ CML, with most patients now having long-term hematological, cytogenetic, and molecular remissions. The drug also has been used in combination with multiagent chemotherapy in the treatment of Ph+ acute lymphoblastic leukemia. This drug also has important activity in gastrointestinal stromal tumors, an otherwise very chemoresistant condition. Dasatinib and nilotinib are similar to imatinib, with activity in certain resistant cases.[18] hiladelphia-positive (Ph+) chronic myelogenous leukemia (CML). Originally synthesized as an inhibitor of platelet derived growth factor, it is also a potent inhibitor of the c-kit tyrosine kinase. Its use has changed the management of patients of Ph+ CML, with most patients now having long-term hematological, cytogenetic, and molecular remissions. The drug also has been used in combination with multi-agent chemotherapy in the treatment of Ph+ acute lymphoblastic leukemia. This drug also has important activity in gastrointestinal stromal tumors, an otherwise very chemoresistant condition. Dasatinib and nilotinib are similar to imatinib, with activity in certain resistant cases.[18]

■ Gefitinib, Erlotinib Hydrochloride, Lapatinib Ditosylate

Gefitinib is a small molecule targeted therapy therapy that has demonstrated a significant survival benefit as a second line treatment in patients with advanced non–small-cell lung cancer.[19] Lapatinib ditosylate, an oral inhibitor of HER-2-NEU, has been recently approved for the treatment of meta-static breast carcinoma in combination with capecitabine.[1,20]

Sunitinib Malate and Sorafenib Tosylate Sunitinib malate and sorafenib tosylate are two new oral small multitargeted molecules with anti-proliferative and antiangiogenic activity attributed to the inhibition of PDGFR, VGEFR, KIT, and LFT3, and in the case of sorafenib, RAF-1. Both drugs have shown activity in advanced renal carcinoma, mainly by inducing stabilization of the disease, and with sunitinib, clinical responses have been seen. These two drugs have displaced IL-2 and interferon as the gold standard for metastatic or advanced renal carcinoma.[21]

■ Bortezomib (Velcade)

Bortezomib, another targeted therapy, is an inhibitor of the 26S proteasome. The 26S proteasome is a ubiquitous multiprotein complex responsible for degrading a variety of regulatory proteins involved in cancer cell proliferation. Bortezomib induces apoptosis in multiple myeloma cells by mechanisms that are not clearly understood. One suggested mechanism of action is inhibition of the proteasomal degradation of I-κβ, a transcription factor for NF-κβ, thus preventing the constitutive activation of NF-κβ. In myeloma cells, NF-κβ is thought to be important for cell proliferation and survival. Bortezomib is currently approved for the treatment of recurrent myeloma,[22] and the drug has been used in conjunction with immunomodulatory agents such as lenalidomide and thalidomide in recurrent and relapsing myeloma patients with-significant responses.[22,23] The drug is also approved for recurrent mantle cell lymphomas and is currently under investigation in other lymphomas and malignancies.[24] Its main toxicity is myelosuppression, in particular thrombocytopenias, neuropathy, rash, fatigue, and abdominal discomfort, with some patients developing hypotension and dehydration. Carfilzomib, a new generation proteasome inhibitor has been associated with congestive heart failure in phase II studies. The incidence of CHF ranged from 3.4% to 6.0% depending on the regimen.[25–27] Association with atrial fibrillation, Hypertension, and supraventricular tachycardia has been reported.[28] It is possible that slowing may decrease the incidence of cardiac events, since most of the happened during the infusion. Ixaxomib, has not been reported to have increased cardiac toxicity.[29]

■ Temsirolimus and Everolimus

Temsirolimus and everolimus are specific inhibitors of mTOR, a signaling protein that regulates cell growth and angiogenesis. The main side effects of these drugs are modest cytopenias, elevation of the triglycerides, occasionally pneumonitis, and fatigue.

These drugs are approved for the treatment of recurrent or advanced renal cancer,[21] and have shown activity in different hematological malignancies such as Hodgkin and non-Hodgkin lymphomas.[15]

HISTONE DEACETYLATION INHIBITORS: VORINOSTAT, DEPSIPEPTIDE

Epigenetic changes regulate the expression of certain genes by regulating a balance between the enzymes that regulate histone deacetylases (HDACs) and histone acetyltransferases (HATs). HDAC inhibitors induce growth arrest, differentiation, or apoptosis in cancer cells.

Vorinostat[30,31] and depsipeptide[25] are both drugs approved for the treatment of recurrent cutaneous T-cell lymphomas. The main side effects of these drugs are nausea, vomiting, fatigue, neutropenia, and thrombocytopenia. Depsipeptide was initially thought to increase QTc prolongation and cardiac arrhythmias; however, appropriate electrolyte replacement has been effective in managing these side effects.

BTK INHIBITORS

BTK inhibitors such as Ibrutinib, Acalabrutinib, they work by inhibiting the Brutton thyroside kinase. Both of these drugs has been associated with increase in atrial fibrillation events, both, in Ibrutinib (3%),[30] and acalabrutinib (3%),[31] associated with enlargement of the atrium as a predisposing factor. An increase in the incidence of bleeding has been associated with these drugs as well.

IMID

Lenalidomide, and thalidomide, drugs with unclear mechanism of action have different toxicity profile, while thromboembolic events are more common in patient receiving thalidomide, The exact mechanism underlying immunomodulatory drug-induced thrombosis is unknown, but it is hypothesized to involve dysregulation of endothelial thrombotic homeostasis via multiple pathways, including upregulation of pro-thrombotic factors, and downregulation of anti-thrombotic factors.[32] In the initial phase II trials, patients treated with thalidomide and dexamethasone demonstrated an incidence of DVT of 7%; when doxorubicin was added to the regimen, the incidence was significantly higher at 27%.[33] In other subsequent studies, the incidence of DVT was 4% or less with single-agent thalidomide; however, when combined with dexamethasone, the incidence of VTE increased to 26% and 34% in combination with multiple other chemotherapies.[34–36] Lenalidomide has also been associated to thromboembolic events, with results of an analysis of two multicenter trials comparing lenalidomide plus dexamethasone to dexamethasone alone showed increased incidence of myocardial infarction (1.98% vs. 0.57%), cerebral vascular events (3.4% vs. 1.7%), deep vein thrombosis (9.1% vs. 4.3%), and pulmonary embolism (4.0% vs. 0.9%).[37] Pomalidomide is the most recently approved IMiD. Recent studies of pomalidomide incorporated mandatory thromboprophylaxis, with resulting 2% incidence of DVT.[38]

PD1 BLOCKING IMMUNOTHERAPY

Immune-checkpoint blocking antibodies have demonstrated objective antitumor responses in multiple tumor types including melanoma, non-small cell lung cancer (NSCLC), Hodgkin's lymphoma, GI tumor (including colon and stomach), Non-Hodgkin's lymphoma, and renal cell cancer. This drugs can cause as a side effect, a plethora of autoimmune effects, including pericarditis, myocarditis, hyperthyroidism due to thyroiditis, with subsequent tachycardia. Among six clinical cancer centers with substantial experience in the administration of immune-checkpoint blocking antibodies, eight cases of immune-related cardiotoxicity after ipilimumab and/or nivolumab/pembrolizumab were identified. Diagnostic findings, treatment and follow-up are reported. A large variety of cardiotoxic events with manifestations such as heart failure, cardiomyopathy, heart block, myocardial fibrosis and myocarditis was documented.[39]

CONCLUSION

It is clear that the practicing oncologist must be knowledgeable about potential side effects of any therapy. In particular, cardiac or cardiovascular toxicity can be substantial, and knowledge continues to evolve as greater experience is documented. Acute side effects are relatively easy to document, especially in the setting of research-driven patient care. However, complete understanding of long-term cardiac toxicity from individual agents and combinations of agents represents an ongoing challenge for oncology. Additionally, as new agents continue to be developed and translated to first-in-man clinical trials, diligent monitoring for toxicity to the cardiovascular system is imperative, as it is clear that even targeted agents have substantial off-target side effects.

REFERENCES

1. Atkinson AJ, Daniels CE, Dedrick RL, et al. *Principles of Clinical Pharmacology*. San Diego, CA: Academic Press; 2001.
2. Ratain MJ, Mick R. Principles of pharmacokinetics and pharmacodynamics. In: Schilsky RI, Milano GA, Ratain MJ, eds. *Principles of Antineoplastic Drug Development and Pharmacology*. New York, NY: Marcel Dekker, Inc.; 1996:123.
3. Sawyer M, Ratain MJ. Body surface as a determinant of pharmacokinetics and drug dosing. *Invest New Drugs*. 2001;19:171–177.
4. Grochow LB, Baraldi C, Noe D. Is dose normalization to weight or body surface area useful in adults? *J Natl Cancer Inst*. 1990;82:323–325.
5. Evans WE, McLeod HL. Pharmacogenomics—drug disposition, drug targets, and side effects. *N Engl J Med*. 2003;348(6):538–549.
6. Zaza G, Cheok M, Krynetskaia N, et al. Thiopurine pathway. *Cancer Epidemiol Biomarkers Prev*. 2006;15(11): 2042–2046.
7. Fujita KI, Sparreboom A. Pharmacogenetics of irinotecan disposition and toxicity: a review. *Curr Clin Pharmacol*. 2010;5(3):209–217.
8. Paiva M, Marques H, Martins A, et al. FcgammaRIIa polymorphism and clinical response to rituximab in non-Hodgkin lymphoma patients. *Cancer Genet Cytogenet*. 2008;183(1):35–40.
9. Weng WK, Negrin RS, Lavori P, Horning SJ. Immunoglobulin G Fc receptor FcgammaRIIIa 158 V/F poly-morphism correlates with rituximab-induced neutropenia after autologous transplantation in patients with non-Hodgkin's lymphoma. *J Clin Oncol*. 2010;28(2):279–284.
10. Lejeune J, Thibault G, Ternant D, et al. Evidence for linkage disequilibrium between Fcgamma RIIIa-V158F and Fcgamma RIIa-H131R polymorphisms in white patients, and for an Fcgamma RIIIa- restricted influence on the response to therapeutic antibodies. *J Clin Oncol*. 2008;26(33):5489–5491.

11. Heist RS, Christiani D. EGFR-targeted therapies in lung cancer: predictors of response and toxicity. *Pharmacogenomics*. 2009;10(1):59–68.

12. Colvin OM, Friedman HS. Alkylating agents. In: DeVita VT, Hellman S, Rosenberg SA, eds. *Cancer Principles and Practice of Oncology*. 7th ed. Philadelphia, PA: Lippincott, Williams, & Wilkins; 2005:332–344.

13. Johnson SW, O'Dwyer PJ. Cisplatin and its analogues. In: DeVita VT, Hellman S, Rosenberg SA, eds. *Cancer Principles and Practice of Oncology*. 7th ed. Philadelphia, PA: Lippincott, Williams & Wilkins; 2005:344–358.

14. Kummar S, Noronha V, Chu E. Antimetabolites. In: DeVita VT, Hellman S, Rosenberg SA, eds. *Cancer Principles and Practice of Oncology*. 7th ed. Philadelphia, PA: Lippincott, Williams, & Wilkins; 2005:358–374.

15. Tay K, Dunleavy K, Wilson WH. Novel agents for B-cell non-Hodgkin's lymphoma: science and promise. *Blood Rev*. 2010;24:69–82.

16. Cunningham D, Humblet Y, Siena S, et al. Cetuximab monotherapy and cetuximab plus irinotecan in irinotecan-refractory metastatic colorectal cancer. *N Engl J Med*. 2004;351:337–345.

17. Bonner JA, Harari PM, Giralt J, et al. Radiotherapy plus cetuximab for locoregionally advanced head and neck cancer: 5-year survival rate from a phase 3 randomised trial, and relation between cetuximab-induced rash and survival. *Lancet Oncol*. 2010;11(1):21–28.

18. Kantarjian HM, Cortes J, La Rosée P, Hochhaus A. Optimizing therapy for patients with chronic myelogenous leukemia in chronic phase. *Cancer*. 2010;116(6): 1419–1430.

19. Gazdar AF. Epidermal growth factor receptor inhibition in lung cancer: the evolving role of individualized therapy. *Cancer Metastasis Rev*. 2010;29(1):37–48.

20. Cameron D, Casey M, Press M, et al. A phase III randomized comparison of lapatinib plus capecitabine versus capecitabine alone in women with advanced breast cancer that has progressed on trastuzumab: updated efficacy and biomarker analyses. *Breast Cancer Res Treat*. 2008;112(3):533–543.

21. Reeves DJ, Liu CY. Treatment of metastatic renal cell carcinoma. *Cancer Chemother Pharmacol*. 2009;64(1):11–25.

22. Thomas SK, Richards TA, Weber DM. Novel agents for relapsed and/or refractory multiple myeloma. *Cancer J*. 2009;15(6):485–493.

23. Laubach JP, Mitsiades CS, Mahindra A, et al. Novel therapies in the treatment of multiple myeloma. *J Natl Compr Canc Netw*. 2009;7(9):947–960.

24. Goy A, Bernstein SH, Kahl BS. Bortezomib in patients with relapsed or refractory mantle cell lymphoma: updated time-to-event analyses of the multicenter phase 2 PINNACLE study. *Ann Oncol*. 2009;20(3):520–525.

25. Duvic M, Vu J. Vorinostat in cutaneous T-cell lymphoma. *Drugs Today (Barc)*. 2007;43(9):585–599.

26. Olsen EA, Kim YH, Kuzel TM, et al. Phase IIb multicenter trial of vorinostat in patients with persistent, progressive, or treatment refractory cutaneous T-cell lymphoma. *J Clin Oncol*. 2007;25(21):3109–3115.

27. Piekarz RL, Frye R, Turner M, et al. Phase II multiinstitutional trial of the histone deacetylase inhibitor romidepsin as monotherapy for patients with cutaneous T-cell lymphoma. *J Clin Oncol*. 2009;27(32):5410–5417.

28. Siegel DS, Martin T, Wang M, et al. A phase 2 study of single-agent carfilzomib (PX-171-003-A1) in patients with relapsed and refractory multiple myeloma. *Blood*. 2012;120:2817–2825.

29. Vij R, Wang M, Kaufman JL, et al. An open-label, single-arm, phase 2 (PX-171-004) study of single-agent carfilzomib in bortezomib-naive patients with relapsed and/or refractory multiple myeloma. *Blood*. 2012;119: 5661–5670.

30. Badros AZ, Vij R, Martin T, et al. Carfilzomib in multiple myeloma patients with renal impairment: pharmacokinetics and safety. *Leukemia*. 2013;27:1707–1714.

31. Atrash S, Tullos A, Panozzo S, et al. Cardiac complications in relapsed and refractory multiple myeloma patients treated with carfilzomib. *Blood Cancer J*. 2015;5:e272.

32. Kumar SK, Berdeja JG, Niesvizky R, et al. Safety and tolerability of ixazomib, an oral proteasome inhibitor, in combination with lenalidomide and dexamethasone in patients with previously untreated multiple myeloma: an open-label phase 1/2 study. *Lancet Oncol*. 2014;15:1503–1512.

33. O'Brien S, Hillmen P, Coutre S, et al. Safety analysis of four randomized controlled studies of Ibrutinib in patients with chronic lymphocytic leukemia/small lymphocytic lymphoma or mantle cell lymphoma. *Clin Lymphoma Myeloma Leuk*. October 2018;18(10):648–657.

34. Byrd JC, Wierda WG, Schuh A, et al. Acalabrutinib monotherapy in patients with relapsed/refractory chronic lymphocytic leukemia: updated results from the Phase 1/2 ACE-CL-001 study. *Blood*. 2017;130:498. Safety and efficacy of acalabrutinib in relapsed/refractory chronic lymphocytic leukemia patients.

35. Li W, Cornell RF, Lenihan D, et al. Cardiovascular complications of novel multiple myeloma treatments. *Circulation*. 2016;133:908–912.

36. Osman K, Comenzo R, Rajkumar SV. Deep venous thrombosis and thalidomide therapy for multiple myeloma. *N Engl J Med*. 2001;344:1951–1952.

37. Weber D, Rankin K, Gavino M, Delasalle K, Alexanian R. Thalidomide alone or with dexamethasone for previously untreated multiple myeloma. *J Clin Oncol*. 2003;21:16–19.

38. Rajkumar SV, Gertz MA, Lacy MQ, et al. Thalidomide as initial therapy for early-stage myeloma. *Leukemia*. 2003;17:775–779.

39. Palumbo A, Rajkumar SV, Dimopoulos MA, et al. Prevention of thalidomide- and lenalidomide-associated thrombosis in myeloma. *Leukemia*. 2007;22:414–423.

40. Lenalidomide: risk of thrombosis and thromboembolism. https://www.gov.uk/drug-safety-update/lenalidomide-risk-of-thrombosis-and-thromboembolism. Accessed on 4/9/2019.

41. Dimopoulos MA, Leleu X, Palumbo A, et al. Expert panel consensus statement on the optimal use of pomalidomide in relapsed and refractory multiple myeloma. *Leukemia*. 2014;28:1573–1585.

42. Heinzerling L, Ott PA, Hodi FS, et al. Cardiotoxicity associated with CTLA4 and PD1 blocking immunotherapy. *J Immunother Cancer*. 2016;4:50.

2 Pharmacology of Cardio-Oncology

Emanuela Salvatorelli ▪ *Pierantonio Menna* ▪ *Giorgio Minotti*

INTRODUCTION

It was not until a couple of decades ago when cardio-oncology was established as an independent discipline that harmonizes and cross fertilizes expertises in the fields of oncology and cardiology.[1] The mission of cardiologists was to identify patients with at increased risk of developing cardiovascular toxicities of antitumor therapies and to advise the cancer expert to not treat at-risk patients or to treat them with less toxic but also less efficacious drugs. The efforts of cardio-oncology teams were mostly focussed on assisting patients during the course of cancer therapy. Strategies for patients' cardiovascular follow up were either lacking or only partly defined as long term survival was achieveable for relatively few patients. The elderly was often given therapies with palliative rather than curative intent.

Things have changed fast and quite dramatically. The pharmacologic framework of cardioncology has become wider and more complex. The pharmacologic portfolio of oncologists and hematologists has expanded immensely. Old fashioned chemotherapeutics are increasingly replaced by, or combined with newer drugs that were developed to target tumor cells while sparing or causing minimal damage to cardiovascular system; regrettably, however, new drugs too seem to induce cardiovascular toxicity of a clinical concern, although this seems to be of a different type what oncologists and hematologists learned about conventional chemotherapeutics. But drugs save lives and many more patients now enjoy long term survival which makes the time ripe for establishing modalities of surveillance tailored to patient characteristics, oncologic history, pharmacodynamics of the new drugs. This having been said, the growing cohorts of adult cancer survivors merge with equally sizeable cohorts of childhood cancer survivors that develop cardiovascular sequelae or other chronic conditions long after cancer diagnosis and treatment. Many such survivors were treated with "old" drugs, which means that surveillance and treatment modalities should be tailored to the pharmacodynamics of those drugs as well. Oncologists, hematologists and cardiologists therefore face a blend of clinical settings that need to be recapitulated under the umbrella of basic and clinical pharmacology.

Here, we do not provide a formal analysis of drugs with frequent or infrequent cardiovascular effects. We would rather introduce the reader to preclinical or clinical pharmacological foundations of cardio-oncology, with a focus on everything that goes from pathophysiology of cardiotoxicity to strategies for drug development and pharmacological approaches to cancer patients in a real world context.

WHAT IS SO SPECIAL ABOUT ANTITUMOR DRUGS AND THE HEART?

Why is the heart so vulnerable by cancer drugs? Cardiomyocytes require that ATP be constantly available. It has been calculated that in 24 hours the heart would produce and consume more ATP than any other organ.[2] There are very little energy stores in the heart, and hence, any chemical or hemodynamic stress that perturbs the balance between ATP production and consumption would intuitively set the stage for cardiac dysfunction. If ATP production ceases ATP levels probably collapse in matter of seconds.[2]

ATP is necessary to support the contractile activity of sarcomeres and the activity of energy-requiring enzymes that govern the contraction-relaxation cycle of heart by maintaining ion gradients. The best known ATP-requiring cardiac ion pump is the sarcoplasmic reticulum calcium ATPase 2a, also referred to as SERCA2a. Systolic contraction requires that calcium be released from the sarcoplasmic reticulum into the cytoplasmic milieu and eventually routed toward the troponin-actin-myosin machinery. Diastolic relaxation requires that calcium be sequestered back into the sarcoplasmic reticulum by SERCA2a. Congestive heart failure (CHF) is typically associated with a reduced re-uptake of cytosolic Ca^{2+} by the sarcoplasmic reticulum, which can be caused by a reduced expression of SERCA2a or by a reduced availability of ATP. This contributes to elevating diastolic $[Ca^{2+}]_i$ and diastolic stiffness, particularly when Ca^{2+} extrusion through the Na^+/Ca^{2+} exchanger is also reduced.[3] On the other hand, if Ca^{2+}-sequestration by SERCA2a is limited by a reduced supply of ATP the Na^+/Ca^{2+} exchanger extrudes higher amounts of Ca^{2+} and systolic rather diastolic dysfunction develops.[3] As simplistic it may sound, a loop that goes from ATP deficiency to systolic or diastolic dysfunction through SERCA2a dysfunction recapitulates clinical phenotypes of heart failure with low or preserved left ventricle ejection fraction (LVEF) in cancer patients. It comes as no surprise that in preclinical models of heart failure viral transfection of the SERCA2a gene into cardiac tissue resulted in improved cardiac contractility and reduced mortality.[4]

By having said that a never-resting pump like the heart shows a continuous demand of ATP, countless mechanisms of cardiotoxicity from anticancer drugs become intuitive.

DISCONNECTIONS BETWEEN PRECLINICAL MECHANISMS AND CLINICAL FACTS

With the prototypic class of cardiotoxic drugs, the anthracyclines, intercalation into mitocondrial DNA (mtDNA) and disruption of genes encoding for key components of oxidative phosphorylation (OXPHOS) chain are very likely to occur.[5] In rats, doxorubicin causes both quantitative and qualitative alterations of mtDNA and OXPHOS chain subunits.[6] In cardiomyocytes, this precedes decrements in ATP levels and contractility.[7] With newer drugs, like the broad family of tyrosine kinase inhibitor (TKI), inhibition of AMP-activated protein kinase (AMPK) should be an obvious mechanism of toxicity or aggravation of it. In fact, in any setting where energy production is challenged or compromised by chemical insults, the normal function of AMPK would be to prevent energy dissipation through protein translation and lipid biosynthesis.[8] Because TKI lacks absolute specificity for their target kinase or kinases.[9] off target inhibition of AMPK would cause ATP to collapse and cardiac dysfunction to develop. Regrettably, however, the picture is considerably more complex. In the case of anthracycline-related disruption of OXPHOS, studies of childhood cancer survivors demonstrate that a compensatory increase of mtDNA copies allows for maintaining normal OXPHOS enzymatic activity. Cardiotoxicity would therefore occur only if competing factors overlap with anthracycline-related injury and dissipate the long-term sustainability of the compensatory mechanism offered by mtDNA extracopies.[10] Mixed findings occurred also for the AMPK story. In some studies of isolated cardiomyocytes the multikinase inhibitor, sunitinib, inhibited AMPK at therapeutically relevant concentrations but this was not enough for cellular levels of ATP to decrease.[11] In other studies, both AMPK inhibition and energy rundown were documented.[12] Regardless of such inconsistencies, sunitinib induced cardiac apoptosis in mice but this only occurred if sympathicomimetic agents were also administered to increase blood pressure.[13] It therefore seems that neither anthracycline disruption of OXPHOS genes nor sunitinib inhibition of AMPK were able to cause cardiotoxicity when considered in isolation. Likewise, studies of cardiovascular events among cancer patients treated with sunitinib showed that LVEF decreased more often when patients carried risk factors like hypertension or pre-existing systolic dysfunction.[14]

Disconnections between preclinical models and clinical facts is a recurrent leitmotiv in cardio-oncology. Imatinib, inhibitor of the Abl kinase of breakpoint cluster region-Abelson kinase (Bcr-Abl) fusion protein encoded by the Philadelphia chromosome (Ph) of leukemic cells, offered unimaginable progresses for treatment of chronic myeloid leukemia (CML). In animal models, imatinib inhibition of Abl caused prolonged endoplasmic reticulum stress, which in turn activated Jun N-terminal kinases (JNKs) known to induce cardiac apoptosis via mitochondrial membrane potential collapse.[8] In early clinical studies imatinib seemed to cause congestive heart failure (CHF) in excess of the 1% incidence characterized in the registration trial.[15] The two findings were apparently bridged by cause-and-effect relations and imatinib was therefore labeled as a cardiotoxic drug with a known mechanism of action. Recent clinical surveys demonstrate that this was not the case. Imatinib cardiotoxicity has been grossly overestimated.[16,17] On the other hand, drugs that were developed to treat patients with imatinib-resistant Bcr-Abl mutations, dasatinib and nilotinib, did not introduce overt concerns about myocardial toxicity. Dasatinib caused primarily pulmonary hypertension and nilotinib caused primarily vascular occlusive events. A drug developed for patients resistant or intolerant to dasatinib and nilotinib, ponatinib, caused even more vascular events than nilotinib.[18] Increasing the potency of Abl inhibitors therefore introduced safety issues other than CHF, which modified the assumption linking Abl inhibition to cardiomyocyte apoptosis and cardiac dysfunction. Because Abl inhibitors can be used for years to treat CML, concerns about long term vascular sequelae have become predominant.

Anthracyclines do not escape disconnections between preclinical hypotyheses and clinical facts. This is both fascinating and frustrating if one appreciates that anthracyclines have been in clinical use for some 40 years now. The antitumor effects of anthracyclines are well defined by their known capability to form a noncleavable ternary complex with DNA and topoisomerase IIα, from which DNA double strand breaks and downstream proapoptotic signals occur.[19] Mechanisms of anthracycline cardiotoxicity are much less defined, presumably because cardiotoxicity builds on a constellation of mechanisms rather than one mechanism in isolation.

Experimental models that help to decipher such complexity are desperately needed. For example, chronic anthracycline administration was shown to inactivate or to reduce expression of SERCA2a,[20] yet transgenic mice that overexpressed SERCA2a proved to be more susceptible rather than more resistant to cardiomyopathy induced by cumulative doses of doxorubicin.[21]

Dose reductions have improved tolerability and long term safety of anthracycline-based cancer therapies in both children-adolescents and adults,[22,23] but given the absence of a firmly established mechanism of cardiotoxicity concerns about long term sequelae should not be ignored. One reason the mechanisms of delayed anthracycline cardiotoxicity are not yet clear is in fact related to limitations of models of cardiovascular toxicity. The effects of chronic anthracycline cardiotoxicity in vivo require weeks to appear and may cause toxicity in only a few drug-treated animals; moreover, adequate studies require large numbers of animals to be monitored for extended periods, increasing costs beyond capacity of a single laboratory. In vitro studies, or short term in vivo studies, are cost convenient and hence more popular but usually evaluate effects that appear within hours or days.[23] A majority of such studies tend to adopt drug concentrations that are of limited relevance to clinical situations. It should therefore come as no surprise that cardiomyocyte apoptosis was seen in acute cardiotoxicity induced by short-term administration of doxorubicin[24,25] but much less so in the progressive cardiotoxicity induced by long-term treatment.[26] By having acknowledged the importance of comorbid conditions like hypertension or pre-existing cardiomyopathy, one should also adopt experimental conditions that included at least one such condition. This might well be accomplished by means of spontaneously hypertensive rats (SHR). In comparison with normotensive rats, SHR show a greater sensitivity to chronic anthracycline treatment and exhibit histologic and functional cardiotoxicity much similar to that seen in cancer patients, including elevations of circulating troponin and decrease of mean arterial pressure.[27] Of particular relevance is the recurrent increase of troponin in these animals. In children small increases of circulating troponin after the first dose of doxorubicin predicted subsequent risk for left ventricular dilatation and wall thinning.[28] In adults, troponin increases predicted later decrements of LVEF in adults.[29] Thus, the SHR model should be preferred to achieve optimal anticipation of clinical situations, but unfortunately, this model is only occasionally exploited. Regulatory bodies and funding agencies pose little attention on these issues. Lack of comorbid conditions is one major flaw of preclinical models of cardiac and vascular toxicity from antitumor drugs.

One more misconception is that anthracycline cardiotoxicity is a matter of cardiomyocyte damage only. Myocytes account for approximately 80% of the cardiac mass but constitute less than 20% of the total cell count. Other cell types, including fibroblasts, endothelial cells, smooth muscle cells, and adipocytes, provide structural and trophic support to the myocytes.[23] Effects of anthracyclines on non-cardiomyocyte cells need to be evaluated. Cardiac endothelial cells and fibroblasts may be more sensitive to the toxic effects of doxorubicin than are cardiomyocytes, suggesting that cardiomyocyte deterioration may be preceded by alterations in matrix composition, paracrine signals, doxorubicin distribution across extracellular fluids and cardiomyocytes.[23,30] Studies of endothelial cells support this concept.[31,32]

CARDIOTOXICITY AND THE ROLE OF NON-CARDIOMYOCYTE CELLS

In approaching mechanisms of cardiotoxicity from any chemotherapeutic one should also consider the role of self replicating cells that in normal conditions are committed to warrant tissue homeostasis, while in pathological conditions serve to replace dying cells and to assist myocardial regeneration.[33] Pressure overload increases the number of cardiac stem cells, which denotes how important they are for the heart to withstand hemodynamically unfauvorable conditions.[34] And accordingly, senescence of cardiac progenitor cells causes or accompanies with heart failure.[35] Cardiac stem cells are potential targets of anthracyclines, which may cause inability of the heart to repopulate apoptotic or necrotic foci.[36] Indirect evidence that this may be the case was provided by post mortem studies of cancer patients who died of CHF induced by anthracycline-containing regimens. The hearts of these patients contained more senescent cardiac progenitor cells than did hearts from age-matched subjects who died of noncardiovascular causes.[37] Innovative methods for exploring cardiotoxicity of candidate anticancer drugs should take vulnerability of these cells in a paramount consideration.

WHAT CAN BE DONE FOR IMPROVING PREDICTIVENESS OF PRECLINICAL MODELS?

■ Regulatory Perspectives

For life-threatening diseases such as cancer, the Food and Drug Administration (FDA) developed the accelerated approval process. The median time from accelerated approval to full approval of oncologic drugs is 3.9 years and the mean time is approximately 4.7 years.[38] These figures denote substantial time savings in terms of earlier availability of drugs to cancer patients, but again, the risk of a post-approval outbreak of toxicity needs to be taken in consideration. The case of ponatib is quite impressive. Ponatinib was granted accelerated approval in December 2012 but was withdrawn from the market in October 2013 as follow up data from phase I and II trials revealed high rates of both arterial and venous thrombotic events. In january 2014 ponatinib was reintroduced in the market and such decision was based on risk–benefit assessment; in fact, ponatinib was effective in otherwise uncurable patients with Philadelphia positive leukemias resistant or intolerant to other TKI or carrying resistance due to T315I gate keeper mutant of Abl-Bcr kinase.[39] Important lessons can be drawn from the ponatinib case. Ponatinib did not cause signals of vascular toxicity in preclinical models,[40] and accordingly, early clinical studies were not designed to include risk mitigation strategies that at least in part might have diminished the occurrence of vascular events.

What can be done for improving predictiveness of cardiovascular toxicity models? There are avenues to be explored but solutions are not yet at sight. One area that needs to be expanded is biomarkers. In most chronic toxicology studies, if performed, biomarkers of cardiac injury are not routinely measured.[41] These should be considered forefront in assessing cardiovascular liability of a clinical candidate in the early stages of its development.[42] Furthermore, in vitro screenings of clinical candidates focus primarily on "functional" cardiotoxicity (e.g., electrophysiological studies) but efforts should be paid to predict and characterize "structural" toxicity as well. Single cell imaging of mitochondrial membrane potential, endoplasmic reticulum integrity, Ca^{2+} transients and membrane permeability should be performed on different cardiac cell lines but this is something that only occasionally can be retrieved from investigational medicinal product dossiers or other regulatory paperworks. The gap is potentially filled by the so-called engineered heart tissue model, a three-dimensional force-generating cardiac tissue model generated from dissociated heart cells and fibrin matrix between flexible silicone posts.[43] A limitation of these models is that acute changes cannot precisely assist a prediction of chronic toxicity, but this can be obviated by 3-D stem cell-based cardiac microtissues/spheroids that allow for repeat drug dosing, simulate cumulative effects, and predict chronic toxicity with a higher level of confidence.[44]

Structural cardiovascular toxicity should also benefit from a wider application of the zebrafish model. In particular, zebrafish can survive in the absence of cardiac output and in the presence of vascular defects for several days, which allows for characterizing abnormalities that would be rapidly fatal to a patient.[42] And finally, there is a need for multicellular models composed of myocytes, fibroblasts, endothelial cells and smooth muscle cells such that an integrated picture of vascular toxicity in cardiac and peripheral tissues is also obtained.

In the era of metabolomics, the problem of inter-species and inter-strain metabolic heterogeneity remains widely open. The metabolic profile of a clinical candidate and its potential to induce cardiovascular toxicity directly or through the action of metabolites may show substantially different in one animal or cellular model as compared to another. The authors developed a translational model of human heart that obviates these pitfalls. The model consists of ex vivo human myocardial samples from which strips are dissected and incubated in plasma added with clinically relevant concentrations of any drug, from anthracyclines to taxanes and others.[45–51] Such samples retain viability and functions for at least 4–5 hours and allow for proper simulations of drug uptake, distribution, metabolisation and efflux. Concurrent changes of mitochondrial electron transport and membrane potential, and release of troponin or other biomarkers, can be investigated. The strips are composed of cardiomyocytes, endothelial cells, fibrocytes and microvasculature, and as such they may prove useful for electron microscopy studies of structural toxicity.

■ Drug Engineering Perspectives

With new drugs, like TKI, lack of an absolute specificity toward a candidate kinase might stimulate reengineering strategies that generate more specific inhibitors. Imatinib fits well in this scenario. Although developed to target the Abl kinase of Bcr-Abl fusion protein, imatinib inhibits also platelet-derived growth factor receptor (PDGFRα/β), mast/stem cell growth factor receptor or tyrosine-protein kinase Kit (c-KIT), and other kinases. By inhibiting PDGFRα/β imatinib shows activity in chronic myelomonocytic and eosinophilic leukemias, while inhibition of c-KIT makes imatinib active in gastrointestinal stromal tumors. Imatinib was granted approval for use in these tumors. Having noticed that the cardiotoxic potential of imatinib was relayed by activated JNKs some investigators felt that reengineering imatinib to prevent JNK activation could be of value for diminishing cardiotoxicity. A redesigned imatinib molecule that spared the Abl kinase was shown to retain c-KIT and JNK inhibition. Pharmacological activities of the new drug were well in keeping with molecular reengineering: the new drug was almost inactive in chronic myeloid leukemia cells, lacked cardiotoxicity in mice, but proved remarkably active in gastrointestinal sarcoma cell lines.[52] The same drug was also active in otherwise imatinib insensitive orthotopic murine models of ovarian cancer, and activity was shown to correlate with inhibition of JNK-1.[53] Although preclinical evidence of imatinib cardiotoxicity did not precisely translate into clinical facts, these studies outlined possible new approaches to changing the safety and spectrum of activity of new chemical entities.

Things may prove more difficult for other drugs. Ponatinib too lacks specificity to Bcr-Abl but inhibits other kinases that possibly contribute to causing vascular events. Off target kinases include vascular endothelial growth factor receptor 2 (VEGFR2), and lessons from angiogenesis inhibitors suggest that inhibition of this kinase may well underlie hypertension and vascular events. On the other hand, some oncologic angiogenesis inhibitors (axitinib, pazopanib, tivozanib) show preclinical activity against Bcr-Abl[T315I] but this occurs at higher concentrations than required for inhibition of VEGFR2.[54-56] These latter findings denote that reengineering ponatinib to retain activity against Bcr-Abl[T315I] but not VEGFR2 might be conceptually feasible and therapeutically advantageous. But preliminary analyses suggest that the two activities may be difficult to separate. All of approved anti CML drugs show equal activity against the two kinases, and this holds true also for a novel compound (PF-114) that was developed to be specific to Bcr-Abl[T315I] (Figure 2-1).[54] Thus, on target inhibition of Bcr-Abl[T315I] seems to be intimately coupled with off target inhibition of VEGFR2, which is consistent with similarities between the ATP-binding site gatekeeper residues of Bcr-Abl[T315I] and VEGFR2 in terms of size and hydrophobicity.[54] With many TKI running in the pipeline, these notions anticipate that the search for ponatinib analogues with improved efficacy and reduced toxicity might prove to be laborious. A thoughtful strategy for improving selectivity and safety of TKI might be to develop fewer TKI targeting the ATP binding pocket and juxtaposed regions, which are highly conserved across human kinases, and to engineer TKI that target less conserved domains at a distance from the ATP site.[57] The latter TKI should demonstrate both increased selectivity and reduced risk of off target toxicities. Concerted actions between basic research scientists, bio-technology and pharmaceutical companies will be needed to achieve this goal.

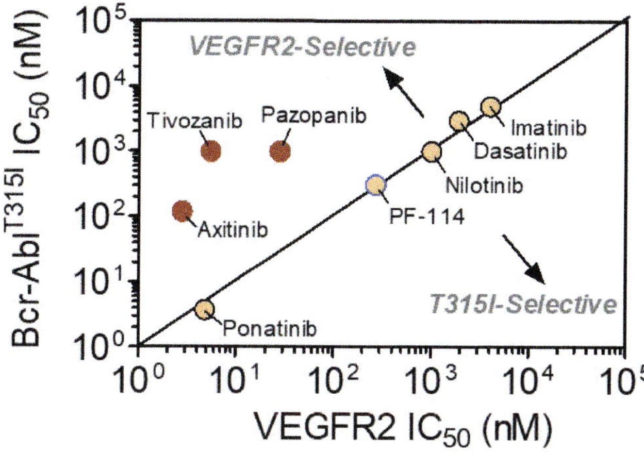

FIGURE 2-1   Dual inhibition of Bcr-Abl[T315I] and VEGFR2 by anti CML TKI and oncologic angiogenesis inhibitors. Symbols above the line of identity refer to oncologic angiogenesis inhibitors that cause greater inhibition of VEGFR2 than Bcr-Abl[T315I]. Antileukemic drugs (ponatinib, nilotinib, dasatinib, imatinib, and the investigational ponatinib analogue, PF-114) are placed on the identity line, i.e., they inhibit Bcr-Abl[T315I] and VEGFR2 with equal potencies. There is no symbol below the line identity, i.e., there is no drug that inhibits Bcr-Abl[T315I] more potently than VEGFR2. (Modified after Gozgit JM, et al., 2015.[54])

PHARMACOLOGICAL APPROACHES TO CLINICAL CARDIO-ONCOLOGY

There are two possible pharmacological approaches to correlate pharmacologic notions to cardio-oncology clinical facts. One approach is exemplified by Table 2-1, which provides a formal though unavoidably incomplete listing of families of drugs with a known or suspected cardiovascular toxicity. The drugs are classified primarily by their mechanisms of action in cancer cells (e.g., alkylators versus topoisomerase inhibitors, TKI versus antibodies), biochemical and molecular mechanisms of cardiac or vascular toxicity, dose dependence of clinical events.[18,51,58-73] This approach emphasizes major differences between anthracyclines (which cause CHF in a dose-dependent manner), other chemotherapeutics (which may or may not induce cardiovascular events in a dose-related manner), antibodies or TKI (which almost uniformly lack a dose dependence of cardiac or vascular effects). Another approach is best known by the Ewer's classification of type 1 versus type 2 agents.[74] Type 1 agents cause irreversible damage that is fingerprinted by histologic lesions and preclude treatment continuation once a clinical event has occurred. Type 2 agents cause reversible dysfunction, do not induce a consistent pattern of histologic lesions, and do not preclude rechallenge. Anthracycline and

TABLE 2-1 Anticancer agents with reported evidence of cardiac and/or vascular toxicity: Classification by families

DRUG FAMILY	CLINICAL MANIFESTATIONS	MECHANISM(S)	DOSE DEPENDENCE
Topoisomerase IIα inhibitors			
Anthracyclines	Primarily systolic dysfunction and CHF	Multifactorial (iron-mediated oxidative stress, ATPase inactivation, altered expression of components of mitochondrial electron transport chain, inhibition of topoisomerase IIβ and DNA damage), resulting in cardiomyocyte necrosis, apoptosis, or necroapoptosis	Typically dose-dependent (e.g., 5%, 15% or 30% risk of CHF after 400, 500 or 600 mg of doxorubicin/m^2, respectively)
Anthracenediones mitoxantrone	Arrhythmias, CHF	Likely related to oxidative stress (albeit with mechanisms different from anthracyclines)	Increased risk with cumulative doses ≥160 mg/m^2
pixantrone[a]	Asymptomatic decrements of LVEF; CHF in patients with continuing cardiomyopathy	Similar to mitoxantrone but substantially attenuated	Not demonstrated
Epipodophyllotoxins etoposide	Ischemia/infarction	Vasospasm?	Not established
Antibiotics			
mitomycin	CHF	Oxidative stress	Increased risk after cumulative doses of ≥ 30 mg/m^2
bleomycin	Pericarditis, ischemic heart disease, lung fibrosis	Likely related to oxidative stress	Studies of testicular cancer patients show that myocardial infarction may occur after one dose as well as years after completion of cumulative regimens
Alkylating agents			
cyclophosphamide	Heart block, tachyarrhythmias, hemorrhagic myopericarditis, CHF	Endothelial capillary damage	Observed at doses of >120–170 mg/kg (CHF may resolve over 3–4 weeks on therapy); anecdotic reports of a toxic synergism with anthracyclines

DRUG FAMILY	CLINICAL MANIFESTATIONS	MECHANISM(S)	DOSE DEPENDENCE
Ifosfamide	Atrial ectopy, bradycardia CHF	Likely similar to cyclophosphamide Loss of striation, fragmentation of ventricular muscle fibers?	Observed at 6.25 to 10 g/m^2 Observed at 10 to 18 g/m^2
cisplatin	Arrhythmias, heart block, CHF, ischemia/ infarction, arterial and venous thromboembolic events	Hypomagnesiemia secondary to nephrotoxicity and tubular defects? Coronary artery fibrosis? Evidence of endothelial dysfunction and platelet activation.	Not firmly established
busulfan	Endocardial fibrosis	Unknown (autoptic case report)	Unknown
Tubuline-active agents			
Vinca alkaloids Vincristine Vinblastine Vinorelbine	Ischemia/infarction	Vasospasm?	Not firmly established (events at below or above 6 mg of vincristine, regardless of a prior cardiac history)
Taxanes Paclitaxel Docetaxel	Arrhythmias, hypotension (more frequent with paclitaxel)	Hypersensitivity reactions (particularly with the paclitaxel vehicle, Cremophor EL)	Not firmly established, attenuated by antihistamines and glucocorticoids. Both paclitaxel and docetaxel may cause vehicle-independent aggravation of the dose-related cardiotoxicity of doxorubicin
Antimetabolites			
Fluoropyrimidines (fluorouracil, capecitabine)	CHF, arrhythmias, ischemia/infarction	Vasospasm	Not firmly established; patients with prior cardiac effects from fluorouracil are at an increased risk for recurrent cardiotoxicity, presumably because of a dose-related accumulation of phosphoramide
Methothrexate	CHF, arrhythmias, ischemia/infarction	Unknown	Unknown
Fludarabine	Hypotension, angina, subacute global left ventricular impairment when used in combination with the alkylating agent, melphalan	Impaired cellular energy metabolism? Impaired removal of concomitant DNA- alkylator adduct formation?	Not established for hypotension or angina; 150 mg/m^2 over 5 days for ventricular dysfunction in patients receiving concomitant melphalan

(continued)

TABLE 2-1 Anticancer agents with reported evidence of cardiac and/or vascular toxicity: Classification by families (*continued*)

DRUG FAMILY	CLINICAL MANIFESTATIONS	MECHANISM(S)	DOSE DEPENDENCE
Cytarabine	Angina, pericarditis with effusion	Unknown	Usually seen with high dose cytarabine (3 g/m² IV over 1 h every 12 h for 12 doses)
Decitabine	Hypertension; left ventricle dysfunction, CHF	Not firmly established; reports of paradoxical correction of hypertension in animal models	Uncertain
Gemcitabine	Atrial fibrillation	Not firmly established	Not demonstrated
Monoclonal antibodies			
Trastuzumab	Left ventricle dysfunction, CHF	Blockade of Erbb2 signalling (reduced energy metabolism and sarcomere turnover, increased vulnerability by oxidants, hyperreactivity to sympathicomimetic agents, and many other mechanisms)	Not demonstrated
Adotrastuzumab emtansine	Left ventricle dysfunction	Probably similar to trastuzumab	Not demonstrated
Bevacizumab	Hypertension, left ventricle dysfunction, CHF, myocardial infarction, arterial thrombosis, venous thromboembolic events	Blockade of VEGF signalling (decreased NO production, rarefaction of microvessels, blockade of cardiac PDGF receptor, contractile dysfunction secondary to hypertension)	Not demonstrated
Tyrosine Kinase Inhibitors[b]			
Lapatinib	Left ventricle dysfunction, CHF	Blockade of Erbb2 signalling	Not demonstrated
Imatinib	Left ventricle dysfunction, heart failure	Inhibition of Abl kinase, endoplasmic reticulum stress, JNKs activation	Not demonstrated (recent metanalyses suggest that cardiac safety issues may have been overestimated)
Dasatinib	Left ventricle dysfunction, CHF, pulmonary arterial hypertension	Inhibition of PDGFRα/β or Src; endothelial oxidative stress dysfunction, and endoplasmic reticulum stress	Not demonstrated

DRUG FAMILY	CLINICAL MANIFESTATIONS	MECHANISM(S)	DOSE DEPENDENCE
-Nilotinib	Occlusive arterial events (peripheral artery disease, coronary artery disease, ischemic cerebrovascular events); hypertension	Not firmly established; possible role for nilotinib-induced insulin resistance and hypercholesterolemia	Not firmly established
Ponatinib	Arterial thrombosis and venous thromboembolic events; hypertension; myocardial infarction	Not firmly established; possible role for inhibition of VEGFR2	Probably dose-dependent; dose reductions prospectively anticipate risk reduction
Ibrutinib	Atrial fibrillation; hypertension	Not firmly established (inhibition of cardiac Bruton's kinase pathways may be involved in atrial fibrillation)	Not demonstrated, but probably dose dependent
Sunitinib	Hypertension, left ventricle dysfunction, CHF	Interference with VEGF/VEGFR signals (decreased NO production, rarefaction of microvessels), blockade of cardiac PDGF receptor, contractile dysfunction secondary to hypertension	Not demonstrated
Sorafenib	Hypertension, left ventricle dysfunction, CHF	Interference with VEGF/VEGFR signals, downregulation of stanniocalcin 1.	Not demonstrated
Axitinib	Hypertension	Probably similar to sunitinib and sorafenib	Not demonstrated
Cabozantinib	Hypertension	Interference with VEGF/VEGFR	Not demonstrated
Pazopanib	Hypertension	Interference with VEGF/VEGFR	Not demonstrated
Regorafenib	Hypertension	Coordinated suppression of NO and stimulation of endothelin-1	Not demonstrated
Trametinib	Hypertension, bradycardia	Not firmly established	Not demonstrated
Ceritinib	Bradycardia	Not firmly established	Unknown
Crizotinib	Bradycardia	Not firmly established	Possibly related to the length of treatment

(continued)

TABLE 2-1 Anticancer agents with reported evidence of cardiac and/or vascular toxicity: Classification by families (*continued*)

DRUG FAMILY	CLINICAL MANIFESTATIONS	MECHANISM(S)	DOSE DEPENDENCE
mTOR inhibitors			
Everolimus Temsirolimus	Hypertension	Not firmly established	Not demonstrated
Angiogenesis inhibitors			
Thalidomide	Bradycardia	Suspected autonomic, autacoid and paracrine mechanisms	Not demonstrated
Lenalidomide	Venous thromboembolism	Possible association of venous thromboembolism with with single-nucleotide polymorphism in NFκB1 (rs3774968) gene	Not firmly established
Proteasome inhibitors			
Bortezomib Carfilzomib	Hypertension, left ventricle dysfunction, CHF	Not firmly established but likely aggravated by pre-existing risk factors	Not firmly established
Differentiating agents			
all-trans retinoic acid	Pulmonary infiltrates during treatment of acute promyelocytic leukemia	Strong associations with leukemic cell CD2 and CD15 expression (leukoagglutination, microvascular occlusion, tissue damage)	Not firmly established (mediated by leukemic cells and influenced by cell count and genotype)
arsenic trioxide	QT prolongation	Altered processing, blockade or inactivation of HERG K+	Not firmly established

[a]Although conventionally grouped with mitoxantrone, pixantrone causes topoisomerase II inhibition that is qualitatively similar but quantitatively more modest; it also shows limited structural interactions with topoisomerase II
[b]All TKI are reported to cause QT prolongation to a variable extent. Clinical evidence and consequences are under scrutiny.
Sources: Modified after Moslehi JJ, Deininger M, 2015[18]; Minotti G et al., 2004[19]; Salvatorelli E, Paz O, et al. 2013[51]; Fernández A et al., 2007[52]; Vivas-Mejia P et al., 2010[53]; Gozgit JM, et al., 2015[54]; Mian AA et al., 2015[55]; Pemovska T et al., 2015[56]; Force T, Kerkelä R, 2008[57]; Menna P et al., 2008[58]; Pettengell R et al., 2012[59]; Moore RA et al., 2011[60]; Togna GI et al., 2000[61]; Montani D et al., 2012[62]; Rea D et al., 2014[63]; Ooi JYY et al., 2014[64]; Narayanan N et al., 2014[65]; Kawabata M et al., 2015[66]; Roodhart JM et al., 2008[67]; Cho YT, Chan CC, 2013[68]; Kaur A et al., 2003[69]; Bagratuni T et al., 2013[70]; Chari A, Hajje D., 2014[71]; Breccia M et al.2008[72]; Ficker E et al., 2004.[73]

the anti-epidermal growth factor receptor (Erbb2) antibody, trastuzumab, would be prototypic type 1 and 2 agents, respectively.

The type 1 versus type 2 agent classification shows obvious clinical implications and yet, some concerns must be scrutinized. This classification was introduced to explain how trastuzumab per se caused moderate and reversible cardiac dysfunction but exacerbated doxorubicin cardiotoxicity when the two drugs were used in combination.[75] It was suggested that by blocking autophosphorylation of Erbb2–Erbb4 heterodimers trastuzumab silenced downstream signals that activated gene expression, cell growth, glucose uptake, and sarcomeric proteins turnover.[76] All such survival-oriented signals may be irrelevant or redundant in the healthy unchallenged heart; however, the very same signals may prove life-saving if cardiomyocytes are challenged by comorbidities or anthracycline stress.[76] This conceptual breakthrough paved the road to assuming that other cytostatic/cytotoxic agents could be classified type 1 agents while new agents, like antibodies or TKI, could be grouped with trastuzumab in the type 2 class of drugs (Table 2-2). Clinical and preclinical evidence seems to support such a generalization. In preclinical settings, sorafenib, per se caused little or no damage to the heart but aggravated mortality of experimental-induced myocardial infarction, as if sorafenib caused trastuzumab-like silencing of survival factors that helped cardiomyocytes to withstand stressor conditions.[77] On a different note, but along similar concepts, we mentioned that sunitinib caused cardiac apoptosis only in mice stressed with sympathicomimetic agents, as if sunitinib per se induced moderate and reversible cardiotoxicity.[13] In clinical settings, bevacizumab aggravated cardiotoxicity of concomitant anthracyclines regardless of blood pressure changes, which was similar to what trastuzumab did in patients receiving concomitant anthracycline.[78] And finally, comprehensive analyses show that cardiovascular events from TKI tend to be reversible, such that treatment could be resumed once hypertension or cardiac dysfunction induced by these drugs resolved spontaneously or was managed by cardiovascular drugs.[14,79] These findings do support the type 1 versus type 2 classification.

Other findings challenge the type 1 versus type 2 classification. This classification rests with the dose dependence and irreversibility of type 1 effects versus the dose independence and reversibility of type 2 effects and yet, not all of type 1 agents cause cardiovascular events in a dose-related manner. Reversible decrements of LVEF or hypertension or arrhythmias may occur with both type 1 and type 2 agents. Prolongation of QT interval is typical of virtually all TKI but the same may also occur for various reasons in patients treated by type 1 multiagent therapies. Arterial thrombosis and venous thromboembolism are irreversible events by definition, introduce a higher risk of recurring events, and may occur with both type 1 and type 2 agents. It is probably safe to conclude that a clear-and-cut separation of type 1 and type 2 events is not always possible (Figure 2-2). We propose that the type 1 versus type 2 classification retains validity in the following settings: i) progressive and irreversible systolic dysfunction from anthracyclines as opposed to transient cardiac dysfunction from most type 2 agents ii), direct myocyte damage by type 1 agents as opposed to perturbations of growth and survival signals by type 2 agents iii), high probability of recurrent cardiac and hemodynamic effects from type 1 agents as opposed to the possibility of rechallenging patients

TABLE 2-2 Anticancer agents with reported evidence of cardiac and/or vascular toxicity: Type 1 versus Type 2 classification

MANIFESTATIONS	TYPE 1	TYPE 2
Clinical course	May stabilize, but subclinical damage persists	Complete or near-to-complete recovery upon withdrawal and/or medication
Dose-dependence	Usually dose-related	Usually dose-independent
Mechanism(s)	See Table 1	Elimination of receptor- and/or kinase-relayed survival factors
Ultrastructure	Usually accompanied by histologic lesions	Inconsistent patterns of histologic lesions
Effect of rechallenge	High probability of recurrent (cumulative) dysfunction	Prevailing evidence for the safety of rechallenge
Effect of late sequential stress	High likelihood of sequential stress-related cardiac dysfunction	Low likelihood of sequential stress-related events at a short-term follow up; concerns about late sequelae at a longer follow up
Synergism with other drugs and/or comorbidities	Established or likely synergism with other type 1 agents and/or comorbidities	May aggravate toxicity of type 1 agents, if administered concomitant; increase cardiac or vascular vulnerability by comorbidities if not adequately controlled

Source: Modified after Menna P et al., 2008.[58]

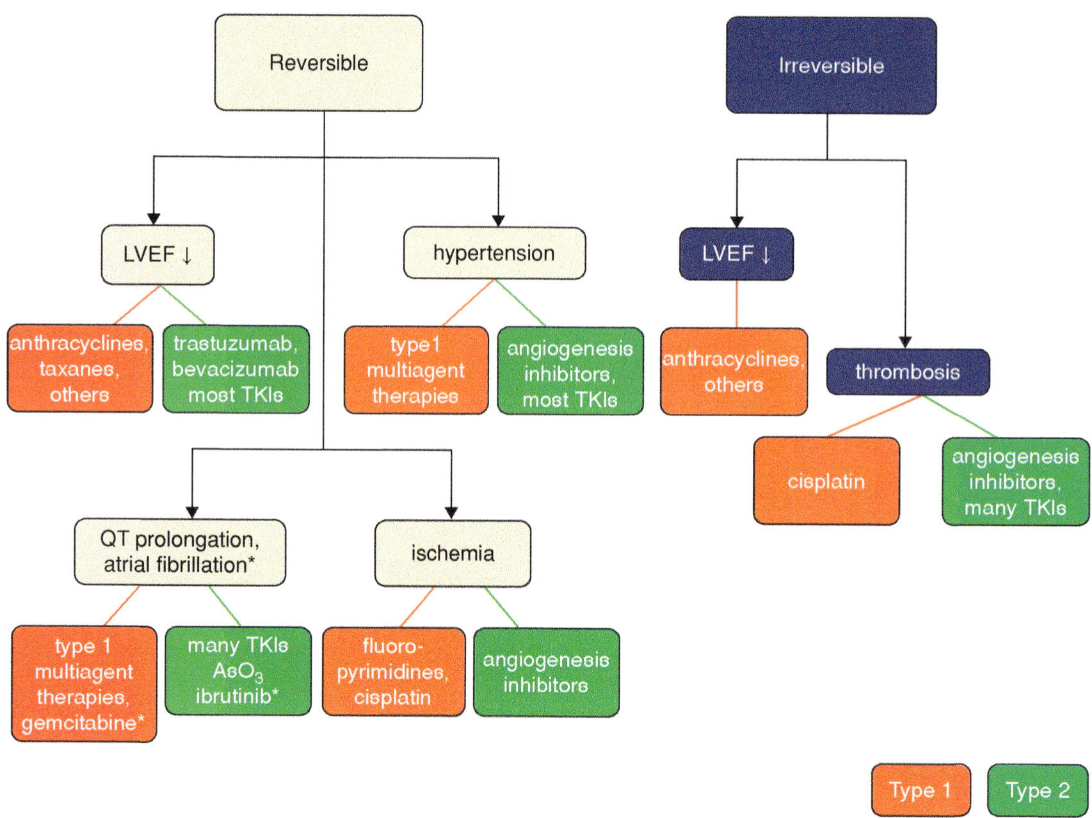

FIGURE 2-2 Reversible and irreversible cardiovascular events from type 1 or type 2 agents. Schematic depiction to show that reversible and irreversible events can under certain circumstances be induced by both type 1 and type 2 agents.

with many type 2 agents iv), exacerbation of type 2 agents toxicity by poorly controlled comorbidities. This latter possibility is nicely illustrated by the fact both catecholamines and angiotensin down-regulate endothelial expression of neuregulin 1, that is the ligand promoting heterodimerization of ErbB-4 with ErbB-4.[32]

Pharmacologic foundations for preventing or treating cardiovascular complications of oncologic therapies will rest with these conceptual pillars.

PHARMACOLOGIC PRINCIPLES OF PRIMARY PREVENTION

The type 1 versus type 2 classification of cardiovascular events (or agents), as described and reassessed above, shows obvious consequences on pharmacologic strategies of primary prevention. Some strategies are specific to patients who are candidate for anthracycline-based treatments, others are less specific and can be applied to patients who are candidates for any type 1 or type 2 agent.

Primary Prevention of Anthracycline Cardiotoxicity

Pharmacokinetic prevention ■ Anthracycline cardiotoxicity can be reduced by interfering with pharmacokinetic, pharmacodynamics, or pharmacogenetic determinants of cardiotoxicity. On pharmacokinetic grounds cardiotoxicity is reduced by replacing bolus administration with slow infusions over 24 to 96 hours. This strategy builds on some established facts. Anthracycline activity correlates with total plasma exposure to anthracyclines (as exemplified by area under curve, [AUC]); in contrast, the risk of developing CHF correlates with peak plasma level of anthracyclines (C_{max}) and their consequent diffusion and accumulation in the heart. Replacing bolus administration with slow infusions does not significantly affect AUC but diminishes C_{max} and anthracycline accumulation in the heart.[19,80] The cardiac safety of slow anthracycline infusions has been documented in numerous studies, even when anthracyclines were administered in cumulative doses otherwise known to induce CHF[19]. The benefit of replacing bolus administration with slow infusions is counterbalanced by disadvantages like patient's prolonged hospitalization and exacerbation of exposure effects like e.g., bone marrow suppression, mucositis, alopecia. Moreover, slow infusions did not prevent delayed cardiomyopathy in survivors of childhood acute lymphoblastic leukemia.[81] Another concern originates from an increased accumulation of DNA oxidized bases in peripheral blood mononuclear cells from breast cancer patients treated by DOX slow infusions.[82] This seems to be a consequence of the prolonged exposure to anthracyclines administered by slow infusion. Should DNA damage occur also in cardiomyocytes, and especially in cardiac stem cells, CHF risk in long term survivors treated by anthracycline slow infusions would increase significantly. Should DNA damage occur also in hematopoietic precursors this might translate into an increased risk of developing second hematologic malignancies.[19]

Anthracycline cardiotoxicity can also be reduced by replacing conventional anthracyclines with liposomal formulations. Two liposomal formulations have been approved for use in some defined clinical indications. One liposomal doxorubicin (Caelyx® in Europe, Doxil® in the United States) has polyethylene glycol embedded in the lipid layer; other formulations of doxorubicin (Myocet®) or daunorubicin (Daunoxome®) adopt uncoated liposomes. Liposomal anthracycline formulations are too big to cross the gap junctions of endothelial linings in the heart and many other healthy tissues.[83] Limited diffusion in extravascular compartments results in higher C_{max} and lower distribution volume and clearance of liposomal formulations as compared to convential anthracyclines but the vast majority of the active drug remains protected within the liposomal vesicle.[84] Liposomal formulations are nonetheless small enough to cross the very irregular and leaky microvasculature that characterizes solid tumors.[19] Following extravasation in tumors, liposomal formulations accumulate by virtue of the insufficient lymphatic drainage and increased interstitial pressure that characterize many tumors. This is the so called Enhanced Permeability and Retention Effect.[84] Moreover, tumor microenvironment destabilizes the liposomal vesicle through a variety of mechanisms that go from low pH to the release of lipases from dying tumor cells or the release of oxidizing agents by tumor-infiltrating inflammatory cells. In the case of uncoated formulations, also the phagocytic cells residing in tumors could metabolize liposomes and release active free anthracycline[84] (Figure 2-3). Preclinical studies showed that liposomal formulations delivered substantial amounts of anthracycline in tumors but not in the heart.[84] In some animal models liposomal formulations actually exposed tumor cells to higher amounts of free anthracycline than conventional formulations did.[84] For many reasons liposomal anthracycline formulations might be considered prototypic examples of "targeted" drugs.

A number of clinical studies demonstrated activity and cardiac tolerability of liposomal anthracyclines,

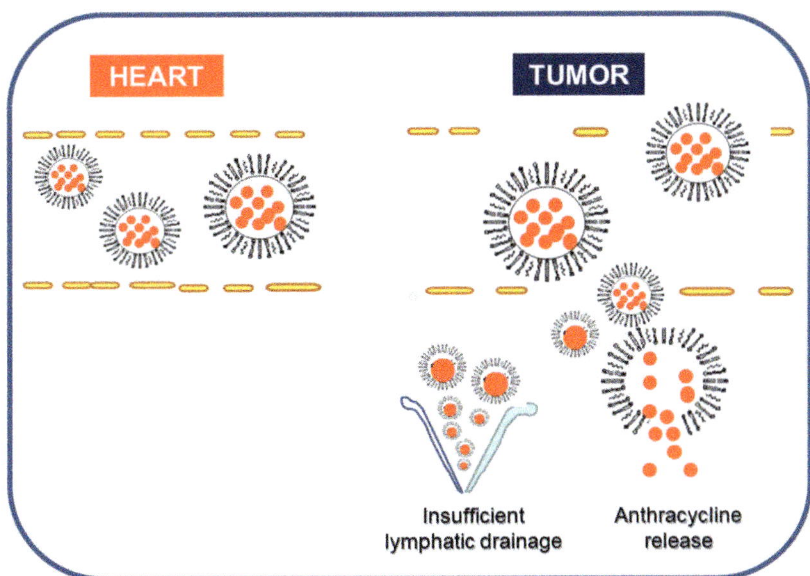

FIGURE 2-3 Tumor-targeted release of active anthracyclines by liposomal formulations. Liposomal formulations are too big to cross the endothelial lining of coronary vessels but are small enough to extravasate through the leaky vasculature of tumors. Once in the tumor interstitium liposomal formulations accumulate due to insufficient lymphatic drainage, the liposomal vesicle destabilizes, and active free anthracycline is released.

and a Cochrane analysis concluded that liposomal anthracyclines were the only formulations with evidence-based reduced cardiotoxicity as compared to doxorubicin.[85] Efficacy and cardiac safety were also documented when uncoated or pegylated liposomal doxorubicin was used in combination with trastuzumab, i.e., under conditions when conventional doxorubicin and trastuzumab synergized and caused unacceptable cardiotoxicity.[86,87] Limited cardiac penetration of liposomal anthracyclines prevented such a toxic synergism. Regrettably, however, liposomal formulations are approved for use in only limited settings (metastatic breast cancer for uncoated liposomal doxorubicin; metastatic breast cancer, advanced/refractory ovarian cancer or multiple myeloma, AIDS related Kaposi's sarcoma, for pegylated liposomal doxorubicin; AIDS related sarcoma for liposomal daunorubicin). All other indications, including the very valuable option of combining liposomal anthracyclines with trastuzumab, remain investigational at this point in time.

Pharmacodynamic prevention ■ A longsought strategy for preventing cardiotoxicity has been to replace a given anthracycline with an equiactive but less cardiotoxic cogener. The number of "less cardiotoxic" analogues keeps growing but after all, unambiguous clinical validation of a "less cardiotoxic" analogue is still lacking. One reason this search has proved so difficult rests with the multifactorial nature of anthracycline cardiotoxicity.

The four main anthracyclines approved for clinical use (doxorubicin, epirubicin, daunourubicin, idarubicin) are composed of a tetracyclic quinone-hydroquinone chromophore, an aminosugar, and a short side chain with a carbonyl group. One-electron reduction of the quinone yields a semiquinone that reduces oxygen to superoxide anion (O_2^{-}) and its dismutation product, hydrogen peroxide (H_2O_2), members of the broad family of reactive oxygen species (ROS) that cause iron-catalyzed oxidative stress in the relatively unprotected heart.[88,89] Two-electron reduction of the side chain carbonyl moiety generates a secondary alcohol metabolite that, in the case of doxorubicin, shows essentially no cardiac clearance and accumulates to form long-lived toxic anthracycline reservoir[90] (Figure 2-4). The latter perpetuates oxidative damage and induces other oxidant stress-independent mechanisms of toxicity like e.g., inhibition of numerous ATPases[91] or inactivation of iron regulatory proteins that control cellular uptake and storage of iron.[92,93]

For each anthracycline, there seems to be a correlation between its clinical cardiotoxicity and the levels of formation of ROS and/or secondary alcohol

metabolite in the heart.[19] However, noticeable exceptions exist. Epirubicin shows a defective conversion to ROS and secondary alcohol metabolite.[45] Epirubicin is said to be clinically more tolerable than doxorubicin but this occurs when the two anthracyclines are given in equal amounts (mg/m^2) and epirubicin shows higher body clearance and reduced antitumor activity. If epirubicin is administered in higher doses to compensate for elimination and to attain the same activity as that of doxorubicin, the risk of cardiotoxicity may increase, particularly for the elderly or patients with competing risk factors.[94] Epirubicin may retain advantages over doxorubicin when anthracyclines are combined with taxanes that cause allosteric stimulation of formation anthracycline secondary alcohol metabolites. In fact, taxanes stimulates formation of doxorubicin metabolite but not of epirubicin metabolite, which may result in an improved cardiac tolerability of epirubicin-taxane regimens as compared to doxorubicin-taxane doublets.[47] Also amrubicin and the novel anthracenedione, pixantrone, show a defective conversion to ROS and/or secondary alcohol metabolite.[50,51] Unfortunately, both drugs are approved for use in limited conditions and systematic clinical comparisons with doxorubicin or other anthracyclines are very limited.[95] Pixantrone was less cardiotoxic than doxorubicin in a Phase II study of patients with newly diagnosed non-Hodgkin lymphoma.[96] Pixantrone was also cardiac tolerable in patients with refractory/relapsed non-Hodgkin lymphoma that had been treated frontline with doxorubicin.[59] Of note, the mechanisms of antitumor activity of pixantrone are substantially different from those of doxorubicin and other anthracenediones, which suggests that pixantrone should not be grouped with anthracycline-like drugs.[97,98]

Other strategies for reducing anthracycline cardiotoxicity were based on the coadministration of drugs or natural compounds that improved cardiomyocytes defenses against oxidative stress. Trials of high dose vitamin E or N-acetylcysteine were uniformly negative.[99,100] Of note, less robust interventions with vitamin E were sufficient to prevent or decrease the incidence of other cardiac events that presumably involved oxidative stress (nonfatal myocardial infarction in patients with coronary atherosclerosis, arrhythmias and reinfarction after aorto-coronary bypass, fatal infarction in smokers).[101] These results could only be interpreted by assuming that antioxidants failed to reach critical levels in cell sanctuaries exposed to oxidative stress. Alternatively, oxidant stress was a unimportant component of anthracycline-related mechanisms of cardiotoxicity.

The only drug that has proven protective in preclinical and clinical settings is dexrazoxane. This is a *bis*-ketopiperazine which diffuses in cardiomyocytes,

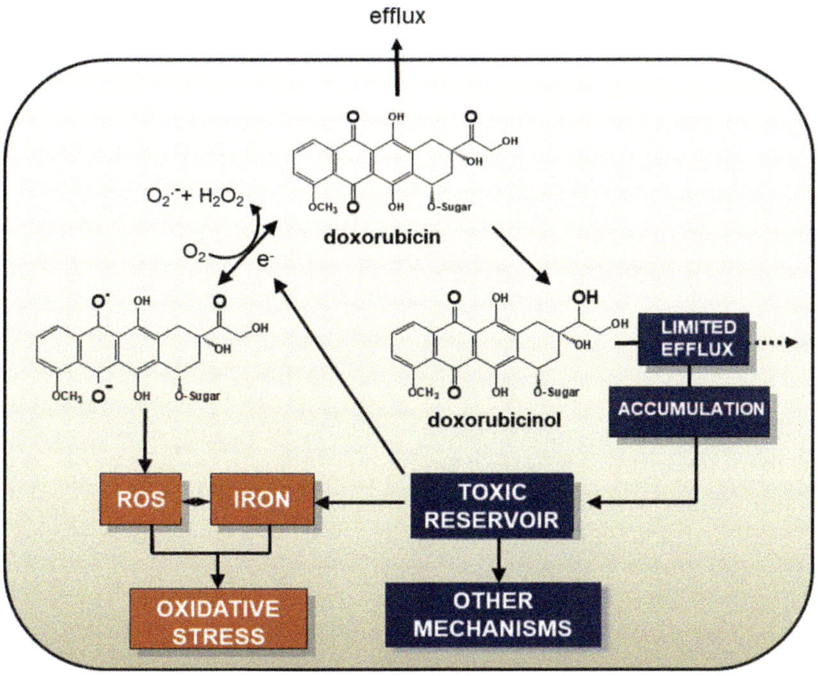

FIGURE 2-4 Metabolic determinants of anthracycline cardiotoxicity. Schematic representation of one-electron reduction of doxorubicin to a semiquinone intermediate (resulting in ROS formation) as opposed to a two-electron reduction of the side chain carbonyl group (resulting in formation of the secondary alcohol metabolite, doxorubicinol). ROS and doxorubicinol may cooperate in inducing cardiotoxicity; doxorubicinol also shows a limited efflux and a tendency to accumulate in a long-lived toxic reservoir. It may also act by mechanisms unrelated to oxidative stree. Boldfaced residues denote the quinone or carbonyl moieties liable to one- or two- electron reduction. This general scheme applies also to epirubicin, daunorubicin, idarubicin. O$_2$·$^-$, superoxide anion; ROS, reactive oxygen species. (Modified after Menna P et al., 2008.[58])

undergoes stepwise hydrolysis of its piperazine rings, and gives a diacid-diamide (code-named ADR 925) that is similar to EDTA and pulls iron away from catalyzing free radical reactions. Myocardial uptake of dexrazoxane is extraordinarily rapid and approaches its maximum level within 1 min, which anticipates a rapid exposure of cardiomyocytes to ADR 529.[102] This having been said, how is it that cardiotoxicity could be prevented by dexrazoxane but not antioxidants? Shouldn't both compounds provide protection were oxidative stress involved? Such a discrepancy can only be put in a context if one surrenders the concept that anthracycline cardiotoxicity is multifactorial by definition and dexrazoxane plays more than one mechanism of protection. A reappraisal of cellular targets of anthracycline may guide this exploration.

The main mechanism of anthracyclines activity in tumor cells rests with the stabilizing of a reaction intermediate in which DNA strands are cut and covalently linked to tyrosine residues of topoisomerase IIα. This reaction impedes DNA resealing and causes accumulation of protein- capped DNA double strand breaks. Topoisomerase IIα-mediated

DNA damage is followed by growth arrest in G1 and G2 and programmed cell death.[19] Whereas topoisomerase IIα is expressed primarily in tumor cells and normal proliferating cells, cardiomyocytes and other quiescent cells express topoisomerase IIβ that is also inhibited by anthracyclines. There is a persuasive evidence that anthracycline inhibition of topoisomerase IIβ inhibition causes DNA double strand breaks and cardiomyocyte death.[103] Thus, topoisomerase IIβ represents a previously unrecognized and probably a major target of anthracycline cardiotoxicity. Dexrazoxane competes for the ATP binding site of topoisomerase IIβ and causes topoisomerase IIβ to assume a closed-clamp configuration that is not permissive to the generation of anthracycline-DNA-topoisomerase IIβ complexes.[104] By so doing, dexrazoxane prevents DNA damage and cardiomyocyte damage.[103,104]

The dexrazoxane-topoisomerase story should not come as a surprise. Dexrazoxane had long been known to bind to topoisomerase IIα as well.[105] It is following these reasonings that one can reconcile the lack of protection by antioxidants with the efficient protection provided by dexrazoxane. Iron chelation and mitigation of oxidative stress is not the only or prevailing mechanism of action of dexrazoxane. Accordingly, there was little or no protection by dexrazoxane analogues that chelated iron but did not inhibit topoisomerases.[106] And in a similar manner, new drugs that were designed to chelate and redox-inactivate iron even more specifically than dexrazoxane did, proved unable to provide equal or better cardiac protection.[107,108]

Regardless of its multiple modes of action, as sketched in Figure 2-5, dexrazoxane was able to prevent anthracycline-related cardiotoxicity in many clinical studies of both childhood and adult cancer patients, often allowing for the administration of anthracycline doses above the threshold associated with risk of CHF.[109] Dexrazoxane was the only drug that granted approval from FDA for use as cardiac protectant in patients exposed to anthracyclines. Regrettably, however, the clinical use of dexrazoxane was limited by just one report of its possible interference with anthracycline activity in metastatic breast cancer.[110] An interference of dexrazoxane with anthracycline activity might, at least in principle, fit in a scenario in which dexrazoxane competed with anthracyclines for topoisomerase IIα but this has never been demonstrated. In contrast, an overwhelming body of clinical studies demonstrates that dexrazoxane did not diminish anthracycline activity.[111] The American Society of Clinical Oncology, Chemotherapy, and Radiotherapy Expert Panel maintained caution and recommended using dexrazoxane only in very limited conditions (e.g., patients who have received more than 300 mg/m² of doxorubicin for metastatic breast cancer and who may benefit from continued anthracycline treatment).[112]

Another controversial issue about dexrazoxane pertains to an increased risk of second malignancies. This was observed in survivors of Hodgkin lymphoma who had received doxorubicin in combination with etoposide. By having considered that both doxorubicin and etoposide and dexrazoxane inhibited topoisomerase IIα, albeit by different mechanisms and with different potencies, it was postulated that combining the three drugs could exceed a threshold above which topoisomerase inhibition caused genetic instability in normal tissues.[113] This report led the European Medicines Agency to conclude that dexrazoxane should not be used in children due to the risk of second malignancies. Two studies of survivors of

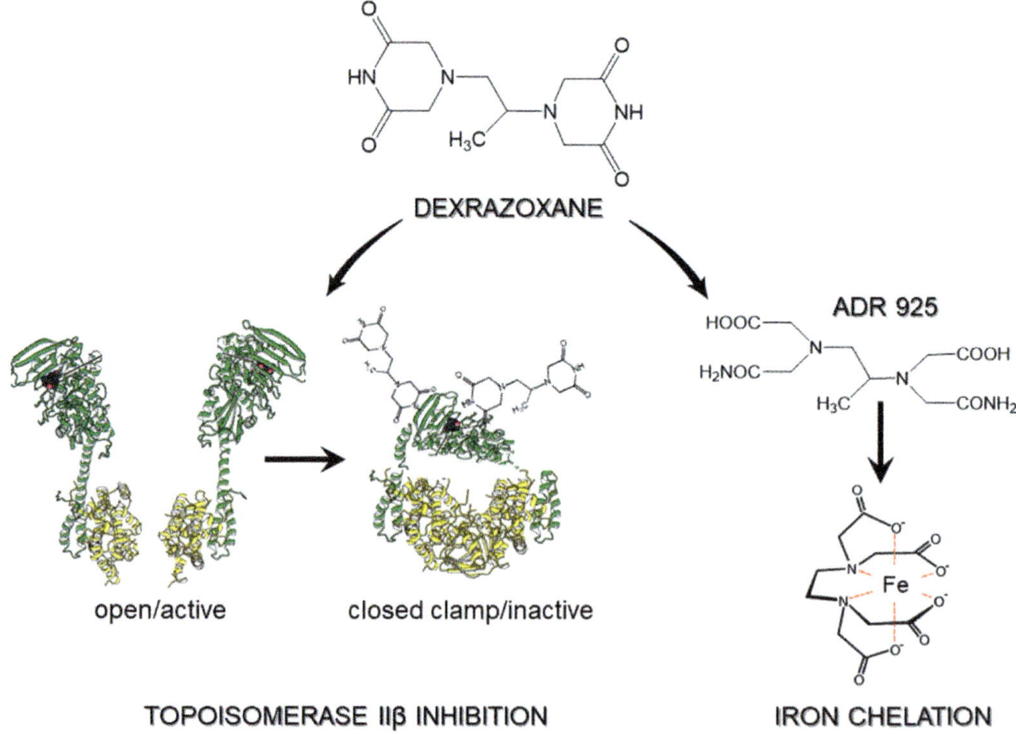

FIGURE 2-5 Mechanisms of action of dexrazoxane. Schematic representation of the two main mechanisms of action of dexrazoxane: inhibition of topisomerase IIβ versus hydrolysis to ADR 925 and iron chelation. (Conceptually adapted from Minotti G, 2004[19], Doroshow JH, 1995[103], Lyu YL, 2007.[104])

childhood acute lymphoblastic leukemia reached opposite conclusions and did not detect an increased risk of second malignancies from dexrazoxane.[114,115] Risk–benefit analyses and pharmacological reasoning strongly support a wider clinical use of dexrazoxane in children adolescents, with the possible exception of clinical settings in which patients received etoposide or etoposide-anthracycline combinations.[116]

Pharmacogenetic prevention ■ Some patients develop CHF after cumulative anthracycline doses that were thought to be safe. This may occur regardless of cardiovascular risk factors but denotes that genetic predisposition is an important factor.[117,118]

A well known example of genetic predisposition pertains to anthracycline secondary alcohol metabolites. This is an instructive story that goes from preclinical evidence to clinical facts. In preclinical studies mice with cardiac-specific overexpression of type 3 carbonyl reductase (CBR) exhibited an increased conversion of doxorubicin to its secondary alcohol metabolite and an accelerated course of development of cardiomyopathy.[119] Conversely, mice with genetic deletion of type 1 carbonyl reductase formed less alcohol metabolite and showed a reduced cardiotoxicity.[120] In clinical settings a retrospective study of childhood cancer survivors, homozygosis for gain-of-function type 3 carbonyl reductase CBR3 V244M G allele contributed to an increased risk of cardiomyopathy associated with low- to moderate-dose anthracyclines, such that no anthracycline dose was "safe" for the predisposed individuals.[121] In individuals with Down syndrome an increased expression of type 1 carbonyl reductase may cause susceptibility to anthracycline-related cardiomyopathy.[122] One limitation of these elegant findings is that only carbonyl reductases were brought into a focus. Anthracycline conversion to secondary alcohol metabolites can in fact be mediated by other enzymes as well. Inhibitor studies suggest that distinct aldehyde reductases may contribute to generate anthracycline secondary alcohol metabolites in the human heart[123] and accordingly, drugs that caused allosteric stimulation of aldehyde reductases were shown to increase the formation of anthracycline secondary alcohol metabolites in human heart. As it was said earlier this was the case of taxanes, which was implicated to explain the higher than expected rates of CHF in breast cancer patients exposed to concomitant administration of doxorubicin and paclitaxel.[46,124,125]

Many other genetic factors may cause an increased risk of cardiotoxicity from anthracyclines. Preliminary results show that high topoisomerase IIβ levels in circulating leukocytes correlate with an individual susceptibility to LVEF decrements after cumulative doxorubicin doses.[126] Excess risk is also caused by reduced expression or genetic variants of drug transporters that contribute to anthracycline elimination (ATP binding cassette proteins of the multidrug resistance proteins family),[127,128] polymorphisms of prooxidant and drug-activating enzymes (NADPH oxidase)[129] or topoisomerase IIβ co-regulating factors (retinoic acid γ receptor)[130] or matrix remodelling enzymes (type 3 hyaluronan synthase).[131] It seems that any single segment of the trajectory that goes from anthracycline disposition to anthracycline activation, DNA damage, and tissue repair is liable to genetic changes that cause an increased susceptibility to anthracyclines. Also mutations associated with familial cardiomyopathy can precipitate anthracycline cardiotoxicity in otherwise asymptomatic patients.[132,133] Unfortunately, genotyping is not routinely performed and cardiac events may occur unexpectedly. On the other hand, recommendations about avoiding anthracyclines or reducing anthracycline dosages in patients with genetic predisposition should be supported by larger prospective studies. The value of genetic screening is therefore uncertain at this point in time.

The pros and cons of primary prevention of anthracycline cardiotoxicity are summarized in Table 2-3.

■ Primary Prevention of Cardiotoxicity from Any Agent

For any chemotherapeutic agent with a known or suspected potential for inducing cardiotoxicity, primary prevention is achieved by measures that rest on common sense at this time in point. Pre-existing comorbidities (hypertension, systolic dysfunction, metabolic disorders) or unfavorable lifestyle choices (smoking, overweight, reduced physical activity) have long been known to increase the risk of cardiotoxicity in patients scheduled to receive anthracyclines.[19] This notion can safely be extended to cardiotoxicity from any other agent and calls for vigorous pharmacological correction of pre-existing comorbidities before chemotherapy was started.[134]

Some reports suggest that cardiovascular drugs should be administered also to patients without risk factors. Significant cardiac protection, measured as preservation or limited decrease of LVEF, was seen in studies of carvedilol (α_1 and β_{1-2} adrenoceptor blocker),[135] nebivolol (β_1 blocker)[136] or carvedilol in combination with the angiotensin converting enzyme inhibitor(s) (ACEI), enalapril.[137] Less protection was seen with metoprolol (β_1 blocker) or enalapril alone.[138] In a recent study the angiotensin II receptor blocker (ARB), candesartan, prevented the decline of LVEF

TABLE 2-3   Primary prevention of anthracycline cardiotoxicity

MEASURE	MECHANISM OF PROTECTION	ANTICIPATED CLINICAL BENEFIT	DISADVANTAGES/ LIMITATIONS
Pharmacokinetic			
Slow infusions	Normal anthracycline AUC but lower C_{max}	Preserved anthracycline activity with reduced risk of cardiotoxicity	Exacerbation of exposure effects, lack of long term cardiac protection in children with acute lymphoblastic leukemia, accumulation of DNA oxidized bases in normal cells
Liposomal formulations	Limited diffusion through the gap junctions of coronary microvasculature	Improved cardiac tolerability; safe administration with concomitant trastuzumab	Mucositis, hand-foot syndrome, high costs, limited approved indications
Pharmacodynamic			
Antioxidants	Mitigation of ROS-mediated mechanisms of cardiotoxicity	Reduced risk of cardiac events	Unproven efficacy (limited cardiac penetration of antioxidants?)
Dexrazoxane	Iron chelation and mitigation of ROS formation/reactivity; inihibition of topoisomerase IIβ-mediated DNA double strand breaks	Prevention of cardiotoxicity in both childhood and adult cancer patients	Interference with anthracycline activity and increased incidence of second malignancies (unconfirmed and/or disproven)
Less cardiotoxic analogues	Reduced activation and toxicity mechanisms	Reduced incidence of CHF?	Not definitely proven; reduced cardiotoxicity of amrubicin and pixantrone in limited approved settings
Pharmacogenetic			
Screening for • CBR3 polymorphisms, topoisomerase IIβ levels and polymorphisms, genetic variants of co-regulating factors • deficiencies, or polymorphisms of drug transporters • polymorphisms of NADPH oxidase • polymorphisms of matrix remodelling enzymes • familial cardiomyopathy mutations	Identification of patients at risk for • altered anthracycline disposition, excess drug activation and/or oxidative stress and/or DNA damage, impaired issue repair	May guide dose adjustments, prophylactic commencement of cardiovascular drugs and/or replacing anthracyclines with nonanthracycline chemotherapeutics	Investigational (information based on retrospective analyses or case reports, lack of prospective clinical trials)

Sources: Modified after reference[95] and based on references.[80–88,94,99–139]

in patients receiving adjuvant anthracycline, with or without subsequent trastuzumab, for the treatment of early breast cancer. Metoprolol was ineffective.[139] Unfortunately, these are limited studies which often focus on marginal decrements of LVEF (e.g., ≥5% by magnetic resonance imaging)[139] or lack long term follow up. Given that LVEF may or may not predict the long term cardiac sequelae of anticancer therapies, the evidence provided by such interventional studies should be interpreted with a due caution.

Primary prevention with cardiovascular drugs merits further consideration with respect to the drug or drugs that were chosen to protect the heart. The rationale for using carvedilol or nebivolol was influenced by precise pharmacodynamic reasonings. In addition to blocking adrenergic receptors, carvedilol diminished ROS formation in isolated cardiomyocytes exposed to doxorubicin.[140] Nebivolol was chosen because it induces endothelial nitric oxide (NO) synthase expression,[141] prevents NO synthase uncoupling and diminishes inappropriate conversion of NO to peroxynitrite.[142] Pleiotropic effects of nebivolol therefore offer vasodilation that was felt to add with hemodynamic effects of β_1 receptor blockade. The available evidence nonetheless suggests that beneficial effects from one β blocker or another ultimately depends on its affinity and selectivity for β_1 receptors $[K_i(\beta_2)/K_i(\beta_1)]$ and consequent effects such as reductions in rate-pressure products and mitigation of myocardial remodeling. This information was obtained in patients exposed to anthracyclines. There is no conceptual obstacle to anticipating beneficial effects also in patients exposed to targeted agents that cause e.g., vasoconstriction and hypertension.

Primary prevention can be done with other drugs as well. An observational clinical cohort study of breast cancer patients treated with anthracyclines suggests that statins could also reduce the risk of CHF.[143] This finding might be reconciled with cardioprotective effects of statins, such as those linked to activation of NO synthase[144] and opening of mitochondrial ATP sensitive potassium channels.[145] Interestingly, however, statin effects were most evident in patients who received other cardiovascular drugs for preexisting risk factors, and hence it remains to be established whether statin effects were coincidental or whether they reflected one or more independent pharmacodynamic mechanisms of cardioprotection.

Each of the aforementioned strategies of primary prevention needs to be scrutinized for risk–benefit balance. Many doctors believe that in patients without risk factors, discomforts from chemotherapy (fatigue, nausea, vomiting) should not be aggravated by class-related effects of cardiovascular drugs (bradicardia, hypotension, fluid retention, cough). Judicious perception of the risk of cardiotoxicity should eliminate this conceptual barrier to primary cardiovascular prevention. On the other hand, many commonly used cardiovascular drugs may alter metabolism and/or transport of anticancer drugs.[134] A risk of harmful pharmacokinetic interactions cannot be ruled out. One can only recommend that in patients without risk factors, cardiovascular drugs were used at "prophylactic" rather than "therapeutic" dosages. Prospective randomized trials are needed to define the efficacy and dose relations of primary prevention with cardiovascular drugs as well as its impact on short and long term efficacy of oncologic treatment. With particular regard to angiogenesis inhibitors we would comment on the possible positive correlation between the oncologic efficacy of these drugs and their ability to induce hypertension through vasoconstriction and microvasculature rarefaction.[144,146,147] Inasmuch as tumor growth, invasion and metastatization, depend on blood supply to cancer cells, one might wonder whether drugs that prevent hypertension through vasodilation could also restore blood supply to tumor cells and diminish oncologic efficacy to some extent. In the absence of studies that explored this issue in depth, common sense and judicious assessment of patient-specific risk–benefit balance must prevail. Drugs that lower blood pressure by controlling cardiac output (β blockers) should at least in principle be preferred over drugs that cause vasodilation (α blockers, ACEI, ARB, dihydropyridine-type Ca^{2+} channel blockers). Again, risk–benefit assessment must prevail.

General concepts of primary prevention of cardiotoxicity from any agent are summarized in Table 2-4.

EMERGING PARADIGMS

■ QT Prolongation

General concepts ■ The QT interval of ECG indicates the total duration of ventricular depolarisation and repolarization. In other words, the QT interval denotes the duration of action potential in ventricular myocytes. Many antitumor drugs can cause prolongation of QT, and in particular, TKI have been recognized or suspected to introduce a measurable risk of QT prolongation.[148,149] Because QT prolongation may result in multifocal ventricular tachiarrhythmias and eventually, in fatal torsade de point (TdP), the FDA requires that QT liability of new drugs be carefully evaluated. This should be done preclinically and in the early

TABLE 2-4   Primary prevention of cardiotoxicity from any agent

MEASURE	MECHANISM OF PROTECTION	ANTICIPATED CLINICAL BENEFIT	DISADVANTAGES/ LIMITATIONS
Pharmacologic correction of comorbidities in high risk patients	Mitigation of cardiovascular, metabolic, and lifestyle risk factors	Reduced incidence of on-treatment cardiac events	none
Coadministration of ACEI, ARB, β-blockers, in low risk patients	Reductions of rate-pressure products and mitigation of cardiac distress; additional pharmacodynamic effects from carvedilol (inhibition of ROS formation) or nebivolol (trophic actions on NO-related pathways that lead to vasodilation)	Improved cardiac tolerability of antitumor agents	Information based on limited studies, need for larger prospective trials; risk of pharmacokinetic interactions of cardiovascular drugs with antitumor drugs (possible but not firmly established); interferences of ACEI, ARB, or dihydropyridine-like Ca^{2+} antagonists with angiogenesis inhibitors (not firmly established)
Statins	Activation of nitric oxide synthase and mitochondrial ATP sensitive potassium channels (preclinical evidence only)	Reduced incidence of CHF	Need for proof of concept studies of low risk patients without concomitant cardiovascular drugs

Sources: Modified after Salvatorelli E et al., 2015[95] and based on Ewer M et al., 2014[134]; Kalay N et al., 2006[135]; Kaya MG et al., 2013[136]; Bosch X et al., 2013[137]; Georgakopoulos P et al., 2010[138]; Gulati G et al., 2016[139]; Spallarossa P et al., 2004[140]; Moen MD et al., 2006[141]; Mason RP et al., 2005[142]; Seicean S et al., 2012[143]; Schmidinger M et al., 2008[144]; Zhao Z et al., 2015[145]; Dahlberg SE et al., 2010[146]; Rautiola J et al., 2016.[147]

stages of clinical development of new pharmacologic entities, according to the nonclinical S7B guidance and the clinical ICH-E14 guideline.[150]

The vast majority of antitumor drugs, and especially TKI, can cause QT prolongation by blocking or causing dysfunction of potassium channels associated with the rapid and slow components of the inwardly rectifying K^+ current (IKr). This results in an abnormally prolonged repolarization. Because part, if not all, of the channel that conducts the rapid component of IKr is encoded by the human Ether-à-go-go Related Gene (hERG) (KCNH2 in the new international gene nomenclature),[151] chemical entities should be probed for the so-called hERG liability[152] (Figure 2-6).

The Comprehensive in vitro Proarrhythmia Assay (CiPA) is a proposal by the FDA and other scientific bodies aimed at revising the nonclinical S7B guidance and replacing the clinical ICH-E14 guidelines. Unfortunately, however, the connection between proarrhythmia and QT prolongation is complex. QT prolongation is a sensitive marker for proarrhythmia but a moderately specific anticipator of cardiac events (i.e., torsadogenic compounds prolong QT but not all QT prolonging drugs are torsadogenic)[149]; therefore, attempts to identifying drugs at risk for inducing TdP have inherent limitations. These caveats having been recognized, the CiPA requires that all new drugs be assessed in multiple and standardized ion channels assays using cell lines that overexpress one channel or the other. Next, ion channel assays should be incorporated in a computational model of cardiac action potential that is calibrated against data from well characterized arrhythmogenic compounds. The results generated *in silico* should eventually be verified in vitro by using induced pluripotent stem cell-derived cardiomyocytes, and in vivo by using telemetry-assisted ECG recordings in rodents. As for the early stages of clinical development, the FDA Interdisciplinary Review Team for QT Studies is in charge of scrutinizing data from clinical trials to waive or call for a "dedicated QT study," a variation of the "thorough QT/QTc Study" that is usually performed in healthy volounteers.[153,154]

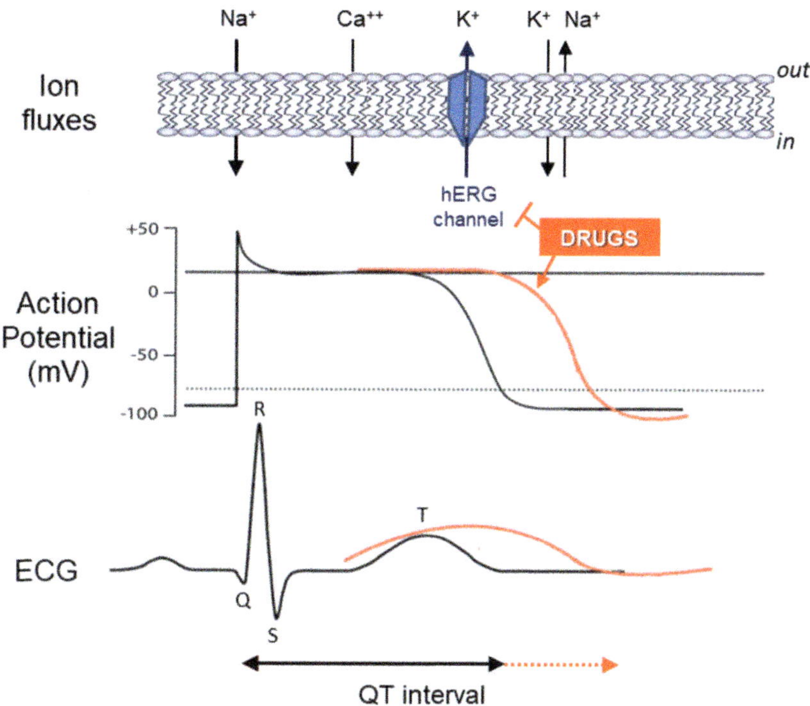

FIGURE 2-6   Prevailing mechanism of QT prolongation by antitumor drugs. Antitumor drugs, and TKI in particular, can prolong QT by blocking or causing dysfunction of potassium channels encoded by the hERG gene (KCNH2 in the new international gene nomenclature).

Dimensions of the problem ■ Methodological issues must be taken in consideration when the actual incidence and torsadogenic potential of QT prolongation are considered. Cardiac repolarization is influenced by heart rate, therefore, the QT tract must be corrected for heart rate. Formulas for heart rate correction of QT have been proposed but each of these formulas (Bazett, Fridericia, Framingham, Hodges) shows limitations. For QTc correction by the Bazett's formula, which is most widely adopted, upper borderline limits have been set at 450 or 470 msec for males or females, respectively.[155] The International Conference on Harmonisation of technical Requirements of Registration of Pharmaceuticals for Human Use (ICHTR) cautions against any QTc prolongation above 500 ms or any ΔQTc change from baseline of >60 ms.[154] Substantial uncertainties about "normal" or "pathologic" QTc intervals nonetheless remain. For example, the Bazett's formula overestimates QT at high heart rates but underestimates it at low heart rates.[156] Either artifact may cause erroneous clinical decisions. High heart rates are quite common in many patients undergoing cancer therapies and are caused by such different factors as anemia or fever. QTc overestimation may lead doctors to adopt unnecessary dose reductions or treatment interruption for these patients. On the other hand, QT underestimation at low heart rates may expose patients to a higher risk of TdP as low heart rates are more torsadogenic than high rates.[148]

Many first- or second-generation TKI have been associated with ΔQTc changes of >60 ms or QTc prolongations above 500 ms; however, relatively few TKI have been reported to cause TdP, and for some of them the actual incidence of TdP is unknown (Table 2-5).[157,158] Absolute and relative risk of severe arrhythmias from TKI therefore remains under scrutiny. It seems that the risk of QTc prolongation is potentially high but the incidence of severe arrhythmias is relatively low. This is even more surprising if one considers that cancer patients are at an increased risk for arrhythmias as compared to healthy controls or nononcologic patients, which is explained by predisposing factors like the underlying disease, treatment-related electrolyte imbalance, concomitant administration of drugs that prolong QTc (Table 2-6).[148] The expertise of doctors in correcting predisposing disturbances or avoiding QT-prolonging medications therefore seems to outweigh the arryhthmogenic risk associated with TKI.[148,157,158]

A very special case: Arsenic trioxide ■ Arsenic trioxide (ATO) has long been used to treat some leukemias. Currently it represents the standard of care for relapsed/refractory acute promyelocytic leukemia (APL) but recent studies led to approving ATO also

TABLE 2-5 Tyrosine kinase inhibitors reportedly associated with QT prolongation

TYROSIN KINASE INHIBITOR	ΔQTC >60 MS (% OF PATIENTS)	QTC >500 MS (% OF PATIENTS)	TORSADE DE POINTES (% OF PATIENTS)
Bosutinib	0.34	0.2	n.a.
Crizotinib	3.5	1.3	n.a.
Dasatinib	0.6–3	<1.4	n.a.
Lapatinib	11	6.1	n.a.
Nilotinib	1.9–4.7	<1.2	n.a.
Pazopanib	n.a.	2	<0.3
Ponatinib	n.a.	n.a.	n.a.
Sorafenib	n.a.	n.a.	n.a.
Sunitinib	1–4	0.5	<0.1
Vandetanib	12–15	4.3-8	reported (unknown %)
Vemurafenib	1.6	1.6	reported (unknown %)

n.a., not available
Sources: Modified and expanded after Shah RR et al., 2013[157]; Strevel EL et al., 2007.[158]

for newly diagnosed low-intermediate risk APL, thus avoiding therapy with cumulative doses of idarubicin.[159,160] The package insert for ATO has a black box warning about TdP; in fact, ATO probably represents the antitumor drug that most consistently introduces a risk of ∅QTc changes of >60 msec or QTc prolongations above 500 ms. ATO binds to, and concentration-dependently inhibits the slow and rapid components of IKr.[161,162] ATO also induces an oxidative inactivation of IKr[161] and can delay IKr protein export from endoplasmic reticulum to the cell surface.[163] All such effects on IKr would recapitulate ATO inhibition of repolarization and prolongation of QTc. Interestingly, however, the type Ib Na^+ channel blocker, lidocaine rescued a patient from long QTc and TdP induced by ATO, which suggests that arrhythmogenic effects of ATO might at least in part be caused also by a prolongation of Na^+-dependent depolarization.[161] Moreover, studies of isolated cells showed that ATO could also activate an ATP-gated K^+ channel, IKATP, that maintains normal repolarization.[162]

Mechanisms of ATO-related arrhythmias are therefore more complex than usually reported. For each patient exposed to antileukemic therapy with ATO the probability of QTc prolongation and risk of TdP may reflect a complex balance between competing factors such as activation of Na^+ dependent depolarization, inhibition of K^+ dependent repolarization, activation of ATP and K' dependent repolarization. How do these facts translate into clinical facts? In a cohort of patients treated for non-APL acute leukemias or myelodisplastic syndrome some 90% of patients showed

Bazett-corrected QT values greater than 470 ms and 65% had QTc above 500 ms.[156] By using alternative rate correction formulas, QTc intervals above 500 ms still were adjudicated in ~30% of patients.[156] In the trial of ATO for the treatment of newly diagnosed low-to-intermediate risk APL, Framingham-corrected prolongations of QTc above 450 msec in males or above 460 msec in females were detected in ~16% of patients.[159] This having been said it is remarkably noticeable that ventricular arrhythmias were very uncommon and canonical TdP did not occur. Most serious QTc prolongations could safely be managed by temporary drug discontinuation, electrolyte repletion, and removal of any concomitant medication that prolonged QTc. Permanent discontinuation of ATO was necessary in one patient only.[159] Similar findings occurred in the trial that probed ATO to treat newly diagnosed high risk APL.[160] As it was said for TKI, there seems to be a discrepancy between the established and potentially life-threatening arrhythmogenic potential of ATO and its apparent cardiac safety in clinical practice or investigational studies. Judicious repletion of potassium and magnesium levels proves more than effective in preventing and managing the risk of serious arrhythmias.[156]

Remarks and perspectives ■ ICH Guidelines were finalized to minimize the risk that oncologic and nononcologic drugs caused post-approval cardiac events attributable to QTc prolongation. Following introduction of these guidelines and their further implementation by CiPA no drug was withdrawn from the market for

TABLE 2-6 **Risk factors for QT prolongation in cancer patients**

RISK FACTORS

Electrolyte imbalance
    Hypokalaemia (<3.5 mEq/L)
    Hypomagnesaemia (<1.6 mg/dL)
    Hypocalcaemia (<8.5 mg/dL)
Treatment-related predisposing toxicities
• nausea and emesis
• diarrhea
• treatment with loop diuretics

Treatment-related hypothyroidism
Concomitant QT-prolonging drugs • Antiarrhythmic (e.g., amiodarone, dronedarone, dofetilide, quinidine, disopyramide, flecainide, procainamide, sotalol, etc.) • Antibiotics (e.g., erythromycin, azithromycin, ciprofloxacin, clarithromycin, levofloxacin, etc.) • Antifungal (fluconazole, itraconazole, ketoconazole, voriconazole) • Antidepressant (e.g., imipramine, doxepine, amitriptyline) • Antipsychotic (chlorpromazine, clozapine, fluphenazine, haloperidol, olanzapine, quetiapine, trifluoperazine, thioridazine, etc.) • Antiemetic (e.g., dolasetron, palonosetron, ondansetron, granisetron, droperidol, etc.) • Antihistamine (diphenhydramine, hydroxyzine, orphenadrine, promethazine, chlorpheniramine)

Source: Modified and expanded after Lenihan DJ et al., 2013.[148]

QT-related proarrhythmia in recent years.[164] This should not be interpreted to conclude that more drugs are being removed from clinical development programs because of concerns about hERG liability. As matter of fact, in 2013, as many as 89% of QT-prolongers were approved for clinical use. Rates of approval were largely irrespective of the QT effect size. FDA approved >80% of drugs that caused QT prolongations of <10 mesc, 10–20 msec, >20 msec (Figure 2-7). The major reason QT prolongers receive an FDA approval rests with risk-benefit assessment. Drugs targeted at otherwise uncurable diseases are deemed to introduce a benefit that outweighs the risk of QT prolongation and related arrhythmias.[164] It goes without saying that such an agreeable philosophy of drug approval requires post-approval surveillance and close collaboration between all involved parties (pharmaceutical companies, doctors, patients). QT prolongation by CDK 4/6 inhibitors, like ribociclib, will greatly benefit from this strategy.

■ Thrombosis and Thromboembolism

Platelet activation and/or hypercoagulation may complicate clinical management of many patients affected by cancer. Predisposing factors can be linked to both the underlying malignancy and the pharmacological treatment. Tumour cells activate the coagulation cascade by synthetizing and releasing procoagulant, antifibrinolytic and pro-aggregation factors, pro-inflammatory cytokines, adhesion molecules.[165] Venous thrombosis and venous thromboembolism (VTE) thus occur quite often in cancer patients and use of indwelling venous catheters introduces an important predisposing factor. Disease-related arterial thrombosis is relatively

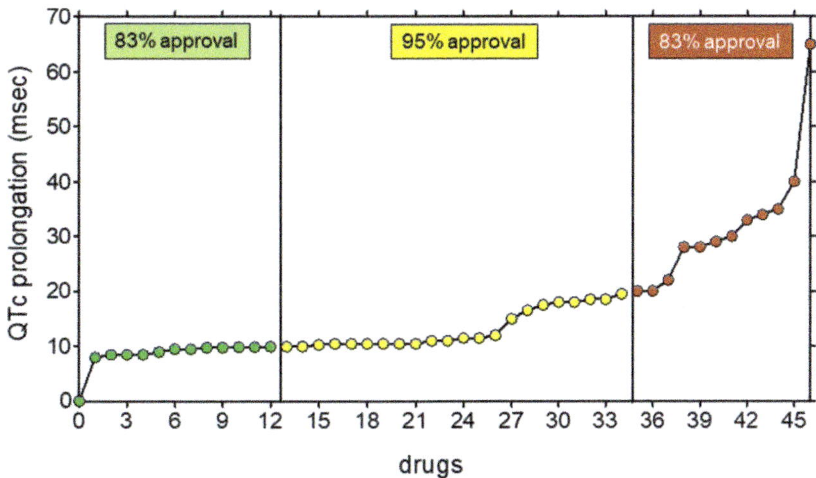

FIGURE 2-7 FDA approval rates of QTc prolonging drugs. Schematic representation of FDA approval rates for oncologic and nononcologic drugs that cause mild (≤10 msec, green symbols), moderate (10–20 msec, yellow symbols) or serious (>20 msec, red symbols) prolongation of QTc. (Modified after Park E, 2014.[164])

less frequent but can seriously complicate the clinical course of patients affected by metastatic pancreatic, breast, colorectal and lung cancers.[166] Venous thrombosis, VTE, and arterial thrombosis are also consequences of certain cancer treatments. Conventional chemotherapeutics, antiangiogenic agents, hormonal agents like e.g., tamoxifen, can cause VTE. On the other hand, Abl inhibitors like nilotinib and ponatinib introduce high rates of both artherial thrombosis event and VTE.

The pharmacologic armamentarium for managing thrombosis and thromboembolism in cancer patients is the same as that available for nononcologic patients. It includes low molecular weight heparins (LMWH), vitamin K antagonists (VKA), new oral anticoagulants (NOACs), antiplatelet agents, but formal guidelines to prescribe cancer patients with one agent or another are lacking. Some pharmacological issues therefore remain unsettled. Given that cancer disease and chemotherapeutics conspire in inducing thrombotic events, should cancer patients be routinely given primary antithrombotic prevention? What are the pharmacological foundations, if any, for choosing between LMWH and VKA or NOAC? Is there a pharmacologic rationale for prescribing antiplatelet agents as primary prevention for patients at risk for TKI-induced arterial thrombosis?

Primary prevention of thromboembolism ▪ Limited but persuasive trial evidence suggests that LMWH might be considered for primary prevention of venous and arterial thrombotic events in cancer patients undergoing chemotherapy for advanced solid tumors. Nadroparin reduced the incidence of thrombotic events in patients undergoing chemotherapy, and did so without introducing an excess risk for major or minor bleeding.[167] Interestingly, post hoc analyses revealed that in patients achieving disease control nadroparin introduced also a measurable survival benefit, which in principle would support an alleged antitumor effect of heparin.[168] Although more data are needed to translate these findings into routine clinical practice, feasibility and efficacy and safety of primary prevention with LMWH seem to be evident. However, all such pros were documented only in high risk patients with advanced solid tumors. Benefit stratification according to tumor type was not characterized. The risk–benefit of primary prevention with LMWH should also be explored in lower risk patients, such as those undergoing adjuvant therapy for early operable tumors.

Choosing between LMWH, VKA, and NOACs ▪ Comparisons between LMWH, VKA, and NOACs for cancer patients are currently limited to clinical trials that explored the efficacy and safety of either agent for preventing recurrent VTE. Following a confirmed episode

of VTE, a 3–6 months course of LMWH was superior to VKA in preventing recurrent VTE in cancer patients and did not introduce an increased risk of mortality or bleeding.[169] With regard to NOACs, there is limited data for their efficacy and safety in cancer patients, and this derives from nononcologic clinical trials that recruited few cancer patients as a special subgroup and for comparison purposes only. Under such limited and well-defined conditions, rivarobaxan (inhibitor of factor Xa) or dabigatran (inhibitor of thrombin) were as effective and safe as warfarin in preventing recurrent VTE.[170,171] A phase IIb placebo-controlled study was designed to evaluate apixaban for prophylaxis of VTE in ambulatory patients who received chemotherapy for the treatment of advanced malignancies. Apixaban safety was encouraging but the sample size was too small to draw conclusions on efficacy.[172]

Given that clinical or random evidence for preferring one agent or another is scant, choosing between LMWH, VKA, or NOAC should be guided by some general considerations on the pharmacologic properties of each anticoagulant and their possible modifications in cancer patients. This is particularly important if NOACs were to be preferred over the other agents in consideration of potential advantages like e.g., fewer pharmacologic interactions and no stringent need for laboratory monitoring and adjustment of the daily dose (Table 2-7). First, by having said that cancer patients are at a higher risk than the general population for thrombosis and thromboembolism, it remains unclear whether the dosing regimens that were approved for NOACs in the general population will show equally protective in cancer patients.[173] Second, some NOACs (apixaban, rivaroxaban) are oxidatively metabolized by cytochrome P4503A, which is also involved in metabolizing many other antitumor drugs; moreover, all NOACs are substrates for the ATP-dependent efflux transporter, P-glycoprotein, that contributes to eliminating drugs via biliary and kidney tubules.[173] Dual pharmacokinetic dependence on P-glycoprotein and cytochrome P4503A is common to many oncologic and nononcologic drugs.[174] Thus, although NOACs are said to engage in fewer drug-drug interactions than VKA, the possibility that such interactions occurred and altered the anticoagulant effect of NOACs should not be excluded a priority. Third, the lack of a standardized laboratory test to monitor the anticoagulant effects of NOACs can be viewed as a double-edged sword. On the one hand, the unnecessity for serial measurement of International Normalized Ratio (INR), which is routine for patients treated with VKA, diminishes patient's psychological distress; on the other hand, however, it does expose doctors and patients to the risk of sudden thrombosis

TABLE 2-7 Advantages and disadvantages of different anticoagulants

	VKA	LMWH	NOACs
Advantages	• Oral bioavailability • Extensive clinical experience • Laboratory test to monitor anticoagulation (INR) • Excess anticoagulation reversed by vitamin K, plasma or concentrates • Safe in kidney impairment	• Rapid onset and offset of anticoagulation • Trial experience in cancer patients • Few drug-drug interactions • Laboratory monitoring not routinely needed	• Oral bioavailability • Rapid onset and offset of anticoagulation • Reportedly few drug-drug interactions • Antidotes available for dabigatran (idarucizumab) and rivaroxaban (andexanet alpha); ciraparantag in development to reverse the effects of rivaroxaban, apixaban, and edoxaban • Laboratory monitoring not routinely needed
Disadvantages	• Slow onset and offset of anticoagulation • Interactions with many drugs and foods • Dose adjustments usually needed • Low therapeutic index • Need for repeat INR	• Parenteral biovailability • Lack of reliable reversal agents • Dose adjustments required in kidney impairment • Need for high level of adherence	• Limited experience in cancer patients • Universal antidote still lacking • Laboratory tests not routinely available (e.g., diluted thrombin time for dabigatran) • Caution advised in patients with kidney impairment • Need for high level of adherence

INR, international normalized ratio
Source: Modified after Short NJ, Connors JM, 2014.[173]

or bleeding caused by unrecognized pharmacokinetic changes. Fourth, and finally, the lack of reversal agents for NOAC was long perceived as a weakness in comparison with VKA, whose effect is reversed by high dose vitamin K. Bleeding complications from NOACs are now manageable by specific antidotes. Andexanet alpha, a synthetic decoy of factor Xa, reverses the effect of rivaroxaban, and the humanized monoclonal antibody, idarucizumab, reverses the effect of dabigatran. The small peptide, ciraparantag, is being developed to reverse the effects of rivaroxaban, apixaban, and edoxaban.[175] The cost effectiveness of such reversal agents should nonetheless to be considered.

Further considerations are needed for the rapid onset and offset of the anticoagulant effect of NOACs. This requires a high level of patient's adherence, particularly when dose adjustments were needed for patients with kidney impairment and reduced drug elimination. All NOACs are in fact characterized by a short elimination half life, usually in the range of 8–17 hours.[173] This translates into a rapid achievement of the anticoagulant effect but also causes, at least in principle, a risk of thrombosis if few daily doses are omitted.

On balance, NOACs represent a novel and important opportunity for cancer patients at risk for thrombosis and VTE but more studies are needed to refine their risk–benefit in different settings like prevention of VTE during chemotherapy or prevention of recurrent VTE once chemotherapy was completed. Moreover, studies are needed that characterize the safety of switching from NOAC to LMWH when disease recurrence requires that chemotherapy be resumed and potential pharmacokinetic interactions with chemotherapeutics may once again occur.

TKI, arterial thrombosis and risk–benefit of antiplatelet agents ■ The high incidence of arterial thrombosis from ponatinib and other Abl inhibitors (e.g., nilotinib) has raised questions about the risk–benefit of primary prevention with aspirin or other antiplatelet agents. Whereas aspirin is more than justified for patients with pre-exisiting vascular disease, little is known about the risk–benefit of inhibiting platelet aggregation in low risk patients. A general recommendation cannot be provided, decisions should be based on a rigorous individualization of risk assessment.[18,176,177] Moreover, risk of thrombosis should be weighed against risk of bleeding associated with disease-related thrombocytopenia and/or possible interferences of ponatinib with platelet function. The precise mechanism or mechanisms of platelet dysfunction induced by ponatinib remain under scrutiny. Ponatinib was said to inhibit kinases of the Src family (LYN, FYN) that mediate early platelet activation;[178] however, the clinical impact of such off target effect on the risk of bleeding has been questioned. According to a single institution experience only a small minority of patients who received ponatinib experienced clinical bleeding, and cause-and-effect relationships between ponatinib and bleeding events could not be demonstrated.[179] It was suggested that bleeding might occur if platelet count was low and patients received concomitant anticoagulants or aspirin or other antiplatelet agents.[179] These premises having been given, all patients prescribed with aspirin or thienopiryridines (clopidogrel, prasugrel) should be carefully monitored for bleeding. Platelet count should be checked periodically, and prophylaxis should be discontinued when platelet count decreases to below e.g., 50.000/μL.[177] In high risk patients with pre-existing peripheral artery disease, concomitant administration of anticoagulants and antiplatelet agents should be avoided or considered with a due caution; in fact, in nononcologic settings, adding oral anticoagulants to antiplatelet therapy in patients with peripheral artery disease did not reduce cardiovascular events but increased the incidence of severe bleeding.[180]

PHARMACOLOGIC PRINCIPLES OF SECONDARY PREVENTION

Clinical symptoms of heart failure and/or ischemic cardiomyopathy may develop on-treatment but also months or years after cancer diagnosis and treatment. This is seen for both childhood and adult cancer patients. Quite evidently the process leading to the so called "late cardiotoxicity" begins as early as the patient is exposed to antitumor drugs but remains subclinical for a length of time that depends on the pathophysiology of each patient and his/her exposure to sequential stressor agents.

As it was mentioned earlier, trial evidence for the efficacy of primary prevention is too limited to form the basis for a general recommendation. Recent studies actually dispel the alleged efficacy of primary prevention with e.g., valsartan.[181] Dexrazoxane is a noticeable exception but regulatory barriers that preclude its clinical use have been described. This having been said, the last chance to protect patients from cardiovascular sequelae of antitumor drugs rests with secondary prevention. This must be guided by laboratory findings of toxicity in otherwise asymptomatic or poorly symptomatic patients.[95] Again, early and late cardiotoxicity intertwin in a pathologic continuum. Secondary prevention can therefore be started during chemotherapy or anytime after completing it.

■ Defining Early Asymptomatic Cardiotoxicity

On-treatment asymptomatic cardiotoxicity might be adjudicated anytime patient's LVEF decreases by >10% and to below 50%.[182] Can this criterion be adopted to guide decisions such as stopping chemotherapy or reducing the dosage of e.g., anthracyclines? The available evidence does not uniformly go in that direction. In some patients LVEF returned to baseline if chemotherapy was stopped but in other patients LVEF normalized also when chemotherapy was continued.[183] This is no surprise if one considers that LVEF may decrease in response to a number factors that have little to do with the process or processes of cardiotoxicity (anemia, infections, transient neurohumoral changes, hydration disorders).[183,184] Decisions about interrupting life-saving antitumor therapies and commencing secondary prevention should better rest with serial measurements that detected a gradual but inexorable deterioration of LVEF. This can only be done in centers that developed collaborations between oncologists and cardiologists; however, there is a lack of evidence-based guidelines that precisely defined when, how often and by which integrative approaches should LVEF be measured during and after treatment. Recommendations have been provided but these should always be interpreted according to patients' characteristics and therapeutic programs.[185]

Secondary prevention might alternatively be guided by biomarkers. These can be used to detect cardiomyocyte necrosis or cardiomyocyte dysfunction due to abnormal ventricle wall tension. Troponin denotes cardiomyocyte necrosis. In blood samples collected after ending chemotherapy infusions, troponin I elevations denoted that oncologic drugs overwhelmed the defense mechanisms of cardiomyocytes and caused formation of necrotic foci systolic dysfunction could build on. Single post-infusion measurements may be informative but complete areas under the curve over 24–72 hours would probably identify the at-risk patients with a higher level of precision.[186] In single institution studies troponin elevations identified patients that subsequently experienced LVEF decrements.[187] Enalapril administration, guided by troponin elevations, prevented LVEF decrements at 1-year follow-up while patients without enalapril protection showed a significant incidence of LVEF decrements to below 50%.[29,187] But the literature reads both positive[188] and negative[181] reports on the association between TnI elevations and risk of systolic dysfunction. Lack of consistency may be due to limitations that are inherent to single institution studies. Multicenter studies that incorporate heterogeneity due to different assays across the participating institutions or adopt a protocol-defined assay are much needed to refine the prognostic value of troponin elevations in real life or trial-like contexts.[189] Concerns were also raised about the characteristics of patients for whom troponin heralded an increased risk of LVEF decrements. In general these were patients who had received several chemotherapy regimens, including high dose protocols with anthracycline and nonanthracycline drugs. Associations between troponin elevations and systolic dysfunction in patients exposed to standard dose chemotherapy, whether anthracycline-based or nonanthracycline, merit more investigations.[189] On balance, many details need to be refined before TnI assay could be recommended to identify at-risk patients and to start heart failure therapy. Technical details include the assay of choice (low-moderate versus high sensitivity TnI), timing of the assay, thresholds for defining TnI elevations (any change over baseline or only elevations above prespecified upper limits of normal), weighing of confounders (kidney dysfunction, unrecognized non-cardiac sources of circulating TnI). Similar inconsistencies and concerns apply to the monitoring of increased levels of circulating BNP or Nt-proBNP, which denote and increased ventricle wall tension.[90,181]

Uncertainties about TnI or natriuretic peptide need to be addressed with no prejudice as the optimization of one or more simple laboratory tests to intercept asymptomatic cardiotoxicity is of obvious value. In cases when biomarkers were monitored and abnormal changes were captured during or after chemotherapy, secondary prevention should be considered as soon as possible. Lessons from childhood cancer survivors clearly demonstrate that the delaying of secondary prevention paves the road to an inexorable progression of cardiac remodelling and function.[190]

■ Pharmacological Correction of Post-Chemotherapy Chronic Health Conditions

Inasmuch as cardiotoxicity often matures asymptomatically and progresses toward clinical symptoms long after cancer diagnosis and treatment, it is imperative that preexisting risk factors be rigorously corrected. Comorbidities correction therefore represents an integral component of primary prevention; however, the availble evidence suggests that chronic health conditions may also mature after cancer treatment. In comparison with age-matched controls, previously healthy survivors of adolescent or adult cancer develop more comorbidities or tend to reducing physical activity.[134,191] For example, in childhood cancer survivors, 10% of 50-year-old patients carry three chronic health conditions, with ~50% and ≥20% cumulative incidence of, respectively, first and second condition. Age-matched siblings would carry only one or two conditions, with ≤20% cumulative incidence of the first condition.[134]

A conspiracy between chronic health conditions and subclinical cardiovascular toxicity from lifelong molecular signatures of antitumor drugs should be taken in consideration. In patients exposed to anthracycline-based regimens, comorbidities that developed after chemotherapy would overlap with the cardiac reservoir of secondary alcohol metabolites.[90] In patients exposed to platinum compounds, comorbidities that developed after chemotherapy would overlap with platinum accumulation in the intima of arteries and exfoliation of endothelial cells.[90,192] It follows that for certain drugs, and especially for the so-called type 1 chemotherapeutics, late cardiovascular sequelae of antitumor therapies would eventually build on a stratification of injuries ("hits") that depend on the characteristics of drugs and the chronic disease that matures after cancer treatment. This is the so-called "multiple-hit hypothesis."[58,193]

This having been recognized, an adequate correction of post-chemotherapy chronic health conditions represents an integral component of secondary prevention. These concepts raise a compelling question: should pharmacological correction of post-chemotherapy chronic health conditions be reshaped according to the characteristics of cancer patients? In other words, should cancer patients be treated earlier or more vigorously than the general population? Here there is a lack of information. In principle, and especially for low risk drugs like e.g., statins, pharmacologic targets should be adjusted as if cancer survivors were high or very high risk patients. LDL Cholesterol should be maintained at <100 mg/dL or <79 mg/dL, respectively, if this were the case.[177] There is no trial evidence to support this notion but retrospective data show that survivors referring to cancer centers tend to accumulate fewer chronic health conditions than survivors referring to other physicians.[194] It is tempting to infer that the benefit from referring to cancer centers reflected a different approach to the pathophysiology of cancer survivors and a higher level of risk perception that cardio-oncology teams may have developed as compared to other caregivers. Much of this information derives from patients treated with anthracyclines and nonanthracycline chemotherapeutics. Less is known about the possible incidence of chronic health conditions in survivors of cancer treated with targeted agents.

■ Pharmacologic Correction of Asymptomatic Diastolic Dysfunction

Secondary prevention should also benefit from studies that identify diastolic dysfunction as the earliest and pharmacologically treatable manifestation of subclinical cardiotoxicity. Several pharmacological reasonings would in fact identify diastolic relaxation as a culprit of cardiotoxicity induced by anthracyclines and nonanthracycline chemotherapeutics. In patients exposed to anthracyclines diastolic relaxation would be impaired by mechanisms that increase cellular levels of Ca^{2+} and prevent myofilament relaxation (inhibition or reduced expression levels SERCA2a, inhibition of the energy processes that assist Ca^{2+} sequestration in mitochondria, inappropriate opening of sarcoplasmic Ca^{2+}-gated Ca^{2+} release channel/ryanodine receptor 2).[19] In patients exposed to nonanthracycline chemotherapeutics, like e.g., fluoropyrimidines, alkylators, tubuline-active alkaloids or taxanes, endothelial dysfunction and interruption of nitric oxide-mediated vasorelaxation would induce subclinical ischemia that also causes Ca^{2+} overload.[195] For patients exposed to trastuzumab, blockade of signaling-driven turnover of sarcomeric proteins, and especially of the giant myofilament protein, titin, would be mechanistically important.[196]

How strong is the evidence for asymptomatic diastolic dysfunction to precede systolic dysfunction and CHF? Asymptomatic survivors of childhood or adolescent cancer often present echocardiographic indices of diastolic dysfunction that precede LVEF decrements or clinical symptoms of CHF.[197–199] Relatively less solid is the evidence for this pattern to occur during and/or shortly after cancer therapy. Limited studies of breast cancer patients who were regularly monitored over 12 months after the last anthracycline administration suggest that the incidence of diastolic dysfunction may be as high as 58%; however, echocardiographic indices of diastolic dysfunction were reversible in 27% of such patients, which suggests that it may be difficult to discriminate between transient abnormalities due to e.g., reversible Ca^{2+} accumulation, and an authentic fixation of diastolic dysfunction.[200] On the other hand, studies of children with hematologic malignancies raise the possibility that early after chemotherapy the right ventricle develops diastolic dysfunction while the left ventricle shows a trend toward asymptomatic systolic dysfunction, which introduces further complexity to consider.[201]

Diastolic dysfunction slowly progresses toward ventricle remodeling if it is left untreated. Canonical CHF or heart failure with normal ejection fraction (HFNEF)[202] may eventually develop. Long standing diastolic dysfunction also progresses toward ischemic disease if it is left untreated. In fact, diastolic stiffness of the ventricle wall increases interstitial pressure and diminishes coronary conductance, eventually inducing a limited oxygen supply to cardiomyocytes.[203] The pathophysiology of diastolic dysfunction therefore embraces all clinical phenotypes of cardiotoxicity (CHF, HFNEF, ischemic disease).

Pharmacotherapy of diastolic dysfunction remains a matter of uncertainties.[204] Common cardiovascular drugs are not specific enough to cure diastolic dysfunction. There are hopes that diastolic dysfunction could be cured with ranolazine, an orally available drug that was approved for the treatment of chronic angina. Ranolazine inhibits the diastolic late inward sodium current (INa,Late). When abnormally activated by ROS or ischemia, as it is in the case of chronic angina, INa,Late causes elevation of intracellular Na^+, which exchanges with extracellular Ca^{2+} via the reverse mode Na^+-Ca^{2+} exchanger. Excess Ca^{2+} entry activates myofilaments, increases ventricle wall stiffness, reduces coronary conductance (Figure 2-8).[195,203] By inhibiting INa,Late ranolazine introduces a positive lusitropic effect that relieves stiffness and improves coronary conductance, eventually breaking

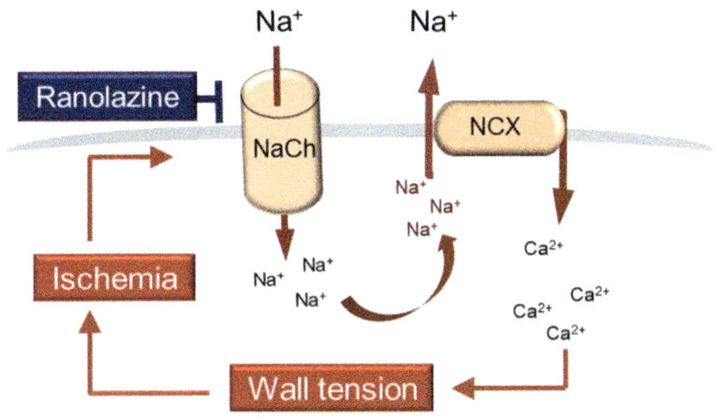

FIGURE 2-8 Ranolazine-inhibitable $I_{Na,Late}$ and its role in diastolic dysfunction and ischemia. $I_{Na,}$Late activation causes elevated intracellular Na+ that exchanges with extracellular Ca2+ via the reverse mode Na+-Ca2+ exchanger. Excess Ca2+ entry causes diastolic wall tension, and the latter causes ischemia that perpetuates $I_{Na,}$Late activation. Ranolazine acts by inhibiting $I_{Na,}$ Late. NaCh, Na+ channel; NCX, Na+-Ca2+ exchanger. (Modified after Minotti G, 2013.[195])

a vicious cycle in which ischemia begets ischemia and diastolic dysfunction begets aggravation of ventricular wall stress. In cancer patients, and regardless of preexisting ischemia, INa,Late might well be activated by anthracycline-induced oxygen consumption and ROS formation. Nonanthracycline chemotherapeutics (fluoropyrimidines, alkylators, tubulin-active vinca alkaloids) would also activate INaLate by perturbing endothelial function and cardiac microvasculature perfusion.[195] Direct evidence that ranolazine inhibits hyperactive INaLate in cancer patients is lacking. Studies of oxidative stress-prone deoxycorticosterone acetate-salt hypertensive mice, which in principle should express a hyperactive INa,Late, suggest that ranolazine might relieve diastolic dysfunction by modulating Ca2+ effects on the contractile apparatus rather than by inhibiting INa,Late.[205] Regardless of such uncertainties, which nonetheless herald a number of ranolazine beneficial effects, a phase IIb study was launched to probe the efficacy and safety of ranolazine versus investigator's choice of other cardiovascular drugs in patients who completed standard dose anthracycline-based or nonanthracycline chemotherapy. The results of this study have not yet been published.

NEW DRUGS AND SCENARIOS

An avalanche of new antitumor drugs will enter clinical practice in the next few years. Newer phenotypes of cardiotoxicity might therefore emerge. For some of the recently approved drugs, like the immune-checkpoint blocking antibodies, ipilimumab and nivolumab and pembrolizumab, immune-mediated cardiotoxicity might become a concern. Cardiotoxic events such as CHF, cardiomyopathy, heart block, myocardial fibrosis, and myocarditis, have been reported for patients receiving these drugs for treatment of melanoma or non-small cell lung carcinoma.[206] Strategies of primary or secondary prevention of cardiotoxicity from these agents are obviously lacking at this point in time. Risk awareness, careful monitoring of patients, and prompt commencement of steroids is the only reasonable strategy to adopt. For other drugs, like ponatinib or the Bruton kinase inhibitor, ibrutinib, the approved dose regimens probably are too high than those required to achieve target inhibition.[39,207] It follows that vascular toxicity from ponatinib or atrial fibrillation from ibrutinib may at least in part depend on plasma and tissue inappropriate exposure to either drug. Dose-related off target effects cannot be ruled out. Once again, this denotes that the current processes of drug approval, including fast track evaluation and accelerated approval, have inherent limitations. Premature conclusions on the best dose regimens to recommend for drug approval add to the list of limitations. Binding decisions to the maximum tolerated dose (MTD) identified in early clinical studies might not be a wise strategy if pharmacodynamic studies demonstrate target inhibition following administration of lower doses.[39,207]

Whereas risk:benefit analysis remains a formidable tool to dissect the pros and cons of using a drug in a patient, the future of cardio-oncology will increasingly rest on pharmacological characterizations of the mechanisms of action of both old and new generation drugs.

REFERENCES

1. Cardinale D. A new frontier: cardio-oncology. *Cardiologia*. 1996;41:887–888.
2. Dyck JR, Lopaschuk GD. AMPK alterations in cardiac physiology and pathology: enemy or ally? *J Physiol*. 2006;574:95–112.
3. Hasenfuss G, Schillinger W, Lehnart SE, et al. Relationship between Na+-Ca2+-exchanger protein levels and diastolic function of failing human myocardium. *Circulation*. 1999;99:641–648.
4. Sikkel MB, Hayward C, MacLeod KT, et al. SERCA2a gene therapy in heart failure: an anti-arrhythmic positive inotrope. *Br J Pharmacol*. 2014;171:38–54.
5. Ashley N, Poulton J. Mitochondrial DNA is a direct target of anti-cancer anthracycline drugs. *Biochem Biophys Res Commun*. 2009;16;378:450–455.

6. Lebrecht D, Walker UA. Role of mtDNA lesions in anthracycline cardiotoxicity. *Cardiovasc Toxicol*. 2007;7:108–113.

7. Maslov MY, Chacko VP, Hirsch GA, et al. Reduced in vivo high-energy phosphates precede adriamycin-induced cardiac dysfunction. *Am J Physiol Heart Circ Physiol*. 2010;299:H332–337.

8. Force T, Krause DS, Van Etten RA. Molecular mechanisms of cardiotoxicity of tyrosine kinase inhibition. *Nat Rev Cancer*. 2007;7:332–344.

9. Hasinoff BB. The cardiotoxicity and myocyte damage caused by small molecule anticancer tyrosine kinase inhibitors is correlated with lack of target specificity. *Toxicol Appl Pharmacol*. 2010;244:190–195.

10. Lipshultz SE, Anderson LM, Miller TL, et al. Impaired mitochondrial function is abrogated by dexrazoxane in doxorubicin-treated childhood acute lymphoblastic leukemia survivors. *Cancer*. 2016;122:946–953.

11. Hasinoff BB, Patel D, O'Hara KA. Mechanisms of myocyte cytotoxicity induced by the multiple receptor tyrosine kinase inhibitor sunitinib. *Mol Pharmacol*. 2008;74:1722–1728.

12. Kerkela R, Woulfe KC, Durand JB, et al. Sunitinib-induced cardiotoxicity is mediated by off-target inhibition of AMP-activated protein kinase. *Transl Sci*. 2009;18:2:15–25.

13. Cheng H, Force T. Molecular mechanisms of cardiovascular toxicity of targeted cancer therapeutics. *Circ Res*. 2010;106:21–34.

14. Ewer MS, Suter TM, Lenihan DJ, et al. Cardiovascular events among 1090 cancer patients treated with sunitinib, interferon, or placebo: a comprehensive adjudicated database analysis demonstrating clinically meaningful reversibility of cardiac events. *Eur J Cancer*. 2014;50:2162–2170.

15. Kerkela R, Grazette L, Yacobi R, et al. Cardiotoxicity of the cancer therapeutic agent imatinib mesylate. *Nature Med*. 2006;12:908–916.

16. Gambacorti-Passerini C, Antolini L, Mahon FX, et al. Multicenter independent assessment of outcomes in chronic myeloid leukemia patients treated with imatinib. *J Natl Cancer Inst*. 2011;103:553–561.

17. Estabragh ZR, Knight K, Watmough SJ, et al. A prospective evaluation of cardiac function in patients with chronic myeloid leukaemia treated with imatinib. *Leuk Res*. 2011;35:49–51.

18. Moslehi JJ, Deininger M. Tyrosine kinase inhibitor–associated cardiovascular toxicity in chronic myeloid leukemia. *J Clin Oncol*. 2015;33:4210–4218.

19. Minotti G, Menna P, Salvatorelli E, et al. Anthracyclines: molecular advances and pharmacologic developments in antitumor activity and cardiotoxicity. *Pharmacol Rev*. 2004;56:185–229.

20. Jeyaseelan R, Poizat C, Baker RK, et al. A novel cardiac-restricted target for doxorubicinCARP, a nuclear modulator of gene expression in cardiac progenitor cells and cardiomyocytes. *J Biol Chem*. 1997;272:22800–22808.

21. Burke BE, Olson RD, Cusack BJ, et al. Anthracycline cardiotoxicity in transgenic mice overexpressing SR Ca2-ATPase. *Biochem Biophys Res Commun*. 2003;303:504–507.

22. Armstrong GT, Chen Y, Yasui Y, et al. Reduction in late mortality among 5-year survivors of childhood cancer. *N Engl J Med*. 2016;74: 833–842.

23. Gianni L, Herman EH, Lipshultz SE, et al. Anthracycline cardiotoxicity: from bench to bedside. *J Clin Oncol*. 2008;26:3777–3784.

24. Arola OJ, Saraste A, Pulkki K, et al. Acute doxorubicin cardiotoxicity involves cardiomyocyte apoptosis. *Cancer Res*. 2000;60:1789–1792.

25. Childs AC, Phaneuf SL, Dirks AJ, et al. Doxorubicin treatment in vivo causes cytochrome C release and cardiomyocyte apoptosis, as well as increased mitochondrial efficiency, superoxide dismutase activity, and Bcl-2:Bax ratio. *Cancer Res*. 2002;62:4592–4598.

26. Zhang J, Clark JR, Herman EH, et al. Doxorubicin-induced apoptosis in spontaneously hypertensive rats: differential effects in heart, kidney and intestine, and inhibition by ICRF-187. *J Mol Cell Cardiol*. 1996;28:1931–1943.

27. Herman EH, el-Hage AN, Ferrans VJ, et al. Comparison of the severity of the chronic cardiotoxicity produced by doxorubicin in normotensive and hypertensive rats. *Toxicol Appl Pharmacol*. 1985;78:202–214.

28. Lipshultz SE, Rifai N, Sallan SE, et al. Predictive value of cardiac troponin T in pediatric patients at risk for myocardial injury. *Circulation*. 1997;96:2641–2648.

29. Cardinale D, Colombo A, Sandri MT, et al. Prevention of high-dose chemotherapy-induced cardiotoxicity in high-risk patients by angiotensin-converting enzyme inhibition. *Circulation*. 2006;114:2474–2481.

30. Wenzel DG, Cosma GN. A model system for measuring comparative toxicities of cardiotoxic drugs for cultured rat heart myocytes, endothelial cells and fibroblasts. II. Doxorubicin, 5-fluorouracil and cyclophosphamide. *Toxicology*. 1984;33:117–128.

31. Zsàry A, Szucs S, Keltai K, et al. Endothelins: a possible mechanism of cytostatics-induced cardiomyopathy. *Leuk Lymphoma*. 2004;45:351–355.

32. Lemmens K, Segers VF, Demolder M, et al. Role of neuregulin-1/ERBB2 signaling in endothelium-cardiomyocyte cross-talk. *J Biol Chem*. 2006;28: 19469–19477.

33. Bearzi C, Rota M, Hosoda T, et al. Human cardiac stem cells. *Proc Natl Acad Sci USA*. 2007;104:14068–14073.

34. Rupp S, Bauer J, von Gerlach S, et al. Pressure overload leads to an increase of cardiac resident stem cells. *Basic Res Cardiol*. 2012;107:252.

35. Cesselli D, Beltrami AP, D'Aurizio F, et al. Effects of age and heart failure on human cardiac stem cell function. *Am J Pathol*. 2011;179:349–366.

36. De Angelis A, Piegari E, Cappetta D, et al. Anthracycline cardiomyopathy is mediated by depletion of the cardiac stem cell pool and is rescued by restoration of progenitor cell function. *Circulation*. 2010;121:276–292.

37. Piegari E, De Angelis A, Cappetta D, et al. Doxorubicin induces senescence and impairs function of human cardiac progenitor cells. *Basic Res Cardiol*. 2013;108:334–357.

38. Johnson JR, Ning YM, Farrell A, et al. Accelerated approval of oncology products: the food and drug administration experience. *J Natl Cancer Inst.* 2011;103: 636–644.

39. Gainor JF, Chabner BA. Ponatinib: accelerated disapproval. *The Oncologist.* 2015;20:847–848.

40. Huang WS, Metcalf CA, Sundaramoorthi R, et al. Discovery of 3-[2-(imidazo[1,2-b]pyridazin-3-yl) ethynyl]-4-methyl-N-{4-[(4-methylpiperazin-1-yl) methyl]-3-(trifluoromethyl) phenyl}benzamide (AP24534), a potent, orally active pan-inhibitor of breakpoint cluster region-abelson (BCR-ABL) kinase including the T315I gatekeeper mutant. *J Med Chem.* 2010;53:4701–4719.

41. Mellor HR, Bell AR, Valentin JP, et al. Cardiotoxicity associated with targeting kinase pathways in cancer. *Toxicol Sci.* 2011;120:14–32.

42. Cross MJ, Berridge BR, Clements PJM. Physiological, pharmacological and toxicological considerations of drug-induced structural cardiac injury. *British J of Pharmacol.* 2015;172: 957–974.

43. Jacob F, Yonis AY, Cuello F, et al. Analysis of tyrosine kinase inhibitor-mediated decline in contractile force in rat engineered heart tissue. *PLOS One.* 2016;11(2):e0145937.

44. Thavandiran N, Dubois N, Mikryukov A, et al. Design and formulation of functional pluripotent stem-cell-derived cardiac microtissues. *Proc Natl Acad Sci USA.* 2013;110: E4698–E4707.

45. Salvatorelli E, Guarnieri S, Menna P, et al. Defective one or two electron reduction of the anticancer anthracycline epirubicin in human heart: relative importance of vesicular sequestration and impaired efficiency of electron addition. *J Biol Chem.* 2006;281: 10990–11001.

46. Salvatorelli E, Menna P, Cascegna S, et al. Paclitaxel and docetaxel stimulation of doxorubicinol formation in the human heart: Implications for cardiotoxicity of doxorubicin-taxane chemotherapies. *J Pharmacol Exp Ther.* 2006;318:424–433.

47. Salvatorelli E, Menna P, Gianni L, et al. Defective taxane stimulation of epirubicinol formation in the human heart: insight into the cardiac tolerability of epirubicin-taxane chemotherapies. *J Pharmacol Exp Ther.* 2007;320:790–800.

48. Salvatorelli E, Menna P, Lusini M, et al. Doxorubicinolone formation and efflux: a salvage pathway against epirubicin accumulation in human heart. *J Pharmacol Exp Ther.* 2009;329:175–184.

49. Salvatorelli E, Menna P, Surapaneni S, et al. Pharmacokinetic characterization of amrubicin cardiac safety in an ex vivo human myocardial strip model. I. Amrubicin accumulates to a lower level than doxorubicin or epirubicin. *J Pharmacol Exp Ther.* 2012a;341: 464–473.

50. Salvatorelli E, Menna P, Gonzalez Paz O, et al. Pharmacokinetic characterization of amrubicin cardiac safety in an ex vivo human myocardial strip model. II. Amrubicin shows metabolic advantages over doxorubicin and epirubicin. *J Pharmacol Exp Ther.* 2012b; 341:474–483.

51. Salvatorelli E, Menna P, Gonzalez Paz O, et al. The novel anthracenedione, pixantrone, lacks redox activity and inhibits doxorubicinol formation in human myocardium: insight to explain the cardiac safety of pixantrone in doxorubicin-treated patients. *J Pharmacol Exp Ther.* 2013;344:467–478.

52. Fernández A, Sanguino A, Peng Z, et al. An anticancer C-Kit kinase inhibitor is reengineered to make it more active and less cardiotoxic. *J Clin Invest.* 2007;117: 4044–4054.

53. Vivas-Mejia P, Benito JM, Fernandez A, et al. c-Jun-NH2-kinase-1 inhibition leads to antitumor activity in ovarian cancer. *Clin Cancer Res.* 2010;16:184–194.

54. Gozgit JM, Song Y, Baker T, et al. Comparative analysis of BCR-ABL and VEGFR2 inhibitory activities of ponatinib, PF-114, and axitinib. *25th Meeting of the European Hematology Association,* June 11–14. 2015;E1075.

55. Mian AA, Rafiei A, Haberbosch I, et al. PF-114, a potent and selective inhibitor of VEGFR2 is active against Philadelphia chromosome-positive (Ph+) leukemias harboring the T315I mutation. *Leukemia.* 2015;29:1104–1114.

56. Pemovska T, Johnson E, Kontro M, et al. Axitinib effectively inhibits Bcr-Abl[T315I] with a distinct binding conformation. *Nature.* 2015;519:102–105.

57. Force T, Kerkelä R. Cardiotoxicity of the new cancer therapeutics- mechanisms of, and approaches to, the problem. *Drug Discov Today.* 2008;13:778–784.

58. Menna P, Salvatorelli E, Minotti G. Cardiotoxicity of antitumor drugs. *Chem Res Toxicol.* 2008;15:1179–1189.

59. Pettengell R, Coiffier B, Narayanan G, et al. Pixantrone dimaleate versus other chemotherapeutic agents as a single-agent salvage treatment in patients with relapsed or refractory aggressive non-Hodgkin lymphoma: a phase 3, multicentre, open-label, randomised trial. *Lancet Oncol.* 2012;13:696–706.

60. Moore RA, Adel N, Riedel E, et al. High incidence of thromboembolic events in patients treated with cisplatin-based chemotherapy: A Large retrospective analysis. *J Clin Oncol.* 2011;25:3466–3473.

61. Togna GI, Togna AR, Franconi M, et al. Cisplatin triggers platelet activation. *Thromb Res.* 2000;99:503–509.

62. Montani D, Bergot E, Günther S, et al. Pulmonary arterial hypertension in patients treated by dasatinib. *Circulation.* 2012;125:2128–2137.

63. Rea D, Mirault T, Cluzeau T, et al. Early onset hypercholesterolemia induced by the 2nd-generation tyrosine kinase inhibitor nilotinib in patients with chronic phase-chronic myeloid leukemia. *Hematologica.* 2014; 99:1197–1203.

64. Ooi JYY, Seymour JF, Keating MJ, et al. Ibrutinib increases the risk of atrial fibrillation, potentially through inhibition of cardiac PI3K-Akt signaling. *Blood.* 2014;124:3829–3830.

65. Narayanan N, Pushpakumar SB, Givvimani S, et al. Epigenetic regulation of aortic remodeling in hyperhomocysteinemia. *FASEB J.* 2014;28:3411–3422.

66. Kawabata M, Umemoto N, Shimada Y, et al. Downregulation of stanniocalcin 1 is responsible for sorafenib-induced cardiotoxicity. *Toxicol Sci*. 2015;143:374–384.

67. Roodhart JM, Langenberg MH, Witteveen E, et al. The molecular basis of class side effects due to treatment with inhibitors of the VEGF/VEGFR pathway. *Curr Clin Pharmacol*. 2008;3:132–143.

68. Cho YT, Chan CC. Cabozantinib-induced hand-foot skin reaction with subungual splinter hemorrhages and hypertension: a possible association with inhibition of the vascular endothelial growth factor signaling pathway. *Eur J Dermatol*. 2013;23:274–275.

69. Kaur A, Yu SS, Lee AJ, et al. Thalidomide-induced sinus bradycardia. *Ann Pharmacother*. 2003;37:1040–1043.

70. Bagratuni T, Kastritis E, Politou M, et al. Clinical and genetic factors associated with venous thromboembolism in myeloma patients treated with lenalidomide-based regimens. *Am J Hematol*. 2013;88:765–770.

71. Chari A, Hajje D. Case series discussion of cardiac and vascular events following carfilzomib treatment: possible mechanism, screening, and monitoring. *BMC Cancer*. 2014;14:915.

72. Breccia M, Latagliata R, Carmosino I, et al. Clinical and biological features of acute promyelocytic leukemia patients developing retinoic acid syndrome during induction treatment with all-trans retinoic acid and idarubicin. *Hematologica*. 2008;93:1918–1920.

73. Ficker E, Kuryshev YA, Dennis AT, et al. Mechanisms of arsenic-induced prolongation of cardiac repolarization. *Mol Pharmacol*. 2004;66:33–44.

74. Suter TM, Ewer MS. Cancer drugs and the heart: importance and management. *Eur Heart J*. 2013;34:1102–1111.

75. Ewer MS, Lippman SM. Type II chemotherapy-related cardiac dysfunction: time to recognize a new entity. *J Clin Oncol*. 2005;23:2900–2902.

76. Peng X, Chen B, Lim CC, et al. The cardiotoxicology of anthracycline chemotherapeutics: translating molecular mechanism into preventative medicine. *Mol Interv*. 2005;5:163–171.

77. Duran JM, Makarewich CA, Trappanese D, et al. Sorafenib cardiotoxicity increases mortality after myocardial infarction. *Circ Res*. 2014;114:1700–1712.

78. D'Adamo DR, Anderson SE, Albritton K, et al. Phase II study of doxorubicin and bevacizumab for patients with metastatic soft-tissue sarcomas. *J Clin Oncol*. 2005; 23:7135–7142.

79. Ewer MS, Ewer SM. Cardiotoxicity of anticancer treatments. *Nat Rev Cardiol*. 2015;12:547–558.

80. El-Kareh AW, Secomb TW. Mathematical model for comparison of bolus injection, continuous infusion, and liposomal delivery of doxorubicin to tumor cells. *Neoplasia*. 2000;2:325–338.

81. Lipshultz SE, Miller TL, Lipsitz SR, et al. Continuous versus bolus infusion of doxorubicin in children with ALL: long-term cardiac outcomes. *Pediatrics*. 2012;130:1003–1011.

82. Doroshow JH, Synold TW, Somlo G, et al. Oxidative DNA base modifications in peripheral blood mononuclear cells of patients treated with high-dose infusional doxorubicin. *Blood*. 2001;97:2839–2845.

83. Seymour LW. Passive tumor targeting of soluble macromolecules and drug conjugates. *Crit Rev Ther Drug Carrier Syst*. 1992;9:135–187.

84. Drummond DC, Meyer O, Hong K, et al. Optimizing liposomes for delivery of chemotherapeutic agents to solid tumors. *Pharmacol Rev*. 1999;51:692–743.

85. van Dalen EC, Michiels, EM, Caron HN, et al. Different anthracycline derivates for reducing cardiotoxicity in cancer patients. *Cochrane Database, Syst. Rev.* 2010;12:CD005006.

86. Cortes J, Di Cosimo S, Climent MA. Nonpegylated liposomal doxorubicin (TLC-D99), paclitaxel, and trastuzumab in HER-2-overexpressing breast cancer: a multicenter phase I/II study. *Clin Cancer Res*. 2009;15:307–314.

87. Rayson D, Suter TM, Jackisch C, et al. Cardiac safety of adjuvant pegylated liposomal doxorubicin with concurrent trastuzumab: a randomized phase II trial. *Ann Oncol*. 2012;23:1780–1788.

88. Doroshow JH. Anthracycline antibiotic-stimulated superoxide, hydrogen peroxide, and hydroxyl radical production by NADH dehydrogenase. *Cancer Res*. 1983;43:4543–4551.

89. Gewirtz DA. A critical evaluation of the mechanisms of action proposed for the antitumor effects of the anthracycline antibiotics adriamycin and daunorubicin. *Biochem Pharmacol*. 1999;57:727–741.

90. Minotti G, Salvatorelli E, Menna P. Pharmacological foundations of cardiooncology. *J Pharmacol Exp Ther*. 2010;334:2–8.

91. Boucek RJ, Olson RD, Brenner DE, et al. The major metabolite of doxorubicin is a potent inhibitor of membrane-associated ion pumps. *J Biol Chem*. 1987;262: 15851–15856.

92. Minotti G, Recalcati S, Mordente A, et al. The secondary alcohol metabolite of doxorubicin irreversibly inactivates aconitase/iron regulatory protein-1 in cytosolic fractions from human myocardium. *FASEB J*. 1998;12:541–552.

93. Minotti G, Ronchi R, Salvatorelli E, et al. Doxorubicin irreversibly inactivates Iron Regulatory Proteins 1 and 2 in cardiomyocytes: evidence for distinct metabolic pathways and implications for iron-mediated cardiotoxicity of antitumor therapy. *Cancer Res*. 2001;61:8422–8428.

94. Ryberg M, Nielsen D, Cortese G, et al. New insight into epirubicin cardiac toxicity: competing risks analysis of 1097 breast cancer patients. *J Natl Cancer Inst*. 2008;100:1058–1067.

95. Salvatorelli E, Menna P, Cantalupo E, et al. The concomitant management of cancer therapy and cardiac therapy. *Biochim Biophys Acta (Biomembranes)*. 2015;1848: 2727–2737.

96. Herbrecht R, Cernohous P, Engert A, et al. Comparison of pixantrone-based regimen (CPOP-R) with doxorubicin-based therapy (CHOP-R) for treatment of diffuse large B-cell lymphoma. *Ann Oncol*. 2013;24:2618–2623.

97. Beeharry N, Di Rora AG, Smith MR, et al. Pixantrone induces cell death through mitotic perturbations and subsequent aberrant cell divisions. *Cancer Biol Ther.* 2015;16:1397–1406.

98. Menna P, Salvatorelli E, Minotti G. Rethinking drugs from chemistry to therapeutic opportunities: pixantrone beyond anthracyclines. *Chem Res Toxicol.* 2016;29:1270–1278.

99. Legha SS, Wang YM, Mackay B, et al. Clinical and pharmacologic investigation of the effects of a-tocopherol on adriamycin cardiotoxicity. *Ann NY Acad Sci.* 1982;393:411–418.

100. Myers C, Bonow R, Palmieri S, et al. A randomized controlled trial assessing the prevention of doxorubicin cardiomyopathy by N-acetylcysteine. *Semin Oncol.* 1983;10 (Suppl.) 53–55.

101. Minotti G, Cairo G, Monti E Role of iron in anthracycline cardiotoxicity: new tunes for an old song? *FASEB J.* 1999;13:199–212.

102. Doroshow JH. Role of reactive-oxygen metabolism in the cardiac toxicity of the anthracycline antibiotics. In: Priebe W (ed.), *Anthracycline Antibiotics: New Analogues, Methods of Delivery, and Mechanisms of Action.* 1995;259–267.

103. Zhang S, Liu X, Bawa-Khalfe T, et al. Identification of the molecular basis of doxorubicin-induced cardiotoxicity. *Nat Med.* 2012;18:1639–1642.

104. Lyu YL, Kerrigan JE, Lin CP, et al. Topoisomerase IIbeta mediated DNA double-strand breaks: implications in doxorubicin cardiotoxicity and prevention by dexrazoxane. *Cancer Res.* 2007;67:8839–8846.

105. Hasinoff BB, Creighton AM, Kozlowska H, et al. Mitindomide is a catalytic inhibitor of DNA topoisomerase II that acts at the bisdioxopiperazine binding site. *Mol Pharmacol.* 1997;52:839–845.

106. Martin E, Thougaard AV, Grauslund M, et al. Evaluation of the topoisomerase II-inactive bisdioxopiperazine ICRF-161 as a protectant against doxorubicin-induced cardiomyopathy. *Toxicology.* 2009;255:72–9.

107. Sterba M, Popelová O, Simunek T, et al. Cardioprotective effects of a novel iron chelator, pyridoxal 2-chlorobenzoyl hydrazone, in the rabbit model of daunorubicin-induced cardiotoxicity. *J Pharmacol Exp Ther.* 2006;319:1336–1347.

108. Popelová O, Sterba M, Sim nek T, et al. Deferiprone does not protect against chronic anthracycline cardiotoxicity in vivo. *J Pharmacol Exp Ther.* 2008;326:259–269.

109. Speyer JL, Green MD, Zeleniuch-Jacquotte A, et al. ICRF-187 permits longer treatment with doxorubicin in women with breast cancer. *J Clin Oncol.* 1992;10:117–127.

110. Swain SM, Whaley FS, Gerber MC, et al. Cardioprotection with dexrazoxane for doxorubicin-containing therapy in advanced breast cancer. *J Clin Oncol.* 1997;15:1318–1332.

111. Swain SM, Vici P. The current and future role of dexrazoxane as a cardioprotectant in anthracycline treatment: Expert panel review. *J Cancer Res Clin Oncol.* 2004;130:1–7.

112. Schuchter LM, Hensley ML, Meropol NJ, et al. 2002 update of recommendations for the use of chemotherapy and radiotherapy protectants: clinical practice guidelines of the American Society of Clinical Oncology. *J Clin Oncol.* 2002;20:2895–2903.

113. Tebbi CK, London WB, Friedman D, et al. Dexrazoxane-associated risk for acute myeloid leukemia/myelodysplastic syndrome and other secondary malignancies in pediatric Hodgkin's disease. *J Clin Oncol.* 2007;25:493–500.

114. Salze WL, Devidas M, Carroll WL, et al. Longterm results of the pediatric oncology group studies for childhood acute lymphoblastic leukemia. *Leukemia.* 2010;24:355–370.

115. Vrooman LM, Neuberg DS, Stevenson KE, et al. The low incidence of secondary acute myelogenous leukemia in children and adolescents treated with dexrazoxane for acute lymphoblastic leukaemia. *Eur J Cancer.* 2011;47:1373–1379.

116. Lipshultz SE, Franco VI, Sallan SE, et al. Dexrazoxane for reducing anthracycline-related cardiotoxicity in children with cancer: an update of the evidence. *Progr Pediatr Cardiol.* 2014;36:39–49.

117. Limat S, Demesmay K, Voillat L et al. Early cardiotoxicity of the CHOP regimen in aggressive non-Hodgkin's lymphoma. *Ann Oncol.* 2003;14:277–281.

118. Yang SC, Chuang MH, Li DK. The development of congestive heart failure and ventricular tachycardia after first exposure to idarubicin in a patient with acute myeloid leukaemia. *Br J Clin Pharmacol.* 2010;69:209–211.

119. Forrest GL, Gonzalez B, Tseng W, et al. Human carbonyl reductase overexpression in the heart advances the development of doxorubicin induced cardiotoxicity in transgenic mice. *Cancer Res.* 2000;60:5158–5164.

120. Olson LE, Bedja D, Alvey SJ, et al. Protection from doxorubicin-induced cardiac toxicity in mice with a null allele of carbonyl reductase 1. *Cancer Res.* 2003;63: 6602–6606.

121. Blanco JG, Sun CL, Landier W, et al. Anthracycline-related cardiomyopathy after childhood cancer: role of polymorphisms in carbonyl reductase genes: a report from the Children's Oncology Group. *J Clin Oncol.* 2012;30:1415–1421.

122. Kalabus JL, Sanborn CC, Jamil RG, Cheng Q, Blanco JG. Expression of the anthracycline-metabolizing enzyme carbonyl reductase 1 in hearts from donors with Down syndrome. *Drug Metab Dispos.* 2010;38:2096–3009.

123. Mordente A, Minotti G, Martorana GE, Silvestrini A, Giardina B, Meucci E. Anthracycline secondary alcohol metabolite formation in human or rabbit heart: biochemical aspects and pharmacologic implications. *Biochem Pharmacol.* 2003;66:989–998.

124. Gianni L, Capri G, Valagussa P, Bonadonna G. Putting taxanes to work in operable breast cancer: a search for selective indications from empirical studies. *Recent Results Cancer Res.* 1998;152:314–322.

125. Minotti G, Saponiero A, Licata S, Menna P, Calafiore AM, Teodori G, Gianni L. Paclitaxel and docetaxel enhance the metabolism of doxorubicin to toxic species in human myocardium. *Clin Cancer Res.* 2001;7:1511–1515.

126. Vejpongsa P, Massey MR, Acholonu SA, et al. Topoisomerase 2b expression in peripheral blood

predicts susceptibility to anthracycline-induced cardiomyopathy (abstr). *Circulation*. 2013;128:A11619.

127. McCaffrey TA, Tziros C, Lewis J, et al. Genomic profiling reveals the potential role of TCL1A and MDR1 deficiency in chemotherapy-induced cardiotoxicity. *Int J Biol Sci*. 2013;9:350–360.

128. Wojnowski L, Kulle B, Schirmer M, et al. NAD(P)H oxidase and multidrug resistance protein genetic polymorphisms are associated with doxorubicin-induced cardiotoxicity. *Circulation*. 2005;112:3754–3762.

129. Reichwagen A, Ziepert M, Kreuz M, et al. Association of NADPH oxidase polymorphisms with anthracycline-induced cardiotoxicity in the RICOVER-60 trial of patients with aggressive CD20(+) B-cell lymphoma. *Pharmacogenomics*. 2015;16:361–372.

130. Aminkeng F, Bhavsar AP, Visscher H, et al. A coding variant in RARG confers susceptibility to anthracycline-induced cardiotoxicity in childhood cancer. *Nat Genet*. 2015;47:1079–1084.

131. Wang X, Liu W, Sun CL, et al. Hyaluronan synthase 3 variant and anthracycline-related cardiomyopathy: a report from the children's oncology group. *J Clin Oncol*. 2014;32:647–653.

132. Shipman KE, Arnold I. Case of epirubicin-induced cardiomyopathy in familial cardiomyopathy. *J Clin Oncol*. 2011;29:537–538.

133. van den Berg MP, van Spaendonck-Zwarts KY, van Veldhuisen DJ, et al. Familial dilated cardiomyopathy: another risk factor for anthracycline-induced cardiotoxicity?. *Eur J Heart Fail*. 2010;12:1297–1299.

134. Ewer M, Gianni L, Pane F, et al. Report on the international colloquium on Cardio-Oncology (Rome, 12–14 March 2014). *Ecancermedicalscience*. 2014;8:433.

135. Kalay N, Basar E, Ozdogru I, et al. Protective effects of carvedilol against anthracycline-induced cardiomyopathy. *J Am Coll Cardiol*. 2006;48:2258–2262.

136. Kaya MG, Ozkan M, Gunebakmaz O, et al. Protective effects of nebivolol against anthracycline induced cardiomyopathy: a randomized control study. *Int J Cardiol*. 2013;167:2306–2310.

137. Bosch X, Sitges M, Rovira M, et al. Enalapril and carvedilol for preventing chemotherapy-induced left ventricular systolic dysfunction in patients with malignant hemopathies: the OVERCOME trial. *J Am Coll Cardiol*. 2013;61:2355–2362.

138. Georgakopoulos P, Roussou P, Matsakas E, et al. Cardioprotective effect of metoprolol and enalapril in doxorubicin-treated lymphoma patients: a prospective, parallel-group, randomized, controlled study with 36-month follow-up. *Am J Hematol*. 2010;85:894–896.

139. Gulati G, Heck SL, Ree AH, et al. Prevention of cardiac dysfunction during adjuvant breast cancer therapy (PRADA): a 2 × 2 factorial, randomized, placebo-controlled, double-blind clinical trial of candesartan and metoprolol. *Eur Heart J*. 2016;37:1671–1680.

140. Spallarossa P, Garibaldi S, Altieri P. Carvedilol prevents doxorubicin-induced free radical release and apoptosis in cardiomyocytes in vitro. *J Mol Cell Cardiol*. 2004;37:837–846.

141. Moen MD, Wagstaff AJ. Nebivolol: a review of its use in the management of hypertension and chronic heart failure. *Drugs*. 2006;66:1389–1409.

142. Mason RP, Kalinowski L, Jacob RF, et al. Nebivolol reduces nitroxidative stress and restores nitric oxide bioavailability in endothelium of black Americans. *Circulation*. 2005;112:3795–3801.

143. Seicean S, Seicean A, Plana JC, et al. Effect of statin therapy on the risk for incident heart failure in patients with breast cancer receiving anthracycline chemotherapy: an observational clinical cohort study. *J Am Coll Cardiol*. 2012;60:2384–2390.

144. Schmidinger M, Zielinski CC, Vogl UM, et al. Cardiac toxicity of sunitinib and sorafenib in patients with metastatic renal cell carcinoma. *J Clin Oncol*. 2008;26:5204–5212.

145. Zhao Z, Cui W, Zhang H, et al. Pre-treatment of a single high-dose of atorvastatin provided cardioprotection in different ischaemia/reperfusion models via activating mitochondrial KATP channel. *Eur J Pharmacol*. 2015;751:89–98.

146. Dahlberg SE, Sandler AB, Brahmer JR, et al. Clinical course of advanced non–small-cell lung cancer patients experiencing hypertension during treatment with bevacizumab in combination with carboplatin and paclitaxel on ECOG 4599. *J Clin Oncol*. 2010;28:949–954.

147. Rautiola J, Donskov F, Peltola K, et al. Sunitinib-induced hypertension, neutropaenia and thrombocytopaenia as predictors of good prognosis in patients with metastatic renal cell carcinoma. *BJU Int*. 2016;117:110–117.

148. Lenihan DJ, Kowey PR. Overview and management of cardiac adverse events associated with tyrosine kinase inhibitors. *Oncologist*. 2013;18:900–908.

149. Shah RR, Morganroth J. Update on cardiovascular safety of tyrosine kinase inhibitors: with a special focus on QT interval, left ventricular dysfunction and overall risk/benefit. *Drug Saf*. 2015;38:693–710.

150. U.S. Department of Health and Human Services Food and Drug Administration Center for Drug Evaluation and Research Center for Biologics Evaluation and Research. E14 clinical evaluation of QT/QTc interval Prolongation and proarrhythmic potential for non-antiarrhythmic. *Drugs*. 2005;1–16.

151. Du F, Babcock JJ, Yu H, et al. Global analysis reveals families of chemical motifs enriched for HERG inhibitors. *PLoS One*. 2015;10:e0118324.

152. Grant AO. Cardiac ion channels. *Circ Arrhythm Electrophysiol*. 2009;2:185–194.

153. Brell JM. Prolonged QTc interval in cancer therapeutic drug development: defining arrhythmic risk in malignancy. *Prog Cardiovasc Dis*. 2010;53:164–172.

154. U.S. Department of Health and Human Services Food and Drug Administration Center for Drug Evaluation and Research Center for Biologics Evaluation and Research. E14 clinical evaluation of QT/QTc interval Prolongation and proarrhythmic potential for non-antiarrhythmic. *Drugs*. 2005;1–16.

155. Yap YG, Camm AJ. Drug induced QT prolongation and torsades de pointes. *Heart*. 2004;89:1363–1370.

156. Roboz GJ, Ritchie EK, Carlin RF, et al. Prevalence, management, and clinical consequences of QT interval prolongation during treatment with arsenic trioxide. *J Clin Ncol* 2014;32:3723–3728.

157. Shah RR, Morganroth J, Shah DR. Cardiovascular safety of tyrosine kinase inhibitors: with a special focus on cardiac repolarisation (QT interval). *Drug Saf.* 2013;36:295–316.

158. Strevel EL, Ing DJ, Siu LL. Molecularly targeted oncology therapeutics and prolongation of the QT interval. *J Clin Oncol.* 2007;25:3362–3371.

159. Lo-Coco F, Avvisati G, Vignetti M, et al. Retinoic acid and arsenic trioxide for acute promyelocytic leukemia. *N Engl J Med.* 2013;369:111–121.

160. Burnett AK, Russell NH, Hills RK, et al. Arsenic trioxide and all-trans retinoic acid treatment for acute promyelocytic leukaemia in all risk groups (AML17): results of a randomised, controlled, phase 3 trial. *Lancet Oncol.* 2015;16:1295–305.

161. Yamazaki K, Terada H, Satoh H, et al. Arrhythmogenic effects of arsenic trioxide in patients with acute promyelocytic leukemia and an electrophysiological study in isolated guinea pig papillary muscles. *Circ J.* 2006;70:1407–1414.

162. Drolet B, Simard C, Roden DM. Unusual effects of a QT prolonging drug, arsenic trioxide, on cardiac potassium currents. *Circulation.* 2004;109:26–29.

163. Ficker E, Kuryshev YA, Dennis AT, et al. Mechanisms of arsenic-induced prolongation of cardiac repolarization. *Mol Pharmacol.* 2004;66:33–44.

164. Park E. The impact of drug-related QT prolongation on FDA regulatory decisions. FDA educational material. 2014.

165. Rickles FR. Mechanisms of cancer-induced thrombosis in cancer. *Pathophysiol Haemost Thromb.* 2006;35:103–110.

166. Zamorano JL, Lancellotti P, Rodriguez Muñoz D, et al; Authors/Task Force Members; ESC Committee for Practice Guidelines (CPG). 2016 ESC Position Paper on cancer treatments and cardiovascular toxicity developed under the auspices of the ESC Committee for Practice Guidelines The Task Force for cancer treatments and cardiovascular toxicity of the European Society of Cardiology (ESC). *Eur Heart J.* 2016;37:2768–2801.

167. Agnelli G, Gussoni G, Bianchini C, et al; PROTECHT Investigators. Nadroparin for the prevention of thromboembolic events in ambulatory patients with metastatic or locally advanced solid cancer receiving chemotherapy: a randomised, placebo-controlled, double-blind study. *Lancet Oncol.* 2009;10:943–949.

168. Barni S, Bonizzoni E, Verso M, et al. The effect of low-molecular-weight heparin in cancer patients: the mirror image of survival? *Blood.* 2014;124:155–156

169. Akl EA, Kahale L, Barba M, et al. Anticoagulation for the long-term treatment of venous thromboembolism in patients with cancer. *Cochrane Database Syst Rev.* 2014;7:CD006650.

170. Prins MH, Lensing AW, Bauersachs R, et al; EINSTEIN Investigators. Oral rivaroxaban versus standard therapy for the treatment of symptomatic venous thromboembolism: a pooled analysis of the EINSTEIN-DVT and PE randomized studies. *Thromb J.* 2013;11:21.

171. Schulman S, Goldhaber SZ, Kearon C, et al. Treatment with dabigatran or warfarin in patients with venous thromboembolism and cancer. *Thromb Haemost.* 2015;114:150–157.

172. Levine MN, Gu C, Liebman HA, et al. A randomized phase II trial of apixaban for the prevention of thromboembolism in patients with metastatic cancer. *J Thromb Haemost.* 2012;10:807–814.

173. Short NJ, Connors JM. New Oral Anticoagulants and the Cancer Patient. *Oncologist.* 2014;19:82–93.

174. Jerling M. Clinical pharmacokinetics of ranolazine. *Clin Pharmacokinet.* 2006;45:469–491.

175. Ruff CT, Giugliano RP, Antman EM. Management of Bleeding With Non-Vitamin K Antagonist Oral Anticoagulants in the Era of Specific Reversal Agents. *Circulation.* 2016;134:248–261.

176. Steegmann JL, Baccarani M, Breccia M et al. LeukemiaNet recommendations for the management and avoidance of adverse events of treatment in chronic myeloid leukaemia. *Leukemia.* 2016;30:1648–1671.

177. Breccia M, Pregno P, Spallarossa P, et al. Identification, prevention and management of cardiovascular risk in chronic myeloid leukaemia patients candidate to ponatinib: an expert opinion. *Ann Hematol.* 2017;96:549.

178. Neelakantan P, Marin D, Laffan M, et al. Platelet dysfunction associated with ponatinib, a new pan BCR-ABL inhibitor with efficacy for chronic myeloid leukemia resistant to multiple tyrosine kinase inhibitor therapy. *Haematologica.* 2012;97:1444.

179. Nazha A, Romo CG, Kantarjian H, et al. The clinical impact of ponatinib on the risk of bleeding in patients with chronic myeloid leukemia. *Haematologica.* 2012;98:e131.

180. Warfarin Antiplatelet Vascular Evaluation Trial Investigators, Anand S, Yusuf S, Xie C, et al. Oral anticoagulant and antiplatelet therapy and peripheral arterial disease. *N Engl J Med.* 2007;357:217–227.

181. Boekhout AH, Gietema JA, Milojkovic Kerklaan B, et al. Angiotensin II-receptor Inhibition with candesartan to prevent trastuzumab-related cardiotoxic Effects in patients with early breast cancer: a randomized clinical trial. *JAMA Oncol.* 2016;2:1030–1037.

182. Cardinale D, Colombo A, Bacchiani G, et al. Early detection of anthracycline cardiotoxicity and improvement with heart failure therapy. *Circulation.* 2015;131:1981–1988.

183. Wouters KA, Kremer LC, Miller TL, et al. Protecting against anthracycline-induced myocardial damage: a review of the most promising strategies. *Br J Haematol.* 2005;131:561–78.

184. Yeh ET, Salvatorelli E, Menna P, Minotti G. What is cardiotoxicity? *Progr Pediatr Cardiol.* 2014;36:3–6.

185. Plana JC, Galderisi M, Barac A, et al. Expert consensus for multimodality imaging evaluation of adult patients during and after cancer therapy: a report from the American Society of Echocardiography and the

European Association of Cardiovascular Imaging. *J Am Soc Echocardiogr*. 2014;27:911–939.

186. Sandri MT, Cardinale D, Zorzino L, et al. Minor increases in plasma troponin I predict decreased left ventricular ejection fraction after high-dose chemotherapy. *Clin Chem*. 2003;49:248–252.

187. Cardinale D, Cipolla CM. *Expert Rev Cardiovasc Ther*. 2016;28:1–3.

188. Sawaya H, Sebag IA, Plana JC, et al. Early detection and prediction of cardiotoxicity in chemotherapy-treated patients. *Am J Cardiol*. 2011;107:1375–1380.

189. Cardinale D, Ciceri F, Latini R, et al. Anthracycline-induced cardiotoxicity: a multicenter randomised trial comparing two strategies for guiding prevention with enalapril: the International CardioOncology Society-one trial. *Eur J Cancer*. 2018;94:126-137.

190. Lipshultz SE, Lipsitz SR, Sallan SE, et al. Long-term enalapril therapy for left ventricular dysfunction in doxorubicin-treated survivors of childhood cancer. *J Clin Oncol*. 2002;20:4517–4522

191. Wilson CL, Stratton K, Leisenring WL, et al. Decline in physical activity level in the Childhood Cancer Survivor Study cohort. *Cancer Epidemiol Biomarkers Prev*. 2014;23:1619–1627.

192. Vaughn DJ, Palmer SC, Carver JR, et al. Cardiovascular risk in long-term survivors of testicular cancer. *Cancer*. 2008;12:1949–1953.

193. Jones LW, Haykowsky MJ, Swartz JJ, et al. Early breast cancer therapy and cardiovascular injury. *J Am Coll Cardiol*. 2007;50:1435–1441.

194. Nathan PC, Ford JS, Henderson TO, et al. Health behaviors, medical care, and interventions to promote healthy living in the Childhood Cancer Survivor Study cohort. *J Clin Oncol*. 2009;27:2363–2373.

195. Minotti G. Pharmacology at work for cardio-oncology: ranolazine to treat early cardiotoxicity induced by antitumor drugs. *J Pharmacol Exp Ther*. 2013;346:343–349.

196. Chen B, Peng X, Pentassuglia L, et al. Molecular and cellular mechanisms of anthracycline cardiotoxicity. *Cardiovasc Toxicol*. 2007;7:114–121.

197. Carver JR, Shapiro CL, Ng A, et al. for the ASCO Cancer Survivorship Expert Panel, American Society of Clinical Oncology clinical evidence review on the ongoing care of adult cancer survivors: Cardiac and pulmonary late effects. *J Clin Oncol*. 2007;25:3991–4007.

198. Altena R, de Haas EC, Nuver J, et al. Evaluation of subacute changes in cardiac function after cisplatin-based combination chemotherapy for testicular cancer. *Br J Cancer*. 2009;100:1861–1866.

199. Pellicori P, Calicchia A, Lococo F, et al. Subclinical anthracycline cardiotoxicity in patients with acute promyelocytic leukemia in long-term remission after the AIDA protocol. *Congest Heart Fail*. 2012;18:217–221.

200. Serrano JM, González I, Del Castillo S, et al. Diastolic dysfunction following anthracycline-based chemotherapy in breast cancer patients: incidence and predictors oncologist. *Oncologist*. 2015;20:864–872.

201. Agha H, Shalaby L, Attia W, et al. Early ventricular dysfunction after anthracycline chemotherapy in children. *Pediatr Cardiol*. 2016;37:537–544.

202. Sanderson JE. HFNEF, HFpEF, HF-PEF, or DHF: what is in an acronym? *J Am Coll Cardiol Heart Fail*. 2014;2:93–94.

203. Hale SL, Shryock JC, Belardinelli L, et al. Late sodium current inhibition as a new cardioprotective approach. *J Mol Cell Cardiol*. 2008;44:954–967.

204. Paulus WJ and van Ballegoij JJ. Treatment of heart failure with normal ejection fraction: an inconvenient truth! *J Am Coll Cardiol*. 2010;55:526–537.

205. Lovelock JD, Monasky MM, Jeong EM, et al. Ranolazine improves cardiac diastolic dysfunction through modulation of myofilament calcium sensitivity. *Circ Res*. 2012;110:841–850.

206. Heinzerling L, Ott PA, Hodi FS, et al. Cardiotoxicity associated with CTLA4 and PD1 blocking immunotherapy. *J Immunother Cancer*. 2016;16:4–50.

207. Bose P, Gandhi VV, Keating MJ. Pharmacokinetic and pharmacodynamic evaluation of ibrutinib for the treatment of chronic lymphocytic leukemia: rationale for lower doses. *Expert Opin Drug Metab Toxicol* 2016;11:1–12.

3 Anthracycline Cardiotoxicity: Clinical Aspects, Recognition, Monitoring, Treatment, and Prevention

Michael S. Ewer

INTRODUCTION AND GENERAL CONSIDERATIONS

Anthracyclines were discovered in 1963, when a red fluorescent dye was isolated from a fermentation broth of the bacteria *Streptomyces peucetius*. This first anthracycline, originally called rubidomycin in France and daunomycin in Italy, subsequently was named daunorubicin, the name by which it is still known today. The agent remains a useful adjunct in the treatment of hematologic malignancies. Later, the 14-hydroxy derivative initially called Adriamycin and later doxorubicin was introduced. Doxorubicin had significant activity against solid tumors and was effective at treating hematologic malignancies.[1] The anthracyclines remain an important group of oncologic agents, and they are still widely used to treat breast cancer, lymphoma, sarcoma, and a variety of other malignancies (Table 3-1). Since the discovery of the first anthracycline, several hundred analogs have been synthesized or isolated from *Streptomyces* bacteria; most have not been of special clinical interest, but a few have entered the therapeutic armamentarium. Others, including those that offered reduced cardiotoxicity, have been studied, but have not enjoyed widespread clinical use.[2,3]

Anthracyclines have a polyaromatic structure bound by a glycoside bond to an aminodeoxypentose, daunosamine. Although anthracyclines demonstrate antimicrobial properties, this characteristic has never been applied clinically, largely because the agents are too toxic. The chemical structures of doxorubicin and one of its more frequently used analogues, epirubicin, are depicted in Figure 3-1 and demonstrate that small alterations in chemical structure affect anthracyclines' properties in clinically important ways. Especially relevant are lipophilicity and pKa of the amino group, characteristics that may influence cellular uptake, the duration of the drug in the cell, protein and lipid binding, and enzymatic and other metabolic interactions.

Anthracyclines' oncologic action has not yet been fully elucidated, but several mechanisms are probably involved. One of the better understood mechanisms is deoxyribonucleic acid (DNA) intercalation, with inhibition of DNA and ribonucleic acid (RNA) synthesis.[4] The interaction of anthracyclines and topoisomerase II also plays a role.[5] Doxorubicin may react directly with cell membranes to alter membrane function.[6]

Doxorubicin, like other anthracyclines and analogues, results in cardiotoxicity characterized by cell injury that progresses to cell death. On the

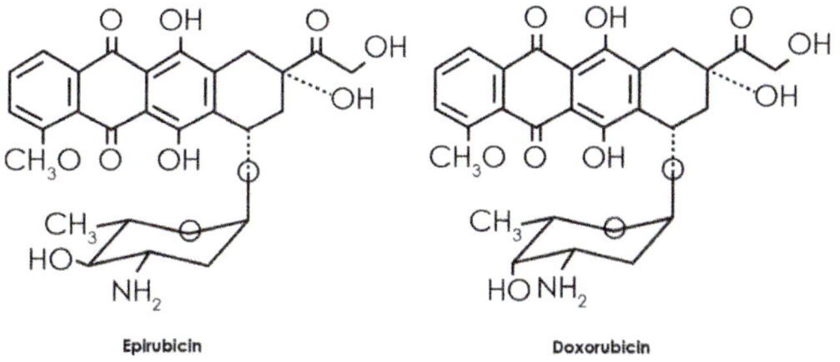

TABLE 3-1 Malignancies commonly treated with doxorubicin

| Breast cancer |
| Malignant lymphoma |
| Soft tissue and bone sarcoma |
| Acute lymphoblastic leukemia |
| Ovarian carcinoma |
| Neuroblastoma |
| Transitional cell bladder carcinoma |
| Thyroid carcinoma |
| Gastric carcinoma |
| Wilm's tumor |
| Bronchogenic carcinoma (small cell) |
| AIDS-related Kaposi's sarcoma |

FIGURE 3-1 Formulae for epirubicin and doxorubicin showing structural similarities.

cellular level the injury, once the threshold of cell death has been reached, is irreversible; thus, this form of cardiotoxicity is related to the lifetime total cumulative dose of the drug. The clinical presentation of doxorubicin-associated cardiotoxicity is similar to other forms of cardiac dysfunction; however, the mechanism and characteristic ultrastructural changes observed on cardiac biopsy material demonstrate that it differs sufficiently from other forms to be considered a separate entity. Anthracycline cardiotoxicity has been termed Type I chemotherapy-related cardiac dysfunction.[7] In contrast, as will be discussed in Chapter 4, Type II chemotherapy-related cardiac dysfunction tends to be much less severe and does not demonstrate anthracycline-like ultrastructural changes; Type II agents may be given for extended periods of time as these agents do not exhibit a cumulative-dose dependent toxicity. These differences are depicted in Table 3-2.

Type I cardiotoxicity is characterized by the presence of free-radical formation.[8] From the perspective of cardiotoxicity, this characteristic is of considerable importance, as anthracyclines can undergo a 1-electron reduction that leads to a semiquinone radical form and gives rise to toxic reactive oxygen species. These radicals may be responsible for lipid peroxidation and DNA breaks.[9,10] In addition, free radical formation may result from doxorubicin-Fe^{3+} complex reduction, which is due to the high affinity of doxorubicin for metal ions.[11] Although free radicals may play a subordinate role in anthracyclines' oncologic effects, little debate exists about the association between free radical formation and anthracycline-associated cardiotoxicity. However, other mechanisms including the fact that topoisomerase 2β is required for anthracycline to induce DNA double-strand breaks and changes in the transcriptome, that leads to mitochondrial dysfunction and generation of reactive oxygen species.[12]

One of the more interesting aspects of anthracyclines' cardiotoxicity is that the predominant mechanisms of oncologic efficacy and cardiac injury are almost certainly different. Therefore, altering the characteristics of the drug itself (the side chain, for example), the biologic environment into which it is administered (the presence of dexrazoxane), or the administration cycle length, which alters the peak plasma levels achieved (continuous infusion schedules), modifies the drug's cardiotoxicity while preserving oncologic efficacy. Were the mechanisms of oncologic efficacy and cardiotoxicity identical, one would need merely to define acceptable cardiac injury levels in the overall population to determine the corresponding cumulative dose of the drug. Because of the different mechanisms, research over the last four decades has been expended to change the ratio of oncologic efficacy to cardiotoxicity.[13] New strategies are still emerging as knowledge of these variables is acquired.

Early animal studies with anthracyclines demonstrated cardiotoxicity, and this was confirmed during

TABLE 3-2   Type I and Type II treatment-related cardiac dysfunction

TYPE I; E.G., DOXORUBICIN AGENTS WITH PRIMARY OR DIRECT TOXICITY TO THE MYOCYTE	TYPE II; E.G., TRASTUZUMAB AGENTS WITHOUT PRIMARY OR DIRECT TOXICITY TO THE MYOCYTE
Cellular death Damage starts with the first administration	Cellular dysfunction
Biopsy changes Typical of anthracyclines)	No typical anthracycline-like biopsy changes
Cumulative dose-related	Not cumulative dose related

Permanent damage
   Myocyte death; bad prognosis
	Predominantly reversible
	   Myocyte dysfunction; good prognosis

Risk factors:
   Combination CT
   Prior/concomitant RT
   Age
   Previous cardiac disease
   Hypertension
	Risk factors:
	   Prior/concomitant anthracyclines or paclitaxel
	   Age
	   Previous cardiac disease
	   Obesity (BMI > 25 kg/m^2)

Source: Modified from Ewer M and Lippman S, 2005.[7]

early clinical trials. The clinical relationship was explored by Von Hoff et al., who subsequently plotted congestive heart failure as a function of cumulative dose in more than 4000 patients who had received the drug according to a 3-week administration schedule.[14,15] As a result of these studies, dosing guidelines emerged; at that time a cumulative dose of approximately 550 mg/m^2 was felt to correlate with a likelihood of congestive heart failure in about 5% of otherwise healthy adults. This 5% guideline for congestive heart failure results in a low rate of severe heart failure and a still lower rate of cardiac death; it also demonstrates that to maximize survival a balance must be found between cardiotoxicity and oncologic effectiveness. While much has been learned about cardiac risk and oncologic benefit, the 5% limit of cardiotoxicity has served clinicians well for more than four decades. However, it is now clear that a cumulative dose of 550 mg/m^2 correlates with a heart failure incidence in excess of 5%; we have come to recognize that doxorubicin is considerably more cardiotoxic than was initially thought, and estimates have been revised upwards.[16]

Patients show considerable variability with regard to cardiotoxicity; some tolerate unusually high doses of doxorubicin, sometimes far in excess of the accepted maximal cardiotoxic cumulative dosages, whereas others develop cardiotoxicity at much lower cumulative dosages. Among those who experience augmented toxicity, no cause can be identified in some, and genetic predisposition is thought to play a role.[17] Others can be grouped according to risk factors.[18] Initially, isolated conditions such as extremes of age, prior exposure of the heart to radiation, pre-existing valvular heart disease, and concomitant use of specific chemotherapeutic agents had been identified as risk factors. Other factors were subsequently added to the list and included increased left ventricular end-diastolic pressure.[19] In general, individuals who have experienced prior cardiac damage of any kind, or who have a diminished threshold for cardiac damage should be considered to be at increased risk for cardiotoxicity. Patients who require anthracyclines for oncologic control and who are deemed to be at increased risk are treated with lower cumulative dosages, although the extent of augmented risk may be difficult to estimate in the case of any given patient.

Non-invasive cardiac testing became the standard for identifying individual patients at risk for unexpected early toxicity, and for monitoring patients during and following anthracycline exposure. Several possible measurements were evaluated, including systolic time intervals and electrocardiographic changes.[20,21] The ejection fraction and the related fractional shortening, a parameter sometimes preferred by pediatric investigators, remains the standard tool for identifying and monitoring these patients. Unfortunately, despite a variety of techniques used to measure these indices, they are sub-optimal indicators of impending cardiac damage. Ejection fraction estimates can detect severe cardiac damage but cannot predict cardiac dysfunction resulting from subsequent treatment cycles. Adding ultrasonic parameters of diastolic function or changes in function with exercise leads to significantly enhanced sensitivity when large groups of patients are considered, but does not have sufficiently predictive value when evaluating individual patients.[22–26]

A host of other parameters have been advocated to increase the ejection fraction's predictive value for quantifying the extent of cardiac damage. Some are based on improved methods for estimating ejection fraction and include 3-dimensional echocardiography, strain rate determination, and magnetic resonance imaging. These techniques may be more accurate but are not able to detect increased risks of impending heart failure at lower cumulative dosages, thereby identifying patients likely to experience cardiac dysfunction in the next 1 or 2 treatment cycles.[27] In addition, despite a considerable number of studies, these techniques do not yet allow optimal anthracycline dosing with significantly reduced cardiotoxicity.[28] (For further discussion of the role of imaging techniques in anthracycline cardiotoxicity, see Chapter 10.)

Quantifying the release of troponin I at the time of anthracycline administration allows an estimate of myocyte death that occurs after administration of the drug and correlates with later toxicity. Knowing that augmented cell death has taken place, as assessed by troponin I elevation, may allow early cardiac intervention in the form of cardioprotection or the use of alternate regimens that are less cardiotoxic.[29–32]

Notwithstanding the potential use of newer imaging techniques and biomarkers, endomyocardial biopsy is the only test that is both sufficiently sensitive to detect early cardiotoxicity and sufficiently specific to avoid over-including patients when toxicity is not a true clinical problem. Electron microscopic evaluation of biopsy specimens can grade the extent of structural changes and can predict the relative risk associated with the next administration. However, the invasive nature of the test, the associated expense, and the potential risk of serious complications such as cardiac perforation, make cardiac biopsy impractical as a standard modality for assessing anthracycline-associated damage. While the technique remains important in evaluating transplant rejection as well as in the evaluation of some forms of cardiomyopathy, it has been largely relegated to use as a research tool with regard to anthracycline cardiotoxicity.[33] Nevertheless, cardiac biopsy has contributed greatly to our knowledge of cardiotoxicity and has allowed us to quantify and compare the relative cardiotoxicities of various anthracyclines. Cardiac biopsy has also allowed investigation of potential cardiotoxicity of new agents as well as the complex interactions of various oncologically active drugs when administered concurrently or sequentially.[7,34-37] The biopsy had been especially important because non-invasive tests for cardiotoxicity were not sufficiently sensitive and specific, and because the biopsy could detect cell damage much earlier than was possible using non-invasive procedures. When comparing the relative toxicities of various anthracyclines, structural alterations of the myocytes at dosages that result in equivalent myelosuppression allowed for the best comparisons. Such data allowed comparisons using a far smaller sample size than would have been possible with non-invasive testing. In the post-biopsy era, comparisons of relative toxicity are much more difficult and require groups of patients that are substantially larger.

Over the past two decades the focus of cardiotoxicity has shifted from treatment to prevention; several strategies have been shown to be clearly cardioprotective. One well-established technique for prevention is administration schedule modification; prolonged infusions are considerably less cardiotoxic than is rapid infusion. Innovative delivery systems such as liposomal formulations also can significantly reduce toxicity; however, the approved oncologic indications for liposomal-encapsulated preparations remain limited. Pharmacologic cardioprotectors have been evaluated, and dexrazoxane, the only agent specifically approved in this group, has been shown to be highly effective at preventing cardiotoxicity; unfortunately, the results of one study suggest that it may alter oncologic efficacy.[38] The agent is approved for use in preventing doxorubicin-associated cardiotoxicity in many countries but is not widely used. It has been used successfully in pediatric patients as well, where cardiotoxicity is a larger problem than it is in adults. Finally, newer agents may be less cardiotoxic when administered in dosages that are of equivalent myelosuppression, and they are the subject of considerable interest and ongoing research.

■ Mechanistic Considerations of Doxorubicin Cardiotoxicity

Several interactions to contribute to the final picture of anthracycline-induced cardiotoxicity; the mechanisms

are complex and not yet fully elucidated. The process is believed to be at least partly due to iron-dependent oxidative stress as it affects cardiac muscle cells. The reduction of the quinone groups on the B ring of the anthracene structure results in a semiquinone radical before reduction to alcohol (in the case of doxorubicin, doxorubicinol). Free radicals induce peroxidation of myocyte membranes and subsequent influx of intracellular calcium.[39-45] Doxorubicin-iron (Fe^{3+}) complexes have a strong affinity for the cardiolipin-rich inner mitochondrial membrane and thus may be able to initiate oxygen radical-mediated, site-specific lipid peroxidation and increased inner membrane permeability.[46-52] Mitochondrial dysfunction is associated with morphologic changes that result in cumulative and irreversible cardiotoxicity and may be due to accumulation and persistence of 8-hydroxyguanosine adducts in cardiac mitochondrial DNA.[53] Sirtuin-3, a mitochondrial protein, restores mitochondrial respiratory chain defects, contributing to cell viability in doxorubicin-exposed patients.[54]

Impaired sequestration of intracellular free calcium ions in individual myocytes, as a result of drug exposure, may lead to diastolic dysfunction and impaired essential fatty acid metabolism.[55,56] High cardiac tissue levels of the doxorubicin alcohol metabolite, doxorubicinol, are associated with functional and morphologic changes consistent with anthracycline lesions, preventing the formation of the reductase pathway that leads to doxorubicinol may decrease anthracyclines' cardiotoxicity but not effectiveness (see also Chapter 1, and the discussion below regarding the pharmacologic prevention of cardiotoxicity).[57,58]

As alluded to above, the mechanisms that induce cardiotoxicity are at variance, at least to some extent, from those associated with oncologic efficacy. This is important with regard to cardioprotection, as the heart may be protected without while oncologic efficacy is preserved. This characteristic applies to doxorubicin as well as other anthracyclines and anthracenediones.[59] It is discussed below in the sections on cardioprotection.

CLINICAL CONSIDERATIONS OF ANTHRACYCLINE TOXICITY

■ Early and Late Doxorubicin Cardiotoxocity

Doxorubicin's cardiac effects were initially categorized into two distinct forms: early and late toxicity.[18,60] Chronic cardiomyopathy, a late manifestation of toxicity that presents as left-ventricular dysfunction or heart failure, has been alluded to above. Heart failure remains at the forefront of cardiac concerns, but early cardiac effects also occur and are of special interest as the natural history of anthracycline-related cardiotoxicity is better understood. Newer data suggest that categorizing toxicity as early or late is no longer a valid concept. Anthracyclines' effect on the heart should be thought of as a damaging insult to the myocyte; the initial cellular injury may be overcome by repair mechanisms, but may also result in myocyte death. When cell loss is sufficiently great, cardiac and vasculature compensatory mechanisms such as remodeling and hypertrophy ensue. In patients for whom compensation cannot be fully achieved, a reduction in systolic function, manifested by a drop in ejection fraction and ultimately congestive heart failure, occurs. The late sequelae may be dramatic in their presentation, but they now are thought to represent an integral part of a continuum initiated early after exposure and continuing, albeit sometimes sub-clinically, indefinitely.

It has been known for many years that the earlier clinical manifestations of cardiac dysfunction manifest, the more severe and more rapidly progressive are the cardiac sequelae. The fact that early cellular damage and subsequent clinical presentations all result from a single event is consistent with this; the more severe the initial damage is, i.e., the greater the initial cell loss, especially if it occurs in the face of decreased baseline reserves, the earlier and more severe will be the clinical presentation of decompensation.[35,61–63]

Early Manifestations of Doxorubicin Cardiotoxicity ■ Early cardiac manifestations of doxorubicin administration are seen with some regularity, and reflect the initial insult. As noted above, the injury may progress to overt cardiomyopathy; these initial manifestations of injury may be sufficiently subtle and often are not considered a serious medical concern.[64] Early signs and symptoms often resolve, albeit with the heart left with increased vulnerability due to diminished reserves.[61] The importance of the initial injury is often underappreciated as it almost never requires treatment. The most common clinical findings seen early after exposure are transient electrocardiographic changes, usually in the form of repolarization changes involving the ST-segment and the T-wave, and dysrhythmia, usually in the form of supraventricular or ventricular ectopy, which is seen often but only rarely is sustained or malignant.[63,65,66] Cases of myocarditis and pericarditis have been reported but are less common and generally self-limited; neither dysrhythmia nor mild transient inflammation constitutes an absolute contraindication for further administration, but monitoring for myocyte apoptosis with troponins is prudent, and clinical assessment of risks and benefits should be considered. Elevated troponins may be a harbinger of

later problems.[67] In rare instances, myocarditis is fulminant and probably represents significant myocardial damage. Such events require clinical correlation but suggest that further anthracycline administration is imprudent.

Not surprisingly, early toxicity is more common in the elderly and is probably related to underlying and unrelated heart disease that exists in the aging population and the associated likelihood of increased oxidative stress and reduced cardiac reserves; age is a well-described risk factor for anthracycline cardiotoxicity. Early toxicity is also more common with large single doses of doxorubicin. To date, no conclusive studies have correlated these early clinical manifestations with late cumulative dose-related cardiotoxicity caused by doxorubicin; however, the recognition of troponin I elevation immediately after treatment and the mathematical relationship between cumulative dosage and heart failure reinforces that early and late expressions of toxicity, including heart failure, result from a single destructive event. Data from Cardinale et al. suggest that troponin levels at the time of the first doxorubicin infusion are predictive of future cardiotoxicity.[29,32,68] Interestingly, the incidence of early manifestations of anthracycline exposure has been reported to be more common with daunorubicin than with doxorubicin.

Late Manifestations of Doxorubicin-Associated Cardiotoxicity ■ Late manifestations of toxicity (the classic form of doxorubicin-associated cardiac dysfunction) are widely known.[15,16] As discussed above, toxicity is related to the cumulative doxorubicin dose, with the injury resulting from the death of myocytes. Troponin release and necrosis on biopsy specimens underscore this fact; therefore, at least on the cellular level, cell death occurs and the damage is permanent. Heart failure treatment alleviates symptoms, may slow progression, and improve metrics, as is demonstrated by noninvasive assessments of ejection fraction, but myocyte death should be thought of as irreversible; ultimately the injury may lead to clinically devastating congestive heart failure that will be described in further detail below.

Doxorubicin cardiotoxicity is a cardiomyopathy that, in its clinical features, is much like congestive cardiomyopathy of other etiologies. Its end result is global cardiac dysfunction that ranges from sub-clinical asymptomatic declines in systolic function to severe and potentially fatal congestive heart failure. The entity is most closely related to the cumulative dose, although other factors that are generally considered risk factors for increased anthracycline-associated cardiotoxicity, clearly influence the degree of damage and presentation of symptoms.[18,60,69,70]

■ Cumulative Dose of Doxorubicin versus Congestive Heart Failure Relationship

The cumulative dose-versus-congestive heart failure relationship, as it is now understood, suggests a mathematical function wherein the curve is virtually horizontal at low cumulative dosages and progresses toward a theoretical limit, which is tangential to the vertical axis at extremely high cumulative dosages (Figure 3-2). The shape of this curve was first empirically derived from clinical data from a large group of patients and later fine-tuned as larger populations and more sophisticated monitoring techniques became available.[15,16] These curves suggest that at low cumulative dosages, congestive heart failure is unusual, but becomes increasingly more likely as dosages increase. Data from Swain et al. and the MD Anderson Cancer Center suggest that doxorubicin is substantially more cardiotoxic than was originally thought. The dose corresponding to an incidence of congestive heart failure risk of 5% should be considered the maximal standard cumulative dose, and, as shown in Figure 3-2, this is now believed to correlate with a cumulative dose of 400 mg/m². When cumulative dosages below 400 mg/m² are used, the likelihood of congestive heart failure for groups of patients falls below 5%. Notwithstanding these curves as they are depicted, we are increasingly seeing late toxicity in some patients, and a further shift of the curve to the left is likely as the methods to detect heart failure become more sensitive, and as clinicians become more aware of treatment-related cardiac injury.[71]

The shape of the doxorubicin-versus-congestive heart failure curve is based on a number of factors. The likelihood of toxicity reflects the sequential residual damage resulting from the total previously administered drug, a consideration that is clearly consistent with both the observed shape and with data from cardiac biopsies.[15,62] Anthracyclines' inherent ability to damage the heart can be mitigated or amplified by cardioprotective or toxicity-intensifying factors. Simply stated, the first anthracycline administration results in damage to the myocyte, and the intensity of that damage is, at least in part, dictated by the magnitude of the injury and the ability of the myocyte to withstand the insult. Myocytes undergo repair, but remain especially vulnerable to sequential stresses, and further exposure results in augmented myocyte injury. The initial injury may be entirely subclinical (i.e., not detectable by non-invasive tests). Each subsequent dose adds a sequential and incremental injury that further damages the heart. Such a relationship is intuitive if damage is considered a destructive force that continues to exert its effect over a period of time and additive to the effects of the previous damage. What remains after each cycle is an ever-smaller number of viable myocytes; the

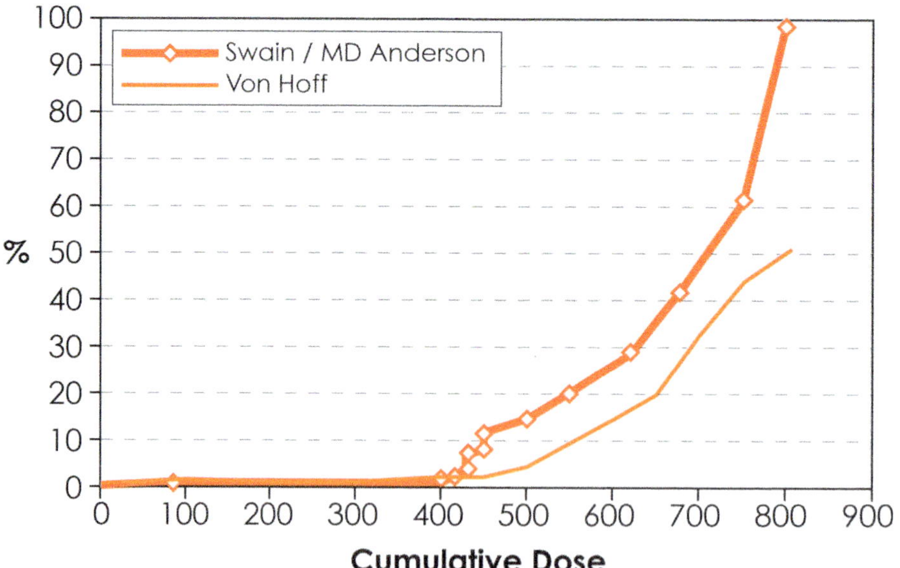

FIGURE 3-2 CHF versus cumulative dose, bolus adriamycin. Curve depicting estimations in the likelihood of developing congestive heart failure as a function of cumulative doxorubicin dose. The solid line depicts the original curve proposed by Von Hoff, the curve with diamonds depicts revised curve based on studies by Swain et al., and of the MD Anderson Cancer Center.[13,16]

ratio of destroyed to remaining myocytes increases with each doxorubicin administration, resulting in the hyperbolic curve when the cumulative dose is plotted against the likelihood of experiencing congestive heart failure (Figure 3-2).

Cell injury that results in death of the myocyte, however, is a threshold effect, whereby initial myocyte damage may not progress to cell death and some cells recover rather than undergo apoptosis. Although this threshold cannot currently be measured, it can be assumed to exist. In reality, the dose-versus-congestive heart failure curve for any individual patient may not be as smooth as that depicted in Figure 3-2, as some cells recover. The evidence of this phenomenon is indirect; the most supportive indicator is that cardiac biopsies regain a normal appearance over time. Additionally, the interval between the administration of doxorubicin and trastuzumab is an important factor in the degree of toxicity seen after trastuzumab exposure; trastuzumab is thought to interfere with cell repair (see Chapter 4 for further discussion of the importance of doxorubicin and trastuzumab timing).[72–74]

Sequential damage can be expressed as a function of the destructive force to the second power: (destructive force)^2, or, in more clinical terms, as (cumulative dose)^2 or (number of cycles)^2 relationship if the cycles are of equal dosages. This relationship presents a reasonable working model. The curve meets the criteria for the broad group of mathematical functions of the type $y = cx^2$, where y denotes the incidence of congestive heart failure and x is a factor related to the cumulative dose or the number of cycles administered. The constant, c, is introduced as a correction factor, whereby the value of c, depends on the anthracycline under question, the dosage administered per cycle, and the units used. In the case of doxorubicin, when x is taken as the number of cycles of 50 mg/m^2 each administered every three weeks, and y is the percent of patients who will demonstrate evidence of congestive heart failure, the correction constant, c, has been calculated on the basis of clinical data and is approximately equal to 1/16. The equation for doxorubicin administered according to the parameters outlined above is $y = x^2/16$.[68] Figure 3-3 depicts the observed incidence of CHF plotted against the cumulative doxorubicin dose, along with the curve of the above equation, showing remarkable congruence.

The Swain, et al. and MD Anderson Cancer Center refinement of the von Hoff curve fits this model well (Figure 3-3).[16] As doxorubicin cardiotoxicity follows such a predictable model, early damage must assume a role of far more importance than has heretofore been appreciated. Methods of predicting who is most vulnerable to doxorubicin cardiotoxicity are important, as are methods of preventing damage during exposure and mitigating ongoing stress following treatment to reduce late expression of toxicity.

The shape of the cumulative doxorubicin dose-versus-cardiotoxicity curve is not related solely to doxorubicin's cellular destruction or dysfunction,

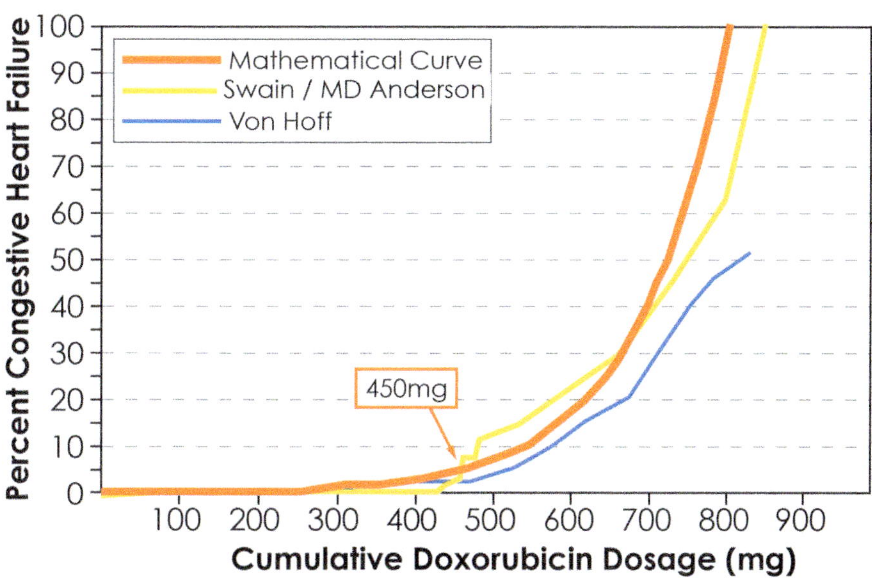

FIGURE 3-3   The Von Hoff curve along with the MD Anderson Cancer Center modification depicting cumulative dose in cycles versus the likelihood of congestive heart failure along with the plot of the mathematical equation $y = x^2/16$. See text for discussion.[68]

regardless of which data group is plotted. The component of damage related to cardiac muscle loss must be integrated into a schema of what happens to undamaged cells in the heart (or other organs affected in similar ways by analogous toxicities) and additional biologic considerations. These factors include compensation by undamaged cardiac tissue, whether by other cardiovascular system components or other body systems, and repair of injured myocardial cells. As with other organs, the heart has considerable reserves and is well designed to compensate for damage. The compensatory mechanisms undoubtedly play a huge role in our inability to detect early cardiac damage by non-invasive techniques.[75] Compensation for early damage at least partly explains the gradual, almost imperceptible rise in the incidence of detectable cardiotoxicity at low cumulative dosages of doxorubicin (Figure 3-2). If the heart had no compensatory capacity, the curve would ascend earlier and more rapidly and probably more closely parallel the changes seen on cardiac biopsy (see below).[35]

A somewhat different relationship appears to be present in young children, in whom cardiac muscle is not yet fully developed; the sequential stress model for developed myocytes and a synergistic mechanism involving developmental impairment of myocytes are probably present in children, for whom the end result is significantly augmented toxicity.[76–79] (See Chapter 20 for further discussion.)

■ CLINICAL RECOGNITION OF CARDIAC DAMAGE

Clinical Signs and Symptoms ■ Heart failure may have a long preclinical course. Patients experiencing doxorubicin-associated cardiac damage usually exhibit minimal symptoms until cardiac damage exceeds the ability for the heart to fully compensate. Depending on the extent of the initial damage, the latency period may be months, years, or decades. The first clinical sign may be a failure of the pulse rate to return promptly to baseline level after mild or moderate exertion. A heart rate that increases unexpectedly with relatively mild exertion is also an early sign of lost cardiac reserve. These early signs are not specific but help to recognize a potential early manifestation of heart failure. More significant losses in cardiac reserve may result in persistent resting tachycardia, but patients may experience only mild objective decreases in their performance status, and many patients remain asymptomatic. New diagnostic tools allow for objective assessment of these early signs.[80]

As reserves are further compromised, increased shortness of breath on exertion or inability to complete tasks that previously had not produced symptoms,

ensues. By this juncture, however, significant damage has already occurred. Difficulty climbing stairs is often the first reported symptom. As cardiac reserves decrease further with additional loss of cardiac muscle, patients become more sedentary and increasingly short of breath. Resting dyspnea, nocturnal dyspnea, orthopnea, fluid retention with weight gain, end-organ dysfunction, electrolyte abnormalities, and a diastolic (S_3) gallop are all manifestations of advanced heart failure of any cause and also are seen in patients with advanced cardiomyopathy that has resulted from an anthracycline.[61]

Non-Invasive Testing ■ No sensitive or specific non-invasive tests exist that reliably predict which patients will develop clinically relevant cardiac sequelae after subsequent doxorubicin cycles. Attempts to add such predictability to non-invasive testing are ongoing and are discussed below; progress has been made in this regard, but the predictive value of non-invasive testing remains problematic.[28]

The suboptimal predictive value of non-invasive tests for anthracycline-associated cardiotoxicity has resulted in considerable confusion. At low cumulative dosages, when the likelihood of a decreased ejection fraction due to anthracycline is small, the likelihood of a false-positive result may exceed the number of true-positives (Figure 3-4A and B). However, when the likelihood of a true-positive result is high, as is the case when high cumulative doxorubicin doses have been administered, false-negative results that do not detect potentially important decreases in ejection fraction are problematic. A statistically valid threshold for positivity that ignores borderline-to-moderate abnormalities and categorizes only markedly abnormal cases as positive tends to minimize false-positive results but is clearly under-inclusive. Such a threshold results in some doxorubicin cardiotoxicity cases going unrecognized and may delay crucial interventions. Clearly, a fixed threshold that excludes most patients with false-positive findings does not solve the clinical dilemma. The problem might be reduced by using a variable threshold for positive results, whereby a higher degree of abnormality is required at low cumulative dosages, where the likelihood of cardiotoxicity is low, and a lower degree of decline from baseline would be needed as the cumulative dose approaches more toxic levels. Such a sliding scale for positivity, while intriguing, would require integration of a number of factors including variations in cycle dose, cycle timing, and risk factor corrections; what would be significant for a given patient might not be so for another. To a great extent, this is not entirely at variance with what we, as effective clinicians, already undertake; we integrate all

(A)

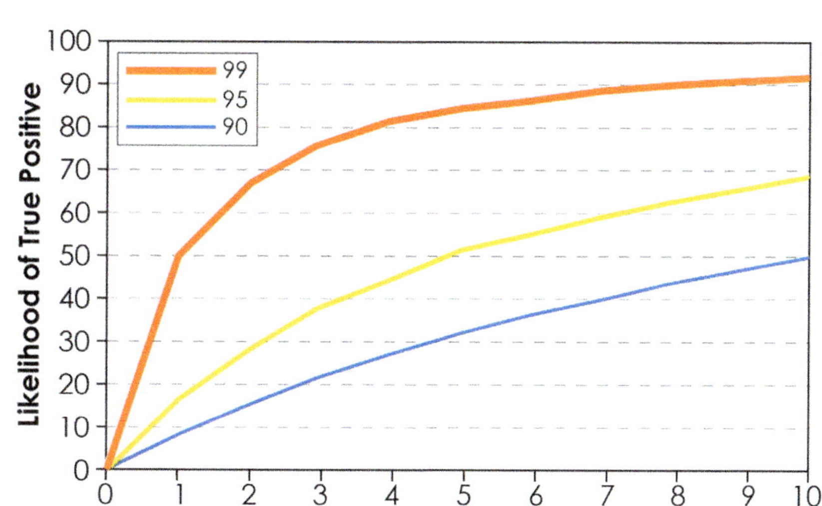

(B)

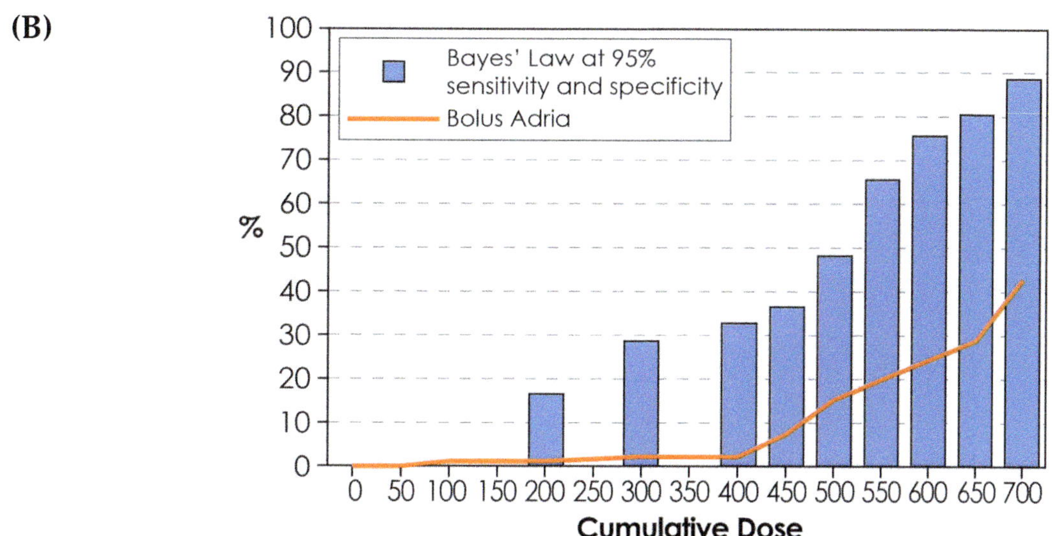

FIGURE 3-4 (A) Bayes' law at different levels of sensitivity/specificity. (B) Likelihood of accurate prediction of adriamycin cardiac toxicity by cumulative dose.

available clinical data to arrive at an individualized probability of disease that we use to guide our interpretation of test results.

Ejection fractions are affected by many factors beyond cardiotoxic agent a patient may be receiving. The non-specific nature of the ejection fraction estimate often makes it difficult to isolate the role of anthracyclines when additional factors as well as the well-recognized variations between and among the individual interpreters. The more common changes that affect ejection fraction are listed in Table 3-3.

Determining the extent of early toxicity by non-invasively screening of large numbers of patients treated with low cumulative doxorubicin doses is ineffective and potentially dangerous because of the high probability of false-positive results exceeding true-positive results; such findings may result in a decision to stop an important treatment regimen on the basis of a false-positive test result.[75]

Non-invasive testing can result in the recognition or confirmation of subclinical abnormalities in selected patients with cardiac damage. Patients may be well served by recognizing such damage at a stage at which treatment is more likely to be beneficial and when further cardiotoxic exposure can be avoided. Early recognition and treatment may allow patients to remain stable from the cardiac standpoint, to enjoy normal activities for longer periods of time, and to maintain a good quality of life despite significant cardiac damage resulting in loss of cardiac reserve.[81]

TABLE 3-3 Factors that may affect ejection fraction estimations in cancer patients

Interobserver variations
Physiologic variations
Metabolic variations
Circadian variations
Variations in stress level
Pathologic variations
Not related to the tumor or its treatment
Hormonal variations
Related to tumor
Blood shunting
Anemia
Hormonal variations
Related to treatment (other than direct anthracycline cardiotoxicity)
Nutritional state
Metabolic state
Hyperadrenergic state
Pharmacologic effects of non-anthracycline cardiosuppressive agents
Pharmacologic effects of medications for sedation or control of side-effects
Anthracycline-associated cardiac dysfunction

Despite the lack of predictive value in screening individual patients, small changes in non-invasive parameters are often pooled for research purposes. When pooled, even small changes in the mean ejection fraction when large numbers of patients are included suggest broader population trends that are essential to understanding the natural history of agents with the propensity to adversely affect cardiac function.[82] They are also vital in comparing the relative cardiotoxicity of various anthracyclines with one another or with other agents. It remains counterproductive to extrapolate highly significant pooled data to individual patients, as doing so may result in incorrect conclusions regarding toxicity and the need to alter or reassess oncologic strategy (Figure 3-4A and B).

Non-Invasive Indices of Left-Ventricular Ejection Fraction. The relationship between the internal measurements of left ventricular chamber size at end-systole and end-diastole may be expressed in a variety of ways. When considered as a linear function, the parameter of fractional shortening is calculated; when these measurements are corrected to express an estimate of intracardiac volume, the ejection fraction is approximated. The left ventricular stroke volume is the difference in volume at end-diastole and end-systole; the ejection fraction is defined by the formula:

$$1-[(\text{end-systolic volume})/(\text{end-diastolic volume})]$$

and expressed as a percentage.

Most experts agree that at least half the blood in the left ventricle at the beginning of systole should be ejected for the value to be considered normal. Theoretically, left ventricular ejection fraction estimates should be the same regardless of the technique used to assess this parameter. Unfortunately, despite considerable improvement in the methods used, non-invasive estimates of left ventricular volume and ejection fraction remain imprecise.

Various cardiac techniques attempt to approximate the ejection fraction, including left ventricular angiography performed as part of a left-heart catheterization, cardiac ultrasonography, nuclear modalities, magnetic resonance imaging, computerized tomography, and positron emission tomography.[83,84] Newer techniques are more accurate, but most doxorubicin patients undergo evaluation using cardiac ultrasound or cardiac blood pool scans; the ejection fraction remains the most widely used parameter, both clinically for single patients and for the evaluation large groups of patients enrolled in clinical trials.

Echo imaging quality depends on several factors. Obese patients and those who have received radiation to the left side of the chest are especially difficult to image adequately. Sonographic contrast enhancers, in the form of microspheres, generally make wall-blood interfaces better defined and allow chamber volume estimates to be made when such assessments would not be otherwise possible.

Ejection fractions are often estimated using nuclear techniques. Cardiac radionuclide imaging, often referred to as multi-gated or MUGA cardiac blood pool scans, are widely accepted.[85] The test is performed by making the blood pool minimally radioactive and accruing counts over the cardiac chambers that can be quantitated and localized. To estimate an ejection fraction from such scans the cardiac cycle must be divided into a finite number of time segments (gating), and the position and location of counts for each time period, as a segmental component of the cardiac cycle, must be stored in a separate area of computer memory to form a discrete cardiac image. Counts are accumulated over several minutes, whereby the counts for each cardiac segment are added to those of the same temporal segment collected from previous cardiac cycles.

The images may then be viewed sequentially in a computer-generated loop that represents the entire cardiac cycle. The numbers of counts in each time segment are summated, and the segments depicting the largest and smallest number of counts represent the end-systolic and end-diastolic images, and are used to calculate an estimation of the ejection fraction. Multi-gated cardiac blood pool scans also provide information on diastolic function. Nuclear studies are generally reproducible; however, cardiac dysrhythmia may make cardiac gating difficult or impossible.

Cardiac perfusion scans provide data on relative uptake for various cardiac vasculature distributions. Significant perfusion defects can be visualized and the extent and location of the injury ascertained. Perfusion scans can estimate ejection fractions but are not suitable for following up patients during or after treatment.[86,87] First-pass nuclear imaging studies do not require gating and provide information on left and right ventricular sizes and volumes; they are increasingly being replaced by more modern techniques. (See Chapter 10 for additional information on nuclear and non-nuclear imaging in cancer patients as methods of estimating ejection fraction.)

Diastolic dysfunction, in which the ventricular chambers do not relax normally, has also been evaluated with respect to doxorubicin cardiotoxicity. Some investigators find diastolic function indices helpful, but others have found little or no advantage over systolic function indices. As technology evolves and measurements become more precise and accurate, diastolic function may prove to be valuable for following selected patients receiving doxorubicin.[22,88] At present, despite interest in diastolic dysfunction as an early marker for anthracycline-related cardiotoxicity, we lack a perspective on how to interpret early changes in diastolic function.[89]

Electrocardiograms. Cancer patients frequently undergo electrocardiography, but its usefulness in doxorubicin follow-up is limited. Nonspecific repolarization abnormalities are considered a manifestation of early injury, but changes involving the ST-segment and T-wave are often related to other etiologies such as electrolyte alterations or ischemia. They have no defined predictive value and they usually resolve promptly, with resolution of the underlying problem. Repolarization changes are not recognized as being a harbinger of later cardiac dysfunction. It is recognized that the mean QRS voltage is reduced in patients with doxorubicin cardiotoxicity.[21] Voltage declines, however, are common in cancer patients and occur for reasons unrelated to anthracycline exposure. Interstitial fluid retention, effusions,

and emphysema, are all associated with this finding, thereby limiting the usefulness of decreased mean QRS voltage as an indicator of anthracycline-related cardiotoxicity.

Dysrhythmia is recognized often in early doxorubicin cardiotoxicity but is seldom a concern in late toxicity unless it occurs as a component of severe heart failure. Conduction abnormalities are also a non-specific finding; they are a manifestation of congestive heart failure but may be related to other factors as well; they are also not helpful as a predictive parameter for following patients receiving doxorubicin.

Other Non-Invasive Studies. Chest roentgenograms are helpful in identifying other causes of symptoms that may be confused with anthracycline-associated congestive heart failure, such as pleural or pericardial effusion or lymphangitic tumor spread. Systolic time intervals and phonocardiography were considered helpful in some early reports on doxorubicin cardiotoxicity but are now only of historical interest.[62]

Biochemical markers of cardiac damage have also been studied in doxorubicin patients. Creatinine phosphokinase, a useful marker of myocardial injury associated with acute ischemia, has not been helpful in identifying patients at increased risk for developing congestive heart failure with additional doxorubicin. Troponin I is a marker of myocyte destruction and has been shown to be elevated after acute anthracycline injury.[29,90] Clear criteria for using this marker have yet to emerge.[26] However troponin I clearly is a marker of cell destruction, confirming that cell injury occurs immediately after anthracycline administration. Interestingly, troponin I elevation levels are generally low and certainly much lower than are seen with myocardial infarction. One possible explanation is that in contrast with acute ischemic injury, in which considerable cell damage takes place over a relatively brief period of time, the rate of cell death resulting from anthracyclines is much more protracted, producing a broader but lower concentration curve for troponins.[29] In addition, in a model using hypertensive rats who received doxorubicin, troponin I elevations were correlated with and preceded histopathologic cardiotoxicity changes.[91] The augmented release of troponin I after anthracycline is gaining acceptance as a marker for identifying patients at risk for late cardiac events; it may aid in stratifying such patients for cardiac monitoring, identify those for whom less cardiotoxic regimens may be better suited, and assist in categorizing some patients into groups for which preventive therapeutic initiatives may be appropriate.[71,73,90] The association between troponin I level and late toxicity likelihood, the optimal time to measure the marker, and the best assay for these measurements have not yet been established. Because troponin I levels indicate recent cell damage, they cannot be used to estimate damage that occurred in the distant past.

Several studies have confirmed that estimates of B-type natriuretic peptide (BNP), a neuro-hormone that is elevated in response to hypervolemia, are useful in diagnosing and monitoring congestive heart failure. In contrast to troponin I, a marker for recent cell death, BNP is elevated when the atrial volume or pressure is increased. Patients with cardiac decompensation often have abnormally high BNP levels. Some researchers have reported finding BNP elevations shortly after anthracycline exposure; this finding suggests that extensive, acute anthracycline injury results in hemodynamic alterations sufficient to cause some degree of chamber dilation or fluid shifts.[92]

Invasive testing for anthracycline-associated myopathy: cardiac biopsy ■ Structural changes that correlate with anthracyclines' functional impairments have been sought. Such changes were identified and quantitated by Margaret Billingham at Stanford University, where the technique of endomyocardial biopsy was refined.[93] Trans-vascular cardiac biopsy was described in the Japanese medical literature in the 1960s; by the late 1970s, cardiac biopsy was used extensively both at Stanford University and The University of Texas MD Anderson Cancer Center to evaluate anthracycline cardiomyopathy.[5,37,94,99] During an era when maximal cumulative anthracycline doses were preferred by many oncologists, cardiac biopsy offered insight into the extent of cardiac damage that non-invasive testing could not provide. The use of unusually high cumulative anthracycline doses has become rare, and their is little need for cardiac biopsy information. At present, cardiac biopsy still plays a role in evaluating anthracycline and other cardiotoxicities in the research setting, but it has been displaced as a routine clinical procedure. However, the biopsy procedure and its role in quantifying anthracycline injury are mentioned briefly.

Biopsy specimens are usually obtained via the right internal jugular vein, allowing access to the right-sided cardiac chambers without having to negotiate venous anatomy curves or lengthy transvenous routes that would be required if other entry sites were used. The vein is entered, and the bioptome is advanced to the apex of the right ventricle, where myocardium specimens are removed. The small tissue fragments, usually 1–2 mm in their largest dimension, are preserved in glutaraldehyde for electron microscopic analysis or formalin for light microscopy. Overall complications are rare but include cardiac perforation by the bioptome, which can result in life-threatening

acute tamponade. Less serious complications include pericarditis, presumably due to some slow leakage of blood into the pericardial space, and complications related to entry in the central vasculature. Transient dysrhythmia, usually in the form of isolated ventricular premature complexes, almost always occurs at the time of tissue removal and results from mechanical stimulation of the myocardium by the bioptome. Late complications were not observed in our series of nearly 2000 biopsies.[97] Entry into the arterial system and biopsy of the left ventricle have also been undertaken but the more invasive left-sided procedure appeared to offer no advantages over right-sided biopsy for identifying anthracycline-associated changes.

Margaret Billingham proposed the first grading scale for doxorubicin toxicity based on morphologic changes seen electron microscopically.[93] The Billingham grading scale included grades 0–3 based on increasingly severe structural abnormalities. The earliest change is increased vacuole formation. More advanced changes include myofibrillar dropout and ultimately necrosis. Later, the Billingham grading scale was modified at The University of Texas MD Anderson Cancer Center to include the intermediate grades 0.5 and 1.5, which allowed for grouping by more subtle criteria without altering the previously established grades.[99] Grading criteria, regardless of which system is used, are based on the number of cells demonstrating abnormalities and the extent of those abnormalities in electron microscopic grids, where changes in vacuole formation, myofibrillar dropout, or necrosis may be seen. Multiple electron-mcroscopic grids are evaluated before the final grade is assigned, as normal cells may abut abnormal ones in any individual grid. The criteria for assigning the various biopsy grades according to Billingham and MacKay grading criteria are provided in Table 3-4; typical pathologic changes are shown in Figure 3-5A through D.

Relationship between cumulative dose, functional change, and structural abnormalities in patients receiving doxorubicin ■ The maximal recommended dose of doxorubicin was initially chosen so that not more than 5% of patients treated at that level would develop clinical evidence of heart failure. It was believed that this threshold represented a rational compromise, reached empirically, that was designed to offer optimal overall survival to patients who required maximal anthracycline exposure for tumor control. It was believed that at higher doses, cardiotoxicity would create more harm for the average patient than would the oncologic benefit achieved by the incremental doxorubicin dosage beyond that point. At lower doses, the risk of decreased tumor destruction may be higher than the

Table 3-4   Morphologic grading scale

MORPHOLOGIC GRADING SYSTEMS FOR ANTHRACYCLINE CARDIOTOXICITY					
	BILLINGHAM SCORING SYSTEM[93,171]		MACKAY SCORING SYSTEM BASED ON THE NUMBER OF CELLS DEMONSTRATING THESE CHARACTERISTICS IN AN ELECTRON MICROSCOPIC GRID[*98,99]		
GRADE		MORPHOLOGIC CHARACTERISTICS	VACUOLES	MYOFIBRILLAR DROPOUT	NECROSIS
0		Normal myocardial ultrastructural morphology	0	0	0
0.5[#]		Not completely normal but no evidence of anthracycline-specific damage	<4	0	0
1		Isolated myocytes affected and/or early myofibrillar loss; damage to <5% of all cells	4–10	<3	0
1.5[#]		Changes similar to grade 1 except damage involves 6%–15% of all cells	<10	3–5	<2
2.0		Clusters of myocytes affected by myofibrillar loss and/or vacuolization, with damage to 16%–25% of all cells	~	6–8	2–5
2.5[#]		Many myocytes (26%–35% of all cells) affected by vacuolization and/or myofibrillar loss			
3.0		Severe, diffuse myocytes damage (>35% of all cells)	~	>8	>5

* Average number of abnormal muscle fibers per grid based on an examination of a minimum of six grids obtained from six blocks.

Grades of 0.5, 1.5, and 2.5 were not included in the original Billingham grading scale.

~ The number of vacuoles does not alter the grade for higher biopsy grades.

incremental reduced risk of congestive failure. At the level at which 5% of patients experience clinically detectable heart failure, devastating cardiac sequelae and cardiac death are acceptably rare; only a small proportion of patients who experience heart failure develop severe cardiac dysfunction or cardiac death. These considerations are evolving in that a lower and less toxic regimens are being used, especially when treating those malignancies where effective alternatives exist.

Early and empiric estimations of the maximal permissible doxorubicin dose were overestimated. As the drug became more widely used, aggressive testing became part of many doxorubicin protocols, and patients underwent cardiac sonographic or nuclear imaging to identify early ejection fraction changes. It was hoped that finding early changes in cardiac function would identify those who developed toxicity early (i.e., at lower cumulative dosages) so that therapy could be changed and further damage avoided. This strategy was largely unsuccessful,

as the non-invasive tests describe function rather than an estimation of actual myocyte damage as is provided by cardiac biopsy. What did emerge from extensive early testing was that cardiotoxicity had been considerably underestimated and that 400 mg/m^2 is a more accurate estimate of the cumulative dose that is correlated with a 5% incidence of congestive heart failure.[16,100,101]

Non-invasive studies of systolic dysfunction are suboptimal on the basis of early false-positive and late false-negative findings, as has been addressed above; we will now review some of the specific problems that interfere with valid cardiac function assessment: (1) lack of reproducibility and variability because of interobserver interpretation, (2) biologic factors other than those in the heart that can affect cardiac function and cause true ejection fraction changes that are not related to anthracycline cardiotoxicity, and (3) other pharmacologic influences that affect cardiac muscle. None of these factors can be isolated; thus, changes in systolic function may be assumed to be multifactorial

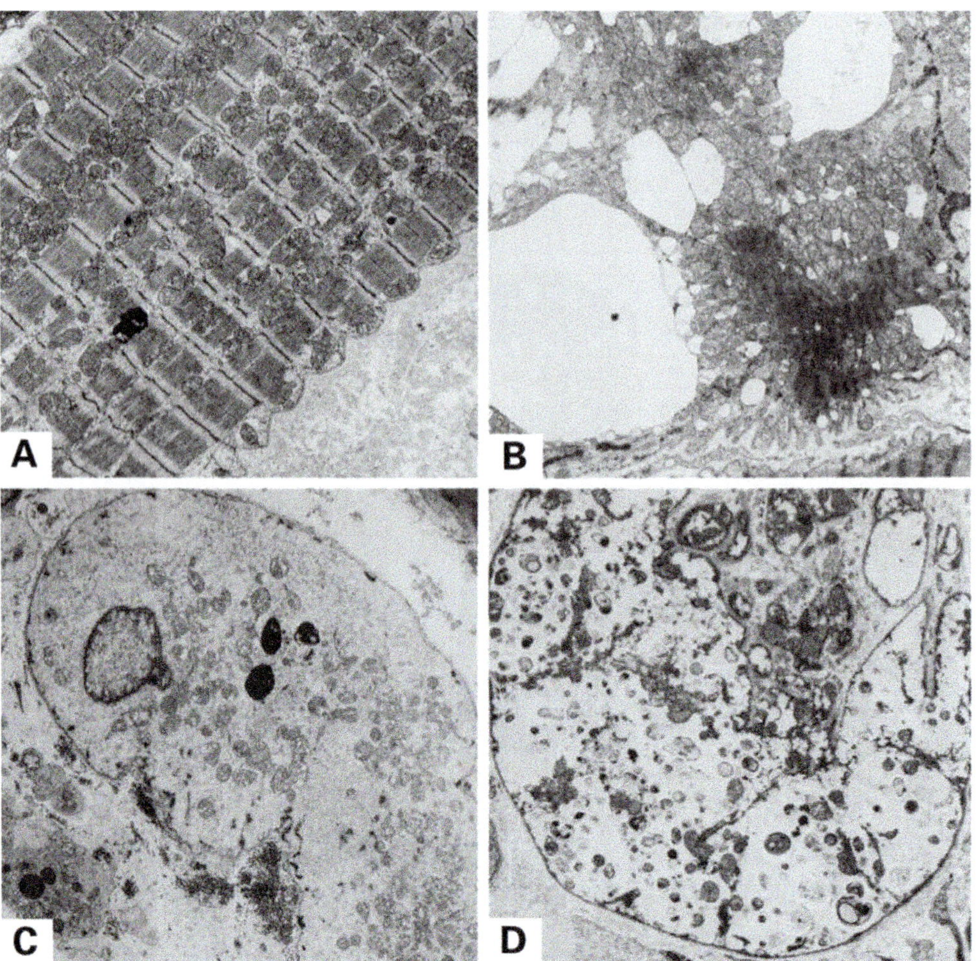

FIGURE 3-5 Typical electron micrographs showing normal myocardium (A), vacuoles (B), myofibrillar dropout (C), and myocardial necrosis (D).

until the true cause is defined. We cannot always precisely estimate how much the ejection fraction has decreased because of anthracycline exposure and how much it has decreased or increased because of other contributing factors. Some of the factors that affect the heart and cardiovascular system are delineated in Table 3-3.

The estimated ejection fraction for any given patient represents a moment in time with regard to systolic function. After a brief interval, the ejection fractions may change; the pulse rate may be different, and the patient may have an altered sympathetic tone. Days later, medications may have been ingested, and the hemoglobin level may be significantly higher or lower because of blood loss or transfusion. Clinicians must not assume that decreases in the ejection fraction are entirely the result of the cardiotoxic drug under consideration, and should consider other possible valid explanations for the change in systolic function. In some instances changes that are unrelated to the anthracycline may

result in premature discontinuation of a highly effective therapeutic regimen.

Despite the difficulty in detecting doxorubicin's effects early, an abundance of data suggest that early damage does take place in adults; the strongest evidence is electron-microscopically detectable morphologic changes at low cumulative doses.[35,102] Interestingly, the characteristic electron microscopic changes described above are seen at cumulative dosages far below those at which clinical cardiac dysfunction is typically found; investigators sought to identify and quantitate these subclinical abnormalities non-invasively. Ejection fractions were an obvious candidate, as they could be determined serially in large groups of patients without invasive interventions. Even though ejection fraction was found to be suboptimal, the studies supplied vital information for preventing toxicity by early and intensive non-invasive monitoring. Some patients had abnormal ejection fractions at lower cumulative dosages than did others, giving rise to the identification of risk factors. In addition, the underappreciated risk of doxorubicin cardiotoxicity was re-evaluated and a downward revision of the maximum prudent cumulative dose was advocated. Paradoxically, even though monitoring should have been beneficial, some patients had no cardiotoxicity but had false-positive ejection fraction decreases at low cumulative doses. These patients were given less cardiotoxic regimens that were less effective than is doxorubicin. Thus, these non-invasive tests were clearly a double-edged sword. The differences in timing between cardiac biopsy changes and the appearance of cardiac symptoms is depicted in Figure 3-6.[35]

Despite limitations to non-invasive tests, guidelines were published to define cardiotoxicity standards based on a threshold of absolute ejection fraction standards from baseline or specific value decreases to a level below normal. In large clinical trials, the factors not related to doxorubicin were at least partly balanced, and mean decreases for the group were probably related to the drug in question. For individual patients, however, the guidelines proved much less useful.

■ Risk Factors for Doxorubicin Cardiotoxicity

As noted above, some patients are more sensitive to doxorubicin than are others.[103] In these patients, the cumulative dose-versus-cardiotoxicity curve (Figure 3-2) is shifted to the left; they have a 5% likelihood of developing congestive heart failure at a cumulative dosage substantially lower than 400 mg/m^2. Among the groups at increased risk are those who have undergone certain non-anthracycline anticancer treatments, including radiation to the heart, extreme young or old age, and varying types of underlying heart disease. These groups are further delineated in Table 3-5. Because anthracycline cardiotoxicity is related to the cumulative dose, any patient who has previously received an anthracycline is at increased risk on the basis of the extent of prior exposure. The cardiotoxicity mechanisms of other potentially cardiotoxic drugs are less clear; when such agents precede anthracycline exposure they may augment toxicity, and when they follow the anthracycline damage persists and plays an important role in subsequent expression of cardiotoxicity. Cyclophosphamide and mitomycin C fall within this group of agents. The interaction of sequentially administered cardiotoxic drugs, especially Type II agents, is discussed in Chapter 4. Radiation injury to the myocardium appears to affect small cardiac vessels and may induce myocarditis; this increased toxicity may be a manifestation of an inability to properly provide substrate to marginally functioning tissue (see Chapter 7 on radiation effects).[104–108] Again, in this setting, sequential stress probably plays an important role.

Underlying heart disease includes an especially interesting group of entities such as aortic stenosis, hypertrophic cardiomyopathy, and systemic hypertension with left ventricular hypertrophy. All of these lead to increased wall stress. The mechanism of doxorubicin's damage has not been fully elucidated, but increased oxidative stress may be a common denominator that is consistent with a decreased reserve of

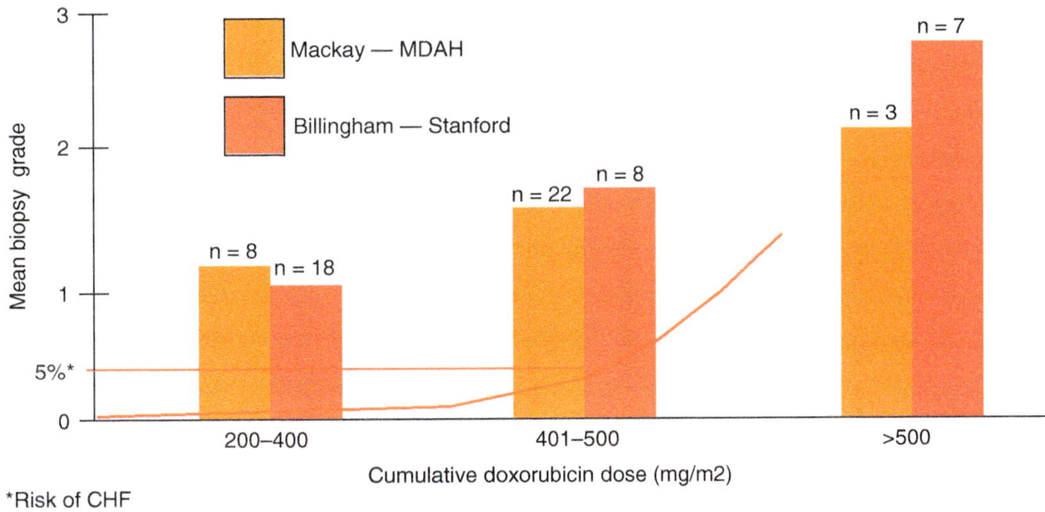

Figure 3-6 Correlation of cardiac biopsy grades with cumulative doxorubicin dose. Doxorubicin was given intravenously every three to four weeks, and biopsy specimens were taken approximately three weeks following the most recent administration. Note that biopsy changes occur at relatively low cumulative dosages. (Adapted from Ewer M et al., 1984.[35])

TABLE 3-5   Risk Factors associated with anthracyclines

- **Any condition that has previously caused damage to the heart**
  Prior anthracycline exposure
  Prior exposure to other cardiotoxic agents
  Geriatric population
  Exposure of the heart to radiation
  Underlying heart disease
  Diabetes
- **Any condition that makes the heart more susceptible to ongoing damage**
  Concomitant exposure to other cardiotoxic agents
  Pediatric population
  Obesity
  Genetic factors

myocardial cells; DNA double-strand breaks caused by activation of topoisomerase II B may be more important than previously thought.[12,109]

Despite extensive interest regarding cardiac risk factors, it is convenient to think of the cardiovascular system rather than specific pathologic entities or conditions. As noted above, any patient who has sustained previous myocardial injury or is at increased susceptibility for ongoing injury is at increased risk for cardiotoxicity associated with anthracyclines. In any event, sequential exposures and stresses are true risk factors, and patients deemed to be at increased risk should be, whenever possible limited with regard to their exposure of anthracyclines. A prudent limitation in exposure may be achieved by reducing the acceptable cumulative doxorubicin dose to about 2/3 the generally-regarded safe dose healthy patients. Even with a 1/3 reduction in cumulative dosage serious cardiac sequelae cannot always be avoided. Increased monitoring with troponin I determinations and modern imaging techniques should be undertaken in patients with increased risk even when the anticipated exposure has been reduced. While there is limited data to support such a recommendation, caution is prudent.[26]

Cardiac Monitoring During Anthracycline Treatment

Because of cardiac reserves and the lack of sensitivity and specificity of non-invasive testing, the value of screening large groups of otherwise healthy and asymptomatic patients for early signs of toxicity when exposed to low or intermediate cumulative dosages of an anthracycline is limited. Non-invasive tests can, however, help recognize or confirm early or developed cardiac dysfunction in patients with early symptoms, and can do so at a stage when interventions are possible and cardiac intervention is most likely to be of benefit. False-positive results are still problematic in these patients, but the likelihood of misinterpreting results is much lower than that in routine surveillance. Below, we describe one possible approach to evaluating patients for cardiotoxicity, based on the author's preferences and experience.

Prior to the initiation of doxorubicin therapy, all patients should be considered for cardiac protective regimens. Newer modalities make protection feasible and cost effective, and indications for cardioprotection should be recognized and accepted broadly. In centers at which cardioprotection is deemed a priority, such as The University of Texas MD Anderson Cancer Center, advanced congestive heart failure due to doxorubicin is unusual, as is the need to modify the chemotherapeutic regimen because of cardiologic concerns once a regimen has been started.

All patients should undergo a baseline measurement of ejection fraction using echocardiography or a nuclear technique. The baseline results are useful for later comparisons and to identify patients with cardiac risk factors who require closer scrutiny with regard to cardiac monitoring. Patients with normal systolic function and no risk factors will usually tolerate up to 400 mg/m^2 of doxorubicin or the maximum recommended cumulative dose of other anthracyclines. Toxicity expressed as heart failure at cumulative doses below 2/3 of the maximal recommended dosage (260–300 mg/m^2 in the case of doxorubicin) is unusual. As noted above, routine non-invasive monitoring below this cumulative dose is not warranted for individual patients without risk factors and without some clinical indication of cardiac dysfunction. In the cumulative dose range from 2/3 to the maximally recommended dose (300–400 mg/m^2 for doxorubicin), patients should be evaluated by obtaining a clinical history and follow-up echocardiogram, either at that time of, or approximately 3 months after, therapy. After treatment, clinical follow-up and annual or biennial estimates of ejection fraction are a reasonable yet not overly burdensome compromise.

Patients with risk factors or poor baseline systolic function often tolerate 2/3 of the maximal recommended cumulative dosage, but alternate non-cardiotoxic regimens should be explored in this population. When undertaken, the reduction should be by reducing the number of cycles, and not by reducing the dose of the individual cycles. Most, albeit not all, patients with risk factors or baseline abnormalities can tolerate reduced exposure with acceptable risk.[70] As the cumulative dose increases above recommended cumulative dosage level, the likelihood of cardiotoxicity, especially in patients deemed to be at increased risk, rises, and non-invasive measurement of the ejection fraction should be performed every one or two cycles thereafter; earlier and more intensive surveillance is prudent in these patients, although strong data to support enhanced surveillance is lacking. By selecting patients in whom cardiac problems are suspected on the basis of clinical assessment, the predictive value of ejection fraction testing rises and approaches useful levels even at intermediate cumulative dosages. For patients with cardiac signs, symptoms, or risk factors, and ejection fraction decreases of >10 percentage points, confirmation is appropriate, as are considerations of less cardiotoxic regimens. In the rare instances in which the drug is deemed oncologically essential, cardiac biopsy may be considered; a biopsy grade ≥ 1.0 is a clear indication to stop and not re-introduce doxorubicin or any other anthracycline; only rarely is cardiac biopsy deemed essential in modern clinical practice.

No perfect algorithm exists for avoiding doxorubicin cardiotoxicity; thus, some patients will ultimately fall outside the norms and will not be protected by these monitoring guidelines. Even with caution, some patients will develop significant cardiotoxicity, and in rare instances, patients will die of doxorubicin-associated congestive heart failure. The goal should be to maximize survival and minimize death from all causes in these patients not just the incidence of death due to cardiotoxicity. To achieve this, the ongoing oncologic benefit must be weighed against the ongoing cardiotoxic risks, and individualized judgments became as important as schemata in clinical decision-making. Avoiding anthracycline cardiotoxicity by limiting exposure and reducing cumulative dosages does not maximize overall survival because of higher recurrence rates or shorter disease-free survival intervals. More widespread use of cardioprotective measures should further decrease the incidence of severe cardiac problems associated with anthracyclines. These guidelines are summarized in Table 3-6.

TABLE 3-6　Cardiac Monitoring of Ejection Fraction in Patients Receiving Anthracyclines[#]

CUMULATIVE DOSE (STANDARD DOXORUBICIN EQUIVALENT) OR TIME AFTER COMPLETION OF DOXORUBICIN	PATIENT WITHOUT RISK FACTORS OR CLINICAL INDICATORS OF CARDIAC DYSFUNCTION	PATIENTS WITH RISK FACTOR OR CLINICAL INDICATORS OF CARDIAC DYSFUNCTION
Baseline	Echo or MUGA	Echo or MUGA
<300 mg/²	Not needed	Echo or MUGA if cardiac concerns arise
300–400 mg/²	Echo or MUGA every 1–2 cycles or if cardiac concerns arise	Echo or MUGA every cycle or if cardiac concerns arise; cardiac risk may be increased[*]
>400 mg/²[*]	Use only with caution. Echo or MUGA every cycle; cardiac risk is increased; consider cardiac biopsy[*]	Use only with caution. Echo or MUGA every cycle; cardiac risk is increased; consider cardiac biopsy[*]
1–3 months following conclusion of anthracycline	Echo or MUGA; perform sooner if cardiac concerns arise	Echo or MUGA; perform sooner if cardiac concerns arise
3 months–5 years following conclusion of anthracycline	Yearly Echo or MUGA (perform sooner if cardiac concerns arise)	Yearly Echo or MUGA (perform sooner if cardiac concerns arise)
>5 years following conclusion of anthracycline	Every 2 years (perform more often if cardiac concerns arise)	Yearly (perform more often if cardiac concerns arise)

[#]These suggestions are for anthracycline cumulative dosages corrected for variations in cardiotoxicity that depend on the agent used, the administration schedule, and cardioprotection. As printed, they apply to doxorubicin administered at a dosage of 50 mg/m² per 3-week cycle, but must be corrected according to the guidelines of Table 3-7 when other administration schedules or other anthracyclines are administered.

[*]Doxorubicin at cumulative dosages of >400 mg/² is associated with cardiotoxicity in more than 5% of those treated. In the case of patients with risk factors known to be associated with increased anthracycline cardiotoxicity this threshold is lower, and may be as low as 300 mg/². In selected cases where doxorubicin is deemed crucial for tumor control at cumulative dosages above these levels careful monitoring is required. In very unusual instances, the judicious scrutiny of cardiac biopsy material may be helpful.

■ Treatment of Established Anthracycline-Associated Cardiac Dysfunction

Potential therapeutic modalities for patients with doxorubicin-associated congestive heart failure include interventions that will: (1) mitigate further cardiac damage, (2) minimize symptoms, (3) reduce afterload and increase cardiac output, and (4) facilitate cell regeneration through stem cell therapy. In some instances, organ transplantation may also be a consideration.

Undoubtedly, the most important consideration in patients who have received an anthracycline and have developed cardiotoxicity is avoiding further anthracycline exposure. As all of the known agents in this group of drugs cause the same form of cardiac damage, switching from one anthracycline to another does not offer protection and may result in relentlessly progressive cardiotoxicity. Anthracycline cardiotoxicity is an absolute contraindication for further anthracycline exposure. When a change from one anthracycline to another is oncologically appropriate, the previously administered cumulative injury of the first agent must be added to the anticipated damage of subsequent agents to arrive at an estimation of the maximally tolerated dose. Guidance is provided in Table 3-7.[100] Changing from one anthracycline to another does not offer cardioprotection from either.

When a patient presents with signs or symptoms consistent with cardiac dysfunction the clinician must determine whether it is heart failure or another abnormality with a similar presentation. If it is heart failure, was it caused by the medication being administered? One important clue is the cumulative anthracycline dose, corrected for protection when cardioprotective regimens have been incorporated (see Table 3-7).[100] The lower the corrected cumulative dosages, the more aggressive must be the search for other causes, bearing in mind that cardiac dysfunction symptoms are often nonspecific and may be caused by lung abnormalities, metastatic disease progression, endocrine abnormalities, infections, neurologic lesions, metabolic disturbances, or blood dyscrasia. As the corrected cumulative dose increases, anthracycline cardiotoxicity becomes more likely and an aggressive hunt for other causes is much less likely to be fruitful.

Once the offending agent has been withdrawn and other causes of the patient's symptoms have been eliminated, the treatment for anthracycline-associated cardiac dysfunction should follow the guidelines for cardiac dysfunction of any cause. The modern approach to treatment has become much more aggressive, the hope being to mitigate further damage resulting from strain and remodeling. Even asymptomatic patients with left-ventricular dysfunction should now be considered for treatment, and the results of major trials suggest that early intervention results in significant benefits.[26,110]

The American College of Cardiology and The American Heart Association, The Heart Failure Society of America, and the European Society of Cardiology have all created guidelines on the treatment of heart failure.[111–113] Diuretics and salt restriction are useful, but hypovolemic states may exist in the cancer patient and patients may need more rigorous oversight. Angiotensin-converting enzyme inhibitors (ACE inhibitors) and angiotensin receptor blockers achieve neurohormonal modification and vasodilation and have shown a benefit in survival in heart failure patients. This fact should apply to the cancer population as well. Beta-adrenergic blocking drugs (β-blockers) have been shown to improve symptoms and prolong survival in patients with symptomatic congestive heart failure. Additionally β-blockers reduce the incidence of dysrhythmia and slow the ventricular rate. These agents are generally introduced as soon as doxorubicin-associated cardiac dysfunction is recognized, and are administered at low doses that are gradually increased as tolerated. They may lead to hypotension as a dose-limiting event, a characteristic of special importance for the cancer patient. Spironolactone can be considered, but careful attention is required to avoid hyperkalemia.[114] Newer approaches such as the "funny current" inhibitor ivabradine may be helpful, but has not been adequately studied in the cancer population.[115]

For patients with advanced heart failure, inotropic agents given by intravenous infusion (dopamine or milrinone) may be helpful as a bridge therapy during the time that it takes for other strategies to become effective. Left-ventricular assist devices, biventricular pacemakers, and implantable defibrillators may also be used selectively.[116] The first may be effective as a bridge to cardiac transplantation and the latter in high-risk patients. Patients with significant heart failure are at increased risk for thromboembolic events, and anti-platelet agents and anti-coagulants should be considered; the risk of bleeding is often increased in cancer patients, and the risk hemorrhage should be considered when the use of these agents is contemplated.

For the rare patient with end-stage heart failure in whom the cancer is cured or in prolonged remission, heart transplantation may be considered; the indications for heart transplantation in cancer patients are gradually becoming broader.[117–119] The stages of heart

TABLE 3-7 Comparison of relative toxicities of different cardiotoxic drugs and dosage schedules

DRUG	SCHEDULE	RELATIVE MYELOSUPPRESSIVE POTENCY OF SINGLE DOSE COMPARED WITH DOXORUBICIN ADMINISTERED BY STANDARD SCHEDULE	APPROXIMATE RELATIVE CARDIOTOXICITY[a]	CARDIOTOXICITY INDEX COMPARED WITH DOXORUBICIN ADMINISTERED BY STANDARD SCHEDULE[b]	RECOMMENDED MAXIMUM DOSE[c] (MG.M²)
Doxorubicin	Rapid infusion	1	1	1	400
Doxorubicin	Weekly	1	0.7	0.7	550
Doxorubicin	24-h infusion	1	0.62	0.62	550
Doxorubicin	48-h infusion	1	0.57	0.57	625[d]
Doxorubicin	96-h infusion	1	0.5	0.5	800–1000[d]
Epirubicin	Rapid infusion	0.67	0.66	0.44	900
Mitoxantrone	Rapid infusion	5	0.5	2.5	160
Daunorubicin	Rapid infusion	0.67	0.75[e]	0.5[e]	800[e]
Idarubicin	Rapid infusion	5	0.53	2.67	150
Pirarubicin	Rapid infusion	1	0.62	0.62	650[e]
Doxorubicin + dexrazoxane	Rapid infusion	1[e]	0.5	0.5[e]	800–1000[e]
Doxorubicin, 300 mg/m² + Dexrazoxane	Rapid infusion	1[e]	0.73[e]	0.73[e]	550[e]

[a]Factor by which the cardiotoxic effects of the cumulative dose of rapid infusion doxorubicin can be compared with the cumulative dose of the agent, combination and schedule listed, when given at an equivalent myelosuppressive dose.

[b]Derived by dividing 400 mg/m², the recommended maximum dose of rapid-infusion doxorubicin, by the recommended maximum dose for the agent in question. The cardiotoxicity index represents a factor by which to multiply the cumulative dose of a drug administered to obtain an approximation of toxicity that might be expected had the resultant amount of doxorubicin been given by rapid infusion. For example, if a cumulative dose of 120 mg/m² mitoxantrone had been administered, the patient would be expected to demonstrate cardiac damage approximately equal to 300 mg/m² of doxorubicin given by rapid infusion (120 × 2.5 = 300). This value is useful when changing from one cardiotoxic regimen to another. When the sum of the products of the indexes and the cumulative doses administered exceeds 400, the risk of clinically significant cardiotoxicity exceeds 5%.

[c]Dose producing clinically significant congestive heart failure in 5% of patients.

[d]Less toxic by endomyocardial biopsy.

[e]Inadequate data.

Source: Ewer M et al. 2017.[172]

failure and the most commonly used therapies are shown in Figure 3-7.[120]

Cardioprotection: The Rationale for Early Cardioprotection

Cardioprotection has two goals. The first goal, which had received a great deal of prior attention, is to allow a larger total cumulative doxorubicin dosage to be given with manageable and acceptable cardiotoxicity; in the modern era excessive anthracycline dosing is unusual. The priority has shifted towards preserving the structural integrity of the heart so that later stresses, both the unavoidable stress of everyday life and the stress of future cardiotoxic interventions, will be better tolerated. The premise that anthracycline toxicity starts with the first exposure is firmly established, and mitigation of this damage forms the basis for cardioprotection. Whatever additional stresses and insults augment the initial damage will be manifested in the form of increased cardiac vulnerability, and it is this end result, perhaps manifested

years later, that cardioprotection is designed to reduce. Of course, further chemotherapy is not the only sequential stress; other insults include viral infections, pregnancy, and non chemotherapeutic toxic exposure (most commonly alcohol) and high-output states that may be related to the malignancy. Cardioprotection spares the myocardium from initial damage, and more normal myocardium can be called upon in response to sequential stresses. Protection provides greater options, without which some later therapeutic strategies become prohibitively risky. The adage that prevention is better than successful treatment is especially relevant for cancer patients treated with anthracyclines. Most patients can undergo some form of cardioprotection; the benefits are significant, and the disadvantages are comparatively small.

Cardioprotection

Five cardioprotection modalities exist that deserve consideration: (1) dose limitation, (2) schedule modification, (3) innovative delivery systems, (4) chemical

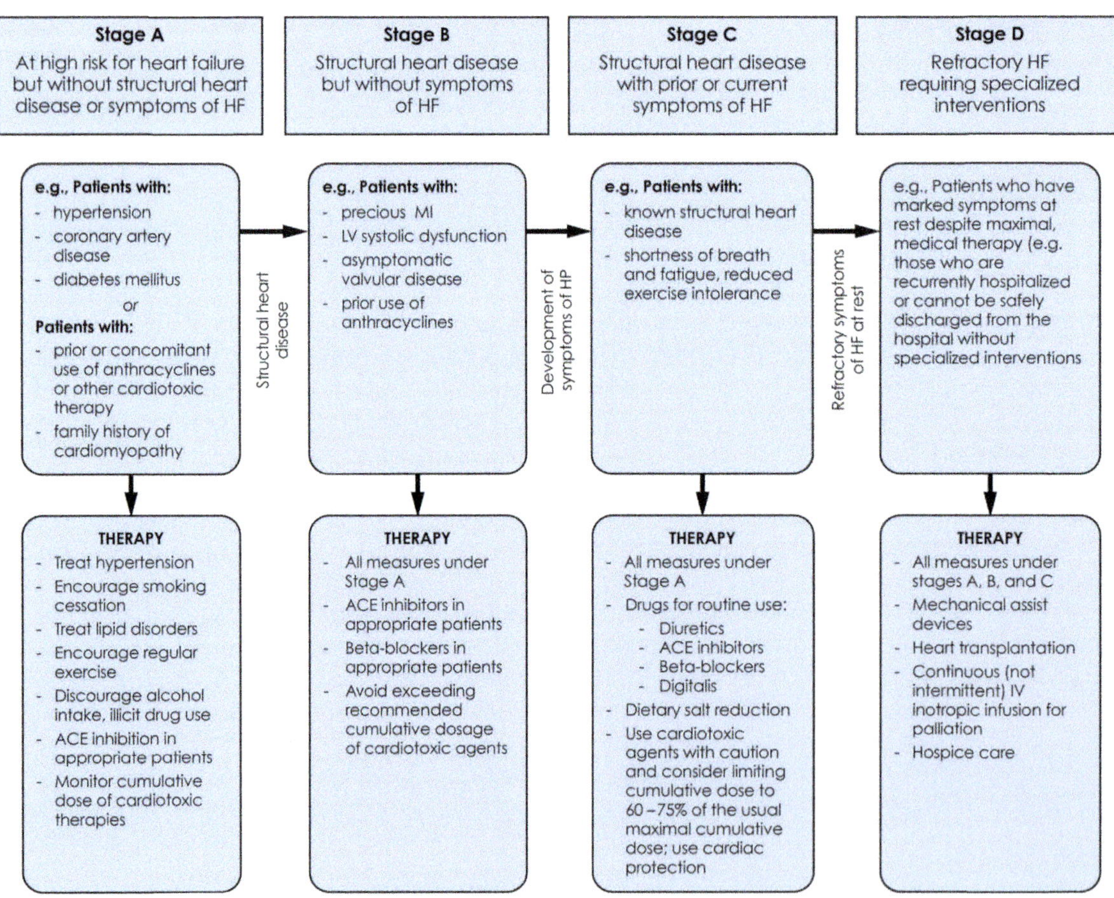

FIGURE 3-7 Stages and suggested management strategies for congestive heart failure. ACE, angiotensin-converting enzyme; ARB, Angiotensin-receptor blocker; IV, intravenous; LV, left ventricle; MI, myocardial infarction. (Adapted and modified from the American College of Cardiology / American Heart Association, 2001.[120])

and pharmacologic cardioprotectors, and (5) use of less toxic doxorubicin analogues.

Dose Limitation ■ Perhaps the simplest strategy for preventing cardiotoxicity is limiting the cumulative dose. As is clear from the cumulative dose-versus-congestive heart failure curve, clinically relevant cardiotoxicity is unusual at dosages below 240–300 mg/m^2 and remains acceptable at what is now considered an intermediate dosage of 300–400 mg/m^2. By maintaining the cumulative dose below these levels, cardiotoxicity remains within the range of <5% for patients who do not have underlying heart disease of risk factors. For patients without risk factors or no cardiac symptoms, a baseline assessment of cardiac reserves is appropriate, but further monitoring is usually not required. Dose limitation may be combined with other strategies, including continuous infusion schedules (see below) and chemical protectors, to treat patients with known risk factors. The disadvantage of this approach is that while cardiotoxicity is unusual, oncologic efficacy may not be optimized. Dose restriction does not allow flexibility with regard to retreatment with potentially cardiotoxic agents in as high a cumulative dose as would be possible with other strategies that actively protect the myocardium rather than merely limiting exposure. Dose limitation is therefore a compromise whereby anticipated, and to some extent predictable, toxicity is balanced against potentially reduced efficacy. In some instances, post-administration cardiac monitoring may be reduced. Notwithstanding these comments, it should be borne in mind that spectrum of toxicity is broad, and these suggestions regarding dose restriction, while reasonable, are not based on prospective trials, hard data, or expert consensus.[26]

Schedule Modification ■ Early and indirect retrospective comparisons revealed that weekly doses of doxorubicin (1/3 of the standard dose administered every week) were considerably less cardiotoxic than were 3-weekly doses.[121] Endomyocardial biopsy assessments of cardiotoxicity demonstrated that an additional 160 mg/m^2 (which is approximately equal to three additional cycles) could be safely given when the drug was administered on a weekly schedule.[122] A direct comparison of the weekly and 3-weekly schedules was undertaken and confirmed these earlier results. The study involved 102 patients with non-small cell lung cancer who were treated with a combination of cyclophosphamide, doxorubicin, and cisplatin and randomly assigned to receive either weekly or 3-weekly doxorubicin. LVEF and endomyocardial biopsy samples were serially evaluated.[122] No significant differences

were found in response rate or survival, although responders treated with weekly doxorubicin experienced a longer response duration. The median dose at which endomyocardial evidence of cardiotoxicity was found was significantly higher for those treated with weekly versus three-weekly doxorubicin. Interestingly, the extent of myelosuppression, alopecia, diarrhea, as well as nausea and vomiting were also reduced with weekly administration.[124] Pharmacologic studies demonstrated that the peak plasma concentration was substantially lower with weekly administration, suggesting that cardiotoxicity may correlate more closely with peak plasma levels, while oncologic efficacy is more closely related to the area under the plasma concentration curve.

It was hypothesized that if the peak plasma level could be reduced further, the likelihood of cardiotoxicity would also be incrementally lower, and this was found to be true. In studies of continuous intravenous infusions of doxorubicin over 48 hours or 72 hours administered every 3 weeks, cardiotoxicity was reduced to the extent that it became difficult to quantitate non-invasively. Ultimately, cardiac biopsies were used to compare these groups and confirmed a substantial decrease in cardiotoxicity. Increased cardioprotection was clearly achieved by longer infusion times. No change in efficacy could be established, and the degree of myelosuppression was not altered. Continuous infusions of doxorubicin administered over 96 hours are even less cardiotoxic, and this is true regardless of whether toxicity is assessed by endomyocardial biopsy or data from pooled cardiac functional studies.[125,126] At cumulative doses of 401–600 mg/m^2 given by rapid infusion (i.e., standard administration), 32% of cardiac biopsies were high-grade (>1.5); however, when the drug was administered as a continuous infusion, the high-grade biopsy rate was reduced to 2%. This was confirmed in a prospective trial in which 82 patients with soft tissue sarcomas (69 evaluable for cardiotoxicity) who were randomly assigned to receive 60 mg/m^2 doxorubicin as a bolus or 72-hour continuous infusion.[127] Cardiotoxicity, defined as a 10% decrease in LVEF, was observed in 61% of rapid infusion patients and occurred at a median cumulative dose of 420 mg/m^2. Only 42% of continuous infusion patients developed cardiotoxicity, and they did so at a median dose of 540 mg/m^2 ($p = 0.0017$). It was not entirely clear whether the two dose schedules were equally effective. A similar decrease in cardiotoxicity was seen with 4-day continuous infusion therapy, and no difference in efficacy was seen in a further randomized trial of 240 patients with soft tissue sarcomas.[128] Extensive experience at MD Anderson Cancer Center and randomized trial evidence strongly suggest that continuous infusion is significantly less cardiotoxic than bolus regimens, at least at the usual dose schedules used for adults, and no loss in oncologic efficacy is observed. The cumulative dose-versus-congestive heart failure curve for rapid infusion, weekly, 48-hour, 72-hour, and 96-hour administrations is depicted in Figure 3-8.[34,129] The limiting factor for infusions beyond 96 is problematic stomatitis. Patients treated with continuous infusions require an in-dwelling central catheters and an infusion pump. Nausea and vomiting have been reported less frequently than when the drug is administered by rapid infusion, and many patients ambulate with their infusion pumps and carry out normal activities and work schedules. Continuous infusion schedules are more expensive than rapid infusions because of the added cost of the infusion pump; the extent of protection is substantial. As shown in Figure 3-8, 96-hour infusions allow about 900 mg/m² of doxorubicin to be given, or about twice the number of cycles for an equivalent level of toxicity that would be expected had the drug been given by standard infusion. The amounts of doxorubicin that can be given in 48-hour and 96-hour infusions are 625 mg/m² and 900 mg/m², respectively (Table 3-7).

Despite dramatic reductions in cardiotoxicity, continuous infusion schedules have not been universally accepted. Many centers find the need for infusion pumps problematic, and some patients prefer to receive their treatment in a single day. Additionally, failure to appreciate the need for cardioprotection from the first exposure to reduce the latter expression of anthracycline toxicity, and failure to consider the advantage of broader future treatment options may impact the use of this cardioprotective strategy. Despite a failure to gain universal acceptance, continuous infusion administration remains among the most successful strategies for reducing cardiotoxicity.

Doxorubicin administered as a continuous infusion has been widely used and studied, but little experience with other anthracyclines given by continuous infusion is available. The benefits of such infusions with other agents, if any, are difficult to determine for a number of reasons: first, the lack of sensitivity and specificity of non-invasive tests make quantification of protection much more difficult than is the case when cardiac ultrastructure is evaluated. In addition, cumulative doses are generally lower now than previously, making subclinical damage harder to identify on non-invasive tests.[130] Given what we know about the structure and metabolism of epirubicin, cardioprotection by continuous infusion administration would be expected to offer some benefit.[131]

Chemical and Pharmacologic Cardioprotectors ■ Several compounds have been studied with the hope that they would be able to mitigate the cardiotoxic properties of anthracyclines. Chemical cardioprotection, as with other strategies to reduce these agents' cardiotoxicity, is based on the premise that the mechanisms that further cardiac damage differ from those of oncologic efficacy. Were this not the case, cardioprotection would come exclusively at the cost of reduced efficacy.[12]

Initial attempts at cardioprotection were based on mechanistic similarities and the similarities in pathologic changes with α-tocopherol (vitamin E) deficiency and doxorubicin cardiotoxicity. Alpha-tocopherol is an important lipid-soluble antioxidant, and it was able to reduce the incidence and severity of the histologic changes observed with doxorubicin cardiotoxicity.[132]

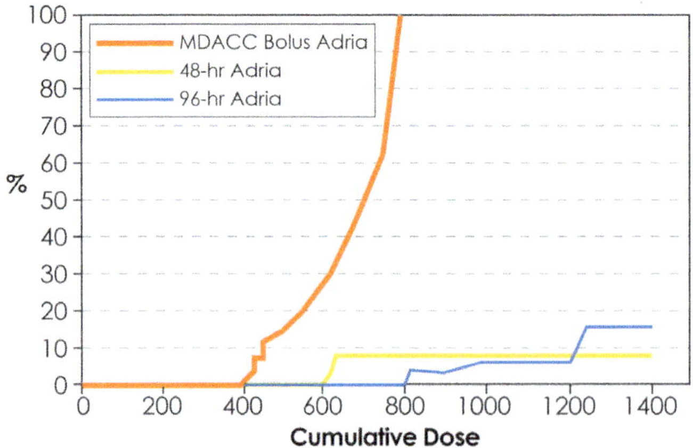

Figure 3-8　Comparison of curves depicting the likelihood of developing congestive heart failure for cumulative doxorubicin dose curves administered by for rapid infusion, 48-hour continuous infusion, and 96-hour infusions. Note that the 96-hour infusion allows about twice the cumulative dose for an equivalent risk of congestive heart failure as dose rapid infusion administration.[34,129]

One of the earlier attempts to protect patients from doxorubicin cardiotoxicity was undertaken by Legha and colleagues, who studied 21 women undergoing combination chemotherapy with 5-fluorouracil, cyclophosphamide, and doxorubicin for metastatic breast cancer and treated with α-tocopherol and evaluated by cardiac biopsy. No significant reduction in toxicity could be demonstrated.[133] Efforts to identify other substances that may selectively reduce the cardiotoxic sequelae of anthracyclines ensued and continue to be explored by several investigators. Among these *N*-acetylcysteine and coenzyme Q10 were studied, but neither entered the clinical armamentarium.[134,135] Other potential cardioprotectors have also been studied.[136]

Dexrazoxane is the one agent that has gained acceptance as a specific cardioprotector in both the United States and Europe. While this agent has a broad pharmacological spectrum (see Table 3-8), its pharmacoprotective quality is of especial interest. Speyer and colleagues performed a randomized controlled clinical trial to determine whether dexrazoxane allows the safe use of doxorubicin at dosages beyond what was previously acceptable.[137,138] Patients who were randomly assigned to receive dexrazoxane underwent two additional cycles of therapy, and 11 of these patients received 1000 mg/m² of doxorubicin without overt cardiotoxicity. Two patients in the dexrazoxane group developed congestive heart failure versus 20 patients in the standard therapy group. Among patients who experienced heart failure, the

extent of the event was considerably lower than that in the non-experimental group. This study also included patients who underwent endomyocardial biopsy at a cumulative dose of 450 mg/m²; in the standard group, 6 of 14 patients had a biopsy grade of 2, whereas in the dexrazoxane group, none of the 16 patients who underwent biopsy had a grade of 2. This study clearly demonstrated the cardioprotection of dexrazoxane, and the response rates were slightly higher in patients who received dexrazoxane (7% vs. 9%).[139]

Two large multicenter, randomized, double-blind, manufacturer-sponsored studies were carried out by Swain and colleagues in metastatic breast cancer patients who had not previously been treated with anthracyclines.[140,141] The objectives were to compare the cardioprotective effectiveness of dexrazoxane with doxorubicin and assess antitumor efficacy as measured by response rate, time to progression, and survival. In both trials, significant cardioprotection was observed among patients in the dexrazoxane arms; however, in the larger trial, the objective response rate was significantly lower in dexrazoxane-treated patients. The conclusions drawn from these trials was that dexrazoxane is cardioprotective, and this was evident for patients who received the drug at the outset of therapy and patients in whom it was started after they had received 300 mg/m² of doxorubicin. Because of the possibility that dexrazoxane interfered with tumor response, the final Food and Drug Administration recommendation was made that dexrazoxane cardioprotection be used "in women with metastatic breast cancer who have received a cumulative doxorubicin dose of 300 mg/m² and who will continue to receive doxorubicin therapy to maintain tumor control."[141]

Knowing what we now know about the cardiotoxicity of anthracyclines, the indication is clearly inappropriate; dexrazoxane is cardioprotective in men, as well as in tumors beyond metastatic breast cancer. As noted above, cardiac damage takes place at the time of administration, and not providing protection until considerable exposure and myocyte damage has already taken place does not maximize cardioprotection. The conclusion that dexrazoxane interferes with oncologic efficacy had not been demonstrated in animal studies or in other clinical trials. Other studies have confirmed the cardioprotective characteristics of dexrazoxane.[143] Dexrazoxane has been used more widely in the pediatric population; there was no effect on event-free survival at 2.5 years in one review, emphasizing that the agent does not detrimentally affect the effectiveness of anthracycline therapy in children.[77]

Dexrazoxane has also been studied in regimens using anthracyclines other than doxorubicin. Trials

TABLE 3-8   Pharmacologic spectrum of dexrazoxane

Pharmacologic spectrum of Dexrazoxane (ICRF-187)
• Prevents spontaneous metastases
• Normalizes tumor neovasculature
• Potentiates radiotherapy
• Potentiates chemotherapy (in both the mouse model and in leukemia patients)
• Blocks cell cycle at G2/M
• Cytoprotective for myocardium, pulmonary epithelium, gastrointestinal tract, and kidney
• Cytoprotective against doxorubicin daunorubicin, bleomycin, mitoxantrone, etoposide, cisplatin
• Does not convert nonresponders to responders, but cytoprotection permits more extensive exploration of the dose-response relationship
• Keeps responders responding

Source: Modified from Hellmann, 1998.[173]

with epirubicin were carried out in breast cancer and sarcoma patients. Dexrazoxane was clearly cardioprotective when given in conjunction with epirubicin.[144,145] Daunorubicin cardioprotection has also been observed. Dexrazoxane has been used to mitigate the injury associated with extravasation of several anthracyclines.[146]

Other pharmacologic strategies for cardioprotection, such as β-adrenergic blockade and angiotensin-converting enzymes, are being studied increasingly in this regard.[30,147,148] While the protective mechanism has not yet been adequately studied, the hypothesis that reducing wall stress at the time of injury is cardioprotective is appealing. Anecdotally, the degree of protection varies, but it is generally less than that achieved by either the use of the more specific cardioprotective agent dexrazoxane or the use of extended, i.e., 48 or 72 hour infusions. Additionally, lowering wall stress and after-load during the post-treatment period is cardioprotective in that it delays or mitigates cardiac remodeling.[149]

Innovative Delivery Systems ■ Liposomal anthracycline formulations are an important option, providing patients with a less cardiotoxic alternative to native doxorubicin. The cardioprotective properties of liposomal doxorubicin have been clearly established and documented in several studies and reviews.[131,150,151] In liposomal preparations cardioprotection is at least partially related to an inhibition of diffusion of the agent from the intravascular space in areas of normal vasculature, as is found in the normal myocardium. Liposomal doxorubicin penetrates vessels more readily in areas of vessel fragility as is encountered in tumors with rapid growth; the liposomal delivery system therefore directs the anthracycline to the tumor and away from the heart.[152]

A wide range of liposomal anthracycline formulations have been evaluated with the goal of improving the therapeutic index of the parent drug. Pegylated liposomal doxorubicin (Doxil®, Janssen, Johnson&Johnson) is the most commonly used preparation in the United States, but liposomal daunorubicin citrate is also available (DaunoXome®, Gilead Science, Inc., San Dimas, CA). Non-pegylated doxorubicin (Myocet®) is approved for use in Canada and Europe. The various liposomal anthracycline preparations are more cardioprotective than is free anthracycline, but these agents should not be considered interchangeable. The differences between pegylated and non-pegylated liposomal doxorubicin include lipid make up, molecular size, plasma concentration, tissue distribution, dosing requirements, and safety profiles.[153] The pharmacokinetics of these agents is sufficiently varied so that they should not be deemed

oncologically equivalent to the native doxorubicin preparation.

Liposomal formulations fall into four general classes on the basis of their physical properties, composition, and drug loading and retention mechanisms. At physiologic PH the primary amino group of doxorubicin is partially protonated and thus positively charged. Class I and II liposomes are formulated to take advantage of the electrostatic binding of doxorubicin to negatively charged phospholipids incorporated into the liposome structure. Class I liposomes contain cardiolipin, and class II liposomes contain phosphatidylserine or phosphatidylglycerol, all naturally occurring negatively charged phospholipids. No class I or class II liposomal formulation is approved for clinical use. Class III liposomal doxorubicin includes non-pegylated liposomal formulations and the agent Myocet. Myocet reduces the peak distribution of the drug to the heart but effectively delivers doxorubicin to tumors.[154] It is usually administered at the same dose and schedule as is free doxorubicin; therefore, it is easier to compare the cardiotoxicity of the two formulations and assess the potential benefit of the liposomal formulation. In animal models, a comparison of the same dose of liposomal doxorubicin and conventional doxorubicin showed that the liposomal formulation was associated with significantly less cardiotoxicity, whereas antitumor efficacy was at least similar to that of the parent molecule. Preclinical studies showed significant cardioprotection, and when used in combination with docetaxel and trastuzumab, non-pegylated liposomal doxorubicin demonstrated acceptable levels of cardiotoxicity.[155–158] Incremental cardioprotection is retained, and this holds true for patients who had previously been treated with conventional doxorubicin prior to their challenge with the liposomal formulation.

Pegylated liposomal doxorubicin is approved in the United States for AIDS-related Kaposi's sarcoma and multiple myeloma and is widely used in Europe to treat metastatic breast cancer and as adjuvant therapy. Cardiac biopsy in a small series of patients with AIDS-related Kaposi's sarcoma who had received pegylated liposomal doxorubicin to cumulative doses of 440–840 mg/m² were evaluated for anthracycline damage and compared with historical controls of patients who had received cumulative doses of 174–671 mg/m² of un-encapsulated doxorubicin. Pegylated liposomal doxorubicin patients had significantly lower biopsy scores than did doxorubicin controls, despite higher achieved cumulative doses of the anthracycline.[36]

Cardiotoxicity resulting from pegylated liposomal doxorubicin was compared with that from free doxorubicin in 509 metastatic breast cancer patients who were randomly assigned to receive pegylated liposomal doxorubicin (50 mg/m² every 4 weeks or doxorubicin 60 mg/m² every 3 weeks). Eighty-five percent of patients had never undergone anthracycline-based therapy. There were no significant differences in the disease-free or overall survival among patients treated with pegylated liposomal doxorubicin and those treated with conventional doxorubicin. Sixteen percent of pegylated liposomal doxorubicin-treated patients continued treatment for more than 9 months compared with only 1% of doxorubicin patients. It is somewhat difficult to make strong conclusions because of differences in the total dose of doxorubicin received (higher in the group that received conventional doxorubicin). Nevertheless, the likelihood of experiencing a cardiac event was three times higher in the doxorubicin arm, implying significantly more tolerance of pegylated liposomal doxorubicin over time with less cardiotoxicity than when conventional doxorubicin was administered.[159] A second randomized trial directly comparing pegylated liposomal doxorubicin with conventional doxorubicin was discontinued early because of excessive cardiotoxicity in the doxorubicin arm.[158,159] Patients received 30 mg/m² of pegylated liposomal doxorubicin or 60 mg/m² of free doxorubicin every three weeks. Each drug was administered in combination with 200 mg/m² of paclitaxel over 1 hour. Thirteen patients were randomly assigned to receive pegylated liposomal doxorubicin with paclitaxel and 10 received conventional doxorubicin with paclitaxel. None of the patients had been treated for metastatic breast cancer or had received prior anthracycline exposure. The overall response rates to the regimens were 69% and 70%. However, cardiotoxicity developed in 6 of the 10 patients given doxorubicin but in none of the patients who received pegylated liposomal doxorubicin.

Available preclinical and clinical data strongly suggest that liposomal doxorubicin reduces the incidence and severity of cumulative dose-related cardiomyopathy associated with conventional anthracycline administration while preserving oncologic efficacy. The degree of cardioprotection (see Table 3-7) suggests that approximately twice the number of cycles of pegylated liposomal doxorubicin results in a similar level of cardiotoxicity to that of the parent compound. In one study, 646 multiple myeloma patients were randomly assigned to receive bortezomid, with or without pegylated liposomal doxorubicin, after being treated with 240 mg/m² of doxorubicin; no difference was noted in the incidence of cardiac events between the two groups.[161] In subsequent phase III study of breast cancer patients, no patients who had received an end-of-treatment cumulative anthracycline dose of 500 mg/ m² or more experienced heart failure. Other formulations may offer different levels of cardioprotection.[162]

■ Special Considerations Regarding Anthracycline Formulations other than Doxorubicin and with Anthracenediones

Doxorubicin remains the most commonly used anthracycline in much of the world. Our knowledge of anthracyclines' cardiac damage mechanisms, myocyte death, functional tests, structural abnormalities, treatment, and surveillance was largely derived from doxorubicin studies. Nevertheless, several other anthracyclines are in common use and should be discussed individually.

Alternate formulations are similar to the parent compound but differ in structure and pharmacodynamics. Therefore, different anthracycline preparations should not be considered entirely interchangeable but as drugs in a single class that share common characteristics. Cardiotoxicity, albeit with considerable variation, is common to all anthracyclines in current use. As shown in Table 3-7, doxorubicin is considered the agent against which cardiotoxicity is compared; this is not a reflection of its potential for increased cardiotoxicity but merely a convenience because so much of the basic and clinical research has been carried out on that agent.

Daunorubicin ■ Daunorubicin (Cerubidine®) is used to treat some forms of leukemia as well as neuroblastoma. Its cardiotoxicity, like that all of anthracyclines, is of the Type I form; the degree of cardiotoxic expression is thought to be less than that of doxorubicin but more than that of epirubicin and idarubicin (see Table 3-7). The recommended maximal cumulative dosage is approximately 800 mg/m²; however, the data on which this is based are not nearly as rigorous as it is for doxorubicin. Considerations related to monitoring and treatment are similar to those suggested above for doxorubicin; dexrazoxane is cardioprotective and that agent may be used to reduce the morbidity associated with extravasation as well.

IDARUBICIN ■ Idarubicin is the 4-demethoxyanthracycline analogue of daunorubicin; it is distributed in Britain and Australia under the trade name Zavedos® and is marketed in the United States as Idamycin®. Idarubicin is used to treat acute myeloid leukemia but has also been used to treat advanced breast cancer, lymphoma, and myelodysplastic syndrome. It exhibits Type I cardiotoxicity, in that the cardiac damage is cumulative dose related. When equivalent myelosuppressive dosages are compared, the agent is less cardiotoxic than doxorubicin.[163,164] Cumulative dosages of more than 150 mg/m^2 are associated with a higher risk of cardiotoxicity; additional information regarding its relative toxicity is provided in Table 3-7. Dexrazoxane provides cardioprotection and is effective in the management of extravasation.

Epirubicin ■ Epirubicin is the 4-prime epimer of doxorubicin. The structural difference is shown in Figure 3-1. Its spectrum of oncologic efficacy is similar to that of doxorubicin, and it is used widely to treat breast cancer, primarily because of its reduced cardiotoxic profile. It is also used to treat lymphoma. Compared with doxorubicin, epirubicin has a higher clearance, shorter terminal half-life, and larger distribution volume.[165]

Direct comparisons of toxicity between doxorubicin and epirubicin are problematic in that they must be made using oncologically equivalent dosages; when expressed in milligrams per meter squared, epirubicin requires a dosage that is approximately 1/3 higher to achieve the same degree of myelosuppression. More meaningful direct comparisons of efficacy, such as time to survival, are much more difficult to quantitate, and similar myelosuppression levels are an achievable compromise. The epirubicin dose per cycle is therefore often 1/3 higher, and even when taking this dosage into account, the likelihood of cardiotoxicity is sufficiently reduced to allow 2–4 additional cycles of chemotherapy to be administered. From the perspective of cardiotoxicity, the mean maximally tolerated cumulative dosage of epirubicin is about 900 mg/m^2, oncologically equivalent to approximately 600 mg/m^2 of doxorubicin, and about 3–4 cycles higher. Modern regimens usually do not require such high anthracyclines doses, but the inherent residual cardiac damage after any number of cycles of epirubicin is thought to be lower than that for oncologically equivalent cumulative doses of doxorubicin; lower toxicity, although not clearly confirmed in the Cochrane Database, has nevertheless been suggested.[131,166]

Epirubicin is frequently used in combination with other agents, and its cardiac-sparing characteristic is maintained; use with paclitaxel results in a lower level of toxicity than does parent compound.[167] Epirubicin cardiotoxicity, analogous to that of doxorubicin, is mitigated by dexrazoxane use. The risk factors for epirubicin cardiotoxicity, cardiac function monitoring, and cardiotoxicity treatment are similar to those described for doxorubicin.

Mitoxantrone and Pixantrone ■ Mitoxantrone is an anthracenedione but not an anthracycline. It is an anti-cancer antibiotic that disrupts DNA and RNA replication; the drug has a narrower spectrum of antineoplastic activity than does doxorubicin. On a milligram-to-milligram basis, mitoxantrone is much more cardiotoxic than doxorubicin, but it is less toxic at equivalent myelosuppressive dosages. It shares the cardiotoxic characteristics of the other Type I treatment-related agents: it demonstrates the biopsy changes associated with anthracyclines and it is cumulative dose related and irreversible on a cellular basis (see Table 3-7). The mechanism of its decreased cardiotoxicity had been thought to be related to its reduced ability to generate oxygen-free radicals, but the results of recent animal studies suggest that mitoxantrone enhances Ca2+ release from the sarcoplasmic reticulum, with apparent enhancement of function. As anthracyclines suppress this function, mitoxantrone may be less cardiotoxic on the basis of enhanced Ca2+ release as well.[168,169] When used sequentially in patients who have undergone prior chemotherapy with an anthracycline, the total cumulative dose of mitoxantrone must be reduced in the manner described for other Type I agents (see above).

Pixantrone is an anthracenedione approved for use in Europe for the treatment of refractory or relapsed non-Hodgkin lymphoma. At the time of this writing the agent is not approved by the U.S. Food and Drug Administration.[3] Pixantrone appears to be an agent with less Type I cardiotoxicity than would be anticipated with doxorubicin.[170]

SUMMARY

Anthracycline-induced cardiotoxicity varies considerably in presentation. The usual measures of systolic function are only useful when the cardiomyopathic process has impaired cardiac function to the extent that real functional decreases in systolic function are not lost in the uncertainties of false-positive and false-negative results of imperfect non-invasive tests.[174] Cardiac damage, as detected by biopsy, occurs earlier than was appreciated initially, and begins with the first administration of the drug. Cardioprotection, therefore, would be helpful if started at the onset of doxorubicin exposure. Finally, as treatment options for heart failure do not replace destroyed myocardial cells, damage prevention is more important than symptom control, and should be a priority for all patients. Prevention is especially important for patients who may need further anti-cancer treatment in the future.

REFERENCES

1. Booser DJ, Hortobagyi GN. Anthracycline antibiotics in cancer therapy: Focus on drug resistance. *Drugs*. 1994;47(2):223–258. doi:10.2165/00003495-199447020-00002

2. Longo M, Della Torre P, Allievi C, et al. Tolerability and toxicological profile of pixantrone (Pixuvri®) in juvenile mice: comparative study with doxorubicin. *Reprod Toxicol*. 2014;46:20–30.

3. Minotti G, Menna P, Salvatorelli E. Do you know Pixantrone? *Chemotherapy*. 2017;62:192–193.

4. Chairs J. *Biophysical chemistry of the daunomycin-DNA interaction. Biophys Chem*. 1990;35:191–202.

5. Gómez HL, Pinto JA, Olivera M, et al. Topoisomerase II-alpha as a predictive factor of response to therapy with anthracyclines in locally advanced breast cancer. *Breast*. 2011;20:39–45.

6. Tritton TR. Immobilized doxorubicin: a tool for separating cell surface from intracellular drug mechanism. *Fed Proc*. 1983;42:184–289.

7. Ewer M, Lippman S. Type II chemotherapy-related cardiac dysfunction: time to recognize a new entity. *J Clin Oncol*. 2005;23:2900–2902.

8. Gianni L, Meyers C. The role of free radical formation in the cardiotoxicity of anthracycline. In: Muggia F, Green M, Speyer J, eds. *Cancer Treatment and the Heart*. Baltimore, MD, The Johns Hopkins University Press; 1992.

9. Sinka BK. Free radicals in anticancer drug pharmacology. *Chem Biol*. 1989;69:293–317.

10. Doroshow JH, Akman S, Chu FF, et al. Role of glutathione-glutathione peroxidase cycle in the Cytotoxicity of the anticancer quinones. *Pharmacol Ther*. 1990;47:359–370.

11. Doroshow J. Doxorubicin-induced cardiac toxicity. *N Engl J Med*. 1991;324:843–845.

12. Veipongsa P, Yeh ET. Topoisomerase 2β: a promising molecular target for primary prevention of anthracycline-induced cardiotoxicity. *Clin Pharmacol Ther*. 2014;95:45–52.

13. Ewer M, Ewer S. Cardiotoxicity of anticancer treatments: what the cardiologist needs to know. *Nat Rev Cardiol*. 2010;7:564–575.

14. Von Hoff D, Rozencweig M, Layard M, Slavik M, Muggia FM. Daunomycin induced cardiotoxicity in children and adults: a review of 110 cases. *Am J Med*. 1997;62:200–208.

15. Von Hoff D, Layard M, Basa P, et al. Risk factors for doxorubicin-induced congestive heart failure. *Ann Intern Med*. 1979;91:710–717.

16. Swain S, Whaley F, Ewer M. Congestive heart failure in patients treated with doxorubicin: a retrospective analysis of three trials. *Cancer*. 2003;97:2869–2879.

17. Mihalcea DJ, Florescu M, Vinereanu D. Mechanisms and genetic susceptibility of chemotherapy-induced cardiotoxicity in patients with breast cancer. *Am J Ther*. 2017;24:e3–e11.

18. Minow R, Benjamin R, Lee E, et al. Adriamycin cardiomyopathy - risk factors. *Cancer*. 1977;39:1397–1402.

19. Curigliano G, Mayer EL, Burstein HJ, Winer EP, Goldhirsch A. Cardiac toxicity from systemic cancer therapy: a comprehensive review. *Prog Cardiovasc Dis*. 2010;53:94–104.

20. Cortes E, Gupta M, Chou C, et al. Adriamycin cardiotoxicity: Early detection by systolic time interval and possible prevention by coenzyme Q10. *Cancer Treat Rep*. 1978;62:887–891.

21. Ali M, Soto A, Maroongroge D, et al. Electrocardiographic changes after Adriamycin chemotherapy. *Cancer*. 1979;43:465–471.

22. Ewer M, Ali M, Gibbs H, et al. Cardiac diastolic function in pediatric patients receiving doxorubicin. *Acta Oncol*. 1994;33:645–649.

23. Stoddard M, Seeger J, Liddell N, et al. Prolongation of isovolumetric relaxation time as assessed by Doppler echocardiography predicts doxorubicin-induced systolic dysfunction in humans. *J Am Coll Cardiol*, 1992;20:62–69.

24. Ewer M. Exercise echocardiography reflects cumulative anthracycline exposure during childhood. *Pediatr Blood Cancer*. 2004;42:554–555.

25. Hauser M, Gibson B, Wilson N. Diagnosis of anthracycline-induced late cardiomyopathy by exercise-spiroergometry and stress echocardiography. *Eur J Pediatr*. 2001;160:601–610.

26. Armenian SH, Lacchetti C, Barac A, et al. Prevention and monitoring of cardiac dysfunction in survivors of adult cancers: American society of clinical oncology clinical practice guideline. *J Clin Oncol*. 2017;35:893–911.

27. Jassal DS, Han SY, Hans C, et al. Utility of tissue Doppler and strain rate imaging in the early detection of trastuzumab and anthracycline mediated cardiomyopathy. *J Am Soc Echocardiogr*. 2009;22:418–424.

28. Walker J, Bhullar N, Fallah-Rad N, et al. The role of 3D echocardiography in breast cancer: comparison with 2D echocardiography, MUGA and cardiac MRI. *J Clin Oncol*. 2010;28:3429–3436.

29. Cardinale A, Sandri M, Martinoni A, et al. Myocardial injury revealed by plasma troponin I in breast cancer treated with high-dose chemotherapy. *Ann Oncol*. 2002;13:710–715.

30. Cardinale D, Colombo A, Lamantia G, et al. Anthracycline-induced cardiomyopathy: clinical relevance and response to pharmacologic therapy. *J Am Coll Cardiol*. 2010;55:213–220.

31. Cardinale D, Colombo A, Torrisi R, et al. Trastuzumab-induced cardiotoxicity: clinical and prognostic implication of troponin I elevation. *J Clin Oncol*. 2010;28:3910–3916.

32. Ewer M, Ewer S. Troponin I provides insight into cardiotoxicity and the anthracycline-trastuzumab interaction. *J Clin Oncol*. 2010;25:3901–3904.

33. Ewer MS, von Hoff DD, Benjamin RS. A historical perspective of anthracycline cardiotoxicity. *Heart Fail Clin*. 2011;3:363–372.

34. Legha S, Benjamin R, Mackay B, et al. Reduction of doxorubicin cardiotoxicity by prolonged continuous intravenous infusion. *Ann Intern Med*. 1982;96:133–139.

35. Ewer M, Ali M, Mackay B, et al. A comparison of cardiac biopsy grades and ejection fraction estimations in patients receiving Adriamycin. *J Clin Oncol*. 1984;2:112–117.

36. Berry G, Billingham M, Alderman E, et al. The use of cardiac biopsy to demonstrate reduced cardiotoxicity in AIDS Kaposi's sarcoma patients treated with pegylated liposomal doxorubicin. *Ann Oncol*. 1998;9:711–716.

37. Ewer M, Ali M. Cardiac biopsy: a review of the procedure, complications and indications. *Prac Cardiol*. 1981;7:143–154.

38. Swain S, Whaley F, Gerber M, et al. Congestive heart failure after doxorubicin containing therapy in advanced breast cancer patients treated with or without dexrazoxane. *Proc Am Soc Clin Oncol*. 1996;15:A536.

39. Gianni L, Corden B, Myers C. The biochemical basis of anthracycline toxicity and antitumor activity. In: Hodgson E, Bend J, Philport R, eds. *Reviews in biochemical toxicology*. Amsterdam, The Netherlands: Elsevier; 1983:1–82.

40. Falcon G, Filippelli W, Mazzarella B, et al. Cardiotoxicity of doxorubicin: effects of 21-aminosteroids. *Life Sci*. 1998;63:1525–1532.

41. Andrieu-Abadie N, Jaffrezou J, Hatem S, et al. L-carnitine prevents doxorubicin-induced apoptosis of cardiac myocytes: role of inhibition of cermide generation. *Faseb J*. 1999;13:1501–1510.

42. Doroshow J. Effect of anthracycline antibiotics on oxygen radical formation in rat heart. *Cancer Res*. 1983;43:460–472.

43. Doroshow J, Locker G, Myers C. Enzymatic defenses of the mouse heart against reactive oxygen metabolites: Alterations produced by doxorubicin. *J Clin Invest*. 1980;65:128–135.

44. Zhang Y, Shi J, Li Y, et al. Cardiomyocyte death in doxorubicin-induced cardiotoxicity. *Arch Immunol Ther Exp*. 2009;57:435–445.

45. Simunek T, Sterba M, Popelova O, et al. Anthracycline-induced cardiotoxicity: overview of studies examining the roles of oxidative stress and free cellular iron. *Pharmacol Rep*. 2009;61:154–171.

46. Hasinoff BB. Chemistry of dexrazoxane and analogues. *Sem Oncol*. 1998;25:3–9.

47. Hasinoff B. Inhibition and inactivation of NADH-cytochrome c reductase activity of bovine heart submitochondrial particles by the iron (III)-adriamycin. *Biochem J*. 1990;265:865–870.

48. Hershko C, Pinson A, Link G. Prevention of anthracycline cardiotoxicity by iron chelation. *Acta Haematol*. 1996;95:87–92.

49. Link G, Tirosh R, Pinson A, et al. Role of iron in the potentiation of anthracycline cardiotoxicity: indentification of heart cell mitochondria as a major site of iron-anthracycline interaction. *J Lab Clin Med*. 1996;127:272–278.

50. Gille L, Nohl H. Analysis of the molecular mechanism of adriamycin-induced cardiotoxicity. *Free Radic Biol Med*. 1997;23:775–782.

51. Herman E, Zang J, Hasinoff B, et al. Comparison of the protective effects against chronic doxorubicin cardiotoxicity and the rates of iron (III) displacement reactions of ICRF-187 and other bisdiketopiperazines. *Cancer Chemother Pharmacol*. 1997;40:400–408.

52. Al-Nasser I. In vivio prevention of adriamycin cardio toxicity by cyclosporin A or FK506. *Toxicology*. 1998;131:175–181.

53. Serrano J, Palmeira C, Kuehl D, et al. Cardioselective and cumulative oxidation of mitochondrial DNA following subchronic doxorubicin administration. *Biochim Biophys Acta*. 1999;1411:201–205.

54. Du, Q, Zhu B, Zhai Q, Yu B. Sirt3 attenuates doxorubicin-induced cardiac hypertrophy and mitochondrial dysfunction via suppression of Bnip3. *Am J Transl Res*. 2017;9:3360–3373.

55. Maeda A, Honda M, Kuramochi T, et al. Doxorubicin cardiotoxicity: diastolic cardiac myocyte dysfunction as a result of impaired calcium handling in isolated cardiac myocytes. *Jpn Circ J*. 1998;62:505–511.

56. Bordoni A, Biagi P, Hrelia S. The impairment of essential fatty acid metabolism as a key factor in doxorubicin-induced damage in cultured rat cardiomyocytes. *Biochem Biophys Acta*. 1999;1440:100–106.

57. Olson R, Mushlin P, Brenner D, et al. Doxorubicin cardiotoxicity may be caused by its metabolite, doxorubicinol. *Proc Natl Acad Sci USA*. 1988;85:3585–3589.

58. Minotti G, Ronchi R, Salvatorelli E, et al. Doxorubicin irreversibly inactivates iron regulatory proteins 1 and 2 in cardiomyocytes: evidence for distinct metabolic pathways and implications for iron-medicated cardiotoxicity of antitumor therapy. *Cancer Res*. 2001;61:8422–8428.

59. Lemez P, Maresova J. Efficacy of dexrazoxane as a cardioprotective agent in patients receiving mitoxantrone-and daunorubicin-based chemotherapy. *Semin Oncol*. 1998;4(suppl 10):61–65.

60. Singal P, Iliskovic N. Doxorubicin-induced cardiomyopathy. *N Engl Med*. 1998;339:900–905.

61. Ali M, Ewer M. *Cancer and the Cardiopulmonary System*. New York, NY: Raven Press; 1984.

62. Bristow M, Mason J, Billingham M, et al. Doxorubicin cardiomyopathy: evaluation by phonocardiography, endomyocardial biopsy, and cardiac catheterization. *Ann Intern Med*. 1978;88:168–175.

63. Lefrak E, Pitha J, Rosenheim S, et al. A clinicopathologic analysis of adriamycin cardiotoxicity. *Cancer*. 1973;32:302–314.

64. Bristow M, Thompson P, Martin R, et al. Early anthracycline cardiotoxicity. *Am J Med*. 1978;65:823–832.

65. Signori E, Guevarra D. Evaluation of cardiac arrhythmias by 24-hour halter monitoring during adriamycin administration (abst). *Proc Am Assoc Cancer Res*. 1981;22:355.

66. Wortman J, Lucas V, Schuster E, et al. Sudden death during doxorubicin administration. *Cancer*. 1979;44:1588–1591.

67. Cardinale D, Biasillo G, Salvatici M, Sandri MT, Cipolla CM. Using biomarkers to predict and to prevent cardiotoxicity of cancer therapy. *Expert Rev Mol Diang.* 2017;17:245–256.

68. Ewer M, Benjamin R. Formulae for predicting the likelihood of developing congestive heart failure following anthracycline chemotherapy: added evidence for early cardiotoxicity. *J Card Fail.* 2005;11:S159. Abstract No. 259.

69. Frei EI. Clinical cancer research: an embattled species. *Cancer.* 1982;50:1979–1982.

70. Ibrahim NK, Hortobagyi GN, Ewer M, et al. Doxorubicin-induced congestive heart failure in elderly patients with metastatic breast cancer, with long-term follow-up: the M.D. Anderson experience. *Cancer Chemother Pharmacol,* 1999;43:471–478.

71. Ewer M, Lenihan D. Left ventricular ejection fraction and cardiotoxicity: is our ear really to the ground? *J Clin Oncol.* 2008;26:1201–1203.

72. Ewer SM, Ewer MS. Cardiotoxicity profile of Trastuzumab. *Drug Saf.* 2008;31:459–467.

73. Ewer S, Ewer M. Anthracycline cardiotoxicity: why are we still interested? *Oncology.* 2009;23:234–235, 239.

74. Ewer MS, Ewer SM. Cardiotoxicity of anticancer treatments. *Nat Rev Cardiol.* 2015;11:620.

75. Ewer M, Gibbs H, Swafford J, et al. Cardiotoxicity in patients receiving trastuzumab (Herceptin): primary toxicity, synergistic or sequential stress, or surveillance artifact? *Semin Oncol.* 1999;26:96–101.

76. Ewer M, Jaffe N, Ried H, et al. Doxorubicin cardiotoxicity in children: comparison of a consecutive divided daily dose administration schedule with single dose (rapid) infusion administration. *Med Pediatr Oncol.* 1998;31:512–515.

77. Lipshultz S, Colan S, Silverman L, et al. Dexrazoxane reduces incidence of doshurxorubicin-associated acute myocardiocyte injury in children with acute lymphoblastic leukemia (ALL.). Proceedings of ASCO; 2002.

78. Lipshultz S, Colan S, Gelber R. Late cardiac effects of doxorubicin therapy for acute lymphoblastic leukemia in childhood. *N Engl J Med.* 1991;324:808–815.

79. Steinherz L, Graham T, Hurwitz R, et al. Guidelines for cardiac monitoring of children during and after anthracycline therapy: report of the cardiology committee of the children's cancer study group. *Pediatrics.* 1992;89:942–949.

80. Mavrogeni S, Koutsogeorgopoulou L, Markousis-Mavrogenis G, et al. Cardiovascular magnetic resonance detects silent heart disease missed by echocardiography in systemic lupus erythematosus. *Lupus.* 2018;27:564–571. doi:10.1177/0961203317731533

81. Petek BJ, Greenman C, Herrmann J, Ewer MS, Jones RL. Cardio-oncology: an ongoing evolution. *Future Oncol.* 2015;11:2059–2066.

82. Herson J. Data and safety monitoring committees in clinical trials. 2nd ed. *Chapman and Hall/CRC (Biostatistics series);* Boca Raton, FL: CRC Press; December 19, 2016:1–191.

83. Higgins C, Holt W, Pflugfelde P, et al. Functional evaluation of the heart with magnetic resonance imaging. *Magn Res Med.* 1988;6:121–139.

84. Jacobson H. Council of scientific affairs of the American medical association: magnetic resonance of the cardiovascular system. *JAMA.* 1988;259:253–259.

85. Ritchie J, Bateman T, Bonow R. Guidelines for clinical use of cardiac radionuclide imaging. Report of the American college of cardiology/American heart association task force on assessment of diagnostic and therapeutic cardiovascular procedures (Committee on radionuclide imaging), developed in association with the American society of nuclear cardiology. *J Am Coll Cardiol.* 1995;25:521–547.

86. Carrio I, Estorch M, Berna L, et al. Assessment of anthracycline-induced myocardial damage by quantitative indium 111 myosin-specific monoclonal antibody studies. *Eur J Nucl Med.* 1991;18:806–812.

87. Dymond D, Elliot A, Stone D. Factors that affect the reproducibility of measurements of left ventricular function from first-pass radionuclide ventriculograms. *Circulation.* 1982;65:311–322.

88. Clements IP, Davis BJ, Wiseman GA. Systolic and diastolic cardiac dysfunction early after the initiation of doxorubicin therapy: significance of gender and concurrent mediastinal radiation. *Nucl Med Commun.* 2002;23:521–527.

89. Radulescu D, Pripon S, Radulescu L, et al. Left ventricular diastolic performance in breast cancer survivors threated with anthracyclines. *Acta Cardiol.* 2008;63:27–32.

90. Cardinale D, Sandri MT, Colombo A, et al. Prognostic value of troponin I in cardiac risk stratification of cancer patients undergoing high-dose chemotherapy. *Circulation.* 2004;109:2749–2754.

91. Herman E, Lipshultz S, Rifai N, et al. Use of cardiac troponin T levels as an indicator of doxorubicin-induced cardiotoxicity. *Can Res.* 1998;38:195–197.

92. Okumura H, Iuchi K, Yoshida T, et al. Brain natriuretic peptide is a predictor of anthracycline-induced cardiotoxicity. *Acta Haematol.* 2000;104:158–163.

93. Billingham M, Bristow M. Endomyocardial biopsy findings in Adriamycin-treated patients. *Proc Am Soc Clin Oncol.* 1976;17:281(Abstr).

94. Sakakibara S, Konno S. Endomyocardial biopsy. *Japan Heart J.* 1962;3:537–543.

95. Mason J. Techniques for right and left ventricular endomyocardial biopsy. *Am J Cardiol.* 1978;41: 887–892.

96. Billingham M, Bristow M. Evaluation of anthracycline cardiotoxicity: predictive ability and functional correlation of endomyocardial biopsy. *Cancer Treat Symp.* 1984;3:71–76.

97. Ewer M, Carrasco C, MacKay B, et al. Cardiac biopsy procedures at a cancer center. *Proc Am Soc Clin Oncol.* 1991;336.

98. Mackay B, Keyes LM, Benjamin RS, et al. Texas society for electron microscopy. *Cardiac Biopsy.* 1981;11: 7–15.

99. Mackay B, Ewer M, Carrasco C, et al. Assessment of anthracycline cardiomyopathy by endomyocardial biopsy. *Ultrastructural Pathology*. 1994;18:203–211.

100. Ewer MS, Ewer SM. Cardiac complications. In: Holland-Frei E, ed. *Cancer Medicine*. 9th ed. Hoboken, NJ: Wiley Blackwell, 2017:1774.

101. Swain S. Adult multicenter trials using dexrazoxane to protect against cardiac toxicity. *Sem Oncol*. 1998;25:43–47.

102. Ewer MS, Vooletich MT, Durand JB, et al. Reversibility of trastuzumab-associated cardiotoxicity: new insights based on clinical course and response to medical treatment. *J Clin Oncol*. 2005;23:7820–7826.

103. Hershman D, McBride R, Eisenberger A, et al. Doxorubicin, cardiac risk factors, and cardiac toxicity in elderly patients with diffuse B-cell non-Hodgkin's lymphoma. *J Clin Oncol*. 2008;26:3159–3165.

104. Myrehaug S, Pintilie M, Tsang R, et al. Cardiac morbidity following modern treatment for Hodgkin lymphoma: supra-additive cardiotoxicity of doxorubicin and radiation therapy. *Leuk Lymphoma*. 2008;49:1486–1493.

105. Guldner L, Haddy N, Pein F, et al. Radiation dose and long term risk of cardiac pathology following radiotherapy and anthracyclin for a childhood cancer. *Radiother Oncol*. 2006;81:47–56.

106. Stewart JR, Fajardo LF. Radiation-induced heart disease: an update. *Prog Cardiovasc Dis*. 1984;27:173–194.

107. Renzi R, Straus K, Glatstein E. Radiation-induced myocardial disease. In: Muggia F, Green M, Speyer J, eds. *Cancer Treatment and the Heart*. Baltimore, MD, The Johns Hopkins University Press; 1992:289–295.

108. Gottdiener J, Appelbaum F, Ferrans V, et al. Cardiotoxicity associated with high dose cyclophosphamide therapy. *Arch Intern Med*. 1981;141:758–763.

109. Veipongsa P, Yeh ET. Prevention of anthracycline-induced cardiotoxicity: challenges and opportunities. *J Am Coll Cardiol*. 2014;64:938–945.

110. Minotti G, Salvatorelli E, Menna P. Pharmacological foundations of cardio-oncology. *J Pharmacol Exp Ther*. 2010;334:2–8.

111. Yancy CW, Jessup M, Bozkurt B, et al. ACCF/AHA guideline for the management of heart failure: a report of the American college of cardiology foundation/American heart association task force on practice guidelines. *J Am Coll Cardiol*. 2013.

112. Lindenfeld J, Alber NM, Boehmer JP, et al. For the Heart Failure Society of America Executive summary HFSA 2010 comprehensive heart failure practice guideline. *J Card Fail*. 2010;16:e1–194.

113. Dickstein K, Choen-Solal A, Filippatos G, et al. for the task force for the diagnosis and treatment of acute and chronic heart failure 2008 of the European Society of Cardiology. *Eur Heart J*. 2008;29:2388–2442.

114. Keefe DL. Anthracycline-induced cardiomyopathy. *Semin Oncol*. 2001;28:2–7.

115. Swedbert K, Komajda M, Bohm M, et al. Ivabradine and outcomes in chronic heart failure (SHIFT): a randomized placebo-controlled study. *Lancet*. 2010;376(9744):875–885.

116. Rickard J, Kumbhani D, Baranowski B, et al. Usefulness of cardiac resynchronization therapy in patients with Adriamycin-induced cardiomyopathy. *Am J Cardiol*. 2010;105:522–526.

117. Armitage JM, Kormor R, Griffith B, et al. Heart transplantation in patients with malignant disease. *J Heart Transplant*. 1990;9:627–629.

118. Christiansen S. Surgical treatment of doxorubicin-induced heart failure. *Thorac Cardiovasc Surg*. 2010;58:8–10.

119. Urbanova D, Bubanska E, Hrebik M, et al. Heart transplant in a childhood leukemia survivor: a case report. *Exp Clin Transplant*. 2010;8:79–81.

120. Hunt S, Baker D, Chin M, et al. ACC/AHA guidelines for the evaluation and management of chronic heart failure in the adult: executive summary: a report of the American College of Cardiology/American Heart Association Task Force on Practice Guidelines (Committee to revise the 1995 guidelines for the evaluation and management of heart failure). *J Am Coll Cardiol*. 2001;38:2101–2113.

121. Torti F. *Weekly Adriamycin*. Columbus, OH: Adria Labs; 1985.

122. Lum B, Svec J, Torti F. Doxorubicin: alteration of dose scheduling as a means of reducing cardiotoxicity. *Drug Intel Clin Pharm*. 1985;19:259–264.

123. Umsawasdi T, Valdivieso M, Booser D, et al. Weekly doxorubicin versus doxorubicin every 3 weeks in cyclophosphamide, doxorubicin, and cisplatin chemotherapy for non-small cell lung cancer. *Cancer*. 1989;64:1995–2000.

124. Valdivieso M, Burgess M, Ewer M, et al. Increased therapeutic index of weekly doxorubicin in the therapy of non-small cell lung cancer: a prospective randomized study. *J Clin Oncol*, 1984;2:207–214.

125. Legha S, Benjamin R, Ewer M, et al. Continuous intravenous infuison of adriamcyin. *Evaluation of its efficacy and toxicity*. In: Ogawa M, Muggia F, Rozencweig M, eds. *Adriamycin. It's Expanding Role in Cancer Treatment*. Amsterdam, The Netherlands: Excerpta Medica; 1984:378–386.

126. Benjamin R, Chawla S, Ewer M. Adriamycin cardiac toxicity - An assessment of approaches to cardiac monitoring and cardioprotection. In: Hacker M, Lazo J, Tritton T, eds. *Organ-Directed Toxicities of Anticancer Therapy*. Leiden, The Netherlands: Martinus Nijhoff; 1987.

127. Casper E, Gaynor J, Hajdu S, et al. A prospective randomized trial of adjuvant chemotherapy with bolus versus continuous infusion of doxorubicin in patients with high-grade extremity soft tissue sarcoma and an analysis of prognostic factors. *Cancer*. 1991;68:1221–1229.

128. Zalupski M, Metch B, Balcerzak S, et al. Phase III comparison of doxorubicin and dacarbazine given by bolus versus infusion in patients with soft-tissue sarcomas: a Southwest Oncology Group study. *J Natl Cancer Inst*. 1991;83:926–932.

129. Hortobagyi G, Frye D, Buzdar A, et al. Decreased cardiac toxicity of doxorubicin administered by continuous

intravenous infusion in combination chemotherapy for metastatic breast carcinoma. *Cancer.* 1989;63:37–45.

130. Sirohi B, A'hern R, Coombes G, et al. A randomised comparative trial of infusional ECisF versus conventional FEC as adjuvant chemotherapy in early breast cancer: the TRAFIC trial. *Ann Oncol.* 2010;21:1623–1629.

131. Van Dalen EC, Michiels EM, Caron HN, Kremer LC. Different anthracycline derivates for reducing cardotoxicity in cancer patients. *Cochrane Database Syst Rev.* 2010; 12(5):CD005006. doi:10.1002/14651858.CD005006.pub3.

132. Myers C, McGuire W, Liss R, et al. *Adriamycin: the role of lipid peroxidation in cardiac toxicity and tumor response. Science* 197:165–167, 1977.

133. Legha S, Wang Y, Mackay B, et al. Clinical and pharmacologic investigation of the effects of a-tocopheral on adriamycin cardiotoxicity. In: Lubin B, Machlin L, eds. *Vitamin E: biochemical, hematological, and clinical aspects.* New York, NY: The New York Academy of Sciences; 1982:411–417.

134. Myers C, Bonow R, Palmeri S, et al. A randomized controlled trial assessing the prevention of doxorubicin cardiomyopathy by N-acetylcysteine. *Semin Oncol.* 1983;10:53–55.

135. Herman E, Ferrans V. Preclinical animal models of cardiac protection from anthracycline-induced cardiotoxicity. *Sem Oncol.* 1998;25:15–21.

136. Van Acker F, Boven E, Kramer K, et al. Frederine, a new and promising protector against doxorubicin-induced cardiotoxicity. *Clin Cancer Res.* 2001;7:1378–1384.

137. Speyer J, Green M, Zeleniuch-Jacquotte A, et al. ICRF-187 permits longer treatment with doxorubicin in women with breast cancer. *J Clin Oncol.* 1992;10:117–127.

138. Speyer J, Wasserheit C. Strategies for reduction of anthracycline cardiac toxicity. *Semin Oncol.* 1998;25: 525–537.

139. Speyer J, Green M, Kramer E, et al. Protective effect of the bispiperazinedione ICRF-187 against doxorubicin-induced cardiac toxicity in women with advanced breast cancer. *N Engl J Med.* 1988;319:745–752.

140. Swain S, Whaley F, Gerber M, et al. Cardioprotection with dexrazoxane for doxorubicin-containing chemotherapy in advanced breast cancer. *J Clin Oncol.* 1997;15:1318–1332.

141. Swain S, Whaley F, Gerber M, et al. Delayed administration of dexrazoxane provides cardioprotection for patients with advanced breast cancer treated with doxorubicin-containing chemotherapy. *J Clin Oncol.* 1997;15:1333–1340.

142. Zinecard (dexrazoxane for injection) prescribing information. https://www.pfizer.com/products/product-detail/zinecard. Accessed October 31, 2017.

143. Popelová O, Sterba M, Hasková P, et al. Dexrazoxane-afforded protection against chronic anthracycline cardiotoxicity in vivo: effective rescue of cardiomyocytes from apoptotic cell death. *Br J Cancer.* 2009;101: 792–802.

144. Venturini M, Michelotti A, Del Mastro L, et al. Multicenter randomized controlled clinical trial to evaluate cardioprotection of dexrazoxane versus no cardioprotection in women receiving epirubicin chemotherapy for advanced breast cancer. *J Clin Oncol.* 1996;14:3112–3120.

145. Lopez M, Vici P, Di Lauro L, et al. Randomized prospective clinical trial of high-dose epirubicin and dexrazoxane in patients with advanced breast cancer and soft tissue sarcomas. *J Clin Oncol.* 16:86–92, 1998.

146. Hasinoff B. The use of dexrazoxane for the prevention of anthracycline extravasation injury. *Expert Opin Investig Drugs.* 2008;17:217–223.

147. Cardinale D, Colombo A, Sandri M, et al. Prevention of high-dose chemotherapy-induced cardiotoxicity in high-risk patients by angiotensin-converting enzyme inhibition. *Circulation.* 2006;114:2474–2481.

148. Kalay N, Basar E, Ozdogru I, et al. Protective effects of carvedilol against anthracycline-induced cardiomyopathy. *J Am Coll Cardiol.* 2006;48:2258–2262.

149. Wittayanukorn S, Qian J, Westrick SC, Billor N, Johnson B, Hansen RA. Prevention of Trastuzumab and Anthracycline-induced cardiotoxicity using angiotensin-converting enzyme inhibitors or β-blockers in older adults with breast cancer. *Am J Clin Oncol.* 2017;41:909–918. doi:10.1097/COC.0000000000000389

150. Ewer M, Martin F, Henderson I, et al. Cardiac Safety of Liposomal Anthracyclines. *Semin Oncol.* 2004; 31: 161–181.

151. Theodoulou M, Hudis C. Cardiac profiles of liposomal anthracyclines: greater cardiac safety versus conventional doxorubicin? *Cancer.* 2004;100:2052–2063.

152. Tardi P, Boman N, Cullis P. *Liposomal doxorubicin. J Drug Target.* 1996;4:129–140.

153. Martin F. Liposome drug products: product evolution and influence of formulation on pharmaceutical properties and pharmacology. *United States Food and Drug Administration.* 2010. http://www.fda.gov/ohrms/dockets/ac/01/slides/3763s2_08_martin/tsld001.htm. Accessed March 31, 2010.

154. Balazsovits J, Mayer L, Bally M, et al. Analysis of the effect of liposome encapsulation on the vesicant properties, acute and cardiac toxicities, and antitumor efficacy of doxorubicin. *Cancer Chemother Pharmacol.* 1989;23:81–86.

155. Mayer L, Bally M, Cullis P, et al. Comparison of free and liposome encapsulated doxorubicin tumor drug uptake and antitumor efficacy in the SC115 murine mammary tumor. *Cancer Lett.* 1990;53:183–190.

156. Kanter P, Bullard G, Ginsberg R, et al. Comparison of the cardiotoxic effects of liposomal doxorubicin (TLC D-99) versus free doxorubicin in beagle dogs. *In Vivo.* 1993;7:17–26.

157. Harris L, Batist G, Belt R, et al. Liposome-encapsulated doxorubicin compared with conventional doxorubicin in a randomized multicenter trial as first-line therapy of metastatic breast carcinoma. *Cancer.* 2002;94:25–36.

158. Venturini M, Bighin C, Puglisi F, et al. A multicentre Phase II study of non-pegylated liposomal doxorubicin in combination with trastuzumab and docetaxel as first-line therapy in metastatic breast cancer. *Breast.* 2010;19:333–338.

159. O'Brian M, Wigler N, Inbar M, et al. Reduced cardiotoxicity and comparable efficacy in a phase III trial of pegylated liposomal doxorubicin HCL (CAELYX/Doxil) versus conventional doxorubicin for first-line treatment of metastatic breast cancer. *Ann Oncol.* 2004;15:440–449.

160. Robert N, Vogel CL, Henderson I, et al. The role of the liposomal anthracyclines and other systemic therapies in the management of advanced breast cancer. *Semin Oncol.* 2004;31:106–146.

161. Orlowski RZ, Nagler A, Sonneveld P, et al. Randomized phase III study of pegylated liposomal doxorubicin plus bortezomib compared with bortezomib alone in relapsed or refractory multiple myeloma: combination therapy improves time to progression. *J Clin Oncol.* 2007;25:3892–3901.

162. Sparano J, Makhson A, Semiglazov V, et al. Pegylated liposomal doxorubicin plus docetaxel significantly improves time to progression without additive cardiotoxicity compared with docetaxel monotherapy in patients with advanced breast cancer previously treated with neoadjuvant-adjuvant anthracycline therapy: results from a randomized phase III study. *J Clin Oncol.* 2009;27:4522–4529.

163. Platel D, Pouna P, Bonoron-Adèle S, et al. Comparative cardiotoxicity of idarubicin and doxorubicin using the isolated perfused rat heart model. *Anticancer Drugs.* 1999;10:671–676.

164. Anderlini P, Benjamin R, Wong F, et al. *Idarubicin cardiotoxicity: a retrospective study in acute myeloid leukemia and myelodysplasia. J Clin Oncol.* 1995;13:2827–2834.

165. Fogli S, Danesi R, Gennari A, et al. Gemcitabine, epirubicin and paclitaxel: pharmacokinetic and pharmacodynamic interactions in advanced breast cancer. *Ann Oncol.* 2002;13:919–927.

166. Gennari A, Salvadori B, Donati S, et al. Cardiotoxicity of epirubicin/paclitaxel-containing regimens: Role of cardiac risk factors. *J Clin Oncol.* 1999;17:3596–3602.

167. Gianni L, Dombernowsky P, Sledge G, et al. Cardiac function following combination therapy with paclitaxel and doxorubicin: an analysis of 657 women with advanced breast cancer. *Ann Oncol.* 2001;12:1067–1073.

168. Faulds D, Balfour J, Chrisp P, et al. Mitoxantrone. A review of its pharmacodynamic and pharmacokinetic properties, and therapeutic potential in the chemotherapy of cancer. *Drugs.* 1991;41:400–449.

169. Chugun A, Uchide T, Tsurimaki C, et al. Mechanisms responsible for reduced cardiotoxicity of mitoxantrone compared to doxorubicin examined in isolated guinea-pig heart preparations. *J Vet Med Sci.* 2008;70:255–264.

170. Herbrecht R, Cernohous P, Engert A, et al. Comparison of pixantrone-based regimen (CPOP-R) with doxorubicin-based therapy (CHOP-R) for treatment of diffuse large B-cell lymphoma. *Ann Oncol.* 2013;24:2618–2623.

171. Billingham M, Mason J, Bristow M, et al. *Anthracycline cardiomyopathy monitored by morphologic changes. Cancer Treat Rep.* 1978;62:865–872.

172. Ewer M, Ewer S, Suter T. Cardiac complication. In: Hong W, Bast R, Hait W, et al., eds. *Cancer Medicine* (9th ed.). Shelton, CT: People's Medical Publishing House; 2017:1932–1948.

173. Hellmann K. Overview and Historical Development of Dexrazoxane. *Semin Oncol.* 1998;25:48–54.

4 Trastuzumab-Associated Cardiotoxicity

Thomas M. Suter ▪ *Michael S. Ewer*

INTRODUCTION

Trastuzumab is a monoclonal antibody that targets human epidermal growth factor receptor 2, or HER2. Initially it was not anticipated that it would cause cardiac dysfunction. However, early reports of significant numbers of both symptomatic and asymptomatic cardiac events led to broad investigations of the cardiac sequelae of this highly effective agent. The drug is approved for the treatment of metastatic as well as adjuvant regimens for HER2 positive breast cancer. It is also approved for the treatment of HER2 overexpressing metastatic gastric cancer and pancreatic cancers. Cardiac events related to trastuzumab now are known to be different from those of the anthracyclines, and extended use of the agent for periods of over ten years has been utilized in selected instances of metastatic breast cancer. This chapter will summarize how this important agent affects the heart and the clinical experience regarding its use.

BASIC SCIENCE CONSIDERATIONS

▪ Epidermal Growth Factor in the Heart: A Complex Signaling System

The epidermal growth factor (EGF) signalling system is present in the human heart and has a multitude of important roles during cardiac development as well with regard to the adult post-mitotic organ. Of the four known ErbB tyrosine kinase receptors (EGFR/ErbB1, ErbB2/HER2, ErbB3, and ErbB4), all are expressed in the fetal myocardium, but only the EGF, ErbB2, and ErbB4 receptors are expressed in postnatal or mature myocytes.[1] EGF ligands can bind to these receptors and induce homo- and heterodimer formation, which induce the autophosphorylation of the cytoplasmic domain of the receptor. Adaptor proteins then bind to the phosphorylated tyrosine receptor and induce a cascade of events, including the activation of small G proteins (Ras, Raf) as well as the stimulation of the mitogen-activated protein kinase (MAPK) and of the phosphoinositide 3-kinase (PI-3 kinase) pathways. The MAPK pathway has several important functions in the myocyte including the hypertrophic response of these cells to different stimuli and sarcomeric organization.[2] Inhibition of MAPK activity, or some of the regulatory proteins, such as MEK1-ERK 1/2, prevents agonist-induced cardiomyocyte hypertrophy and reduces activation of the cardiac-enriched transcription factor GATA4, a key regulator of many structural proteins in the myocardium.[3] GATA4 depletion is also an early event in anthracycline cardiotoxicity, which might explain, at least in part, the multiplicative cardiotoxic effect of ErbB2 inhibitors when used simultaneously with anthracyclines.[4,5]

Several EGF ligands are secreted in the heart, including neuregulins (NRGs, in different splice forms) and EGF, and play a major role in the endothelial cell–myocyte crosstalk. These ligands are both transmembrane proteins, are soluble, and have diverse affinities to myocyte EGF and ErbB4 receptors. ErbB2 has no known ligand but can activate downstream signaling by forming heterodimers with either EGF or ErbB4 receptors and inhibition of ErbB2 receptor activity with monoclonal antibodies; this attenuates downstream signaling.[6] The interaction between ligands and receptors is dynamically regulated and likely plays an important role in the maintenance and function of the myocardium.

▪ Role of the EGF Signaling System During Cardiac Development and Myocardial Stress

The importance of the EGF signaling system in the heart has been shown in several experimental settings, although the exact mechanism of trastuzumab-associated cardiotoxicity has not yet been established. NRG, ErbB2, and ErbB4 receptors are essential in the developing heart, and mice, deficient of either ligands or receptors, die in midgestation with virtually identical cardiac malformations.[7–9] Disruption of the NRG signaling system leads to impaired ventricular trabeculation, abnormal heart valve formation, and malformation of the cardiac conduction system.[10–12]

In the adult heart, NRG signaling mediates synthesis and stabilization of structural proteins and attenuates myocyte cell death.[1] ErbB2-deficient adult mice are viable and initially demonstrate no overt pathologic phenotype. However, over time, these animals develop features of dilated cardiomyopathy with left ventricular dysfunction and dilation and are more susceptible to increased cardiac stress, such as aortic banding.[13,14] Ventricular cardiac myocytes from these ErbB2-deficient mice are also more sensitive to anthracycline toxicity than wild-type cells, and these data demonstrate that ErbB2 signaling is important for normal cardiac function, particularly during episodes of cardiac stress.[14]

The subcellular mechanism of the protective effect of EGF signaling in the adult heart remains controversial. Whereas some data indicate that NRG-ErbB2 signaling is important for stress-induced attenuation of myocyte apoptosis, other experiments show that NRG signaling attenuates anthracycline-induced structural damage of contractile proteins (Figure 4.1).[6,14] However, clinical observation of several investigators suggests that trastuzumab-associated cardiotoxicity is frequently reversible, favoring a subcellular mechanism that is distinct from other chemotherapy-induced myocardial damage.[5]

CLINICAL CONSIDERATIONS

■ The Trastuzumab-Anthracycline Interaction

As will be seen from the clinical data presented below, trastuzumab, when administered in the absence of an anthracycline, has a very low level of cardiotoxicity; the inherent or independent cardiotoxicity of trastuzumab is seldom of clinical concern, and should be distinguished from the more profound and potentially more serious cardiac dysfunction associated with the concomitant or sequential use of trastuzumab and any of the anthracyclines (see Chapter 3). Review of data from the various trials provides four intriguing observations: 1) much (although not all) of the observed cardiotoxicity associated with trastuzumab administered following an anthracycline is reversible.[15] 2) Even in instances where transient cardiotoxicty has been observed, many patients go on to

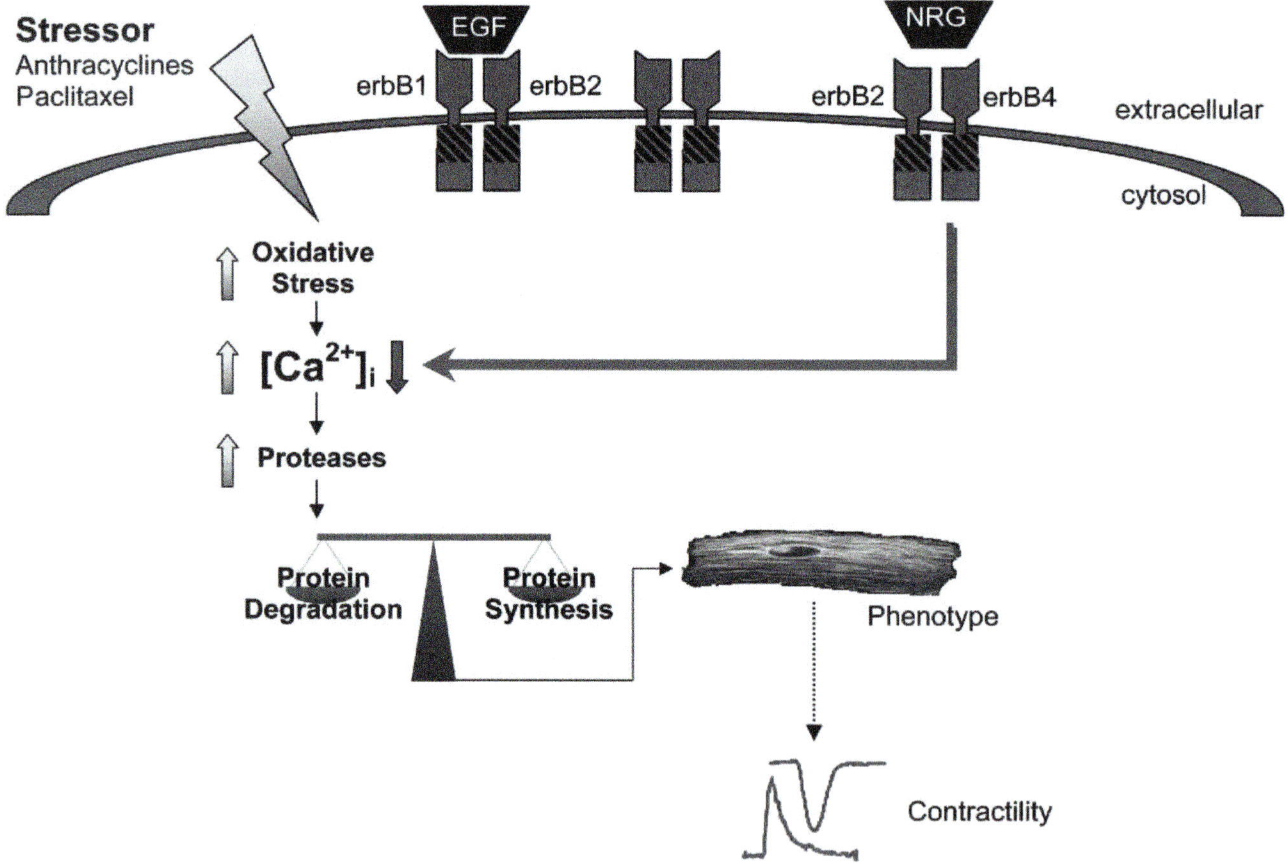

FIGURE 4-1 Possible mechanisms of trastuzumab-associated cardiotoxicity. Cardiac stressors, such as anthracyclines, increase myocardial oxidative stress, leading to an increase in cytosolic calcium concentration and to an activation of proteases. The consecutive activation of protein degradation induces changes in the tertiary structure of the contractile proteins, leading to contractile dysfunction. Neuregulin (NRG), a ligand of the ErbB receptors, attenuates these stress-induced changes, and inhibition of this system worsens anthracycline-induced cardiac changes.[6,35] EGF, epidermal growth factor.

receive additional trastuzumab for months or years following the event, and do so with low instances of cardiac adverse events. This observation excludes a cumulative-dose related form of toxicity that is clearly present with the anthracyclines. 3) There appears to be a temporal relationship between the time of anthracycline administration related to the time of trastuzumab administration, and 4) The reported risk factors for anthracycline cardiotoxicity and for that of trastuzumab are remarkably similar, suggesting some interaction despite a clear difference in the mechanism of cardiotoxicity that results from the administration of these agents.[16] These observations have led to the concept of an alternate, or Type II treatment-related cardiac dysfunction in contrast to that associated with the anthracyclines (Type I) and to a plausible, albeit not yet scientifically proven, hypothesis regarding the trastuzumab-anthracycline interaction.[17]

Based on the discussion of anthracycline associated damage presented in Chapter 3, we understand that myocyte damage following anthracycline exposure starts with the initial exposure. Some of the injured myocytes go on to experience cell death, a phenomenon well-evidenced from endomyocardial biopsy observation. Alternately, a collection of myocytes may undergo cell repair, and the repair process for the entire cohort appears to extend over a considerable, albeit not fully defined, period of time. It is hypothesized that when exposed to a stressful or toxic environment some cells that might, under more favorable conditions, recover, fail to do so. Under prolonged myocardial stress or impaired or inhibited recovery pathways, the probability of cell recovery is diminished; some cells that under more favorable conditions might recover fail to do so.

It is during the vulnerable period following anthracycline administration that trastuzumab often enters the scene. It has been demonstrated that damaged myocytes have increased binding capacity for trastuzumab, but beyond that, it is also known that the myocyte needs the very pathways blocked by trastuzumab for some forms of cell repair.[18] Consequently it is the anthracycline injury that is augmented, superimposed on any inherent trastuzumab-induced impairment of the functioning of myocyte contractile elements. Interestingly, in the absence of other agents, trastuzumab, in vitro, does not result in myocyte death.[19]

Several observations support this hypothesis. First, following the vulnerable post-anthracycline period when the myocytes have either recovered or have been replaced within the matrix, and are no longer vulnerable, trastuzumab can be given for long periods of time without undo effect on the stable myocardium. More relevant is the intriguing finding that cardiac

dysfunction appears to be maximal when an anthracycline is given concurrently with trastuzumab. This was the case in the pivotal study performed in patients with metastatic disease, where the rate of New York Heart Association heart failure of grade III or IV was found to be 19%.[20] In trials where the interval between the anthracycline was approximately three weeks, the rate of cardiac failure was about 3%, and in the case of the Herceptin Adjuvant trial (HERA), where the duration between the agents was 89 days, the rate of heart failure was below 1%. This data is depicted in Figure 4-2.[16] Additionally, heart biopsies studied three weeks following exposure to anthracyclines are abnormal, but biopsies studied much later fail to demonstrate myocyte abnormalities; the abnormal cells have regained a morphologically normal appearance or have been eliminated and presumably replaced by the fibrous network. Finally, the risk factors that have

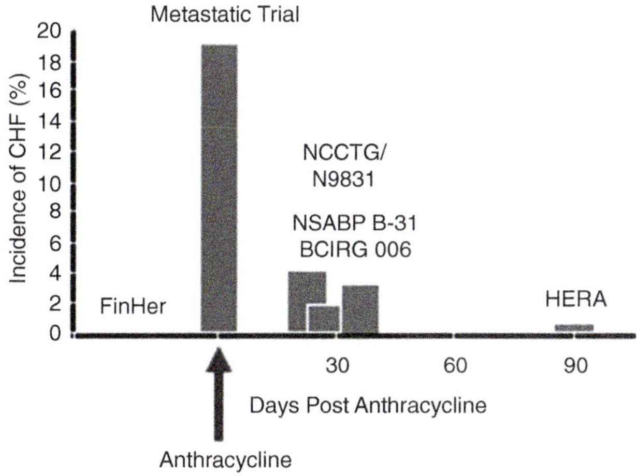

FIGURE 4-2 Incidence of congestive heart failure (CHF) in patients on adjuvant trials that included an anthracycline and trastuzumab. The arrow depicts the time of anthracycline administration; trastuzumab was started concurrently in the metastatic trial, approximately three weeks after anthracycline administration in the National Surgical Adjuvant Breast and Bowel Project B-31 trial (NSABP B-31), the North Central Cancer Treatment Group (NCCTG N9831) and the Breast Cancer International Research Gropu 006 trial (BCIRG-006). In the Herceptin Adjuvant trial (HERA) there was a mean delay of 89 days between the last anthracycline administration and the start of trastuzumab. In the FinHer trial trastuzumab was administered prior to the anthracycline. Tote the high rate of CHF observed when administration was concurrent, a much lower rate when the interval between anthracycline and trastuzumab was about 21 days, and a value approaching the level seen when no prior anthracycline was administered when the interval was extended to 89 days. See also Figure 4-3. (Modified from Ewer M and Ewer S, 2010.[16])

been identified for anthracyclines and for trastuzumab show considerable overlap, despite the fact that some of the classic anthracycline risks either are not applicable to patients who are receiving trastuzumab, or have not been studied in the latter populations. For both groups of drugs, the risks may be summarized as anything that has caused previous damage to myocyte, or anything that increases the likelihood of damage to the myocyte upon exposure (see also Chapter 3).

TRASTUZUMAB-ASSOCIATED CARDIOTOXICITY IN CLINICAL TRIALS

Although it has been known since the late 1980s that the cardiac myocytes express EGF and ErbB receptors, the preclinical testing of the monoclonal antibody against ErbB2/HER2 trastuzumab did not reveal any cardiac side effects.[21] Consequently, the early clinical trials, in which trastuzumab was used as a single agent or in combination with chemotherapy did not formally monitor cardiac function.[20,22] However, continued safety monitoring after regulatory approval of the drug for use in HER2-positive patients with metastatic breast cancer revealed a troubling safety signal for cardiotoxicity. This initiated a retrospective analysis of the adverse events of all pivotal trials with trastuzumab which indicated that the use of the drug was associated with a significant incidence of symptomatic congestive heart failure (CHF).[5] These early data are summarized in Table 4-1. The rate of symptomatic heart failure was particularly high in patients who were concurrently treated with trastuzumab and anthracyclines. Patients treated with trastuzumab alone had a moderate risk of developing symptomatic heart failure. However, it is important to note that the majority of these patients were pretreated with anthracyclines. The incidence of asymptomatic cardiac dysfunction was difficult to assess because most of the asymptomatic patients were not examined using the usual left ventricular functional tests such as echocardiography or multiple gated cardiac blood-pool scans (MUGA).

The clinical manifestation of patients with trastuzumab-associated heart failure was similar to other forms of heart failure. Their typical signs and symptoms included dyspnea on exertion, pulmonary edema, peripheral edema, and cardiomegaly.[20] Although the reported incidence may include some degree of artifact based on how heart failure was defined and measured, the numbers resulted in considerable concern.[23]

■ Cardiac Safety of Trastuzumab in the Adjuvant Trials

Cardiac data from the trials in metastatic disease prompted a more careful, systematic, and prospective assessment of cardiac function in the adjuvant trials of trastuzumab. Four large prospective, randomized, multicenter adjuvant clinical trials of trastuzumab in HER2-positive breast cancer patients are presently under way: the National Surgical Adjuvant Breast and Bowel Project (NSABP) B-31, the North Central Cancer Treatment Group (Intergroup), the HERceptin Adjuvant (HERA) trial, and the Breast Cancer International Research Group (BCIRG) 006.[24,25] Two of these trials, the NSABP B-31 and the Intergroup N9831, were designed to investigate the safety and efficacy of adjuvant anthracycline and cyclophosphamide followed by paclitaxel plus concurrent or sequential

TABLE 4-1 Retrospective analysis of cardiac side effects of trastuzumab in the pivotal metastatic breast cancer trials: Incidence of symptomatic heart failure and cumulative doses of anthracyclines

	TRASTUZUMAB ALONE	TRASTUZUMAB AND PACLITAXEL	PACLITAXEL	TRASTUZUMAB AND ANTHRACYCLINES/ CYCLOPHOSPHAMIDE	ANTHRA CYCLINES
Symptomatic heart failure, %	8.5	8.8	4.2	28	9.6
Heart failure NYHA III–IV, %	5	4	1	19	3
Anthracycline, median dose, mg/m²	316	245	245	347	346
Number of patients	213	91	95	143	135

NYHA, New York Heart Association.

weekly trastuzumab (Figure 4-2). The HERA trial (BIG01-01/BO16348) examines the effect of 3-weekly trastuzumab monotherapy either for 1 or 2 years after completion of adjuvant chemo- and radiotherapy (see Figure 4-2). In spring 2005, a joint interim efficacy analysis of the NSABP B-31 and Intergroup N9831 trial and an interim efficacy analysis of the HERA trial were presented. Trastuzumab and chemotherapy led to a 52% reduction in disease recurrence and a 33% improved survival compared with chemotherapy alone.[26] Similarly, in the HERA trial, trastuzumab led to a 46% improved disease-free survival.[24]

Because the cardiotoxicity of trastuzumab was a major concern in these trials, external independent data monitoring committees regularly reviewed safety data and the incidence of cardiac events. Three interim analyses were performed after a pre-specified number of patients (NSABP B-31 and NCCTG N9831: 100, 300, and 500; HERA 300, 600, and 900) were enrolled in the trial for 6 months. If an absolute difference of more than 4% in the primary cardiac end point (symptomatic heart failure New York Heart Association [NYHA] III or IV or cardiac death) between the trastuzumab-containing regiment and the control arm had been detected, the trials would have been stopped. None of the three trials reached this point, although the Intergroup trial was temporarily halted.[27] In the NSABP B-31 and Intergroup N9831 trials, clinical evaluation and left ventricular ejection fraction (LVEF), measured either by echocardiography or MUGA scanning, were performed at baseline, after completion of anthracycline/cyclophosphamide and paclitaxel, and 3 and 18 months after randomization (see Figure 4-3). In the HERA trial, similar cardiac assessments were performed prior to and 3, 6, and 12 months after randomization (see Figure 4-2). Patients receiving 2 years of trastuzumab were evaluated after

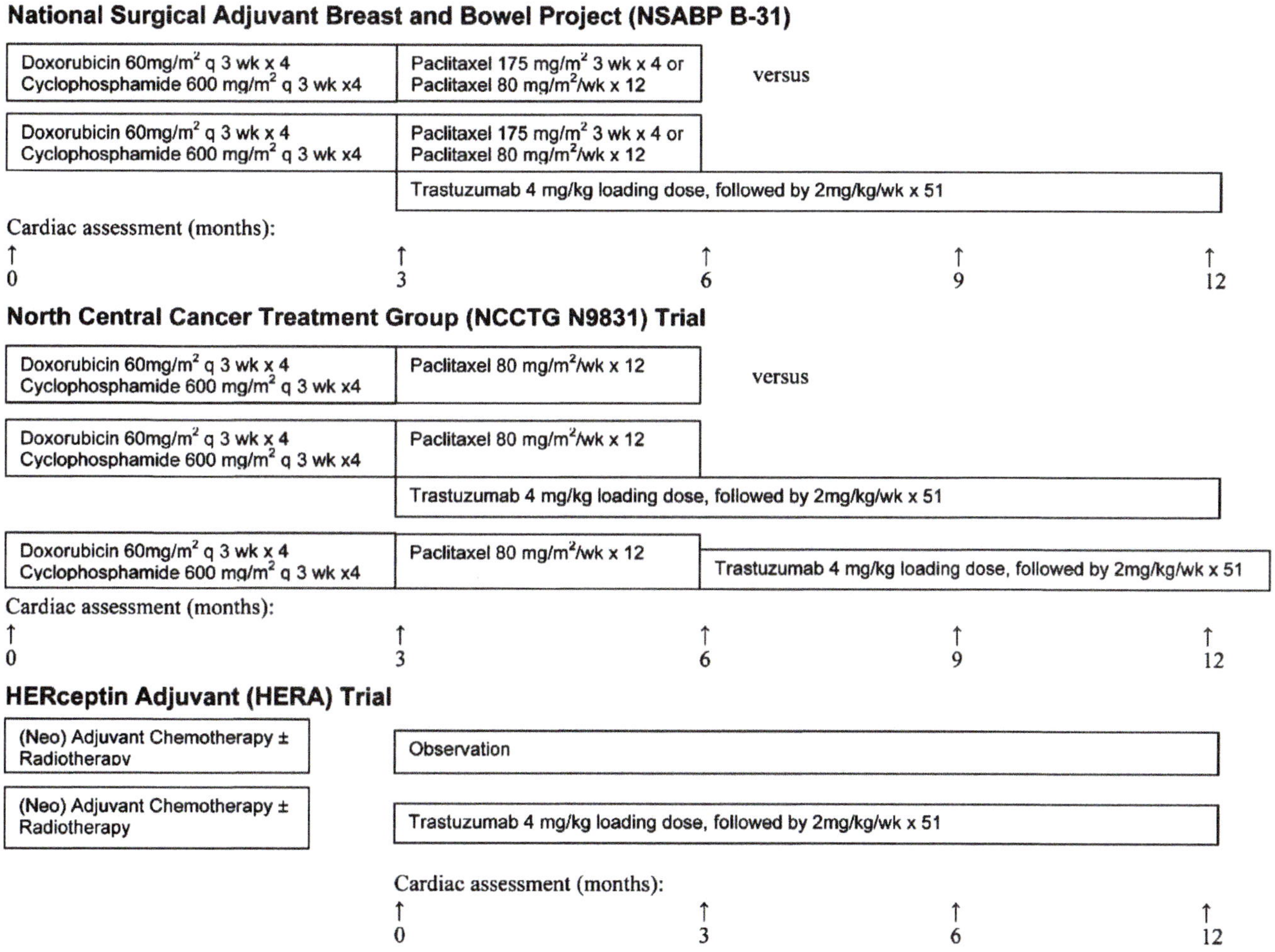

National Surgical Adjuvant Breast and Bowel Project (NSABP B-31)

| Doxorubicin 60mg/m^2 q 3 wk x 4
Cyclophosphamide 600 mg/m^2 q 3 wk x4 | Paclitaxel 175 mg/m^2 3 wk x 4 or
Paclitaxel 80 mg/m^2/wk x 12 | versus |

| Doxorubicin 60mg/m^2 q 3 wk x 4
Cyclophosphamide 600 mg/m^2 q 3 wk x4 | Paclitaxel 175 mg/m^2 3 wk x 4 or
Paclitaxel 80 mg/m^2/wk x 12 |
| Trastuzumab 4 mg/kg loading dose, followed by 2mg/kg/wk x 51 |

Cardiac assessment (months):

0   3   6   9   12

North Central Cancer Treatment Group (NCCTG N9831) Trial

| Doxorubicin 60mg/m^2 q 3 wk x 4
Cyclophosphamide 600 mg/m^2 q 3 wk x4 | Paclitaxel 80 mg/m^2/wk x 12 | versus |

| Doxorubicin 60mg/m^2 q 3 wk x 4
Cyclophosphamide 600 mg/m^2 q 3 wk x4 | Paclitaxel 80 mg/m^2/wk x 12 |
| Trastuzumab 4 mg/kg loading dose, followed by 2mg/kg/wk x 51 |

| Doxorubicin 60mg/m^2 q 3 wk x 4
Cyclophosphamide 600 mg/m^2 q 3 wk x4 | Paclitaxel 80 mg/m^2/wk x 12 | Trastuzumab 4 mg/kg loading dose, followed by 2mg/kg/wk x 51 |

Cardiac assessment (months):

0   3   6   9   12

HERceptin Adjuvant (HERA) Trial

| (Neo) Adjuvant Chemotherapy ±
Radiotherapy | Observation |

| (Neo) Adjuvant Chemotherapy ±
Radiotherapy | Trastuzumab 4 mg/kg loading dose, followed by 2mg/kg/wk x 51 |

Cardiac assessment (months):

0   3   6   12

FIGURE 4-3   Graphic representation of three adjuvant trials of trastuzumab in patients with breast cancer presented during the 2005 annual meeting of the American Society of Clinical Oncology. The North Central Cancer Treatment Group N9831 was a three-arm trial comparing paclitaxel alone with trastuzumab and paclitaxel concomitantly and trastuzumab and paclitaxel subsequently. Cardiac assessment indicates cardiac clinical evaluation and measurement of left ventricular ejection fraction.[22–24]

24 months and compared to the one-year cohort. Disease-free survival was the same for the two groups, however decreases in ejection fraction were more common in the two-year cohort although New York Heart Association class III or IV events with a drop of at least 10 percentage points to a value below 50% were only slightly higher in the 2-year group (0.8% vs. 1.0%).[28] Trastuzumab was held for individual patients in the NSABP B-31 and Intergroup N9831 trials if the LVEF dropped more than 10% to a level below the lower limit of normal or more than 15% if the LVEF remained within normal limits. If a reassessment of LVEF after 4 weeks showed cardiac dysfunction within these limits, trastuzumab was permanently discontinued. Similarly, for patients in the HERA trial, trastuzumab treatment was stopped if the LVEF dropped to a level below 45% or more than 10 percentage points and to a level within the range of 45% to 49%.

The NSABP B-31 Intergroup N9831 trials included a provision only to randomize patients to receive trastuzumab or placebo if, following completion of the anthracycline/ cyclophosphamide components of the trial, their LVEF remained above the lower limit of normal or had not dropped more than 15%. Similarly, the HERA trial required a baseline LVEF of ≥ 55% prior to randomization to trastuzumab. The BCIRG 006 trial used cardiotoxicity thresholds similar to those of the NSABP; here, too, the threshold to curtail the enrolment into the trial was a 4% difference between the arms, and this threshold was not achieved.

In the NSABP B-31 trial, 19.9% of the patients who started trastuzumab stopped treatment because of cardiac dysfunction. Of the remaining patients, 4% treated concomitantly with paclitaxel and trastuzumab developed severe CHF compared with 0.6% who were treated with paclitaxel alone (Table 4-2); 15.9% of patients in the combined paclitaxel-trastuzumab arm had an asymptomatic drop in the LVEF.[26] Similarly, in the Intergroup trial, 3.3% of patients who were treated concomitantly with paclitaxel and trastuzumab developed severe CHF, whereas if trastuzumab was given sequentially after paclitaxel, only 2.2% of patients developed severe CHF.[27] The incidence of asymptomatic LVEF drop was similar to that in the NSABP B-31 trial. The investigators of the HERA trial reported an incidence of 0.5% severe CHF and a 7.1% asymptomatic LVEF drop in their trastuzumab-treated patients, despite the fact that 68% of the patients had received adjuvant anthracycline treatment albeit many with epirubicin that may be slightly less cardiotoxic than doxorubicin.

These data indicate that the combination of paclitaxel and trastuzumab leads to a significant risk of trastuzumab-associated cardiotoxicity and that sequential treatment appears to be safer than concomitant treatment with these two drugs. Based on the data from the pivotal trials of trastuzumab in metastasizing

TABLE 4-2 Cardiac safety data from three adjuvant trastuzumab trials

	NSABP B-31		NCCTG N9831 INTERGROUP			HERA TRIAL	
	Paclitaxel	*Trastuzumab Weekly and Paclitaxel*	*Paclitaxel*	*Trastuzumab Weekly Sequential to Pacitaxel*	*Trastuzumab Weekly Concomitant with Pacitaxel*	*Observation*	*Trastuzumab 3-Weekly*
Cardiac death	1	0	0	1	1	1	0
Severe (NYHA III–IV) heart failure, % (range)	0.6	4.0	0 (0–0.7)	2.2 (1.2–3.8)	3.3 (2.0–5.1)	0 (0–0.2)	0.5 (0.3–1.0)
Asymptomatic LVEF drop, % (below LLN or < 50%)	UK	15.9	6 and 5	14	17	2.2	7.1
Number of patients	811	846	544 and 549	582	602	1736	1,677

CI, confidence interval; HERA, HERceptin Adjuvant Trial; LLN, lower limit of normal; LVEF, left ventricular ejection fraction; NCCTG, North Central Cancer Treatment Group; NSABP, National Surgical Adjuvant Breast and Bowel Project; NYHA, New York Heart Association.

breast cancer, the combination of trastuzumab with paclitaxel appears to be safer than the combination with anthracyclines. The NSABP-Intergroup and HERA trials can only be cautiously compared because the treatment scheme, definition of cardiotoxicity, and adjuvant chemotherapy were significantly different in these trials. A number of unanswered questions remain that are of considerable importance with regard to the cardiotoxicity of trastuzumab: does intense monitoring of cardiac function that may result in early recognition of ejection fraction declines and early intervention have any clinical relevance? Furthermore, is there any strategy that mitigates the cardiac events of this agent? And lastly, because the mechanism of trastuzumab cardiotoxicity is different from that of anthracyclines, what is the true natural history of cardiotoxicity in these patients?

Risk Factors for Cardiotoxicity

The retrospective analysis of the pivotal trials led to the identification of several risk factors for trastuzumab-associated cardiotoxicity.[5,28] In a multivariate analysis, they included the concomitant use of anthracyclines, previous anthracycline exposure, age > 50 years, and NYHA dyspnea class greater than class II before enrolment in the trial (Table 4-3). Interestingly, these risk factors seem to be similar to those of anthracycline-induced cardiotoxicity (see Table 4-3).[29] While numerous risk factors have been identified for anthracyclines as well as trastuzumab, it is becoming increasingly clear that cellular injury in the absence of prior anthracycline exposure is limited. Many now feel for the sequential use of trastuzumab following anthracyclines, the cardiac risk factors are the same as those for anthracyclines, and comprise any entity that either has previously caused myocyte destruction, or that increases the cellular damage upon toxic exposure.[16]

Several estimates of cardiotoxicity for patients receiving trastuzumab monotherapy shed additional light on this issue. In the pivotal trial, when trastuzumab was given weekly as second- or third-line monotherapy, 6.0% to 8.5% of patients experienced some degree of cardiac dysfunction, whereas in the first-line monotherapy trial, 2.6% of patients had cardiac dysfunctional abnormalities.[22,30] In a recent phase II trial with trastuzumab administered 3-weekly, the incidence of cardiac dysfunction, defined as an LVEF drop of $\geq$ 15% and/or an LVEF < 50%, was 16%, but only 1 of the 103 patients had trastuzumab-associated symptomatic heart failure. These data again indicate with high probably the single most important risk factor for trastuzumab-associated cardiotoxicity is combination chemotherapy with prior exposure to an anthracycline.

TABLE 4-3 Risk factors for trastuzumab- and doxorubicin-induced cardiotoxicity: One retrospective analysis of the pivotal trials

Trastuzumab
Previous or concomitant anthracyclines[1]
Age > 50 yr[1]
Previous cardiac disease[1]
Hyperlipidemia[1]
Doxorubicin
Combination chemotherapy
Previous or concomitant mediastinal radiotherapy
Age > 70 yr
Previous cardiac disease
Hypertension
Whole-body hyperthermia

Source: Adapted from Suter T, Procter M, van Veldhuisen DJ, 2004.[24]

In the three adjuvant trials presented in spring 2005, the incidence of severe CHF was relatively low (see Table 4-2). There was a trend to a higher occurrence of symptomatic CHF in patients receiving trastuzumab concomitantly with paclitaxel compared with the patient who received trastuzumab sequentially after paclitaxel in the Intergroup trial, again suggesting that combination chemotherapy is an important risk factor for trastuzumab-associated cardiotoxicity. These data also indicate that not only anthracyclines but also paclitaxel can lead to cardiotoxicity in combination with trastuzumab. The incidence of an asymptomatic drop in the LVEF was between 5% and 6% in the paclitaxel group and increased to 14% to 17% in the group treated with paclitaxel and trastuzumab (see Table 4-2). Furthermore, the analysis of the NSABP B-31 data revealed that, similar to the data from the pivotal trial, age > 50 years and left ventricular dysfunction prior to treatment with trastuzumab are risk factors for trastuzumab-associated cardiotoxicity.[26]

Outcome of cardiotoxicity ■ Based on the available data, it is generally believed that trastuzumab-associated cardiotoxicity is distinctly different from the form of chemotherapy-related cardiac dysfunction associated with the anthracyclines.[17] For example, doxorubicin-induced cardiotoxicity is clearly dose related, and strategies to reduce oxidative stress during anthracycline therapy prevent or attenuate myocardial damage.[31,32] Trastuzumab-associated cardiotoxicity seems to be dose independent, and myocardial structural changes, at least in vitro, appear to be on the level of the contractile proteins (myofibrils).[6] In contrast, anthracyclines cause dose-dependent myocardial cell death by inducing apoptosis and necrosis at a higher concentration. Since the heart is a post mitotic organ with only very limited capacity of regeneration, anthracycline-related cardiotoxicity is frequently not reversible. In contrast, 80% of patients with trastuzumab-associated cardiotoxicity in the pivotal trials had significant improvement of the cardiac dysfunction when treated with drugs commonly used for heart failure (angiotensin-converting enzyme [ACE] inhibitors, digoxin).[5] In addition, most of the time, improvement in the cardiac function occurred irrespective of whether trastuzumab was continued or withdrawn.

Similar observations were made by Ewer and colleagues in 38 women with trastuzumab-related cardiac dysfunction followed over a 4-year period.[15] Almost all of these patients had recovery of the LVEF after withdrawal of trastuzumab; although most were treated for heart failure, this was not the case in six of these patients, suggesting that the role of treatment in reversing cardiac dysfunction remains uncertain and the recovery without specific treatment for heart failure does occur. Of these women, 25 were re-challenged to trastuzumab while still on heart failure medications. Only three (12%) women had recurrent left ventricular dysfunction (Figure 4-4). These data suggest that trastuzumab-associated cardiotoxicity is frequently reversible, particularly if myocardial stress factors are eliminated or controlled. This also suggests that the ErbB-NRG system is a modulator of myocardial stress and that inhibition of the ErbB-NRG signaling system during episodes of elevated cardiac stress (such as chemotherapy) could have a deleterious effect on myocardial function (Figure 4-1).

More recent trials have incorporated trastuzumab with other agents intending to increase overall oncologic efficacy. In the Cleopatra trial pertuzumab, a HER2/neu receptor antagonist, was added to a trastuzumab + docetaxel regimen. Interestingly, cardiac adverse events were less common in the group treated with both anti-HER2 agents (all grades of left ventricular systolic dysfunction was 8.3% and 3.8% in the placebo and pertuzumab arm respectively).[33] In the BERENICE trial, pertuzumab and trastuzumab were given after either dose-dense doxorubicin and cyclophosphamide or fluorouracil, epirubicin, and cyclophosphamide. While the event rate was higher in the dose-dense doxorubicin cohort, no new safety signals were identified when using the two anti HER2 agents.[34]

Monitoring and treatment guidelines and future perspectives ■ Prior to trastuzumab therapy, patients should be carefully evaluated for cardiovascular risk factors and cardiac disease. Patients whose tumors exhibit the HER2/neu marker should be considered for cardioprotective regimens when anthracyclines form part of the treatment plan or could do so in the future (see Chapter 3). The pretreatment evaluation should include a detailed medical history, a physical examination, an electrocardiogram and either an echocardiogram or a nuclear imaging study to evaluate cardiac systolic function. If the LVEF is lower than the lower limit of normal (i.e., usually <50 or, in some centers 55%), the risk-benefit ratio of treatment with trastuzumab or the intended combination, especially if an anthracycline forms part of this combination, should be carefully considered. This is especially important in the adjuvant setting and in patients who are older than 60 years.

Less cardiotoxic than the combination of trastuzumab and anthracyclines but still problematic

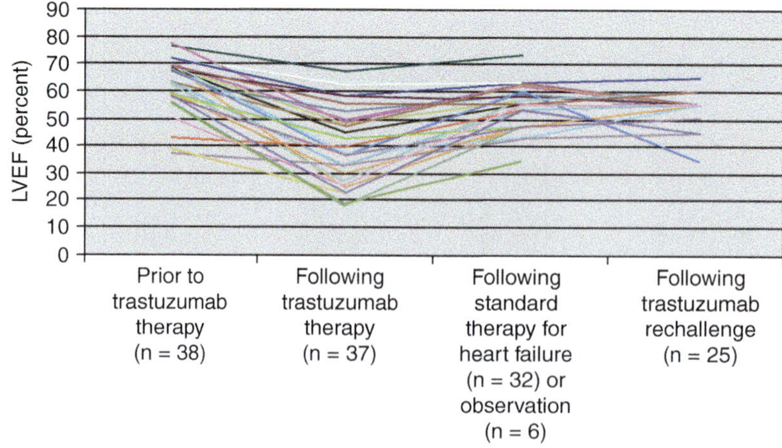

FIGURE 4-4 Plot of 38 patients who developed trastuzumab-related cardiac dysfunction showing baseline left ventricular ejection fraction (LVEF), LVEF following development of cardiac dysfunction, and after a recovery period, and for 25 patients who were rechallenged, LVEF following rechallenge. (Reproduced with permission from Ewer MS Vooletich MT, Durand JB, et al., 2005.[15])

is the concomitant treatment of trastuzumab and paclitaxel. Throughout the treatment period, patients at risk should be monitored for signs and symptoms of cardiac dysfunction and heart failure. In patients who develop heart failure, trastuzumab treatment may be halted temporarily, and left ventricular function should be evaluated. If left ventricular function is found to be below the lower limit of normal, treatment with ACE inhibitors and β-blockers should be considered and the risk-benefit ratio for continuing trastuzumab treatment should be assessed. Limited data from observational studies, however, suggest that continued trastuzumab treatment might be justifiable in patients with trastuzumab-associated cardiac dysfunction; symptomatic patients, should be treated with ACE inhibitors and β-blockers, and these agents may also be helpful in asymptomatic patients who have experienced a significant drop in ejection fraction.

The data presently available also suggest that an important pathophysiologic mechanism for trastuzumab-associated cardiotoxicity is the inhibition of MAPK. Future therapeutic approaches that inhibit the ErbB2 signaling pathway should therefore be expected to have similar cardiac side effects, regardless of how the signaling pathway is inhibited (i.e., ErbB antibodies, tyrosine kinase inhibitors, Ras/Raf inhibitors). Furthermore, newer strategies to improve the efficacy of ErbB-targeted therapies are to inhibit not only EGFR or ErbB2 but also multiple ErbB receptors. However, the cardiac side effects of these approaches remain unknown, and cardiac monitoring is prudent with these multiple or pan-ErbB approaches.

Trastuzumab in combination with other anti-HER2 therapies ■ Trastuzumab has been combined with other anti-HER2 agents in a number of clinical trials. In the Cleopatra trial, pertuzumab was given with trastuzumab plus doctaxel, and progression-free survival was significantly increased (18.7 vs. 12.4 months; p<0.001) for patients on dual anti-HER2 therapy. There was considerable concern that adding a second anti-HER2 agent would significantly increase cardiotoxicity. Curiously, the incidence of cardiac events was lower in the combination group.[33] The criteria used in the Cleopatra trial was a decline in left ventricular ejection fraction of 10 percentage points or more from baseline to a value below 50%. This threshold was met in 6.6% of the trastuzumab-treated patients and in 3.8% of patients who received the combination. Recovery to a value of > 50% was seen in 72% in the trastuzumab arm and 86.7% in the combination arm. Some of the reported events may have been false-positive results, as 77% of the patients were studied by cardiac ultrasound, known to be an imperfect modality.[36]

In the ALTTO trial comparing 1 year of anti-HER2 therapy with lapatinib, trastuzumab, or their use in sequence or combination. The incidence of primary cardiace end points was low: 1% for lapatinib + trastuzumab, 0.5% for trastuzumab followed by lapatinib, and 0.9% for trastuzumab without lapatinib.[37] Additional results related to the ALTTO trial are anticipated. In the Berenice trial, pertuzumab, trastuzumab, and standard anthracycline- and taxane-based chemotherapy was evaluated. In patients who received trastuzumab and pertuzumab, the incidence grade III/IV cardiac events was 1.5%. The authors concluded that no new safety signals were identified.[34]

ACKNOWLEDGMENTS

This work was supported in part by the Swiss Science Foundation SNF 3231-054985.98/1, an unrestricted grant for basic research from F. Hoffmann La Roche International LTD, and the DeVigier Foundation, all to T.M.S.

REFERENCES

1. Zhao YY, Sawyer DR, Baliga RR, et al. Neuregulins promote survival and growth of cardiac myocytes. Persistence of ErbB2 and ErbB4 expression in neonatal and adult ventricular myocytes. *J Biol Chem*. 1998;273:10261–10269.
2. Clerk A, Michael A, Sugden P. Stimulation of the p38 mitogen-activated protein kinase pathway in neonatal rat ventricular myocytes by the G protein-coupled receptor agonists, endothelin-1 and phenylephrine: a role in cardiac myocyte hypertrophy? *J Cell Biol*. 1998;142(2):523–535.
3. Liang F, Lu S, Gardner D. Endothelin-dependent and -independent components of strain-activated brain natriuretic peptide gene transcription require extracellular signal regulated kinase and p38 mitogen-activated protein kinase. *Hypertension*. 2000;35(1 pt 2):188–192.
4. Aries P, Paradis P, Lefebvre C, Schwartz RJ, Nemer M. Essential role of GATA-4 in cell survival and drug-induced cardiotoxicity. *Proc Natl Acad Sci USA*. May 4, 2004;101(18):6975–6980.
5. Suter T, Cook-Bruns N, Barton C. Cardiotoxicity associated with trastuzumab (Herceptin) therapy in the treatment of metastatic breast cancer. *Breast*. 2004;13:173–183.
6. Sawyer D, Zuppinger C, Miller TA, Eppenberger HM, Suter TM. Modulation of anthracycline-induced myofibrillar disarray in rat ventricular myocytes by neuregulin-1beta and anti-erbB2: potential mechanism for trastuzumab-induced cardiotoxicity. *Circulation*. 2002;105(13):86–92.
7. Gassman H, Meadows R, Baker L, Metastatic tumors of the heart. *Am J Med*. 1955;19:357–365.

8. Lee KF, Simon H, Chen H, Bates B, Hung MC, Hauser C. Requirement for neuregulin receptor erbB2 in neural and cardiac development. *Nature*. November 1995;378:394–398.

9. Meyer D, Birchmeier C. Multiple essential functions of neuregulin in development. *Nature*. 1995;378:386–390.

10. Goldhirsch A, Gelber RD, Piccart-Gebhart MJ, et al. 2 year versus 1 year of adjuvant trastuzumab for HER2-positive breast cancer (HERA: an open-label, randomized controlled trial. *Lancet*. 2013;382:1021–1028.

11. Camenisch T, Schroeder JA, Bradley J, Klewer SE, McDonald JA. Heart-valve mesenchyme formation is dependent on hyaluronan-augmented activation of ErbB2-ErbB3 receptors. *Nat Med*. 2002;8:850–855.

12. Rentschler S, Zander J, Meyers K, et al. Neuregulin-1 promotes formation of the murine cardiac conduction system. *Proc Natl Acad Sci USA*. 2002;99:10464–10469.

13. Ozcelik C, Erdmann B, Pilz B, et al. Conditional mutation of the ErbB2 (HER2) receptor in cardiomyocytes leads to dilated cardiomyopathy. *Proc Natl Acad Sci USA*. 2002;99:8880–8885.

14. Crone S, Zhao YY, Fan L, et al. ErbB2 is essential in the prevention of dilated cardiomyopathy. *Nature Med*. 2002;8:459–465.

15. Ewer M, Vooletich MT, Durand JB, et al. Reversibility of trastuzumab-telated cardiotoxicity: new insights based on clinical course and response to medical treatment. *J Clin Oncol*. 2005;23:7820–7827.

16. Ewer M, Ewer S. Cardiotoxicity of anticancer treatments: what the cardiologist needs to know. *Nat Rev Cardiol*. 2010;7:564–575.

17. Ewer M, Lippman S. Type II chemotherapy-related cardiac dysfunction: time to recognize a new entity. *J Clin Oncol*. 2005;23(13):2900–2902.

18. de Korte M, de Vries EG, Lub-de Hooge MN, et al. 111Indium-trastuzumab visualises myocardial human epidermal growth factor receptor 2 expression shortly after anthracycline treatment but not during heart failure: a clue to uncover the mechanisms of trastuzumab-related cardiotoxicity. *Eur J Cancer*. 2007;43:2046–2051.

19. Ewer M, Ewer S. Troponin I provides insight into cardiotoxicity and the anthracycline-trastuzumab interaction. *J Clin Oncol*. 2010;28:3901–3904.

20. Slamon D, Leyland-Jones B, Shak S, et al. Use of chemotherapy plus a monoclonal antibody against HER2 for metastatic breast cancer that overexpresses HER2. *N Engl J Med*. 2001;344(11):783–792.

21. Komuro I, Kurabayashi M, Takaku F, Yazaki Y. Expression of cellular oncogenes in the myocardium during the developmental stage and pressure-overloaded hypertrophy of the rat heart. *Circ Res*. 1988;62:1075–1079.

22. Cobleigh MA, Vogel CL, Tripathy D, et al. Multinational study of the efficacy and safety of humanized anti-HER2 monoclonal antibody in women who have HER2-overexpressing metastatic breast cancer that has progessed after chemotherapy for metastatic disease. *J Clin Oncol*. 1999;17(9):2639–2648.

23. Ewer M, Gibbs HR, Swafford J, Benjamin RS. Cardiotoxicity in patients receiving trastuzumab (Herceptin): primary toxicity, synergistic or sequential stress, or surveillance artifact? *Semin Oncol*. 1999;26(suppl 12):96–101.

24. Suter T, Procter M, van Veldhuisen DJ, et al. Trastuzumab-associated cardiac adverse effects in the herceptin adjuvant trial. *J Clin Oncol*. 2007;25:3859–3865.

25. Perez E, Rodeheffer R. Clinical cardiac tolerability of trastuzumab. *J Clin Oncol*. 2004;22:322–329.

26. Tan-Chiu E, Yothers G, Romond E, et al. Assessment of cardiac dysfunction in a randomized trial comparing doxorubicin and cyclophosphamide followed by paclitaxel, with or without trastuzumab as adjuvant therapy in node-positive, human epidermal growth factor receptor 2-overexpressing breast cancer: NSABP B31. *J Clin Oncol*. 2005;23:7811–7819.

27. Perez E, Romond EH, Suman VJ, et al. NCCTG N9831: May 2005 update. Paper Presented at: The annual meeting of the American Society of Clinical Oncology 23, 2005, Orlando, FL, ASCO Annual Meeting Proceedings.

28. Cook-Burns N. Retrospective analysis of the safety of Herceptin immunotherapy in metastatic breast cancer. *Oncology*. 2001;61(suppl 2):58-66.

29. Singal P, Iliskovic N. Doxorubicin-induced cardiomyopathy. *N Engl Med*. 1998;339:900–905.

30. Desai A, Vogelzang NJ, Rini BI, et al. A high rate of venous thromboembolism in a multi-institutional phase II trial of weekly intravenous gemcitabine with continous infusion fluorouracil and daily thalidomide in patients with metastatic renal cell carcinoma. *Cancer*. 2002;95:1629–1636.

31. Lipshultz S, Rifai N, Dalton VM, et al. The effect of dexrazoxane on myocardial injury in doxorubicin-treated children with acute lymphoblastic leukemia. *N Engl J Med*. 2004;351:145–153.

32. O'Brian M, Wigler N, Inbar M, et al. Reduced cardiotoxicity and comparable efficacy in a phase III trial of pegylated liposomal doxorubicin HCL (CAELYX/Doxil) versus conventional doxorubicin for first-line treatment of metastatic breast cancer. *Ann Oncol*. 2004;15:440–449.

33. Swain SM, Ewer MS, Cortes J, et al. Cardiac tolerability of pertuzumab plus trastuzumab plus docetaxel in patients with HER2-positive metastatic breast cancer in CLEOPATRA: a randomized, double-blind, placebo-controlled phase III study. *Oncologist*. 2013;18:257–264.

34. Swain SM, Ewer MS, Viale G, et al. Pertuzumab, trastuzumab, and standard anthracycline-and taxane-based chemotherapy for the neoadjuvant treatment of patients with HER2-ositive localized breast cancer (BERENICE): a phase II, open-label, multicenter, multinational cardiac safety study. *Ann Oncol*. 2018;29:646–653.

35. Lim C, Zuppinger C, Guo X, et al. Anthracyclines induce calpain-dependent titin proteolysis and necrosis in cardiomyocytes. *J Biol Chem*. 2004;279:8290–8299.

36. Ewer MS, Herson J. False positive cardiotoxicity events in cancer-related clinical trials: risks related to imperfect noninvasive parameters. *Chemotherapy*. 2019; (in press).

37. Moreno-Aspitia A, Holmes EM, Jackisch C, et al. Updated results from the phase III ALTTO trial (BIG 2-06; NCCTG [Alliance] N063D) comparing one year of anti-HER2 therapy with lapatinib alone (L), trastuzumab alone (T), their sequence (T→L) or their combination (L+T) in the adjuvant treatment of HER2-positive early breast cancer. *J Clin Oncol*. 2017;35,(15,suppl):502-502.

5 Mechanisms of Anti-HER2 Cardiotoxicity: Interference with Neuregulin-1 Cardioprotective Signaling

Zarha Vermeulen ■ Vincent Segers ■ Gilles W. De Keulenaer

INTRODUCTION

The introduction of trastuzumab for the treatment of ErbB2-amplified breast tumors in 1998, and the subsequent observation of coincident heart failure, led to the accidental discovery of protective ErbB2 signaling in cardiovascular physiology. The combined role of ErbB2 in malignant tumor growth and in compensatory processes in the heart positions ErbB2 at the crossroad between cancer and chronic heart failure. Hence, pharmacological inhibition of ErbB2 as treatment for cancer may lead to ventricular dysfunction, and systemic activation of ErbB2 as treatment for heart failure may induce malignancy.

The complexity of ErbB2 signaling in physiological and oncological conditions is better understood now than it was 15 years ago. Overwhelming evidence indicates that the principles of ErbB2 signaling in physiological conditions, e.g., in the regulation of cardiac function, are fundamentally different from those in cancer cells.[1] This finding suggests that it may be feasible to specifically interfere with either physiological or tumor cell ErbB2 signaling to activate ErbB2 signaling in patients with heart failure without increasing the risk of cancer, and to inhibit ErbB2 signaling in patients with cancer without increasing the risk of heart failure. Smart drug design developed in a stepwise fashion has now provided at least seven separate anti-ErbB2 cancer drugs, together with a few molecules that activate physiological ErbB2 signaling and are used to treat heart failure. Each of these drugs interferes with ErbB2 in a unique way. In this review, we present a comprehensive overview of these developments at the crossroad between cancer and heart failure. We will address the biology of ErbB signaling in cancer and cardiac cells, the regulatory aspects of the neuregulin 1 (NRG-1)/ErbB system in heart failure, and the working mechanisms of various anti-HER2 drugs and their degree of cardiotoxicity.

ERBB2 SIGNALING IN CANCER

In many types of cancer cells, ErbB2 is amplified by increased gene transcription. Tumor growth is vitally dependent on ErbB2 amplification, a process called *oncogene addiction*. ErbB2 belongs to the family of human epidermal growth factor (EGF) receptors consisting of EGFR (ErbB1), ErbB2, ErbB3, and ErbB4 (Figure 5-1). Unlike the other members of this family, ErbB2 has no known ligand but instead has an open conformation. Hence, it is constitutively active, continuously exposing a dimerization arm for interaction with another ErbB family member (heterotypic ErbB signaling). In cancer cells, amplified ErbB2 binds to ErbB3 in an uncontrolled and at least partially ligand-independent way, forming an oncogenic ErbB2/ErbB3 complex (Figure 5-2).[2] In this complex, after phosphorylation of ErbB3 tyrosine residues by the ErbB2 kinase, ErbB3 interacts with the regulatory p85 subunit of phosphoinositide 3-kinase (PI3K) without the need for any adaptor proteins.[3] This interaction results in robust activation of the PI3K/Akt pathway and intense cell growth, positioning ErbB3 as the key node in oncogenic ErbB2 signaling. This scenario is found in 20% to 30% of invasive breast carcinomas and in substantial numbers of ovarian, gastric, and bladder cancers.

ErbB2 has been the main therapeutic target within the ErbB2/ErbB3 oncogenic unit. The goal of ErbB2-targeted therapy is to interrupt PI3K/Akt signaling and thus to stop cell proliferation and to induce cell apoptosis. Clinical introduction of this strategy with the humanized anti-ErbB2 antibody trastuzumab has been successful, but chronic treatment has been disturbed by unforeseen problems, namely the development of tumor drug resistance and the induction of cardiac dysfunction and heart failure.[4] These drawbacks have forced the design of next-generation anti-ErbB2 drugs.

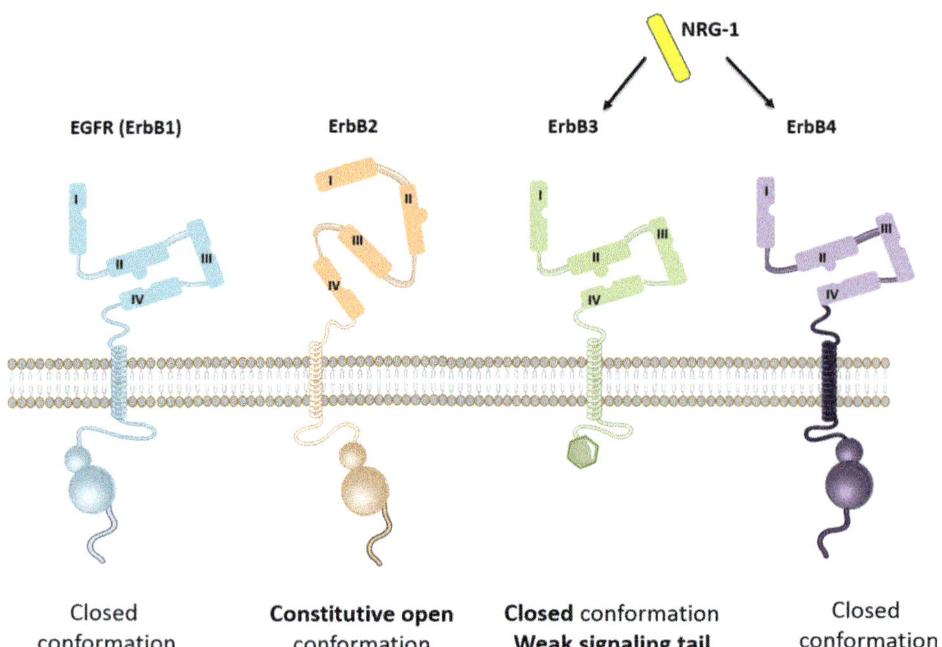

FIGURE 5-1 ErbB receptors. The human epidermal growth factor receptor family consists of EGFR (ErbB1), ErbB2, ErbB3, and ErbB4. ErbB receptors share high homology in the extracellular domain and the kinase domain. However, ErbB3 lacks tyrosine kinase activity, and ErbB2 has no known ligand; instead, it has a constitutive open conformation, which continuously exposes a dimerization arm for interaction with another ErbB family member.

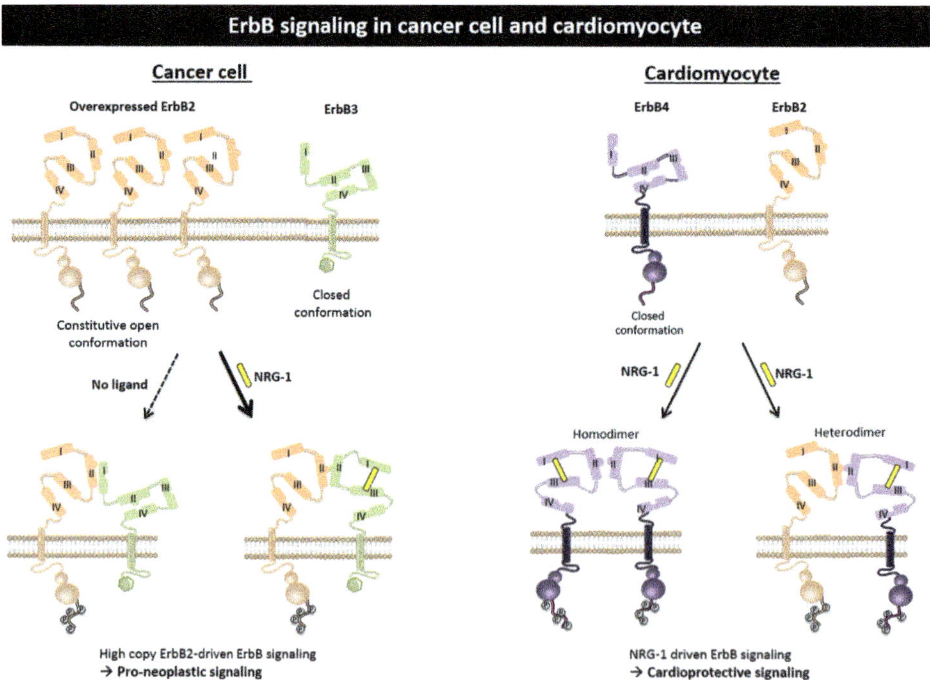

FIGURE 5-2 ErbB signaling in ErbB2-overexpressing breast cancer cells and in cardiomyocytes Left. Oncogenic signaling in breast cancer cells can be mediated by the overexpression of ErbB2. Amplified ErbB2 triggers predominantly ligand-independent oncogenic ErbB2/ErbB3 heterodimers, and this triggering leads to the phosphorylation of specific tyrosines in the tail region of the receptors, the activation of downstream proteins, and pro-neoplastic signaling. Right. In adult cardiomyocytes, the binding of NRG-1 to ErbB4 induces a switch from a closed to an open receptor conformation, thereby exposing a dimerization arm (domain II). Ligand-activated ErbB4 results in the formation of either ErbB2/ErbB4 heterodimers or ErbB4/ErbB4 homodimers, and these complexes lead to the phosphorylation of specific tyrosines in the tail region, the activation of downstream proteins, and cardioprotective signaling cascades.

A first challenge has been to intercept biological escape routes leading to anti-ErbB2 drug resistance. Recent evidence suggests that upregulation of ErbB3 is crucially involved in the process.[5] ErbB3 mRNA transcription is negatively controlled by ErbB2 signaling, a finding explaining why ErbB3 is upregulated during the suppression of ErbB2 signaling.[6] Enhanced ErbB3 forms new oncogenic complexes with residually active ErbB2, thereby maintaining oncogenic signaling and endorsing anti-ErbB2 drug resistance.[3] This mechanism is especially intense when autocrine or paracrine NRG-1 is available in the tumor.[7] When NRG-1 binds to ErbB3, it switches to an open conformation, boosting the dimerization of ErbB3 with remaining active ErbB2. Thus, if drug resistance is to be avoided, it seems compulsory to combine specific anti-ErbB2 therapy with anti-ErbB3 interventions, or to engineer bispecific anti-ErbB drugs that inhibit both ErbB2 and ErbB3 in a combined fashion.

A second challenge has been to avoid anti-ErbB2 cardiotoxicity. As elaborated below, ErbB2 signaling is important for cardiac physiology, especially in conditions of cardiac overload and injury. However, as opposed to ErbB2 signaling in tumor cells, cardiac ErbB2 signaling is critically ligand (NRG-1)-dependent. This finding suggests that, as long as anti-ErbB2 treatment does not interfere with ligand-dependent ErbB2 signaling, its cardiac profile is safe.[1]

ERBB2 SIGNALING IN THE HEART

Myocardial ErbB2 signaling remains elementary for preserving ventricular function throughout life, as shown by the ventricular dysfunction that develops in mice in which the Erbb2 gene is conditionally silenced after birth.[8,9] Myocardial ErbB2 becomes part of an endothelium-controlled NRG-1/ErbB4 signaling axis in which NRG-1, secreted from cardiac endothelial cells, binds to the ErbB4 of cells in the myocardial tissue (Figure 5-2).[1] The expression of ErbB3 seems to be absent or at least less prominent in most cardiac cells, unlike cancer cells, and no physiological function of ErbB3 has been found in adult cardiac physiology. Ligand binding to ErbB4 leads to a switch from a closed conformation to an open conformation, the exposure of a dimerization arm in subdomain II, the subsequent formation of ErbB4/ErbB2 heterodimers, increased ErbB4/ErbB2 tyrosine kinase activity, and the transphosphorylation of the ErbB cytoplasmic signaling tails (Figure 5-2). Although ErbB2 is the preferred dimerization partner of ligand-activated ErbB4, NRG-1 may also induce the formation of ErbB4 homodimers (homotypic ErbB signaling), and as such may signal in an ErbB2-independent manner. The relative contribution of NRG-1 to both homotypic and heterotypic signaling is unknown, and it is also not known whether the relative contribution of homodimer and heterodimer signaling may change in certain conditions. Experiments with

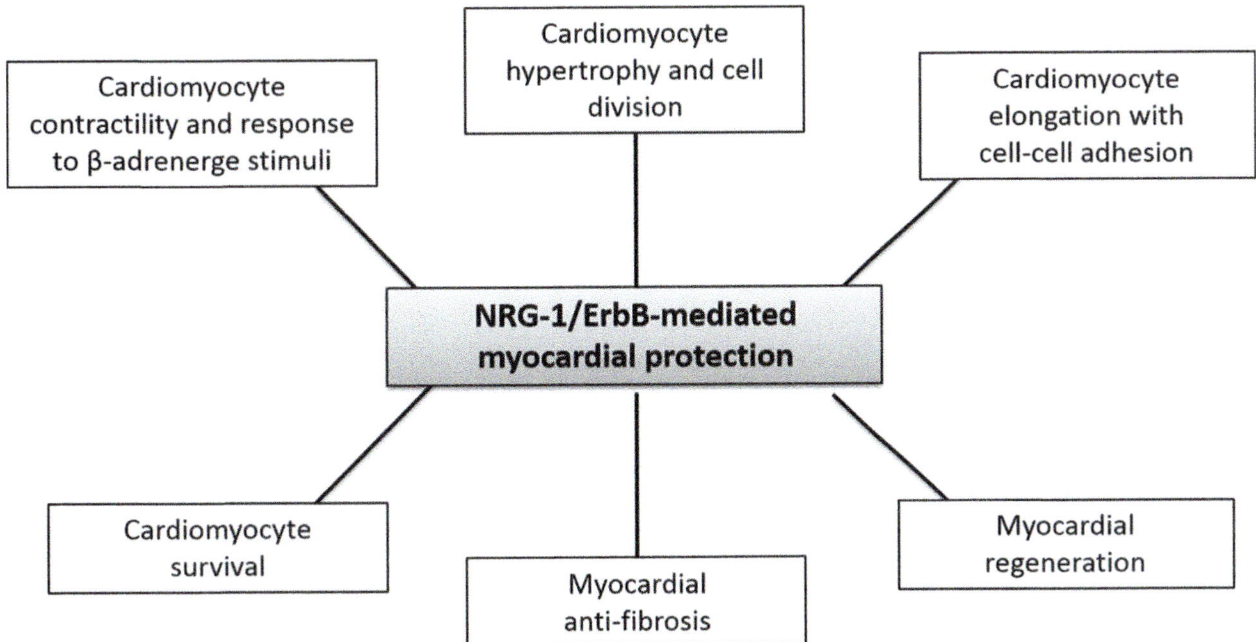

FIGURE 5-3 Cardioprotective effects of NRG-1/ErbB signaling. Antiapoptotic pathways, hypertrophic and even mitotic growth, cell elongation with improved cell-cell adhesion, and reduced sensitivity to adrenergic stimulation may all contribute to NRG-1 -mediated cardioprotection. NRG-1 also promotes myocardial regeneration and antifibrotic effects.

bivalent NRG-1 have nevertheless shown that homotypic NRG-1 signaling through ErbB4/ErbB4 homodimers may suffice for cardioprotection.[10]

The NRG-1/ErbB signaling axis is activated in heart failure and compensates for maladaptive processes that lead to progression of cardiac dysfunction, at least during early stages of the syndrome (Figure 5-3).[8,11] NRG-1 has been used in many animal models of heart failure and is currently being tested in a phase III clinical trial involving patients with heart failure with reduced ejection fraction (Tables 5-1 and 5-2).[9] In these trials, NRG-1 has been administered as an EGF-domain fragment of recombinant human (rh)NRG-1β or as an Ig domain–containing version of NRG-1β known as glial growth factor 2 (GGF2), usually by intravenous infusions during a short interval, thereby triggering reverse cardiac remodeling and functional improvement.

A concern during systemic treatment with these ErbB4 ligands is to stimulate tumor growth. As explained above, tumor growth in ErbB2-amplified cells results from the partially ligand-independent formation of ErbB2/ErbB3 oncogenic complexes. Therefore, at first glance, NRG-1 should not induce oncogenic complexes, and the risk of inducing malignancy should be limited. However, NRG-1 also binds to ErbB3, forcing it into an open conformation, which is more prone to form new oncogenic complexes. In this scenario, NRG-1 may advance tumor growth, promote tumor resistance, or both during treatment with anti-ErbB2 therapies.

TABLE 5-1   Administration of rhNRG-1 in animal models of heart failure

MODEL	SPECIES	TREATMENT	OUTCOME	REF
MI	Rat	10 µg/kg/day i.v. for 5 or 10 days, 1 week or 2 months after LAD ligation	Improved LV structure and dysfunction Increased angiogenesis Improved survival rates	Liu et al.[30]
MI	Mouse	2.5 µg per mouse i.p. for 12 weeks, 1 week after LAD	Improved LV structure and dysfunction Increased myocardial regeneration	Bersell et al.[31]
MI	Rat	5 µg/kg/h i.v. for 7 days, 8 weeks after LAD ligation	Improved LV structure and dysfunction	Gu et al.[32]
MI	Rat	10 µg/kg/day i.v. for 10 days, 4 weeks after LAD ligation	Improved LV structure and dysfunction Decreased mitochondrial dysfunction Decreased apoptosis Decreased oxidative stress	Guo et al.[33]
MI	Rat	Infarcted area injected with rhNRG-1–carrying lentivirus	Decreased apoptosis Increased angiogenesis	Xiao et al.[34]
MI	Swine	0.67 mg/kg i.v. every 2 days for 4 weeks, 1 week after MI	Improved LV dysfunction Decreased fibrosis	Galindo et al.[35]
I/R	Rat	1, 2, 4, or 8 µg/kg i.v. for 20 minutes before I/R	Improved LV structure Decreased apoptosis Decreased infarct size	Fang et al.[36]
Myo-carditis	Mouse	30 µg/kg/day i.v. for 5 days	Improved LV structure and dysfunction Decreased necrosis Improved survival rates	Liu et al.[30]

MODEL	SPECIES	TREATMENT	OUTCOME	REF
Doxo-induced CM	Rat	20 μg/kg/day i.v. for 5 days, 4 weeks after first administration of doxo	Improved LV structure and dysfunction Decreased necrosis Improved survival rates	Liu et al.[30]
Doxo-induced CM	Mouse	0.75 mg/kg/day s.c. for 3-5 days, 1 day before administration of doxo	Improved LV structure and dysfunction Improved survival rates Decreased apoptosis Preserved cardiac troponins	Bian et al.[37]
Pacing-induced CM	Dog	3 μg/kg/day i.v. for 5 days with continuous pacing, 3 weeks after initiation of rapid pacing	Improved LV dysfunction	Liu et al.[30]
Pacing-induced CM	Rhesus monkey	3 μg/kg/day i.v. for 10 days	Improved LV dysfunction Increased myosin heavy chain α	Li et al.[38]
Type 1 DCM	Mouse	10 μg/kg i.v. every 2 days for 2 weeks, 12 weeks after STZ injection	Improved LV structure and dysfunction Decreased apoptosis Decreased fibrosis	Li et al.[39]
Type 1 DCM	Mouse	5 sites of the LV injected with rhNRG-1–carrying lentivirus, 12 weeks after STZ injection	Improved LV structure and dysfunction Decreased apoptosis Decreased fibrosis	Li et al.[40]

rhNRG-1, recombinant human neuregulin-1; MI, Myocardial infarction; i.v., intravenous; LAD, left anterior descending artery; LV, left ventricle; i.p., intraperitoneal; I/R, ischemia/reperfusion; doxo, doxorubicin; s.c., subcutaneous; CM, cardiomyopathy; DCM, diabetic cardiomyopathy; STZ, streptozotocin.

TABLE 5-2 Clinical trials with rhNRG-1 as treatment for heart failure

DESCRIPTION	DOSAGE	OUTCOME	REF
Phase II, randomized, double-blind, multicenter, background therapy–based, placebo-controlled, parallel-group study	0.3, 0.6, or 1.2 μg/kg for 10-hour i.v. infusion, 10 consecutive days	Improved and sustained LVEF% and decreased LVEDV and LVESV 30 and 90 days after treatment	Gao et al.[41]
Single-center, prospective, non-randomized, open-label study	Initial dose of 1.2 μg/kg for 6 hours 0.6, 1.2, or 2.4 μg/kg for 12-hour i.v. infusion, 10 consecutive days	Acute increase in CO Improvement in LVEF%	Jabbour et al.[42]

rhNRG-1, recombinant human neuregulin-1; i.v., intravenous; LVEF%, % left ventricle ejection fraction; LVEDV, left ventricle end-diastolic volume; CO, carbon monoxide; LVESV, left ventricle end-systolic volume.

TRASTUZUMAB, THE FIRST ERBB2-TARGETED DRUG: HOW DOES IT WORK, WHERE DOES IT FAIL?

■ The clinical picture

Trastuzumab is an effective treatment for ErbB2-overexpressing breast cancer in the adjuvant, neoadjuvant, and metastatic settings. Adding conventional chemotherapeutic agents increases the overall response to trastuzumab. In the adjuvant setting, treatment with trastuzumab is given for one year; this treatment schedule is based on the results of several phase III trials. In the first human trials of trastuzumab, however, an unexpected cardiac toxicity was identified: 27% of patients receiving trastuzumab concurrently with anthracycline-containing chemotherapy developed either asymptomatic cardiomyopathy or clinical heart failure, whereas these complications occurred in only 7% of patients receiving anthracycline chemotherapy alone.12,13 Fortunately, in many cases, the cardiac dysfunction was asymptomatic, and additional clinical trials indicated that, in the absence of concomitant anthracycline treatment, the incidence of cardiac dysfunction was relatively low during treatment with trastuzumab and was generally transient after completion of therapy. In addition, the cardiac risks were outweighed overall by the potent anticancer effects of trastuzumab treatment.[14]

Trastuzumab (Herceptin) is a monoclonal antibody that binds to subdomain IV of ErbB2 (Figure 5-4). This binding disrupts ligand-independent ErbB2/ErbB3 interactions in ErbB2-amplified cells and subsequently impedes PI3K/Akt activity.[4,15] However, it

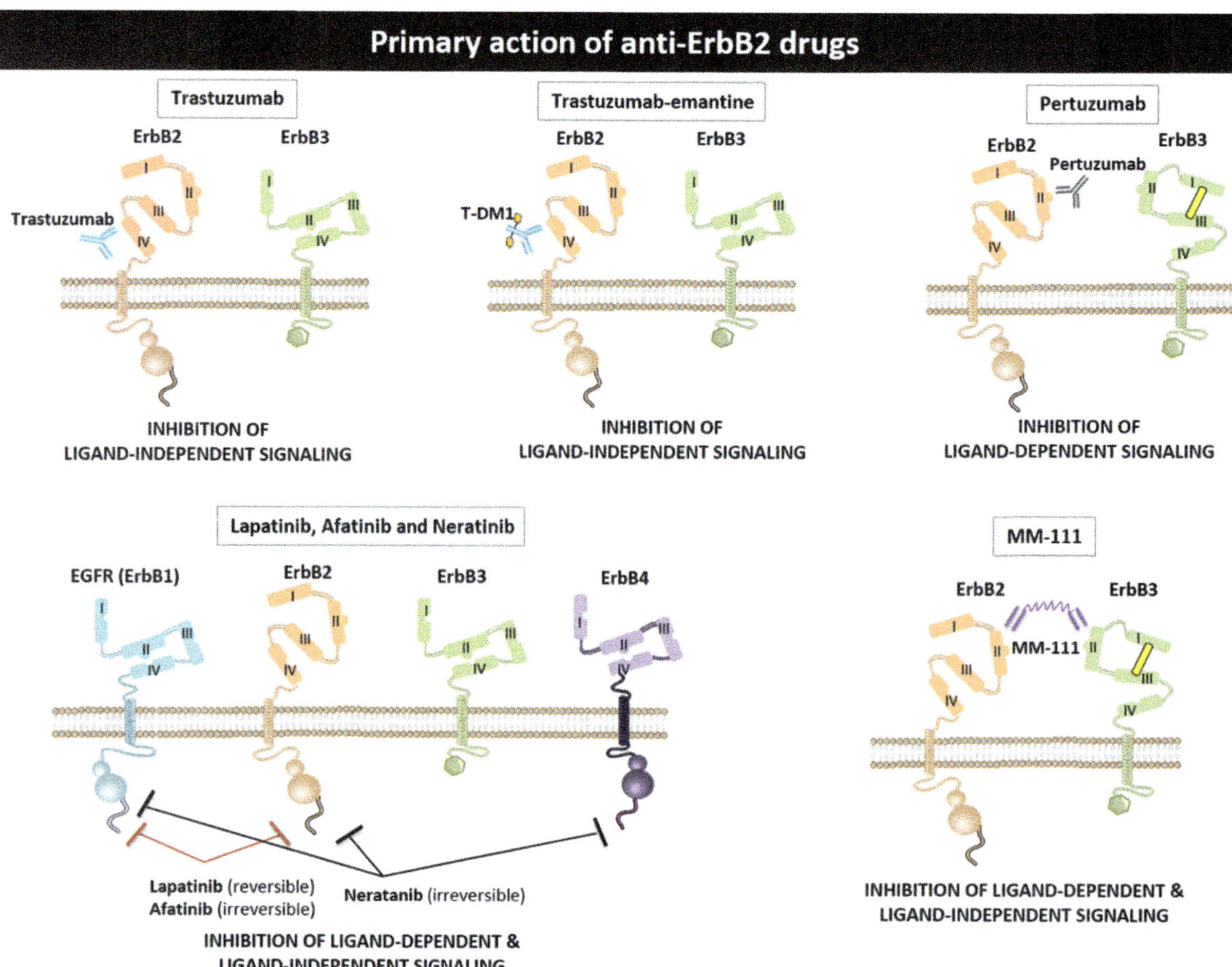

FIGURE 5-4   Trastuzumab resistance. Trastuzumab provides an ErbB3 escape route for the development of tumor resistance. When it inhibits ErbB2 signaling, ErbB3 expression will be upregulated to form new oncogenic complexes with ErbB2, especially when NRG-1 or another ErbB3 ligand is available to open its conformation. Consistently, both the upregulation of ErbB3 mRNA and the concentration of NRG-1 in the tumor predict trastuzumab drug resistance.

remains unknown whether this is the only mechanism responsible for trastuzumab's in vivo cancer-inhibiting actions. Other proposed mechanisms include increased endocytotic destruction of ErbB2, reduced shedding of the extracellular domain of ErB2, and immune activation by recruiting Fc-competent immune effector cells and other components of antibody-dependent cell-mediated cytotoxicity (ADCC).[4]

The monoclonal humanized nature of trastuzumab explains why this antibody can be studied only in human cells; for this reason it has long remained unclear whether trastuzumab also interferes with NRG-1–dependent physiological ErbB signaling in the heart. Recently, however, using human fetal cardiomyocytes, Fedele and coworkers showed that trastuzumab indeed inhibited the formation of NRG-1-induced ErbB4/ErbB2 complexes.[16] This observation most likely explains why trastuzumab's cardiac toxicity occurs primarily when it is administered simultaneously with anthracyclines. Indeed, NRG-1/ErbB signaling in the heart is part of a stress-activated compensatory system: this signaling plays a modest role in physiological conditions but is indispensable in the injured heart, e.g., during ischemia or exposure to cardiotoxic agents such as anthracyclines.[17,18]

Another disadvantage of trastuzumab's working mechanism is that it provides an ErbB3 escape route for the development of tumor resistance. Indeed, upon inhibition of ErbB2 signaling, ErbB3 expression is upregulated and forms new oncogenic complexes with ErbB2, especially when NRG-1 or another ErbB3 ligand is available to open its conformation. Consistently, both the upregulation of ErbB3 mRNA and the concentration of NRG-1 in tumors predict trastuzumab drug resistance (Figure 5-5).[3]

Accordingly, trastuzumab effectively inhibits malignant signaling in ErbB2-overexpressing tumor cells, but it has the disadvantages of interfering with NRG-1/ErbB2 signaling in the heart, an interference that becomes harmful during co-treatment with anthracyclines, and of allowing an ErbB3-dependent escape route for drug resistance through the upregulation of ErbB3 and the formation of ligand-induced ErbB2/ErbB3 oncogenic complexes.

HOW DO NEXT-GENERATION ERBB2 ANTAGONISTS DIFFER FROM TRASTUZUMAB?

During the past decade we have witnessed the introduction of several new drugs targeting ErbB2 in cancer. These drugs include new monoclonal

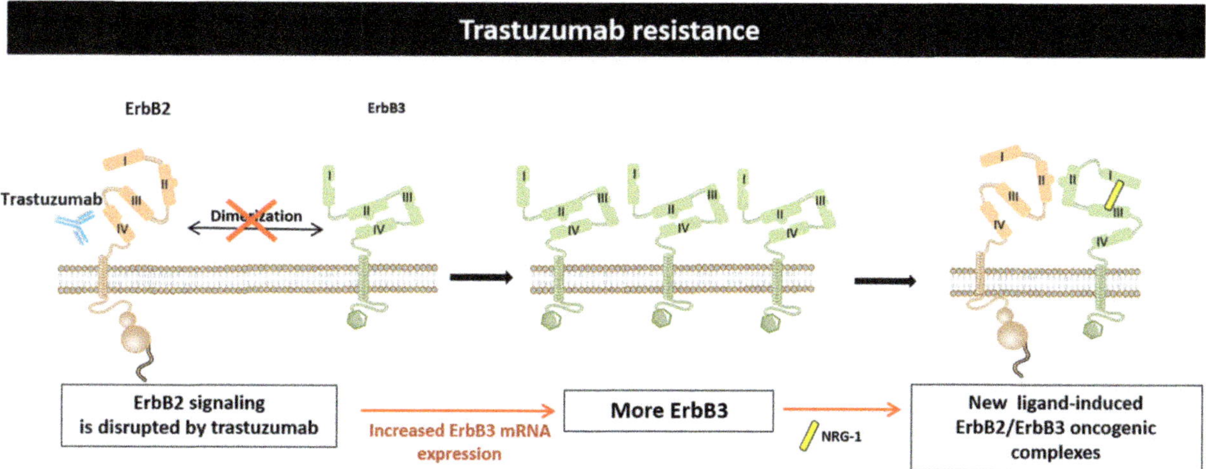

FIGURE 5-5 Primary actions of current ErbB2 inhibitors. Trastuzumab is a humanized monoclonal antibody to subdomain IV of ErbB2. This antibody leads to the inhibition of ligand-independent ErbB2 signaling. Trastuzumab-emtansine is an antibody conjugate consisting of the monoclonal antibody trastuzumab linked to the cytotoxic agent emtansine, an antimicrotubule drug. Pertuzumab is a humanized monoclonal antibody to subdomain II of the dimerization arm of ErbB2. Pertuzumab leads to inhibition of ligand-induced ErbB2 signaling. Lapatinib is a small-molecule tyrosine kinase inhibitor of EGFR (ErbB1) and ErbB2. Afatinib and neratinib are second-generation irreversible tyrosine kinase inhibitors. Afatinib is highly selective for EGFR/ErbB1 and ErbB2, whereas neratinib also inhibits ErbB4. Tyrosine kinase activity is blocked independently of whether this activity is ligand-induced. MM-111 is a bispecific antibody and a polypeptide fusion protein of two human single-chain variable fragment (scFv) antibodies linked to modified human serum albumin. MM-111 forms a trimeric complex with ErbB2 and ErbB3 and inhibits ligand-dependent ErbB2 and ErbB3 signaling.

antibodies against ErbB2 (pertuzumab, MM-111), oral small-molecule ErbB tyrosine kinase inhibitors (lapatinib, afatinib, neratinib), and an antibody-drug conjugate of trastuzumab combined with a cytotoxic agent, emtansine. Each of these molecules has a specific mode of action at the level of the ErbB receptors, hence uniquely influencing ligand-dependent and ligand-independent ErbB signaling (Figure 5-4). Specific activity profiles allow prediction of their effect on tumor growth, the potential for development of drug resistance, and their interference with physiological NRG-1–induced ErbB signaling in the heart and other organs. In the next paragraphs we describe these profiles, and they are summarized in Table 5-3.

■ Trastuzumab-Emtansine

Trastuzumab-emtansine (also known as T-DM1) is an antibody conjugate consisting of the monoclonal antibody trastuzumab linked to the cytotoxic agent

TABLE 5-3 Action of various ERBB2 antagonists on cancer cells, on ligand (NRG-1)-induced signaling, and on cardiac function

AGENT	TUMOR CELLS		CARDIAC CELLS	
	INHIBITORS			
	Anticancer mechanism of action	*Secondary resistance*	*Effect on NRG-1 signaling*	*Level of cardiotoxicity*
Trastuzumab	Inhibition of ErbB2/ErbB3 dimerization by binding domain IV of the ErbB2 receptor	Yes	Inhibits heterotypic ErbB2/ErbB4 signaling, but not homotypic ErbB4/ErbB4 signaling	Trastuzumab monotherapy:[12,43] 7%Trastuzumab with anthracyclines:[13] 27%
Trastuzumab-emtansine (T-DM1)	Trastuzumab activity combined with intracellular delivery of a microtubule depolymerization agent (emtansine)	Unknown	Inhibits heterotypic ErbB2/ErbB4 signaling, but not homotypic ErbB4/ErbB4 signaling	T-DM1 monotherapy:[44] <2%
Pertuzumab	Inhibition of ErBb2/ErbB3 dimerization by binding domain II of the ErbB2 receptor	No	Inhibits heterotypic ErbB2/ErbB4 signaling, but not homotypic ErbB4/ErbB4 signaling	Pertuzumab monotherapy:[45] <7%
Lapatinib	Reversible tyrosine kinase inhibitor of EGFR/ErbB1 and ErbB2	Yes[46]	Inhibits heterotypic ErbB2/ErbB4 signaling, but not homotypic ErbB4/ErbB4 signaling	Lapatinib monotherapy:[47] <2%
Neratinib	Irreversible tyrosine kinase inhibitor of EGFR/ErbB1, ErbB2, and ErbB4	Unknown	Inhibits heterotypic ErbB2/ErbB4 signaling but not homotypic ErbB4/ErbB4 signaling	None reported[48,49]
Afatinib	Irreversible tyrosine kinase inhibitor of EGFR/ErbB1 and ErbB2	Unknown	Inhibits heterotypic ErbB2/ErbB4 signaling, but not homotypic ErbB4/ErbB4	None reported[50,51]
MM-111	A bispecific molecule targeting the ErbB2/ErbB3 heterodimer, forming an inactive complex	Unknown	No binding in the heart given absence of ErbB2/ErbB3 heterodimers	None

emtansine (Figure 5-4B). Trastuzumab targets ErbB2-positive tumors, whereas emtansine is a highly potent antimicrotubule drug.[19] This toxic effect is restricted to ErbB2-expressing cells and results in very little neuropathy and no hair loss.[20] T-DM1 has a better overall safety profile than trastuzumab. Its administration resulted in no clinically significant cardiotoxicity among patients previously treated with trastuzumab and a taxane.[21] Obviously, T-DM1 has never been tested in combination with anthracyclines.

■ Pertuzumab

The clinical picture ■ *Compared with placebo plus trastuzumab plus docetaxel, the combination of pertuzumab plus trastuzumab plus docetaxel, when used as first-line treatment for ErbB2-positive metastatic breast cancer, significantly prolongs progression-free survival. In the phase III randomized, double-blind, multinational CLEOPATRA trial, pertuzumab plus trastuzumab did not increase the incidence of cardiac toxic effects.[22] The combination of pertuzumab plus anthracyclines has not been tested.*

Pertuzumab is a monoclonal antibody binding to subdomain II of ErbB2, interfering specifically with ligand-induced ErbB2 dimerization (Figure 5-4).[1] This mechanism of action makes pertuzumab the perfect drug to be combined with trastuzumab, because it will complementarily inhibit the formation of ligand-induced ErbB2/ErbB3 oncogenic complexes arising after the upregulation of ErbB3 by trastuzumab.[15] This phenomenon most likely explains the success of the combination of trastuzumab and pertuzumab in clinical use: the survival of patients with metastatic breast cancer was prolonged when pertuzumab was added to therapy with trastuzumab and anthracyclines.[23]

In contrast to trastuzumab, pertuzumab will also interfere with physiological ligand-induced ErbB2 signaling, thereby potentially abrogating the protective actions of NRG-1 in the heart.[15] In fact, ErbB2 signaling may be abrogated more efficiently in non-amplified ErbB2 cells than in tumor cells, given the lower number of ERBB2 copies in non-amplified cells. However, pertuzumab does not impede ligand-induced homotypic signaling through ErbB4 homodimers. It seems plausible that, in the presence of pertuzumab and the reduced availability of ErbB2's dimerization arms, physiological NRG-1 signaling will shift toward ErbB4 homodimers. Pertuzumab may thus merely modify but not inhibit physiological ErbB signaling activity. These phenomena may explain why, in clinical trials, pertuzumab has emerged as a safe drug, associated with little or no cardiac toxicity.

■ Lapatinib

The clinical picture ■ *Lapatinib is generally reserved for late-stage treatment, and only in combination with capecitabine, for women with ErbB2-positive breast cancer that has progressed after previous chemotherapy with anthracycline, taxanes, and trastuzumab. When lapatinib is administered in combination with capecitabine, reversible decreases in left ventricular function occur.[24]*

Lapatinib is a small-molecule intracellular and reversible ErbB2 and EGFR/ErbB1 tyrosine kinase inhibitor (Figure 5-4).[1] As such, compared with trastuzumab, lapatinib has the advantage of inhibiting the phosphorylation of ErbB3 by ErbB2 in the oncogenic complex, independently of whether this complex was formed in a ligand-dependent or a ligand-independent manner. Hence, treatment with lapatinib alone leaves little room for the development of drug resistance through ligand-induced ErbB2/ErbB3 oncogenic complexes, thereby mimicking the combination of trastuzumab plus pertuzumab. Nevertheless, recent studies indicate that ErbB3 is upregulated in lapatinib-treated cells and that it may still form ErbB2/ErbB3 complexes with residually active ErbB2.[25]

With regard to its effect on physiological NRG-1/ErbB signaling, lapatinib clearly abrogates ligand-induced ErbB2 signaling, hence potentially interfering with NRG-1–induced signaling. Like pertuzumab, however, lapatinib should not interfere with ligand-induced ErbB4/ErbB4 homotypic signaling, a fact that may explain why lapatinib is associated with little or no cardiac toxicity.[26]

Afatinib and neratinib are second-generation irreversible tyrosine kinase inhibitors. Afatinib is highly selective for EGFR/ErbB1 and ErbB2, whereas neratinib also inhibits ErbB4, thus carrying the risk of blocking both homotypic and heterotypic signaling (Figure 5-4). Phase I and II trials have found that no clinically significant cardiac dysfunction is associated with afatinib and neratinib. These early cardiac safety data are promising.[26]

■ MM-111

MM-111 is a new bispecific antibody and polypeptide fusion protein consisting of two human single-chain variable fragment (scFv) antibodies linked to modified human serum albumin (Figure 5-4). The resulting molecule, MM-111, forms a trimeric complex with ErbB2 and ErbB3; in preclinical models it inhibits ErbB3 signaling and exhibits antitumor activity that is dependent on the overexpression of ErbB2.[25] By its design, MM-111 blocks the activity of ligand-dependent and ligand-independent ErbB2/ErbB3 complexes in tumor cells, hence recapitulating the effect achieved by combining trastuzumab and pertuzumab or lapatinib, albeit in a completely different manner. A recent study demonstrated that the ability of MM-111 to inhibit ligand-activated ErbB3 phosphorylation is superior to that of pertuzumab, and that the combination of MM-111 with trastuzumab more effectively inhibits tumor cell growth than does the combination of pertuzumab plus trastuzumab.[25] The underlying reason for this superiority is that pertuzumab merely indirectly inhibits ErbB3 activation by precluding ErbB2 dimerization. In tumor cells with a high number of copies of ERBB2, the inhibition of ErbB2 by pertuzumab may be incomplete. By contrast, MM-111 directly inactivates ErbB3.

An important advantage of MM-111 is its specific binding to ErbB2/ErbB3 complexes. Because these complexes are absent from or occur in small numbers in the heart with few or no physiological effects, it is very unlikely that MM-111 interferes with the physiological function of NRG-1 in the heart. Accordingly, at least from this perspective, the cardiotoxic profile of MM-111 should be safe.

CARDIOTOXICITY OF ANTI-ERBB2 SIGNALING: A MANIFESTATION OF CARDIAC ENDOTHELIAL IMPAIRMENT?

In the heart, most anti-ErbB2 drugs inhibit or at least modify ligand-dependent ErbB2 signaling, which is a factor underlying their potential cardiotoxicity. As explained above, MM-111 is an exception to this rule: by design it prefers tumor cells, not cardiac cells, because no ErbB2/ErbB3 heterodimers are present in the heart. Inhibition of ligand-dependent ErbB2 signaling by the other anti-ErbB3 drugs interferes with the physiological effects of NRG-1 in the heart, thereby creating a state of cardiac endothelial dysfunction.[27] NRG-1 is secreted by endothelial cells, and it also induces nitric oxide synthesis.[28] Hence, inhibition of NRG-1 signaling may affect multiple cardiac endothelial pathways. This pharmacologically induced endothelial impairment by anti-ErbB2 drugs may explain why cardiovascular risk factors such as

arterial hypertension and obesity, which also impair endothelial function, aggravate the risk of trastuzumab-induced cardiomyopathy.[27]

THE REVERSE SIDE OF THE COIN: CAN WE ACTIVATE ERBB SIGNALING TO TREAT HEART FAILURE WITHOUT INCREASING THE RISK OF CANCER?

As explained above, increased tissue concentrations of ErbB3 ligands, such as NRG-1, promote the formation of oncogenic ErbB2/ErbB3 heterodimers in ErbB2-amplified tumors and, as such, may initiate or accelerate tumor growth. This phenomenon creates a potential drawback in the use of NRG-1 to treat chronic diseases such as heart failure.

In an attempt to design a translationally relevant ErbB agonist for the treatment of chronic diseases such as heart failure, Griffith and Lee created bivalent NRG-1β (NN).[10,29] NN is a ligand of both ErbB3 and ErbB4 and drives particular homotypic interactions at the expense of others, thus leading to signaling and phenotypic outcomes that differ from those achieved with their native, monovalent counterparts. In tumor cells, NN drives a stable homotypic association of ErbB3, which traps ErbB3, keeping it away from undesirable oncogenic signaling with ErbB2. The kinase activity of ErbB3 is weak; therefore, ErbB3 homodimers cannot activate downstream signaling pathways (Figure 5-6, left panel). NN consistently induces antineoplastic or cytostatic responses in cancer cells.[10] In cardiac cells, NN predominantly promotes homotypic association of ErbB4, thereby reducing signaling through ErbB2/ErbB4 heterodimers (Figure 5-6, right panel). The differences in the mechanisms of action of monovalent NRG-1 and bivalent NN are summarized in Table 5-4. Subsequent studies have shown that NN significantly attenuates doxorubicin-induced cardiac dysfunction, a finding indicating that ErbB4 homodimer signaling suffices for cardioprotection or, alternatively, that enough ErbB2/ErbB4 signaling remains to support normal activity.[10]

Accordingly, given that the pro-neoplastic potential of NN is lower than that of recombinant human neuregulin 1 (rhNRG-1), NN has demonstrated translational potential for the treatment of chronic diseases such as heart failure, with no increased risk of the induction of cancer.

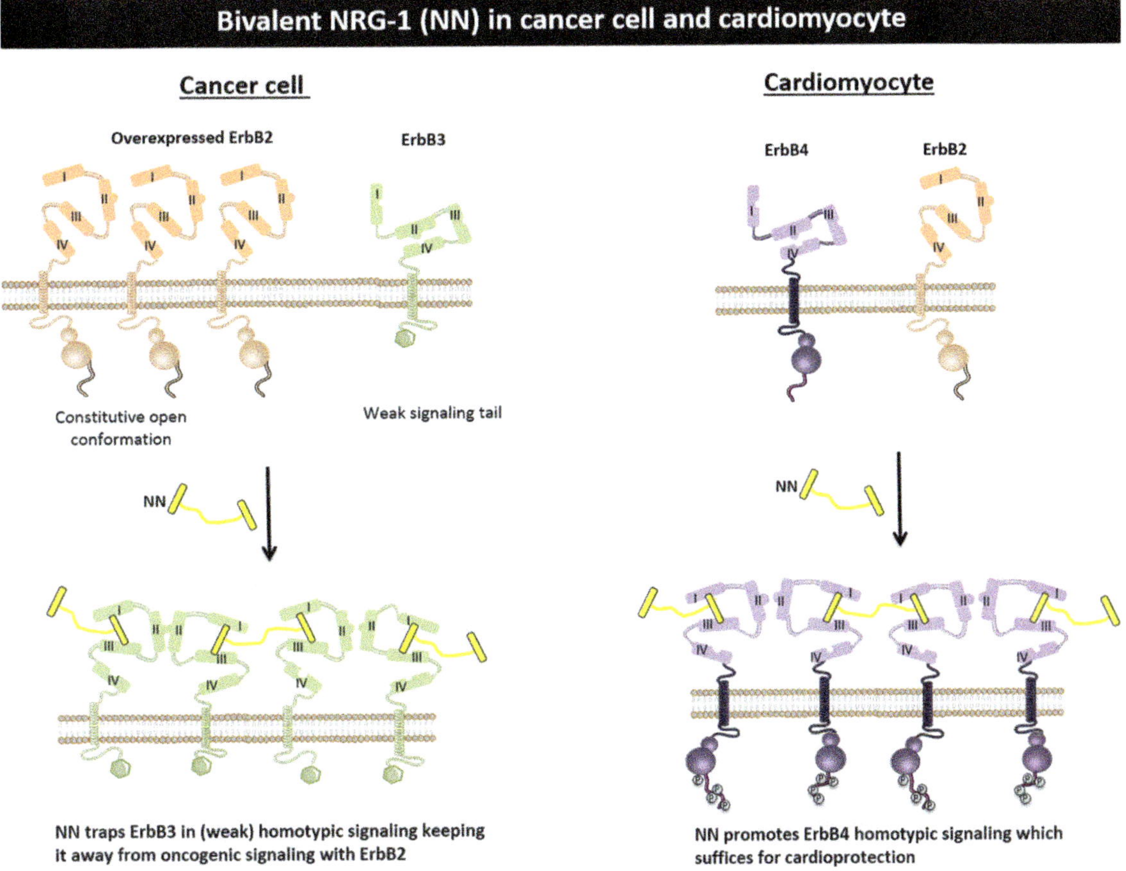

FIGURE 5-6 The effect of bivalent NRG-1β (NN) on ErbB2-overexpressing breast cancer cells and cardiomyocytes. Left: In tumor cells, NN drives a stable homotypic association of ErbB3, which traps ErbB3, keeping it away from undesirable oncogenic signaling with ErbB2. ErbB3 exerts weak kinase activity; therefore, hence ErbB3 homodimers are incapable of activating downstream signaling pathways. Consistently, NN induces antineoplastic or cytostatic responses in cancer cells. Right: In cardiac cells, NN predominantly promotes homotypic association of ErbB4, but signaling through ErbB2/ErbB4 heterodimers is reduced. ErbB4 homotypic signaling seems to be sufficient for cardioprotective signaling.

TABLE 5-4 Differences between monovalent NRG-1 and bivalent NRG-1 in mechanism of action

AGENT	TUMOR CELLS	CARDIAC CELLS
	ACTIVATORS	
	Mechanism of action	*Mechanism of action*
Neuregulin-1 (NRG-1)	NRG-1 stimulation may increase malignant potential of ErbB3-expressing cancer cells by inducing ErbB2 and ErbB3 heterotypic interactions	NRG-1 exerts cardioprotective effects by inducing ErbB2/Erbb4 heterotypic and ErbB4/ErbB4 homotypic interactions, initiating downstream signaling in cardiomyocytes
Bivalent NRG-1 (NN)	NN decreases migration, inhibits proliferation, and increases apoptosis in ErbB-expressing cancer cells by trapping ErbB3 for weak or non-signaling homotypic interactions	NN exerts cardioprotective effects via through ErbB4 homotypic signaling

CONCLUSIONS

The crucial position of ErbB2 at the crossroad between cancer and heart failure has made it an attractive therapeutic target in both oncology and cardiology. Increases in knowledge about ErbB2 and smart drug design have gradually led to the development of therapeutic agents that can target ErbB2 signaling in the appropriate cell type, allowing their safe use for patients with cancer and heart failure. These drugs are increasingly being introduced into the clinical setting, and the results of their use will indicate whether they can live up to the expectations of clinicians.

REFERENCES

1. De Keulenaer GW, Doggen K, Lemmens K. The vulnerability of the heart as a pluricellular paracrine organ: lessons from unexpected triggers of heart failure in targeted ErbB2 anticancer therapy. *Circ Res.* 2010;106(1):35–46.
2. Holbro T, Beerli RR, Maurer F, Koziczak M, Barbas CF 3rd, Hynes NE. The ErbB2/ErbB3 heterodimer functions as an oncogenic unit: ErbB2 requires ErbB3 to drive breast tumor cell proliferation. *Proc Natl Acad Sci USA.* 2003;100(15):8933–8938.
3. Schoeberl B, Pace EA, Fitzgerald JB, et al. Therapeutically targeting ErbB3: a key node in ligand-induced activation of the ErbB receptor-PI3K axis. *Sci Signal.* 2009;2(77):ra31.
4. Hudis CA. Trastuzumab—mechanism of action and use in clinical practice. *N Engl J Med.* 2007;357(1):39–51.
5. Sergina NV, Rausch M, Wang D, et al. Escape from HER-family tyrosine kinase inhibitor therapy by the kinase-inactive HER3. *Nature.* 2007;445(7126):437–441.
6. Garrett JT, Olivares MG, Rinehart C, et al. Transcriptional and posttranslational up-regulation of HER3 (ErbB3) compensates for inhibition of the HER2 tyrosine kinase. *Proc Natl Acad Sci USA.* 2011;108(12):5021–5026.
7. Ritter CA, Perez-Torres M, Rinehart C, et al. Human breast cancer cells selected for resistance to trastuzumab in vivo overexpress epidermal growth factor receptor and ErbB ligands and remain dependent on the ErbB receptor network. *Clin Cancer Res.* 2007;13(16):4909–4919.
8. Lemmens K, Doggen K, De Keulenaer GW. Role of neuregulin-1/ErbB signaling in cardiovascular physiology and disease: implications for therapy of heart failure. *Circulation.* 2007;116(8):954–960.
9. Odiete O, Hill MF, Sawyer DB. Neuregulin in cardiovascular development and disease. *Circ Res.* 2012;111(10):1376–1385.
10. Jay SM, Murthy AC, Hawkins JF, et al. An engineered bivalent neuregulin protects against doxorubicin-induced cardiotoxicity with reduced proneoplastic potential. *Circulation.* 2013;128(2):152–161.
11. Lemmens K, Doggen K, De Keulenaer GW. Activation of the neuregulin/ErbB system during physiological ventricular remodeling in pregnancy. *Am J Physiol.* 2011;300(3):H931–H942.
12. Seidman A, Hudis C, Pierri MK, et al. Cardiac dysfunction in the trastuzumab clinical trials experience. *J Clin Oncol.* 2002;20(5):1215–1221.
13. Slamon DJ, Leyland-Jones B, Shak S, et al. Use of chemotherapy plus a monoclonal antibody against HER2 for metastatic breast cancer that overexpresses HER2. *N Engl J Med.* 2001;344(11):783–792.
14. Bellinger AM, Arteaga CL, Force T, et al. Cardio-oncology: How new targeted cancer therapies and precision medicine can inform cardiovascular discovery. *Circulation.* 2015;132(23):2248–2258.
15. Junttila TT, Akita RW, Parsons K, et al. Ligand-independent HER2/HER3/PI3K complex is disrupted by trastuzumab and is effectively inhibited by the PI3K inhibitor GDC-0941. *Cancer Cell.* 2009;15(5):429–440.
16. Fedele C, Riccio G, Malara AE, D'Alessio G, De Lorenzo C. Mechanisms of cardiotoxicity associated with ErbB2 inhibitors. *Breast Cancer Res Treat.* 2012;134(2):595–602.
17. Hedhli N, Huang Q, Kalinowski A, et al. Endothelium-derived neuregulin protects the heart against ischemic injury. *Circulation* 2011;123(20):2254–2262.
18. Liu FF, Stone JR, Schuldt AJ, et al. Heterozygous knockout of neuregulin-1 gene in mice exacerbates doxorubicin-induced heart failure. *Am J Physiol* 2005;289(2):H660–H666.
19. Lambert JM, Chari RV. Ado-trastuzumab Emtansine (T-DM1): an antibody-drug conjugate (ADC) for HER2-positive breast cancer. *J Med Chem.* 2014;57(16):6949–6964.
20. Eisenstein M. Medicine: Eyes on the target. *Nature.* 2015;527(7578):S110–S112.
21. Hurvitz SA, Kakkar R. The potential for trastuzumab emtansine in human epidermal growth factor receptor 2 positive metastatic breast cancer: latest evidence and ongoing studies. *Ther Adv Med Oncol.* 2012;4(5):235–245.
22. Swain SM, Baselga J, Kim SB, et al. Pertuzumab, trastuzumab, and docetaxel in HER2-positive metastatic breast cancer. *N Engl J Med.* 2015;372(8):724–734.
23. Cortés J, Fumoleau P, Bianchi GV, et al. Pertuzumab monotherapy after trastuzumab-based treatment and subsequent reintroduction of trastuzumab: activity and tolerability in patients with advanced human epidermal growth factor receptor 2-positive breast cancer. *J Clin Oncol.* 2012;30(14):1594–1600.
24. Cameron D, Casey M, Press M, et al. A phase III randomized comparison of lapatinib plus capecitabine versus capecitabine alone in women with advanced breast cancer that has progressed on trastuzumab: updated efficacy and biomarker analyses. *Breast Cancer Res Treat.* 2008;112(3):533–543.
25. McDonagh CF, Huhalov A, Harms BD, et al. Antitumor activity of a novel bispecific antibody that targets the ErbB2/ErbB3 oncogenic unit and inhibits heregulin-induced activation of ErbB3. *Mol Cancer Ther.* 2012;11(3):582–593.

26. Sendur MA, Aksoy S, Altundag K. Cardiotoxicity of novel HER2-targeted therapies. *Curr Med Res Opin.* 2013;29(8):1015–1024.

27. Sandoo A, Kitas GD, Carmichael AR. Endothelial dysfunction as a determinant of trastuzumab-mediated cardiotoxicity in patients with breast cancer. *Anticancer Res.* 2014;34(3):1147–1151.

28. Lemmens K, Fransen P, Sys SU, Brutsaert DL, De Keulenaer GW. Neuregulin-1 induces a negative inotropic effect in cardiac muscle: role of nitric oxide synthase. *Circulation.* 2004;109(3):324–326.

29. Jay SM, Kurtagic E, Alvarez LM, et al. Engineered bivalent ligands to bias ErbB receptor-mediated signaling and phenotypes. *J Biol Chem.* 2011;286(31):27729–27740.

30. Liu X, Gu X, Li Z, et al. Neuregulin-1/erbB-activation improves cardiac function and survival in models of ischemic, dilated, and viral cardiomyopathy. *J Am Coll Cardiol.* 2006;48(7):1438–1447.

31. Bersell K, Arab S, Haring B, Kühn B. Neuregulin1/ErbB4 signaling induces cardiomyocyte proliferation and repair of heart injury. *Cell.* 2009;138(2):257–270.

32. Gu X, Liu X, Xu D, et al. Cardiac functional improvement in rats with myocardial infarction by up-regulating cardiac myosin light chain kinase with neuregulin. *Cardiovasc Res.* 2010;88(2):334–343.

33. Guo YF, Zhang XX, Liu Y, Duan HY, Jie BZ, Wu XS. Neuregulin-1 attenuates mitochondrial dysfunction in a rat model of heart failure. *Chin Med J (Engl).* 2012;125(5):807–814.

34. Xiao J, Li B, Zheng Z, et al. Therapeutic effects of neuregulin-1 gene transduction in rats with myocardial infarction. *Coron Artery Dis.* 2012;23(7):460–468.

35. Galindo CL, Kasasbeh E, Murphy A, et al. Anti-remodeling and anti-fibrotic effects of the neuregulin-1β glial growth factor 2 in a large animal model of heart failure. *J Am Heart Assoc.* 2014;3(5):e000773.

36. Fang SJ, Wu XS, Han ZH, et al. Neuregulin-1 preconditioning protects the heart against ischemia/reperfusion injury through a PI3K/Akt-dependent mechanism. *Chin Med J.* 2010;123(24):3597–3604.

37. Bian Y, Sun M, Silver M, et al. Neuregulin-1 attenuated doxorubicin-induced decrease in cardiac troponins. *Am J Physiol.* 2009;297(6):H1974–H1983.

38. Li J, Gu XH, Duan JC, Zeng L, Li Y, Wang L. [Effects of recombined human neuregulin on the contractibility of cardiac muscles of rhesus monkeys with pacing-induced heart failure]. *Sichuan Da Xue Xue Bao Yi Xue Ban.* 2007;38(1):105–108.

39. Li B, Zheng Z, Wei Y, et al. Therapeutic effects of neuregulin-1 in diabetic cardiomyopathy rats. *Cardiovasc Diabetol.* 2011;10:69.

40. Li B, Xiao J, Li Y, Zhang J, Zeng M. Gene transfer of human neuregulin-1 attenuates ventricular remodeling in diabetic cardiomyopathy rats. *Exp Ther Med.* 2013;6(5):1105–1112.

41. Gao R, Zhang J, Cheng L, et al. A Phase II, randomized, double-blind, multicenter, based on standard therapy, placebo-controlled study of the efficacy and safety of recombinant human neuregulin-1 in patients with chronic heart failure. *J Am Coll Cardiol.* 2010;55(18):1907–1914.

42. Jabbour A, Hayward CS, Keogh AM, et al. Parenteral administration of recombinant human neuregulin-1 to patients with stable chronic heart failure produces favourable acute and chronic haemodynamic responses. *Eur J Heart Fail.* 2011;13(1):83–92.

43. Suter TM, Procter M, van Veldhuisen DJ, et al. Trastuzumab-associated cardiac adverse effects in the herceptin adjuvant trial. *J Clin Oncol.* 2007;25(25):3859–3865.

44. Verma S, Miles D, Gianni L, et al. Trastuzumab emtansine for HER2-positive advanced breast cancer. *N Engl J Med.* 2012;367(19):1783–1791.

45. Lenihan D, Suter T, Brammer M, Neate C, Ross G, Baselga J. Pooled analysis of cardiac safety in patients with cancer treated with pertuzumab. *Ann Oncol.* 2012;23(3):791–800.

46. D'Amato V, Raimondo L, Formisano L, et al. Mechanisms of lapatinib resistance in HER2-driven breast cancer. *Cancer Treat Rev.* 2015;41(10):877–883.

47. Perez EA, Koehler M, Byrne J, Preston AJ, Rappold E, Eser MS. Cardiac safety of lapatinib: pooled analysis of 3689 patients enrolled in clinical trials. *Mayo Clin Proc.* 2008;83(6):679–686.

48. Burstein HJ, Sun Y, Dirix LH, et al. Neratinib, an irreversible ErbB receptor tyrosine kinase inhibitor, in patients with advanced ErbB2-positive breast cancer. *J Clin Oncol.* 2010;28(8):1301–1307.

49. Segovia-Mendoza M, González-González ME, Barrera D, Diaz L, Garcia-Becerra R. Efficacy and mechanism of action of the tyrosine kinase inhibitors gefitinib, lapatinib and neratinib in the treatment of HER2-positive breast cancer: preclinical and clinical evidence. *Am J Cancer Res.* 2015;5(9):2531–2561.

50. Lin NU, Winer EP, Wheatley D, et al. A phase II study of afatinib (BIBW 2992), an irreversible ErbB family blocker, in patients with HER2-positive metastatic breast cancer progressing after trastuzumab. *Breast Cancer Res Treat.* 2012;133(3):1057–1065.

51. Yap TA, Vidal L, Adam J, et al. Phase I trial of the irreversible EGFR and HER2 kinase inhibitor BIBW 2992 in patients with advanced solid tumors. *J Clin Oncol.* 2010;28(25):3965–3972.

6 Checkpoint Inhibitors

Lavanya Kondapalli ▪ *Rupal O'Quinn* ▪ *Joseph R. Carver*

INTRODUCTION

According to Merriam-Webster, the immune system is "the bodily system that protects the body from foreign substances, cells, and tissues by producing the immune response and that includes especially the thymus, spleen, lymph nodes, special deposits of lymphoid tissue (as in the gastrointestinal tract and bone marrow), macrophages, lymphocytes including the B cells and T cells, and antibodies."[1] This network enables the body to recognize and defend itself against bacteria, viruses, and substances that appear foreign and harmful, such as cancer. The most important cells involved in the immune process are T cells or T lymphocytes that act as scavengers to detect and fight infection and disease, and B cells that produce antibodies.

T cells have receptors on their surface. Other cells, called antigen-presenting cells (APCs), can attach to these receptors and activate the T cell to target and destroy cancer. Immune checkpoints are inhibitory proteins that prevent this immune response from attacking normal cells or, in other words, prevent the body from attacking itself, a process known as autoimmunity. T-cell proliferation is an early part of the immune response occurring in the lymph nodes, whereas much of the actual suppression occurs in peripheral tissue, processes that Buchbinder and Desai have termed the *priming* phase in lymph nodes and the *effector* phase in peripheral tissue.[2] Two immune checkpoints, cytotoxic T lymphocyte–associated antigen 4 (CTLA-4), which is present in the lymph nodes, and programmed cell death 1 (PD-1) protein, which is found in peripheral tissue, have important implications for cancer and cancer treatment.[3–5]

To avoid antitumor immunity, cancer cells adapt and create an immunosuppressive environment by co-opting and manipulating immune checkpoints to evade immune system attack. These cancer cells can bind to CTLA-4 to reduce T-cell activation or can aberrantly express PD-1, which allows them to bind to T cells, causing downregulation and T-cell apoptosis, thereby facilitating their own (cancer cell) survival.[6]

The development of immune checkpoint inhibitors (ICPI) targeting CTLA-4 and PD-1 has created a successful new strategy in anticancer therapy. These immune checkpoint inhibitors interfere with the ability of cancer cells to evade T cell–mediated death. Currently, six checkpoint inhibitors are approved by the U.S. Food and Drug Administration (FDA): one CTLA-4 inhibitor, ipilimumab, and five PD-1/programmed cell-death ligand 1 (PD-L1) pathway inhibitors: nivolumab, pembrolizumab, atezolizumab, avelumab, and durvalumab. Others are under development. Although checkpoint inhibitors have led to disease remission, they are also associated with immune-related adverse events. Many of these events are treatable, although rare and serious cardiac adverse events, such as fulminant myocarditis resulting in death, have been reported.[7] In this chapter we will present an overview of the mechanism of action of the currently available checkpoint inhibitors, discuss their potential for cardiac adverse events, and propose a management strategy for recognizing and managing cardiotoxicity.

ROLE OF IMMUNE CHECKPOINTS IN NORMAL IMMUNITY

T cells or T lymphocytes are white blood cells that help protect against infection, and it is understood that the immune system can mount a cytotoxic response to kill cancer cells.[8] Figure 6-1 presents a simplified schematic illustrating the normal response.

Antigen is presented to the T cell by APCs. Costimulation of the T-cell receptor (TCR) and CD28 on the T cell and of the major histocomptability complex (MHC) and B7 on the APC leads to T-cell activation and proliferation and to interleukin 2 (IL-2) secretion and an immune response.[6]

Before and during the initial T-cell activation, a potential checkpoint (CTLA-4) is dormant. After activation, intracellular CTLA-4 moves to the cell surface and is upregulated to provide a negative feedback loop that prevents damage to normal tissue. It then binds with B7 on the APC. This inhibitory signaling leads to T-cell anergy, apoptosis, and decreased IL-2 production, as illustrated in Figure 6-2.[2–6]

Another checkpoint occurs in peripheral tissues engaging PD-1, which is expressed on T cells, and the associated programmed cell death ligand 1 (PD-L1) or programmed cell death ligand 2 (PD-L2), both of which are expressed by APCs on cancer cells (Figure 6-3).

The end result of engaging these two checkpoints is downregulation of the immune response with dampening of the immune system response.

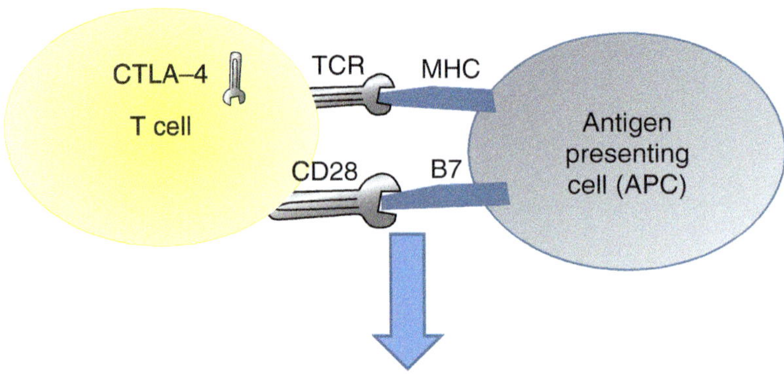

FIGURE 6-1 T-Cell activation and proliferation. APC, antigen-presenting cell; CTLA-4, cytotoxic T lymphocyte–associated antigen 4; MHC, major histocompatibility complex; TCR, T-cell receptor.

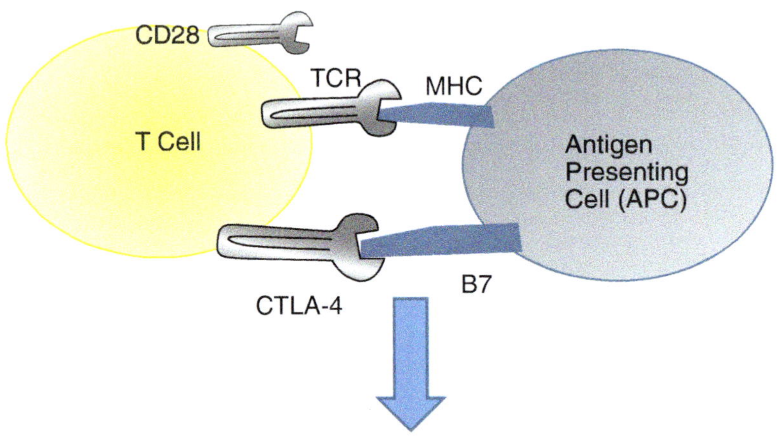

FIGURE 6-2 T-cell inactivation. APC, antigen-presenting cell; CTLA-4, cytotoxic T lymphocyte–associated antigen 4; MHC, major histocompatibility complex; TCR, T-cell receptor.

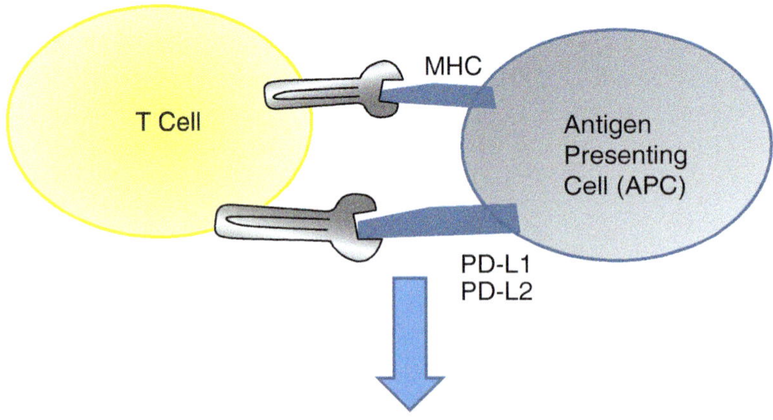

FIGURE 6-3 T cell inactivation. APC, antigen-presenting cell; CTLA-4, cytotoxic T lymphocyte–associated antigen 4; MHC, major histocompatibility complex; PD-1, programmed cell death 1; PD-L1, programmed cell death ligand 1; TCR, T-cell receptor.

ROLE OF CHECKPOINTS IN CANCER

As previously mentioned, cancer cells can co-opt the CTLA-4 and PD-L1/PD-L2 checkpoints to reduce the immune response and evade destruction by the immune system.

■ Targeting Checkpoints to Treat Cancer

Because tumor cells can manipulate checkpoints to prevent their own T cell–mediated death, checkpoints are an attractive target of anticancer therapy. CTLA-4 and PD-L1 blockade can increase the number of activated T cells to yield an antitumor response. The first checkpoint inhibitors developed were monoclonal antibodies that targeted CTLA-4. By inhibiting the binding of CTLA-4 to APCs via B7-1 (CD80)/B7-2 (CD 86), checkpoint inhibitors promote the immune activity of T cells. Antibodies that inhibit the production of PD-1 and the PD-L1 ligand have also been developed, and they result in increased cytokine production and T cell–mediated death of the cancer cell.[4,6]

CLINICALLY AVAILABLE CHECKPOINT INHIBITORS OF CTLA-4

■ Ipilimumab

Ipilimumab (Yervoy) is a human immunoglobulin G1 (IgG1) monoclonal antibody that blocks CTLA-4. In phase III randomized clinical trials in 2011, ipilimumab was the first FDA-approved checkpoint inhibitor and the first systemic therapy to show a long-term survival benefit that was durable in 10%–20% of patients with advanced melanoma.[9–11] As adjuvant therapy for patients with resected metastatic melanoma, ipilimumab resulted in a 64% survival benefit compared with a 54.4% survival benefit with placebo.[12] Clinical trials for other solid malignancies, including non-small-cell lung, prostate, and pancreatic cancer, are under way.

CLINICALLY AVAILABLE CHECKPOINT INHIBITORS OF PD-1

■ Pembrolizumab

Pembrolizumab (Keytruda) is a monoclonal antibody that binds to PD-1. Pembrolizumab is currently approved by the FDA for treating melanoma, non-small-cell lung cancer, squamous cell cancer of the head and neck, and classic Hodgkin lymphoma. The KEYNOTE-001 study treated 411 advanced malignant melanoma patients with pembrolizumab and followed them up for a median of 18 months. The treatment response rate was 34%, and the median overall survival time was 25.9 months. The response rate was maintained for 81% of the responding patients.[13]

Another study used pembrolizumab to treat 495 patients with non-small-cell lung cancer. The objective response rate was 19.4%, and the median duration of response was 12.5 months. The median duration of progression-free survival was 3.7 months, and the median duration of overall survival was 12.0 months.[14] These studies demonstrated a durable overall benefit.

■ Nivolumab

Nivolumab (Opdivo) is a human IgG4 monoclonal antibody that blocks the PD-1 receptor. Nivolumab has a wide range of approved indications, including the treatment of unresectable or metastatic melanoma, metastatic non-small-cell lung cancer, advanced renal cell cancer, relapsed or refractory classic Hodgkin lymphoma, recurrent or metastatic head and neck cancer, locally advanced or metastatic urothelial cancer, and microsatellite instability-high or mismatch repair–deficient metastatic colorectal cancer. Nivolumab is also approved in combination with ipilimumab to treat unresectable or metastatic melanoma. The Checkmate 066 trial randomly assigned 418 patients with previously untreated melanoma without the BRAF mutation to receive either nivolumab or dacarbazine. The response rate was 72.9% (95% confidence interval [CI], 65.5–78.9; P<0.001) for the nivolumab group and 42.1% (95% CI, 33.0–50.9; P<0.001) for the dacarbazine group (hazard ratio for death, 0.42; 99.79% CI, 0.25–0.73; P<0.001).[15] The randomized double-blind phase 3 CheckMate 067 trial randomly assigned 945 previously untreated patients with unresectable stage III or IV melanoma to receive (in a 1:1:1 ratio) nivolumab alone, nivolumab plus ipilimumab, or ipilimumab alone. Nivolumab alone or with ipilimumab was associated with significantly longer progression-free survival times, and combination therapy was more effective than either drug alone for treating patients with PD-1–negative tumors.[16] Similarly, a double-blind trial used a combination of ipilimumab and nivolumab to treat 142 patients with previously untreated metastatic melanoma. The treatment resulted in a significantly higher objective-response rate and a longer progression-free survival time than did ipilimumab alone.[17]

CLINICALLY AVAILABLE CHECKPOINT INHIBITORS OF PD-L1

■ Atezolizumab

Atezolizumab (Tecentriq) is a monoclonal antibody against PD-L1. It was the first FDA-approved anti–PD-L1 checkpoint inhibitor. Currently, it is approved for the treatment of locally advanced or metastatic urothelial cancer and metastatic non-small-cell lung cancer. A multicenter phase 2 trial using atezolizumab to treat 385 patients with advanced or metastatic urothelial carcinoma found an overall response rate of 15%.[18]

■ Avelumab

Avelumab (Bavensio) is a fully human monoclonal antibody against PD-L1. Currently, it is approved for metastatic Merkel cell carcinoma and locally advanced or metastatic urothelial carcinoma that has progressed after platinum-based chemotherapy. Approval was based on two Avelumab in Non-Small Cell Lung Cancer (JAVELIN) trials that treated 1738 patients with an overall response rate of 30%.[19–20]

■ Durvalumab

Durvalumab (Imfinzi) is a human IgG1 monoclonal antibody that blocks PD-L1 and prevents its binding to PD-1 and CD80. Currently, durvalumab is approved for unresectable or metastatic urothelial carcinoma that has progressed after platinum-based chemotherapy.

Approval was based on one single-arm trial involving 182 patients. The confirmed objective response rate, as assessed by blinded independent central review per **Response Evaluation Criteria in Solid Tumors** (RECIST) 1.1, was 17.0% (95% CI, 11.9–23.3).[21,22]

Figure 6-4 illustrates the currently available immune checkpoint inhibitors.

ADMINISTRATION

All approved checkpoint inhibitors are administered as intravenous infusions. For patients with baseline cardiac disease for whom fluid volume is a concern, it is important to know the relative volume of fluid infused for each drug, as illustrated in Table 6-1.

IMMUNE-RELATED ADVERSE EVENTS

■ Common Adverse Events

Unrestrained T-cell activation with immune checkpoint blockade translates into antitumor responses but can also lead to toxicity. Checkpoint inhibitors are associated with immune-related adverse events

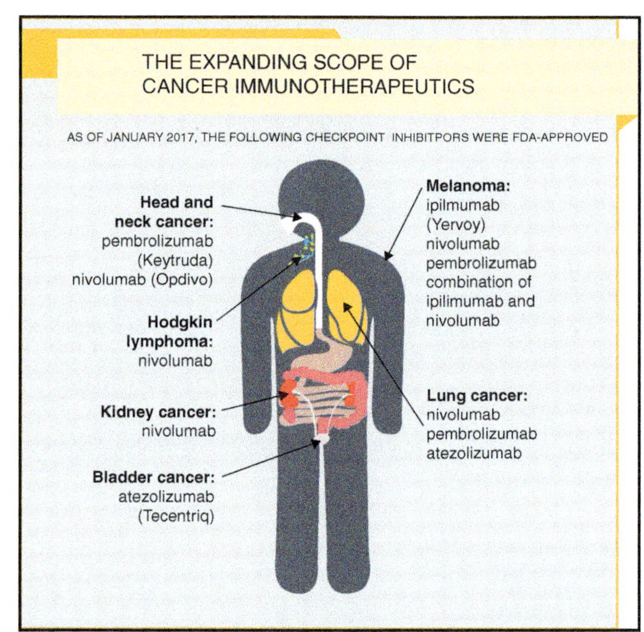

FIGURE 6-4   The available checkpoint inhibitors.

Table 6-1   Checkpoint inhibitor administration

CHECKPOINT INHIBITOR	AMOUNT OF FLUID	INFUSION TIME
Ipilimumab	100 cc NSS* or 5% dextrose	90 min
Pembrolizumab	50 cc NSS	30 min
Nivolumab	50 cc NSS	60 min
Atezolizumab	250 cc NSS	60 min for first dose, 30 min thereafter if well tolerated
Avelumab	250 cc NSS or 0.45 NSS	60 min
Durvalumab	250 cc NSS	60 min

*NSS=0.9%

NSS, normal saline solution

(irAEs) that may occur in as many as 72% of patients and can affect every organ system of the body, as illustrated in Figure 6-4.[23,24] PD-1–blocking antibodies have a more favorable safety profile than do CTLA-4–blocking antibodies, probably because of where they work: PD-1 blockade occurs primarily in the periphery, i.e., within the tumor microenvironment, whereas CTLA-4 blockade occurs mainly in lymphoid tissue. This difference in location helps to explain the quantitative differences in the adverse-effect profiles of ipilimumab and the anti–PD-1 or anti–DL-1 drugs. The most frequent adverse events reported with both classes of checkpoint inhibitors are mild fatigue, rash, pruritus, diarrhea, and colitis. Given the pervasive nature of checkpoints in the immune system, irAEs may occur in every organ system (Figure 6-5). For example, depending on the drug used, the following irAEs have been reported: pneumonitis, colitis, hepatitis, pancreatitis, endocrinopathies (thyroid, pituitary insufficiency, adrenal insufficiency, Type 1 diabetes as a consequence of the immune attack on the beta cells of the pancreas), nephritis, ocular inflammation, dermatologic reactions (reticular lesions, erythematous maculopapular rash, mucositis, Stevens-Johnson syndrome, toxic epidermal necrolysis), and a variety of musculoskeletal/rheumatologic issues (myositis, arthralgia, rheumatoid arthritis, polymyalgia rheumatica, psoriatic arthritis, vasculitis, sicca syndrome) and neurological reactions (encephalitis, myasthenia gravis, Guillain-Barré syndrome), as well as severe infusion reactions that can cause systemic collapse.

Immune-related adverse events are typically grade 1 or 2 and are usually reversible with early recognition and appropriate treatment, often not necessitating drug discontinuation.[18,25–27]

Dermatologic toxicity is frequent and occurs early, usually during the first weeks after initiation of treatment. Organ toxicity (liver, gastrointestinal, lung) occurs later (6–8 weeks) after treatment initiation, and endocrinopathies are more common after the second month of treatment.[28] Another curious phenomenon associated with these drugs is the late onset of toxicity after completion of treatment.[29] Among the irAEs, dermatologic toxicity is most common and occurs with the earliest onset. Colitis is associated with the highest clinical impact; its onset occurs weeks later than that of dermatitis.[4,25,26,28,29]

The severity of adverse events is graded according to the National Cancer Institute's Common Terminology Criteria for Adverse Events (CTCAE), version 4.[30] In general, treatment is temporarily withheld for grade 1 or 2 (mild to moderate) reactions and can be discontinued for severe or life-threatening reactions (grade 3 or 4). Because these irAEs arise from an enhanced immunologic response, reactive immunosuppression with high-dose corticosteroids has been the first step in pharmacologic management. Because all of the checkpoint inhibitors have long elimination half-lives, ranging from 15 to 25 days,[31] the occurrence of an irAE establishes a potentially prolonged period of risk that requires surveillance and treatment until the drugs are totally eliminated. A recently published collaborative position paper outlined in detail the management of irAEs associated with the blockade of an immune checkpoint.[32]

Cardiac Adverse Events

In the clinical trials that led to FDA approval of ipilimumab, cardiac events were uncommon, occurring in fewer than 1% of all treated patients.[7] An analysis of phase 3 trials involving 5,347 patients found 10 (0.19%) reported cases of cardiovascular toxicity.[33] A pharmacovigilance registry at Gustave Roussy, which enrolled 388 patients over an 18-month period, listed only one cardiac event (atrial fibrillation) and no cases of heart failure or heart block.[34] As a result, cardiac monitoring has not been routinely recommended for patients undergoing treatment with these agents. However, in clinical practice, checkpoint inhibitors have been associated with potentially fatal, although rare, cardiac events.[7,12,16,34–39] Table 6-2 shows a compilation of reported checkpoint inhibitor–mediated cardiac events.[7,12,16,25,34–51]

NON-CARDIAC SIDE EFFECTS OF IMMUNE CHECKPOINT INHIBITOR THERAPY

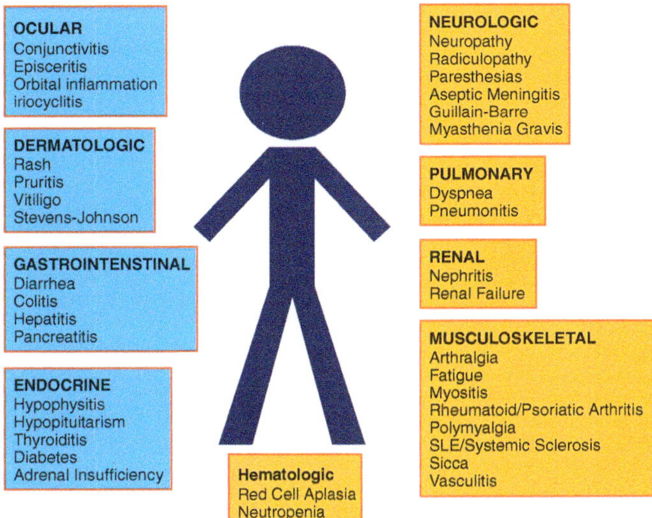

FIGURE 6-5 Noncardiac side effects of immune checkpoint inhibitor therapy.

Table 6-2 Overview of reported cardiac irAEs

TUMOR TYPE	TREATMENT	ONSET (WEEKS)	EVENT	OUTCOME	REF
Melanoma	IPI	16	Myocarditis		Voskens[18]
Melanoma	IPI	NR	Myocardits	Death	Eggermont[22]
Melanoma	IPI	12	Takotsubo/SVT/VT		Geisler[23]
Melanoma	IPI (prior PEMBRO)	15	Myocarditis/VA		Laubli[24]
Melanoma	IPI	21	Pericarditis		Yun[25]
Melanoma	IPI	NR	CA	Death	Larkin[11]
Melanoma	IPI/NIVO	12 days 15 days	Chest pain, fatigue, myalgia, Myocarditis AVB, VT	Death Death	Johnson[26]
Melanoma	IPI/NIVO IPI IPI IPI IPI IPI PEMBRO IPI	22 12 4 22 31 5 20 5	Myocarditis,thyroiditis/ hypophysitis Cardiomyopathy Myocardial fibrosis, Hepatitis CHF, colitis, hypophysitis Myocarditis, Uveitis Myocarditis CA, ?Takotsubo, AF, BBB Myocarditis, Hepatitis	Death Death Death	Heinzerling[2,7]
Melanoma	IPI/NIVO	3	Chest pain, Myocarditis,	Hospice	Mehta[28]
Melanoma	NIVO	8	Myocarditis		Takadoro[29]
Melanoma	NIVO	NR	Myocarditis, AF		Koelzer[30]
Melanoma	IPI	18	Myocarditis , chest pain, AF, VT	Death	Roth[31]
Melanoma	PEMBRO	10 7 2 2-5 17	Angina Sinus tach (Thyroid) HBP AF-then Myocarditis/VF Asystole, ?Takaotsubo	Death	Zimmer[32]
NSCLC	NIVO	18	Myocarditis		Semper[33]
NSCLC	NIVO	3	Myocarditis, AV Block, BBB		Gibson[40]
Melanoma	IPI/NIVO	10 days	Myocarditis, BBB, AV Block		Jain[35]
Relapsed CML	IPI	7 days 15 days	Colitis (7 days of steroids) Myocarditis , AVB, BBB, Myositis	Death	Berg[36]
Melanoma	NIVO	2	Myocarditis, AVB, Myositis	Death	Behling[37]
Sarcoma	IPI/NIVO	2	Myocarditis, AVB, Myositis		Reddy[38]
NSCLC	NIVO	7 days 7 days	CHF (steroids-2 month taper) Rechallenge Myocarditis		Chuahan[34]

TUMOR TYPE	TREATMENT	ONSET (WEEKS)	EVENT	OUTCOME	REF
uNSCLC	NIVO	24 days 6	New DM Myocarditis, VT	Death	Matson[39]
NSCLC	DURV	NR	MI (5),CA (1), CHF (4), pericardial effusion (2), HBP (1), VT (1)		Antonio[67]

IPI, ipilimumab; PEMBRO, pembrolizimab; NIVO, nilumab; DURV, durvalumab; AF, atrial fibrillation; AVB, A-V block; BBB, bundle branch block; CA, cardiac arrest; CHF,congestive heart failure; HBP, hypertension; MI, myocardial infarction; VT, ventricular tachycardia; VF, ventricular fibrillation; NR, not reported.

It is very possible that cardiotoxicity has been underreported in clinical trials because of nuances in the recognition and adjudication of toxicity (an adverse event may be reported as a toxicity, e.g., a patient presents with heart block, and that condition is coded rather than the underlying or precipitating myocarditis) and because coexisting but subtle cardiotoxicity may have been missed (see below).

The presentation of cardiac toxicity is highly variable and may take the form of any of the following (of note, QT prolongation has not been a problem):

1. Classic heart failure with some combination of progressive dyspnea, weight gain, edema, and fatigue.

2. Conduction system disease as detected by electrocardiogram (ECG) and including new atrioventricular (AV) block, bundle branch block, or both. These changes are often asymptomatic and, when new, may be a harbinger of future overt myocarditis.

3. Palpitations, atrial and ventricular arrhythmias (atrial fibrillation [AF], ventricular tachycardia [VT], ventricular fibrillation [VF]), cardiac arrest with or without full-blown myocarditis, or incessant electrical instability that may be hemodynamically significant.

4. Chest and arm pain upon infusion. Consistently, coronary arteriography has shown no evidence of obstructive epicardial coronary artery disease (CAD), although several case reports of Takotsubo stress cardiomyopathy have been published.

5. Pericarditis with chest pain, typical ECG changes, and associated pericardial effusion. This may be isolated inflammation and may occur in the absence of myocarditis.

6. Aggravation of underlying hypertension, CAD, and baseline compensated heart failure.

The onset of cardiac irAEs is highly variable; they can occur at any time from the day after the initial infusion to 32 weeks after the initiation of treatment. These events have been reported by patients taking ipilimumab, pembrolizumab, nivolumab, or durvalumab. Early ECG findings may be new conduction abnormalities, new resting sinus tachycardia, or nonspecific changes in ST or T waves. The ECG may appear normal early in the course of treatment and may not show a clinically significant reduction in left ventricular (LV) systolic function. Consistently, troponin or N-terminal pro-brain natriuretic peptide (NT-proBNP) concentrations are elevated and may be the first markers of the development of cardiomyopathy or myocarditis.[33,36,46] There is no association between the risk for irAEs and the underlying malignancy.

One consistent finding has been that cardiac toxicity occurs more frequently when drugs are used in combination and typically occurs earlier after treatment initiation than does toxicity associated with monotherapy. An analysis of Bristol-Myers Squibb corporate databases up to April 2016 showed that the incidence of myocarditis was 0.09% among 20,594 patients being treated with nivolumab, ipilimumab, or both.[7] The combination of nivolumab and ipilimumab was associated with more-frequent and more-severe cases of myocarditis than was nivolumab alone.[7] Curiously, isolated myocarditis with no other noncardiac immune toxicity is unusual. In the cases reported, noncardiac irAEs may accompany myocarditis, but there is no consistent association between immune toxicities.

The actual incidence of cardiac irAEs may be historically underestimated. Because cardiac biomarkers are not routinely measured and ECGs are not routinely performed during checkpoint inhibitor therapy, it is possible that asymptomatic cases of cardiac toxicity have been missed, especially when they occur in the setting of other immune-mediated toxicity. In such cases, immune-mediated toxicity becomes the clinical focus of treatment and actually has a dual benefit: treating the primary issue and managing the possibly unrecognized cardiac immune toxicity. In this scenario, subtle cardiac symptoms, such as fatigue, also improve with the administration of high-dose steroids and the withdrawal of checkpoint inhibitors. Given the potential severity of cardiac irAEs, clinicians must have a heightened suspicion for them and should evaluate patients for cardiac causes when they present with noncardiac toxicities of checkpoint therapy.

The following case report illustrates several important clinical features of checkpoint inhibitor cardiac toxicity.

A 53-year-old woman was found to have metastatic ovarian cancer. She completed neoadjuvant chemotherapy with carboplatin/paclitaxel, followed by hysterectomy/oophorectomy. She then underwent two cycles of adjuvant pembrolizumab. Ten days after her last infusion of pembrolizumab, she presented with transient facial droop and slurred speech and was admitted for management of suspected stroke. Magnetic resonance imaging (MRI) of the brain showed no acute lesion. Troponin T levels were elevated at 0.653 ng/mL, and creatine kinase (CK) activity was 1319 U/L; these levels were believed to be related to pembrolizumab administration. Echocardiogram showed a left ventricular ejection fraction (LVEF) of 55%. The patient was treated with prednisone (2 mg/kg daily) for pembrolizumab-induced cranial nerve neuropathy and asymptomatic myocarditis as indicated by the elevated levels of cardiac biomarkers.

Symptoms improved promptly but returned after rapid tapering of the steroid dosage. The patient was readmitted with chest pain and shortness of breath. Electrocardiogram showed a new left bundle branch block. Telemetry indicated hemodynamically stable ventricular tachycardia, and a repeat ECG showed that LVEF had decreased to 35%. Creatinine kinase activity and troponin levels continued to trend higher. Coronary arteriography demonstrated no epicardial obstructive coronary artery disease. The patient declined myocardial biopsy. The results of cardiac MRI were consistent with a diagnosis of myocarditis. In spite of treatment with metoprolol, captopril, 1 mg/kg steroids IV, and antiarrhythmic therapy with dofetilide, lidocaine, and amiodarone, she experienced persistent ventricular tachycardia.

Electrical instability prompted treatment with high-dose steroids (1000 mg/day for 3 days), and ventricular tachycardia promptly ceased. The prednisone dosage was reduced to 2 mg/kg per day; however, 1 day after the reduction of this maintenance dose, the arrhythmia returned. Troponin levels continued to be elevated.

Although the medical literature contained conflicting efficacy data for infliximab (5 mg/kg), the patient was treated with this monoclonal antibody because of its efficacy in treating immune-mediated colitis. This treatment

resulted in cessation of ventricular tachycardia. The patient was discharged with a maintenance dosage of steroids (2 mg/kg per day) and an external defibrillator vest. In the subsequent 2 months, the ventricular tachycardia did not return, troponin levels trended down, the steroid dosage was slowly tapered, and use of the defibrillator vest was discontinued. A repeat echocardiogram showed that LVEF had returned to the baseline level of 55%. Troponin remained elevated for 9 months.

This case illustrates the following points:

1. Biomarkers of cardiac damage, i.e., elevated troponin levels, may precede clinical heart failure.

2. LVEF may be normal early in the clinical course despite biomarker evidence of active inflammation.

3. The primary clinical presentation may be conduction disease and ventricular arrhythmias rather than symptomatic heart failure.

4. Cardiac and noncardiac irAEs may be present.

5. The duration of risk after the withdrawal of checkpoint inhibitors was lengthy because of the prolonged half-life of`` this class of agents.

6. There is a need for aggressive anti-inflammatory management that may include immune suppression beyond that offered by high-dose steroids.

7. Most important, this case demonstrates that, with aggressive management, myocarditis can resolve; it also demonstrates the crucial role of serial measurements of troponin levels as monitors of patient status.

POTENTIAL MECHANISMS OF CARDIOTOXICITY

Simplistically, irAEs occur as a result of uncontrolled activation of the immune system. Myocarditis is an inflammatory disease of the myocardium diagnosed by histologic evidence of inflammatory infiltrates within the myocardium. These infiltrates are associated with myocyte degeneration and necrosis of nonischemic origin ($\geq$ 14 leukocytes per mm^2, including up to 4 monocytes per mm^2 with $\geq$ 7 CD3$^+$ T lymphocytes per mm^2).[52]

Although the behavior of checkpoint inhibitor–mediated myocarditis has not been clinically confirmed, it seems to be similar to the behavior of giant cell myocarditis, with predominant and incessant ventricular tachyarrhythmia and rapidly progressive myocardial dysfunction.

Endocardial biopsies have consistently shown dense lymphocytic infiltration with predominantly CD8+ PD-1− T cells (Figure 6-5). The most comprehensive evaluation to date of the mechanism underlying checkpoint inhibitor–mediated myocarditis was reported by Johnson et al.[7] who described findings from two patients with fatal fulminant myocarditis. They found a high frequency of shared TCR sequences among cardiac, skeletal, and tumor-shared antigens. Because T cells targeted a shared antigen, the selectivity of the enhanced T-cell responses between muscle, myocardium, and tumor and, ultimately, the development of lethal autoimmune myocarditis and myositis were presumed to be low (Figure 6-6).

PD-L1 is expressed in the heart. In an experimental model of autoimmune myocarditis, mice lacking PD-1 exhibited more myocardial inflammation, higher levels of serum markers of myocardial damage, and more infiltration of inflammatory cells than did wild-type mice. They were also more likely than wild-type mice to experience dilated cardiomyopathy. Murine models suggest that PD-1 plays an important role in protecting the heart from T cell–mediated damage and that disruption of the gene encoding for PD-1 leads to cardiomyopathy.[53,54]

With improved recognition of cardiac irAEs and data from additional endomyocardial biopsies, the mechanisms underlying cardiac irAEs will be better understood and will ideally lead to the development of cardioprotective strategies.

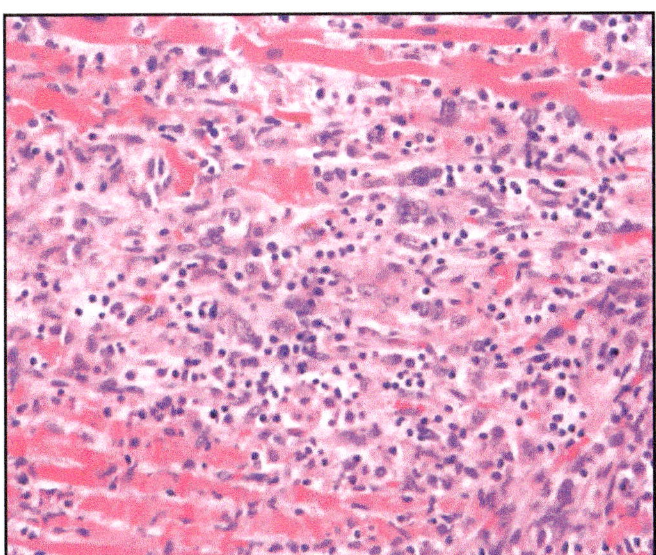

FIGURE 6-6 Immune checkpoint inhibitor myocarditis. Hematoxylin and eosin (H&E) stained lymphocytic infiltration of the myocardium.

IMMUNE CHECKPOINT INHIBITORS AMONG PATIENTS WITH PREEXISITNG IMMUNE OR CARDIAC DISEASE AND RECHALLENGE

■ Use for Patients with Preexisting Immune Disease

The immune checkpoint inhibitors frequently cause immune-related toxicity. Most clinical trials have excluded patients with baseline organ dysfunction, such as immune and cardiac disorders. Surprisingly, these trials rarely exclude patients with cardiac exclusion, save for the generalized condition of "impaired" organ function. Therefore, we may assume that patients with underlying and compensated cardiac disease were, at least to some degree, included in these clinical trials. Their inclusion leads to the question of how safe these checkpoint inhibitors are for patients with preexisting immune and cardiac disease, because these inhibitors are prescribed for patients in a more comprehensive clinical setting outside clinical trials. Will these agents work against the malignancy? Will they exacerbate the underlying immune or cardiac disease? And will they be associated with an exaggerated profile of irAEs, especially for patients with immune disease?

With a focus on preexisting immune disease, Johnson et al. performed a retrospective review of melanoma patients treated at 9 academic medical centers between January 2012 and August 2015. Thirty patients with a variety of preexisting immune disease (rheumatoid arthritis, psoriasis, inflammatory bowel disease, lupus, thyroiditis, multiple sclerosis) were treated with ipilimumab. Thirteen (43%) of the thirty were also being treated with immunosuppressive therapy when melanoma treatment was initiated. The melanoma response rate was 20% (consistent with response rates reported for other populations). Eight patients (27%) experienced an exacerbation of their autoimmune disorder, and 10 patients (33%) experienced a reversible grade 3 to 5 irAE. Of special interest, fifteen patients (50%) actually experienced neither a flare nor a new irAE. One patient with baseline psoriasis died of presumed immune-related colitis after a one-week delay before symptoms were reported.[55]

■ Rechallenge

Rechallenge is defined as re-exposure to the same or different ICPI after prior development of irAE. A study by Menzies et al. included 67 advanced melanoma patients who had a prior non-cardiac irAE when treated with ipilimumab. They had an objective response rate of 40%. Two (3%) patients had recurrence of the same irAE and 23 (34%) experienced a new irAE (21% were grade 3–4) and 8 (12%) discontinued treatment. There were no treatment related deaths. There were no cardiac irAEs.[56]

Pollack and colleagues[57] studied the safety of anti–PD-1 rechallenge among 80 patients who had experienced significant irAEs (pneumonitis, colitis, hepatitis) from combined CTLA-4 and PD-1 blockade. No patients had prior cardiac irAEs. Fourteen (18%) experienced recurrent irAEs at a median of 14 days after resumption of therapy. Colitis was less likely to recur than were other AEs. Other toxicities occurred in 17 patients (21%). There was no correlation with the schedule of steroid taper, the severity of the initial irAE, or the use of additional immunosuppressive therapy. The authors' conclusion was that patients with preexisting immune disease who discontinue CTLA-4/PD-1 blockade for severe irAEs experienced relatively high rates of recurrent or new toxicities with rechallenge.

■ Use for Patients with Preexisting Cardiac Disease

Similar questions apply regarding the safety and risk of irAE cardiotoxicity among patients treated with immune checkpoint inhibitors who had pretreatment cardiac disease.[58,59] In a series of 27 patients with organ dysfunction (renal, hepatic, cardiac) at baseline before the initiation of anti–PD-L1 therapy, Kanz et al. found that 11 patients had baseline cardiac dysfunction due to ischemia, a history of alcohol consumption, hypertension, or previous exposure to tyrosine kinase inhibitors. LVEF ranged from 10% to 45% in this group. The authors found no irAEs leading to obvious worsening of cardiac function. Four of the patients had reversible volume overload and congestive heart failure that responded to diuresis; all of these complications occurred within the first 12 weeks of treatment and did not recur after adjustment of the diuretic doseage.[58] Because all of the patients responded to diuresis alone and were able to continue anti–PD-L1 therapy, it is less likely that severe inflammation was the culprit.

The issue is not as clear as is depicted above. Of the eight patients with cardiac irAEs fully described by Heinzerling,[34] only one had no pretreatment cardiac disease. Of the seven remaining patients, three had CAD (2 had previously experienced myocardial infarctions), one had dilated cardiomyopathy, one had hypertension alone, and three had peripheral artery disease (PAD). Myocarditis outcome is most likely not related to baseline cardiac disease. The four patients who survived had more clinically significant baseline cardiac disease than the three patients who died; those three patients had either no cardiac disease, isolated PAD, or hypertension (Table 6-3). Similarly, the two fatal cases of myocarditis reported by Johnson et al had no baseline cardiac disease.[7]

Table 6-3 Baseline cardiac disease with cardiac irAEs

BASELINE CARDIAC DISEASE	TREATMENT	EVENT	OUTCOME	REF
None None	IPI/NIVO	Chest pain, fatigue, myalgia, Myocarditis AVB, VT	Death Death	Johnson[26]
CAD-prior MI, HBP, PAD	IPI/NIVO	Myocarditis, thyroiditis/hypophysit		Heinzerling[27]
Dilated Cardiomyopathy	IPI	Cardiomyopathy		Heinzerling[27]
None	IPI	Myocardial fibrosis, Hepatitis	Death	Heinzerling[27]
CAD-prior MI, AF,VF with ICD	IPI	CHF, colitis,hypophysitis		Heinzerling[27]
None	IPI/vemurafenib	Myocarditis , chest pain, uveitis		Heinzerling[27]
PAD	IPI	Myocarditis	Death	Heinzerling[27]
CAD	PEMBRO	Ca, ?Takotsubo, AF, BBB		Heinzerling[27]
HBP	IPI	Myocarditis, hepatitis	Death	Heinzerling[27]

IPI, ipilimumab; PEMBRO, pembrolizimab; NIVO, nilumab; DURV, durvalumab; AF, atrial fibrillation; AVB, A-V block; BBB, bundle branch block; CA, cardiac arrest; CHF, congestive heart failure; VT, ventricular tachycardia; VF, ventricular fibrillation; NR, not reported

We can conclude that the existence of prior cardiac disease is not a major risk factor for the development of cardiac irAEs for the following reasons:

1. Patients with baseline cardiac disease or uncontrolled risk factors were included, not excluded, from the pre-approval trials

2. The real world mix and prevalence of co-existent cardiac disease in the cancer population is high (congestive heart failure 9.7%, previous myocardial infarction 2.0%)

3. 3)The pre-approval cardiac irAE event rate was <1%.[60]

It is therefore more likely that pretreatment cardiac disease neither predicts nor increases the risk of cardiac irAEs after checkpoint inhibitor therapy, because neither patients with no baseline cardiac disease nor patients with preexisting cardiac disease exhibited augmented vulnerability related to CAD, PAD, or a reduction in LVEF. Similar to the experience in patients with pre-existing autoimmune disease, clinicians can consider re-challenge with ICPIs in patients with prior ICPI-induced severe irAEs with typical response rates, but with an increased frequency of exacerbated or new irAEs.[55–57] Safe administration includes individual decision based on their cancer and performance status, the availability of alternative ctreatment options and the grade of the prior toxicity coupled with vigilant monitoring and collaboration with the appropriate medical specialist. There are no data for rechallenge in patients who experienced prior cardiac irAEs. However, until more conclusive evidence exists, monitoring algorithms should include, at least, extra vigilance in detecting any subtle hints of cardiac deterioration among patients with preexisting cardiac disease.

■ Safety of Immune Checkpoint Inhibitors for Cardiac Transplant Patients

Another important issue related to checkpoint inhibitors arises when augmented rejection occurs after checkpoint inhibitor immune therapy among patients who have undergone solid organ transplant.[61,62] Because cardiac transplant patients require lifetime immunosuppression, and because skin cancers, including melanoma and Merkel cell lymphoma, are among the most common cancers occurring after cardiac transplant,[63] it is not surprising that a recent publication reported cardiac allograft rejection after anti–PD-1 therapy (nivulomab) for metastatic squamous cell skin carcinoma.[62] However, anti–CTLA-4 therapy (ipilimumab) for solid organ transplant patients may not result in graft rejection and may be better tolerated.[64] This difference between the two treatments may be related to the crucial role of PD-1 in protecting patients against chronic allograft rejection.[23]

Although no recommendations have been developed, our Heart Failure and Transplantation team treats cardiac transplant patients who require immune checkpoint inhibitor treatment in a manner similar to their treatment of patients with posttransplant lymphoproliferative disorder (PTLD): by reducing but not discontinuing antirejection therapy, with close monitoring of the cancer and of myocardial function. Anti–CTLA-4 treatment may be safer than anti–PD-L therapy.[64]

MANAGEMENT OF IMMUNE CHECKPOINT CARDIOTOXICITY

For health care providers, the most important principle for managing irAEs is prompt recognition and immunosuppression proportional to the severity of the event(s). For patients, awareness of potential cardiac toxicity and prompt reporting of subtle symptoms is crucial. For both, close monitoring is the key.

When cardiac toxicity is suspected or recognized, the culprit drug should be discontinued. The administration of high-dose steroids should be considered and implemented early for suspected immune-mediated cardiac toxicity. Because the triad of rapidly progressive conduction disease, fatal arrhythmias, and cardiogenic shock commonly exists, heightened surveillance and monitoring are vital; a low threshold for monitoring patients in an intensive care unit should exist. Patients should undergo testing that includes ECG, echo imaging, measurement of NT-proBNP concentrations, and serial testing of troponin concentrations. Persistent elevation of troponin levels is an excellent marker of an ongoing cardiac inflammatory response.

Coronary arteriography should be performed to exclude CAD as the cause of the clinical presentation. Standard aggressive cardiac care should otherwise be implemented and may entail inotropic support, temporary pacing, and even consideration of advanced heart failure therapies. If myocarditis is suspected and CAD is excluded, endomyocardial biopsy should be considered at the time of catheterization because this test is the gold standard for diagnosis. Cardiac MRI, with late gadolinium enhancement similar to that used for non–immune-mediated myocarditis, provides complimentary information and is a substitute for biopsy when patients decline biopsy or when biopsy would be unsafe (e.g., for patients with severe thrombocytopenia).

Given the morbidity rates associated with myocarditis in general, early consultation about advanced interventions, including cardiac transplant, is prudent. Temporary mechanical support with ventricular assist device(s) or extracorporeal membrane oxygenation should be considered for patients with rapidly progressive hemodynamic instability.[65,66] Other immunosuppressive therapies, including antithymocyte globulin (ATG), mycophenolate mofetil (Cellcept), and infliximab (Remicade), have achieved variable success.[27] A proposed algorithm for treatment is presented in Figure 6-7.

MONITORING FOR CARDIOTOXICITY

Currently, there are no guidelines for cardiac monitoring of patients being treated with checkpoint inhibitors. However, a baseline ECG for all patients before initiation of treatment and an echocardiogram for patients older than 65 years with a history of cardiac disease or with cardiac risk factors will be useful in detecting baseline abnormalities in rhythm and conduction and in assessing biventricular function. These test results are crucial, as illustrated by the following case.

A 78-year-old woman was referred for suspected myocarditis after completing 3 cycles of ipilimumab for locally advanced refractory malignant melanoma. She presented with mild dyspnea on exertion, and ECG showed a "new" left bundle branch block. Her oncologist discontinued immune checkpoint therapy. Laboratory tests showed an LVEF of 50%, no detectable circulating troponin, and an NT-proBNP concentration of 400 pg/mL. Cardiac MRI showed no evidence of myocarditis. After an exhaustive search, it was found that an ECG obtained 7 years previously showed left bundle branch block. Ipilimumab was restarted with no further toxicity, and the tumor regressed.

This case illustrates the importance of baseline data in preventing treatment interruption and excessive cardiac testing. It also shows that not all dyspnea is cardiac in origin.

Depending on the degree of detected baseline cardiac abnormality, more-vigilant cardiac monitoring during treatment may be warranted. A baseline cardiac assessment is also helpful in discerning whether a new symptom is due to the checkpoint inhibitor or to the progression of preexisting cardiac disease as a result of the stress of the cancer and its treatment, the interruption of baseline maintenance cardiac medication because of an intervening non-cardiac toxicity (e.g., hyperthyroidism and tachycardia), or a non-cardiac cause. Because troponin can be a marker of early myocardial damage that has progressed to myocyte apoptosis, baseline and serial pre-cycle monitoring of troponin concentrations can be considered, similar to routine monitoring of thyroid function, which is part of the current standard of care.

During active treatment, common subtle complaints, such as fatigue, any unexplained weight

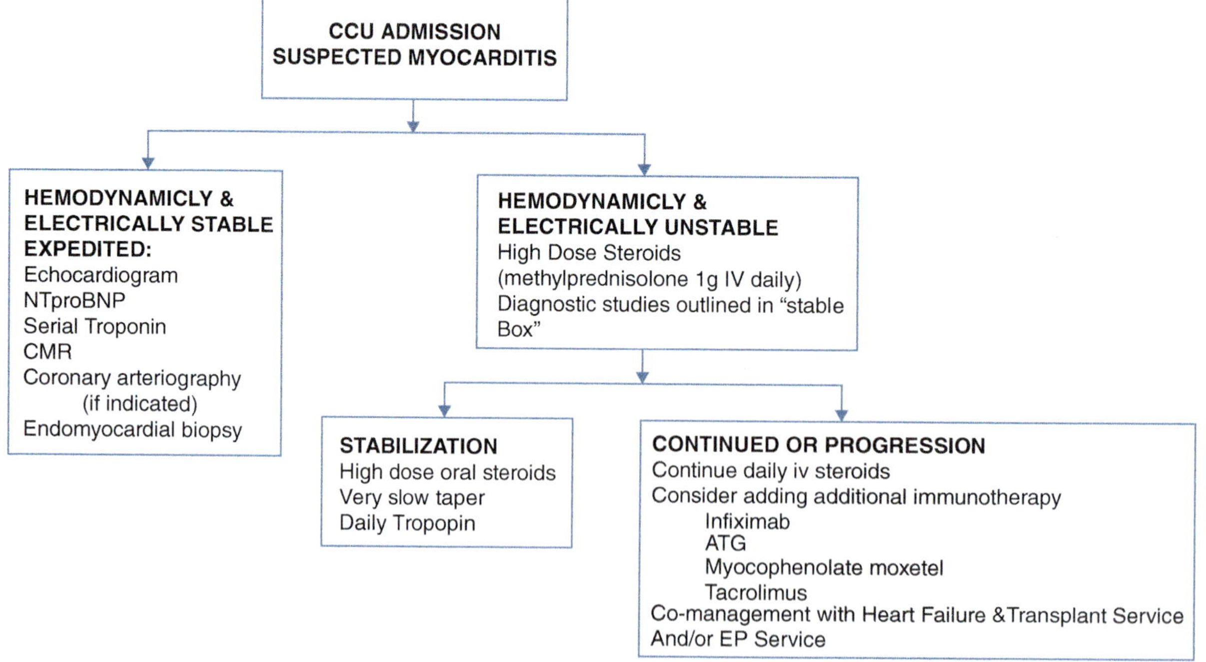

FIGURE 6-7 A proposed algorithm for treatment of checkpoint inhibitor cardiac toxicity.

gain, an increase in resting heart rate, or breathlessness, should trigger prompt repetition of the baseline studies. When non-cardiac irAEs are encountered, serum troponin concentrations should be measured, at a minimum.

A proposed algorithm for monitoring is presented in Figure 6-8.

Currently, we have no understanding of which patients may be at high risk of immune-mediated cardiotoxicity. Currently, it is not clear that preexisting cardiac disease, underlying autoimmune disease, the type of tumor being treated, or the immune checkpoint inhibitor chosen predicts the development of cardiotoxicity. As with other cardiomyopathies (pregnancy-associated and dilated cardiomyopathy), a genetic predisposition[67] to immune-mediated cardiotoxicity may be discovered. One theme is consistently present: with low penetrance, combinations of anti-CTLA-4 and anti-PD1 drugs increase the risk of cardiotoxicity and should increase awareness of and vigilance in detecting cardiac complications of therapy.

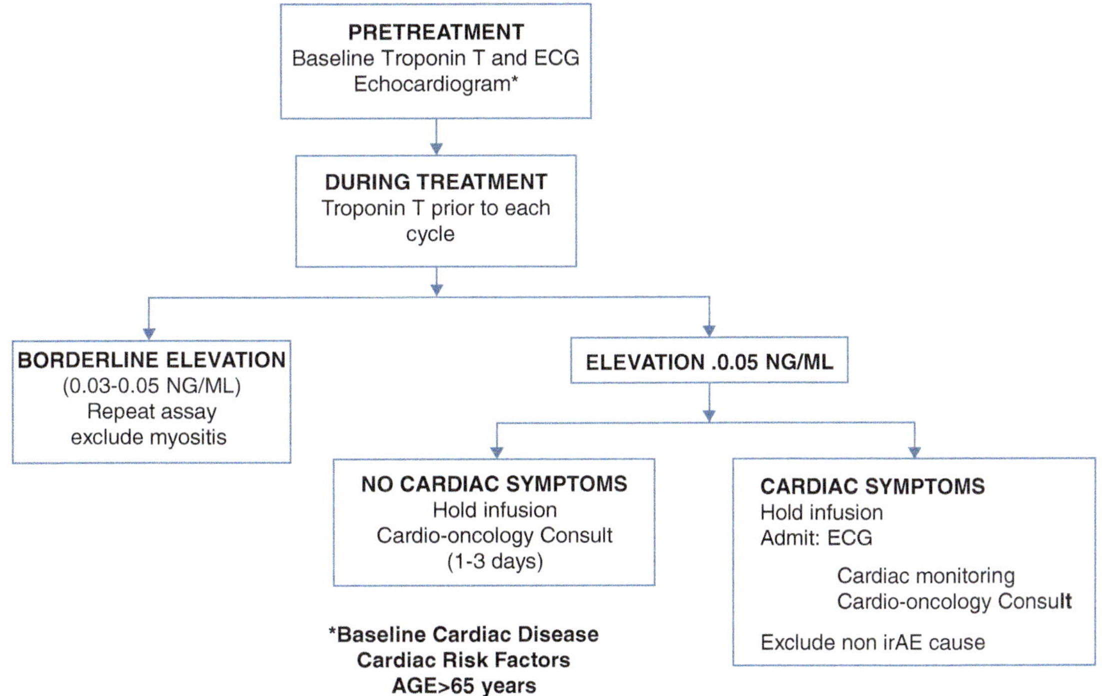

FIGURE 6-8   A proposed algorithm for monitoring of checkpoint inhibitor therapy.

Table 6-4   Major take-home points: cardiac irAEs

- The risk of cardiac toxicity is low (most likely <1%) but when it occurs, the incidence of fatal myocarditis appears to be 30% in reported cases.
- The risk of cardiac irAEs increases sequentially from anti-PD-1 to anti-CTL-4 to combinations.
- The occurrence of cardiac ieAEs can be as short as the first days after initiating therapy to at least 32 weeks and may even occur after treatment completion.
- It is usual to have co-existing noncardiac irAEs present.
- Myocarditis onset is more often insidious with a wide spectrum of presentation.
- Pre-existing cardiac disease is probably not a risk factor for development of cardiac irAEs but may suggest more vigilant monitoring for cardiotoxicity and more vigilance about fluid status during treatment.
- It appears that the earlier the onset the more aggressive and more often fatal is the disease.
- Treatment is based on early recognition, high dose immunosuppression with steroids with a prolonged taper in responding patients coupled with optimized evidence-based heart failure treatment.
- In selected cases, rechallenge is possible after recovery from cardiotoxicity.

CONCLUSION

In summary, checkpoint inhibitors offer exciting opportunities and promising results in the management of a variety of cancers. However, the success of these drugs in treating cancer comes at the cost of immune-mediated adverse events. Important concerns are enumerated in Table 6-4.

Although rare, the cardiac irAEs reported in the medical literature can be fatal. Clinicians managing the care of patients who are being treated with checkpoint inhibitors must be cognizant of the potential for these cardiac events and must have a low threshold for cardiac evaluation and prompt intervention with anti-inflammatory drugs. These therapies will probably be approved as treatment for other cancers, probably in combination with other therapies, such as chimeric antigen receptor (CAR) T cells, tyrosine kinase inhibitors, vascular endothelial growth factor (VEGF) inhibitors, and proteasome inhibitors. Therefore, we need a full understanding of how these drugs and combinations will change the cardiotoxicity spectrum.[68] Current knowledge suggests that cardio-oncology and cardio-oncologists will play an expanding and increasingly important role.

REFERENCES

1. Merriam-Webster. Immune system. https://www.merriam-webster.com/dictionary/immune system. Accessed May 14, 2018.
2. Buchbinder EI, Desai A. CTLA-4 and PD-1 pathways: similarities, differences, and implications of their inhibition. *Am J Clin Oncol*. 2016;39(1):98–106.
3. Goodman A, Patel SP, Kurzrock R. PD-1PD-L1 immune checkpoint blockade in B-cell lymphomas. *Nat Rev Clin Oncol*. 2017;14(4):203–219.
4. Postow MA, Callahan MK, Wolchok JD. Immune checkpoint blockade in cancer therapy. *J Clin Oncol*. 2015;33(17):1974–1982.
5. Luke JJ, Ott PA. PD-1 pathway inhibitors: the next generation of immunotherapy for advanced melanoma. *Oncotarget*. 2015;6(6):3479–3492.
6. Fong L, Small EJ. Anti-cytotoxic T-lymphocyte antigen-4 antibody: the first in an emerging class of immunomodulatory antibodies for cancer treatment. *J Clin Oncol*. 2008;26(32):5275–5283.
7. Johnson DB, Balko JM, Compton ML, et al. Fulminant myocarditis with combination immune checkpoint blockade. *N Eng J Med*. 2016;375(18):1749–1755.
8. Ribas A. Adaptive immune resistance: how cancer protects from immune attack. *Cancer Discov*. 2015;5(9):915–919.
9. Hodi FS, O'Day SJ, McDermott DF, et al. Improved survival with ipilimumab in patients with metastatic melanoma. *N Engl J Med*. 2010;363(8):711–723.
10. Robert C, Thomas L, Bonarenko I, et al. Ipilimumab plus dacarbazine for previously untreated metastatic melanoma. *N Engl J Med*. 2011;364(26):2517–2526.
11. Wolchok JD, Weber JS, Maio M, et al. Four year survival rates for patients with metastatic melanoma who received ipilimumab in phase II clinical trials. *Ann Oncol*. 2013;24(8):2174–2180.
12. Eggermont AM, Chiarion-Sileni V, Grob JJ, et al. Adjuvant ipilimumab versus placebo after complete resection of high-risk stage III melanoma (EORTC 18071): a randomized, double-blind, phase 3 trial. *Lancet Oncol*. 2015;16(5):522–530.
13. Robert C, Schachter J, Long GV, et al. KEYNOTE-006 Investigators. Pembrolizumab versus ipilimumab in advanced melanoma. *N Engl J Med*. 2015;372(26):2521–2532.
14. Garon EB, Riuzi NA, Hui R, et al. KEYNOTE-001 Investigators. Pembrolizumab for the treatment of non-small-cell lung cancer. *N Engl J Med*. 2015;372(21):2018–2028.
15. Robert C, Long GV, Brady B, et al. Nivolumab in previously untreated melanoma without BRAF mutation. *N Engl J Med*. 2015;372(4):320–330.
16. Larkin J, Chiarion-Sileni V, Gonzalez R, et al. Combined nivolumab and ipilimumab or monotherapy in untreated melanoma. *N Engl J Med*. 2015;373(1):23–34.
17. Postow MA, Chesney J, Pavlick AC, et al. Nivolumab and ipilimumab versus ipilimumab in untreated melanoma. *N Engl J Med*. 2015;372(21):2006–2017.
18. Rosenberg JE, Hoffman-Censits J, Powles T, et al. Atezolizumab in patients with locally advanced and metastatic urothelial carcinoma who have progressed following treatment with platinum-based chemotherapy: a single arm, multicentre, phase 2 trial. *Lancet*. 2016;387(10031):1909–1920.
19. Kaufman HL, Russell J, Hamid O, et al. Avelumab in patients with chemotherapy-refractory metastatic Merkel cell carcinoma: a multicentre, single-group, open-label, phase 2 trial. *Lancet Oncol*. 2016;17(10);1374–1385.
20. Apolo AB, Infante JR, Hamid O, et al. Safety, clinical activity, and PD-L1 expression of avelumab (MSB0010718C), an anti-PD-L1 antibody, in patients with metastatic urothelial carcinoma from the JAVELIN Solid Tumor phase 1b trial. *J Clin Oncol*. 2016;34(suppl 2):367.
21. Powles T, O'Donnell PH, Massard C, et al. Updated efficacy and tolerability of durvalumab in locally advanced or metastatic urothelial carcinoma. *J Clin Oncol*. 2017;35(suppl 6):286.
22. Massard C, Gordon MS, Sharma S, et al. Safety and efficacy of durvalumab (MED14736), an anti-programmed cell death ligand-1 immune checkpoint inhibitor, in patients with advanced urothelial bladder cancer. *J Clin Oncol*. 2016;34(26):3119–3125.
23. Tanaka K, Albin MJ, Yuan X, et al. PDL1 is required for peripheral transplantation tolerance and protection from chronic allograft rejection. *J Immunol*. 2007;179(8):5204–5210.

24. Hahn AW, Gill DM, Agarwal N, Maughan BL. PD-1 checkpoint inhibition: Toxicities and management. *Urol Oncol*. 2017;35(12):701–707.

25. Voskens CJ, Goldinger SM, Loquai C, et al. The price of tumor control: an analysis of rare side effects of anti CTLA-4 therapy in metastatic melanoma. *PLOS ONE*. 2013;8(1):e53745.

26. Di Giacomo AM, Biagioli M, Maio M. The emerging toxicity profiles of anti-CTLA-4 antibodies across clinical indications. *Semin Oncol*. 2010;37(5):499–507.

27. Gangadhar TC, Vonderheide RH. Mitigating the toxic effects of anticancer immunotherapy. *Nat Rev Clin Oncol*. 2014;11(2):91–99.

28. Villadolid J, Amin A. Immune checkpoint inhibitors in clinical practice: update on management of immune-related toxicities. *Transl Lung Cancer Res*. 2015;4(5):560–575.

29. Weber JS, Kähler KC, Hauschild A. Management of immune-related adverse events and kinetics of response with ipilimumab. *J Clin Oncol*. 2012;30(21):2691–2697.

30. National Institutes of Health; National Cancer Institute. Common Terminology Criteria for Adverse Events (CTCAE). Version 4.03. June 14, 2010. https://www.eortc.be/services/doc/ctc/CTCAE_4.03_2010-06-14_QuickReference_5x7.pdf. Accessed May 14, 2018.

31. Postel-Vinay S, Aspeslagh S, Lanoy E, Robert C, Soria JC, Marabelle A. Challenges of phase 1 clinical trials evaluating immune checkpoint-targeted antibodies. *Ann Oncol*. 2016;27(2):214–224.

32. Champiat S, Lambotte O, Barreau E, et al. Management of immune checkpoint blockade dysimmune toxicities: a collaborative position paper. *Ann Oncol*. 2016;27(4):559–574.

33. Ederhy S, Voisin AL, Champiat S. Myocarditis with immune checkpoint blockade. *N Engl J Med*. 2017;376(3):290–291.

34. Heinzerling L, Ott PA, Hodi FS, et al. Cardiotoxicity associated with CTLA4 and PD1 blocking immunotherapy. *J Immunother Cancer*. 2016;4:50.

35. Roth ME, Muluneh B, Jensen B, Madamanchi C, Lee CB. Left ventricular dysfunction after treatment with ipilimumab for metastatic melanoma. *Am J Ther*. 2016;23(6):e1925–e1928.

36. Zimmer L, Goldinger SM, Hofmann L, et al. Neurological, respiratory, musculoskeletal, cardiac and ocular side effects of anti-PD-1 therapy. *Eur J Cancer*. 2016;60:210–225.

37. Berg DD, Vaduganathan M, Nohria A, et al. Immune-related fulminant myocarditis in a patient receiving ipilimumab therapy for relapsed chronic myelomonocytic leukaemia. *Eur J Heart Fail*. 2017;19(5):682–685.

38. Matson DR, Accola MA, Rehrauer WM, Corliss RF. Fatal myocarditis following treatment with the PD-1 inhibitor nivolumab. *J Forensic Sci*. 2017;63(3):954–957.

39. Behling J, Kaes J, Münzel T, Grabbe S, Loquai C. New-onset third-degree atrioventricular block because of autoimmune-induced myositis under treatment with anti-programmed cell death-1 (nivolumab) for metastatic melanoma. *Melanoma Res*. 2017;27(2):155–158.

40. Geisler BP, Raad RA, Esaian D, Sharon E, Schwartz DR. Apical ballooning and cardiomyopathy in a melanoma patient treated with ipilimumab: a case of takotsubo-like syndrome. *J Immunother Cancer*. 2015;3:4.

41. Läubli H, Balmelli C, Bossard M, Pfister O, Glatz K, Zippelius A. Acute heart failure due to autoimmune myocarditis under pembrolizumab treatment for metastatic melanoma. *J Immunother Cancer*. 2015;3:11.

42. Yun S, Vincelette ND, Mansour I, Hariri D, Motamed S. Late onset ipilimumab-induced pericarditis and pericardial effusion a rare but life threatening complication. *Case Rep Oncol Med*. 2015;2015:794842.

43. Mehta A, Gupta A, Hannallah F, Koshy T, Reimold S. Myocarditis as an immune-related adverse event with ipilimumab/nivolumab combination therapy for metastatic melanoma. *Melanoma Res*. 2016;26(3):319–320.

44. Tadokoro T, Keshino E, Makiyama A, et al. Acute lymphocytic myocarditis with anti-PD-1 antibody nivolumab. *Circ Heart Fail*. 2016;9(10). doi:10.1161/CIRCHEARTFAILURE.116.003514.

45. Koelzer VH, Rothschild SI, Zihler D, et al. Systemic inflammation in a melanoma patient treated with immune checkpoint inhibitors – an autopsy study. *J Immunother Cancer*. 2016;4:13.

46. Semper H, Muehlberg F, Schulz-Menger J, Allewelt M, Grohé C. Drug-induced myocarditis after nivolumab treatment in a patient with PDL1–negative squamous cell carcinoma of the lung. *Lung Cancer*. 2016;99:117–119.

47. Chauhan A, Burkeen G, Houranieh J, Arnold S, Anthony L. Immune checkpoint-associated cardiotoxicity: case report with systematic review of literature. *Ann Oncol*. 2017;28(8):2034–2038.

48. Jain V, Bahia J, Mohebtash M, Barac A. Cardiovascular complications associated with novel cancer immunotherapies. *Curr Treat Options Cardiovasc Med*. 2017;19(5):36.

49. Reddy N, Moudgil R, Lopez-Mattei JC, et al. Progressive and reversible conduction disease with checkpoint inhibitors. *Can J Cardiol*. 2017;33(10):e13–e1335.e15.

50. Gibson R, Delaune J, Szady A, Markham M. Suspected immune myocarditis and cardiac conduction abnormalities with nivolumab therapy for non-small cell lung cancer. *BMJ Case Rep*. July 20, 2016;2016. doi:10.1136/bcr-2016–216228.

51. Antonia SJ, Villegas A, Daniel D, et al. PACIFIC Investigators. Durvalumab after chemotherapy in stage III non-small-cell lung cancer. *N Engl J Med*. 2017;377(20):1919–1929.

52. Caforio AL, Parkuweit S, Arbustini E, et al. Current state of knowledge on aetiology, diagnosis, management, and therapy of myocarditis: a position statement of the European Society of Cardiology Working Group on Myocardial and Pericardial Diseases. *Eur Heart J*. 2013;34(33):2636–2648.

53. Tarrio ML, Grabie N, Bu DX, Sharpe AH, Lichtman AH. PD-1 protects against inflammation and myocyte damage in T cell-mediated myocarditis. *J Immunol*. 2012;188(10):4876–4884.

54. Nishimura H, Okazaki T, Tanaka Y, et al. Autoimmune dilated cardiomyopathy in PD-1 receptor-deficient mice. *Science*. 2001;291(5502):319–322.

55. Johnson DB, Sullivan RJ, Ott P, et al. Ipilimumab therapy in patients with advanced melanoma and preexisting autoimmune disorders. *JAMA Oncol*. 2016;2(2):234–240.

56. Menzies AM, Johnson DB, Ramanujam VG, et al. Anti-PD-1 therapy in patients with advanced melanoma and preexisting autoimmune disorders or major toxicity with ipilimumab. *Ann Oncol*. 2017;28(2):368–376.

57. Pollack MH, Betof A, Dearden H, et al. Safety of resuming anti-PD-1 in patients with immune-related adverse events (irAEs) during combined anti-CTLA-4 and anti-PD-1 in metastatic melanoma. *Ann Oncol*. 2018;29(1):250–255.

58. Kanz BA, Pollack MH, Johnpulle R, et al. Safety and efficacy of anti-PD-1 in patients with baseline cardiac, renal, or hepatic dysfunction. *J Immunother Cancer*. 2016;4:60.

59. Johnson DB, Sullivan RJ, Menzies AM. Immune checkpoint inhibitors in challenging populations. *Cancer*. 2017;123(11):1904–1911.

60. Edwards BK, Noone AM, Mariotto AB, et al. Annual Report to the Nation on the status of cancer, 1975–2010, featuring prevalence of comorbidity and impact on survival among persons with lung, colorectal, breast, or prostate cancer. *Cancer*. 2014;120(9):1290–1314.

61. Lipson EJ, Bagnasco SM, Moore, J, et al. Tumor regression and allograft rejection after administration of anti-PD-1. *N Engl J Med*. 2016;374(9):896–898.

62. Owonikoko TK, Kumar M, Yang S, et al. Cardiac allograph rejection as a complication of PD-1 checkpoint blockade for cancer immunotherapy: a case report. *Cancer Immunol Immunother*. 2017;66(1):45–50.

63. Ilyas M, Sharma A. Clinical finings, treatments and outcomes of transplant recipients with metastatic skin cancer. *ARC J Dermatol*. 2017;2(1):1–10.

64. Lipson EJ, Bodell MA, Kraus ES, Sharfman WH. Successful administration of ipilimumab to two kidney transplantation patients with metastatic melanoma. *J Clin Oncol*. 2014;32(19):e69–e71.

65. Varricchi G, Galdiero MR, Marone G, et al. Cardiotoxicity of immune checkpoint inhibitors. *ESMO Open*. 2017;2(4):e000247.

66. Wang DY, Okoye GD, Neilan TG, Johnson DB, Moslehi JJ. Cardiovascular toxicities associated with cancer immunotherapies. *Curr Cardiol Rep*. 2017;19(3):21.

67. van Spaendonck-Zwarts KY, Posafalvi A, van den Berg MP, et al. Titin gene mutations are common in families with both peripartum cardiomyopathy and dilated cardiomyopathy. *Eur Heart J*. 2014;35(32):2165–2173.

68. Ali AK, Watson DE. Pharmacovigilance assessment of immune-mediated reactions reported for checkpoint inhibitor cancer immunotherapies. *Pharmacotherapy*. 2017;37(11):1383–1390.

7 Effects of Radiation Therapy on the Cardiovascular System

David J. Cutter ■ Carolyn W. Taylor ■ Kazem Rahimi ■ Paul McGale ■ Vanessa Ferreira ■ Matthew Burrage ■ Sindu Vivekanandan ■ Maria Hawkins ■ Sarah C. Darby

INTRODUCTION

Radiation therapy is a vital component of modern cancer management. During the course of their treatment more than half of cancer patients receive radiotherapy, three quarters of these with curative intent. The potential for long-lasting adverse effects of radiation on normal tissues has been known since the dawn of radiation oncology, and the concept of achieving tumour control while minimizing normal tissue damage has been a fundamental principle of radiotherapy since the 1930s.[1] Following this principle, techniques of radiation therapy have been progressively developed over decades, for example through alteration of the total dose administered, reduction in the volumes treated, and by improved shielding of the normal tissues at risk by a number of technical advances. These developments have been made in order to minimize the possibility of adverse effects from normal tissue damage while maximizing the efficacy of the treatment.

The first case-report of an effect of X-rays on the heart was published in 1897, only 2 years after the discovery of this form of electromagnetic radiation by Wilhelm Röntgen.[2] Further evidence of cardiovascular injury as a result of ionizing irradiation began to accumulate throughout the first half of the twentieth century, mainly in the form of further case reports. However, during this period the cardiovascular system was generally considered relatively resistant to radiation-induced injury and little consideration was given to avoidance of the heart during thoracic radiotherapy. It was not until the 1960s that detailed reports of the pathological changes seen in patients treated with radiotherapy for Hodgkin lymphoma including doses of >30 Gray (Gy) to the heart,[3] established radiation-induced cardiovascular disease as a distinct entity. Over the next two decades, continued follow-up of large series of Hodgkin lymphoma patients started to provide quantitative information of the cardiovascular risks of these higher risks of radiotherapy.[4] But it was still thought that cardiovascular disease was not induced by cardiac radiation doses of <30 Gy. Over the last twenty years new evidence from several independent sources has revealed that cardiovascular risks are also increased by lower doses of radiation. For example, in patients treated for breast cancer rates of major coronary events following radiotherapy were found to increase linearly with the mean dose to the heart by 7.4% per Gy, with no apparent threshold.[5] Similar results have been reported following treatment of Hodgkin lymphoma.[6] In childhood cancer survivors, radiation doses of <15 Gy to the heart have been shown to increase the risk of cardiac mortality[7] and morbidity.[8] Additionally following irradiation for peptic ulcer disease[9] and in exposed atomic bomb survivors[10,11] cardiac mortality was increased by heart doses of <5 Gy. The details of the mechanisms[12] and dose-volume response relationships[13] for the various types of radiation-induced cardiovascular disease (RICD) are being actively researched and there is much to be learned about how these risks may interact with other factors, such as cardiotoxic anthracycline chemotherapy, or conventional cardiovascular risk factors. Current research into radiation effects on the cardiovascular system is seeking to clarify these issues in order that such effects may be understood, predicted and, hopefully, avoided in the future.

Late adverse effects of radiation therapy, especially those that are potentially fatal such as cardiovascular disease, attain particular importance in situations where a cure is likely, such as with early breast cancer or Hodgkin lymphoma. This importance seems set to increase into the future due to improvements in the treatment of cancer. A recent study in the UK concluded that by 2008 approximately 3% of the population, including 12% of those over 65 years of age, were cancer survivors.[14] The equivalent number of total cancer survivors in the United States is predicted to reach 19 million by 2020. A substantial proportion of these survivors will have received radiation therapy that may have involved irradiation of the cardiovascular system. Although modern radiotherapy techniques undoubtedly deliver lower doses to normal tissues such as the heart than in previous decades, some degree of cardiovascular radiation exposure remains inevitable. Cancer survivors may, therefore, be at increased risk of cardiovascular disease as a consequence and knowledge regarding this is of considerable importance.

PATHOLOGY, CLINICAL MANIFESTATIONS, AND TREATMENT OF RADIATION-RELATED CARDIOVASCULAR DISEASE

The pathology of radiation-induced injury to the human cardiovascular system is non-specific to radiation, but radiation-related cardiovascular disease (RRCD) does demonstrate consistent morphological patterns. The pathological changes most often described in human specimens are late changes observed months or years after irradiation to at least 30 Gy. Earlier effects and the cellular and molecular mechanisms of pathogenesis have been more extensively described in animal models and are detailed in the subsequent section. The typical patterns of radiation-induced cardiovascular disease, how they present to the clinician and how they are treated are best described according to the anatomic structures affected.

■ Coronary Artery Disease

Radiation-related coronary artery disease (CAD) described in human cases is essentially morphologically indistinguishable from age-related atherosclerotic coronary artery disease. Some differences with more smooth muscle loss from the media and greater adventitial fibrosis than non-irradiated controls were described in one case series,[15] but this observation has not been repeated. More recently a large pathological study of irradiated arteries from asymptomatic human subjects examined within 10 years of radiotherapy suggests qualitative and quantitative differences between radiation-induced changes and age-related atherosclerosis, with variations in intima-media wall thickness and collagen, proteoglycan and inflammatory cell contents.[16] Animal models also suggest that radiation-induced disease may be more prone to rupture and subsequent thrombotic complications.[17] The anatomical distribution of radiation-related CAD differs from age-related disease with a predisposition for sections of the coronary arteries that absorbed the highest radiation dose.[18] For example isolated coronary ostial narrowing, while rare in spontaneous CAD, has been reported following irradiation for Hodgkin lymphoma (HL) where the proximal coronary arteries typically receive a high dose.[19] Similarly the left anterior descending coronary artery is more commonly diseased than would be expected in the general population following tangential irradiation of the left breast, where this artery receives a high dose.[20,21] These differences aside, a pathological assessment of the underlying cause of CAD may be extremely difficult, especially in older patients with other cardiac risk factors. Coronary artery disease has been observed in patients irradiated at a young age with no other conventional cardiac risk factors (Figure 7-1).[22] In the face of such cases it

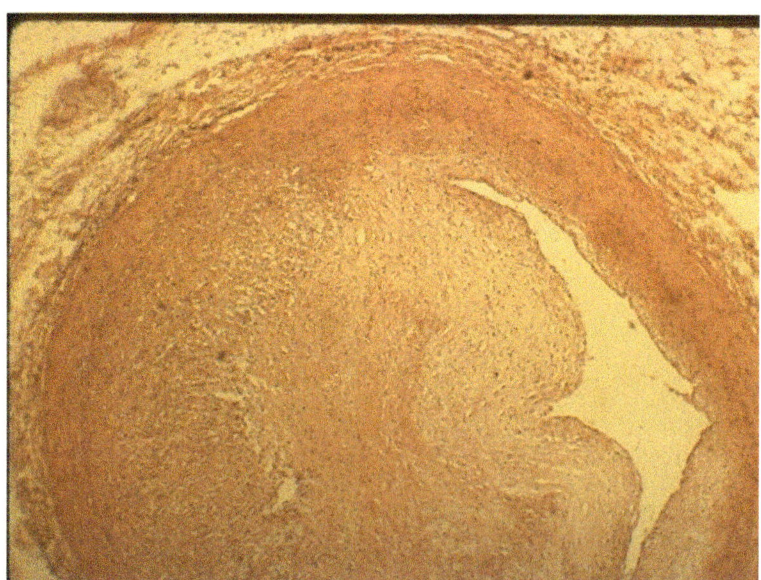

FIGURE 7-1 Left anterior descending coronary artery in a 16-year-old boy, one year after receiving 40 Gy mantle radiotherapy for Hodgkin disease. Myo-intimal proliferation has considerably narrowed the lumen. Fatal cases like this, in a patient who had no cardiac risk factors other than radiation illustrate that the morphology of arterial disease due to radiation is essentially no different from that of age-related atherosclerosis. Hematoxylin & Eosin. (Reproduced with permission from Fajardo LF, 2005.[22])

is difficult to argue that radiation is not causative, and this conclusion is supported by data from both randomised trials and epidemiological studies.

Apart from a younger age of onset and an absence of conventional cardiovascular risk factors the clinical presentation of radiation-related coronary artery disease does not differ substantially to that due to other causes. One possible difference is that radiation-related damage to the autonomic nervous system innervating the heart may, in theory, cause "silent" ischaemia where patients present atypically without chest pain, such as has been commonly observed in patients with diabetic neuropathy. The medical treatment for radiation-related CAD does not currently differ from that used for other CAD. Risk factors, such as smoking, hypertension and hypercholesterolaemia, are known to increase the risk of CAD above that of radiation-alone,[23–25] and therefore early and aggressive management of these risk factors should be recommended in patients with a history of cardiac irradiation or established radiation-related CAD.[26] Surgical treatment with coronary artery bypass grafting (CABG) can be successful for radiation-related CAD but may be complicated by associated mediastinal fibrotic tissue damage from irradiation, which may make surgery technically more challenging. Concomitant myocardial and pulmonary fibrosis may also increase the risk of perioperative morbidity. The internal mammary artery is commonly used as a donor artery for CABG and may also have been within the irradiation volume making it also vulnerable to radiation damage, but available evidence suggests that this artery may still be used safely if patent at the time of the procedure.[27] Prior to CABG for radiation-related CAD it is vital that a thorough assessment of all aspects of cardiac function is undertaken, as it not uncommon for radiation-related CAD to co-exist with other radiation-related cardiac complications such as pericardial or valvular disease. Any synchronous pathology that is likely to require future intervention with cardiac surgery should be considered at the same time as CABG, as later procedures through the irradiation field will become increasingly difficult due to radiation-induced and surgical scarring.[26] Although immediate outcomes following CABG for radiation-related CAD may be good, late survival may be limited by death from cardiorespiratory causes and recurrent or second malignancies.[28,29] The immediate complication rate and prognosis following surgery is associated with the extent of radiotherapy received, with patients who received extensive mediastinal irradiation, e.g., for Hodgkin lymphoma, at greatest risk.[30] These patients more frequently have radiation-induced restrictive pulmonary dysfunction that accounts for some of the increased risk.[31] In patients otherwise at lower surgical risk, mortality may be higher in those with lower left ventricular global longitudinal strain pre-operatively.[32]

■ Cardiomyopathy

The characteristic change seen in the myocardium following high dose irradiation is diffuse interstitial fibrosis with proliferation of bands of collagen separating and replacing myocytes, occurring in patches of varying size and distribution (Figure 7-2).[33] Fibrosis has been reported to be more frequent in the left ventricle in some series[3] and in the right ventricle in others.[15] It is possible that the observed distribution of fibrosis in these cases has more to do with the distribution of radiation dose received rather than any intrinsic difference in sensitivity between the left and right ventricles. Diffuse fibrosis has, however, been rarely observed in the atria. There is no accompanying cellular or fibrinous exudates and little or no necrosis evident. Occasionally calcification of myocytes has been seen, suggesting that previous necrosis secondary to ischemia may occasionally occur. An increase in the ratio of type I to type III collagen has been reported[34] that is thought to decrease myocardial compliance and contribute to diastolic dysfunction.

Clinically evident radiation-related cardiomyopathy is rare following radiation alone except following irradiation of large volumes of the myocardium to high doses (>30 Gy), which is unusual for most radiotherapy regimens since the 1970s. It is more common nowadays to see clinically evident cardiomyopathy primarily due to anthracycline chemotherapy (see Chapter 3) and perhaps exacerbated by irradiation. In individual cases the manifestations seen depend on the dose and volume of cardiac irradiation, the presence or absence of anthracycline toxicity, and the age of the patient at irradiation. Irradiation of a large volume of the myocardium to a high dose (even in the absence of cardiotoxic chemotherapy) may lead to a restrictive cardiomyopathy due to widespread fibrosis, which may occur in combination with constrictive pericardial disease and other radiation-associated heart disease. The combination of anthracyclines and radiotherapy more commonly produces a progressive dilated cardiomyopathy. Irradiation at a young age, while the heart is still growing and developing may increase the risk of a restrictive pattern of disease. Subclinical radiation-related myocardial

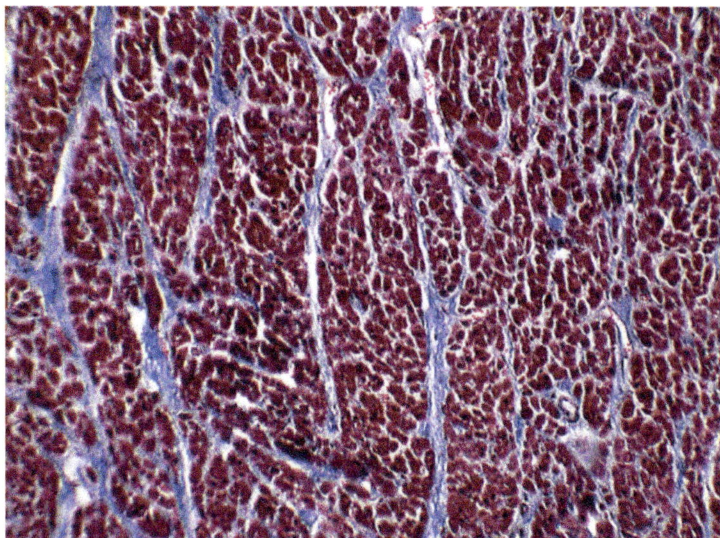

FIGURE 7-2 Fatal diffuse myocardial fibrosis several years after irradiation for Hodgkin disease. Whereas normally there should be very little collagen among the dark red myocytes, this heart muscle is criss-crossed by multiple bands of blue collagen. Gomori trichrome. (Reproduced with permission from Darby SC et al., 2010.[33])

damage is much more common than clinically evident cardiomyopathy. Asymptomatic diastolic dysfunction, detected by echocardiography, has been linked with an increased risk of later cardiac events[35] indicating that, while not clinically evident, such changes may still be clinically relevant. The microvasculature of the myocardium is known to be damaged by relatively small volumes of cardiac irradiation as demonstrated by nucleotide imaging, but the clinical significance of these findings is currently unknown.[36]

Treatment for radiation-related cardiomyopathy is as for other causes of heart failure. Systolic dysfunction is treated with angiotensin-converting enzyme (ACE) inhibitors, beta-blockers and aldosterone antagonists as normally indicated. There is no evidence that the treatment of subclinical systolic or diastolic dysfunction due to radiation with, for example, ACE inhibitors improves prognosis. However, given that subclinical abnormalities can be identified and that a proportion of patients progress to develop clinical heart failure, there is a potential window for pharmacological intervention in this condition. For patients with end-stage heart failure, orthotopic heart transplant is technically possible, but is undertaken with caution with respect to case selection due to the high risk of peri-operative complications and poor long-term survival in these patients due to cardiorespiratory disease, renal disease (due to immunosuppressive drugs) and second malignancies.[37,38]

Valvular Heart Disease

Pathological series have described diffuse or focal fibrotic thickening of the endocardium covering the chambers and valves of the heart, with associated late calcification, in a substantial proportion of patients following mediastinal irradiation. No inflammatory changes or neovascularization has been identified.[15,39] The lesions described are non-specific to radiation and could have been caused by a number of other aetiologies including, for example, rheumatic fever; however epidemiological evidence suggests that radiation is a causative factor in valvular heart disease (VHD) following mediastinal irradiation. The pathogenesis is not clearly understood but is thought to be essentially fibrogenic in keeping with late radiation effects in a variety of tissues.[40] Recently it has been shown that radiation induces an osteogenic phenotype in human aortic valve interstitial cells,[41] which may give a mechanistic insight into the calcification that is seen.

Radiation-related VHD is often a very late complication of RT with a median time to diagnosis of 22–23 years,[13,23] although an epidemiological study of breast cancer survivors has demonstrated an increased risk of VHD just 5–9 years after diagnosis.[42] The incidence is higher for left-sided heart valves (mitral and aortic) than right-sided valves (tricuspid and pulmonary), with calcification typically affecting the mitral-aortic curtain.[43] It has been suggested that this is due to greater haemodynamic stresses present within the higher pressure left ventricle.[15]

Valvular stenosis is more common than regurgitation,[23] although both occur and may often co-exist.[44] Subvalvular stenosis due to fibrosis of the mural endocardium may occur, but is rare.[26] Valvular damage from radiation is progressive and the severity of calcification[44] and dysfunction[13,45] has been shown to worsen over time.

When valvular dysfunction is severe enough to warrant surgical intervention, outcomes are often good except in the presence of constrictive pericarditis or cardiomyopathy.[46] Valve replacement should perhaps be preferred to repair, as repairs appear to have limited durability when performed on irradiated structures.[47] Alternatively a percutaneous approach, e.g., transcatheter aortic valve replacement or mitral valve repair, may be preferable in those with mediastinal fibrosis or a circumferentially calcified ("porcelain") aorta secondary to radiation exposure, where surgery may be contraindicated.[48,49]

■ Pericardial Disease

The characteristic change seen in the pericardium late after irradiation is fibrosis and thickening of the fibrous layers. Both the parietal and visceral pericardium may be affected, but the outer parietal pericardium tends to be more severely affected, with the fibrous layer of the anterior aspect increasing from <1mm (normal) up to 8mm.[33] The external adipose layer is extensively replaced by a dense, irregular proliferation of collagen (Figure 7-3).[22] Although this fibrotic process may progress to constriction it is uncommon to see adhesions between the parietal and visceral pericardium, in contrast to other causes of pericardial disease. A second characteristic feature is the presence of a fibrinous exudate both on the inner surface of the parietal pericardium and within the fibrous layer itself. This type of stromal or interstitial exudate is typical of delayed radiation injury in a variety of tissues. A cellular inflammatory infiltration is scanty at the delayed stage with only modest numbers of lymphocytes. Granulocytes are only seen in the presence of associated infection, tumour or trauma.[50] Many cases are associated with pericardial effusion that tends to be protein rich (up to 6mg/100ml), but may be variable both in volume and in the speed with which it accumulates.[51]

Historically, radiation-related pericardial disease (RRPD) was the first manifestation of radiation-related cardiac disease to be documented following mediastinal irradiation for HL. During the 1960s and 1970s, pericarditis was reported in 25%–60% of patients treated for HL with mediastinal RT.[52] Due to changes in RT techniques the incidence of RRPD has fallen and it is now relatively rare.[53,54] Irradiation of the pericardium can cause acute and/or chronic pericarditis, often with associated pericardial effusion, and may result in pericardial constriction. Radiation-induced acute pericarditis occurs several weeks following RT. It can occasionally occur earlier, during the course of treatment, in which case it is usually related to the irradiation of a large tumour adjacent to the heart

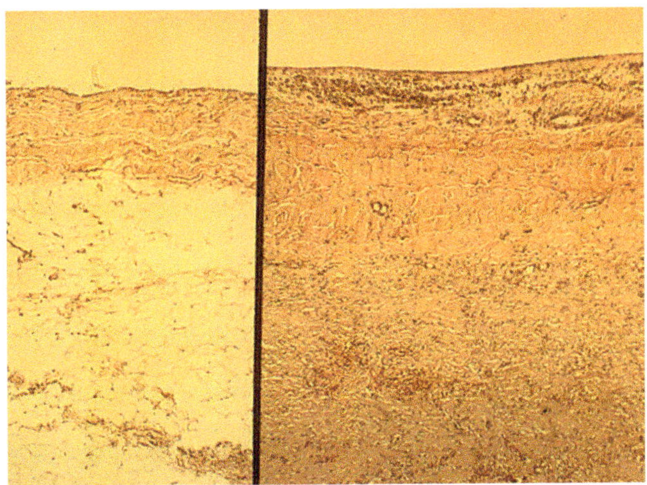

FIGURE 7-3 Perpendicular sections of human pericardium. The left image illustrates the normal parietal pericardium with a thin, uniform fibrous layer that faces the heart (upper), and an outer layer of adipose tissue (lower). The right image is a typical example of irradiated pericardium, 17 months after 67 Gy. The adipose tissue has been replaced by dense fibrous tissue that actually extended well below the limits of this micrograph. Hematoxylin & Eosin. (Reproduced with permission from Fajardo LF, 2005.[22])

where inflammation and necrosis of the tumour due to RT directly irritates the pericardium. Later-onset radiation-induced chronic pericarditis may occur following an initial episode of acute pericarditis or may occur without prior manifestations. The clinical presentation of radiation-related pericarditis is similar to that due to other causes, with pleuritic chest pain, tachycardia, fever, pericardial friction rub and ECG changes. Echocardiography or other imaging may demonstrate an associated pericardial effusion. Alternative aetiologies for any pericardial thickening or effusion such as malignant effusion, infection or hypothyroidism (which may be induced by thyroid irradiation) should be excluded before making a diagnosis of RRPD. Radiation-related constrictive pericardial disease presents as that due to other aetiologies with symptoms of heart failure.

The majority of cases of radiation-induced pericarditis resolve spontaneously and are usually managed symptomatically with non-steroidal anti-inflammatory drugs. Colchicine may be beneficial as adjunctive therapy, while glucocorticoids may be associated with recurrent pericarditis and should be reserved for specific aetiologies such as autoimmune or uraemic pericarditis.[55] Occasionally an associated pericardial effusion may accumulate quickly enough to cause cardiac tamponade and necessitate urgent pericardiocentesis to prevent acute compromise of cardiac function and death. Persistent or recurrent effusion large enough to cause symptoms may be managed by pericardiocentesis, pericardial window formation or surgical pericardiectomy. Mild constrictive disease may be managed medically in the first instance, for example with diuretics for oedema, although it has been argued that early sub-total pericardiectomy may prevent the progression to more severe constrictive disease.[56] Severe pericardial constriction may be managed with total pericardiectomy, although the prognosis is significantly worse for radiation-induced constrictive pericarditis than for non-radiation-induced disease, presumably partially due to concomitant underlying cardiomyopathy and coronary artery disease.[57,58]

■ Conduction System Abnormalities

Fibrotic scars have been found post-mortem within or near to the location of conduction pathways in patients who had received mediastinal irradiation. Those scars may not be caused directly by radiation however, as they are nonspecific and often seen in combination with other manifestations of radiation-related heart disease. The myocardial cells that comprise the conduction system are presumably just as vulnerable to the consequences of radiation-induced microvascular or macrovascular damage as other parts of the myocardium, and such damage could indirectly result in fibrotic scarring.

A wide variety of conduction defects have been described following mediastinal irradiation. These include supraventricular arrhythmias, junctional disorders (including all degrees of heart block), prolonged QTc interval and ventricular defects (such as bundle branch blocks and ventricular ectopic beats).[26] The more severe radiation-related conduction defects tend to occur concomitantly with other forms of radiation-related heart disease such as CAD.[59] Persistent invariant tachycardia has also been described and is presumed to be secondary to damage to the autonomic nerves that normally regulate heart rate.[60] Minor ECG abnormalities, such as T-wave changes, have been described acutely post-irradiation, but appear to resolve spontaneously without clinical consequence.[61]

There are no specific recommendations for the treatment of radiation-related conduction abnormalities and they are usually managed as would be otherwise clinically indicated, for example with pacemaker implantation for symptomatic or high-grade atrioventricular block.[26]

■ Cerebrovascular Disease

Vessels of all sizes within the cerebrovasculature are sensitive to the effects of radiation. The smallest vessels (arterioles and capillaries) are the most vulnerable with radiation-induced endothelial cell injury leading to thrombotic occlusion and ischaemia, which may result in cerebral necrosis.[62] Medium and large-sized vessels exhibit a chronic occlusive vasculopathy with vascular wall thickening, atherosclerotic disease and stenosis.[63,64] In addition to effects on the cerebral vasculature, irradiation of the aortic arch, coronary arteries and heart may also increase the risk of developing cerebrovascular disease.[65]

The type of cerebrovascular disease varies depending on the vessels irradiated, the radiation dose and the age at irradiation. High dose irradiation of brain can result in cerebral radionecrosis usually presenting within the first year following RT,[66] the symptoms depending on the extent and location of the necrosis. Irradiation of larger vessels in the head and neck increases the risk of transient ischaemic attacks (TIAs) and stroke.[67] The clinical presentation of radiation–related TIAs and strokes mimics those due to naturally occurring atheromatous disease, although patients often present at a younger age than expected for cerebrovascular disease due to other causes, with less concurrent vascular disease at other sites, with fewer conventional atherosclerotic risk factors and there may be pathophysiological differences in plaque composition.[68] Greater vessel tortuosity has also been reported in radiation-related disease.[69] In a Dutch study, 36% of ischaemic events occurring following irradiation to the neck and chest for Hodgkin lymphoma were observed to be of cardiac origin,[65] suggesting that radiation-related damage to the heart including arrhythmias, myocardial dysfunction, valvular disease and endocardial damage may predispose to intra-cardiac thrombosis and embolism. In contrast to cerebral radionecrosis, TIAs and strokes tend to occur late after RT with a median interval of >15 years,[65,70] but the range is wide occurring from 1 to 22 years after treatment.[71] A syndrome of stroke-like migraine attacks after RT ("SMART" syndrome) has recently been described,[72] the presumed pathophysiology of which is also vascular damage and dysfunction.[73] Cranial irradiation in childhood may also cause abnormal development of the cerebral vasculature, leading to a vasculopathy with similar appearance to primary Moyamoya syndrome with netlike vessels and transdural anastomoses.[74] The adverse cognitive effects of cranial irradiation during childhood are also thought to be due, in part, to small vessel damage.[75]

Management of cerebral radionecrosis may be conservative, with corticosteroid therapy alone, but often requires surgery for the management of raised intracranial pressure or rapid control of symptoms. The management of radiation-related TIA and stroke is generally as for other causes. No adequate trials have been performed to assess the use of standard medical treatment options in this special circumstance. The roles of anti-platelet agents and statins, for example, remain unclear. Experience has demonstrated that intervention for carotid artery stenosis as for indications in non-radiation-related disease can be successful. Both open carotid surgery[76] and angioplasty with stenting[77] have been used for radiation-related disease. An open operation in a previously irradiated neck may result in a higher frequency of complications (cranial nerve injuries, wound complications, and increased use of interposition grafting)[68] and may be more technically difficult due to disease situated more proximally in the common carotid artery.[78] Carotid artery stenting has been reported to lead to a higher rate of re-stenosis in radiation-related disease in some studies[79] but not in all.[68] As the number of patients with radiation-related disease is insufficient to conduct a randomised

trial of open surgery versus carotid artery stenting, is has been svuggested that the most appropriate management should be decided by experts with adequate experience on an individual basis.[80]

■ Peripheral Vascular Disease

The entire arterial tree is sensitive to the late effects of radiation and, although less well studied than cardiac damage and cerebrovascular disease, radiation-related peripheral vascular disease (PVD) has also been described. The pathological lesions in small and medium arteries are similar to age-related atherosclerosis. Distinguishing features are that they occur in atypical sites, in clear relation with known volumes of irradiation and with a severity of disease in contrast to the rest of the individual's (unirradiated) vasculature. For larger arteries damage to the vasa vasorum, which supplies the arterial wall, becomes a more prominent pathological finding, resulting in ischaemic lesions of the vessel wall itself with characteristic features that distinguish this radiation-related injury from spontaneous atherosclerosis.[81]

Clinical examples of radiation-related PVD include; subclavian and axillary stenosis following neck irradiation,[23,82] renal and superior mesenteric artery stenosis following abdominal irradiation,[83,84] iliac and femoral disease following pelvic irradiation,[85,86] and femoral and popliteal disease following RT for osteosarcoma.[87] The clinical manifestations depend on the site and severity of the disease and include upper and lower extremity ischaemia, renal hypertension and mesenteric ischaemia. The venous system is generally thought less sensitive to damage from irradiation but may also suffer late adverse effects, most commonly stenosis complicated by thrombosis.[88]

When vascular intervention is required, it has been suggested that percutaneous procedures may be preferred to open surgery due to the technical difficulties that arise though operating within a surgical field that may be scarred and fibrotic due to the late effects of radiotherapy.[89] However open surgical revascularization has been performed with good results[90] and the management of individual cases is best decided by a vascular surgeon with some experience of the condition. As for all forms radiation-related cardiovascular disease, good control of cardiovascular risk factors, such as smoking cessation, hypertension, diabetes and hypercholesterolemia should be maintained, and anti-platelet therapy considered based on the severity of disease.[89]

CELLULAR AND MOLECULAR MECHANISMS OF RADIATION-RELATED CARDIOVASCULAR DISEASE

In contrast to the acute adverse effects of irradiation, where depletion of rapidly proliferating cells through cell death is the predominant mechanism of damage, the late adverse effects of irradiation arise through a wider variety of mechanisms.[91] The pathogenesis involves the interaction of various tissue components and multiple cell types including the endothelium, parenchyma, stroma, and immune system. Late adverse effects on the cardiovascular system are no exception and, although it is generally accepted that the main target in radiation-related cardiovascular disease is the endothelial cell (EC), the pathogenesis cannot be simply explained in terms of depletion of this cell type. There is experimental evidence that a range of cellular and molecular regulatory systems and mechanisms contribute to the development of RRCD. These mechanisms are summarised in this section.

■ Endothelial Damage and Dysfunction

The endothelial cells (ECs) that line the vasculature are thought to be the primary target for all forms of microvascular and macrovascular RRCD.[33] Although the heart valve leaflets are avascular, they are also covered in endocardium composed of ECs, which represents a target of irradiation[92] and may contribute to the development of fibrosis and calcification seen in radiation-related valve dysfunction. Rather than simply lining the vasculature and acting as a selectively permeable barrier, the vascular endothelium has many functions including the control of vascular tone and blood flow and the regulation of immune, inflammatory, thrombotic and coagulation responses.[93] Therefore the response of ECs to irradiation is central to understanding the mechanisms that underlie RRCD.

Much of the experimental evidence regarding the EC response to irradiation in the context of radiation-related heart disease pertains to microvascular damage within the myocardium. During animal experiments performed in the 1960s, it was observed using light microscopy that radiation damage to the heart muscle was preceded by alteration in capillary ECs.[94,95] These changes were later extensively described at the ultrastructural level using electron microscopy.[96] In response to irradiation, ECs swell and develop blebbing and extrusions. Vascular permeability is increased due to increased pinocytotic transport and widening of gap junctions, with transudation of serum components into the vessel wall causing subendothelial oedema. Leukocyte adhesion and extravasation and platelet sequestration are also seen. There is thickening of the basement membrane and foci of EC detachment cause exposure of the subendothelium. There is an increased proliferation of the remaining ECs, but this is inadequate to maintain microvascular function.[97] The end result of these observed changes is functional and physical capillary loss with narrowing, thrombosis, occlusion and a reduction in capillary density. This leads to parenchymal ischaemia initiating and exacerbating tissue injury with myocardial cell death and subsequent fibrosis.

While the pattern of endothelial response to irradiation described above has been recognized for more than 40 years, it is only more recently that the cellular and molecular mechanisms underlying this response are being elucidated through a combination of in vitro and animal experiments. The main pathways and processes thought to be involved are illustrated in Figure 7-4. While the details are not yet fully understood, an increasing volume of data is beginning to form a more coherent picture of the cellular and molecular radiobiology underlying RRCD.

■ Cytokine Activation, Inflammation and Increased Vascular Permeability

Endothelial activation by irradiation is known to result in the up-regulation of cellular adhesion molecules and cytokines, and the disruption of normal vascular permeability. These combine to produce a dysfunctional endothelium where resultant inflammation and oedema contribute to tissue damage.

Studies involving irradiation of ECs up to 20 Gy, both in vitro[98–103] and in vivo,[104,105] have reported dose-related elevations in the expression of the adhesion molecules ICAM-1, VCAM-1, PECAM-1, P-selectin and E-selectin. These molecules are known to mediate the rolling, adhesion and transmigration of leukocytes through the endothelium. The precise results vary between different experimental systems, apparently with the origin of the ECs, suggesting that the response may vary between different types of vessels and vascular beds. There is strong evidence that the induction of ICAM-1 by radiation is regulated by nuclear factor kappa-beta (NF-κβ).[106] More recently, activation of the NF-κβ signalling pathway has been shown to result in sustained inflammation in irradiated human arteries.[107]

The dose-dependent up-regulation of pro-inflammatory cytokines, including IL-6, IL-8, tumour necrosis factor-α (TNF-α) and monocyte chemotactic protein-1 (MCP-1) has been observed following endothelial cell

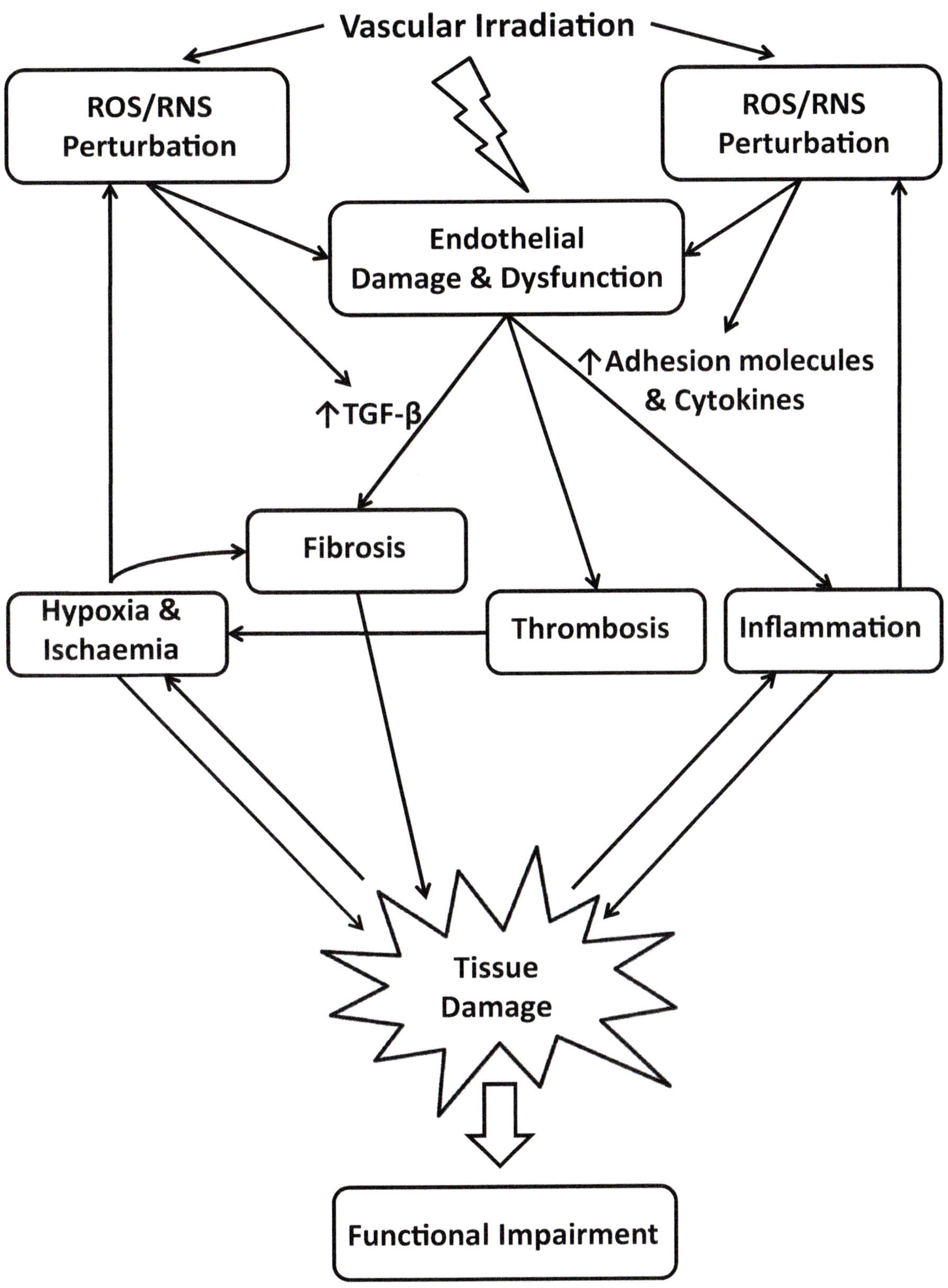

FIGURE 7-4 A diagram of the major processes thought to be involved in the pathogenesis of radiation-related cardiovascular damage (ROS, reactive oxygen species; RNS, reactive nitrogen oxide species; TGF-β, transforming growth factor-beta).

irradiation.[108,109] These are chemo-attractant to leukocytes and are also known to induce endothelial activation and proliferation.[110]

Irradiation of the endothelium results in dysregulation of its barrier function resulting in tissue oedema and contributing to local haemoconcentration and stasis of blood flow.[111] In vitro irradiation of cultured monolayers of ECs has been shown to affect the structure of the cytoskeleton, the organization of actin microfilaments and the integrity of intracellular junctions in a dose-dependent manner, with cells originating from the microvasculature being more severely affected than those from larger vessels.[112,113] A link between radiation-induced activation of the Rho/Rho-associated protein kinase (ROCK) pathway in endothelial cells and cytoskeletal remodelling and increased permeability has been demonstrated in vitro.[112] In vivo, changes in microvascular permeability have been observed within hours of irradiation in rodent models with leucocyte infiltration and fibrin accumulation in the perivascular tissues.[114]

In contrast to experiments utilizing higher doses mentioned above, studies of low dose irradiation of ECs in the range 0.3 to 0.7 Gy have been associated with reductions in leukocyte adhesion molecules[115–117] and varying radiation doses have been shown to have differential effects on cytokine expression.[118] It is therefore possible that the endothelial inflammatory response may vary qualitatively as well as quantitatively depending on radiation dose.

The inflammatory infiltrates produced by the above processes cause tissue injury through the release of proteases and reactive oxygen species (ROS) from activated phagocytes, and also contribute to tissue fibrosis as discussed below.

■ Thrombosis, Abnormal Coagulation and Altered Vascular Tone

Endothelial cells are central to the control of platelet adhesion, coagulation, fibrinolysis and vascular tone.[119] Impairment of this control can cause occlusion of the vascular lumen and impaired perfusion leading to hypoxia, oxidative stress and ischaemic tissue damage.

In response to injury, including radiation-induced damage, a number of prothrombotic changes are known to occur. Molecular responses reported following endothelial irradiation include the increased release of von Willebrand factor in both in vitro[120,121] and in vivo[122,123] experimental systems. Inhibition of the production of prostacycline (PGI$_2$), which normally functions as a potent inhibitor of platelet aggregation, has also been observed following 2 Gy irradiation of in vitro preparations of human endothelial cells.[124] These changes result in increased platelet recruitment to the vessel wall and the promotion of platelet aggregation and thrombus formation with the consequent release of platelet-derived mediators. EC death and detachment, with exposure of the basement membrane components, also contributes to platelet adhesion activation, and aggregation.

Endothelial cells normally express a number of surface molecules with anti-coagulant properties, including thrombomodulin (TM). In an in vivo model, irradiation of rat gut microvasculature resulted in a dose-dependent deficiency in TM due to inhibition of synthesis by mediators released by platelets adherent to the activated endothelium. This leads to the accumulation of thrombin, which, as well as being a powerful coagulant also has inflammatory and fibrogenic effects.[125] Activity of tissue factor (also known as factor III), an important initiator of the coagulation cascade, has been shown to be increased following EC irradiation.[126] Apoptotic ECs are also known to be pro-coagulant.[127] The normally pro-fibrinolytic properties of ECs are disrupted following irradiation[128] and the release of tissue plasminogen activator (tPA) is decreased.[129] The sum consequence of these changes is coagulation and fibrin deposition contributing to vascular occlusion.

Endothelial dysfunction is also characterised by an imbalance in vascular tone with a reduction in the availability of nitric oxide (NO) and other vasodilators, such as PGI$_2$, and an increase in the levels of vasoconstrictors such as endothelin-1, thromboxane A$_2$ and angiotensin-II.[93] NO-mediated relaxation of arteries has been shown to be impaired following irradiation in animal models[130,131] and in humans.[132,133] Changes in vascular tone may lead to altered blood flow causing reduced perfusion and worsening tissue hypoxia. In addition, NO and PGI$_2$ not only affect vascular tone but also inhibit platelet aggregation and have tPA-like properties, thus their reduction also contributes to thrombosis and coagulation.

■ Hypoxia and Oxidative Stress

There is a growing body of evidence that tissue hypoxia and chronic oxidative stress drive a variety of radiation-induced late effects.[134,135] Oxidative stress is postulated to play a role in the initiation and/or perpetuation of non-radiation induced cardiovascular conditions, including atherosclerosis and cardiac fibrosis,[136] and most classical cardiovascular risk factors contribute to oxidative stress.[137] It is therefore likely that oxidative stress also contributes to radiation-induced cardiovascular late effects.

The molecular mechanisms underlying oxidative stress are beginning to be understood in terms of an imbalance between reactive oxygen and nitrogen oxide species. Reactive oxygen species (ROS), such as superoxide ($O_2^{\cdot-}$), hydrogen peroxide (H_2O_2) and hydroxyl radicals ($^{\cdot}OH$) are continuously generated by normal aerobic cell metabolism. These are usually neutralised by anti-oxidant enzymes, such as superoxide dismutase (SOD) and catalase, or dietary anti-oxidants, such as vitamin C and E, to prevent the oxidative damage of proteins, deoxyribonucleic acid (DNA) and lipids. Reactive nitrogen oxide species (RNS) also play a role in physiological and pathophysiological processes. These include the free radical nitrogen oxide ($^{\cdot}NO$) and other RNS formed by the reaction of $^{\cdot}NO$ with oxygen or $O_2^{\cdot-}$. $^{\cdot}NO$ is synthesised by the enzyme nitrogen oxide synthase (NOS), which is found in a variety of cells and tissues including the vascular endothelial cells.[134] Under normal conditions the production and destruction of ROS and RNS remain in balance. In some pathological circumstances however the mechanisms maintaining this balance are disrupted, creating a cellular state known as oxidative stress.

Irradiation of biological material produces an immediate burst of ROS generation due to the direct ionization of water and other target molecules. However, the quantity of ROS produced in this fashion is minute compared to that produced by normal cell activity[138] and prolonged cellular production of ROS/RNS has been observed days after irradiation.[134] It seems likely that it is perturbation of normal cellular functioning, rather than direct production of reactive species by radiation, which causes oxidative stress in these circumstances. There are several postulated mechanisms by which this could occur including radiation-induced inflammation, hypoxia and mitochondrial dysfunction.

The inflammatory processes initiated by irradiation, as described above, result in increased levels of ROS, which are produced by activated phagocytes such as macrophages. Irradiation-induced endothelial damage and dysfunction lead to microvascular thrombosis and reduced capillary density, resulting in reduced tissue perfusion, hypoxia and further ROS production. Both of these processes can be self-perpetuating in the absence of normal physiological controls as ROS can cause tissue damage and further inflammation and decreased levels of NO, due to degradation by superoxide or a reduction in NOS activity, can cause further endothelial dysfunction.

There are several results from animal experiments supporting the involvement of these mechanisms in the context of RRCD. Cardiac irradiation of a rat model resulted in activation of anti-oxidant pathways, with decreased vitamin E and increased SOD and glutathione peroxidise, and an associated decline in cardiac function.[139] Total body irradiation of rats resulted in a reduction in endothelial NOS activity and structural and functional cardiac degeneration.[140] Xanthine oxidase (XO) activation, and increased superoxide production, resulting in endothelial dysfunction and increased vascular stiffness has also been observed in rat aorta following irradiation.[131,141] In addition, a number of animal experiments investigating anti-oxidant strategies to ameliorate endothelial or cardiovascular effects of irradiation have met with some success[142] lending further weight to the concept that oxidative stress is involved in the pathogenesis of RRCD.

Mitochondria are the primary site of ROS and RNS following irradiation,[143] and damage and dysfunction of endothelial mitochondria has been linked to the development of non-radiation-related cardiovascular disease.[144] Recently, proteomic analyses of cardiac mitochondria following in vivo irradiation of mouse hearts with doses of 0.2 and 2 Gy revealed persistent alterations in oxidative function and mitochondrial cytoskeletal proteins 4 weeks following irradiation.[145] There was also evidence of enhanced ROS production in the mitochondria irradiated to 2 Gy.

Taken together these findings support the theory that inflammation, hypoxia and mitochondrial dysfunction with resultant free-radical production produce chronic oxidative stress that contributes to late normal tissue damage within the cardiovascular system.

■ Fibrosis

Radiation-induced fibrosis is a process central to late adverse effects of radiation treatment in many organs, including the skin, lung, gut and liver.[146] The pathogenesis is complex and remains incompletely understood, but has been likened to a "wound that does not heal" with an abnormal perpetual activation of repair signalling by cytokines thought to be key.[147] Myocardial fibrosis was described decades ago as a component of radiation-induced heart disease both in experimental animal models and in post-mortem studies of humans.[148] An increase in the ratio of type I to type III collagen has been reported in irradiated myocardium from human autopsy studies, which is thought to decrease myocardial compliance and contribute to diastolic dysfunction.[34] As well as interfering with the mechanical function of the heart, fibrosis may also affect electrophysiological function further reducing cardiac efficiency.[149]

Radiation is known to trigger fibroblasts and other progenitors (e.g., vascular smooth muscle cells)[150] to differentiate into post-mitotic functional myofibroblasts resulting in the increased collagen and extracellular matrix deposition that characterises tissue fibrosis.[151] Experiments in cell culture models suggest that radiation doses as low as 1 Gy may be able to stimulate the fibrogenic process.[152] A greater understanding of the cellular and molecular mechanisms underlying radiation-induced fibrosis has developed over the last decade.

Transforming growth factor-β1 (TGF-β1) effects[153] mediated by the SMAD pathway[154] play a pivotal role in radiation-induced fibrosis. TGF-β1 is activated by release from a latent form bound to the extracellular matrix, both directly by irradiation and also indirectly through endothelial cell damage and perturbation of the ROS/RNS balance.[155] TGF-β1 activation has been observed following irradiation by doses as low as 0.1 Gy.[156] Studies of the TGF-β1/SMAD pathway have been performed in a variety of tissues including the skin, gut and lung, and there is good evidence that TGF-β1 is also involved in the fibrotic processes seen in radiation-related heart disease. In rats the expression of TGF-β1 mRNA has been shown to increase within 1 day of cardiac irradiation and remain elevated for at least 3 months subsequently, during which time cardiac fibrosis is seen to develop.[157] Over-expression of TGF-β1 leads to an increase in pro-collagen mRNA, the precursor of collagen production.[157,158] Administration of pentoxifylline (PTX) and vitamin E to suppress this up-regulation reduces the appearance of cardiac fibrosis, both in the myocardium and the walls of coronary arteries.[146,159] Conversely, administration of a TGF-β1-inducing compound worsens radiation-induced cardiac fibrosis.[160] In humans, a recent study of women previously irradiated for breast cancer suggested an association between a TGF-β1 genetic polymorphism (TGF-β1 29C>T) and subsequent cardiovascular disease risk (HR = 1.76, 95% CI 0.99-3.26, p = 0.06), but it could be that this effect is independent of radiotherapy as there was not sufficient power to test for any interaction.[161]

As well as the involvement of the TGF-β/SMAD pathway, the Rho/ROCK pathway has more recently been demonstrated to be activated in fibrotic irradiated tissues.[162] ROCKs, the downstream regulators of Rho GTPases, are involved in the regulation of cell motility and morphology through action on the cytoskeleton. This is thought to result in fibrogenic changes in cell phenotype. Activation of this pathway been demonstrated to occur following irradiation in both cultured mouse cardiomyocytes in vitro and in the heart and lungs of mice in vivo, where it was associated with cardiac hypertrophy and a decline in left ventricular (LV) function. Inhibition of the pathway with statins (which inhibit Rho) or the ROCK inhibitor Y-27632, protected against cardiac fibrosis.[163]

The best characterised downstream target of TGF-β1 signalling is connective tissue growth factor (CTGF), a protein that promotes fibroblast proliferation and extracellular matrix production. After the initiation of fibrogenic processes, and despite very low TGF-β1 levels, CTGF induction persists via activation of the Rho/ROCK pathway, independent of SMAD signalling, in an auto-feedback mechanism.[164] It has therefore been suggested that initiation of fibrosis may occur through SMAD pathway signalling but, even following removal of the initial stimulus, it is maintained through the Rho/ROCK/CTGF cascade.

Experimental rat models have suggested a regulatory role for mast cells in the pathogenesis of myocardial fibrosis. Mast cell deficient rats were observed to suffer more severe post-irradiation collagen deposition and a greater reduction of cardiac function in response to cardiac irradiation when compared to normal controls.[165] Mast cells are known to express a wide range of mediators, including pro- and anti-fibrotic factors that may affect tissue deposition of collagen and collagen cross-linking through effects on cardiac fibroblasts. It has been suggested that mast cells may interact with the cardiac endothelin system during response to irradiation,[166] which has also been implicated in the pathophysiology of non-radiation-related cardiovascular disease.[167] The cardiac sensory nervous system signalling through neuro-peptide mediators including calcitonin gene related peptide (CGRP), substance P and neuropeptide Y may also play a role in these interactions.[160]

In addition to those described above there is a long list of further fibrogenic factors that can activate fibroblasts in response to tissue injury, including IL-4, IL-13, basic fibroblast growth factor (bFGF), platelet-derived growth factor (PDGF) and insulin-like growth factor (IGF).[40] PDGF inhibitors have been shown to inhibit pulmonary fibrosis secondary to irradiation in mice,[168] but the significance of these other mediators in cardiac radiation fibrosis is currently unknown.

■ Renin-Angiotensin-Aldosterone System

The renin-angiotensin-aldosterone (RAA) system is established as a key endocrine and paracrine component in the regulation of blood volume, arterial blood pressure and cardiovascular function.[169] It is known to have an important pathophysiological role in many forms of cardiovascular disease. The significance of this role has been confirmed by a number of clinical trials demonstrating the benefits of down-regulating the RAA system, using angiotensin converting enzyme (ACE) inhibitors or angiotensin receptor (AR) blockers, in hypertension, ischaemic heart disease and heart failure.

More recently additional functions of the RAA system have been recognised, including tissue homeostasis and response to injury,[170] which may be relevant to the pathogenesis of radiation-induced late effects. The involvement of the RAA system has been demonstrated in animal-models of radiation-induced nephropathy, pulmonary fibrosis and late brain injury.[171] ACE inhibitors appear to decrease the risk of radiation damage at doses that do not affect blood pressure and molecular types without a free-radical scavenging thiol group are also effective. Therefore it has been proposed that they may act locally and through non-anti-oxidant mechanisms. What these exact mechanisms may be are currently unknown, but the effects of the RAA system at a molecular and cellular level are wide ranging and there are several routes through which it could be involved. For example, angiotensin II (Ang II) is recognised as having many non-haemodynamic effects, acting as a pro-inflammatory mediator and growth factor, participating in transcriptional regulation via NF-κβ and exerting effects through the endothelin-1 and Rho pathways.[172] Importantly it is known that local Ang II enhances TGF-β1 expression,[173] an important signal in fibrosis following irradiation as described above. Ang II also alters cell function by increasing the generation of ROS,[171] which could contribute to chronic oxidative stress. It therefore seems likely that the RAA system is involved in the pathogenesis of radiation-induced heart disease and there is some experimental evidence to support this hypothesis. For example, in rat models the RAA system is activated following local heart irradiation by single doses of 15 Gy, with systemic increases in the levels of Ang II and aldosterone[174] and local increases in the cardiac expression of ACE and AR type 1.[158] Also, the ACE inhibitor captopril reduced myocardial fibrosis and prevented capillary density loss after cardiac irradiation of in rats, although it did not protect function.[175] Interestingly, mast cell chymases are a main converter of Angiotensin I to AngII other than ACE and the RAA system may also interact with the endothelin and cardiac nervous systems, demonstrating again the interrelated nature of the candidate systems thought to be involved in the pathogenesis of RRCD.[160]

Endothelial Cell Death, Compensatory Proliferation and Repair

As well as endothelial damage and dysfunction, EC death and compensatory EC proliferation are known to play a role in radiation-induced vascular effects. It is thought that EC death occurs mainly through delayed mitotic death. It has been suggested that early radiation-induced apoptosis may also play a role,[176,177] but this mechanism remains controversial.[178] The paradigm-shift away from the target-cell hypothesis towards cytokine networks[179] suggests that that sub-lethal EC damage and dysfunction as discussed above is more important in the pathogenesis of radiation-related cardiovascular disease than EC death.

Radiation dose-dependent loss of alkaline phosphatase activity (an endothelial marker) prior to capillary loss and subsequent myocardial degeneration has been observed in irradiated animal models.[180] Compensatory EC proliferation and subsequent myocardial degeneration was seen only in the areas of focal enzyme loss. The mechanistic significance of loss of alkaline phosphatase activity in this circumstance remains unclear, but it is known to be involved in EC proliferation and regulation of microvascular blood flow by dephosphorylating extracellular nucleoside phosphates.[181]

Irradiation has been demonstrated to inhibit re-endotheliolization and angiogenesis,[182] reducing the regenerative capacity of the vasculature. Concomitant irradiation of bone marrow may also impair the production of endothelial progenitor cells (EPCs)[183] that would normally contribute to repair.[184] Recently reported experiments utilizing mouse and human-cultured EPCs have demonstrated that their irradiation results in functional defects, mediated by p53 activation and vascular endothelial growth factor (VEGF) suppression, leading to attenuated vascular regeneration.[185] The importance of damage of these endothelial repair mechanisms to the development of RRCD is yet to be confirmed.

Mechanisms of Radiation-Related Atherosclerosis

Much of the laboratory investigation into the endothelial mechanisms underlying the vascular effects of irradiation has concentrated on ECs in culture or on the microvasculature, largely because of the technical difficulties of studying larger vessels. There is good experimental evidence, however, that radiation is a risk factor for macrovascular, as well as microvascular, damage. Commonly used laboratory animals tend to be relatively resistant to atherosclerosis and investigators have therefore needed to utilise atherosclerosis prone models. For example irradiation has been shown to cause atherosclerosis in hypercholesterolaemic rabbits[186,187] and apolipoprotein-E negative (ApoE(-/-)) mice.[17,188–190] The EC is thought to still represent the primary target, with the initial events being endothelial damage, monocyte adhesion and transmigration into the vessel wall. These are then activated into lipid ingesting macrophages forming foam cells and fatty streaks, the earliest stage of atheroma formation.[191] Sustained inflammation within irradiated human arterial walls has recently been demonstrated[107] analogous to the type of on-going inflammatory process that is thought to underlie spontaneous atherosclerosis.[192] Both microvascular and macrovascular radiation-related damage likely combine to cause clinical disease in the heart.[33]

DNA Damage

Irradiation is known to cause damage to DNA both directly and via the production of free radicals. However the extent to which DNA damage is responsible for the cardiovascular late effects of radiotherapy, is not known. It has been theorised that the risk and severity of adverse normal tissue responses may depend on an underlying genetically determined DNA repair capacity.[193] Against this suggestion in the context of RRCD is that the classical molecular radiobiology of DNA strand breaks leading to cell depletion does not appear to play a predominant role in what is understood of the mechanisms described above. Results from immunohistochemical staining of irradiated human arteries indicate that an important early step in endothelial activation, NF-κβ activation, is present in virtually every single cell of the arterial wall,[137] making it unlikely that the cause was DNA-damage in each separate cell. It is much more likely that either an original DNA-damage signal is propagated between cells by a "bystander effect"[194] or that the initiating signal is some other stressor, such as oxidative stress. These observations bring into question the logic of using classic radiobiological models, such as the linear quadratic model, to describe dose-responses for late effects cardiovascular effects, as this is based on an assumption that DNA-damage is the underlying mechanism.

One cardiovascular disease in which DNA damage, in the form of somatic mutation, has been recognized is atherosclerosis. Proliferating smooth muscle cells in atherosclerotic plaques have been shown to be monoclonal and these clones could, in theory, be initiated or propagated by irradiation.[195] Genetic instability in age-related human atherosclerotic plaques has also been described.[196] Additionally radiation damage to telomeres within ECs may trigger cells into senescence, initiating atherosclerosis.[191] Low doses of radiation are known to induce persistent genetic instability, suggesting a mechanism by which the pathogenic pathways of age-related and radiation-related atherosclerosis may interact.

Direct Radiation Damage to Myocardiocytes

Although the generally held view is that myocardiocyte death and subsequent myocardial fibrosis is secondary to microvascular damage and ischaemia, there are experimental findings that suggest direct death of myocardial cells secondary to high-dose irradiation (>30 Gy) with replacement fibrosis may occur.[197,198] There are however differences in the degree of myocardial degeneration seen between different species and strains of experimental animal, and whether this mechanism is apparent in humans or at the doses and fractionations used in therapeutic radiotherapy is uncertain. Studies of biomarkers of myocardial damage (e.g., high sensitivity troponin) have revealed some evidence of direct damage during or immediately after radiotherapy,[199] but it remains most likely that the development of cardiovascular disease in the long term occurs through indirect pathways involving other cells types, rather than solely through a direct effect on cardiomyocytes themselves.

Abscopal Effects

It is possible that cardiovascular risk may be elevated by indirect or abscopal effects, i.e., "off target" effects as a consequence of irradiation of tissues other than those comprising the organ in which the late effects are expressed clinically. There are many theoretical mechanisms by which this could occur, for example; renal irradiation causing hypertension,[200,201] systemic inflammatory or immune effects,[202–206] effects on lipid metabolism[207,208] and endocrine effects including diabetes,[209,210] hypothyroidism, hyperparathyroidism[211] and growth hormone deficiency.[212,213] There is some experimental evidence in rats demonstrating cardiac abnormalities following total body irradiation that did not occur with localised thoracic irradiation to the same dose[141] and degenerative cardiac changes have been observed in mice following brain irradiation.[214] However it remains uncertain whether and to what extent these possible abscopal effects of irradiation affect cardiovascular risk in humans.

Conclusion

While the pathogenesis of RRCD is clearly complicated and remains incompletely understood, advances in cellular and molecular radiobiology have led to an improved understanding of the mechanisms underlying this important late effect of radiation therapy.

It can be anticipated that further technical advances, perhaps utilizing newer techniques such as radiogenomics[137,161] and radioproteomics,[145,215] will continue to improve our knowledge over the coming years. For example, profiling by microarray has recently been used to characterise gene expression in irradiated human arteries versus controls from the same individual and has revealed over-representation of genes associated with angiogenesis, coagulation, and inflammation in the irradiated vessels and suggested a role for the HOXA9 homeobox transcription factor in the regulation of NF-$\kappa\beta$ activation.[137] The primary clinical motivation for understanding these mechanisms is that it opens potential opportunities to reduce or avoid the adverse effects of radiation on the cardiovascular system by pharmacological intervention. This concept has already resulted in a substantial number of animal experiments and studies using cultured human cells where drugs have been used in an effort to ameliorate radiation damage. A small number of clinical trials in patients have also been performed,[216-219] but such agents remain largely experimental and are yet to establish any role in clinical practice. It may be hoped that, in the future, the combination of advances in radiotherapy planning and delivery with the development of pharmacological interventions, both based on improved radiobiological understanding, may improve outcomes in cancer survivors by reducing the negative impact of RRCD.

RADIATION-RELATED HEART DISEASE FOLLOWING BREAST CANCER TREATMENT

▪ Randomized Data

Radiotherapy has been given to women with breast cancer for more than 50 years and it is currently recommended for a substantial proportion of such women. Overviews of the randomized trials of radiotherapy for breast cancer from the Early Breast Cancer Trialists' Collaborative Group (EBCTCG) have shown that in suitable women, radiotherapy reduces the risk of recurrence by a substantial amount and reduces breast cancer mortality by a moderate amount, ignoring deaths from other causes. The absolute 15-year reductions in breast cancer mortality were around 4% from radiotherapy after breast conserving surgery based on 10,801 women in 17 randomized trials[220] and around 7% from radiotherapy after mastectomy for node positive disease, based on 3131 women in 22 trials.[221] Most of the breast cancer radiotherapy regimens in these trials involved some unwanted irradiation of normal tissues, including the heart, and the EBCTCG analyses have shown that the beneficial effect of the radiotherapy on breast cancer mortality was offset by an increase in mortality from heart disease.[222]

▪ Observational Data

In observational studies where the women receiving radiation have not been selected at random, comparison of irradiated and unirradiated women may give misleading answers.[223] However, regimens used to treat left-sided cancers usually deliver a higher cardiac radiation dose than those used to treat right-sided cancers.[224] So comparison of heart disease rates between women irradiated for left-sided breast cancer and women irradiated for right-sided breast cancer may provide information on the extent to which the risk of heart disease has been increased as a result of the radiotherapy. There is little confounding in this comparison as most factors causing heart disease will not differ in women with left and right-sided breast cancer.[225] This was shown in a study of 35,000 women treated for breast cancer during 1976–2006;[42] in unirradiated women heart disease incidence did not vary according to laterality.

Two factors should be taken into account when comparing heart disease rates in women with left and right-sided breast cancer. First, the comparison is only informative if laterality does not affect the decision to give radiotherapy or the technique used, as was the case until the 2000s. Since the year 2000, concerns about radiation-induced heart disease in some countries have resulted in a tendency to avoid radiotherapy in women with left breast cancer, so left versus right cardiac mortality ratios for patients treated since 2000 may reflect patient selection rather than the effect of radiotherapy. Second, the left versus right comparison gives information on the risks of higher versus lower radiation dose, not the risks of radiotherapy versus no radiotherapy. This is because irradiation of right-sided breast cancer usually involves some cardiac exposure,[226] which may result in some cardiac hazard therefore the increase in the risk of heart disease associated with radiotherapy is likely to be higher than the left versus right cardiac mortality ratios.

Heart disease rates in women irradiated for left-sided and right-sided breast cancers have been reported in several populations of women: Studies of cardiac mortality after breast cancer radiotherapy are summarised in Table 7-1[24,225,227-247] and studies of incident heart disease in Table 7-2.[24,25,42,228,231,237,240,243,248-252]

TABLE 7-1 Observational studies comparing heart disease mortality in women irradiated for left-sided breast cancer with women irradiated for right-sided breast cancer

STUDY*	NUMBER WOMEN**	YEARS OF IRRADIATION	FOLLOW-UP (YEARS) MEAN OR MEDIAN	NUMBER OF DEATHS FROM HEART DISEASE		MORTALITY RATE RATIO LEFT VERSUS RIGHT
				Left-sided cancer	Right-sided cancer	
USA Wright et al.[227]	66,687	1990–1999	16	2,256	2,248	0.97 (0.92–1.03)
USA Boero et al.[228]	29,102	2000–2009	<10	619	572	1.08 (0.96–1.21)
USA Ye et al.[229]	2,796	1990–1997	14	60	85	0.70 (0.51–0.97)
British Columbia Chan et al.[230]	5,334	1990–1998	14	117	115	0.99 (0.77–1.27)
Netherlands Boekel et al.[231]	10,468	1989–2004	8	11[a]	13[a]	0.70 (0.31–1.56)
Norway Tjessem et al.[232]	1,566	1975–1991	>20	NS	NS	0.93 (0.52–1.66)
USA Henson et al.[233]	5,58,871	1973–2008	7	3,117	2,743	1.08 (1.03–1.14)
France Bouillon et al.[234]	4,456	1954–1984	28	85	61	1.56 (1.27–1.90)
Switzerland Bouchardy et al.[235]	1,245	1980–2004	8	8	11	0.7 (0.3–1.6)
USA Gutt et al.[236]	41[¶]	1980–1994	10	4	2	4.2 (0.9–20.9)
Netherlands Borger et al.[237]	1,601	1980–1993	16	14[b]	5[b]	2.35 (0.85–6.50)
Canada Marhin et al.[238]	7,447	1984–2000	8	52	47	1.07 (0.72–1.59)
UK Roychoudhuri et al.[239]	20,871 (53% irradiated)	1971–1988	18	130[c]	101[c]	1.23 (0.95–1.60)
Canada Paszat et al.[240]	6,680	1982–1988	>13	47[b]	42[b]	1.07 (0.65–1.72)
USA Harris et al.[24]	961	1977–1994	12	17	10	1.67 (0.78–3.62)
USA Darby et al.[225]	1,15,165	1973–2001	6	1,756	1,434	1.16 (1.08–1.24)
USA Giordano et al.[241]	27,283	1973–1989	9	1,218[c]	996[c]	1.16 (1.07–1.26)

STUDY*	NUMBER WOMEN**	YEARS OF IRRADIATION	FOLLOW-UP (YEARS) MEAN OR MEDIAN	NUMBER OF DEATHS FROM HEART DISEASE		MORTALITY RATE RATIO LEFT VERSUS RIGHT
Sweden Darby et al.[242]	89,407 (~33% irradiated)	1970–1996	8	2,492[c]	2,199[c]	1.06 (1.00–1.12)
Canada Vallis et al.[243]	2,128	1982–1988	10	8[b]	6[b]	1.31 (0.46–3.76)
Canada Paszat et al.[244]	3,006	1982–1987	8	30[b]	14[b]	2.10 (1.11–3.95)
USA Paszat et al.[245]	47,948	1973–1992	7	NS	NS	1.17 (1.01–1.36)
USA Nixon et al.[246]	745	1968–1986	>12	9	9	1.3 ($p = 0.29$)
Sweden Rutqvist et al.[247]	54,617 (~50% irradiated)	1970–1985	9	1,803[b]	1,566[b]	1.09 (1.02–1.17)

* Some studies include overlapping data. For example Henson 2013, Darby 2005, Giordano 2005 and Paszat 1998 all include women registered on the SEER cancer registry.
**100% irradiated unless indicated.
¶Radiotherapy given for ductal carcinoma in situ.
[a]Cardiovascular disease
[b]Myocardial infarction
[c]Ischemic heart disease
NS, Not stated
Studies with fewer than 5 events in any of the above categories are excluded.

TABLE 7-2 Observational studies comparing incidence of heart disease in women irradiated for left-sided breast cancer with women irradiated for right-sided breast cancer

STUDY	NUMBER WOMEN**	YEAR OF IRRADIATION	FOLLOW-UP (YEARS) MEAN OR MEDIAN	NUMBER OF EVENTS		INCIDENCE RATE RATIO LEFT VERSUS RIGHT
				Left-sided cancer	Right-sided cancer	
USA Boero et al.[228]	29,102	2000–2009	<10	NS	NS	1.05 (0.98–1.13)[b]
Netherlands Boerman et al.[248]	229	1970–2007	~9	NS	NS	0.7 (0.3–1.4)[a]
Netherlands Boekel et al.[231]¶	10,468	1989–2004	8	73[a]	65[a]	0.94 (0.67–1.32)[a]
				31[c]	33[c]	0.78 (0.48–1.27)[c]
				10[d]	10[d]	0.83 (0.34–2.03)[d]
Denmark/ Sweden McGale et al.[42]	34,825	1976–2006	8	2,275	2,016	1.08 (1.02–1.15)

(continued)

TABLE 7-2 Observational studies comparing incidence of heart disease in women irradiated for left-sided breast cancer with women irradiated for right-sided breast cancer (*continued*)

STUDY	NUMBER WOMEN**	YEAR OF IRRADIATION	FOLLOW-UP (YEARS) MEAN OR MEDIAN	NUMBER OF EVENTS		INCIDENCE RATE RATIO LEFT VERSUS RIGHT
				878[c]	712[c]	1.18 (1.07–1.30)[c]
				310[d]	315[d]	0.95 (0.81–1.11)[d]
Netherlands Borger et al.[237]	1,601	1980–1993	16	139[a]	85[a]	1.38 (1.05–1.81)[a]
				73[c]	44[c]	1.35 (0.93–1.98)[c]
Netherlands Hooning et al.[25]	4,414 (86% irradiated)	1970–1986	18	122[b]	117[b]	0.98 (0.77–1.25)[b]
				184[d]	167[d]	1.03 (0.84-1.26)[d]
USA Doyle et al.[249]	25,653	1992–2000	10	NS	NS	0.99 (0.87–1.11)[b]
Canada Paszat et al.[240]	6,680	1982–1988	>13	72[b]	49[b]	1.42 (0.92–2.17)[b]
USA Pinder et al.[250]	43,338 (44% irradiated)	1992–2002	5	NS	NS	1.04 (0.97–1.10)[d]
USA Harris et al.[24]	961	1977–1994	12	30[b]	9[b]	3.1 (1.5–6.5)[b]
USA Patt et al.[251]	16,270	1986–1993	10	1,780	1,668	1.06 (0.99–1.14)
				808[d]	764[d]	1.05 (0.95–1.17)[d]
Canada Vallis et al.[243]	2,128	1982–1988	10	26[b]	23[b]	1.11 (0.64–1.93)[b]
Sweden Rutqvist et al.[252]	684	1976–1987	9	5[b]	7[b]	0.77 (0.25–2.42)[b]

**100% irradiated unless indicated
[¶]Radiotherapy given for ductal carcinoma in situ
[a]Cardiovascular disease
[b]Myocardial infarction
[c]Ischemic heart disease
[d]Congestive heart failure
NS, Not stated
Studies with fewer than 5 events in any of the above categories are excluded.

Studies of cardiac mortality after breast cancer radiotherapy ■ Around a million women worldwide irradiated since the 1950s have been included in 23 studies in which cardiac mortality in women irradiated for left-sided breast cancer was compared with that for women irradiated for right-sided breast cancer. The cardiac mortality ratio left versus right was greater than one in 17 of the 23 studies, and in 8 of them the increase was statistically significant. In one recent study, the left versus right cardiac mortality ratio was significantly less than one: 0.70 (0.51–0.97).[229] Inter-study variation in the left-right cardiac mortality ratio is likely to arise from differing study follow-up times, radiotherapy techniques and cardiac endpoints.

The largest study, involving more around 6,000 cardiac deaths, was based on data from the U.S. Surveillance Epidemiology and End Results (SEER) cancer registry.[233] The left versus right cardiac mortality ratio was 1.08 (1.03–1.14). The study demonstrated very clearly the increasing cardiac risk with increasing time since diagnosis. For women irradiated during 1973–1982 the cardiac mortality ratios, left-sided versus right-sided during time-periods <10, 10–14, 15–19 and 20+ years since diagnosis, were 1.19 (1.03–1.38),

1.35 (1.05–1.73), 1.64 (1.26–2.14) and 1.90 (1.52–2.37) respectively (2p for trend: <0.001). There was some evidence of a reduced hazard for women diagnosed more recently. Inevitably, however, information on the possible long-term risks associated with modern radiotherapy regimens is not yet available.

Studies of incident heart disease after breast cancer radiotherapy ■ Around 150,000 women irradiated since the 1970s have been included in 13 studies that compared incidence of heart disease in women irradiated for left-sided breast cancer with women irradiated for right-sided breast cancer. The left versus right ratio of incident heart disease varied from 0.7 to 3.1 but was elevated in most studies. Variation in this ratio is probably due to differences in the populations studied and treatments involved, as in the studies of cardiac mortality. In addition, four studies of incident heart disease included only women over 65 years old at the time of their radiotherapy[228,249–251] and one study only included women who were also treated with anthracycline-based chemotherapy.[250]

The largest study included 35,000 women who received radiotherapy for breast cancer during 1976–2006 and were followed to 2006.[42] For irradiated women, the incidence ratio, left-sided versus right-sided, was raised for all heart diseases combined (1.08, 95% CI 1.02–1.15, $p = 0.01$). It was also raised for the individual diagnoses of ischaemic heart disease (1.18, 95% CI 1.07–1.30, $p = 0.001$), pericarditis (1.61, 95% CI 1.06–2.43, $p = 0.03$), and valvular heart disease (1.54, 95% CI 1.11–2.13, $p = 0.009$). Three other studies have investigated the left versus right ratio of valvular heart disease. In the first,[251] the left-versus right ratio of valve disease in 16,270 women who received radiotherapy between 1986 and 1993 when aged >65 years was 1.07 (0.89–1.30), based on 465 events. In the second,[24] the left versus right ratio of valve disease in 961 women irradiated between 1977 and 1994 was 0.85 (0.6–1.3) based on 90 events. The third study only included 8 events.[231] These differences in left versus right ratios of valve disease are likely to be due to differences in radiotherapy techniques: Some radiotherapy techniques used in the 1970s and 80s included the valves in the radiotherapy fields and others did not.

■ Variation in Risk with Cardiac Dose

A few studies have investigated the relationship between the risk of heart disease and the type of breast cancer radiotherapy used. First, a case-cohort study of women irradiated for breast cancer in Ontario, Canada between 1982 and 1988[240] included detailed information on the sites irradiated and the

radiotherapy fields used. The risk of myocardial infarction was increased by the use of internal mammary radiotherapy, left breast radiotherapy and the size of the left breast boost field, all of which increase radiation dose to the heart. A similar finding was reported by Hooning et al.[25] who studied 4414 women irradiated in the Netherlands between 1970 and 1986 and found that the risk of myocardial infarction was greatest for women who received internal mammary irradiation in the 1970s. These findings suggest that the use of radiotherapy regimens or fields that delivered higher heart doses increased the risk of myocardial infarction relative to regimens that delivered lower heart doses.

The dose-response relationship based on the largest number of cardiac events was a population-based case-control study, including nearly 1000 incident cases of ischaemic heart disease after breast cancer radiotherapy.[5] The rate of major coronary events rates increased approximately linearly with mean heart dose, by 7.4% per Gy (95% CI 2.9-14.5; p<0.001) with no apparent threshold (Figure 7-5). The increase started within 5 years of radiotherapy and continued into the third decade. The percentage increase in major coronary events per Gy was similar in women with and without cardiac risk factors at the time of radiotherapy. It did not differ significantly according to any other patient or tumour characteristics for which information was available, or according to other cancer treatments that the women had received.

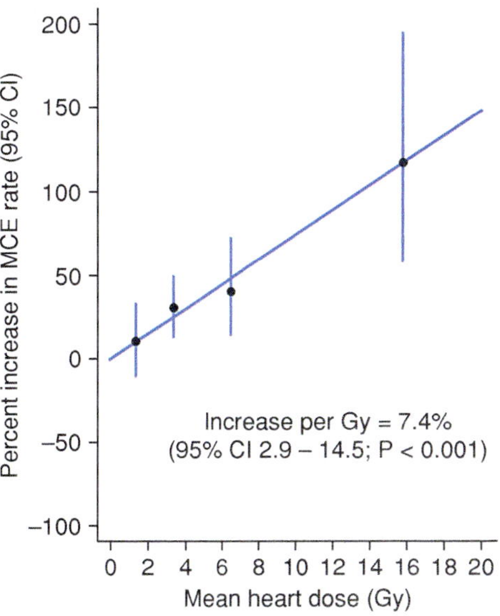

FIGURE 7-5 Percent increase in rate of major coronary events (MCEs) according to mean heart dose in Gy. Gradient based on dose estimates for individual women. Points based on categories of women; vertical lines are 95% confidence intervals (CI). (Reproduced with permission from Darby SC et al., 2013.[5])

Estimates of the absolute risks of radiation-related ischaemic heart disease are needed to help oncologists plan each individual woman's treatment. These risks can then be balanced against the absolute benefits of radiotherapy. The absolute increase in cardiac risk from radiotherapy for an individual is given by her background cardiac risk in the absence of radiotherapy multiplied by the percentage increase in risk arising from radiotherapy. Thus absolute radiation-related risks are greater for women with pre-existing cardiac risk factors than for other women. For a woman aged 50 with no pre-existing cardiac risk factors, radiotherapy involving a mean heart dose of 3 Gy would increase her 30-year risk of having at least one acute coronary event from 4.5% to 5.4%, i.e., an absolute risk from radiotherapy of about 0.9% percentage points (Figure 7-6), provided that she did not die of other causes first. If she had a cardiac risk factor before her radiotherapy, a mean heart dose of 3 Gy would increase her risk of an acute coronary event from 8.0% to 9.7%, i.e., an absolute risk from radiotherapy of about 1.7% percentage points (Figure 7-6), again provided that she did not die of other causes first.

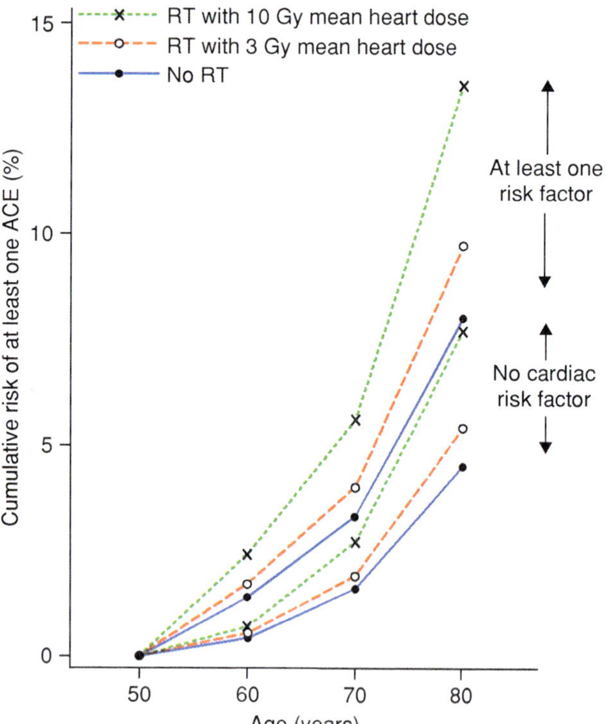

FIGURE 7-6 Cumulative risk of at least one acute coronary event (ACE, i.e., a non-fatal or fatal MCE, or unstable angina) for a 50-year old woman according to mean heart dose from breast cancer radiotherapy [RT], and presence or not of at least one cardiac risk factor. Note: Cumulative risks do not take competing risks from other causes into account. (Reproduced with permission from Darby SC et al., 2013.[5])

The population-based dose-response relationship in Figure 7-5 can be used to provide reassurance for many women that their absolute risk of ischaemic heart disease from breast cancer radiotherapy is likely to be very small compared with their likely absolute benefit. For example, for a typical 50 year old woman with no cardiac risk factors, radiotherapy after breast conserving surgery may on average reduce her absolute 15-year risk of dying from breast cancer by a few percent.[220] If she receives a dose of 3 Gy mean heart dose from her left breast radiotherapy, her absolute 30-year risk of having an acute coronary event as a result of the radiotherapy would be less than 1% (Figure 7-6).[5] So for her, the benefit from radiotherapy far outweighs the risk. For other women, for example those for whom adequate coverage of the target tissue cannot be achieved without a high heart dose or for those with prior heart disease, the dose-response relationship can be used to identify the minority of women for whom the risk-benefit ratio is less favourable. In these women, consideration may be given to reducing cardiac radiation dose to reduce the radiation-related cardiac risk.

■ Trends in Cardiac Exposure from Breast Cancer Radiotherapy

Radiotherapy practice has changed markedly over the past few decades. In the 1950s to the 1970s, exposure of the heart from breast cancer radiotherapy was greater than in subsequent decades for two main reasons. First, techniques were designed to treat wide areas of the breast, chest wall and regional nodes therefore field sizes were often large. Second, radiotherapy planning and treatment equipment were limited in their ability to identify and avoid normal tissues such as the heart and lungs. Since the 1980s, use of tangential fields with the medial border on midline has increased (Figure 7-7).[253] This field arrangement is designed to minimize irradiation of the heart and lungs. In the 1990s, CT-based 3-dimensional radiotherapy planning for breast cancer started to be used. This enables estimation of dose to normal tissues and customization of the fields to ensure optimal coverage of the breast or chest wall and regional lymph nodes and the minimization of dose to normal tissues such as the heart.

A review of worldwide heart doses in breast cancer radiotherapy published between 2003 and 2013 has shown that, on average, the mean heart dose worldwide in 496 regimens reported in 167 studies was 5.4 Gy in left-sided radiotherapy and 3.3 Gy in right-sided radiotherapy.[226] Heart dose varied considerably from woman to woman even for similar regimens delivered in the same hospital. Nevertheless there were also some clear

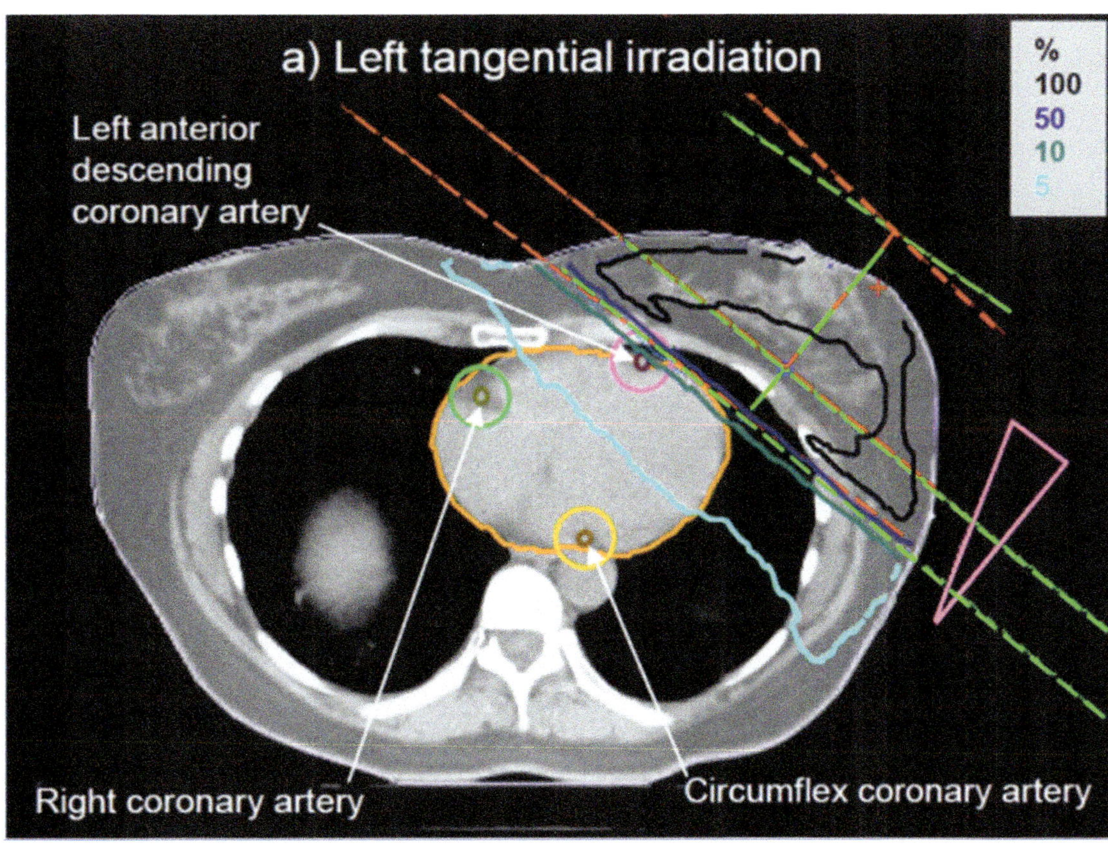

FIGURE 7-7 Dose distribution from 6 MV tangential irradiation typically used in the 2000s. The heart is outlined in orange. The coronary arteries are outlined and a radial margin of 1 cm has been added to each [Taylor 2008]. (Reproduced with permission from Taylor CW et al., 2008.[235])

systematic factors that affected it. These included laterality, radiotherapy technique and irradiation of the internal mammary lymph nodes. Since 2013, three large studies have shown that irradiating the internal mammary lymph nodes improves survival in node-positive breast cancer.[254–256] These results are likely to increase internal mammary irradiation, which may further increase cardiac exposure. Ongoing work aims to develop and implement cardiac-sparing radiotherapy techniques.[226]

Injury to Cardiac Structures after Breast Cancer Radiotherapy

Several studies have investigated which cardiac structures are injured after breast cancer radiotherapy. Myocardial injury has been demonstrated in myocardial perfusion studies that show that perfusion defects, i.e., ischaemic areas of the heart muscle, occur preferentially in the part of the left ventricle that was included in the radiotherapy fields.[36] This suggests that radiotherapy may damage the microvasculature in the left ventricle. The clinical importance of these perfusion defects is unclear. Very few of the

women with injury subsequently developed left ventricular dysfunction, and none had major coronary events. Similarly studies using Doppler echocardiography[257,258] have demonstrated subclinical abnormalities in left ventricular function within 14 months of radiotherapy in the parts of the heart muscle that received >3 Gy. Further follow-up of these studies is needed to determine the proportion of defects that eventually result in cardiac events. Disease of the main coronary arteries following breast cancer has been demonstrated in two angiography studies that show that coronary artery disease tends to occur in areas of high radiation dose.[20,21]

Ongoing research on radiation-induced heart disease after breast cancer radiotherapy includes further studies that will relate the radiation dose distribution in the heart with the spatial location of subsequent cardiac damage. In addition, epidemiological studies will be performed to estimate the effects of breast cancer radiotherapy in women who also receive anthracycline chemotherapy, and to estimate dose-response relationships for valvular heart disease and heart failure after breast cancer radiotherapy.

RADIATION-RELATED HEART DISEASE FOLLOWING HODGKIN LYMPHOMA TREATMENT

The adverse effects of incidental irradiation of the cardiovascular system during radiation therapy were first conclusively illustrated in patients who had received mediastinal radiotherapy for Hodgkin Lymphoma (HL). Although earlier case reports and smaller series had been published prior, the first large series was of patients treated at Stanford University between 1964 and 1972.[53] This paper describes 377 patients treated for HL with mantle radiotherapy alone to doses of at least 35 Gy (mean midline dose to the mediastinum of 44.1 Gy). 49 patients (13%) developed pericarditis at a median interval of 9 months following treatment (range 0 to 85 months). The proportion developing pericarditis was shown to increase with the whole-pericardial dose from 7% (14/198) at <6 Gy to 50% (7/14) at >30 Gy. In contrast, those patients treated with subcarinal shielding above a dose of 30 Gy had a pericarditis risk of only 2.5% (2/79).

■ Cardiac Mortality in Hodgkin Lymphoma Survivors

The larger cohort studies (>1000 patients) reporting mortality from cardiac causes following treatment for HL in adults are summarized in Table 7-3.[4,259–266] Further follow-up of the Stanford University cohort after the initial publication, expanded to 2232 patients treated between 1960 and 1991,[4] revealed that the relative risk (RR) cardiac deaths from all causes fell from 5.3 (3.1–7.5) prior to the introduction of subcarinal shielding to 1.4 (0.6–2.9) afterwards. However, the rate of fatal myocardial infarction was not significantly reduced with subcarinal shielding (RR, 3.7 vs. 3.4). The likely explanation for this is that the proximal coronary arteries still receive a substantial radiation dose with the use of the subcarinal shielding, whereas the pericardium and myocardium are relatively spared with this technique, resulting in a reduction in deaths from pericardial and myocardial disease, but not from coronary artery disease.

The more recent study of 4401 patients within 8 consecutive EORTC trials from 1964 to 2000,[259] found no statistically significant excess of cardiac deaths. This is in contrast to a study of the 4 earlier EORTC trials alone (1964 to 1986) that found an elevated risk of death from myocardial infarction.[267] A study of 6552 paediatric and adolescent HL patients treated when aged 0 to 21 years between 1973 and 2007 found a cumulative incidence of cardiac-specific mortality of 5% at 30-years following diagnosis.[265] There was, however, a decrease in cardiac mortality in recent decades, and radiotherapy use was not independently associated with cardiac mortality on multivariable analysis. A recent reduction in cardiovascular mortality was also observed in a study of 19,781 patients treated when aged 20 to 49 years between 1990 and 2011 with a 7% decrease in cardiovascular mortality per year of diagnosis.[266] Similarly a population-based study from Sweden of 5462 HL patients treated when aged 19 to 80 years between 1973 and 2006, reported excess deaths from diseases of the circulatory system in HL survivors to have declined continually since the mid-1980s.[268] The reasons for these observed reductions in cardiac death in HL patients treated more recently may be several-fold; reductions in the background rates of cardiac mortality, effect of shorter follow-up in more recent cohorts and changes in cardiac radiation and anthracycline exposures could all contribute. Although cardiovascular causes of death may be decreasing among HL survivors treated more recently, they still represent the third most common cause of death in this population ranked only behind HL and second malignancies. The historically observed several-fold increase in cardiovascular mortality for HL survivors versus an age- and sex-matched population is substantially higher than the increases seen in breast cancer survivors. This difference is likely real, and due to a younger age at treatment and a higher cardiac radiation dose and volume in the HL patients compared to those with breast cancer.

■ Cardiac Morbidity of Hodgkin Lymphoma Survivors

As well as an increased risk of cardiac mortality, HL survivors also exhibit considerable non-fatal cardiac morbidity. A number of studies have investigated this and a selection of the largest and most recent are summarized in Table 7-4.[23,269–273] The most comprehensive studies of cardiac morbidity following HL treatment to date have been performed on a cohort of patients from the Netherlands.[269,273] The strengths of these studies include prolonged and almost complete follow-up, radiotherapy and chemotherapy treatment data, information on cardiovascular risk factors, general practitioner- and cardiologist-reported outcomes, and incidence rates for cardiovascular disease from the general population with which to compare results. Of the 2524 patients in this cohort, 81% received mediastinal radiotherapy and the cumulative incidence of any cardiovascular disease at 40 years was 50%. Hazard ratios for ischaemic heart disease, valvular heart disease and congestive heart failure were all increased with

TABLE 7-3 Larger cohort studies (>1000 patients) reporting mortality from cardiac causes following treatment for HL

COUNTRY; STUDY	NUMBER OF PATIENTS	YEARS OF IRRADIATION	AGE AT TREATMENT IN YEARS (RANGE)*	TREATMENT	FOLLOW UP IN YEARS (RANGE)*	RISK OF CARDIAC OR MI DEATH
USA (SEER): Al-Kindi et al.[266]	19,781	1990–2011	32 (20 to 49)	Radiotherapy 40% Chemotherapy not known	Not given	6.5% of deaths from cardiovascular disease (3rd most common cause)
USA (SEER); Amini et al.[265]	6,552	1973–2007	17 (0 to 21)	Radiotherapy 56% Chemotherapy not known	12 (0 to 40)	Cumulative incidence = 5.0% at 30 years) Not associated with radiotherapy use on multivariable analysis (HR = 1.18, $p = 0.452$)
Sweden; Eloranta et al.[268]	5,462	1973–2006	Median not given (19 to 80)	Not specified	Not specified	14.8% of deaths from circulatory disease Excess mortality from circulatory disease decreasing since mid-1980s
Belgium, France & Netherlands; Favier et al.[259] 2009	4,401	1964–2000	34 (mean) (15 to 69)	Radiotherapy alone 36% Combined treatment 64% Radiotherapy included the mediastinum in c.90%, to >36 Gy in all Chemotherapy included anthracyclines in >75%	7.8 (not specified)	5% of deaths from cardiovascular disease (3rd commonest cause but not significantly in excess)

(continued)

TABLE 7-3 Larger cohort studies (>1000 patients) reporting mortality from cardiac causes following treatment for HL (*continued*)

COUNTRY; STUDY	NUMBER OF PATIENTS	YEARS OF IRRADIATION	AGE AT TREATMENT IN YEARS (RANGE)*	TREATMENT	FOLLOW UP IN YEARS (RANGE)*	RISK OF CARDIAC OR MI DEATH
United Kingdom; Swerdlow et al.[260]	7,033	1967–2000	76% <45 years (not specified)	Radiotherapy 72% Chemotherapy >99% Radiotherapy known to be supradiaphragmatic in 69% Chemotherapy included anthracyclines in 27%	11.1 (not specified)	SMR for death from MI = 2.5 (2.1–2.9)
Netherlands; Aleman et al.[261]	1,261	1965–1987	26 (≤41)	Radiotherapy 97% Chemotherapy 77% (including salvage treatments)	17.8 (not specified)	RRs for death from cardiovascular disease (excluding cerebrovascular): Males = 6.0 (4.1–8.4) Females = 7.3 (0.9–12.4)
USA (Boston) ; Ng et al.[262]	1,080	1969–1997	25 (3 to 50)	Radiotherapy alone 64% Chemotherapy alone 4% Combined treatment 32% Radiotherapy supradiaphragmatic in 94% to a median dose of 36 Gy Chemotherapy included anthracyclines in 44%	12 (not specified)	SMR for cardiac death = 3.2 (1.9–5.2)
Mexico; Aviles et al.[264]	2,980	1975–1995	All >18 years 62% <40 years (not specified)	Radiotherapy alone 3% Chemotherapy alone 37% Combined treatment 60% Radiotherapy included the mediastinum in >90%, to >30 Gy in 74% Chemotherapy included anthracyclines in >75%	14.6 (5 to 24)	SMR for cardiac death = 29.8 (15.6–46.8)

COUNTRY; STUDY	NUMBER OF PATIENTS	YEARS OF IRRADIATION	AGE AT TREATMENT IN YEARS (RANGE)*	TREATMENT	FOLLOW UP IN YEARS (RANGE)*	RISK OF CARDIAC OR MI DEATH
USA (Stanford); Hancock et al. 1993	2,232	1960–1991	29 (mean) (2 to 82)	Radiotherapy alone 43% Chemotherapy alone 5% Combined treatment 53% Radiotherapy included mediastinum in >90%, to >40 Gy in 79% Chemotherapy included anthracyclines in 16%	9.5 (mean)	SMR for cardiac death = 3.1 (2.4–3.7)
USA and Canada; Boivin et al.[263]	4,665	1940–1985	Majority <40 (not specified)	Not specified	7 (mean)	SMR for death from MI = 2.6 (1.1–5.9)

[a]Median unless otherwise stated
HR, Hazard Ratio; SMR, Standardized Mortality Ratio; MI, Myocardial Infarction.

TABLE 7-4 Summary of studies of incidence of heart disease following radiotherapy for Hodgkin lymphoma

STUDY	NUMBER OF PATIENTS	YEARS OF TREATMENT	AGE AT TREATMENT IN YEARS[a] (RANGE)	TREATMENT	FOLLOW UP IN YEARS (RANGE)	FINDINGS
Netherlands; Van Nimwegen et al.[269]	2524	1965–1995	27.3 (up to 51)	CMT 64% RT alone 30% CT alone 6% 81% received mediastinal RT 30% received anthracyline	20.3 (5 to 47)	40-year cumulative incidence of any cardiovascular disease = 49.5% (95% CI = 46.6%–52.4%). 51.4% of those affected developed ≥2 events. For mediastinal RT: HR for IHD = 2.7 (95% CI, 2.0–3.7) HR for VHD = 6.6 (95% CI, 4.0–10.8) HR for CHF = 2.7 (95% CI, 1.6–4.48) For anthracycline CT: HR for VHD = 1.5 (95% CI, 1.1–2.1) HR for CHF = 3.0 (95% CI, 1.9-4.7)
EORTC-LYSA; Maraldo et al.[270]	6039	1964–2004	30 (IQR 23 to 40)	CMT 64% RT alone 23% CT alone 11% Median MHD = 23.3 Gy (IQR 7.8 to 26.2) 67% received anthracycline	9 (IQR 6 to 14)	25-year cumulative incidence of cardiovascular disease = 42.3% (10% VHD, 8.4% arrhythmia, 7.1% CHF, 6.0% IHD, 10.8% others) HR for RT: 1.015 [95% CI 1.006–1.024] per 1 Gy MHD HR for anthracycline = 1.077 [95% CI, 1.021-1.137] per 50mg/m^2
Boston, USA; Galper et al.[271]	1279	1969–1998	25 (3 to 93)	RT alone 61% CMT 39% Median mid-mediastinal radiation dose = 40 Gy (range 15-53 Gy) CT not specified	14.7	5-, 10-, 15-, 20- and 25-year cumulative incidence rates of cardiac events were 2.2%, 4.5%, 9.6%, 16% and 23.2%. SIR for CABG = 3.19 (95% CI, 2.83–3.55) SIR for PTCA = 1.55 (95% CI, 1.39–1.71) SIR for a pacemaker or AICD = 1.90 (95% CI, 1.70–2.21) SIR for valve surgery = 9.19 (95% CI, 8.07–10.31) SIR for pericardial surgery = 12.91 (95% CI, 10.61–15.21)

(continued)

TABLE 7-4 Summary of studies of incidence of heart disease following radiotherapy for Hodgkin lymphoma (*continued*)

STUDY	NUMBER OF PATIENTS	YEARS OF TREATMENT	AGE AT TREATMENT IN YEARS[a] (RANGE)	TREATMENT	FOLLOW UP IN YEARS (RANGE)	FINDINGS
Canada; Myrehaug et al.[272]	615	1988–2000	29 (13 to 81)	CMT 49% RT alone 32% CT alone 13% RT included mediastinum in 81% to 30–35 Gy CT included anthracycline in all cases	11.8 (0.1 to 17)	HR for cardiac hospitalization (versus matched local population): Mediastinal radiotherapy alone = 1.82 (p = 0.038) Mediastinal radiotherapy and anthracycline = 2.77 ($p < 0.0001$) Anthracycline and no radiotherapy = 0.82 (p = 0.7)
Netherlands; Aleman et al.[273]	1474	1965–1995	25.7 (up to 40)	CMT 67% RT alone 28% CT alone 5% Radiotherapy included mediastinum in 84% to 30–40 Gy CT included anthracycline in 44%	18.7 (not specified)	SIR for AP = 4.1 SIR for MI = 3.6 SIR for CHF = 4.9 11% had valvular disorders (no reference rate available)
Florida, USA; Hull et al.[23]	415	1962–1998	25 (4 to 75)	CMT 62% RT alone 38% RT included the mediastinum in >90% to 33 Gy (median) CT not specified	11.2 (2.1 to 36.3)	10.4% CAD (at a median of 9 years after RT) 6.2% valvular disease (at a median of 22 years after RT) O/E for CABG or PCI = 1.63 (95% CI 0.98-2.28) O/E for valve surgery = 8.42 (95% CI 3.20–13.65)

[a]Median
IQR, Inter-Quartile Range; CMT, Combined modality Therapy; RT, Radiotherapy; CT, Chemotherapy; IHD, Ischaemic heart disease; VHD, Valvular heart disease; CHF, Congestive heart failure; IQR, Interquartile range; PTCA, percutaneous transluminal coronary angioplasty; AICD, automatic implantable cardioverter defibrillator.

mediastinal radiotherapy (see Table 7-4). Exposure to anthracycline chemotherapy was also associated with increased risks. The highest relative risks were seen for patients treated before 25 years of age, but substantial absolute excess risks were also observed for patients treated at older ages. 51% of patients experienced multiple events.[269] In the earlier study including many of the same patients, the authors concluded that HL treatment was the cause of 66%–88% of the cardiac disease diagnosed within the cohort.[273]

■ Radiation Dose-Response Relationships for Cardiac Morbidity

Case-control studies nested within the Dutch cohort described above have recently given more detailed information regarding the dose-response relationships between radiation dose to the heart and/or cardiac substructures and the risk of individual cardiac morbidities. A study of valvular heart disease showed that risk increased more than linearly with radiation dose to the heart valves.[13] For mean doses to the affected valve(s) of less than or equal to 30, 31–35, 36–40, and more than 40 Gy, VHD rates increased by factors of 1.4, 3.1, 5.4, and 11.8, respectively compared with unirradiated individuals (P_{trend} <0.001). (Figure 7.8b) A study of coronary heart disease showed that, in contrast to VHD, the risk increased linearly with mean radiation dose to the heart by 7.4% per Gy (95% CI, 3.3% to 14.8%) (Figure 7-8a).[6] The increased risk per Gy is remarkably similar to that seen following treatment for breast cancer.[5] A third study of congestive heart failure again revealed the suggestion of a more than linear increase with radiation dose to the heart. For mean doses to the heart of 1-20, 21–25, 26–30 and ≥31 Gy, CHF rates increased by factors of 1.43, 1.03, 2.78 and 4.16 respectively compared with unirradiated individuals (P_{trend} = 0.002) (Figure 7-8c).[274] Exposure to anthracycline-containing chemotherapy also increased the rate of CHF by 2.83 (95%CI: 1.43–5.59), with no evidence of interaction with radiation dose.

■ Evolution of Radiotherapy Techniques for Hodgkin Lymphoma

There has been considerable change in techniques of radiation therapy for HL over the past 40 years including reductions in field size, total dose and fraction size and the introduction of higher beam energies, beam weighting and subcarinal shielding. More recently, advanced techniques such as involved node radiotherapy,[275] intensity-modulated and deep-inspiration breath hold radiotherapy have reduced cardiac exposure yet further.[276] Dosimetric studies have demonstrated lower cardiac doses for these techniques and predicted consequent reductions in the risk of cardiac morbidity and mortality.[277,278] Proton beam therapy also has potential to reduce cardiac dose when compared to conventional photon-based radiotherapy.[279] It remains unclear, however, whether these new techniques will abolish the increased risk of treatment-induced heart disease entirely, due to the continued use of anthracyclines as a component of combined modality therapy and uncertainty over whether there is a threshold dose below which cardiac risk is not elevated. Primarily due to concerns over the incidence of late radiation-induced effects, including cardiac disease, the use of radiotherapy for the treatment of HL has declined substantially over recent years. This is despite evidence from randomized trials demonstrating that the omission of radiotherapy, even guided by functional imaging to identify patients with the most favourable prognosis, increases the relapse rate of HL.[280,281] Additionally, large observational studies have demonstrated superior overall survival associated with radiotherapy use as part of combined-modality therapy compared to treatment with chemotherapy alone.[282,283] Further work is therefore required to assess the cardiac safety of contemporary radiation therapy for Hodgkin lymphoma.

■ Radiation-Related Heart Disease Following Childhood Cancer Treatment

More than 80% of children diagnosed with cancer are expected to survive longer than 5 years from diagnosis with modern therapy.[284] This success rate has led to an increasing recognition of the late adverse effects of treatment among survivors, including cardiovascular morbidity and mortality, and an increasing effort to avoid such effects. The two treatments that primarily cause cardiovascular toxicity following the treatment of childhood cancer are anthracyclines, as described in Chapter 3, and radiotherapy.

Studies of mortality and cause of death in childhood cancer survivors consistently reveal a significantly elevated risk of cardiovascular mortality (Table 7-5).[285–294] Estimates of this risk vary from approximately 2- to 10-times that expected in the general population depending on the cohort studied. Most cohorts do not have access to individual treatment data and do not therefore attempt to assess the proportion of this risk that may be due to radiotherapy treatment. Where available, the relative risk of cardiovascular death has been observed to be 2 to 3-fold higher in those given RT versus those not.[286,287] But, as mentioned in the section on radiation-induced

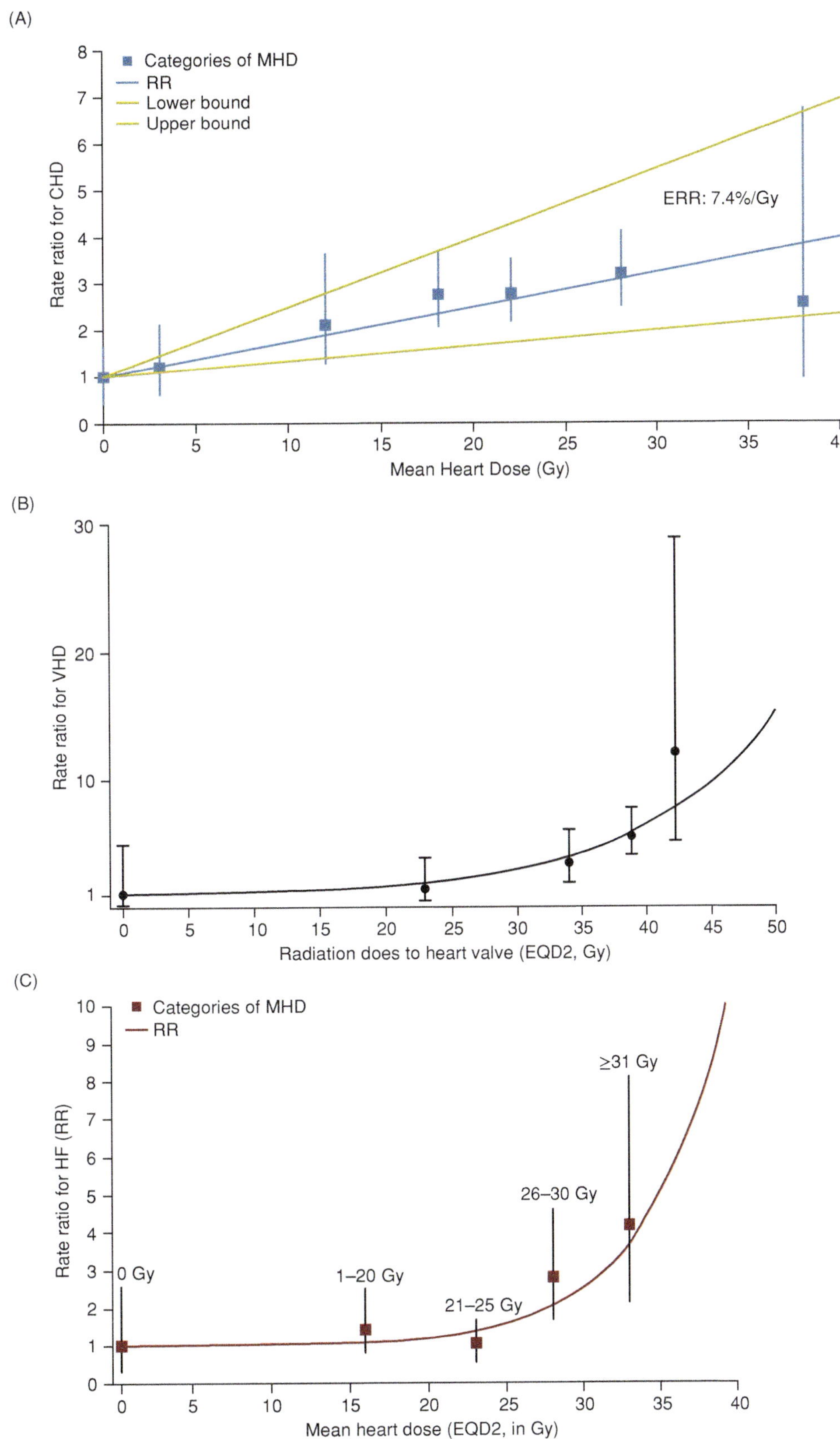

FIGURE 7-8 Rate ratios (RR) for (A) coronary heart disease (CHD), (B) valular heart disease (VHD) and (C) heart failure (HF) following radiotherapy for Hodgkin lymphoma by mean heart dose (MHD) radiation dose to affected heart valve measured in Gray (Gy).

TABLE 7-5 Summary of studies reported cardiovascular mortality following treatment for childhood cancers

STUDY	NUMBER OF PATIENTS	YEARS OF DIAGNOSIS	FOLLOW-UP (YEARS)	CARDIOVASCULAR SMR (95% CI)	RR (95%CI) RT VS. NO RT
BCCSS, UK; Fidler et al.[285]	34,489	1940–2006	15.2	3.8 (3.4 to 4.3)	Not given
CCSS, USA; Mertens et al.[286]	20,483	1970–1986	(not specified)	7.0 (5.9 to 8.2) (excluding cerebrovascular deaths)	3.3 (2.0–5.5)
BCCSS, UK; Reulen et al.[287]	17,981	1940–1991	24.3	3.9 (3.4 to 4.6)	1.9 (1.2–3.0)
Nordic; Moller et al.[288]	13,711	1960–1989	14.7	5.8 (4.2 to 7.6) (excluding cerebrovascular deaths)	Not given
Finland; Kero et al.[289]	5,352	1966–2004	(not specified)	4.3 (3.0 to 5.6)	Not given
Scotland, Brewster et al.[290]	5,229	1981–2003	(not specified)	2.4 (1.4 to 3.9)	Not given
Switzerland; Schindler et al.[291]	3,965	1976–2007	17.5 (mean)	12.7 (7.8 to 20.7)	Not given
Canada; MacArthur et al.[292]	2,354	1970–1995	15 (mean)	9.69 (4.19 to 19.1)	Not given
St Jude, USA; Hudson et al.[293]	2,053	1962–1983	24.7 (1963–1970) 14.2 (1971–1983)	6 (1.7 to 15.0) (excluding cerebrovascular deaths)	Not given
Amsterdam; Cardous-Ubbink et al.[294]	1,378	1966–1996	16.1	5.64 (1.16 to 16.5)	Not given

[a]Median unless stated
[b]Those age 0–19 years.
SMR, Standardized Mortality Ratio; RR, Relative Risk; RT, Radiation Therapy.

cardiovascular disease in breast cancer, one must be cautious of drawing unqualified conclusions from observational studies, as any observed difference may be substantially affected by other characteristics of the group chosen to receive radiotherapy, as well as the effect of RT itself.[223]

As well as being at an increased risk of cardiovascular death, cardiovascular morbidity has been demonstrated to be a substantial problem in survivors of childhood cancer. The U.S. Childhood Cancer Survival Study (CCSS) compared the frequency of chronic health conditions in 14,358 survivors to 3,899 siblings and found elevated risks of congestive heart failure (HR = 5.9, 95% CI 3.4 to 9.6), myocardial infarction (HR = 5.0, 95% CI 2.3 to 10.4), pericardial disease

(HR = 6.3, 95% CI 3.3–11.9) and valvular abnormalities (RR = 4.8, 95% CI 3.1 to 7.6).[295] Cardiac irradiation of >15 Gy resulted in a 2- to 5-fold relative risk of these cardiac abnormalities in irradiated versus unirradiated survivors. In addition to symptomatic morbidity, survivors of childhood cancer have been demonstrated to have a substantial incidence of sub-clinical toxicity.[296]

Much of the data regarding the effect of radiation therapy on the cardiovascular system of children treated for cancer has come from patients treated as children and adolescents for Hodgkin lymphoma. For example, in a series of 635 children and adolescents treated with mediastinal radiotherapy at Stanford University, between 1961 and 1991 at a mean age of 15.4, the relative risk of cardiac death was 29.6 (95% CI 16.0 to 49.3) and of death from acute MI was 41.5 (95% CI 18.1 to 82.1).[297] An analysis of 4 similar studies of cardiac mortality following irradiation for childhood lymphoma yielded a pooled SMR of 28.4.[298] The patients who died of cardiac causes in these series all received >40 Gy of mediastinal radiotherapy. Since those children were treated the radiation doses received by the heart have undoubtedly reduced, with reductions in the total dose administered, cardiac shielding, alterations in the volumes treated and the development of radiotherapy techniques. The risk of late cardiac toxicity has also presumably decreased, but there is a lack of knowledge regarding the dose-response relationship and the extent of the residual risk is uncertain. There is some evidence that the excess risk had decreased in recent decades,[285] but it remains unclear how much this is due to changes radiotherapy and how much is due to changes chemotherapy, particularly anthracycline, use. It is evident, however, that lower radiation doses to the heart (15–30 Gy) such as in use today, particularly in combination with anthracyclines, can cause an increase in clinically significant cardiac morbidity in childhood cancer survivors.[295]

There have only been limited attempts to establish more formal dose–response relationships between cardiac radiotherapy dose and cardiac morbidity and mortality in survivors of childhood cancer. In a study of ventricular function,[299] detailed cardiac evaluations were performed upon 229 patients a mean of 18 years after they had received anthracycline for the treatment of solid childhood malignancies between 1968 and 1985. For the 120 (52%) who had received radiotherapy, individualized retrospective estimates of cardiac radiation dose were made. Twenty-four patients (10%) were found to have clinical cardiac failure and a further 65 (28%) were found to have asymptomatic cardiac dysfunction, such as fractional shortening of <25%, an ejection fraction of <50% or end systolic wall stress of >100kd/cm2 measured on ECHO. Following adjustment for cumulative anthracycline dose, age at treatment, sex, and attained age, there remained dose-response relationships between mean heart dose and cardiac failure (excess relative risk [EER] per 1 Gy = 19%, 95% CI -2% to 50%) and mean heart dose and asymptomatic cardiac dysfunction (EER per 1 Gy = 35%, 9% CI -0.5% to 120%). The difference in risk was substantial at lower doses with a cumulative incidence of cardiac failure of 18% in those who received >3.5 Gy mean heart dose and 9% in those who received less or no radiotherapy. Other more recent studies have again demonstrated an increasing risk of asymptomatic myocardial dysfunction or cardiac failure with increasing radiation dose.[300–302] A recent study has also demonstrated a radiation-associated risk of valvular heart disease in childhood cancer survivors,[303] with the risk increasing by an odds ratio of 1.33 per 10 Gy to the heart region. Childhood cancer survivors

are also known to be at an increased risk of ischaemic heart disease with radiation doses to the heart of >15 Gy, although a dose-response has not been defined in this patient group. A study of cardiac mortality involved a joint French and British cohort of 4122 5-year survivors of childhood cancer, with individualized cardiac radiation doses for the 70% that received radiotherapy.[7] Despite only 21 cardiac deaths within the cohort, analysis revealed evidence of a dose-response relationship below 15 Gy mean heart dose with an ERR of 60% per Gy (95% CI 20%–250%). The ERR per Gy found in this cohort is higher than that seen in adult cancers due mainly to the low background rate of cardiac death in childhood and perhaps a greater use of, and sensitivity to, cardiotoxic chemotherapy within childhood cancer.

Despite some evidence that excess cardiac mortality in childhood cancer survivors may be decreasing in patients treated more recently,[285] late cardiac toxicity following treatment for childhood cancer remains an important clinical problem. This is due both to the historical cohorts of survivors treated with regimens that are known to be cardiotoxic who are now entering middle age, and the increased proportion of modern childhood cancer patients who are now expected to achieve long-term survival and who may still be at future risk despite adaptions in management aimed at reducing the toxicity of treatment. Greater knowledge regarding the cardiac risks of modern radiotherapy for childhood cancer, and how these interact with systemic therapies, is therefore required. An on-going large scale collaborative European study; "PanCareSurFup,"[304] has been designed to provide further information regarding the dose-response relationships for radiation-related cardiovascular disease following childhood cancer treatment. A further international collaboration, "PENTEC" (Pediatric Normal Tissue Effects in the Clinic) aims to provide summary reports on issues relating to the quantification of radiation dose effects in children treated for cancer, including cardiovascular effects.[305] Such knowledge could help treatment schedules to be further modified in future to minimize morbidity in survivors, and could also direct appropriate surveillance for cardiac late effects allowing early diagnosis and intervention when such problems arise.

RADIATION-RELATED HEART DISEASE FOLLOWING ESOPHAGEAL CANCER TREATMENT

Definitive chemoradiotherapy (dCRT)[306,307] and neo-adjuvant CRT (nCRT)[308] have been introduced to improve survival rates in locally advanced esophageal cancer (EC) achieving a median survival of 48·6 months (95% CI 32·1-65·1) in the nCRT group.

CRT may result in appreciable morbidity, including cardiac toxicity due to the close proximity of these tumors to the heart. The impact of cardiac irradiation was previously thought not to be clinically relevant in these patients due to the poor prognosis of locally advanced EC and the expected prolonged latency of radiation related heart disease (RRHD). However, with the advent of new therapies and increasing long-term survival, RRHD following EC treatment is now being reported in the literature and is of increasing relevance.

Large epidemiological studies have shown the risk of heart disease related death is significantly higher in those who received radical radiotherapy as part of their treatment (HR 1.62, p<0.0001) and that this effect is seen as soon as 8 months following treatment.[309] Cardiac effects of nCRT are especially important as they could have direct implications on anesthetic and operative risks and management. Radiation modalities resulting in lower normal tissue doses have been shown to be an independent predictor of fewer post-operative cardiopulmonary complications.[310]

A recent review demonstrated that 10.8% (range: 5%–44%) of EC patients treated with radiotherapy experience ≥ grade 3 cardiopulmonary toxicity and that most events occur within 26.1–57 months.[311] The actual rates may be higher due to under-reporting of cardiac morbidity in older trials because, at this time, the potential importance of cardiotoxicity was not considered. The most frequently observed toxicities were pericardial effusions, cardiac ischaemia and heart failure.[311] It is difficult, however, to determine appropriate dosimetric parameters to predict and/or minimize these effects as the radiation techniques and toxicity end points assessed in these studies are diverse.

■ Pericarditis and Pericardial effusions

A retrospective review of 57 EC patients reported 5 patients had non-malignant pericardial effusions (PCE) after CRT and found that large fraction size (3.5 Gy) and biologically adjusted mean and maximum heart doses of >27.1 and >47.0 Gy, respectively, were predictive of pericarditis.[312] In another larger study of 101 EC patients who received definitive CRT, the mean time to onset of PCE was 5.3 months, with a crude incidence rate of 27.7%.[313] They identified that a mean pericardium dose of >26.1 Gy and V30 (the percentage volume of pericardium receiving more than 30 Gy) >46% were associated with PCE. A follow up study confirmed mean pericardium dose and V45 as well as V30 as predictive values for PCE in EC patients after CRT.[314] A more recent study of 60 patients with EC who underwent definitive CRT at

60 Gy in 30 fractions had a PCE rate of 52.2% and pericardial V30 >41.6% was significantly associated with PCE.[315] Another study of 143 EC patients treated with CRT (>50 Gy) found 38.5% developed PCE at a median 3.5 months (Range 0.2–9.9) but, in contrast, a lower dosimetric parameter of V10 of >72.8% was identified as the most influential factor.[316] A further study including 127 patients found that women were at a significantly greater risk of PCE than men for the same cardiac dose.[317]

■ Myocardial and Microvascular Damage

Tripp et al. observed a statistically, but not clinically, significant reduction in median left ventricular ejection fraction (LVEF) (59% to 54%) 6 weeks after CRT using multiple-gated acquisition cardiac scans in EC patients receiving CRT, but did not observe any significant association between radiation-dose to the heart, left ventricle, or left anterior descending artery.[318] This is in line with the results of another small retrospective study of 15 patients treated with CRT at 45-50 Gy in 25 fractions in the preoperative setting that also saw a decrease in LVEF in 12 of 15 patients.[319] The median left ventricular ejection fraction fell from 63% to 58% a median of 32 days post completion of treatment. Again, there was no correlation between heart dose and reduction in LVEF. A decline in ejection fraction from 64% to 40% precluded surgery in one patient, but otherwise no clinically significant morbidity was observed albeit with no prolonged follow-up. Further evidence of radiotherapy inducing acute impairment of left ventricular function arises from another study that demonstrated subclinical changes in systolic and diastolic function on echocardiography and NT-proBNP elevation following nCRT but not neo-adjuvant chemotherapy only.[320] Hatakenaka et al. also studied patients treated with CRT using cardiac magnetic resonance imaging and found left ventricle function impaired from an early treatment-stage.[321] LVEF decreased irrespective of left ventricle dose, but more prominently in a group receiving high LV-dose, as early as 1 to 3 days after completing CRT. Heart rate increased significantly in patients receiving high LV-dose, which is consistent with findings of Zhang et al. who used 99mTc-methoxyisobutylisonitrile (MIBI) single photon emission computed tomography (SPECT) gated myocardial perfusion imaging (GMPI) to demonstrate new myocardial perfusion defects in 8/18 patients receiving nCRT and also observed a significant increase in heart rate that they suggested may represent compensation for the decrease in the LVEF. V37–V40 was significantly higher in the patients with the new perfusion defects.[322] At doses greater than 40 Gy, the wall motion (WM), wall thickening (WT), end-diastolic perfusion (EDP) and end-systolic perfusion (ESP) decreased significantly. Gayed et al. also used GMPI and found perfusion abnormalities and inferior left ventricular wall ischaemia more in irradiated patients than non-irradiated patients, especially in areas of the ventricular wall receiving more than 45 Gy, but functional parameters (left ventricular ejection fraction, end diastolic, and systolic) did not differ significantly.[323] The observed changes were not predictive of future cardiac complications.[324] Konski et al. also found reduced 18F-Fluorodeoxyglucose (FDG) uptake on FDG-Positron emission tomography (PET) in the myocardium shortly after treatment with a significant association between the V20, V30 and V40 of the heart and symptomatic cardiac toxicity.[325] Takanami et al. investigated changes in myocardial fatty acid metabolic impairment caused by CRT in 12 EC patients who underwent SPECT/CT using 1-123 beta-methyl-p-iodophenylpentadecanoic acid (BMIPP).[326] At 3-month post-CRT, myocardial BMIPP uptake was significantly correlated with left ventricle V40, and heart V40 and V60. However, there were no statistically significant correlations at 1-year post-CRT suggesting that in the long term after CRT, myocardial metabolism might be affected by factors other than the radiation dose to the heart and highlights need for careful planning of timing of investigations in dosimetric studies. Clinically significant functional defects or symptomatic cardiac disease were not demonstrated in these imaging studies. However, a study using cardiac MRI in EC survivors[327] demonstrated late gadolinium enhancement indicative of myocardial fibrosis in cardiac segments receiving more than 40 Gy, suggesting prolonged effects on the myocardium that may partially explain the increase in cardiac disease demonstrated in epidemiological studies of EC survivors. Even a short term impairment of left ventricular function could impact the incidence of postoperative cardiovascular and pulmonary morbidity after esophagectomy in patients receiving nCRT, so is an important factor to consider in these patients.

■ Other Cardiac Effects Following Esophageal Cancer Treatment

Pericardial disease and effects on the myocardium and microvasculature are the most common reported radiation-related effects reported in EC survivors. Other conditions reported include ischaemic heart disease[328] and dysrhythmias.[311,329] The risk depended on V45, V50, and V55 with the lowest significant cut-off values of 15%, 10%, and 5%, respectively. High-dose and large heart volume irradiation increased the risk of symptomatic cardiac disease in long-term survivors highlighting the importance of using modern radiotherapy techniques to minimize heart irradiation while escalating tumor dose.

■ Future of Esophageal Cancer Radiotherapy

To improve outcomes for EC treated with CRT in the future, modification of radiotherapy techniques will need to take account of cardiopulmonary toxicity. Incorporation of more sophisticated radiotherapy techniques such as intensity modulated radiation therapy (IMRT) in comparison to 3D conformal radiotherapy (3D-CRT) have shown the potential to reduce heart dose, limit post-operative complications and therefore improve survival.[310,330,331] Proton beam therapy (PBT) can be used to further reduce heart dose but clinical experience with PBT is currently limited. In 62 EC patients treated with PBT, there were few severe toxicities and encouraging clinical outcomes.[331] Wang et al. showed lower post-operative complications with PBT.[310] A recent review summarized single institution experiences of reduced heart and substructure doses, lower toxicities, and post-operative complications with PBT in comparison to 3DCRT and IMRT.[332] Prospective randomized trials comparing PBT to 3DCRT and IMRT would be useful to confirm these benefits.

RADIATION-RELATED HEART DISEASE FOLLOWING LUNG CANCER TREATMENT

In an attempt to improve the poor prognosis associated with lung cancer, radiotherapy and chemoradiotherapy (CRT) has been delivered post-operatively and definitively. Due to the proximity of these tumours to the heart, high doses of radiation are delivered to the heart but, largely due to poor prognosis, there is very little data available regarding cardiac toxicity following radiotherapy for lung cancer.

Patients with lung cancer often have substantial shared risk factors for both thoracic malignancy and cardiac disease, particularly smoking.[333,334] Consequently, patients treated with thoracic radiation are often at high risk for treatment-independent, cardiovascular disease and would therefore be expected to be at high absolute risk for radiation-related heart disease (RRHD). As symptoms of cardiac dysfunction such as dyspnea overlap with lung cancer symptoms and death rates are high, cardiac morbidity and cardiac-specific mortality may be under reported. So care must be taken to minimize the adverse cardiac effects of radiation that might otherwise negate the anticipated survival benefits. Similar arguments apply to the improvements in survival seen with CRT for limited stage small cell lung cancer,[335] as well as non-small cell lung cancer (NSCLC).

Although there is no direct evidence of heart irradiation impacting survival in lung cancer, there is suggestive evidence. For example, in a study of 34,209 patients aged over 65 years with stages I–IV NSCLC treated with radiotherapy, chemotherapy or CRT from the Surveillance, Epidemiology, and End Results (SEER) database who were free of cardiac disorders at diagnosis,[336] there were significant associations between the use of chemotherapy and radiotherapy and the risks of developing ischemic heart disease, conduction disorders, cardiac dysfunction, and heart failure. The risk of cardiac dysfunction and ischemic heart disease was higher when radiation was administered to the left lung compared to the right lung suggesting an association between cardiac radiation dose and risk.

■ Post-Operative Radiotherapy (PORT)

PORT studies in NSCLC have alluded to the lower overall survival associated with PORT being partly due to increased cardiac toxicity. A systemic review and meta-analysis in 1998[337] analysed nine randomized controlled trials including a total of 2128 patients with stage I–IIIA NSCLC who were randomized to surgery alone versus surgery plus PORT of 30 Gy to 60 Gy in 10 to 30 fractions. An absolute detriment of 7% in overall survival at 2 years was seen with PORT (55% vs. 48%). The deaths due to non-cancer causes among the patients treated with PORT was 19% compared to 11% in the surgery only group, suggesting that treatment-related toxicity may be responsible for this deficit. Detailed analysis of one included trial that randomized 728 patients with completely excised NSCLC to receive either PORT at a total dose of 60 Gy or observation revealed 27.5% deaths in the PORT group versus 11% in the control group were due to non-cancer causes.[338] The most frequent cause of non-cancer death in the PORT group was cardiac causes that resulted in 26% of the deaths. There was a significant trend for less overall survival detriment with higher nodal stage, the hazard ratio for patients with N2 disease treated with radiotherapy being 0.96. As there is no rationale for why PORT would be less toxic for N2 disease compared to N0-N1, one must conclude that an increase in non-cancer deaths following radiotherapy is being offset by a greater oncological benefit within this group where the risk of cancer recurrence is highest.

The potential for cardiac toxicity to negate possible benefit from PORT is also supported by a single institution series of 98 patients treated in Turkey between 1994 and 2004.[339] The majority of these patients were treated using cobalt-60 based techniques rather than modern conformal megavoltage radiotherapy. The median survival was significantly lower for patients with left-sided compared to right-sided tumours (25 months versus 100 months), and the authors postulate that this discrepancy may be explained by greater cardiac toxicity from irradiation of the left thorax. A similar finding of poorer prognosis for left-sided tumours was reported in a series of 155 patients from Roswell Park, although this finding was not statistically significant (HR = 1.3, 95% CI 0.91–2.03).[340] Only 25% of this cohort received adjuvant radiotherapy.

Further supportive evidence comes from an analysis of the SEER database.[341] The risk of death from heart disease was examined in 6,148 patients with surgically treated NSCLC, 58% of whom had received PORT between 1983 and 1993 and were followed up until 2005. PORT was significantly associated with an increased risk of death from heart disease (hazard ratio [HR], 1.30; 95% confidence interval [95% CI], 1.04–1.61; p = 0.0193). However, this excess of cardiovascular toxicities after PORT was only observed in the cohort of patients treated between 1983 and 1988 but not in the cohort of patients treated from 1989 to 1993 (HR, 1.49; 95% CI, 1.11–2.01 [p = 0.0090], HR, 1.08; 95% CI, 0.79–1.48 [p = 0.6394] respectively), which could reflect the impact of more modern radiotherapy techniques utilized in the second half of the 1990s (i.e., treatment planning with 3 dimensional conformal radiotherapy and higher energy radiation delivered by linear accelerator instead of Cobalt-60). They also observed that PORT was not associated with heart disease mortality for patients who had tumors located in right upper lobe regardless of their period of diagnosis supporting higher cardiac dose being associated with increased cardiac mortality. Modelling studies also suggest that there may be improvements in local control and overall survival with the use of modern PORT following chemotherapy and surgery.[342]

■ Definitive Chemoradiotherapy (CRT)

The standard of care for locally-advanced inoperable NSCLC is CRT. For more than 30 years, the accepted "standard" RT dose is 60–66 Gy in 1·8–2·0 Gy fraction sizes established by the Radiation Therapy Oncology Group (RTOG) 7301 trial.[343] However, local failure rates at these doses remain high with poor overall survival (OS). Therefore, there has been much interest in radiotherapy dose escalation to the tumor to increase therapeutic gain. Though biological modelling and meta-analysis of clinical trials has suggested a tumor dose–response,[344,345] the clinical benefit of high dose radiation remains controversial. Many prospective phase I/II studies suggested that concurrent chemoradiotherapy (CRT) up to 74 Gy was safe and RT dose escalation may improve local control and OS, e.g., Landau et al.[346] But this approach has been challenged by the results from the phase III randomized CRT trial, RTOG 0617 that showed lower survival with 74 Gy compared to 60 Gy in 2 Gy per fraction, despite no significant difference in local failure, distant metastases, progression free survival (13% difference in survival at 2 years (44.6% vs. 57.6%).[347] They noted that a high heart volume receiving ≥5 Gy (V5) and ≥30 Gy (V30) was significantly associated with the poorer survival seen in the 74 Gy arm, though specific heart toxicity outcomes were not tracked. In this trial, the dose escalation was not carried out isotoxically respecting normal tissue dose constraints and though the protocol suggested dose–volume constraints for the heart, compliance was poor.

More detailed clinical evidence for cardiac irradiation impacting survival in lung cancer is starting to emerge. In a retrospective study of 250 inoperable patients with stage I–III or recurrent NSCLC with no previous cardiac disease who received definitive CRT, 84% were found to die without cardiac event while 15% developed cardiac disease, mostly supraventricular tachycardia and myocardial infarctions.[348] Although there was a trend for worse survival in the group of patients with doses to the left ventricle above 14.5 Gy, they did not find a significant correlation between high mean-dose to left ventricle, both ventricles or whole heart and cardiac toxicity defined as having a cardiac event after radiotherapy. Further exploration of other cardiac substructures and dose-volume parameters is required.

■ Future of Lung Cancer Radiotherapy

Modern radiotherapy modalities with image-guided targeting and inverse planning demonstrate better heart sparing.[349] Analysis of the RTOG0617 trial found IMRT reduced radiation doses to the heart and lungs, reduce radiation pneumonitis, and improves quality of life compared to conventional 3D conformal radiation therapy.[350] Virtual clinical studies have shown the dosimetric advantages of proton-based radiation therapy over photon-based radiation therapy in sparing the heart and delivering higher radiation doses to the tumor in patients with locally advanced NSCLC, particularly with intensity modulated proton therapy (IMPT).[351] A consensus statement on proton therapy in NSCLC suggests that proton therapy may potentially result in reduced long-term medical costs because of reduced toxicities.[352] The question of whether proton beam therapy is able to improve overall survival is being addressed in a randomized phase III trial, RTOG 1308. A total of 560 inoperable Stage II-IIIB NSCLC patients are being randomized to photon or proton

chemoradiotherapy; the dose delivered is 70 Gy using either modality, with the option to decrease to as low as 60 Gy if the dose constraints to the organs at risk cannot be met.[353] These studies may demonstrate whether a reduction heart dose and consequently in radiation-related heart disease could contribute to an improved outcome in patients with NSCLC.

RADIATION-RELATED HEART DISEASE FOLLOWING TREATMENT FOR TESTICULAR CANCER

Testicular cancer is the most common cancer in men aged 15–45 and the treatment is curative in the majority of cases. Due to the exceptionally high cure rates and relatively young age of the patients, it is important to consider treatment related morbidities including cardiovascular disease, as these may result in life-threatening illness in these patients. Although largely replaced by chemotherapy in modern treatment regimens, radiotherapy is a highly effective treatment for seminoma. In the past, prophylactic mediastinal irradiation was used and recognized to be related to an increased incidence of heart disease at a median dose of 24 Gy.[354] A lack of a proven survival benefit and recognition of the potential cardiac complications led to a marked reduction in the use of prophylactic mediastinal irradiation by the mid-1980s. Infra-diaphragmatic radiotherapy, however, remained standard practice.

The largest study of cause of death in survivors of testicular cancer identified 38,907 patients from 14 cancer registries across Scandinavia and North America from 1943 to 2002.[355] After a median follow-up of 10 years, patients who were younger than 35 years at diagnosis and were treated with radiotherapy alone in 1975 or later had a higher mortality from circulatory diseases (standardized mortality ratio (SMR) = 1.70, 95% CI = 1.21 to 2.31) compared to the general population, whereas those treated at 35 years or above did not (SMR = 0.88, 95% CI = 0.76 to 1.01). This is consistent with the finding that younger age at irradiation has been associated with increased risk of cardiovascular complications following radiotherapy for both HL and breast cancer.[356] The majority of the patients (estimated >80%) treated with radiotherapy during this period would have received infra-diaphragmatic irradiation only and would therefore have received only modest radiation dose to the heart. Another large study with a longer median follow up of 19 years also showed the patients receiving chemotherapy and radiotherapy or chemotherapy alone had a higher risk of MI (HR4.8 and 3.1 respectively) compared to normal controls.[357]

A more recent retrospective review of 251 patients with stage I and II seminioma, treated with adjuvant megavoltage radiotherapy at The Mayo Clinic between 1972 and 2009, found a major cardiac event (MCE, myocardial infarction, coronary artery bypass grafting or stenting, valve replacement) incidence of 19% at a median follow-up of 19 years in stage II patients.[358] The median infradiaphragmatic dose was 30.7 Gy. 50% (before 1989) received prophylactic mediastinal radiotherapy (median dose 20.5 Gy). For stage I disease treated with adjuvant radiotherapy to paraaortic nodes or ipsilateral pelvic nodes (median dose 25.5 Gy) the MCE incidence was 12% at 20 years, an annual risk of 0.6% in comparison to 0.4% that would be expected from the Framingham study.[359]

The finding that infra-diaphragmatic radiotherapy in the absence of mediastinal irradiation increases the risk of cardiovascular mortality was previously demonstrated in a cohort of 477 seminoma patients treated at the MD Anderson Cancer Centre with megavoltage radiotherapy between 1951 and 1999.[360] The SMR for cardiac deaths beyond 15 years of follow-up of patients receiving infra-diaphragmatic radiotherapy was 1.95 (99% CI 1.07 to 3.28), but was not significantly elevated before 15 years, emphasizing the typical latency of the effect on increased risk of cardiac mortality as seen in other cancers.[225] Another analysis of 992 patients with testicular tumours treated in the UK between 1982 and 1992, when only 8.3% of patients received mediastinal radiotherapy, demonstrated a significantly increased risk of a cardiac event with radiotherapy alone (RR = 2.40, 95% CI 1.04 to 5.45, p = 0.036).[200] This risk remained elevated when the patients who received mediastinal radiotherapy were excluded from the analysis, in the presence or absence of chemotherapy, and after adjustment for age at treatment. After a median follow-up of 10 years, 9.6% of patients treated with infradiaphragmatic radiotherapy had experienced a cardiac event, compared to 3.7% of patients treated with orchidectomy alone. Mean dose received by the heart in this cohort was estimated to have been 0.75 Gy, with only 14% of the cardiac volume receiving over 0.9 Gy. Another study, focussing on organ dose calculation, estimated the average heart dose from RT with an equally weighted anteroposterior (AP) and posteroanterior (PA) modified "dog-leg" field when prescribed 30 Gy was 0.59 Gy, and when prescribed 36 Gy was 0.69 Gy.[361] So, the doses delivered the heart are very small and alone would seem unlikely account for the observed elevation in risk of cardiac toxicity, suggesting the possibility of an abscopal effect. It has been suggested that radiation nephropathy due to the irradiation of renal tissue, leading to hypertension and a consequent increase in the risk of cardiac disease may be partly responsible. The proposed mechanisms of indirect effect on heart after infradiaphragmatic radiotherapy include direct parenchymal damage, small vessel sclerosis, and renal artery stenosis.[362] Also the self-perpetuating process of endothelial inflammation initiated by radiotherapy can confer adverse risk to the whole cardiovascular system, rather than just the parts directly irradiated. Ionizing radiation can cause a rise in reactive oxygen species triggering lipid oxidation, damage of the endothelium and activation of nuclear factor (NF)-B, a transcriptional factor involved in the local inflammatory responses. Accordingly, survivors treated with radiotherapy have been found to have elevated systemic levels of inflammatory markers (CRP and soluble CD40 ligand) up to 20 years after treatment, compared to patients treated with surgery alone and/or chemotherapy, which provides further support for a potential indirect abscopal effect on the heart.[202] However, another larger study of 2707 that explored cardiac morbidity not mortality in testicular cancer survivors, while confirming mediastinal radiotherapy as a risk factor for cardiac morbidity, failed to demonstrate a statistically significant increased risk following infra-diaphragmatic radiotherapy alone (HR = 1.2, 95% CI 0.9 to 1.7) despite a median follow-up of 17.6 years.[363] As well as greater numbers and prolonged follow-up, this study also adjusted for other risk factors. Additionally a large, population-based study of 9193 mean diagnosed with stage I seminoma demonstrated no increased risk of cardiovascular mortality following radiotherapy (SMR = 0.89; 95% CI, 0.76–1.04), which was received by 78% of patients.[364] So whether infra-diaphragmatic radiotherapy for seminoma may increase cardiac risks, and whether it does so via a direct or indirect effect on the heart, remains controversial.

RADIATION-RELATED HEART DISEASE FOLLOWING TREATMENT FOR OTHER CANCERS

In addition to the specific sections on malignancies above, there are a number of other circumstances in which therapeutic irradiation may cause cardiac toxicity. An example is total body irradiation (TBI) used as part of conditioning regimens prior to bone marrow transplantation, typically for haematological malignancies. During TBI the entire cardiovascular system typically receives a fractionated radiation dose of 10–15 Gy. TBI is often combined with conventional and high dose chemotherapy that is also potentially cardiotoxic (for example anthracyclines and cyclophosphamide) and it is difficult to establish the contribution of TBI to an observed elevation in cardiac risk following such treatment. There is some evidence that the addition of TBI may increase toxicity, for example plasma BNP levels have been observed to be higher in patients receiving TBI compared to those that did not.[365] Due to the prolonged latency of radiation-induced cardiac effects in this dose range and the lack of detailed long-term follow-up, it is possible that there may be a substantial burden of late cardiac morbidity and mortality that continues to develop for decades following treatment.[366] Another example is thymoma, which, although rare, has a good prognosis such that adjuvant radiotherapy must be performed with sufficient care to avoid unnecessary toxicity to normal tissues, including the heart and great vessels. This principle is of extra importance for the stages of thymoma where the benefit of adjuvant radiotherapy remains controversial.[367] The recent recognition that lower radiation doses may cause late cardiac disease, has even raised the question whether radiation doses from prophylactic breast bud irradiation should be considered when studying cardiac morbidity from androgen suppression therapy for prostate cancer.[368] With a profusion of examples of potential harm, it becomes obvious that the issue of effects of radiation therapy on the cardiovascular system is not simply one affecting management of a few tumour types, but should be a general concern of radiation oncologists and the cardiologists that they work alongside.

DETECTION AND MONITORING OF RADIATION-RELATED HEART DISEASE

A considerable problem in the study and management of patients at risk of radiation-induced heart disease is that there is often prolonged latency from irradiation to the development of symptomatic disease. Sub-clinical disease may be difficult to detect without specialist investigation and the clinical significance of such disease is uncertain. There remains a need to develop tools that can provide early surrogate markers for those at risk of later clinical cardiac events, and efficient methods of management to reduce the risk for those identified. Effective early surrogate markers would help to ensure that the patients at greatest risk receive adequate follow-up and, if necessary, intervention. They would also allow the cardiovascular safety of current and evolving radiotherapy techniques to be assessed within a practical timescale. A range of imaging techniques and blood biomarkers have been investigated, but no technique has yet become established as a routine clinical screening tool for RIHD.

■ Imaging Techniques

Nuclear Medicine Imaging ■ A number of studies have utilized nuclear scintigraphy to assess myocardial perfusion and function in patients treated with radiotherapy. These studies have mainly involved patients with Hodgkin lymphoma (Table 7-6)[54,369–374] and breast cancer (Table 7-7),[375–384] but those with other malignancies such as oesophageal[322,385] and lung cancer[324] have also been studied. The results of these studies can appear contradictory with the prevalence of myocardial perfusion defects varying widely between studies, e.g., from 0% to 85% in patients who received radiotherapy for Hodgkin lymphoma and 0% to 76% in patients who received radiotherapy for left-sided breast cancer. The reasons for this are several and include the lower sensitivity of planar scintigraphy versus single photon emission computed tomography (SPECT), the use of different radioligands, entry criteria, time points of scans and radiotherapy techniques, and differing amounts of chemotherapy exposure. Despite this variation in the frequency of observed perfusion abnormalities it is obvious that they do develop following cardiac irradiation in a proportion of patients treated with radiotherapy for Hodgkin lymphoma and breast cancer. Although the results of SPECT scanning are predictive of later cardiac events in patients with age-related ischemic heart disease,[386,387] whether they are of prognostic utility for radiation-induced heart disease is unproven.

The largest series to have used SPECT scanning to study RIHD in breast cancer, consists of 160 patients who received radiotherapy for left-sided breast cancer at Duke University from 1998.[378] This prospective series demonstrated a volume-dependent incidence of perfusion defects occurring within 2 years of radiotherapy for left-sided breast cancer. Where <5% of the left ventricle was included within the radiation field the incidence of new perfusion defects was 10%–20%, compared to 50%–60% when >5% was irradiated. Perfusion defects were associated with the presence of wall motion abnormalities at 6 months following RT. Observed changes in ejection fraction were not associated with the presence of perfusion defects. Continued follow-up of a proportion (44/160) of this cohort to 3–6 years[36] has not yet revealed an association between perfusion defects and declines in cardiac function. There have not yet been any clinical cardiac events (myocardial infarction or congestive cardiac failure) within this cohort to suggest that the observed perfusion abnormalities are predictive of such events following breast irradiation, but there was a suggestion that cardiac symptoms were more common in those who developed new perfusion defects[388] and the follow-up time is short compared to the usual latency of RRHD.

Table 7-6 Summary of studies of nuclear myocardial perfusion following radiotherapy for Hodgkin lymphoma

STUDY	NO. ASSESSED (TOTAL COHORT)	YEARS OF RT	TIMING OF SCANS AFTER RT	TYPE OF SCAN AND ISOTOPE(S) USED	MYOCARDIAL PERFUSION DEFECTS
Heidenreich et al.[369]	274 (of 294)	1960–1995	Mean 15 years (SD 7 years)	SPECT ^{99m}Tc-tetrofosmin for stress images ^{201}Tl for rest images	18% (49/274) Fixed in 6% (17/274) Stress-induced in 12% (32/274)
Girinsky et al.[370]	42 (of 49)	1980s	Median 6.3 years (Range 2.3–17.3 years)	SPECT ^{201}Tl	78% (32/41) (During further follow-up to a median of 13.5 years after RT, 9 cardiac events were observed but perfusion defects where not predictive)
Glanzmann et al.[371]	100 (of 112)	1964–1992	Not specified	SPECT ^{99m}Tc-sestamibi	7% (7/100) "Definitely abnormal" in 4% (4/100)
Constine et al.[372]	38 (of 50)	1964–1994	Mean 9.1 years (SD 7.5 years)	SPECT ^{99m}Tc-sestamibi or ^{201}Tl	5% (2/38)
Savage et al.[373]	12 (of 16)	1967–1985	Mean 9.3 years (SD 6.3 years)	Planar ^{201}Tl	0% (0/12)
Gustavsson et al.[374]	23 (of 26)	1967–1977	Median 15 years (Range 4–20 years)	SPECT ^{201}Tl	61% (14/23) "Definitely abnormal" in 9% (2/23)
Morgan et al.[54]	25	Pre-1980	Mean 9.3 years (SD 2.3 years)	Planar ^{201}Tl	0% (0/25)

RT, Radiation Therapy; SD, Standard deviation; SPECT, single photon emission computed tomography.

Table 7-7 Summary of studies of nuclear myocardial perfusion imaging following radiotherapy for breast cancer

STUDY	NO. ASSESSED (LATERALITY, RT)	YEARS OF RT	TIMING OF SCANS*	TYPE OF SCAN AND ISOTOPE(S) USED	MYOCARDIAL PERFUSION DEFECTS
Eftekhari et al.[375]	71 (35 L-sided, 36 R-sided)	2010–2012	Prospective 6 months after RT	SPECT 99mTc-sestamibi	42.9% (15/25) L-sided vs. 16.7% (6/36) R-sided (Odds ratio = 1.46, $p = 0.02$) Abnormalities in apical and anterolateral segments
Sioka et al.[376]	46 (28 L-sided, MHD 7.7 Gy)	1998–2010	Retrospective Median 40 months after RT (Range 6 to 263 months)	SPECT 99mTc-tetrofosmin	Abnormalities in summed stress score in 54%, 44% and 33% of L-sided, R-sided, and controls respectively. More abnormality in left-sided versus controls ($p = 0.0001$)

STUDY	NO. ASSESSED (LATERALITY, RT)	YEARS OF RT	TIMING OF SCANS*	TYPE OF SCAN AND ISOTOPE(S) USED	MYOCARDIAL PERFUSION DEFECTS
Tzonevska et al.[377]	56 (46 L-sided with heart in field, 10 R-sided)	(not specified)	Retrospective Mean 18 months after RT	SPECT ^{99m}Tc-sestamibi	20% (11/56) overall 24% (11/46) of L-sided vs. 0% (0/10) of R-sided patients ($p<0.001$)
Marks et al.[378]	114 (all L-sided) (160 up to 2006)	1998–2001	Prospective Baseline pre-RT 6-monthly for 2 years	SPECT ^{99m}Tc-sestamibi or ^{99m}Tc-tetrofosmin	27% (21/77), 29% (16/55), 38% (13/34) and 42% (11/26) had new defects at 6, 12, 18 and 24 months after RT
Seddon et al.[379]	36 (24 L-sided with 1cm of heart in field, 12 R-sided)	1987–1995	Retrospective Median 6.7 years for L-sided (IQR 5.8–8.8 years) Median 8.3 years for R-sided (IQR 6.3–10.1)	SPECT ^{99m}Tc-tetrofosmin	53% (19/36) overall 71% (17/24) of L-sided vs. 17% (2/12) of R-sided patients ($p = 0.002$)
Hojris et al.[380]	17 (all L-sided, 10 received RT)	1982–1990	Retrospective Median 7.9 years after RT (Range 6–12.2 years)	SPECT ^{99m}Tc-sestamibi	47% (8/17) overall 40% (4/10) of irradiated patients 57% (4/7) of un-irradiated patients
Gustavsson et al.[381]	90 (34 L-sided, 33 R-sided, 23 no RT)	1978–1983	Retrospective Median 13 years after RT (Range 10–17 years)	SPECT ^{99m}Tc-sestamibi or ^{99m}Tc-tetrofosmin	7% (6/90) overall 12% (4/34) L-sided vs. 6% (2/33) R-sided 0% (0/23) un-irradiated patients
Cowen et al.[382]	17 (all L-sided)	1987–1993	Retrospective Mean 4.8 years (SD 0.55 years)	Planar ^{201}Tl	0% (0/17)
Gyenes et al.[383]	12 (all L-sided)	1993–1994	Prospective Baseline pre-RT Mean 1.1 years after RT (Range 0.7–1.9 years)	SPECT ^{99m}Tc-sestamibi	50% (6/12) new defects
Gyenes et al.[384]	37 (20 L-sided RT, 17 R-sided or no RT)	1971–1976	Retrospective Mean 18.7 years after RT	SPECT ^{99m}Tc-sestamibi	14% (5/37) overall 25% (5/20) of L-sided RT vs. 0% (0/17) of R-sided or no RT patients ($p < 0.05$)

RT, Radiation Therapy; SD, Standard deviation; SPECT, single photon emission computed tomography; L-sided, Left-sided; R-sided, Right-sided.
*Prospective = Patients recruited to the study prior to RT; Retrospecitve = Patients recruited to the study after RT.

The largest series utilizing SPECT scanning following irradiation for Hodgkin lymphoma was undertaken at Stanford University.[369] It consists of 294 patients who had received ≥35 Gy to the mediastinum a mean of 15 years prior to the cardiac evaluation in the study. Despite an entry criteria of no known IHD, evaluation with a combination or stress echocardiography, SPECT and ECG led to the diagnosis of asymptomatic coronary artery stenosis of >50% in 7.5% (22/294) of participants. Eight of these went on to undergo CABG. The patients were followed for a median of 6.5 years subsequent to initial evaluation, and a total of 69 non-fatal cardiac events or deaths occurred. Affected patients were more likely to have had ischemia on prior stress imaging (23% versus 13%, p = 0.02). This study indicates that MPI may form some part of a screening programme for patients who have received high doses of mediastinal radiotherapy. However, the sensitivity and specificity of nuclear scintigraphy alone for CAD were only 65% and 11% respectively and combination with other investigations is necessary to identify false negative tests correctly and refute false positives. A high rate of positive SPECT examinations (89%), were found to be false positive for the presence of CAD on further evaluation. A possible explanation for this high false positive rate is that mediastinal irradiation may often cause microvascular damage and perfusion defects in the absence of macrovascular disease.

FDG-PET has not been used as a tool to study RIHD prospectively, but incidental increased uptake in the myocardium has been noted following radiotherapy for oesophageal cancer.[389] The areas of increased uptake were observed to correspond to the heart regions irradiated. Subsequent SPECT in a proportion of those with increased uptake revealed perfusion defects in the same locations. It is thought that increased uptake may reflect microvascular damage, as the metabolism of myocardial cells is known to shift from using fatty acids to glucose as an energy source under ischemic conditions. FDG-PET does not seem to offer any advantages over the imaging modalities discussed above for the specific detection of RIHD. It may result in incidental findings requiring further cardiac investigation when used for other indications, for example oncological follow-up.

Alternative SPECT tracers to those detailed in Tables 7-6 and 7-7 have occasionally been used to image cardiac injury after irradiation, for example 111In-antimyosin and 123I-meta-iodobenzylguanidine (123I-MIBG). These studies are interesting in that they apparently raise the possibility of imaging mechanisms of damage other than endothelial cell injury. 111In-antimyosin antibody binds to intracellular myosin only following damage to the sarcolemma and increased uptake following irradiation as has

been demonstrated[390] suggests that the integrity of myocytes may have been compromised. Uptake of 123I-MIBG reflects the function of myocardial adrenergic neurones. Decreased myocardial washout following irradiation has been found,[391] suggesting that abnormalities of sympathetic innervation of the heart may also be involved. In addition a recent study in esophageal cancer patients[326] demonstrated that myocardial fatty acid metabolism was progressively impaired during and after chemoradiotherapy using the tracer I-123β-methyl-iodophenyl pentadecanoic acid (BMIPP). These studies suggest that nuclear medicine techniques that measure functions other than myocardial perfusion may be useful in the investigation of RRHD.

Echocardiography ■ Transthoracic echocardiography (ECHO) provides real-time non-invasive imaging of cardiac anatomy and function. It is commonly used in the surveillance for anthracycline and trastuzumab induced cardiac toxicity, but has also proven useful in the detection of radiation-induced abnormalities. It can be used to assess four manifestations of RIHD; pericardial disease, valvular disease, myocardial dysfunction and coronary artery disease.

A number of studies have been performed following mediastinal RT for HL, at mean mediastinal doses of >35 Gy, that identified a substantial prevalence of such manifestations (Table 7-8).[35,44,60,374,392–395] The majority of the abnormalities identified were asymptomatic, and not of clinical relevance at the time of diagnosis, but their frequency has led to recommendations for screening with ECHO within this patient group. There is some evidence that ECHO may be of potential clinical benefit in screening for valvular disease. A study of ECHO in 294 patients who had received mediastinal RT for HL[44] demonstrated a substantial incidence of clinically significant valvular disease (6% at 20 years following radiotherapy). Amongst those irradiated 20 years or more previously, the number needed to screen to detect a candidate for endocarditis prophylaxis was only 1.6 (95% CI 1.3 to 1.9). The same study also found mild to moderate asymptomatic diastolic dysfunction in 14% of those screened, substantially higher than would be expected in the general population.[35] The clinical significance of these findings is uncertain but, in that study, those with diastolic dysfunction were more likely to have stress-induced ischemia than those without (23% versus 11%, p = 0.008) and they also had a worse event-free survival (HR = 1.66, 95% CI 1.06–2.4).[35] This result is consistent with other studies that have demonstrated diastolic dysfunction to be a marker of poor prognosis for non-radiation associated cardiac disease.[396] Stress ECHO has also proven potentially useful as part of a strategy to detect asymptomatic CAD in patients who

Table 7-8 Summary of echocardiographic studies following irradiation for Hodgkin lymphoma

STUDY	NUMBER	YEARS OF RT	AGE AT TREATMENT IN YEARS (RANGE)	TREATMENT RECEIVED	FOLLOW-UP IN YEARS	AGE AT STUDY IN YEARS	PERICARDIAL DISEASE ON ECHO	VALVULAR DISEASE ON ECHO	LEFT VENTRICULAR FUNCTION ON ECHO
Heidenreich et al.[35,44]	294	Not specified	Not specified	100% MRT (mean 43 Gy, SD = 0.3 Gy) 56% (165) chemotherapy (proportion containing anthracyclines not specified)	Median 15.0 (SD = 7.0)	Mean 42.0 (SD = 9.0)	Pericardial thickening in 21% (62/294) Pericardial effusion in 3% (10/294) No evidence of constrictive pericarditis	AR in 26% (77/294) MR in 39% (115/294) TR in 16% (47/294) PR in 7% (20/294) (≥mild regurgitation) AS in 4% (13/294)	36% (95/263) had reduced fractional shortening (<30%). Decreasing ventricular mass with time from irradiation. 14% (40/282) had diastolic dysfunction.
Adams et al.[60]	48	1970 to 1990	Median 16.5 (6.4 to 35.0)	100% MRT (median 40 Gy, range 27 to 51.7 Gy) 44% (21) chemotherapy 8% (4) with anthracyclines	Median 14.3 (range = 5.9 to 27.5)	Median 31.9 (range = 18.7 to 49.5)	Not reported	AR in 19% (9/47) MR in 21% (10/47) TR in 26% (10/39) PR in 3% (1/39) (≥mild regurgitation) AS in 6% (3/47) MS in 2% (1/47)	12% (5/43) had systolic dysfunction. 37% (16/43) had diastolic dysfunction.

(*continued*)

TABLE 7-8 Summary of echocardiographic studies following irradiation for Hodgkin lymphoma (*continued*)

STUDY	NUMBER	YEARS OF RT	AGE AT TREATMENT IN YEARS (RANGE)	TREATMENT RECEIVED	FOLLOW-UP IN YEARS	AGE AT STUDY IN YEARS	PERICARDIAL DISEASE ON ECHO	VALVULAR DISEASE ON ECHO	LEFT VENTRICULAR FUNCTION ON ECHO
Lund et al.[320]	116	1980 to 1988	Not specified	100% MRT (Mean 40.6 Gy, SD 1.4) 66% (76) chemotherapy 40% (46) with anthracyclines	Median 9.0 (range = 5.0 to 13.0)	Mean 37.0 (SD = 7.0)	Pericardial thickening in 15% (18/116) No evidence of constrictive pericarditis	AR in 27% (31/116) MR in 23% (27/116) TR in 32% (37/116) PR in 25% (29/116) (≥mild regurgitation) No stenosis reported	No evidence of systolic or diastolic dysfunction.
Glanzmann et al.[393]	112	1964 to 1992	Mean 31.1 (10.1 to 58.0)	100% MRT (93% of cases between 30 and 42 Gy) 40% (45) chemotherapy 24% (27) with anthracyclines	Median 10.4 (range = 1.3 to 27.4)	Mean 41.5 (range = 22.1 to 70.0)	Pericardial thickening or effusion in 7% (8/112)	AR in 4% (4/112) MR in 8% (9/112) (≥mild regurgitation) AS/sclerosis in 19% (21/112) MS/sclerosis in 14% (16/112) No clinically significant tricuspid or pulmonary valve disease	2% (2/112) had systolic dysfunction. No evidence of diastolic dysfunction (0/39).

TABLE 7-8 Summary of echocardiographic studies following irradiation for Hodgkin lymphoma (*continued*)

STUDY	NUMBER	YEARS OF RT	AGE AT TREATMENT IN YEARS (RANGE)	TREATMENT RECEIVED	FOLLOW-UP IN YEARS	AGE AT STUDY IN YEARS	PERICARDIAL DISEASE ON ECHO	VALVULAR DISEASE ON ECHO	LEFT VENTRICULAR FUNCTION ON ECHO
Kreuser et al.[394]	49	1982 to 1990	Median 35 (15 to 38)	63% (31) MRT 100% chemotherapy All with anthracyclines	Median 5.4 (range = 2.0 to 10.0)	Median 39.0 (range = 29.0 to 65.0)	Pericardial thickening in 39% (19/40)	Valvular thickening in 43% (21/49) No evidence of valvular stenosis	18% (9/49) had reduced fractional shortening. 14% (7/49) had reduced ejection fraction. No evidence of diastolic dysfunction.
Gustavsson et al.[374]	25	1967 to 1977	Median 24 (6 to 33)	100% MRT (mean 40 Gy, range = 35 to 43 Gy) None received chemotherapy	Median 15 (range = 4 to 20)	Median 38 (range = 21 to 45)	No pericardial effusion. Pericardial thickening not reported. 1 patient had surgery for constriction prior to the study.	Valvular thickening in 40% (10/25) AR in 4% (1/25) MR in 36% (9/25) TR in 88% (22/25) PR in 35% (7/20) (≥mild regurgitation) No evidence of valvular stenosis	44% (11/25) had systolic dysfunction. 50% (12/24) had diastolic dysfunction.
Pohjola-Sintonen et al.[395]	28	Not specified	Not specified	100% MRT (mean 38.4 Gy, range = 21.5 to 47 Gy) None received chemotherapy	Mean 8.6 (range = 5 to 14)	Mean 31.9 (range = 12 to 38 years)	Pericardial effusion in 38% (10/26) 2 patients underwent partial pericardiectomy	Aortic sclerosis in 8% (2/26) Pulmonary stenosis in 12% (3/26)	8% (2/26) had systolic dysfunction.

MRT, Mediastinal Irradiation; AR, Aortic regurgitation; SD, Standard Deviation; MR, Mitral regurgitation; TR, Tricuspid regurgitation; PR, Pulmonary regurgitation; AS, Aortic Stenosis; MS, Mitral stenosis.

have previously received mediastinal irradiation for Hodgkin lymphoma, with a sensitivity and specificity for this investigation in isolation of 59% and 89% respectively.[369]

Conventional echocardiography can detect changes in systolic function, although by conventional measures such as fractional shortening the observed differences following irradiation are only slight compared to unirradiated controls.[35] Studies using newer tissue Doppler ECHO techniques have been able to demonstrate changes in systolic function not detected by conventional techniques. For example strain rate imaging (SRI) has been used to measure regional decreases in systolic function, just 2 months following radiotherapy for breast cancer, in a distribution topographically related to areas of the myocardium receiving greater than 3 Gy (Figure 7-9).[397] These changes have been shown to persist for up to 14 months following radiotherapy but have not yet been related to any clinical events.[258] Tissue Doppler imaging has also been used to detect subclinical systolic and diastolic dysfunction in survivors of Hodgkin lymphoma.[398] The use of these newer ECHO techniques may well increase sensitivity for the detection of myocardial dysfunction following irradiation. Whether this increased sensitivity will result in a useful tool to predict future cardiac events remains unproven.

Coronary Computed Tomographic (CT) Angiography and CT Calcium Scores ■ Coronary Computed Tomographic Angiography (CCTA) has been used in the assessment of asymptomatic patients following mediastinal radiotherapy for Hodgkin lymphoma. The first large study reported was of 119 patients treated for Hodgkin lymphoma during childhood at a median age of 7 years (range 2 to 18 years).[399] This study found a 16% prevalence (19/119) of asymptomatic CAD at a mean of 9.5 years (range 2 to 31 years) after treatment, including critical stenoses in 2 patients. Among those who received mediastinal radiotherapy the prevalence was 24% (14/59) and those who had received a mediastinal dose > 20 Gy were found to have a 6.8 fold increased risk of having a coronary artery abnormality compared to those receiving a lower dose ($p = 0.009$). A subsequent study of 179 patients all treated with radiotherapy in adulthood at a median age of 29 years (range 22 to 41 years) revealed a very similar prevalence of coronary artery disease of 26% (46/179) at a median of 11.6 years (range 2.1 to 40.2 years) after treatment.[400] In this study the mean radiation dose to the coronary artery origin was significantly associated with CAD. A similar prevalence of CAD has been reported in two smaller studies.[401,402] It has previously been noted that the degree of CAD seen in these studies was unusually severe for asymptomatic individuals.[403] It is possible that such

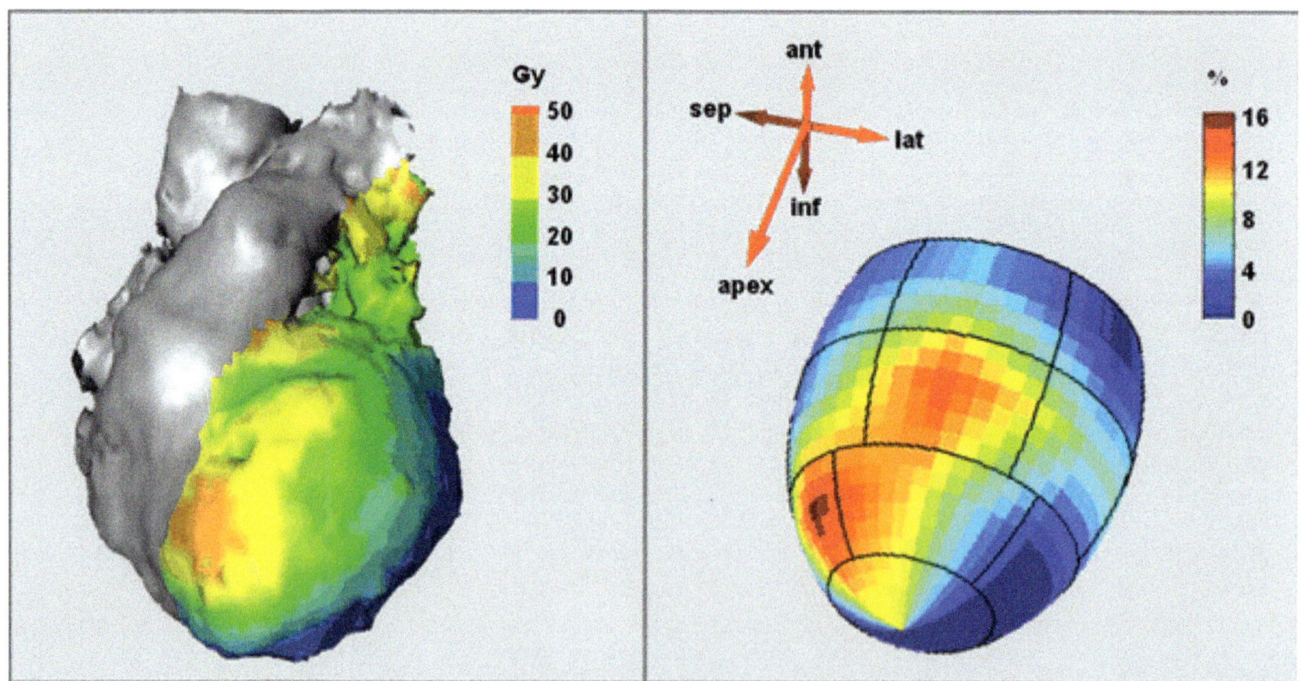

FIGURE 7-9   The left panel shows a 3D CT reconstruction of the surface of the heart with the left ventricle colour-coded according to the radiation dose received. The right panel shows a 3D model of the left ventricle displaying a colour-coded change in systolic function (absolute decrease in peak longitudinal strain at 2 months after RT versus baseline). (Adapted with permission from Jurcut R et al., 2007.[397])

patients may only be asymptomatic due to radiation-induced nerve damage or reduced exercise capacity.

The use of CCTA has yet to be fully validated as a screening tool for asymptomatic irradiated patients. CCTA offers the advantage of sensitivity and, unlike stress testing, will diagnose a proportion of patients with early coronary artery disease before they develop hemodynamically significant stenosis. The disadvantage of this sensitivity is that further tests are often required to assess the significance of any positive findings. Further disadvantages of CCTA include the radiation exposure from the investigation, the use of intravenous iodinated contrast and difficulty in studying patients with higher heart rates. The latter problem may be substantial in patients who have received mediastinal irradiation as it is recognized that such patients often have radiation-induced vagal dysfunction leading to an elevated and invariant heart rate.[60] Further studies are needed to define the role of CCTA (and other available modalities) as part of cardiovascular screening in patients following cardiac radiation exposure.

Cardiovascular Magnetic Resonance Imaging ■ Cardiovascular magnetic resonance (CMR) is an excellent noninvasive tool for examining the heart without exposure to ionizing radiation. It is the most accurate and reproducible imaging method for serial assessment of ventricular volumes, mass, and global and regional ventricular function.[404] Strain imaging (using tagged or feature-tracking CMR) provides local myocardial wall strain, twist, and torsion in three dimensions and can detect mild or subclinical systolic and diastolic dysfunction as early biomarkers of cardiotoxicity.[405] Advantages of CMR over echocardiography include the ability to image any desired plane, superior accuracy and reproducibility,[406] and, importantly, multi-parametric tissue characterisation capabilities. Late gadolinium enhancement imaging can differentiate ischemic from non-ischemic heart disease via characteristic patterns.[407] CMR perfusion imaging with vasodilator stress (e.g., adenosine or dipyridamole) can identify myocardial ischemia due to radiation-induced macrovascular coronary artery stenosis.[408] Newly developed pixel-wise perfusion maps allow quantification of myocardial blood flow and volume, and may detect early microvascular and endothelial dysfunction.[409] Advanced tissue characterisation using novel T1- and T2-mapping allows quantification of tissue T1 and T2 relaxation times on a pixel-wise level and are highly sensitive to detecting subtle abnormalities.[410] They are especially useful in assessing myocardial inflammation,[411] which may include immune checkpoint inhibitor myocarditis

and radiation-induced injury. Extracellular volume quantification derived from pre- and post-contrast T1-mapping may act as a surrogate marker for diffuse myocardial fibrosis, a characteristic histological change seen in cardiac radiation-toxicity. CMR parametric mapping is deemed one of six most innovative imaging methods in heart failure by the European Society of Cardiology[412] and has demonstrated utility in detecting early and even subclinical changes in a number of cardiac diseases.[410] CMR also allows evaluation of radiation-induced pericardial disease, including pericardial inflammation, thickening, adhesions, calcification, effusions, and constrictive physiology.[413] CMR is an excellent tool for cardiac phenotyping and exploration of disease mechanisms through its multi-parametric ability to assess cardiac structure and function, inflammation and oedema, perfusion, necrosis, and focal and diffuse fibrosis. Additionally, myocardial energetics and metabolism may be studied using MR spectroscopy[414] and novel dynamic nuclear polarization techniques[415]; metabolic imaging may become an important component in studying the pathophysiology of cardiotoxicity related to cancer therapies. Although most widely studied in the assessment of chemotherapy-related cardiotoxicity, the clinical and research potential of CMR in RRHD is increasingly recognised as it becomes more widely available and incorporated into cardio-oncology clinical trials.

■ Blood Biomarkers

The use of serum biomarkers represents an attractive strategy for the detection and monitoring of cardiotoxicity due to the relatively non-invasive sampling process, low cost and low inter-observer variability in interpretation. Biomarkers have been investigated extensively with respect to anthracycline-induced cardiotoxicity. They have also been studied in the context of RT treatment.

Troponins ■ Concentrations of cardiac troponins are known to relate to acute myocardial damage. In the context of radiation-related heart disease this marker was first studied in a series of 50 patients receiving whole breast radiotherapy for early stage left-sided breast cancer.[416] No elevations of cardiac troponin T (cTnT) were found during treatment despite a proportion of the myocardium lying within the radiotherapy field that was treated to a dose of 45–46 Gy. Since then multiple studies in various cancer types including lung cancer, mesothelioma, oesophageal cancer and breast cancer, utilizing both cTnT and cardiac troponin I (cTnI), have given variable results (Table 7-9).[199,258,320,365,416–424] When statistically

Table 7-9 Summary of studies of cardiac blood biomarkers after radiation therapy (RT)

REFERENCE	DISEASE(S)	TREATMENT	NO. OF PATIENTS	BIOMARKERS MEASURED	TIMING OF MEASUREMENTS	FINDINGS
Skytta et al.[199]	Breast (left)	RT (no CT)	58	Hs-cTnT BNP	Baseline, during and at end of RT	Elevation of hs-cTnT ($>30\%$) in 12/58 (21%). Those with elevation has higher whole heart ($p = 0.02$) and left ventricle doses ($p = 0.03$). No significant change in BNP.
Lund et al.[321]	Oesophageal	CRT (17) or CT (23)	40	NT-proBNP	Baseline and 4-6 weeks after RT	NT-proBNP increased following CRT ($p = 0.05$) but not after CT ($p > 0.99$).
Haj Mohammed et al.[417]	Oesophageal	CRT	23	cTnT NT-pro-BNP	Baseline and weekly during RT	cTnT significantly increased at week 5 ($p<0.001$). No significant change in NT-pro-BNP.
Gomez et al.[418]	Mainly mesothelioma	RT (18) or CRT (7)	25	cTnI BNP	Baseline, during and 1-2 months after RT	cTnI increased in 2/25 (8%) and then normalized. Increases in BNP observed but not associated with heart RT dose or time from baseline.

TABLE 7-9 Summary of studies of cardiac blood biomarkers after radiation therapy (RT) (*continued*)

REFERENCE	DISEASE(S)	TREATMENT	NO. OF PATIENTS	BIOMARKERS MEASURED	TIMING OF MEASUREMENTS	FINDINGS
Erven et al.[258]	Breast	RT and CT	75 (51 left-sided)	cTnT	Baseline, at end of RT, 8 and 14 months after RT	Mean cTnT levels elevated following RT for left-sided patients ($p = 0.04$).
D'Errico et al.[419]	Breast (left)	RT	30	NT-proBNPcTnI	5 to 22 months after RT	NT-proBNP significantly higher in the RT group compared to matched pre-RT controls ($p = 0.03$). No significant change in cTnI.
Nellessen et al.[420]	Mainly lung	RT and CT	25	cTnI BNP	Baseline and weekly during RT	Small but significant increases in cTnI and BNP during treatment ($p < 0.05$).
Kozak et al.[421]	Mainly lung	CRT (6 RT only)	30	cTnT CK-MB NT-proBNP	Baseline, 2 weeks, end of RT	No elevations observed.
Jingu et al.[422]	Oesophageal	RT	197	BNP MMP-3	Cross-sectional. Grouped by timing in respect to RT.	BNP increased more than 9 months from RT. High BNP and MMP-3 were associated with increased uptake in myocardium on FDG-PET.

(*continued*)

TABLE 7-9 Summary of studies of cardiac blood biomarkers after radiation therapy (RT) (*continued*)

REFERENCE	DISEASE(S)	TREATMENT	NO. OF PATIENTS	BIOMARKERS MEASURED	TIMING OF MEASUREMENTS	FINDINGS
Masuko et al.[365]	Haematological	SCT (TBI in 10)	15	BNP	Baseline and 3-monthly after	BNP significantly higher after TBI. BNP peaked within 6 months and declined thereafter in most, although some peaked late.
Wondergem et al.[423]	Hodgkin lymphoma (73) Breast (48)	RT	121	ANP	9-10 years after RT	ANP was elevated in patients compared to controls. Patients with clinical symptoms had higher levels compared to asymptomatic patients.
Hall KS et al.[424]	Breast	CT and RT	105	ProANP	Baseline and up to 3 years after treatment	ProANP levels were related to epirubicin dose and left-sided breast irradiation.
Hughes-Davies et al.[416]	Breast	RT	50	cTnT	Baseline and during RT	No elevation observed.

CT, Chemotherapy; CRT, Chemo-radiotherapy; Hs-cTnT, High-sensitivity Cardiac Troponin T; BNP, Brain Natriureteric Peptide; NT-proBNP, N-Terminal pro-Brain Natriuretic Peptide; cTnT, Cardiac Troponin T; cTnI, Cardiac Troponin I; CK-MB, Creatinine Kinase-MB; MMP-3, Matrix Metalloproteinase-3; ANP, Atrial Natriuretic Peptide.

significant increases have been reported they have been small and sometimes below the validated quantification level for the assay used.[258] More recently, a high-sensitivity assay for cardiac troponin T (hs-cTnT) has become available[425] and this has been demonstrated to be elevated following radiotherapy for breast cancer.[199] In this study of 58 women with left-sided breast cancer or DCIS who received radiotherapy 21% had an elevation in hs-cTnT of ≥30% from baseline and these women had a significantly higher whole heart dose (4.0 Gy versus 2.8 Gy, $p = 0.02$) and left ventricular dose (6.7 Gy versus 4.5 Gy, $p = 0.03$). It is possible that these elevations are due to radiation-induced endothelial damage and dysfunction leading to microvascular ischaemia and myocyte damage. Although the absolute levels are low and the clinical significance is uncertain, measurable troponin levels have been demonstrated to indicate a worse cardiac prognosis in other conditions.[426]

Natriuretic Peptides ■ Natriuretic peptides are released from myocytes in response to hemodynamic stress rather than as a consequence of direct myocardial damage. Brain natriuretic peptide (BNP) is an endogenous peptide produced initially by ventricular cardiomyocytes as a pre-pro-peptide, which is cleaved into a precursor molecule that is stored in secretory granules (proBNP). Upon release, proBNP is further cleaved by a specific protease into an inactive N-terminal fraction (NT-proBNP) and BNP (the active hormone). BNP and NT-pro-BNP have both been validated as markers that can improve the accuracy of clinical diagnosis of heart failure and predict for poor outcome following the diagnosis of heart failure. They are also useful in the screening of asymptomatic subjects who may be at risk of heart failure, such as the elderly or diabetics.[426] A study of patients who received radiotherapy for oesophageal cancer[422] demonstrated that levels of BNP were significantly increased 9 months after the start of radiotherapy, especially in patients who had high FDG accumulation on PET scanning within irradiated myocardium. This study also measured matrix metalloproteinase 3 (MMP-3), a peptide associated with cardiac remodelling, and found levels were higher in patients with abnormal myocardial FDG uptake, suggesting that high levels may be associated with microvascular damage secondary to irradiation. BNP was also studied in 15 patients receiving stem cell transplantation (SCT) for haematological malignancies.[365] In patients receiving total body irradiation of 13.2 Gy, BNP levels were significantly higher than those receiving no irradiation. BNP levels peaked on average 5.4 months after SCT and 46.7% of patients (7/15) had abnormally high levels more than 6 months following SCT. Although there were no clinical cardiac events in the irradiated

group, the persistent elevation suggests some level of persistent sub-clinical cardiac stress. NT-pro-BNP has been measured and not found to be elevated in some studies of patients receiving radiotherapy for thoracic cancers,[417,421] possibly as the last measurements were taken on completion of RT, whereas other studies[320,365,422] have demonstrated that it may take some time for the marker to become significantly elevated following radiotherapy. Similarly, a study in breast cancer[419] found elevation in NT-pro-BNP 5-22 months following radiotherapy whereas a study that measured BNP on completion of RT did not find any elevation.[199]

Two other natriuretic peptides have been measured in patients receiving radiotherapy. Atrial natriuretic peptide (ANP) was measured in a group of 121 patients who had received radiotherapy for Hodgkin lymphoma and breast cancer an average of 9–10 years previously.[423] Levels of ANP were found to be higher in those who had received radiotherapy compared to 67 unirradiated controls. Levels were also higher in the Hodgkin lymphoma patients than in the breast cancer patients, consistent with them having had a greater volume of cardiac tissue irradiated, and in those patients with cardiac symptoms compared to symptomatic patients. Pro-atrial natiruretic peptide (proANP) was measured in 105 women receiving chemotherapy and radiotherapy for breast cancer.[424] The elevated levels were shown to be related to anthracycline dose and were also higher following left-sided irradiation versus right-sided.

Other blood markers may also give an indication of future cardiovascular risk from radiotherapy. For example, in a study of 589 testicular cancer survivors,[202] those who had received radiotherapy had higher levels of CRP and CD40 ligand, which are markers of inflammation and endothelial dysfunction that may be related in the long term to cardiovascular risk. Other novel biomarkers of inflammation, endothelial activation and damage, microRNAs and microparticles are also being used to prospectively study the effect of radiation on the heart in breast cancer patients.[428]

The inherent practical advantages of blood biomarkers are such that if the exact predictive value of a marker, or set of markers, could be ascertained to be useful then they would form a valuable tool in the monitoring of patients after potentially cardiotoxic radiotherapy regimens. A potential disadvantage of blood biomarkers is that the result is highly dependent on the timing of the assay and, as yet, not enough is known about how the levels of such markers may vary with time following irradiation. None of the studies described above has contained sufficient follow-up or numbers of cardiac events to allow validation of such a marker and none are in routine clinical use for this indication.

Electrocardiography

A variety of electrocardiogram (ECG) changes have been described following irradiation. These include a substantial incidence (35%) of non-specific T-wave abnormalities within 6 months of completion of radiotherapy for left breast cancer, even when only a relatively small volume of the heart received a dose a of >20 Gy.[429] These changes, however, are not of functional significance and have not been demonstrated to be predictive of an increased risk of later cardiac events. A wide range of late conduction abnormalities have been recorded as described in the section on clinical manifestations, especially in patients who have received higher doses (>30 Gy) to larger cardiac volumes (e.g., mantle irradiation for Hodgkin lymphoma). As electrocardiography is a cheap and non-invasive investigation, it therefore seems reasonable to routinely perform ECGs on patients who have received substantial cardiac irradiation as part of clinical follow-up, even if only to document existing but clinically non-significant abnormalities for future reference. A more precise role of ECG in surveillance post-cardiac irradiation has, however, not been defined.

Genetic Susceptibility

The inherent radiosensitivity of normal tissues is well recognized to be subject to genetic variation.[430] Such variation may well modulate cardiovascular risk following radiotherapy. Radiation-induced skin telangiectasia following breast cancer radiotherapy has been associated with certain genetic variations in the ataxia-telangiectasia mutated (ATM) gene and cardiovascular risk.[431,432] And genetic variation in the in TGFβ-1 gene has been associated with cardiovascular disease risk after radiotherapy for breast cancer.[161] The identification of further such genetic associations may, in future, allow the pre-treatment identification of patients at increased susceptibility to radiation-induced cardiovascular toxicity, thus enabling individualization of treatment decision, the targeting of preventative strategies and guidance of the need for post-treatment monitoring.

CONCLUSION

Radiation-induced cardiovascular disease represents a substantial burden to an ever increasing population of cancer survivors. Over the last 50 years the manifestations of RRHD have been described

and the major risk factors identified (Table 7-10).[4–6, 13,20,24,25,224,225,260,272,273,295,297,312,378,433–438] The risk factors for radiation-induced stroke and peripheral vascular disease are not so well studied, but are likely to be similar.

Although these risk factors have been identified in broad terms, there remains much that needs to be learnt before these principles can be put to practical use. Precise dose-volume-response relationships between radiation and cardiovascular end-points have not yet been produced. There remains a practical need to clarify these dose-response relationships so that the risks of radiation administered to the cardiovascular system during modern RT can be accurately predicted. These risks could then be weighed against the expected clinical benefits of current and future RT regimens facilitating their use and development. There is, in addition, a need to establish how radiation may interact with other therapies to increase risk, particularly those that are already known to be cardiotoxic, for example anthracyclines and tyrosine kinase inhibitors. The long term cardiac risks of other newer systemic therapies, and possible interactions with RT, are also not yet known. This is especially important given the increasing use of multimodality treatments in modern cancer management. Furthermore, a quantitative assessment of how the risk of RICD is altered by patient-dependant rather than treatment dependant factors, for example conventional cardiovascular risk factors and genetic susceptibility, is also required. This knowledge will inform individualized clinical decisions on a case-by-case basis in a manner that is currently not possible.

The surveillance of patients at risk of RICD and the treatment of patients with RICD remain in their infancy. Although many studies have documented substantial clinical and subclinical radiation-induced cardiovascular disease in a variety of cancer survivors, effective strategies of management are not well developed. The treatment of clinical disease is largely based on that used for similar conditions with differing underlying aetiologies and may not be optimal. The risk of progression and potential later clinical significance of sub-clinical disease is not well studied and there are, as yet, no treatments specific for the primary or secondary prevention of RICD.

In order to fill these gaps in our knowledge co-operative research will be required between a wide range of disciplines, including pathology, radiobiology, radiation oncology, diagnostic radiology, cardiology and epidemiology. It is only through such multi-disciplinary research that quality of life in cancer survivors will be optimized in the future.

Table 7-10 Postulated risk factors for radiation-induced heart disease

RISK FACTORS	WHAT IS KNOWN	REFERENCES
Treatment-Related Risk Factors		
Total radiation dose	Risk increases with increasing dose	Darby et al.,[5] van Nimwegen et al.,[6] Mulrooney et al.[295]
Radiation dose per fraction	Risk increases with dose per fraction	Martel et al.,[312] Cosset al.[432]
Irradiated volume	Risk increases with volume of heart irradiated	Marks et al.,[378]Gagliardi et al.[433]
Structures irradiated	Risk of certain endpoints may be related to irradiation of certain structures (e.g., LAD)	Hancock et al.,[4] Cutter et al.,[13] Correa et al.[20]
Use of chemotherapy	Risk increases with chemotherapy, especially anthracyclines but also others (e.g., vinca alkaloids)	Swerdlow et al.,[260] Myrehaug et al.,[272] Aleman et al.,[273] Shapiro et al.[434]
Other aspects of radiation technique	Risk affected by cardiac shielding, beam energy, number of fields treated per day, lack of inhomogeneity correction etc.	Hancock et al.,[4] Taylor et al.,[224] Vordermark et al.[435]
Patient-Related Risk Factors		
Age at irradiation	Relative risk increases with decreasing age especially <35 years, but absolute risk increases with increasing age and elevated relative risks have been documented for patients irradiated in their 60s	Hancock et al.,[4] Darby et al.,[225] Swerdlow et al.,[260] Hancock et al.[297]
Cardiovascular risk factors	Radiation-related risk increases with smoking, hypertension, diabetes, obesity, abnormal lipids and family history	Harris et al.,[24] Hooning et al.,[25] Myrehaug et al.,[272] King et al.[436]
Pre-existing cardiovascular disease	Risk higher in patients with pre-existing heart disease	Darby et al.,[5] Myrehaug et al.[437]
Gender	Relative risk higher in females compared to males, but absolute risk higher in males	
Race	Relative risk following treatment in childhood higher in patients of black/African descent compared to whites	
Other Risk Factors		
Period of time since exposure	Risk tends to increase with time from exposure and may not be apparent for 10 years or more. Risk remains elevated for at least 20 years from exposure and perhaps up to 50 years.	Hancock et al.,[4] Darby et al.,[225] Swerdlow et al.[260]

LAD, Left anterior descending (coronary artery).

REFERENCES

1. Holthusen H. Erfahrungen über die Verträglichkeitsgrenze für Röntgen-strahlen and deren Nutzanwendung zur Verhütung von Schäden. *Strahlentherapie.* 1936;57:254–269.

2. Selwyn AP. The cardiovascular system and radiation. *Lancet.* July 16, 1983;2(8342):152–154.

3. Cohn KE, Stewart JR, Fajardo LF, Hancock EW. Heart disease following radiation. *Medicine.* May 1967;46(3):281–298.

4. Hancock SL, Tucker MA, Hoppe RT. Factors affecting late mortality from heart disease after treatment of Hodgkin's disease. *JAMA.* October 27, 1993;270(16):1949–1955.

5. Darby SC, Ewertz M, McGale P, et al. Risk of ischemic heart disease in women after radiotherapy for breast cancer. *N Engl J Med*. March 14, 2013;368(11):987–998.

6. van Nimwegen FA, Schaapveld M, Cutter DJ, et al. Radiation dose-response relationship for risk of coronary heart disease in survivors of Hodgkin Lymphoma. *J Clin Oncol*. January 20, 2016;34(3):235–243.

7. Tukenova M, Guibout C, Oberlin O, et al. Role of cancer treatment in long-term overall and cardiovascular mortality after childhood cancer. *J Clin Oncol*. March 10, 2010;28(8):1308–1315.

8. Haddy N, Diallo S, El-Fayech C, et al. Cardiac diseases following childhood cancer treatment: cohort study. *Circulation*. January 5, 2016;133(1):31–38.

9. Carr ZA, Land CE, Kleinerman RA, et al. Coronary heart disease after radiotherapy for peptic ulcer disease. *Int J Radiat Oncol, Biol, Phys*. March 1, 2005;61(3):842–850.

10. Shimizu Y, Kodama K, Nishi N, et al. Radiation exposure and circulatory disease risk: Hiroshima and Nagasaki atomic bomb survivor data, 1950-2003. *BMJ*. 2010;340:b5349.

11. Ozasa K, Takahashi I, Grant EJ. Radiation-related risks of non-cancer outcomes in the atomic bomb survivors. *Ann ICRP*. Jun. 2016;45:253–261.

12. Tapio S. Pathology and biology of radiation-induced cardiac disease. *J Radiat Res*. September 2016;57(5):439–448.

13. Cutter DJ, Schaapveld M, Darby SC, et al. Risk of valvular heart disease after treatment for Hodgkin lymphoma. *J Natl Cancer Inst*. April 2015;107(4).

14. Maddams J, Brewster D, Gavin A, et al. Cancer prevalence in the United Kingdom: estimates for 2008. *Br J Cancer*. August 4, 2009;101(3):541–547.

15. Brosius FC, 3rd, Waller BF, Roberts WC. Radiation heart disease. Analysis of 16 young (aged 15 to 33 years) necropsy patients who received over 3,500 rads to the heart. *Am J Med*. March 1981;70(3):519–530.

16. Russell NS, Hoving S, Heeneman S, et al. Novel insights into pathological changes in muscular arteries of radiotherapy patients. *Radiother Oncol*. September 2009;92(3):477–483.

17. Stewart FA, Heeneman S, Te Poele J, et al. Ionizing radiation accelerates the development of atherosclerotic lesions in ApoE-/- mice and predisposes to an inflammatory plaque phenotype prone to hemorrhage. *Am J Pathol*. February 2006;168(2):649–658.

18. Moignier A, Broggio D, Derreumaux S, et al. Coronary stenosis risk analysis following Hodgkin lymphoma radiotherapy: a study based on patient specific artery segments dose calculation. *Radiother Oncol*. December 2015;117(3):467–472.

19. Waqar S, Jutley R, Mount R, Sarkar P. Bilateral coronary ostial disease following mediastinal irradiation: a case report. *Cases J*. 2009;2:7792.

20. Correa CR, Litt HI, Hwang WT, Ferrari VA, Solin LJ, Harris EE. Coronary artery findings after left-sided compared with right-sided radiation treatment for early-stage breast cancer. *J Clin Oncol*. July 20, 2007;25(21):3031–3037.

21. Nilsson G, Holmberg L, Garmo H, et al. Distribution of coronary artery stenosis after radiation for breast cancer. *J Clin Oncol*. February 1, 2012;30(4):380–386.

22. Fajardo LF. The pathology of ionizing radiation as defined by morphologic patterns. *Acta Oncol*. 2005;44(1):13–22.

23. Hull MC, Morris CG, Pepine CJ, Mendenhall NP. Valvular dysfunction and carotid, subclavian, and coronary artery disease in survivors of hodgkin lymphoma treated with radiation therapy. *JAMA*. December 3, 2003;290(21):2831–2837.

24. Harris EE, Correa C, Hwang WT, et al. Late cardiac mortality and morbidity in early-stage breast cancer patients after breast-conservation treatment. *J Clin Oncol*. September 1, 2006;24(25):4100–4106.

25. Hooning MJ, Botma A, Aleman BM, et al. Long-term risk of cardiovascular disease in 10-year survivors of breast cancer. *J Natl Cancer Inst*. March 7, 2007;99(5):365–375.

26. Heidenreich PA, Kapoor JR. Radiation induced heart disease: systemic disorders in heart disease. *Heart*. March 2009;95(3):252–258.

27. Brown ML, Schaff HV, Sundt TM. Conduit choice for coronary artery bypass grafting after mediastinal radiation. *J Thorac Cardiovasc Surg*. November 2008;136(5):1167–1171.

28. Handa N, McGregor CG, Danielson GK, et al. Coronary artery bypass grafting in patients with previous mediastinal radiation therapy. *J Thorac Cardiovasc Surg*. June 1999;117(6):1136–1142.

29. Wu W, Masri A, Popovic ZB, et al. Long-term survival of patients with radiation heart disease undergoing cardiac surgery: a cohort study. *Circulation*. April 9, 2013;127(14):1476–1485.

30. Chang AS, Smedira NG, Chang CL, et al. Cardiac surgery after mediastinal radiation: extent of exposure influences outcome. *J Thorac Cardiovasc Surg*. February 2007;133(2):404–413.

31. Desai MY, Karunakaravel K, Wu W, et al. Pulmonary fibrosis on multidetector computed tomography and mortality in patients with radiation-associated cardiac disease undergoing cardiac surgery. *J Thorac Cardiovasc Surg*. August 2014;148(2):475–481. e473.

32. Chirakarnjanakorn S, Popovic ZB, Wu W, et al. Impact of long-axis function on cardiac surgical outcomes in patients with radiation-associated heart disease. *J Thorac Cardiovasc Surg*. June 2015;149(6):1643–1651. e1641–e1642.

33. Darby SC, Cutter DJ, Boerma M, et al. Radiation-related heart disease: current knowledge and future prospects. *Int J Radiat Oncol, Biol, Phys*. March 1, 2010;76(3):656–665.

34. Chello M, Mastroroberto P, Romano R, Zofrea S, Bevacqua I, Marchese AR. Changes in the proportion of types I and III collagen in the left ventricular wall of patients with post-irradiative pericarditis. *Cardiovasc Surg*. April 1996;4(2):222–226.

35. Heidenreich PA, Hancock SL, Vagelos RH, Lee BK, Schnittger I. Diastolic dysfunction after mediastinal irradiation. *Am Heart J*. November 2005;150(5):977–982.

36. Prosnitz RG, Hubbs JL, Evans ES, et al. Prospective assessment of radiotherapy-associated cardiac toxicity

in breast cancer patients: analysis of data 3 to 6 years after treatment. *Cancer*. October 15, 2007;110(8):1840–1850.

37. Uriel N, Vainrib A, Jorde UP, et al. Mediastinal radiation and adverse outcomes after heart transplantation. *J Heart Lung Transplant*. March 2010;29(3):378–381.

38. Saxena P, Joyce LD, Daly RC, et al. Cardiac transplantation for radiation-induced cardiomyopathy: the Mayo Clinic experience. *Ann Thorac Surg*. December 2014;98(6):2115–2121.

39. Veinot JP, Edwards WD. Pathology of radiation-induced heart disease: a surgical and autopsy study of 27 cases. *Hum Pathol*. August 1996;27(8):766–773.

40. Yarnold J, Brotons MC. Pathogenetic mechanisms in radiation fibrosis. *Radiother Oncol*. October 2010;97(1):149–161.

41. Nadlonek NA, Weyant MJ, Yu JA, et al. Radiation induces osteogenesis in human aortic valve interstitial cells. *J Thorac Cardiovasc Surg*. December 2012;144(6):1466–1470.

42. McGale P, Darby SC, Hall P, et al. Incidence of heart disease in 35,000 women treated with radiotherapy for breast cancer in Denmark and Sweden. *Radiother Oncol*. August 2011;100(2):167–175.

43. Brand MD, Abadi CA, Aurigemma GP, Dauerman HL, Meyer TE. Radiation-associated valvular heart disease in Hodgkin's disease is associated with characteristic thickening and fibrosis of the aortic-mitral curtain. *J Heart Valve Dis*. September 2001;10(5):681–685.

44. Heidenreich PA, Hancock SL, Lee BK, Mariscal CS, Schnittger I. Asymptomatic cardiac disease following mediastinal irradiation. *J Am Coll Cardiol*. August 20, 2003;42(4):743–749.

45. Wethal T, Lund MB, Edvardsen T, et al. Valvular dysfunction and left ventricular changes in Hodgkin's lymphoma survivors. A longitudinal study. *Br J Cancer*. August 18, 2009;101(4):575–581.

46. Handa N, McGregor CG, Danielson GK, et al. Valvular heart operation in patients with previous mediastinal radiation therapy. *Ann Thorac Surg*. June 2001;71(6):1880–1884.

47. Crestanello JA, McGregor CG, Danielson GK, et al. Mitral and tricuspid valve repair in patients with previous mediastinal radiation therapy. *Ann Thorac Surg*. September 2004;78(3):826–831; discussion 826–831.

48. Dijos M, Reynaud A, Leroux L, et al. Efficacy and follow-up of transcatheter aortic valve implantation in patients with radiation-induced aortic stenosis. *Open Heart*. 2015;2(1):e000252.

49. Franzen O, Baldus S, Rudolph V, et al. Acute outcomes of MitraClip therapy for mitral regurgitation in high-surgical-risk patients: emphasis on adverse valve morphology and severe left ventricular dysfunction. *Eur Heart J*. June 2010;31(11):1373–1381.

50. Stewart JR, Fajardo LF. Radiation-induced heart disease: an update. *Prog Cardiovasc Dis*. November-December 1984;27(3):173–194.

51. Stewart JR, Fajardo LF, Gillette SM, Constine LS. Radiation injury to the heart. *Int J Radiat Oncol, Biol, Phys*. March 30, 1995;31(5):1205–1211.

52. Schultz-Hector S. Radiation-induced heart disease: review of experimental data on dose response and pathogenesis. *Int J Radiat Biol*. February 1992;61(2):149–160.

53. Carmel RJ, Kaplan HS. Mantle irradiation in Hodgkin's disease. An analysis of technique, tumor eradication, and complications. *Cancer*. June 1976;37(6):2813–2825.

54. Morgan GW, Freeman AP, McLean RG, Jarvie BH, Giles RW. Late cardiac, thyroid, and pulmonary sequelae of mantle radiotherapy for Hodgkin's disease. *Int J Radiat Oncol, Biol, Phys*. November 1985;11(11):1925–1931.

55. Imazio M, Bobbio M, Cecchi E, et al. Colchicine in addition to conventional therapy for acute pericarditis: results of the COlchicine for acute PEricarditis (COPE) trial. *Circulation*. September 27, 2005;112(13):2012–2016.

56. Morton DL, Glancy DL, Joseph WL, Adkins PC. Management of patients with radiation-induced pericarditis with effusion: a note on the development of aortic regurgitation in two of them. *Chest*. September 1973;64(3):291–297.

57. Bertog SC, Thambidorai SK, Parakh K, et al. Constrictive pericarditis: etiology and cause-specific survival after pericardiectomy. *J Am Coll Cardiol*. April 21, 2004;43(8):1445–1452.

58. George TJ, Arnaoutakis GJ, Beaty CA, Kilic A, Baumgartner WA, Conte JV. Contemporary etiologies, risk factors, and outcomes after pericardiectomy. *Ann Thorac Surg*. August 2012;94(2):445–451.

59. Orzan F, Brusca A, Gaita F, Giustetto C, Figliomeni MC, Libero L. Associated cardiac lesions in patients with radiation-induced complete heart block. *Int J Cardiol*. May 1993;39(2):151–156.

60. Adams MJ, Lipsitz SR, Colan SD, et al. Cardiovascular status in long-term survivors of Hodgkin's disease treated with chest radiotherapy. *J Clin Oncol*. August 1, 2004;22(15):3139–3148.

61. Strender LE, Lindahl J, Larsson LE. Incidence of heart disease and functional significance of changes in the electrocardiogram 10 years after radiotherapy for breast cancer. *Cancer*. March 1, 1986;57(5):929–934.

62. Yoshii Y. Pathological review of late cerebral radionecrosis. *Brain Tumor Pathol*. 2008;25(2):51–58.

63. Dorresteijn LD, Kappelle AC, Scholz NM, et al. Increased carotid wall thickening after radiotherapy on the neck. *Eur J Cancer*. May 2005;41(7):1026–1030.

64. Cheng SW, Ting AC, Ho P, Wu LL. Accelerated progression of carotid stenosis in patients with previous external neck irradiation. *J Vasc Surg*. February 2004;39(2):409–415.

65. De Bruin ML, Dorresteijn LD, van' Veer MB, et al. Increased risk of stroke and transient ischemic attack in 5-year survivors of Hodgkin lymphoma. *J Natl Cancer Inst*. July 1, 2009;101(13):928–937.

66. Ruben JD, Dally M, Bailey M, Smith R, McLean CA, Fedele P. Cerebral radiation necrosis: incidence, outcomes, and risk factors with emphasis on radiation parameters and chemotherapy. *Int J Radiat Oncol, Biol, Phys*. June 1, 2006;65(2):499–508.

67. Plummer C, Henderson RD, O'Sullivan JD, Read SJ. Ischemic stroke and transient ischemic attack after head and neck radiotherapy: a review. *Stroke*. September 2011;42(9):2410–2418.

68. Ravin RA, Gottlieb A, Pasternac K, et al. Carotid artery stenting may be performed safely in patients with radiation therapy-associated carotid stenosis without increased restenosis or target lesion revascularization. *J Vasc Surg*. September 2015;62(3):624–630.

69. Derubertis BG, Hynecek RL, Kent KC, Faries PL. Carotid tortuosity in patients with prior cervical radiation: increased technical challenge during carotid stenting. *Vasc Endovascular Surg*. October 2011;45(7):619–626.

70. Bowers DC, Liu Y, Leisenring W, et al. Late-occurring stroke among long-term survivors of childhood leukemia and brain tumors: a report from the Childhood Cancer Survivor Study. *J Clin Oncol*. November 20, 2006;24(33):5277–5282.

71. Dorresteijn LD, Kappelle AC, Boogerd W, et al. Increased risk of ischemic stroke after radiotherapy on the neck in patients younger than 60 years. *J Clin Oncol*. January 1, 2002;20(1):282–288.

72. Black DF, Bartleson JD, Bell ML, Lachance DH. SMART: stroke-like migraine attacks after radiation therapy. *Cephalalgia*. September 2006;26(9):1137–1142.

73. Kerklaan JP, Lycklama a Nijeholt GJ, Wiggenraad RG, Berghuis B, Postma TJ, Taphoorn MJ. SMART syndrome: a late reversible complication after radiation therapy for brain tumours. *J Neurol*. June 2011;258(6):1098–1104.

74. Ullrich NJ, Robertson R, Kinnamon DD, et al. Moyamoya following cranial irradiation for primary brain tumors in children. *Neurology*. March 20, 2007;68(12):932–938.

75. Merchant TE, Conklin HM, Wu S, Lustig RH, Xiong X. Late effects of conformal radiation therapy for pediatric patients with low-grade glioma: prospective evaluation of cognitive, endocrine, and hearing deficits. *J Clin Oncol*. August 1, 2009;27(22):3691–3697.

76. Leseche G, Castier Y, Chataigner O, et al. Carotid artery revascularization through a radiated field. *J Vasc Surg*. August 2003;38(2):244–250.

77. Harrod-Kim P, Kadkhodayan Y, Derdeyn CP, Cross DT, 3rd, Moran CJ. Outcomes of carotid angioplasty and stenting for radiation-associated stenosis. *AJNR Am J Neuroradiol*. August 2005;26(7):1781–1788.

78. Hassen-Khodja R, Kieffer E. Radiotherapy-induced supra-aortic trunk disease: early and long-term results of surgical and endovascular reconstruction. *J Vasc Surg*. August 2004;40(2):254–261.

79. Fokkema M, den Hartog AG, Bots ML, van der Tweel I, Moll FL, de Borst GJ. Stenting versus surgery in patients with carotid stenosis after previous cervical radiation therapy: systematic review and meta-analysis. *Stroke*. March 2012;43(3):793–801.

80. Dorresteijn LD, Vogels OJ, de Leeuw FE, et al. Outcome of carotid artery stenting for radiation-induced stenosis. *Int J Radiat Oncol, Biol, Phys*. August 1, 2010;77(5):1386–1390.

81. Zidar N, Ferluga D, Hvala A, Popovic M, Soba E. Contribution to the pathogenesis of radiation-induced injury to large arteries. *J Laryngol Otol*. October 1997;111(10):988–990.

82. Atabek U, Spence RK, Alexander JB, Pello MJ, Camishion RC. Upper extremity occlusive arterial disease after radiotherapy for breast cancer. J Surg Oncol. March 1992;49(3):205–207.

83. Saka B, Bilge AK, Umman B, et al. Bilateral renal artery stenosis after abdominal radiotherapy for Hodgkin's disease. *Int J Clin Prac*. April 2003;57(3):247–248.

84. Patel DA, Kochanski J, Suen AW, Fajardo LF, Hancock SL, Knox SJ. Clinical manifestations of noncoronary atherosclerotic vascular disease after moderate dose irradiation. *Cancer*. February 1, 2006;106(3):718–725.

85. Moutardier V, Christophe M, Lelong B, Houvenaeghel G, Delpero JR. Iliac atherosclerotic occlusive disease complicating radiation therapy for cervix cancer: a case series. *Gynecol Oncol*. March 2002;84(3):456–459.

86. Melliere D, Becquemin JP, Berrahal D, Desgranges P, Cavillon A. Management of radiation-induced occlusive arterial disease: a reassessment. *J Cardiovasc Surg*. June 1997;38(3):261–269.

87. Saliou C, Julia P, Feito B, Renaudin JM, Fabiani JN. Radiation-induced arterial disease of the lower limb. *Ann Vasc Surg*. March 1997;11(2):173–177.

88. Zhou W, Bush RL, Lin PH, Lumsden AB. Radiation-associated venous stenosis: endovascular treatment options. *J Vasc Surg*. Jul 2004;40(1):179–182.

89. Jurado JA, Bashir R, Burket MW. Radiation-induced peripheral artery disease. *Catheter Cardiovasc Interv*. Octobrer 1, 2008;72(4):563–568.

90. Andros G, Schneider PA, Harris RW, Dulawa LB, Oblath RW, Salles-Cunha SX. Management of arterial occlusive disease following radiation therapy. *Cardiovasc Surg*. April 1996;4(2):135–142.

91. Dorr W. Pathogenesis of normal tissue side effects. In: Joiner MC, Van der Kogel AJ, eds. *Basic Clinical Radiobiology*. 4th ed. London: Hodder Arnold; 2009:169–190.

92. Fajardo LF, Berthrong M, Anderson RE. Cardiovascular system. *Radiation Pathology*. New York, NY: Oxford University Press; 2001:165–192.

93. Gaugler M-H. A unifying system: does the vascular endothelium have a role to play in multi-organ failure following radiation exposure? *Br J Radiol*. 2005;(suppl 27):100–105.

94. Morgenroth K, Jr., Junge-Hulsing G, Hauss WH. [On the changes of rat heart following selective x-ray irradiation]. *Strahlentherapie*. August 1967;133(4):610–620.

95. Fajardo LF, Stewart JR. Experimental radiation-induced heart disease. I. Light microscopic studies. *Am J Pathol*. May 1970;59(2):299–316.

96. Khan MY, Ohanian M. Radiation-induced cardiomyopathy: II. An electron microscopic study of myocardial microvasculature. *Am J Pathol*. January 1974;74(1):125–136.

97. Lauk S, Trott KR. Endothelial cell proliferation in the rat heart following local heart irradiation. *Int J Radiat Biol*. May 1990;57(5):1017–1030.

98. Hallahan D, Clark ET, Kuchibhotla J, Gewertz BL, Collins T. E-selectin gene induction by ionizing radiation is independent of cytokine induction. *Biochem Biophys Res Commun*. December 26, 1995;217(3):784–795.

99. Hallahan D, Kuchibhotla J, Wyble C. Cell adhesion molecules mediate radiation-induced leukocyte adhesion

to the vascular endothelium. *Cancer Res.* November 15, 1996;56(22):5150–5155.

100. Gaugler MH, Squiban C, van der Meeren A, Bertho JM, Vandamme M, Mouthon MA. Late and persistent up-regulation of intercellular adhesion molecule-1 (ICAM-1) expression by ionizing radiation in human endothelial cells in vitro. *Int J Radiat Biol.* August 1997;72(2):201–209.

101. Heckmann M, Douwes K, Peter R, Degitz K. Vascular activation of adhesion molecule mRNA and cell surface expression by ionizing radiation. *Exp Cell Res.* January 10, 1998;238(1):148–154.

102. Quarmby S, Hunter RD, Kumar S. Irradiation induced expression of CD31, ICAM-1 and VCAM-1 in human microvascular endothelial cells. *Anticancer Res.* September–October 2000;20(5B):3375–3381.

103. Khaled S, Gupta KB, Kucik DF. Ionizing radiation increases adhesiveness of human aortic endothelial cells via a chemokine-dependent mechanism. *Radiat Res.* May 2012;177(5):594–601.

104. Hallahan DE, Virudachalam S. Ionizing radiation mediates expression of cell adhesion molecules in distinct histological patterns within the lung. *Cancer Res.* June 1, 1997;57(11):2096–2099.

105. Tsujino K, Kodama A, Kanaoka N, Maruta T, Kono M. Expression of pulmonary mRNA encoding ICAM-1, VCAM-1, and P-selectin following thoracic irradiation in mice. *Radiat Med.* July-August 1999;17(4):283–287.

106. Hallahan DE, Virudachalam S, Kuchibhotla J. Nuclear factor kappaB dominant negative genetic constructs inhibit X-ray induction of cell adhesion molecules in the vascular endothelium. *Cancer Res.* December 1, 1998;58(23):5484–5488.

107. Halle M, Gabrielsen A, Paulsson-Berne G, et al. Sustained inflammation due to nuclear factor-kappa B activation in irradiated human arteries. *J Am Coll Cardiol.* March 23, 2010;55(12):1227–1236.

108. Van Der Meeren A, Squiban C, Gourmelon P, Lafont H, Gaugler MH. Differential regulation by IL-4 and IL-10 of radiation-induced IL-6 and IL-8 production and ICAM-1 expression by human endothelial cells. *Cytokine.* November 1999;11(11):831–838.

109. Fedorocko P, Egyed A, Vacek A. Irradiation induces increased production of haemopoietic and proinflammatory cytokines in the mouse lung. *Int J Radiat Biol.* April 2002;78(4):305–313.

110. Li A, Dubey S, Varney ML, Dave BJ, Singh RK. IL-8 directly enhanced endothelial cell survival, proliferation, and matrix metalloproteinases production and regulated angiogenesis. *J Immunol.* March 15, 2003;170(6):3369–3376.

111. Peterson LM, Evans ML, Thomas KL, Graham MM. Vascular response to fractionated irradiation in the rat lung. *Radiat Res.* August 1992;131(2):224–226.

112. Gabrys D, Greco O, Patel G, Prise KM, Tozer GM, Kanthou C. Radiation effects on the cytoskeleton of endothelial cells and endothelial monolayer permeability. *Int J Radiat Oncol, Biol, Phys.* December 1, 2007;69(5):1553–1562.

113. Waters CM, Taylor JM, Molteni A, Ward WF. Dose-response effects of radiation on the permeability of endothelial cells in culture. *Radiation Res.* September 1996;146(3):321–328.

114. Molla M, Panes J. Radiation-induced intestinal inflammation. *World J Gastroenterol.* June 14, 2007;13(22):3043–3046.

115. Kern PM, Keilholz L, Forster C, Hallmann R, Herrmann M, Seegenschmiedt MH. Low-dose radiotherapy selectively reduces adhesion of peripheral blood mononuclear cells to endothelium in vitro. *Radiother Oncol.* March 2000;54(3):273–282.

116. Roedel F, Kley N, Beuscher HU, et al. Anti-inflammatory effect of low-dose X-irradiation and the involvement of a TGF-beta1-induced down-regulation of leukocyte/endothelial cell adhesion. *Int J Radiat Biol.* August 2002;78(8):711–719.

117. Hildebrandt G, Maggiorella L, Rodel F, Rodel V, Willis D, Trott KR. Mononuclear cell adhesion and cell adhesion molecule liberation after X-irradiation of activated endothelial cells in vitro. *Int J Radiat Biol.* April 2002;78(4):315–325.

118. Hosoi Y, Miyachi H, Matsumoto Y, et al. Induction of interleukin-1beta and interleukin-6 mRNA by low doses of ionizing radiation in macrophages. *Int J Cancer.* October 20, 2001;96(5):270–276.

119. Ruggeri ZM. Platelets in atherothrombosis. *Nat Med.* November 2002;8(11):1227–1234.

120. Sporn LA, Rubin P, Marder VJ, Wagner DD. Irradiation induces release of von Willebrand protein from endothelial cells in culture. *Blood.* August 1984;64(2):567–570.

121. Verheij M, Dewit LG, Boomgaard MN, Brinkman HJ, van Mourik JA. Ionizing radiation enhances platelet adhesion to the extracellular matrix of human endothelial cells by an increase in the release of von Willebrand factor. *Radiat Res.* February 1994;137(2):202–207.

122. van Kleef E, Verheij M, te Poele H, Oussoren Y, Dewit L, Stewart F. In vitro and in vivo expression of endothelial von Willebrand factor and leukocyte accumulation after fractionated irradiation. *Radiat Res.* October 2000;154(4):375–381.

123. Boerma M, Kruse JJ, van Loenen M, et al. Increased deposition of von Willebrand factor in the rat heart after local ionizing irradiation. *Strahlenther Onkol.* February 2004;180(2):109–116.

124. Allen JB, Sagerman RH, Stuart MJ. Irradiation decreases vascular prostacyclin formation with no concomitant effect on platelet thromboxane production. *Lancet.* November 28, 1981;2(8257):1193–1196.

125. Wang J, Zheng H, Ou X, Fink LM, Hauer-Jensen M. Deficiency of microvascular thrombomodulin and up-regulation of protease-activated receptor-1 in irradiated rat intestine: possible link between endothelial dysfunction and chronic radiation fibrosis. *Am J Pathol.* June 2002;160(6):2063–2072.

126. Verheij M, Dewit LG, van Mourik JA. The effect of ionizing radiation on endothelial tissue factor activity and its cellular localization. *Thromb Haemost.* May 1995;73(5):894–895.

127. Bombeli T, Karsan A, Tait JF, Harlan JM. Apoptotic vascular endothelial cells become procoagulant. *Blood*. April 1, 1997;89(7):2429–2442.

128. Henderson BW, Bicher HI, Johnson RJ. Loss of vascular fibrinolytic activity following irradiation of the liver—an aspect of late radiation damage. *Radiat Res*. September 1983;95(3):646–652.

129. Ts'ao C, Ward WF. Acute radiation effects on the content and release of plasminogen activator activity in cultured aortic endothelial cells. *Radiat Res*. February 1985;101(2):394–401.

130. Soloviev AI, Tishkin SM, Parshikov AV, Ivanova IV, Goncharov EV, Gurney AM. Mechanisms of endothelial dysfunction after ionized radiation: selective impairment of the nitric oxide component of endothelium-dependent vasodilation. *Br J Pharmacol*. March 2003;138(5):837–844.

131. Soucy KG, Lim HK, Benjo A, et al. Single exposure gamma-irradiation amplifies xanthine oxidase activity and induces endothelial dysfunction in rat aorta. *Radiat Environ Biophys*. June 2007;46(2):179–186.

132. Sugihara T, Hattori Y, Yamamoto Y, et al. Preferential impairment of nitric oxide-mediated endothelium-dependent relaxation in human cervical arteries after irradiation. *Circulation*. August 10, 1999;100(6):635–641.

133. Beckman JA, Thakore A, Kalinowski BH, Harris JR, Creager MA. Radiation therapy impairs endothelium-dependent vasodilation in humans. *J Am Coll Cardiol*. March 1, 2001;37(3):761–765.

134. Robbins ME, Zhao W. Chronic oxidative stress and radiation-induced late normal tissue injury: a review. *Int J Radiat Biol*. April 2004;80(4):251–259.

135. Spitz DR, Azzam EI, Li JJ, Gius D. Metabolic oxidation/reduction reactions and cellular responses to ionizing radiation: a unifying concept in stress response biology. *Cancer Metastasis Rev*. August-December 2004;23(3–4):311–322.

136. Takano H, Zou Y, Hasegawa H, Akazawa H, Nagai T, Komuro I. Oxidative stress-induced signal transduction pathways in cardiac myocytes: involvement of ROS in heart diseases. *Antioxid Redox Signal*. December 2003;5(6):789–794.

137. Halle M, Hall P, Tornvall P. Cardiovascular disease associated with radiotherapy: activation of nuclear factor kappa-B. *J Intern Med*. May 2011;269(5):469–477.

138. Mikkelsen RB, Wardman P. Biological chemistry of reactive oxygen and nitrogen and radiation-induced signal transduction mechanisms. *Oncogene*. September 1, 2003;22(37):5734–5754.

139. Benderitter M, Maingon P, Abadie C, et al. Effect of in vivo heart irradiation on the development of antioxidant defenses and cardiac functions in the rat. *Radiat Res*. October 1995;144(1):64–72.

140. Baker JE, Fish BL, Su J, et al. 10 Gy total body irradiation increases risk of coronary sclerosis, degeneration of heart structure and function in a rat model. *Int J Radiat Biol*. December 2009;85(12):1089–1100.

141. Soucy KG, Lim HK, Attarzadeh DO, et al. Dietary inhibition of xanthine oxidase attenuates radiation-induced endothelial dysfunction in rat aorta. *J Appl Physiol (1985)*. May 2010;108(5):1250–1258.

142. Leborgne L, Pakala R, Dilcher C, et al. Effect of antioxidants on atherosclerotic plaque formation in balloon-denuded and irradiated hypercholesterolemic rabbits. *J Cardiovasc Pharmacol*. October 2005;46(4):540–547.

143. Leach JK, Van Tuyle G, Lin PS, Schmidt-Ullrich R, Mikkelsen RB. Ionizing radiation-induced, mitochondria-dependent generation of reactive oxygen/nitrogen. *Cancer Res*. May 15, 2001;61(10):3894–3901.

144. Davidson SM. Endothelial mitochondria and heart disease. *Cardiovasc Res*. October 1, 2010;88(1):58–66.

145. Barjaktarovic Z, Schmaltz D, Shyla A, et al. Radiation-induced signaling results in mitochondrial impairment in mouse heart at 4 weeks after exposure to X-rays. *PLOS ONE*. 2011;6(12):e27811.

146. Liu H, Xiong M, Xia YF, et al. Studies on pentoxifylline and tocopherol combination for radiation-induced heart disease in rats. *Int J Radiat Oncol, Biol, Phys*. April 1, 2009;73(5):1552–1559.

147. Martin M, Lefaix J, Delanian S. TGF-beta1 and radiation fibrosis: a master switch and a specific therapeutic target? *Int J Radiat Oncol, Biol, Phys*. May 1, 2000;47(2):277–290.

148. Fajardo LF, Stewart JR. Cardiovascular radiation syndrome. *N Engl J Med*. August 13, 1970;283(7):374.

149. Aiba T, Tomaselli GF. Electrical remodeling in the failing heart. *Curr Opin Cardiol*. January 2010;25(1):29–36.

150. Milliat F, Francois A, Isoir M, et al. Influence of endothelial cells on vascular smooth muscle cells phenotype after irradiation: implication in radiation-induced vascular damages. *Am J Pathol*. October 2006;169(4):1484–1495.

151. Rodemann HP, Bamberg M. Cellular basis of radiation-induced fibrosis. *Radiother Oncol*. May 1995;35(2):83–90.

152. Herskind C, Rodemann HP. Spontaneous and radiation-induced differentiation of fibroblasts. *Exp Gerontol*. September 2000;35(6–7):747–755.

153. Anscher MS. Targeting the TGF-beta1 pathway to prevent normal tissue injury after cancer therapy. *Oncologist*. 2010;15(4):350–359.

154. Attisano L, Wrana JL. Signal transduction by the TGF-beta superfamily. *Science*. May 31, 2002;296(5573):1646–1647.

155. Bentzen SM. Preventing or reducing late side effects of radiation therapy: radiobiology meets molecular pathology. *Nat Rev Cancer*. September 2006;6(9):702–713.

156. Ehrhart EJ, Segarini P, Tsang ML, Carroll AG, Barcellos-Hoff MH. Latent transforming growth factor beta1 activation in situ: quantitative and functional evidence after low-dose gamma-irradiation. *FASEB J*. October 1997;11(12):991–1002.

157. Kruse JJ, Zurcher C, Strootman EG, et al. Structural changes in the auricles of the rat heart after local ionizing irradiation. *Radiother Oncol*. March 2001;58(3):303–311.

158. Ferreira-Machado SC, Rocha Nde N, Mencalha AL, et al. Up-regulation of angiotensin-converting enzyme and angiotensin II type 1 receptor in irradiated rats. *Int J Radiat Biol*. October 2010;86(10):880–887.

159. Boerma M, Roberto KA, Hauer-Jensen M. Prevention and treatment of functional and structural radiation injury in the rat heart by pentoxifylline and alpha-

tocopherol. *Int J Radiat Oncol, Biol, Phys.* September 1, 2008;72(1):170–177.

160. Boerma M, Hauer-Jensen M. Potential targets for intervention in radiation-induced heart disease. *Curr Drug Targets.* November 2010;11(11):1405–1412.

161. Hilbers FS, Boekel NB, van den Broek AJ, et al. Genetic variants in TGFbeta-1 and PAI-1 as possible risk factors for cardiovascular disease after radiotherapy for breast cancer. *Radiother Oncol.* January 2012;102(1):115–121.

162. Bourgier C, Haydont V, Milliat F, et al. Inhibition of Rho kinase modulates radiation induced fibrogenic phenotype in intestinal smooth muscle cells through alteration of the cytoskeleton and connective tissue growth factor expression. *Gut.* March 2005;54(3):336–343.

163. Monceau V, Pasinetti N, Schupp C, Pouzoulet F, Opolon P, Vozenin MC. Modulation of the Rho/ROCK pathway in heart and lung after thorax irradiation reveals targets to improve normal tissue toxicity. *Curr Drug Targets.* November 2010;11(11):1395–1404.

164. Haydont V, Riser BL, Aigueperse J, Vozenin-Brotons MC. Specific signals involved in the long-term maintenance of radiation-induced fibrogenic differentiation: a role for CCN2 and low concentration of TGF-beta1. *Am J Physiol Cell Physiol.* June 2008;294(6):C1332–C1341.

165. Boerma M, Wang J, Wondergem J, et al. Influence of mast cells on structural and functional manifestations of radiation-induced heart disease. *Cancer Res.* April 15 2005;65(8):3100–3107.

166. Boerma M, Hauer-Jensen M. Preclinical research into basic mechanisms of radiation-induced heart disease. *Cardiol Res Prac.* October 4, 2010;2011.

167. Miyauchi T, Masaki T. Pathophysiology of endothelin in the cardiovascular system. *Annu Rev Physiol.* 1999;61:391–415.

168. Abdollahi A, Li M, Ping G, et al. Inhibition of platelet-derived growth factor signaling attenuates pulmonary fibrosis. *J Exp Med.* March 21, 2005;201(6):925–935.

169. Lavoie JL, Sigmund CD. Minireview: overview of the renin-angiotensin system—an endocrine and paracrine system. *Endocrinology.* June 2003;144(6):2179–2183.

170. Duprez DA. Role of the renin-angiotensin-aldosterone system in vascular remodeling and inflammation: a clinical review. *J Hypertens.* June 2006;24(6):983–991.

171. Robbins ME, Diz DI. Pathogenic role of the renin-angiotensin system in modulating radiation-induced late effects. *Int J Radiat Oncol, Biol, Phys.* January 1, 2006;64(1):6–12.

172. Suzuki Y, Ruiz-Ortega M, Lorenzo O, Ruperez M, Esteban V, Egido J. Inflammation and angiotensin II. *Int J Biochem Cell Biol.* June 2003;35(6):881–900.

173. Lijnen PJ, Petrov VV, Fagard RH. Induction of cardiac fibrosis by angiotensin II. *Methods Find Exp Clin Pharmacol.* December 2000;22(10):709–723.

174. Wu R, Zeng Y. Does angiotensin II-aldosterone have a role in radiation-induced heart disease? *Med Hypotheses.* March 2009;72(3):263–266.

175. Yarom R, Harper IS, Wynchank S, et al. Effect of captopril on changes in rats' hearts induced by long-term irradiation. *Radiat Res.* February 1993;133(2):187–197.

176. Paris F, Fuks Z, Kang A, et al. Endothelial apoptosis as the primary lesion initiating intestinal radiation damage in mice. *Science.* July 13, 2001;293(5528):293–297.

177. Cho CH, Kammerer RA, Lee HJ, et al. Designed angiopoietin-1 variant, COMP-Ang1, protects against radiation-induced endothelial cell apoptosis. *Proc Natl Acad Sci USA.* April 13 2004;101(15):5553–5558.

178. Schuller BW, Rogers AB, Cormier KS, et al. No significant endothelial apoptosis in the radiation-induced gastrointestinal syndrome. *Int J Radiat Oncol, Biol, Phys.* May 1, 2007;68(1):205–210.

179. Stewart FA, Dorr W. Milestones in normal tissue radiation biology over the past 50 years: from clonogenic cell survival to cytokine networks and back to stem cell recovery. *Int J Radiat Biol.* July 2009;85(7):574–586.

180. Schultz-Hector S, Balz K. Radiation-induced loss of endothelial alkaline phosphatase activity and development of myocardial degeneration. An ultrastructural study. *Lab Invest.* August 1994;71(2):252–260.

181. Schultz-Hector S, Trott KR. Radiation-induced cardiovascular diseases: is the epidemiologic evidence compatible with the radiobiologic data? *Int J Radiat Oncol, Biol, Phys.* January 1, 2007;67(1):10–18.

182. Soucy KG, Attarzadeh DO, Ramachandran R, et al. Single exposure to radiation produces early anti-angiogenic effects in mouse aorta. *Radiat Environ Biophys.* August 2010;49(3):397–404.

183. Urbich C, Dimmeler S. Endothelial progenitor cells: characterization and role in vascular biology. *Circ Res.* August 20, 2004;95(4):343–353.

184. Hristov M, Weber C. Endothelial progenitor cells in vascular repair and remodeling. *Pharmacol Res.* August 2008;58(2):148–151.

185. Lee MO, Song SH, Jung S, et al. Effect of ionizing radiation induced damage of endothelial progenitor cells in vascular regeneration. *Arterioscler Thromb Vasc Biol.* February 2012;32(2):343–352.

186. Vos J, Aarnoudse MW, Dijk F, Lamberts HB. On the cellular origin and development of atheromatous plaques. A light and electron microscopic study of combined X-ray and hypercholesterolemia-induced atheromatosis in the carotid artery of the rabbit. *Virchows Arch B Cell Pathol Incl Mol Pathol.* 1983;43(1):1–16.

187. Pakala R, Leborgne L, Cheneau E, et al. Radiation-induced atherosclerotic plaque progression in a hypercholesterolemic rabbit: a prospective vulnerable plaque model? *Cardiovasc Radiat Med.* July-September 2003;4(3):146–151.

188. Gabriels K, Hoving S, Seemann I, et al. Local heart irradiation of ApoE(-/-) mice induces microvascular and endocardial damage and accelerates coronary atherosclerosis. *Radiother Oncol.* December 2012;105(3):358–364.

189. Yu T, Parks BW, Yu S, et al. Iron-ion radiation accelerates atherosclerosis in apolipoprotein E-deficient mice. *Radiat Res.* June 2011;175(6):766–773.

190. Hoving S, Heeneman S, Gijbels MJ, et al. Single-dose and fractionated irradiation promote initiation and progression of atherosclerosis and induce an inflammatory plaque phenotype in ApoE(-/-) mice. *Int J Radiat Oncol, Biol, Phys.* July 1, 2008;71(3):848–857.

191. Stewart FA, Seemann I, Hoving S, Russell NS. Understanding radiation-induced cardiovascular damage and strategies for intervention. *Clin Oncol (R Coll Radiol)*. October 2013;25(10):617–624.

192. Hansson GK. Inflammation, atherosclerosis, and coronary artery disease. *N Engl J Med*. April 21, 2005;352(16):1685–1695.

193. Rube CE, Fricke A, Wendorf J, et al. Accumulation of DNA double-strand breaks in normal tissues after fractionated irradiation. *Int J Radiat Oncol, Biol, Phys*. March 15, 2010;76(4):1206–1213.

194. Morgan WF, Sowa MB. Non-targeted bystander effects induced by ionizing radiation. *Mutat Res*. March 1, 2007;616(1–2):159–164.

195. Weakley SM, Jiang J, Kougias P, et al. Role of somatic mutations in vascular disease formation. *Expert Rev Mol Diagn*. March 2010;10(2):173–185.

196. Hatzistamou J, Kiaris H, Ergazaki M, Spandidos DA. Loss of heterozygosity and microsatellite instability in human atherosclerotic plaques. *Biochem Biophys Res Commun*. August 5, 1996;225(1):186–190.

197. Khan MY. Radiation-induced cardiomyopathy. I. An electron microscopic study of cardiac muscle cells. *Am J Pathol*. October 1973;73(1):131–146.

198. McChesney SL, Gillette EL, Powers BE. Radiation-induced cardiomyopathy in the dog. *Radiat Res*. January 1988;113(1):120–132.

199. Skytta T, Tuohinen S, Boman E, Virtanen V, Raatikainen P, Kellokumpu-Lehtinen PL. Troponin T-release associates with cardiac radiation doses during adjuvant left-sided breast cancer radiotherapy. *Radiat Oncol*. July 10, 2015;10:141.

200. Huddart RA, Norman A, Shahidi M, et al. Cardiovascular disease as a long-term complication of treatment for testicular cancer. *J Clin Oncol*. April 15, 2003;21(8):1513–1523.

201. Sasaki H, Wong FL, Yamada M, Kodama K. The effects of aging and radiation exposure on blood pressure levels of atomic bomb survivors. *J Clin Epidemiol*. October 2002;55(10):974–981.

202. Wethal T, Kjekshus J, Roislien J, et al. Treatment-related differences in cardiovascular risk factors in long-term survivors of testicular cancer. *J Cancer Surviv*. March 2007;1(1):8–16.

203. Hakoda M, Kasagi F, Kusunoki Y, et al. Levels of antibodies to microorganisms implicated in atherosclerosis and of C-reactive protein among atomic bomb survivors. *Radiat Res*. August 2006;166(2):360–366.

204. Hayashi T, Kusunoki Y, Hakoda M, et al. Radiation dose-dependent increases in inflammatory response markers in A-bomb survivors. *Int J Radiat Biol*. February 2003;79(2):129–136.

205. Hayashi T, Morishita Y, Kubo Y, et al. Long-term effects of radiation dose on inflammatory markers in atomic bomb survivors. *Am J Med*. January 2005;118(1):83–86.

206. Kusunoki Y, Hayashi T. Long-lasting alterations of the immune system by ionizing radiation exposure: implications for disease development among atomic bomb survivors. *Int J Radiat Biol*. January 2008;84(1):1–14.

207. Wong FL, Yamada M, Sasaki H, Kodama K, Hosoda Y. Effects of radiation on the longitudinal trends of total serum cholesterol levels in the atomic bomb survivors. *Radiat Res*. June 1999;151(6):736–746.

208. Baba T, Amasaki Y, Soda M, et al. Fatty liver and uric acid levels predict incident coronary heart disease but not stroke among atomic bomb survivors in Nagasaki. *Hypertens Res*. September 2007;30(9):823–829.

209. Meacham LR, Sklar CA, Li S, et al. Diabetes mellitus in long-term survivors of childhood cancer. Increased risk associated with radiation therapy: a report for the childhood cancer survivor study. *Arch Intern Med*. August 10, 2009;169(15):1381–1388.

210. Kleinerman RA, Weinstock RM, Mabuchi K. High-dose abdominal radiotherapy and risk of diabetes mellitus. *Arch Intern Med*. September 13, 2010;170(16):1506–1507.

211. Fujiwara S, Sposto R, Shiraki M, et al. Levels of parathyroid hormone and calcitonin in serum among atomic bomb survivors. *Radiat Res*. January 1994;137(1):96–103.

212. Link K, Moell C, Garwicz S, et al. Growth hormone deficiency predicts cardiovascular risk in young adults treated for acute lymphoblastic leukemia in childhood. *J Clin Endocrinol Metab*. October 2004;89(10):5003–5012.

213. Heikens J, Ubbink MC, van der Pal HP, et al. Long term survivors of childhood brain cancer have an increased risk for cardiovascular disease. *Cancer*. May 1, 2000;88(9):2116–2121.

214. Yang VC, Kao CH, Ting WH, Chen KY, Chiang BN. Late effects in mouse heart after 60Co gamma-irradiation of the brain: an ultrastructural study. *Int J Radiat Biol*. June 1990;57(6):1225–1241.

215. Azimzadeh O, Scherthan H, Sarioglu H, et al. Rapid proteomic remodeling of cardiac tissue caused by total body ionizing radiation. *Proteomics*. August 2011;11(16):3299–3311.

216. Andreassen CN, Grau C, Lindegaard JC. Chemical radioprotection: a critical review of amifostine as a cytoprotector in radiotherapy. *Semin Radiat Oncol*. January 2003;13(1):62–72.

217. Cohen EP, Bedi M, Irving AA, et al. Mitigation of late renal and pulmonary injury after hematopoietic stem cell transplantation. *Int J Radiat Oncol, Biol, Phys*. May 1, 2012;83(1):292–296.

218. Delanian S, Lefaix JL. The radiation-induced fibroatrophic process: therapeutic perspective via the antioxidant pathway. *Radiother Oncol*. November 2004;73(2):119–131.

219. Gothard L, Cornes P, Earl J, et al. Double-blind placebo-controlled randomised trial of vitamin E and pentoxifylline in patients with chronic arm lymphoedema and fibrosis after surgery and radiotherapy for breast cancer. *Radiother Oncol*. November 2004;73(2):133–139.

220. Darby S, McGale P, Correa C, et al. Effect of radiotherapy after breast-conserving surgery on 10-year recurrence and 15-year breast cancer death: meta-analysis of individual patient data for 10,801 women in 17 randomised trials. *Lancet*. November 12, 2011;378(9804):1707–1716.

221. McGale P, Taylor C, Correa C, et al. Effect of radiotherapy after mastectomy and axillary surgery on 10-year recurrence and 20-year breast cancer mortality: meta-analysis of individual patient data for 8135 women in 22 randomised trials. *Lancet*. June 21, 2014;383(9935):2127–2135.

222. Clarke M, Collins R, Darby S, et al. Effects of radiotherapy and of differences in the extent of surgery for early breast cancer on local recurrence and 15-year survival: an overview of the randomised trials. *Lancet*. December 17, 2005;366(9503):2087–2106.

223. McGale P, Cutter D, Darby SC, Henson KE, Jagsi R, Taylor CW. Can observational data replace randomized trials? *J Clin Oncol*. September 20, 2016;34(27):3355–3357.

224. Taylor CW, Nisbet A, McGale P, Darby SC. Cardiac exposures in breast cancer radiotherapy: 1950s-1990s. *Int J Radiat Oncol, Biol, Phys*. December 1, 2007;69(5):1484–1495.

225. Darby SC, McGale P, Taylor CW, Peto R. Long-term mortality from heart disease and lung cancer after radiotherapy for early breast cancer: prospective cohort study of about 300,000 women in US SEER cancer registries. *Lancet Oncol*. August 2005;6(8):557–565.

226. Taylor CW, Wang Z, Macaulay E, Jagsi R, Duane F, Darby SC. Exposure of the heart in breast cancer radiation therapy: a systematic review of heart doses published during 2003 to 2013. *Int J Radiat Oncol, Biol, Phys*. November 15, 2015;93(4):845–853.

227. Wright GP, Drinane JJ, Sobel HL, Chung MH. Left-sided breast irradiation does not result in increased long-term cardiac-related mortality among women treated with breast-conserving surgery. *Ann Surg Oncol*. April 2016;23(4):1117–1122.

228. Boero IJ, Paravati AJ, Triplett DP, et al. Modern radiation therapy and cardiac outcomes in breast cancer. *Int J Radiat Oncol, Biol, Phys*. March 15, 2016;94(4):700–708.

229. Ye JC, Yan W, Christos P, Nori D, Chao KS, Ravi A. Second cancer, breast cancer, and cardiac mortality in stage T1aN0 breast cancer patients with or without external beam radiation therapy: a national registry study. *Clin Breast Cancer*. February 2015;15(1):54–59.

230. Chan EK, Woods R, Virani S, et al. Long-term mortality from cardiac causes after adjuvant hypofractionated vs. conventional radiotherapy for localized left-sided breast cancer. *Radiother Oncol*. January 2015;114(1):73–78.

231. Boekel NB, Schaapveld M, Gietema JA, et al. Cardiovascular morbidity and mortality after treatment for ductal carcinoma in situ of the breast. *J Natl Cancer Inst*. August 2014;106(8).

232. Tjessem KH, Johansen S, Malinen E, et al. Long-term cardiac mortality after hypofractionated radiation therapy in breast cancer. *Int J Radiat Oncol, Biol, Phys*. October 1, 2013;87(2):337–343.

233. Henson KE, McGale P, Taylor C, Darby SC. Radiation-related mortality from heart disease and lung cancer more than 20 years after radiotherapy for breast cancer. *Br J Cancer*. January 15, 2013;108(1):179–182.

234. Bouillon K, Haddy N, Delaloge S, et al. Long-term cardiovascular mortality after radiotherapy for breast cancer. *J Am Coll Cardiol*. January 25, 2011;57(4):445–452.

235. Bouchardy C, Rapiti E, Usel M, et al. Excess of cardiovascular mortality among node-negative breast cancer patients irradiated for inner-quadrant tumors. *Ann Oncol*. March 2010;21(3):459–465.

236. Gutt R, Correa CR, Hwang WT, et al. Cardiac morbidity and mortality after breast conservation treatment in patients with early-stage breast cancer and pre-existing cardiac disease. *Clin Breast Cancer*. October 2008;8(5):443–448.

237. Borger JH, Hooning MJ, Boersma LJ, et al. Cardiotoxic effects of tangential breast irradiation in early breast cancer patients: the role of irradiated heart volume. *Int J Radiat Oncol, Biol, Phys*. November 15, 2007;69(4):1131–1138.

238. Marhin W, Wai E, Tyldesley S. Impact of fraction size on cardiac mortality in women treated with tangential radiotherapy for localized breast cancer. *Int J Radiat Oncol, Biol, Phys*. October 1, 2007;69(2):483–489.

239. Roychoudhuri R, Robinson D, Putcha V, Cuzick J, Darby S, Moller H. Increased cardiovascular mortality more than fifteen years after radiotherapy for breast cancer: a population-based study. *BMC Cancer*. 2007;7:9.

240. Paszat LF, Vallis KA, Benk VM, Groome PA, Mackillop WJ, Wielgosz A. A population-based case-cohort study of the risk of myocardial infarction following radiation therapy for breast cancer. *Radiother Oncol*. March 2007;82(3):294–300.

241. Giordano SH, Kuo YF, Freeman JL, Buchholz TA, Hortobagyi GN, Goodwin JS. Risk of cardiac death after adjuvant radiotherapy for breast cancer. *J Natl Cancer Inst*. March 16, 2005;97(6):419–424.

242. Darby S, McGale P, Peto R, Granath F, Hall P, Ekbom A. Mortality from cardiovascular disease more than 10 years after radiotherapy for breast cancer: nationwide cohort study of 90 000 Swedish women. *BMJ*. February 1, 2003;326(7383):256–257.

243. Vallis KA, Pintilie M, Chong N, et al. Assessment of coronary heart disease morbidity and mortality after radiation therapy for early breast cancer. *J Clin Oncol*. February 15, 2002;20(4):1036–1042.

244. Paszat LF, Mackillop WJ, Groome PA, Schulze K, Holowaty E. Mortality from myocardial infarction following postlumpectomy radiotherapy for breast cancer: a population-based study in Ontario, Canada. *Int J Radiat Oncol, Biol, Phys*. March 1, 1999;43(4):755–762.

245. Paszat LF, Mackillop WJ, Groome PA, Boyd C, Schulze K, Holowaty E. Mortality from myocardial infarction after adjuvant radiotherapy for breast cancer in the surveillance, epidemiology, and end-results cancer registries. *J Clin Oncol*. August 1998;16(8):2625–2631.

246. Nixon AJ, Manola J, Gelman R, et al. No long-term increase in cardiac-related mortality after breast-conserving surgery and radiation therapy using modern techniques. *J Clin Oncol*. April 1998;16(4):1374–1379.

247. Rutqvist LE, Johansson H. Mortality by laterality of the primary tumour among 55,000 breast cancer patients

from the Swedish Cancer Registry. *Br J Cancer*. June 1990;61(6):866–868.

248. Boerman LM, Berendsen AJ, van der Meer P, Maduro JH, Berger MY, de Bock GH. Long-term follow-up for cardiovascular disease after chemotherapy and/or radiotherapy for breast cancer in an unselected population. *Support Care Cancer*. July 2014;22(7):1949–1958.

249. Doyle JJ, Neugut AI, Jacobson JS, et al. Radiation therapy, cardiac risk factors, and cardiac toxicity in early-stage breast cancer patients. *Int J Radiat Oncol, Biol, Phys*. May 1, 2007;68(1):82–93.

250. Pinder MC, Duan Z, Goodwin JS, Hortobagyi GN, Giordano SH. Congestive heart failure in older women treated with adjuvant anthracycline chemotherapy for breast cancer. *J Clin Oncol*. September 1, 2007;25(25):3808–3815.

251. Patt DA, Goodwin JS, Kuo YF, et al. Cardiac morbidity of adjuvant radiotherapy for breast cancer. *J Clin Oncol*. October 20, 2005;23(30):7475–7482.

252. Rutqvist LE, Liedberg A, Hammar N, Dalberg K. Myocardial infarction among women with early-stage breast cancer treated with conservative surgery and breast irradiation. *Int J Radiat Oncol, Biol, Phys*. January 15, 1998;40(2):359–363.

253. Taylor CW, Povall JM, McGale P, et al. Cardiac dose from tangential breast cancer radiotherapy in the year 2006. *Int J Radiat Oncol, Biol, Phys*. October 1, 2008;72(2):501–507.

254. Whelan TJ, Olivotto IA, Parulekar WR, et al. Regional nodal irradiation in early-stage breast cancer. *N Engl J Med*. July 23, 2015;373(4):307–316.

255. Thorsen LB, Offersen BV, Dano H, et al. DBCG-IMN: a population-based cohort study on the effect of internal mammary node irradiation in early node-positive breast cancer. *J Clin Oncol*. February 1, 2016;34(4):314–320.

256. Poortmans PM, Collette S, Kirkove C, et al. Internal mammary and medial supraclavicular irradiation in breast cancer. *N Engl J Med*. July 23, 2015;373(4):317–327.

257. Erven K, Jurcut R, Weltens C, et al. Acute radiation effects on cardiac function detected by strain rate imaging in breast cancer patients. *Int J Radiat Oncol, Biol, Phys*. April 1, 2011;79(5):1444–1451.

258. Erven K, Florian A, Slagmolen P, et al. Subclinical cardiotoxicity detected by strain rate imaging up to 14 months after breast radiation therapy. *Int J Radiat Oncol, Biol, Phys*. April 1, 2013;85(5):1172–1178.

259. Favier O, Heutte N, Stamatoullas-Bastard A, et al. Survival after Hodgkin lymphoma: causes of death and excess mortality in patients treated in 8 consecutive trials. *Cancer*. April 15, 2009;115(8):1680–1691.

260. Swerdlow AJ, Higgins CD, Smith P, et al. Myocardial infarction mortality risk after treatment for Hodgkin disease: a collaborative British cohort study. *J Natl Cancer Inst*. February 7, 2007;99(3):206–214.

261. Aleman BM, van den Belt-Dusebout AW, Klokman WJ, Van't Veer MB, Bartelink H, van Leeuwen FE. Long-term cause-specific mortality of patients treated for Hodgkin's disease. *J Clin Oncol*. September 15, 2003;21(18):3431–3439.

262. Ng AK, Bernardo MP, Weller E, et al. Long-term survival and competing causes of death in patients with early-stage Hodgkin's disease treated at age 50 or younger. *J Clin Oncol*. April 15, 2002;20(8):2101–2108.

263. Boivin JF, Hutchison GB, Lubin JH, Mauch P. Coronary artery disease mortality in patients treated for Hodgkin's disease. *Cancer*. March 1, 1992;69(5):1241–1247.

264. Aviles A, Neri N, Cuadra I, Alvarado I, Cleto S. Second lethal events associated with treatment for Hodgkin's disease: a review of 2980 patients treated in a single Mexican institute. *Leuk Lymphoma*. October 2000;39(3–4):311–319.

265. Amini A, Murphy B, Cost CR, Garrington TP, Greffe BS, Liu AK. Cardiac mortality in children and adolescents with Hodgkin's lymphoma: a surveillance, epidemiology and end results analysis. *J Adolesc Young Adult Oncol*. June 2016;5(2):181–186.

266. Al-Kindi SG, Abu-Zeinah GF, Kim CH, et al. Trends and disparities in cardiovascular mortality among survivors of Hodgkin lymphoma. *Clin Lymphoma Myeloma Leuk*. December 2015;15(12):748–752.

267. Henry-Amar M, Hayat M, Meerwaldt JH, et al. Causes of death after therapy for early stage Hodgkin's disease entered on EORTC protocols. EORTC Lymphoma Cooperative Group. *Int J Radiat Oncol, Biol, Phys*. November 1990;19(5):1155–1157.

268. Eloranta S, Lambert PC, Sjoberg J, Andersson TM, Bjorkholm M, Dickman PW. Temporal trends in mortality from diseases of the circulatory system after treatment for Hodgkin lymphoma: a population-based cohort study in Sweden (1973 to 2006). *J Clin Oncol*. April 10, 2013;31(11):1435–1441.

269. van Nimwegen FA, Schaapveld M, Janus CP, et al. Cardiovascular disease after Hodgkin lymphoma treatment: 40-year disease risk. *JAMA Intern Med*. June 2015;175(6):1007–1017.

270. Maraldo MV, Giusti F, Vogelius IR, et al. Cardiovascular disease after treatment for Hodgkin's lymphoma: an analysis of nine collaborative EORTC-LYSA trials. *Lancet Haematol*. November 2015;2(11):e492–e502.

271. Galper SL, Yu JB, Mauch PM, et al. Clinically significant cardiac disease in patients with Hodgkin lymphoma treated with mediastinal irradiation. *Blood*. January 13, 2011;117(2):412–418.

272. Myrehaug S, Pintilie M, Tsang R, et al. Cardiac morbidity following modern treatment for Hodgkin lymphoma: supra-additive cardiotoxicity of doxorubicin and radiation therapy. *Leuk Lymphoma*. August 2008;49(8):1486–1493.

273. Aleman BM, van den Belt-Dusebout AW, De Bruin ML, et al. Late cardiotoxicity after treatment for Hodgkin lymphoma. *Blood*. March 1, 2007;109(5):1878–1886.

274. van Nimwegen FA, Ntentas G, Darby SC, et al. Risk of heart failure in survivors of Hodgkin lymphoma: effects of cardiac exposure to radiation and anthracyclines. *Blood*. April 20, 2017;129(16):2257–2265.

275. Girinsky T, van der Maazen R, Specht L, et al. Involved-node radiotherapy (INRT) in patients with early Hodgkin lymphoma: concepts and guidelines. *Radiother Oncol*. June 2006;79(3):270–277.

276. Aznar MC, Maraldo MV, Schut DA, et al. Minimizing late effects for patients with mediastinal Hodgkin lymphoma: deep inspiration breath-hold, IMRT, or both? *Int J Radiat Oncol, Biol, Phys.* May 1, 2015;92(1):169–174.

277. Maraldo MV, Brodin NP, Vogelius IR, et al. Risk of developing cardiovascular disease after involved node radiotherapy versus mantle field for Hodgkin lymphoma. *Int J Radiat Oncol, Biol, Phys.* July 15, 2012;83(4):1232–1237.

278. Maraldo MV, Brodin NP, Aznar MC, et al. Estimated risk of cardiovascular disease and secondary cancers with modern highly conformal radiotherapy for early-stage mediastinal Hodgkin lymphoma. *Ann Oncol.* August 2013;24(8):2113–2118.

279. Hoppe BS, Flampouri S, Li Z, Mendenhall NP. Cardiac sparing with proton therapy in consolidative radiation therapy for Hodgkin lymphoma. *Leuk Lymphoma.* August 2010;51(8):1559–1562.

280. Radford J, Illidge T, Counsell N, et al. Results of a trial of PET-directed therapy for early-stage Hodgkin's lymphoma. *N Engl J Med.* April 23, 2015;372(17):1598–1607.

281. Andre MP, Girinsky T, Federico M, et al. Early positron emission tomography response-adapted treatment in stage I and II hodgkin lymphoma: final results of the randomized EORTC/LYSA/FIL H10 trial. *J Clin Oncol.* March 14, 2017:JCO2016686394.

282. Parikh RR, Grossbard ML, Harrison LB, Yahalom J. Early-stage classic Hodgkin lymphoma: the utilization of radiation therapy and its impact on overall survival. *Int J Radiat Oncol, Biol, Phys.* November 1, 2015;93(3):684–693.

283. Olszewski AJ, Shrestha R, Castillo JJ. Treatment selection and outcomes in early-stage classical Hodgkin lymphoma: analysis of the National Cancer Data Base. *J Clin Oncol.* February 20, 2015;33(6):625–633.

284. Gatta G, Botta L, Rossi S, et al. Childhood cancer survival in Europe 1999-2007: results of EUROCARE-5-a population-based study. *Lancet Oncol.* January 2014;15(1):35–47.

285. Fidler MM, Reulen RC, Winter DL, et al. Long term cause specific mortality among 34 489 five year survivors of childhood cancer in Great Britain: population based cohort study. *BMJ.* September 1, 2016;354:i4351.

286. Mertens AC, Liu Q, Neglia JP, et al. Cause-specific late mortality among 5-year survivors of childhood cancer: the Childhood Cancer Survivor Study. *J Natl Cancer Inst.* October 1, 2008;100(19):1368–1379.

287. Reulen RC, Winter DL, Frobisher C, et al. Long-term cause-specific mortality among survivors of childhood cancer. *JAMA.* July 14, 2010;304(2):172–179.

288. Moller TR, Garwicz S, Perfekt R, et al. Late mortality among five-year survivors of cancer in childhood and adolescence. *Acta Oncol.* 2004;43(8):711–718.

289. Kero AE, Jarvela LS, Arola M, et al. Late mortality among 5-year survivors of early onset cancer: a population-based register study. *Int J Cancer.* April 1, 2015;136(7):1655–1664.

290. Brewster DH, Clark D, Hopkins L, et al. Subsequent mortality experience in five-year survivors of childhood, adolescent and young adult cancer in Scotland: a population based, retrospective cohort study. *Eur J Cancer.* October 2013;49(15):3274–3283.

291. Schindler M, Spycher BD, Ammann RA, Ansari M, Michel G, Kuehni CE. Cause-specific long-term mortality in survivors of childhood cancer in Switzerland: A population-based study. *Int J Cancer.* July 15, 2016;139(2):322–333.

292. MacArthur AC, Spinelli JJ, Rogers PC, Goddard KJ, Abanto ZU, McBride ML. Mortality among 5-year survivors of cancer diagnosed during childhood or adolescence in British Columbia, Canada. *Pediatr Blood Cancer.* April 2007;48(4):460–467.

293. Hudson MM, Jones D, Boyett J, Sharp GB, Pui CH. Late mortality of long-term survivors of childhood cancer. *J Clin Oncol.* June 1997;15(6):2205–2213.

294. Cardous-Ubbink MC, Heinen RC, Langeveld NE, et al. Long-term cause-specific mortality among five-year survivors of childhood cancer. *Pediatr Blood Cancer.* June 2004;42(7):563–573.

295. Mulrooney DA, Yeazel MW, Kawashima T, et al. Cardiac outcomes in a cohort of adult survivors of childhood and adolescent cancer: retrospective analysis of the Childhood Cancer Survivor Study cohort. *BMJ.* December 8, 2009;339:b4606.

296. Pihkala J, Happonen JM, Virtanen K, et al. Cardiopulmonary evaluation of exercise tolerance after chest irradiation and anticancer chemotherapy in children and adolescents. *Pediatrics.* May 1995;95(5):722–726.

297. Hancock SL, Donaldson SS, Hoppe RT. Cardiac disease following treatment of Hodgkin's disease in children and adolescents. *J Clin Oncol.* July 1993;11(7):1208–1215.

298. van der Pal HJ, van Dalen EC, Kremer LC, Bakker PJ, van Leeuwen FE. Risk of morbidity and mortality from cardiovascular disease following radiotherapy for childhood cancer: a systematic review. *Cancer Treat Rev.* May 2005;31(3):173–185.

299. Guldner L, Haddy N, Pein F, et al. Radiation dose and long term risk of cardiac pathology following radiotherapy and anthracyclin for a childhood cancer. *Radiother Oncol.* October 2006;81(1):47–56.

300. van der Pal HJ, van Dalen EC, van Delden E, et al. High risk of symptomatic cardiac events in childhood cancer survivors. *J Clin Oncol.* May 1, 2012;30(13):1429–1437.

301. Armstrong GT, Joshi VM, Ness KK, et al. Comprehensive echocardiographic detection of treatment-related cardiac dysfunction in adult survivors of childhood cancer: results from the St. Jude Lifetime Cohort Study. *J Am Coll Cardiol.* June 16, 2015;65(23):2511–2522.

302. Chow EJ, Chen Y, Kremer LC, et al. Individual prediction of heart failure among childhood cancer survivors. *J Clin Oncol.* February 10, 2015;33(5):394–402.

303. van der Pal HJ, van Dijk IW, Geskus RB, et al. Valvular abnormalities detected by echocardiography in 5-year survivors of childhood cancer: a long-term follow-up study. *Int J Radiat Oncol, Biol, Phys.* January 1, 2015;91(1):213–222.

304. Feijen EA, Font-Gonzalez A, van Dalen EC, et al. Late cardiac events after childhood cancer: methodological

aspects of the pan-european study panCareSurFup. *PLOS ONE*. 2016;11(9):e0162778.

305. Pediatric Normal Tissue Effects in the Clinic (PENTEC). Available at https://www.pentecradiation.org/. Accessed February 18, 2019.

306. Crosby T, Hurt CN, Falk S, et al. Chemoradiotherapy with or without cetuximab in patients with oesophageal cancer (SCOPE1): a multicentre, phase 2/3 randomised trial. *Lancet Oncol*. June 2013;14(7):627–637.

307. Conroy T, Galais MP, Raoul JL, et al. Definitive chemoradiotherapy with FOLFOX versus fluorouracil and cisplatin in patients with oesophageal cancer (PRODIGE5/ACCORD17): final results of a randomised, phase 2/3 trial. *Lancet Oncol*. March 2014;15(3):305–314.

308. van Hagen P, Hulshof MC, van Lanschot JJ, et al. Preoperative chemoradiotherapy for esophageal or junctional cancer. *N Engl J Med*. May 31 2012;366(22):2074–2084.

309. Frandsen J, Boothe D, Gaffney DK, Wilson BD, Lloyd S. Increased risk of death due to heart disease after radiotherapy for esophageal cancer. *J Gastrointest Oncol*. October 2015;6(5):516–523.

310. Wang J, Wei C, Tucker SL, et al. Predictors of postoperative complications after trimodality therapy for esophageal cancer. *Int J Radiat Oncol, Biol, Phys*. August 1, 2013;86(5):885–891.

311. Beukema JC, van Luijk P, Widder J, Langendijk JA, Muijs CT. Is cardiac toxicity a relevant issue in the radiation treatment of esophageal cancer? *Radiother Oncol*. January 2015;114(1):85–90.

312. Martel MK, Sahijdak WM, Ten Haken RK, Kessler ML, Turrisi AT. Fraction size and dose parameters related to the incidence of pericardial effusions. *Int J Radiat Oncol, Biol, Phys*. January 1, 1998;40(1):155–161.

313. Wei X, Liu HH, Tucker SL, et al. Risk factors for pericardial effusion in inoperable esophageal cancer patients treated with definitive chemoradiation therapy. *Int J Radiat Oncol, Biol, Phys*. March 1, 2008;70(3):707–714.

314. Fukada J, Shigematsu N, Takeuchi H, et al. Symptomatic pericardial effusion after chemoradiation therapy in esophageal cancer patients. *Int J Radiat Oncol, Biol, Phys*. November 1, 2013;87(3):487–493.

315. Tamari K, Isohashi F, Akino Y, et al. Risk factors for pericardial effusion in patients with stage I esophageal cancer treated with chemoradiotherapy. *Anticancer Res*. December 2014;34(12):7389–7393.

316. Hayashi K, Fujiwara Y, Nomura M, et al. Predictive factors for pericardial effusion identified by heart dose-volume histogram analysis in oesophageal cancer patients treated with chemoradiotherapy. *Br J Radiol*. February 2015;88(1046):20140168.

317. Tait LM, Meyer JE, McSpadden E, et al. Women at increased risk for cardiac toxicity following chemoradiation therapy for esophageal carcinoma. *Pract Radiat Oncol*. October-December 2013;3(4):e149–e155.

318. Tripp P, Malhotra HK, Javle M, et al. Cardiac function after chemoradiation for esophageal cancer: comparison of heart dose-volume histogram parameters to multiple gated acquisition scan changes. *Dis Esophagus*. 2005;18(6):400–405.

319. Mukherjee S, Aston D, Minett M, Brewster AE, Crosby TD. The significance of cardiac doses received during chemoradiation of oesophageal and gastro-oesophageal junctional cancers. *Clin Oncol (R Coll Radiol)*. May 2003;15(3):115–120.

320. Lund M, Alexandersson von Dobeln G, Nilsson M, et al. Effects on heart function of neoadjuvant chemotherapy and chemoradiotherapy in patients with cancer in the esophagus or gastroesophageal junction—a prospective cohort pilot study within a randomized clinical trial. *Radiat Oncol*. 2015;10:16.

321. Hatakenaka M, Yonezawa M, Nonoshita T, et al. Acute cardiac impairment associated with concurrent chemoradiotherapy for esophageal cancer: magnetic resonance evaluation. *Int J Radiat Oncol, Biol, Phys*. May 1, 2012;83(1):e67–e73.

322. Zhang P, Hu X, Yue J, et al. Early detection of radiation-induced heart disease using (99m)Tc-MIBI SPECT gated myocardial perfusion imaging in patients with oesophageal cancer during radiotherapy. *Radiother Oncol*. May 2015;115(2):171–178.

323. Gayed IW, Liu HH, Yusuf SW, et al. The prevalence of myocardial ischemia after concurrent chemoradiation therapy as detected by gated myocardial perfusion imaging in patients with esophageal cancer. *J Nucl Med*. November 2006;47(11):1756–1762.

324. Gayed I, Gohar S, Liao Z, McAleer M, Bassett R, Yusuf SW. The clinical implications of myocardial perfusion abnormalities in patients with esophageal or lung cancer after chemoradiation therapy. *Int J Cardiovasc Imaging*. June 2009;25(5):487–495.

325. Konski A, Li T, Christensen M, et al. Symptomatic cardiac toxicity is predicted by dosimetric and patient factors rather than changes in 18F-FDG PET determination of myocardial activity after chemoradiotherapy for esophageal cancer. *Radiother Oncol*. July 2012;104(1):72–77.

326. Takanami K, Arai A, Umezawa R, et al. Association between radiation dose to the heart and myocardial fatty acid metabolic impairment due to chemoradiation-therapy: Prospective study using I-123 BMIPP SPECT/CT. *Radiother Oncol*. April 2016;119(1):77–83.

327. Umezawa R, Ota H, Takanami K, et al. MRI findings of radiation-induced myocardial damage in patients with oesophageal cancer. *Clin Radiol*. December 2014;69(12):1273–1279.

328. Morota M, Gomi K, Kozuka T, et al. Late toxicity after definitive concurrent chemoradiotherapy for thoracic esophageal carcinoma. *Int J Radiat Oncol, Biol, Phys*. September 1, 2009;75(1):122–128.

329. Ogino I, Watanabe S, Iwahashi N, et al. Symptomatic radiation-induced cardiac disease in long-term survivors of esophageal cancer. *Strahlenther Onkol*. June 2016;192(6):359–367.

330. Kole TP, Aghayere O, Kwah J, Yorke ED, Goodman KA. Comparison of heart and coronary artery doses associated with intensity-modulated radiotherapy versus three-dimensional conformal radiotherapy for distal esophageal cancer. *Int J Radiat Oncol, Biol, Phys*. August 1, 2012;83(5):1580–1586.

331. Lin SH, Komaki R, Liao Z, et al. Proton beam therapy and concurrent chemotherapy for esophageal cancer. *Int J Radiat Oncol, Biol, Phys.* July 1, 2012;83(3):e345–e351.

332. Chuong MD, Hallemeier CL, Jabbour SK, et al. Improving outcomes for esophageal cancer using proton beam therapy. *Int J Radiat Oncol, Biol, Phys.* May 1, 2016;95(1):488–497.

333. Aarts MJ, Aerts JG, van den Borne BE, Biesma B, Lemmens VE, Kloover JS. Comorbidity in patients with small-cell lung cancer: trends and prognostic impact. *Clin Lung Cancer.* July 2015;16(4):282–291.

334. Kravchenko J, Berry M, Arbeev K, Kim Lyerly H, Yashin A, Akushevich I. Cardiovascular comorbidities and survival of lung cancer patients: Medicare data based analysis. *Lung Cancer.* April 2015;88(1):85–93.

335. Lally BE, Geiger AM, Urbanic JJ, et al. Trends in the outcomes for patients with limited stage small cell lung cancer: an analysis of the Surveillance, Epidemiology, and End Results database. *Lung Cancer.* May 2009;64(2):226–231.

336. Hardy D, Liu CC, Cormier JN, Xia R, Du XL. Cardiac toxicity in association with chemotherapy and radiation therapy in a large cohort of older patients with non-small-cell lung cancer. *Ann Oncol.* September 2010;21(9):1825–1833.

337. Postoperative radiotherapy in non-small-cell lung cancer: systematic review and meta-analysis of individual patient data from nine randomised controlled trials. PORT Meta-analysis Trialists Group. *Lancet.* July 25, 1998;352(9124):257–263.

338. Dautzenberg B, Arriagada R, Chammard AB, et al. A controlled study of postoperative radiotherapy for patients with completely resected nonsmall cell lung carcinoma. Groupe d'Etude et de Traitement des Cancers Bronchiques. *Cancer.* July 15, 1999;86(2):265–273.

339. Karakoyun-Celik O, Yalman D, Bolukbasi Y, Cakan A, Cok G, Ozkok S. Postoperative radiotherapy in the management of resected non-small-cell lung carcinoma: 10 years' experience in a single institute. *Int J Radiat Oncol, Biol, Phys.* February 1, 2010;76(2):433–439.

340. Ramnath N, Demmy TL, Antun A, et al. Pneumonectomy for bronchogenic carcinoma: analysis of factors predicting survival. *Ann Thorac Surg.* May 2007;83(5):1831–1836.

341. Lally BE, Detterbeck FC, Geiger AM, et al. The risk of death from heart disease in patients with nonsmall cell lung cancer who receive postoperative radiotherapy: analysis of the Surveillance, Epidemiology, and End Results database. *Cancer.* August 15, 2007;110(4):911–917.

342. Billiet C, Decaluwe H, Peeters S, et al. Modern post-operative radiotherapy for stage III non-small cell lung cancer may improve local control and survival: a meta-analysis. *Radiother Oncol.* January 2014;110(1):3–8.

343. Perez CA, Pajak TF, Rubin P, et al. Long-term observations of the patterns of failure in patients with unresectable non-oat cell carcinoma of the lung treated with definitive radiotherapy. Report by the Radiation Therapy Oncology Group. *Cancer.* June 1, 1987;59(11):1874–1881.

344. Partridge M, Ramos M, Sardaro A, Brada M. Dose escalation for non-small cell lung cancer: analysis and modelling of published literature. *Radiother Oncol.* April 2011;99(1):6–11.

345. Ramroth J, Cutter DJ, Darby SC, et al. Dose and fractionation in radiation therapy of curative intent for non-small cell lung cancer: meta-analysis of randomized trials. *Int J Radiat Oncol, Biol, Phys.* 2016 Nov 15;96(4):736-747.

346. Landau DB, Hughes L, Baker A, et al. IDEAL-CRT: a phase 1/2 trial of isotoxic dose-escalated radiation therapy and concurrent chemotherapy in patients with stage II/III non-small cell lung cancer. *Int J Radiat Oncol, Biol, Phys.* August 1, 2016;95(5):1367–1377.

347. Bradley JD, Paulus R, Komaki R, et al. Standard-dose versus high-dose conformal radiotherapy with concurrent and consolidation carboplatin plus paclitaxel with or without cetuximab for patients with stage IIIA or IIIB non-small-cell lung cancer (RTOG 0617): a randomised, two-by-two factorial phase 3 study. *Lancet Oncol.* February 2015;16(2):187–199.

348. Schytte T, Hansen O, Stolberg-Rohr T, Brink C. Cardiac toxicity and radiation dose to the heart in definitive treated non-small cell lung cancer. *Acta Oncol.* October 2010;49(7):1058–1060.

349. Ming X, Feng Y, Liu H, Zhang Y, Zhou L, Deng J. Cardiac exposure in the dynamic conformal arc therapy, intensity-modulated radiotherapy and volumetric modulated arc therapy of lung cancer. *PLOS ONE.* 2015;10(12):e0144211.

350. Chun SG. Outcomes of intensity modulated and 3D-conformal radiotherapy for stage III non-small-cell lung cancer in NRG oncology/RTOG 0617. *Paper presented at: 16th World Conference in Lung Cancer;* 2015; Denver, CO.

351. Zhang X, Li Y, Pan X, et al. Intensity-modulated proton therapy reduces the dose to normal tissue compared with intensity-modulated radiation therapy or passive scattering proton therapy and enables individualized radical radiotherapy for extensive stage IIIB non-small-cell lung cancer: a virtual clinical study. *Int J Radiat Oncol, Biol, Phys.* June 1, 2010;77(2):357–366.

352. Chang JY, Jabbour SK, De Ruysscher D, et al. Consensus statement on proton therapy in early-stage and locally advanced non-small cell lung cancer. *Int J Radiat Oncol, Biol, Phys.* May 1, 2016;95(1):505–516.

353. Giaddui T, Chen W, Yu J, et al. Establishing the feasibility of the dosimetric compliance criteria of RTOG 1308: phase III randomized trial comparing overall survival after photon versus proton radiochemotherapy for inoperable stage II-IIIB NSCLC. *Radiat Oncol.* 2016;11:66.

354. Lederman GS, Sheldon TA, Chaffey JT, Herman TS, Gelman RS, Coleman CN. Cardiac disease after mediastinal irradiation for seminoma. *Cancer.* August 15, 1987;60(4):772–776.

355. Fossa SD, Gilbert E, Dores GM, et al. Noncancer causes of death in survivors of testicular cancer. *J Natl Cancer Inst.* April 4, 2007;99(7):533–544.

356. Adams MJ, Hardenbergh PH, Constine LS, Lipshultz SE. Radiation-associated cardiovascular disease. *Crit Rev Oncol Hematol.* January 2003;45(1):55–75.

357. Haugnes HS, Wethal T, Aass N, et al. Cardiovascular risk factors and morbidity in long-term survivors of

testicular cancer: a 20-year follow-up study. *J Clin Oncol.* October 20, 2010;28(30):4649–4657.

358. Hallemeier CL, Pisansky TM, Davis BJ, Choo R. Long-term outcomes of radiotherapy for stage II testicular seminoma—the Mayo Clinic experience. *Urol Oncol.* November 2013;31(8):1832–1838.

359. Hallemeier CL, Choo R, Davis BJ, Leibovich BC, Costello BA, Pisansky TM. Excellent long-term disease control with modern radiotherapy techniques for stage I testicular seminoma—the Mayo Clinic experience. *Urol Oncol.* January 2014;32(1):24 e21–e26.

360. Zagars GK, Ballo MT, Lee AK, Strom SS. Mortality after cure of testicular seminoma. *J Clin Oncol.* February 15, 2004;22(4):640–647.

361. Mazonakis M, Berris T, Lyraraki E, Damilakis J. Radiation therapy for stage IIA and IIB testicular seminoma: peripheral dose calculations and risk assessments. *Phys Med Biol.* March 21, 2015;60(6):2375–2389.

362. Fossa SD, Aass N, Winderen M, Bormer OP, Olsen DR. Long-term renal function after treatment for malignant germ-cell tumours. *Ann Oncol.* February 2002;13(2):222–228.

363. van den Belt-Dusebout AW, de Wit R, Gietema JA, et al. Treatment-specific risks of second malignancies and cardiovascular disease in 5-year survivors of testicular cancer. *J Clin Oncol.* Oct 1, 2007;25(28):4370–4378.

364. Beard CJ, Travis LB, Chen MH, et al. Outcomes in stage I testicular seminoma: a population-based study of 9193 patients. *Cancer.* August 1, 2013;119(15):2771–2777.

365. Masuko M, Ito M, Kurasaki T, et al. Plasma brain natriuretic peptide during myeloablative stem cell transplantation. *Intern Med.* 2007;46(9):551–555.

366. Leiper AD. Late effects of total body irradiation. *Arch Dis Child.* May 1995;72(5):382–385.

367. Lim YJ, Kim E, Kim HJ, et al. Survival impact of adjuvant radiation therapy in Masaoka stage II to IV thymomas: a systematic review and meta-analysis. *Int J Radiat Oncol, Biol, Phys.* April 1, 2016;94(5):1129–1136.

368. Nieder C, Pawinski A, Andratschke NH, Molls M. Can prophylactic breast irradiation contribute to cardiac toxicity in patients with prostate cancer receiving androgen suppressing drugs? *Radiat Oncol.* 2008;3:2.

369. Heidenreich PA, Schnittger I, Strauss HW, et al. Screening for coronary artery disease after mediastinal irradiation for Hodgkin's disease. *J Clin Oncol.* January 1, 2007;25(1):43–49.

370. Girinsky T, Cordova A, Rey A, Cosset JM, Tertian G, Pierga JY. Thallium-201 scintigraphy is not predictive of late cardiac complications in patients with Hodgkin's disease treated with mediastinal radiation. *Int J Radiat Oncol, Biol, Phys.* December 1, 2000;48(5):1503–1506.

371. Glanzmann C, Kaufmann P, Jenni R, Hess OM, Huguenin P. Cardiac risk after mediastinal irradiation for Hodgkin's disease. *Radiother Oncol.* January 1998;46(1):51–62.

372. Constine LS, Schwartz RG, Savage DE, King V, Muhs A. Cardiac function, perfusion, and morbidity in irradiated long-term survivors of Hodgkin's disease. *Int J Radiat Oncol, Biol, Phys.* November 1, 1997;39(4):897–906.

373. Savage DE, Constine LS, Schwartz RG, Rubin P. Radiation effects on left ventricular function and myocardial perfusion in long term survivors of Hodgkin's disease. *Int J Radiat Oncol, Biol, Phys.* September 1990;19(3):721–727.

374. Gustavsson A, Eskilsson J, Landberg T, et al. Late cardiac effects after mantle radiotherapy in patients with Hodgkin's disease. *Ann Oncol.* September 1990;1(5):355–363.

375. Eftekhari M, Anbiaei R, Zamani H, et al. Radiation-induced myocardial perfusion abnormalities in breast cancer patients following external beam radiation therapy. *Asia Ocean J Nucl Med Biol.* Winter 2015;3(1):3–9.

376. Sioka C, Exarchopoulos T, Tasiou I, et al. Myocardial perfusion imaging with (99 m)Tc-tetrofosmin SPECT in breast cancer patients that received postoperative radiotherapy: a case-control study. *Radiat Oncol.* November 8, 2011;6:151.

377. Tzonevska A, Tzvetkov K, Parvanova V, Dimitrova M. 99mTc-MIBI myocardial perfusion scintigraphy for assessment of myocardial damage after radiotherapy in patients with breast cancer. *J BUON.* October-December 2006;11(4):505–509.

378. Marks LB, Yu X, Prosnitz RG, et al. The incidence and functional consequences of RT-associated cardiac perfusion defects. *Int J Radiat Oncol, Biol, Phys.* September 1, 2005;63(1):214–223.

379. Seddon B, Cook A, Gothard L, et al. Detection of defects in myocardial perfusion imaging in patients with early breast cancer treated with radiotherapy. *Radiother Oncol.* July 2002;64(1):53–63.

380. Hojris I, Andersen J, Overgaard M, Overgaard J. Late treatment-related morbidity in breast cancer patients randomized to postmastectomy radiotherapy and systemic treatment versus systemic treatment alone. *Acta Oncol.* 2000;39(3):355–372.

381. Gustavsson A, Bendahl PO, Cwikiel M, Eskilsson J, Thapper KL, Pahlm O. No serious late cardiac effects after adjuvant radiotherapy following mastectomy in premenopausal women with early breast cancer. *Int J Radiat Oncol, Biol, Phys.* March 1, 1999;43(4):745–754.

382. Cowen D, Gonzague-Casabianca L, Brenot-Rossi I, et al. Thallium-201 perfusion scintigraphy in the evaluation of late myocardial damage in left-side breast cancer treated with adjuvant radiotherapy. *Int J Radiat Oncol, Biol, Phys.* July 1, 1998;41(4):809–815.

383. Gyenes G, Fornander T, Carlens P, Glas U, Rutqvist LE. Myocardial damage in breast cancer patients treated with adjuvant radiotherapy: a prospective study. *Int J Radiat Oncol, Biol, Phys.* November 1, 1996;36(4):899–905.

384. Gyenes G, Fornander T, Carlens P, Rutqvist LE. Morbidity of ischemic heart disease in early breast cancer 15–20 years after adjuvant radiotherapy. *Int J Radiat Oncol, Biol, Phys.* March 30, 1994;28(5):1235–1241.

385. Umezawa R, Takase K, Jingu K, et al. Evaluation of radiation-induced myocardial damage using iodine-123 beta-methyl-iodophenyl pentadecanoic acid scintigraphy. *J Radiat Res.* September 2013;54(5):880–889.

386. Schinkel AF, Elhendy A, van Domburg RT, et al. Incremental value of exercise technetium-99m tetrofosmin myocardial perfusion single-photon emission computed tomography for the prediction of cardiac events. *Am J Cardiol*. February 15, 2003;91(4):408–411.

387. Jain D, Lessig H, Patel R, et al. Influence of 99mTc-tetrofosmin SPECT myocardial perfusion imaging on the prediction of future adverse cardiac events. *J Nucl Cardiol*. July-August 2009;16(4):540–548.

388. Yu X, Prosnitz RR, Zhou S, et al. Symptomatic cardiac events following radiation therapy for left-sided breast cancer: possible association with radiation therapy-induced changes in regional perfusion. *Clin Breast Cancer*. August 2003;4(3):193–197.

389. Jingu K, Kaneta T, Nemoto K, et al. The utility of 18F-fluorodeoxyglucose positron emission tomography for early diagnosis of radiation-induced myocardial damage. *Int J Radiat Oncol, Biol, Phys*. November 1, 2006;66(3):845–851.

390. Ricart Y, Petriz L, Prat L, et al. ^{111}In-Antimyosin myocardial scintigraphy in patients undergoing mediastinum or whole-body irradiation [abstract]. *Paper presented at: European Assocaition of Nuclear Medicine Congress*; August 23–26, 1992; Lisboa, Portugal.

391. Valdes Olmos RA, ten Bokkel Huinink WW, Dewit LG, Hoefnagel CA, Liem IH, van Tinteren H. Iodine-123 metaiodobenzylguanidine in the assessment of late cardiac effects from cancer therapy. *Eur J Nucl Med*. April 1996;23(4):453–458.

392. Lund MB, Ihlen H, Voss BM, et al. Increased risk of heart valve regurgitation after mediastinal radiation for Hodgkin's disease: an echocardiographic study. *Heart*. June 1996;75(6):591–595.

393. Glanzmann C, Huguenin P, Lutolf UM, Maire R, Jenni R, Gumppenberg V. Cardiac lesions after mediastinal irradiation for Hodgkin's disease. *Radiother Oncol*. January 1994;30(1):43–54.

394. Kreuser ED, Voller H, Behles C, et al. Evaluation of late cardiotoxicity with pulsed Doppler echocardiography in patients treated for Hodgkin's disease. *Br J Haematol*. August 1993;84(4):615–622.

395. Pohjola-Sintonen S, Totterman KJ, Salmo M, Siltanen P. Late cardiac effects of mediastinal radiotherapy in patients with Hodgkin's disease. *Cancer*. July 1, 1987;60(1):31–37.

396. Bella JN, Palmieri V, Roman MJ, et al. Mitral ratio of peak early to late diastolic filling velocity as a predictor of mortality in middle-aged and elderly adults: the Strong Heart Study. *Circulation*. April 23, 2002;105(16):1928–1933.

397. Jurcut R, Ector J, Erven K, Choi HF, Voigt JU. Radiotherapy effects on systolic myocardial function detected by strain rate imaging in a left-breast cancer patient. *Eur Heart J*. December 2007;28(24):2966.

398. Alehan D, Sahin M, Varan A, Yildirim I, Kupeli S, Buyukpamukcu M. Tissue Doppler evaluation of systolic and diastolic cardiac functions in long-term survivors of Hodgkin lymphoma. *Pediatr Blood Cancer*. February 2012;58(2):250–255.

399. Kupeli S, Hazirolan T, Varan A, et al. Evaluation of coronary artery disease by computed tomography angiography in patients treated for childhood Hodgkin's lymphoma. *J Clin Oncol*. February 20, 2010;28(6):1025–1030.

400. Girinsky T, M'Kacher R, Lessard N, et al. Prospective coronary heart disease screening in asymptomatic Hodgkin lymphoma patients using coronary computed tomography angiography: results and risk factor analysis. *Int J Radiat Oncol, Biol, Phys*. May 1, 2014;89(1):59–66.

401. Daniels LA, Krol AD, de Graaf MA, et al. Screening for coronary artery disease after mediastinal irradiation in Hodgkin lymphoma survivors: phase II study of indication and acceptancedagger. *Ann Oncol*. June 2014;25(6):1198–1203.

402. Mulrooney DA, Nunnery SE, Armstrong GT, et al. Coronary artery disease detected by coronary computed tomography angiography in adult survivors of childhood Hodgkin lymphoma. *Cancer*. November 15, 2014;120(22):3536–3544.

403. Rademaker J, Schoder H, Ariaratnam NS, et al. Coronary artery disease after radiation therapy for Hodgkin's lymphoma: coronary CT angiography findings and calcium scores in nine asymptomatic patients. *AJR Am J Roentgenol*. July 2008;191(1):32–37.

404. Walsh TF, Hundley WG. Assessment of ventricular function with cardiovascular magnetic resonance. *Cardiol Clin*. February 2007;25(1):15–33, v.

405. Scatteia A, Baritussio A, Bucciarelli-Ducci C. Strain imaging using cardiac magnetic resonance. Heart Fail Rev. July 2017;22(4):465-76.

406. Bellenger NG, Burgess MI, Ray SG, et al. Comparison of left ventricular ejection fraction and volumes in heart failure by echocardiography, radionuclide ventriculography and cardiovascular magnetic resonance; are they interchangeable? *Eur Heart J*. August 2000;21(16):1387–1396.

407. Mahrholdt H, Wagner A, Judd R, et al. Delayed enhancement cardiovascular magnetic resonance assessment of non-ischaemic cardiomyopathies. *Eur Heart J*. August, 2005;26(15):1461-1474.

408. Gerber BL, Raman SV, Nayak K, et al. Myocardial first-pass perfusion cardiovascular magnetic resonance: history, theory, and current state of the art. *J Cardiovasc Magn Reson*. April 28, 2008;10:18.

409. Kellman P, Hansen S, Nielles-Vallespin S, et al. Myocardial perfusion cardiovascular magnetic resonance: optimized dual sequence and reconstruction for quantification. *J Cardiovasc Magn Reson*. April 7, 2017;19(1):43.

410. Messroghli D, Moon J, Ferreira V, et al. Clinical recommendations for cardiovascular magnetic resonance mapping of T1, T2, T2* and extracellular volume: A consensus statement by the Society for Cardiovascular Magnetic Resonance (SCMR) endorsed by the European Association for Cardiovascular Imaging (EACVI). *J Cardiovasc Magn Reson*. October 9, 2017;19(1):75.

411. Ferreira V, Schulz-Menger J, Holmvang G, et al. Cardiovascular Magnetic Resonance in Nonischemic

Myocardial Inflammation: Expert Recommendations. *J Am Coll Cardiol*. December 18, 2018;72(24):3158-3176.

412. Celutkiene J, Plymen C, Flachskampf F, et al. Innovative imaging methods in heart failure: a shifting paradigm in cardiac assessment. Position statement on behalf of the Heart Failure Association of the European Society of Cardiology. *Eur J Heart Fail*. December, 2018;20(12):1615-1633.

413. Karamitsos T, Francis J, Myerson S, et al. The role of cardiovascular magnetic resonance imaging in heart failure. *J Am Coll Cardiol*. October 6, 2009;54(15):1407-1424.

414. Hudsmith LE, Neubauer S. Magnetic resonance spectroscopy in myocardial disease. *JACC Cardiovasc Imaging*. January 2009;2(1):87–96.

415. Rider OJ, Tyler DJ. Clinical implications of cardiac hyperpolarized magnetic resonance imaging. J Cardiovasc Magn Reson. October 8, 2013;15(1):93.

416. Hughes-Davies L, Sacks D, Rescigno J, Howard S, Harris J. Serum cardiac troponin T levels during treatment of early-stage breast cancer. *J Clin Oncol*. October 1995;13(10):2582–2584.

417. Haj Mohammad N, Kamphuis M, Hulshof MC, et al. Reduction of heart volume during neoadjuvant chemoradiation in patients with resectable esophageal cancer. *Radiother Oncol*. Januaty 2015;114(1):91–95.

418. Gomez DR, Yusuf SW, Munsell MF, et al. Prospective exploratory analysis of cardiac biomarkers and electrocardiogram abnormalities in patients receiving thoracic radiation therapy with high-dose heart exposure. *J Thorac Oncol*. October 2014;9(10):1554–1560.

419. D'Errico MP, Grimaldi L, Petruzzelli MF, et al. N-terminal pro-B-type natriuretic peptide plasma levels as a potential biomarker for cardiac damage after radiotherapy in patients with left-sided breast cancer. *Int J Radiat Oncol, Biol, Phys*. February 1, 2012;82(2):e239–e246.

420. Nellessen U, Zingel M, Hecker H, Bahnsen J, Borschke D. Effects of radiation therapy on myocardial cell integrity and pump function: which role for cardiac biomarkers? *Chemotherapy*. 2010;56(2):147–152.

421. Kozak KR, Hong TS, Sluss PM, et al. Cardiac blood biomarkers in patients receiving thoracic (chemo)radiation. *Lung Cancer*. December 2008;62(3):351–355.

422. Jingu K, Nemoto K, Kaneta T, et al. Temporal change in brain natriuretic Peptide after radiotherapy for thoracic esophageal cancer. *Int J Radiat Oncol, Biol, Phys*. December 1, 2007;69(5):1417–1423.

423. Wondergem J, Strootman EG, Frolich M, Leer JW, Noordijk EM. Circulating atrial natriuretic peptide plasma levels as a marker for cardiac damage after radiotherapy. *Radiother Oncol*. March 2001;58(3):295–301.

424. Hall KS, Wiklund T, Erikstein B, et al. Effects of dose-intensive chemotherapy and radiotherapy on serum n-terminal proatrial natriuretic peptide in high-risk breast cancer patients. *Breast Cancer Res Treat*. June 2001;67(3):235–244.

425. Giannitsis E, Kurz K, Hallermayer K, Jarausch J, Jaffe AS, Katus HA. Analytical validation of a high-sensitivity cardiac troponin T assay. *Clin Chem*. February 2010;56(2):254–261.

426. Cramer G, Bakker J, Gommans F, et al. Relation of highly sensitive cardiac troponin T in hypertrophic cardiomyopathy to left ventricular mass and cardiovascular risk. *Am J Cardiol*. April 1, 2014;113(7):1240–1245.

427. Braunwald E. Biomarkers in heart failure. *N Engl J Med*. May 15, 2008;358(20):2148–2159.

428. Jacob S, Pathak A, Franck D, et al. Early detection and prediction of cardiotoxicity after radiation therapy for breast cancer: the BACCARAT prospective cohort study. *Radiat Oncol*. April 7, 2016;11:54.

429. Lindahl J, Strender LE, Larsson LE, Unsgaard A. Electrocardiographic changes after radiation therapy for carcinoma of the breast. Incidence and functional significance. *Acta Radiol Oncol*. 1983;22(6):433–440.

430. Barnett GC, West CM, Dunning AM, et al. Normal tissue reactions to radiotherapy: towards tailoring treatment dose by genotype. *Nat Rev Cancer*. February 2009;9(2):134–142.

431. Tanteles GA, Whitworth J, Mills J, et al. Can cutaneous telangiectasiae as late normal-tissue injury predict cardiovascular disease in women receiving radiotherapy for breast cancer? *Br J Cancer*. August 4, 2009;101(3):403–409.

432. Tanteles GA, Murray RJ, Mills J, et al. Variation in telangiectasia predisposing genes is associated with overall radiation toxicity. *Int J Radiat Oncol, Biol, Phys*. November 15, 2012;84(4):1031–1036.

433. Cosset JM, Henry-Amar M, Pellae-Cosset B, et al. Pericarditis and myocardial infarctions after Hodgkin's disease therapy. *Int J Radiat Oncol, Biol, Phys*. July 1991;21(2):447–449.

434. Gagliardi G, Lax I, Rutqvist LE. Partial irradiation of the heart. *Semin Radiat Oncol*. July 2001;11(3):224–233.

435. Shapiro CL, Hardenbergh PH, Gelman R, et al. Cardiac effects of adjuvant doxorubicin and radiation therapy in breast cancer patients. *J Clin Oncol*. November 1998;16(11):3493–3501.

436. Vordermark D, Seufert I, Schwab F, et al. 3-D reconstruction of anterior mantle-field techniques in Hodgkin's disease survivors: doses to cardiac structures. *Radiat Oncol*. April 20, 2006;1:10.

437. King V, Constine LS, Clark D, et al. Symptomatic coronary artery disease after mantle irradiation for Hodgkin's disease. *Int J Radiat Oncol, Biol, Phys*. November 1, 1996;36(4):881–889.

438. Myrehaug S, Pintilie M, Yun L, et al. A population-based study of cardiac morbidity among Hodgkin lymphoma patients with preexisting heart disease. *Blood*. September 30, 2010;116(13):2237–2240.

Syed Wamique Yusuf

INTRODUCTION

Amyloidosis is a condition in which protein aggregates are deposited in various tissues in bundles of β-sheet fibrillar protein.[1] More than 30 separate precursor proteins exhibit a propensity to form amyloid fibrils.[2] In 1838 a German botanist named Matthias Schleiden coined the term *amyloid* to describe a normal amylaceous constituent of plants; to describe a human affliction, the term was first used by Rudolph Virchow in 1854.[3] An early description of primary amyloidosis was reported by Samuel Wilks in 1856, when he published the case report of a man with lardaceous viscera in whom the changes were not related to syphilis, tuberculosis, osteomyelitis, or other osseous disease.[3]

INCIDENCE AND PREVALANCE

In the general population, systemic amyloidosis is a rare disease; a population-based study performed in Olmsted County, Minnesota, found an incidence of approximately 8.9 per million person-years.[4] The prevalence of this condition increases with increasing age. A Swedish study found that the incidence of nonhereditary amyloidosis was 8.29 per million person-years; the incidence was highest at a diagnostic age of more than 65 years.[5] The prevalence of senile cardiac amyloidosis is approximately 10% among persons older than 80 years and 50% among those older than 90 years.[6] The amyloid type and the severity of organ involvement are prognostically important. Hence, every effort should be made to diagnose the condition early and to accurately classify it.[7]

CLASSIFICATION OF AMYLOIDOSIS

The classification of amyloidosis is based on the nature of the precursor plasma protein that forms the fibril deposits.[8] According to this classification, the amyloid protein is designated A and is followed by the protein designation in abbreviated form with no space after the first letter A. For example, amyloidosis due to the deposition of abnormal immunoglobulin light chains is abbreviated as AL.

CLINICAL CONDITIONS ASSOCIATED WITH AL AND AA AMYLOIDOSIS

The AL type of amyloidosis is commonly associated with immunocyte (plasma cell) dyscrasia, whereas the AA (amyloid amyloidosis) type usually occurs as a complication of a chronic inflammatory process.[9–11]

■ AL Amyloidosis

AL amyloidosis is the most common variety and affects approximately 70% of amyloidosis patients.[12] In AL amyloidosis, the precursor protein is either the kappa or the lambda immunoglobulin light chain. Patients with this variant usually present when they are in the fifth to sixth decades of life, although they may present as early as the third decade.[13] The clinical picture depends on the organs involved, but cardiac involvement is sometimes the only presenting feature and occurs in most cases.[12,13] Echocardiographic abnormalities (see below) are present in nearly two-thirds of the patients at the time of diagnosis.[12]

■ AA Amyloidosis

In the AA type of amyloidosis, the abnormal AA protein is derived from the circulating acute-phase reactant serum amyloid A (SAA), which is synthesized in hepatocytes; cytokines such as interleukin (IL)-1 and IL-6 play an important role in its production. AA amyloidosis has been associated with rheumatoid arthritis, inflammatory bowel disease, and other chronic inflammatory conditions.[11] It primarily affects the kidney; cardiac involvement is rare.[11]

■ Hereditary Amyloidosis

Mutations in several genes, such as fibrinogen and apolipoprotein A1 and A2, have been associated with hereditary amyloidosis. The most common variant of hereditary amyloidosis, however, is ATTR. The amyloid precursor protein is a mutated transthyretin (TTR), which in its normal form binds thyroxine and retinol in the serum. ATTR is associated with neuropathy and cardiac involvement.[14,15]

The long-term prognosis depends on the genetic variant and the degree of cardiac and other organ involvement. Symptoms vary and can range from those similar to cardiac AL amyloidosis to less-systemic effects, such as peripheral and autonomic neuropathy.[16] Other organs, including spleen and kidney, may also be involved.[16]

Senile Systemic Amyloidosis

Wild-type TTR amyloidosis (ATTR or WTTA), also known as senile systemic amyloidosis, is a disease of the elderly caused by the deposition of amyloid fibrils derived from wild-type TTR, a transport protein produced in the liver and the choroid plexus. In senile systemic amyloidosis, the TTR molecule may have a normal structure, a finding indicating that a mechanism other than amino acid substitution is also important in the fibrillogenesis associated with TTR amyloidosis.[17] Senile ATTR is mainly a cardiac disease, most common among men older than 70 years; it presents as cardiomyopathy with heart failure.[18,19] The other clinically significant extracardiac manifestation is carpal tunnel syndrome, which may precede the development of congestive heart failure (CHF).[18,19] The natural history is not well understood, but data suggest a median survival time of approximately 6 years after presentation.[20] This survival time is significantly better than that of patients with AL amyloidosis.[20]

Isolated Atrial Amyloidosis

In isolated atrial amyloidosis (IAA), amyloid fibrils are linearly deposited along the atria. The incidence of isolated atrial amyloid deposits increases with age, with an incidence of 75% among patients aged 51 to 60 years and 86% among those aged 81 to 90 years.[21] The disease may affect atrial conduction, and it increases the risk of atrial fibrillation.[22,23]

CLINICAL MANIFESTATIONS OF VARIOUS TYPES OF AMYLOID PROTEIN

The amyloid protein may be deposited in various organs, leading to organ-specific manifestations. Any type of amyloid protein can affect the cardiac structure, but the two types of amyloid protein that commonly infiltrate the heart are immunoglobulin light-chain (AL or primary systemic) amyloid and TTR amyloid.

Cardiac involvement is a prominent feature of AL amyloidosis,[13] whereas in AA amyloidosis involvement of the heart is rare.[11] Cardiac amyloidosis may affect the myocardium or valves and can result in cardiomyopathy, CHF, coronary heart disease, valvular heart disease, arrhythmia, or heart block. Amyloid protein can also be deposited on the valves, and amyloid of a yet unknown fibril type is also commonly found in explanted cardiac valves.[24,25]

Primary involvement of the myocardium leads to restrictive cardiomyopathy and diastolic heart failure. Later in the course of the disease, systolic failure ensues as well. Thus, symptoms are mostly related to exercise intolerance, fatigue, breathlessness, and, occasionally, syncope or presyncope. Exertional dyspnea is the most common symptom.[13] Syncope may be due to heart block, arrhythmias, or autonomic dysfunction.[26] Among patients with AL amyloidosis, stress-precipitated syncope is associated with poor survival rates because of sudden and presumed arrhythmic cardiac death.[26] A study of 26 patients with syncope found that the median survival time after diagnosis was significantly shorter (2 months) for patients with stress-related syncope than for patients with non–stress-related syncope (13 months).[26] Rarely, the patient may present with a stroke associated with atrial fibrillation, an arrhythmia found in approximately 10% of patients with cardiac AL amyloidosis.[26]

Rarely, angina pectoris may be the first cardiac manifestation of systemic amyloidosis.[27] Among patients with this condition, the results of coronary angiography may be normal, showing only an abnormality of coronary flow reserve.[27] One study of AL amyloidosis found that approximately 25% of patients had chest pain and that most of those who underwent catheterization (> 75%) had no epicardial coronary artery disease.[13] Chest pain among these patients may be due to small-vessel disease, because amyloidosis is known to infiltrate the intramyocardial vessels. Histologic examination of the coronary arteries of patients with AL amyloidosis shows variable degrees of diffuse stenosis of the small coronary arteries by amyloid deposition that occurs mainly in the media of the vessel, although the epicardial vessels appear normal or nearly normal.[28] Even among patients with no significant obstructive intramural coronary amyloidosis, approximately 50% or more exhibit microscopic changes in the myocardial ischemia.[29]

Other clinical characteristics of systemic amyloidosis include nephrotic syndrome, autonomic neuropathy (postural hypotension, diarrhea), cutaneous involvement (telangiectasia, periorbital ecchymosis), vascular involvement causing bleeding (cutaneous, such as periorbital, gastrointestinal), soft-tissue infiltration (carpal tunnel syndrome, macroglossia), pleural involvement (pleural effusion), and bowel involvement (malnutrition, diarrhea, cachexia).[13] The presence of systemic features of amyloidosis should prompt a search for cardiac involvement, because fewer than 5% of patients with AL amyloidosis involving the heart exhibit evidence of isolated heart disease.[13]

Cardiac Examination

Examination of the heart during the early stages of cardiac amyloidosis may yield normal results or may show only sinus tachycardia. In individual cases, orthostatic hypotension and atrial arrhythmias may also be present. Later in the course of the disease, cardiac findings include signs of right-sided heart failure, such as lower-extremity edema, hepatomegaly, splenomegaly, ascites, and especially elevated jugular venous pressure, with rapid and prominent x and y descent. Late in the course of the disease, when systolic function decreases, a third heart sound may be heard. A regurgitation murmur may be present as the result of primary valvular involvement with amyloid; it may also be functional in nature. Pleural effusion may be present, caused either by worsening cardiac congestion or by direct amyloid infiltration of the pleural surface.

DIAGNOSTIC APPROACH

The diagnosis of cardiac amyloidosis should be considered for patients who present with cardiomyopathy with unexplained left ventricular (LV) hypertrophy as demonstrated by echocardiography, particularly in the setting of conditions known to be associated with amyloidosis. Although there may be no clinical features that differentiate senile cardiac amyloidosis from the AL type, the absence of abnormal M protein in serum and urine, in addition to the presence of cardiac amyloidosis among patients older than 60 years with no extracardiac manifestation of primary amyloidosis, raises the possibility of senile systemic amyloidosis (senile cardiac amyloidosis).

Patients with systemic amyloid involvement (e.g., proteinuria or gastrointestinal involvement) should undergo a cardiac evaluation, including baseline electrocardiography (ECG), echocardiography, and levels of biomarkers (brain natriuretic peptide [BNP] and troponin). Among patients for whom the clinical suspicion of cardiac amyloidosis is high, the next step is to establish a diagnosis by performing cardiac biopsy. When obtaining a biopsy specimen is not possible, a biopsy of the subcutaneous abdominal fat can be substituted.[30]

Cardiac magnetic resonance imaging (MRI) is also a very useful test in the evaluation of patients with clinical suspicion of cardiac amyloidosis.[31] Because the treatment approach differs for each subtype, hence, the next logical step is to ascertain the type of amyloidosis. Because AL amyloidosis is the most common type, the next step is to search for plasma cell dyscrasia by immunofixation electrophoresis of the serum and urine, or to perform a bone marrow biopsy with immunohistochemical staining of plasma cells for kappa or lambda light chains.[10] The bone marrow biopsy will also help exclude myeloma or other conditions, such as Waldenstrom macroglobulinemia, as the cause of amyloidosis. If the results of these tests are normal, the next step, even in the absence of a family history of amyloidosis, is to test for a mutant TTR protein in the serum, a mutant TTR gene in the genomic DNA, or both.[10] The various amyloid subtypes can be identified by laser microdissection of the amyloid plaques followed by mass spectrometry–based proteomic analysis. Specific cardiac investigations are briefly discussed below.

INVESTIGATIONS

Serum Biomarkers

Serum N-terminal pro-BNP (NT-proBNP) is a sensitive marker of cardiac involvement and a predictor of the prognosis of patients with AL amyloidosis.[32,33] Some data suggest that the NT-proBNP concentration is correlated with LV wall thickness and LV ejection fraction (LVEF) in ATTR amyloidosis.[34]

Serum troponins (I or T) are detectable in ATTR amyloidosis, but their role in risk stratification or determining the type of amyloidosis has not been established.[35] Similarly, cardiac troponins (cTn) are a powerful predictor of survival for patients with AL amyloidosis; cardiac troponin T (cTnT) appears to be a better predictor of survival than cardiac troponin I (cTnI).[36] A study that involved 261 patients with biopsy-proven AL amyloidosis found that the median survival time after diagnosis for patients with detectable cTnT was 6 months and that of patients with detectable cTnI was 8 months, whereas the median survival time for patients with undetectable cTnT was 22 months and that for patients with undetectable cTnI was 21 months.[36] Troponin and NT-proBNP are independent predictors of survival for patients with AL amyloidosis and can be incorporated into a simple prognostic staging system.[37]

Electrocardiography

ECG abnormalities are helpful in differentiating cardiac amyloidosis from other conditions, such as hypertension, that lead to hypertrophic heart disease. Characteristically, the ECG abnormality of low-voltage complexes (<5 mm on all limb leads and <10 mm on precordial leads) with poor R-wave progression is present in as many as half of patients with AL amyloidosis.[38] Other characteristic ECG abnormalities are pseudoinfarct pattern (47%) and atrial fibrillation (20%).[39] ECG may also show biatrial enlargement. Left bundle branch

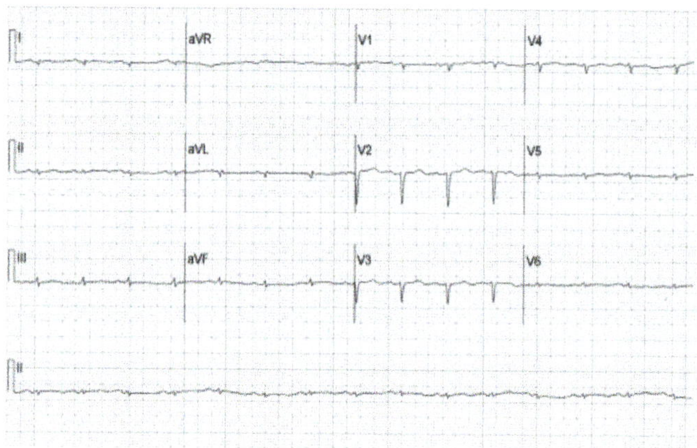

FIGURE 8-1 A 12-lead electrocardiogram showing low voltage and pseudoinfarct in a patient with cardiac amyloidosis.

block is seen among 40% of patients with wild-type ATTR but is rare among those with AL (4%).[40] Holter ECG monitoring detects asymptomatic arrhythmias in a number of patients. One study using Holter monitoring found supraventricular dysrhythmia in 37% of patients and ventricular dysrhythmia in 47%.[41]

ECG can also detect low voltage associated with other conditions, such as obesity, emphysema, hypothyroidism, and pericardial effusion. However, ECG findings of low voltage in conjunction with echocardiographic findings of LV hypertrophy in a patient's systemic amyloidosis should prompt a clinical suspicion of cardiac amyloidosis.

A study in which low voltage (56% of cases) and pseudoinfarct pattern (60%) were the most common ECG findings showed that, when ECG detects low voltage and echocardiography shows an intraventricular septum thickness of more than 1.98 cm, the diagnosis of cardiac amyloidosis can be made with a sensitivity of 72% and a specificity of 91%.[42] Figure 8-1 shows low voltage and a pseudoinfarct pattern on a 12-lead ECG of a patient with cardiac amyloidosis.

■ Echocardiography

Echocardiography is the most common imaging technique used to evaluate patients for suspected cardiac amyloidosis. Findings are characteristic in advanced disease and have both diagnostic and prognostic significance, but they are harder to appreciate earlier in the course of the disease.[43–45]

The echocardiographic characteristics of cardiac amyloidosis are a thick-walled ventricle with a speckled appearance of the myocardium, valve thickening, small LV chamber size, and biatrial enlargement. Small pericardial effusions and signs of elevated filling pressures (pleural effusions, dilated vena cava) caused by restrictive diastolic filling may also be seen (Figure 8-2).[46] Although the data on which these echocardiographic features are based are derived from the AL population, similar findings have been reported among patients with TTR amyloid cardiomyopathy.[20]

Increased wall thickness is still the principal diagnostic feature of cardiac amyloidosis. According to an international consensus panel of experts in amyloid disease, interventricular septal thickness of 12 mm, in the absence of other causes of hypertrophy, is the echocardiographic criterion that determines cardiac involvement among patients with AL systemic amyloidosis.[47] This single threshold, however, fails to account for sex-specific differences in normal wall thickness.[48] Intracardiac thrombus may be present in as many as 27% of patients with cardiac amyloidosis, with the highest prevalence in the AL type.[49]

In the early stages of cardiac amyloidosis, the LV systolic function is preserved. However, in the later stages systolic function is reduced; right ventricular (RV) dilation is associated with a poor prognosis.[50] Valves are also affected, with valvular thickening and regurgitation.[50,51]

Advanced echocardiographic techniques reveal more details about the underlying pathology and mechanical abnormalities.[52,53] Strain and strain rate imaging may help differentiate cardiac amyloidosis from hypertrophic cardiomyopathy.[54,55] Typically, basal movement is much more restricted than apical movement in amyloidosis; this difference in restriction is not found in true myocardial hypertrophy.[56] Longitudinal mechanical function is often severely impaired among patients with cardiac amyloidosis, and tissue Doppler imaging studies have shown decreased diastolic velocities in patients with cardiac AL amyloidosis.[57] Recently, radial strain has been shown to distinguish patients with cardiac AL amyloidosis from healthy control subjects.[58] Longitudinal strain and strain rate are reduced among patients with AL amyloidosis, even before heart failure or LV dysfunction is diagnosed.[59] Similar findings have been reported among ATTR patients, with a characteristic bull's-eye strain pattern derived from speckle tracking, consistent with a lower basal longitudinal strain than that found in the apex.[55]

■ Cardiac Catheterization with Hemodynamic Assessment

Cardiac catheterization with hemodynamic assessment is particularly useful in equivocal cases, in which it helps differentiate restrictive amyloid heart disease from a constrictive physiology. When the cardiac involvement

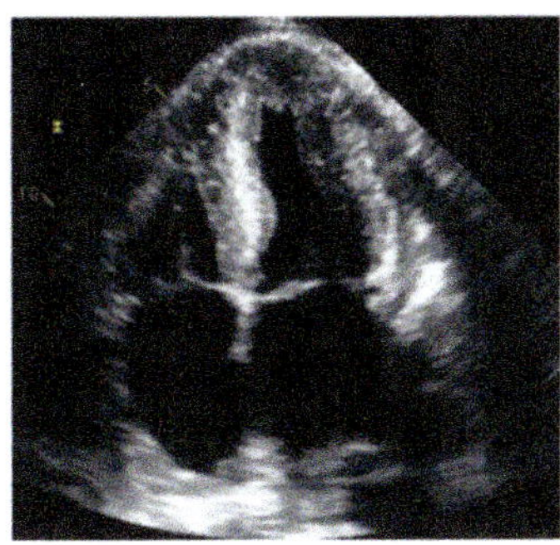 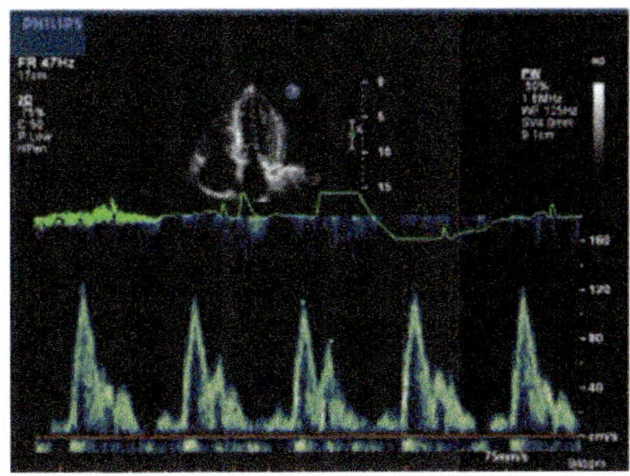

FIGURE 8-2   (A) Echocardiogram (4 chamber view) showing dilated atria and ventricular hypertrophy. (B) Mitral inflow showing a restrictive pattern in a patient with amyloidosis.

is mild and occurs in the initial phase of the disease, the intracardiac hemodynamics may be normal, but as the disease progresses the hemodynamics become increasingly consistent with a restrictive physiology. Both atrial pressures are elevated, but more significantly in the left than the right. Right atrial pressure tracings show prominent x and y descents.[60]

Simultaneous left- and right-heart catheterization will show elevated LV end-diastolic pressure exceeding that in the RV by at least 7 mmHg.[61] A dip and plateau waveform is commonly present but is not an invariable finding,[61] because this waveform can also be seen with constrictive physiology. Restrictive cardiomyopathy exhibits a concordant decrease in LV and RV pressures during inspiration, whereas constrictive pericarditis exhibits ventricular discordance with an increase in RV pressure and a decrease in LV pressure during inspiration.[62] Pulmonary hypertension with a peak systolic pulmonary pressure higher than 50 mmHg, a value not usually seen with constriction, may also be seen with the restrictive pattern of cardiac amyloidosis.

Cardiovascular Magnetic Resonance Imaging

Cardiac magnetic resonance imaging (MRI) is a very useful tool for diagnosing cardiac amyloidosis and for differentiating that entity from other cardiomyopathies.[31,63] Various ischemic and nonischemic cardiomyopathies exhibit a different and characteristic delayed-enhancement pattern on cardiac MRI after the administration of a gadolinium-based contrast agent.[64] In amyloidosis, the pattern typically shows global subendocardial late enhancement.[31]

Cardiac MRI is also helpful in differentiating amyloidosis from other causes of LV hypertrophy, such as hypertension-related LV hypertrophy and hypertrophic cardiomyopathy, which may not always be

detected by other imaging modalities, such as echocardiography.[65-67] Compared with endomyocardial biopsy, which is the gold standard for diagnosing cardiac amyloidosis, delayed-enhancement cardiac MRI detects cardiac amyloidosis with a sensitivity of 80%, a specificity of 94%, a positive predictive value of 92%, and a negative predictive value of 85%.[66]

Nuclear Scintigraphy

Various nuclear imaging modalities are used to diagnose cardiac amyloidosis.[68] Uptake of [99mTc]-3, 3-diphosphono-1,2-propanodicarboxylic acid ([99mTc]-DPD) in particular may help detect the disease.[68] In a small study using N-[*methyl*-[11C]]2-(4'-methylaminophenyl)-6-hydroxybenzothiazole ([11C]-PIB) with positron emission tomography (PET)/computed tomography (CT) to study systemic amyloidosis affecting the heart, myocardial [11C]-PIB uptake was evident in all patients with cardiac amyloidosis but not in healthy volunteers.[69] In addition, [99mTc]-DPD scintigraphy is useful in differentiating TTR amyloidosis and monoclonal AL amyloidosis in patients with established cardiac amyloidosis.[70] That study found that all patients with TTR-related cardiac amyloidosis exhibited intense [99mTc]-DPD uptake in the heart, with deposition in both the RV and the LV in every case, whereas for patients with AL cardiac amyloidosis there was no appreciable deposition of [99mTc]-DPD in the cardiac region, and only 45% of cases exhibited mild cardiac uptake.[70]

Endomyocardial Biopsy

Endomyocardial biopsy is considered the gold standard for the diagnosis of cardiac amyloid deposition.[71] In general, because cardiac amyloidosis is a uniform process, the results of series of endomyocardial biopsies are basically 100% sensitive in detecting the disease.[72] Light microscopy with Congo red staining detects amorphous pink deposits that yield apple-green birefringence under polarized light.[73]

To differentiate amyloid deposits from other hyaline deposits, such as collagen and fibrin, Congo red stain is commonly used. Under ordinary light this stain imparts a red or pink color to the tissue, but under cross-polarized light microscopy it yields an apple-green birefringence.[9] Sulfated Alcian blue is an alternative stain with high specificity for amyloid deposits.[73]

■ Fat Pad Biopsy

For patients with a clinical suspicion of cardiac amyloidosis, a fat pad biopsy may be considered. This test has a sensitivity of more than 80% for AL amyloidosis.[74]

TREATMENT

Management of cardiac amyloidosis requires a prompt diagnosis of the type of amyloid disease, because amyloid deposition can progress rapidly within the myocardial tissue.[43] Patients are best cared for by a multidisciplinary team with close collaboration between oncologists, cardiologists, nursing staff, and other members of the team. This approach allows better care of concomitant diseases such as myeloma, nephrotic syndrome, and neuropathy or gastrointestinal symptoms; such care is essential to the general well-being of the patient.

■ Treatment of Cardiac Manifestations

Treatment of angina ■ Angina should be treated with standard antianginal medications, albeit with cautious use of beta blockers and calcium channel blockers. In a small group of patients with AL amyloidosis, chest pain on exertion was promptly relieved by nitrates but frequently recurred despite long-term use of these drugs.[28,75] Because of the recurrence of chest pain despite long-term administration of nitrates, some clinicians have advocated the use of antianginal medications such as nicorandil; intracoronary injection of this drug in a population without amyloidosis was found to cause a dose-dependent increase in coronary flow velocity and a decrease in coronary vascular resistance.[76] In one reported case, recurrent angina with ECG changes developed despite the use of diltiazem and nicorandil.[77]

Sufficient data are not available to allow any firm recommendations about the ideal medication for patients with angina related to amyloidosis, but nitrates seem to be the logical initial choice. Newer antianginal medications such as ranolazine may be helpful for patients who do not respond to standard antianginal medications.

Treatment of congestive heart failure ■ CHF is treated with standard heart failure medications, such as diuretics, angiotensin-converting enzyme (ACE) inhibitors, aldosterone antagonists, and beta blockers, although the administration of these medications has not been systematically studied in any large group of patients with amyloid cardiomyopathy.

ACE inhibitors should be used cautiously because they may cause or exacerbate postural hypotension. The administration of these drugs should begin at a low initial dose, which should be increased in small increments; dose escalation should be carried out gradually and cautiously.

Calcium channel blockers should also be used cautiously to treat patients with amyloidosis, because these drugs have been reported to precipitate and worsen heart failure even in the presence of normal LVEF.[78] Discontinuing the administration of verapamil in one case was followed by clinical and echocardiographic improvement with normalization of LV systolic function.[78]

Salt restriction and fluid management are important because, as a result of the infiltrative process, the hearts of patients with amyloidosis are often stiff, with restrictive physiology, and are sensitive to both preload and after-load changes. Daily self-reported weights and dose adjustment of diuretics are often helpful; however, resistant pleural fluid may be a sign of pleural amyloid deposit and not of isolated elevated left-sided filling pressures. Small doses of diuretics should be used, and hypotension should be avoided. Peripheral edema can be treated by the use of compression stockings. Digoxin should be avoided, because it avidly binds to amyloid fibrils.[79]

■ Use of Pacemakers and Defibrillators

The indications for the use of pacemakers and defibrillators are the same as those for the general population.[80] However, when the heart is extensively involved with amyloid tissue, the successful insertion of a pacemaker may still not be life-saving. Similarly, the prophylactic implantation of a cardioverter-defibrillator may not be beneficial, because most patients die as a result of progressive heart failure, culminating in electromechanical dissociation.[81]

Treatment of End-Stage Heart Failure

The treatment of end-stage heart failure is challenging, with limited options for assistive devices and cardiac transplant. Some centers have treated a small number of selected patients with heart transplant followed by autologous stem cell transplant.[82] Heart transplant is the last option, because the recurrence of amyloid deposition in transplanted hearts has been reported.[83]

Treatment of AL Amyloidosis

Treating patients with AL amyloidosis by using a combination of oral melphalan and dexamethasone is associated with a 67% response rate and low treatment-related mortality rates (4%). This treatment is considered the standard of care for patients not eligible for high-dose chemotherapy and autologous hematopoietic stem cell transplant (auto-HCT).[84,85] However, this combination has achieved relatively disappointing outcomes for patients with advanced cardiac involvement.[86] Immunomodulatory imide drugs (IMiDs) are a relatively new class of drugs, including thalidomide, lenalidomide, and pomalidomide. These agents have demonstrated substantial activity against AL amyloidosis when given in combination with dexamethasone, with or without alkylating agents. IMiD-based combinations have achieved response rates ranging from 40% to 70% among patients with AL amyloidosis.[87–90] However, the onset of response is relatively slow, and the risk of cardiac and renal toxicity remains relatively high.[91,92]

The proteasome inhibitor bortezomib has been the most promising of all of the newer agents for treating AL amyloidosis. Bortezomib, in combination with cyclophosphamide and dexamethasone, has been associated with the highest response rates seen so far (> 80%) and with a rapid onset of response.[93,94] High-dose melphalan and auto-HCT have been associated with higher response rates (> 75%) and longer survival times (> 4 years) for selected patients with AL amyloidosis who are eligible for this therapy.[95]

The best long-term survival time was seen among patients for whom auto-HCT achieved a complete remission.[96] This treatment was previously associated with high treatment-related mortality rates (> 10%), but these rates have been reduced substantially in the past several years because of better patient selection.[97,98]

The availability of cardiac biomarker assays (NT-ProBNP, troponin T, and troponin I) has been an important advance in stratifying patients by early or advanced cardiac disease. These assays may also be helpful in patient selection and in predicting the outcome of auto-HCT.[99,100]

Treatment of Transthyretin Cardiac Amyloidosis

Although treatment data are available for AL amyloidosis, such data are lacking for TTR amyloidosis. An attractive option would be to use an agent that would either clear the TTR amyloidosis or stabilize it early in the course of the disease.

Some of the drugs that are currently being evaluated in ongoing or recently completed clinical trials are tafamidis (disease-modifying agent that stabilizes TTR amyloidosis), diflunisal (a nonsteroidal agent), doxycycline/tauroursodeoxycholic acid (combination of doxycycline, an antibiotic, and tauroursodeoxycholic acid [TUDCA], a biliary acid), ISIS-TTRRX (an antisense therapy that suppress TTR mRNA expression), and ALN-TTR01 and ALN-TTR02 (systemically delivered RNA interference therapies designed to suppress the expression of TTR protein and to prevent amyloid formation).[101,102] Recently, ALN-TTR01 and ALN-TTR02 were shown to suppress the production of both mutant and nonmutant forms of TTR.[103]

Because variant TTR is produced largely in the liver, one option for the treatment of hereditary amyloidosis is liver transplant or, in selected cases, combined heart and liver transplant.[101,102] Although orthotopic liver transplant appears to be the only definite treatment that potentially eliminates the source of mutant TTR, it also has its limitations. Only 20% of patients with familial amyloid polyneuropathy experienced an improvement in the disease after orthotopic liver transplant, whereas the remaining patients reported no change or a progression of their cardiovascular disease.[104] Another study of the clinical outcome of patients with familial amyloid polyneuropathy associated with the TTR alanine 60 variant found that cardiac amyloidosis progressed among patients who underwent orthotropic liver transplant, and only half of the patients survived for more than 5 years.[34]

Because senile systemic amyloidosis typically presents when patients are at an advanced age, cardiac transplant is rarely an option for these patients. However, cardiac transplant has been used to treat selected cases of wild-type (senile) TTR cardiac amyloidosis.[105]

PROGNOSIS

Cardiac amyloidosis is associated with various prognoses, depending on the presence of other disease and the concomitant involvement of other organs. Among patients with primary amyloidosis, cardiac involvement is associated with a poorer outcome, and most deaths are cardiac-related.[106] Among patients with primary (AL) amyloidosis, the most common cause of death is cardiac as the result of either sudden cardiac death or CHF.[13]

The median survival time of a group of 232 patients after a diagnosis of AL amyloidosis was 1.08 years (range, 0.83–1.25 years), and the median survival time from the date of the index ECG was 0.50 years (range, 0.42–0.66 years).[13] That study found that among patients with CHF the median survival time after diagnosis was 0.75 years (range, 0.59–1.00 years), a significantly shorter survival time than that experienced by patients with heart involvement but no CHF (2.34 years; range, 1.58–2.92 years).[13] Among patients with systemic amyloidosis, elevated troponin and BNP levels are predictors of mortality and hence also provide important prognostic information.[37]

Patients with both senile systemic amyloidosis and cardiac amyloidosis, although they may be older and may exhibit a thicker LV wall, appear to have a survival advantage and a better prognosis than patients with AL amyloidosis involving the heart.[20] Amyloid infiltration may discordantly affect the geometry of the ventricles; when the RV is dilated to a greater extent than the LV, the patient's prognosis is poor, with a median survival time of only 4 months.[50]

The prognosis of patients with amyloidosis may improve in the future, because therapy targeting the removal of amyloid protein from the tissues has recently shown promising results. A recent study (which did not include patients with clinical evidence of cardiac involvement) found that treating patients with (R)-1-[6-[(R)-2-carboxy-pyrrolidin-1-yl]-6-oxo-hexanoyl] pyrrolidine 2-carboxylic acid (CPHPC), followed by humanized monoclonal IgG1 anti–serum amyloid P (SAP) antibody, triggered clearance of amyloid deposits from the liver and other tissues.[107]

In patients with transthyretin amyloid cardiomyopathy, use of tafamidis was associated with reduction in all causes of mortality and cardiovascular hospitalization, in addition to significantly reducing the decline in functional capacity and quality of life.[108]

REFERENCES

1. Merlini G, Bellotti V. Molecular mechanisms of amyloidosis. *N Engl J Med*. 2003;349(6):583–596.
2. Sipe JD, Benson MD, Buxbaum JN, et al. Nomenclature 2014: amyloid fibril protein and clinical classification of the amyloidosis. *Amyloid*. 2014;21(4):221–224.
3. Kyle RA. Amyloidosis: a convoluted story. *Br J Haematol*. 2001;114(3):529–538.
4. Kyle RA, Linos A, Beard CM, et al. Incidence and natural history of primary systemic amyloidosis in Olmsted County, Minnesota, 1950 through 1989. *Blood*. 1992;79:1817–1822.
5. Hemminki K, Li X, Försti A, Sundquist J, Sundquist K. Incidence and survival in non-hereditary amyloidosis in Sweden. *BMC Public Health*. 2012;12:974.
6. Pomerance A. Senile cardiac amyloidosis. *Br Heart J*. 1965;27(5):711–718.
7. Dubrey SW, Hawkins PN, Falk RH. Amyloid diseases of the heart: assessment, diagnosis, and referral. *Heart*. 2011;97(1):75–84.
8. Nomenclature of amyloid and amyloidosis. WHO-IUIS Nomenclature Sub-Committee. *Bull World Health Organ*. 1993;71(1):105–112.
9. Cotran RS, Kumar V, Collins T, Robbins SL. *Robbins Pathologic Basis of Disease*. Philadelphia, PA: Saunders; 1999.
10. Falk RH, Comenzo RL, Skinner M. The systemic amyloidoses. *N Engl J Med*. 1997;337(13):898–909.
11. Dubrey SW, Cha K, Simms RW, Skinner M, Falk RH. Electrocardiography and Doppler echocardiography in secondary (AA) amyloidosis. *Am J Cardiol*. 1996;77(4): 313–315.
12. Kyle RA, Gertz MA. Primary systemic amyloidosis: clinical and laboratory features in 474 cases. *Semin Hematol*. 1995;32(1):45–59.
13. Dubrey SW, Cha K, Anderson J, et al. The clinical features of immunoglobulin light-chain (AL) amyloidosis with heart involvement. *QJM*. 1998;91(2):141–157.
14. Jacobson DR, Pastore RD, Yaghoubian R, et al. Variant-sequence transthyretin (isoleucine 122) in late-onset cardiac amyloidosis in black Americans. *N Engl J Med*. 1997;336(7):466–473.
15. Falk RH. The neglected entity of familial cardiac amyloidosis in African Americans. *Ethn Dis*. 2002;12(1):141–143.
16. Lachmann HJ, Booth DR, Booth SE, et al. Misdiagnosis of hereditary amyloidosis as AL (primary) amyloidosis. *N Engl J Med*. 2002;346(23):1786–1791.
17. Westermark P, Sletten K, Johansson B, Cornwell GG 3rd. Fibril in senile systemic amyloidosis is derived from normal transthyretin. *Proc Natl Acad Sci U S A*. 1990;87(7):2843–2845.
18. Dubrey SW, Falk RH. Amyloid heart disease. *Br J Hosp Med (Lond)*. 2010;71(2):76–82.
19. Cornwell GG 3rd, Murdoch WL, Kyle RA, Westermark P, Pitkänen P. Frequency and distribution of senile cardiovascular amyloid. A clinicopathologic correlation. *Am J Med*. 1983;75(4):618–623.
20. Ng B, Connors LH, Davidoff R, Skinner M, Falk RH. Senile systemic amyloidosis presenting with heart failure: a comparison with light chain-associated amyloidosis. *Arch Intern Med*. 2005;165(12):1425–1429.
21. Steiner I, Hájková P. Patterns of isolated atrial amyloid: a study of 100 hearts on autopsy. *Cardiovasc Pathol*. 2006;15(5):287–290.
22. Leone O, Boriani G, Chiappini B, et al. Amyloid deposition as a cause of atrial remodelling in persistent valvular atrial fibrillation. *Eur Heart J*. 2004;25(14):1237–1241.

23. Röcken C, Peters B, Juenemann G, et al. Atrial amyloidosis: an arrhythmogenic substrate for persistent atrial fibrillation. *Circulation*. 2002;106(16):2091–2097.

24. Kristen AV, Schnabel PA, Winter B, et al. High prevalence of amyloid in 150 surgically removed heart valves—a comparison of histological and clinical data reveals a correlation to atheroinflammatory conditions. *Cardiovasc Pathol*. 2010;19(4):228–235.

25. Iqbal S, Reehana S, Lawrence D. Unique type of isolated cardiac valvular amyloidosis. *J Cardiothorac Surg*. 2006;1:38.

26. Chamarthi B, Dubrey SW, Cha K, Skinner M, Falk RH. Features and prognosis of exertional syncope in light-chain associated AL cardiac amyloidosis. *Am J Cardiol*. 1997;80(9):1242–1245.

27. Al Suwaidi J, Velianou JL, Gertz MA, et al. Systemic amyloidosis presenting with angina pectoris. *Ann Intern Med*. 1999;131(11):838–841.

28. Hongo M, Yamamoto H, Kohda T, et al. Comparison of electrocardiographic findings in patients with AL (primary) amyloidosis and in familial amyloid polyneuropathy and anginal pain and their relation to histopathologic findings. *Am J Cardiol*. 2000;85(7):849–853.

29. Neben-Wittich MA, Wittich CM, Mueller PS, Larson DR, Gertz MA, Edwards WD. Obstructive intramural coronary amyloidosis and myocardial ischemia are common in primary amyloidosis. *Am J Med*. 2005;118(11):1287.

30. Libbey CA, Skinner M, Cohen AS. Use of abdominal fat tissue aspirate in the diagnosis of systemic amyloidosis. *Arch Intern Med*. 1983;143(8):1549–1552.

31. Maceira AM, Joshi J, Prasad SK, et al. Cardiovascular magnetic resonance in cardiac amyloidosis. *Circulation*. 2005;111(2):186–193.

32. Nordlinger M, Magnani B, Skinner M, Falk RH. Is elevated plasma B-natriuretic peptide in amyloidosis simply a function of the presence of heart failure? *Am J Cardiol*. 2005;96(7):982–984.

33. Palladini G, Campana C, Klersy C, et al. Serum N-terminal pro-brain natriuretic peptide is a sensitive marker of myocardial dysfunction in AL amyloidosis. *Circulation*. 2003;107(19):2440–2445.

34. Sattianayagam PT, Hahn AF, Whelan CJ, et al. Cardiac phenotype and clinical outcome of familial amyloid polyneuropathy associated with transthyretin alanine 60 variant. *Eur Heart J*. 2012;33(9):1120–1127.

35. Suhr OB, Anan I, Backman C, et al. Do troponin and B-natriuretic peptide detect cardiomyopathy in transthyretin amyloidosis? *J Intern Med*. 2008;263(3):294–301.

36. Dispenzieri A, Kyle RA, Gertz MA. et al. Survival in patients with primary systemic amyloidosis and raised serum cardiac troponins. *Lancet*. 2003;361(9371):1787–1789.

37. Dispenzieri A, Gertz MA, Kyle RA, et al. Serum cardiac troponins and N-terminal pro-brain natriuretic peptide: a staging system for primary systemic amyloidosis. *J Clin Oncol*. 2004;22(18):3751–3757.

38. Cheng ZW, Tian Z, Kang L, et al. Electrocardiographic and echocardiographic features of patients with primary cardiac amyloidosis [Chinese]. *Zhonghua Xin Xue Guan Bing Za Zhi*. 2010;38(7):606–609.

39. Murtagh B, Hammill SC, Gertz MA, Kyle RA, Tajik AJ, Grogan M. Electrocardiographic findings in primary systemic amyloidosis and biopsy-proven cardiac involvement. *Am J Cardiol*. 2005;95(4):535–537.

40. Rapezzi C, Merlini G, Quarta CC, et al. Systemic cardiac amyloidoses: disease profiles and clinical courses of the 3 main types. *Circulation*. 2009;120(13):1203–1212.

41. Falk RH, Rubinow A, Cohen AS. Cardiac arrhythmias in systemic amyloidosis: correlation with echocardiographic abnormalities. *J Am Coll Cardiol*. 1984;3(1):107–113.

42. Rahman JE, Helou EF, Gelzer-Bell R, et al. Noninvasive diagnosis of biopsy-proven cardiac amyloidosis. *J Am Coll Cardiol*. 2004;43(3):410–415.

43. Kristen AV, Perz JB, Schonland SO, et al. Rapid progression of left ventricular wall thickness predicts mortality in cardiac light-chain amyloidosis. *J Heart Lung Transplant*. 2007;26(12):1313–1319.

44. Koyama J, Falk RH. Prognostic significance of strain Doppler imaging in light-chain amyloidosis. *JACC Cardiovasc Imaging*. 2010;3(4):333–342.

45. Migrino RQ, Mareedu RK, Eastwood D, Bowers M, Harmann L, Hari P. Left ventricular ejection time on echocardiography predicts long-term mortality in light chain amyloidosis. *J Am Soc Echocardiogr*. 2009;22(12):1396–1402.

46. Selvanayagam JB, Hawkins PN, Paul B, Myerson SG, Neubauer S. Evaluation and management of the cardiac amyloidosis. *J Am Coll Cardiol*. 2007;50(22):2101–2110.

47. Gertz MA, Comenzo R, Falk RH, et al. Definition of organ involvement and treatment response in immunoglobulin light chain amyloidosis (AL): a consensus opinion from the 10th International Symposium on Amyloid and Amyloidosis, Tours, France, 18–22 April 2004. *Am J Hematol*. 2005;79(4):319–328.

48. Lang RM, Bierig M, Devereux RB, et al. Recommendations for chamber quantification: a report from the American Society of Echocardiography's Guidelines and Standards Committee and the Chamber Quantification Writing Group, developed in conjunction with the European Association of Echocardiography, a branch of the European Society of Cardiology. *J Am Soc Echocardiogr*. 2005;18(12):1440–1463.

49. Feng D, Syed IS, Martinez M, et al. Intracardiac thrombosis and anticoagulation therapy in cardiac amyloidosis. *Circulation*. 2009;119(18):2490–2497.

50. Patel AR, Dubrey SW, Mendes LA, et al. Right ventricular dilation in primary amyloidosis: an independent predictor of survival. *Am J Cardiol*. 1997;80(4):486–492.

51. Siqueira-Filho AG, Cunha CL, Tajik AJ, Seward JB, Schattenberg TT, Giuliani ER. M-mode and two-dimensional echocardiographic features in cardiac amyloidosis. *Circulation*. 1981;63(1):188–196.

52. Park SJ, Miyazaki C, Bruce CJ, Ommen S, Miller FA, Oh JK. Left ventricular torsion by two-dimensional speckle tracking echocardiography in patients with diastolic

dysfunction and normal ejection fraction. *J Am Soc Echocardiogr*. 2008;21(10):1129–1137.

53. Porciani MC, Cappelli F, Perfetto F, et al. Rotational mechanics of the left ventricle in AL amyloidosis. *Echocardiography*. 2010;27(9):1061–1068.

54. Kusunose K, Yamada H, Iwase T, et al. Images in cardiovascular medicine. Cardiac magnetic resonance imaging and 2-dimensional speckle tracking echocardiography in secondary cardiac amyloidosis. *Circ J*. 2010;74(7):1494–1496.

55. Sun JP, Stewart WJ, Yang XS, et al. Differentiation of hypertrophic cardiomyopathy and cardiac amyloidosis from other causes of ventricular wall thickening by two-dimensional strain imaging echocardiography. *Am J Cardiol*. 2009;103(3):411–415.

56. Maciver DH, Townsend M. A novel mechanism of heart failure with normal ejection fraction. *Heart*. 2008;94(4): 446–449.

57. Koyama J, Ray-Sequin PA, Davidoff R, Falk RH. Usefulness of pulsed tissue Doppler imaging for evaluating systolic and diastolic left ventricular function in patients with AL (primary) amyloidosis. *Am J Cardiol*. 2002;89(9):1067–1071.

58. Bellavia D, Pellikka PA, Abraham TP, et al. Evidence of impaired left ventricular systolic function by Doppler myocardial imaging in patients with systemic amyloidosis and no evidence of cardiac involvement by standard two-dimensional and Doppler echocardiography. *Am J Cardiol*. 2008;101(7):1039–1045.

59. Koyama J, Ray-Sequin PA, Falk RH. Longitudinal myocardial function assessed by tissue velocity, strain, and strain rate tissue Doppler echocardiography in patients with AL (primary) cardiac amyloidosis. *Circulation*. 2003;107(19):2446–2452.

60. Tyberg TI, Goodyer AV, Hurst VW 3rd, Alexander J, Langou RA. Left ventricular filling in differentiating restrictive amyloid cardiomyopathy and constrictive pericarditis. *Am J Cardiol*. 1981;47(4):791–796.

61. Swanton RH, Brooksby IA, Davies MJ, Coltart DJ, Jenkins BS, Webb-Peploe MM. Systolic and diastolic ventricular function in cardiac amyloidosis. Studies in six cases diagnosed with endomyocardial biopsy. *Am J Cardiol*. 1977; 39(5):658–664.

62. Nishimura RA, Carabello BA. Hemodynamics in the cardiac catheterization laboratory of the 21st century. *Circulation*. 2012;125(17):2138–2150.

63. Germans T, Nijveldt R, Brouwer WP, et al. The role of cardiac magnetic resonance imaging in differentiating the underlying causes of left ventricular hypertrophy. *Neth Heart J*. 2010;18(3):135–143.

64. Shah DJ, Judd RM, Kim RJ. Technology insight: MRI of the myocardium. *Nat Clin Pract Cardiovasc Med*. 2005;2(11):597–605.

65. Mahrholdt H, Wagner A, Judd RM, Sechtem U, Kim RJ. Delayed enhancement cardiovascular magnetic resonance assessment of non-ischaemic cardiomyopathies. *Eur Heart J*. 2005;26(15):1461–1474.

66. Vogelsberg H, Mahrholdt H, Deluigi CC, et al. Cardiovascular magnetic resonance in clinically suspected cardiac amyloidosis: noninvasive imaging compared to endomyocardial biopsy. *J Am Coll Cardiol*. 2008;51(10):1022–1030.

67. Karamitsos TD, Piechnik SK, Banypersad SM, et al. Noncontrast T1 mapping for the diagnosis of cardiac amyloidosis. *JACC Cardiovasc Imaging*. 2013;6(4):488–497.

68. Chen W, Dilsizian V. Molecular imaging of amyloidosis: will the heart be the next target after the brain? *Curr Cardiol Rep*. 2012;14(2):226–233.

69. Antoni G, Lubberink M, Estrada S, et al. In vivo visualization of amyloid deposits in the heart with 11C-PIB and PET. *J Nucl Med*. 2013;54(2):213–220.

70. de Haro-del Moral FJ, Sánchez-Lajusticia A, Gómez-Bueno M, Garcia-Pavía P, Salas-Antón C, Segovia-Cubero J. Role of cardiac scintigraphy with ^{99}mTc-DPD in the differentiation of cardiac amyloidosis subtype. *Rev Esp Cardiol (Engl Ed)*. 2012;65(5):440–446.

71. Kieninger B, Eriksson M, Kandolf R, et al. Amyloid in endomyocardial biopsies. *Virchows Arch*. 2010;456(5): 523–532.

72. Ardehali H, Qasim A, Cappola T, et al. Endomyocardial biopsy plays a role in diagnosing patients with unexplained cardiomyopathy. *Am Heart J*. 2004;147(5):919–923.

73. Pomerance A, Slavin G, McWatt J. Experience with the sodium sulphate-Alcian Blue stain for amyloid in cardiac pathology. *J Clin Pathol*. 1976;29(1):22–26.

74. Ansari-Lari MA, Ali SZ. Fine-needle aspiration of abdominal fat pad for amyloid detection: a clinically useful test? *Diagn Cytopathol*. 2004;30(3):178–181.

75. Mueller PS, Edwards WD, Gertz MA. Symptomatic ischemic heart disease resulting from obstructive intramural coronary amyloidosis. *Am J Med*. 2000;109(3):181–188.

76. Hongo M, Takenaka H, Uchikawa S, Nakatsuka T, Watanabe N, Sekiguchi M. Coronary microvascular response to intracoronary administration of nicorandil. *Am J Cardiol*. 1995;75(4):246–250.

77. Yamano S, Motomiya K, Akai Y, et al. Primary systemic amyloidosis presenting as angina pectoris due to intramyocardial coronary artery involvement: a case report. *Heart Vessels*. 2002;16(4):157–160.

78. Pollak A, Falk RH. Left ventricular systolic dysfunction precipitated by verapamil in cardiac amyloidosis. *Chest*. 1993;104(2):618–620.

79. Rubinow A, Skinner M, Cohen AS. Digoxin sensitivity in amyloid cardiomyopathy. *Circulation*. 1981;63(6): 1285–1288.

80. Epstein AE, DiMarco JP, Ellenbogen KA, et al. 2012 ACCF/AHA/HRS focused update incorporated into the ACCF/AHA/HRS 2008 guidelines for device-based therapy of cardiac rhythm abnormalities: a report of the American College of Cardiology Foundation/American Heart Association Task Force on Practice Guidelines and the Heart Rhythm Society. *J Am Coll Cardiol*. 2013;61(3):e6–e75

81. Kristen AV, Dengler TJ, Hegenbart U, et al. Prophylactic implantation of cardioverter-defibrillator in patients with severe cardiac amyloidosis and high risk for sudden cardiac death. *Heart Rhythm*. 2008;5(2):235–240.

82. Sack FU, Kristen A, Goldschmidt H, et al. Treatment options for severe cardiac amyloidosis: heart transplantation combined with chemotherapy and stem cell

transplantation for patients with AL-amyloidosis and heart and liver transplantation for patients with ATTR-amyloidosis. *Eur J Cardiothorac Surg*. 2008;33(2):257–262.

83. Dubrey SW, Burke MM, Khaghani A, Hawkins PN, Yacoub MH, Banner NR. Long term results of heart transplantation in patients with amyloid heart disease. *Heart*. 2001;85(2):202–207.

84. Palladini G, Perfetti V, Obici L, et al. Association of melphalan and high-dose dexamethasone is effective and well tolerated in patients with AL (primary) amyloidosis who are ineligible for stem cell transplantation. *Blood*. 2004;103(8):2936–2938.

85. Palladini G, Russo P, Nuvolone M, et al. Treatment with oral melphalan plus dexamethasone produces long-term remissions in AL amyloidosis. *Blood*. 2007;110(2):787–788.

86. Dietrich S, Schönland SO, Benner A, et al. Treatment with intravenous melphalan and dexamethasone is not able to overcome the poor prognosis of patients with newly diagnosed systemic light chain amyloidosis and severe cardiac involvement. *Blood*. 2010;116(4):522–528.

87. Palladini G, Perfetti V, Perlini S, et al. The combination of thalidomide and intermediate-dose dexamethasone is an effective but toxic treatment for patients with primary amyloidosis (AL). *Blood*. 2005;105(7):2949–2951.

88. Wechalekar AD, Goodman HJ, Lachmann HJ, Offer M, Hawkins PN, Gillmore JD. Safety and efficacy of risk-adapted cyclophosphamide, thalidomide, and dexamethasone in systemic AL amyloidosis. *Blood*. 2007;109(2):457–464.

89. Dispenzieri A, Lacy MQ, Zeldenrust SR, et al. The activity of lenalidomide with or without dexamethasone in patients with primary systemic amyloidosis. *Blood*. 2007;109(2):465–470.

90. Kumar SK, Hayman SR, Buadi FK, et al. Lenalidomide, cyclophosphamide, and dexamethasone (CRd) for light-chain amyloidosis: long-term results from a phase 2 trial. *Blood*. 2012;119(21):4860–4867.

91. Specter R, Sanchorawala V, Seldin DC, et al. Kidney dysfunction during lenalidomide treatment for AL amyloidosis. *Nephrol Dial Transplant*. 2011;26(3):881–886.

92. Tapan U, Seldin DC, Finn KT, et al. Increases in B-type natriuretic peptide (BNP) during treatment with lenalidomide in AL amyloidosis. *Blood*. 2010;116(23):5071–5072.

93. Mikhael JR, Schuster SR, Jimenez-Zepeda VH, et al. Cyclophosphamide-bortezomib-dexamethasone (CyBorD) produces rapid and complete hematologic response in patients with AL amyloidosis. *Blood*. 2012;119(19):4391–4394.

94. Venner CP, Lane T, Foard D, et al. Cyclophosphamide, bortezomib, and dexamethasone therapy in AL amyloidosis is associated with high clonal response rates and prolonged progression-free survival. *Blood*. 2012;119(19):4387–4390.

95. Skinner M, Sanchorawala V, Seldin DC, et al. High-dose melphalan and autologous stem-cell transplantation in patients with AL amyloidosis: an 8-year study. *Ann Intern Med*. 2004;140(2):85–93.

96. Cibeira MT, Sanchorawala V, Seldin DC, et al. Outcome of AL amyloidosis after high-dose melphalan and autologous stem cell transplantation: long-term results in a series of 421 patients. *Blood*. 2011;118(16):4346–4352.

97. Gertz MA, Lacy MQ, Dispenzieri A, et al. Trends in day 100 and 2-year survival after auto-SCT for AL amyloidosis: outcomes before and after 2006. *Bone Marrow Transplant*. 2011;46(7):970–975.

98. Sanchorawala V, Skinner M, Quillen K, Finn KT, Doros G, Seldin DC. Long-term outcome of patients with AL amyloidosis treated with high-dose melphalan and stem-cell transplantation. *Blood*. 2007;110(10):3561–3563.

99. Dispenzieri A, Gertz MA, Kyle RA, et al. Prognostication of survival using cardiac troponins and N-terminal pro-brain natriuretic peptide in patients with primary systemic amyloidosis undergoing peripheral blood stem cell transplantation. *Blood*. 2004;104(6):1881–1887.

100. Madan S, Kumar SK, Dispenzieri A, et al. High-dose melphalan and peripheral blood stem cell transplantation for light-chain amyloidosis with cardiac involvement. *Blood*. 2012;119(5):1117–1122.

101. Ruberg FL, Berk JL. Transthyretin (TTR) cardiac amyloidosis. *Circulation*. 2012;126(10):1286–1300.

102. Ando Y, Coelho T, Berk JL, et al. Guideline of transthyretin-related hereditary amyloidosis for clinicians. *Orphanet J Rare Dis*. 2013;8:31.

103. Coelho T, Adams D, Silva A, et al. Safety and efficacy of RNAi therapy for transthyretin amyloidosis. *N Engl J Med*. 2013;369(9):819–829.

104. Herlenius G, Wilczek HE, Larsson M, Ericzon BG; Familial Amyloidotic Polyneuropathy World Transplant Registry. Ten years of international experience with liver transplantation for familial amyloidotic polyneuropathy: results from the Familial Amyloidotic Polyneuropathy World Transplant Registry. *Transplantation*. 2004;77(1):64–71.

105. Dubrey SW, Burke MM, Hawkins PN, Banner NB. Cardiac transplantation for amyloid heart disease: the United Kingdom experience. *J Heart Lung Transplant*. 2004;23(10):1142–1153.

106. Kyle RA, Gertz MA, Greipp PR, et al. A trial of three regimens for primary amyloidosis: colchicine alone, melphalan and prednisone, and melphalan, prednisone, and colchicine. *N Engl J Med*. 1997;336(17):1202–1207.

107. Richards DB, Cookson LM, Berges AC, et al. Therapeutic clearance of amyloid by antibodies to serum amyloid P component. *N Engl J Med*. 2015;373(12):1106–1114.

108. Maurer MS, Schwartz JH, Gundapaneni B, et al. Tafamidis treatment for patients with transthyretin amyloid cardiomyopathy. *New Engl J Med*. 2018;379:1007-1016.

9 Cardiac Arrhythmias in the Cancer Patient

Asif Jafferani ■ *Syed Wamique Yusuf* ■ *Steven M. Ewer*

Cardiac arrhythmias are a common problem facing today's cancer patients and, when present, can affect quality of life and complicate treatment of their malignancies. The presentation of cardiac rhythm disturbances spans a spectrum from asymptomatic incidental findings to harbingers of terminal disease or even sudden cardiac death. Patients can also suffer secondary complications of their arrhythmia, such as heart failure, syncope-related trauma and stroke from atrial fibrillation. Arrhythmias may be directly related to a patient's malignancy, its treatment, or may occur as the result of unrelated and often preexisting medical problems. Although the electrocardiographic (ECG) representation of the arrhythmia may have the same appearance in patients with and without cancer, malignancy can influence the incidence, clinical presentation and management of arrhythmias. This chapter looks at the more frequent arrhythmias seen in cancer patients and some of the attributes that distinguish arrhythmia in patients with and without cancer.

Arrhythmia, both related and not related to cancer, is often transient. Normal sinus rhythm revealed on a single ECG tracing does not exclude the possibility of a latent and potentially serious paroxysmal rhythm disturbance. Even without obvious arrhythmias detected on initial evaluation, a rhythm disturbance should be more thoroughly pursued when patients present with suggestive clinical scenarios.

The initial approach to arrhythmias is similar for patients with and without cancer. Analysis of cardiac rhythm, however, may be more complicated in cancer patients because these patients often have exaggerated respiratory variations of the electrical axis, augmented variation in the RR interval, and cycle-dependent changes in QRS voltage that can be confused with arrhythmia. Such changes may be due to chronic lung disease, pleural or pericardial effusions, pulmonary resection, or radiation to the chest with damage to the lungs.

CHARACTERIZATION OF ARRHYTHMIA

Although cardiac arrhythmias are traditionally categorized according to their electrical mechanism, it can also be conceptually useful to distinguish them by etiology. Arrhythmias of primary cardiac origin arise from abnormalities within cardiac structures themselves. Secondary arrhythmias, in contrast, are related to systemic metabolic abnormalities without evidence for structural heart disease. Overlap can of course occur; a heart that has been severely weakened by the malignancy or its treatment may be more sensitive to metabolic or environmental derangements.

Primary arrhythmias encompass disturbances that arise from cardiac and pericardial structures and include mechanical abnormalities, structural abnormalities, and local metabolic sequelae of primary cardiac disease. Primary arrhythmias may be caused by focal or diffuse abnormalities: focal abnormalities are those that involve one or more discrete and localized areas of the myocardium, such as tumor or infarction; diffuse abnormalities can be found throughout the heart and include cardiomyopathy and infiltrative processes such as cardiac amyloidosis. Ischemic heart disease, elevated intracardiac pressure and wall stress, dilated cardiomyopathy, and fibrosis related to aging are all common causes of primary arrhythmia in both cancer patients and those without malignancy. A number of other abnormalities, however, are more likely to be found in patients with cancer and include primary or metastatic cardiac tumors, amyloid infiltration, pericardial disease, and chemotherapy-related cardiomyopathy. Chest radiation can also contribute to primary arrhythmias related to endomyocardial fibrosis, myopericarditis or accelerated coronary artery disease.

Secondary arrhythmias arise without identifiable structural cardiac or localized metabolic abnormalities. Precipitating causes include toxic reactions to drugs, increased sympathetic tone, surgery, hypoxia, mediator release, and other derangements of metabolism, including electrolyte abnormalities. Early cardiotoxic effects of chemotherapy should be considered when aggressive antitumor therapy is temporally related to arrhythmias. When serious arrhythmias are encountered during cancer treatment, modification of therapy may need to be considered. Treatments other than antineoplastic drugs that are commonly employed in the care of cancer patients may also cause arrhythmia; among these are antibiotics, psychotropic medications, and radiation. Some of these associations are discussed below.

SUPRAVENTRICULAR ARRHYTHMIAS

The supraventricular arrhythmias originate above the level of the AV node and are summarized in Table 9-1. Supraventricular arrhythmias may be sustained or intermittent and usually result in tachycardia. Symptoms are related to the ventricular rate, the duration of the arrhythmia, and the degree to which cardiac output is compromised. Symptoms can include episodic palpitations, neck fullness, chest pain, diaphoresis, dyspnea, congestive heart failure, lightheadedness and syncope. It is not uncommon for patients to be misdiagnosed as experiencing panic attacks well before the arrhythmia, the true culprit, is discovered.

Supraventricular arrhythmias are more commonly encountered in cancer patients. Mostly in the form of atrial fibrillation and paroxysmal supraventricular tachycardia, these rhythms are a reflection of

TABLE 9-1 Summary of supraventricular tachycardias

	ATRIAL RATE (BPM)	ATRIAL MORPHOLOGY	CONDUCTION	VENTRICULAR RATE	RESPONSE TO VAGAL MANEUVERS	THERAPY
Sinus tachycardia	> 100, usually < 160	Normal P wave (upright in lead 2)	1:1	Same as atrial; gradual onset and termination	Gradual slowing or none	Treatment of underlying cause
PSVT (AVRT and AVNRT)	150–250	Usually not seen. Inverted P wave may be seen just after QRS.	1:1	Same as atrial; sudden onset and termination	Conversion to NSR or none	Adenosine and other AV nodal blockers
Atrial flutter	240–350	Sawtooth baseline; usually inverted in 2, 3, and aVF	Freq. 2:1; higher block with therapy; 1:1 rare	Often 140–160 bpm	Geometric slowing (e.g., 150 to 100 or 75 bpm) or none	AV nodal blockers, cardioversion
Atrial fibrillation	> 350	Variable coarse to fine grossly irregular activity	Variable	Usually > 120 bpm if untreated	Slowing or none	AV nodal blockers, cardioversion, type IC or III antiarrhythmias
Atrial tachycardia with block	120–220	Usually upright in 2, 3, aVF, particularly when due to digoxin	Variable; 2:1 most common	Variable depending on conduction	Geometric slowing	Same as AF if not digoxin toxic. Phenytoin, potassium, or digoxin antibody if toxic.
MAT	> 100, usually > 120	Varying morphology; 3 or more P-wave morphologies occurring in 30 s	Often 1:1 with occasional blocked beats	Rapid and irregular	Usually none	AV nodal blockers other than digoxin; treatment of underlying cause

AV, atrioventricular; AVNRT, atrioventricular nodal reentrant tachycardia; AVRT, atrioventricular reentry tachycardia; bpm, beats per minute; MAT, multifocal atrial tachycardia; NSR, normal sinus rhythm; PSVT, paroxysmal supraventricular tachycardia.

significant multisystem organ disease, various hemodynamic stressors, increased catecholamine states, metabolic perturbations, an older patient population, and an overall disruption of physiologic homeostasis. Atrial fibrillation has been associated with elevated C-reactive protein levels in the general population,[1] suggesting that systemic inflammatory states may play a causative role in this arrhythmia. Similar data have been shown specifically for cancer patients; a study of surgical patients with colorectal carcinoma found a threefold increase in the incidence of atrial fibrillation compared with controls, despite a lack of structural heart disease or any obvious other risk factors.[2] Systemic inflammation was the presumed mechanism. Along the same line of reasoning, supraventricular arrhythmias have been found to be associated with high-dose chemotherapy and stem cell transplantation.[3] A variety of anti-cancer therapies can precipitate atrial fibrillation.[4] These include gemcitabine, docetaxel, alemtuzumab, 5-fluorouracil, and interleukin-2; and although direct cardiotoxicity cannot be ruled out, systemic inflammation likely plays a role. Ibrutinib, not only increases the risk of atrial fibrillation, but also increases the bleeding risk, which poses great clinical challenges when establishing the risk-benefit ratio of anticoagulation for stroke prophylaxis in these patients. In three randomized phase 3 trials of ibrutinib, the incidence of atrial fibrillation was between 5%–7%[5]; however, more recently rates as high as 12% have also been reported.[6] In one study of 56 patients who developed atrial fibrillation during ibrutinib therapy for chronic lymhocytic leukemia, approximately 14% also experienced grade 3–4 bleeding complication.[7] Supraventricular arrhythmias, including atrial fibrillation are seen with higher incidence in association with hematopoietic stem cell transplantation and lead to increasing patient hospitalization costs, morbidity and mortality.[8] Even radiation distant from the heart has been implicated in a series of patients treated for cervical cancer.[9]

Once inflammation has been localized closer to the heart, the incidence of atrial fibrillation and other supraventricular arrhythmias is even higher. Intracardiac tumors such as primary cardiac lymphoma and cardiac metastases often present with such arrhythmias. Mediastinal tumors have likewise been implicated.[10,11] In a series of patients with esophagectomy for cancer, postoperative atrial fibrillation was present in 25% of cases and was associated with an increased risk of morbidity and mortality.[12] Atrial fibrillation is often associated with acute pulmonary embolism and pericarditis. These conditions occur frequently in the cancer patient, particularly thromboembolic disease with any adenocarcinoma and

pericarditis with malignancies that tend to metastasize to the pericardium (i.e., breast and ovarian cancers) or that are treated with radiation to the chest.

Among the patients with the highest incidence of supraventricular arrhythmias are those postoperative from lung resection for primary lung cancer. Several studies have shown the risk of arrhythmia to be about 30%, with atrial fibrillation accounting for most of the cases.[13,14] Those patients with concomitant chronic obstructive pulmonary disease developed arrhythmias in 59% of cases.[13] Other important risk factors include age, the extent of resection, and preexisting cardiac disease. Although the arrhythmia contributed to longer hospitalizations, there was no appreciable effect on long-term morbidity or mortality.[15,16] Treatment with a limited course of amiodarone has been shown to be safe and effective,[17,18] but an isolated case of acute pulmonary toxicity has been reported in this population.[19] Dronedarone may ultimately prove to be a less toxic (albeit somewhat less effective) alternative to amiodarone. Strategies for prophylaxis of higher-risk patients have also been investigated, and diltiazem has been shown to be superior to digoxin for this purpose.[14]

■ Sinus Tachycardia

Sinus tachycardia is often overlooked, despite being among the most clinically significant of the arrhythmias. It is almost exclusively a secondary arrhythmia. P waves are present and are identical in morphology to those seen in normal sinus rhythm. One of the key features of sinus tachycardia is its gradual onset and termination, which, when observed, help distinguish this rhythm from paroxysmal supraventricular tachycardia. Causes of sinus tachycardia among cancer patients are usually readily apparent and include pain, anxiety, fever, anemia, hypovolemia, hypotension and pulmonary embolism. Since sinus tachycardia is an appropriate physiologic response to stress, treatment of this arrhythmia (e.g., with beta-blockers) is usually not warranted and, indeed, may be counterproductive. Unexplained sinus tachycardia remains one of the most concerning clinical findings, and this is especially true in cancer patients. An aggressive search for the underlying cause is necessary.

■ Atrial Premature Complexes

The simplest and most common supraventricular arrhythmia is the isolated atrial premature complex (APC). APCs are identified by early P waves that typically differ in morphology from those that originate from the sinus node. The QRS complex is usually narrow and similar in morphology to normally originating beats. Most premature atrial complexes are benign and asymptomatic and are found in a significant portion of the normal population. Unless the associated palpitations trouble a patient, they do not require treatment. In the cancer patient, APCs are frequently seen following administration of chemotherapy, at times of stress, and as a manifestation of a hyperadrenergic state. They may also be seen with high-output states that occur in cancer patients and that include anemia, AV shunting of blood through tumors, large tumor burdens, and hyperthyroidism.

■ Paroxysmal Supraventricular Tachycardia

Although composed of several different arrhythmias, it is useful to consider this group as a whole because they share several mechanistic and clinical features. As their name implies, they are episodic, and, in contrast to sinus tachycardia, they start and terminate abruptly. With rare exceptions, ventricular rates are between 100 and 300 bpm. They are regular and typically manifest with narrow QRS complex, but some arrhythmias in this category will present as wide-complex tachycardias owing to aberrant conduction. In these instances, the distinction between supraventricular and ventricular tachycardia can be difficult, but certain ECG features can help clarify the nature of the arrhythmia (see below).

Reentrant paroxysmal supraventricular tachycardias include AV nodal reentry, AV reentry, and the much less common sinus node or atrial reentry. These individual entities are considered briefly below. The shared mechanism of this group involves an abnormal conduction system, which consists of two (or more) parallel conducting pathways that differ in their fundamental properties (i.e., conduction velocity and refractory period). This then allows the possibility of anterograde conduction through one pathway and retrograde conduction through another, thus creating a closed circuit for "reentry." The two limbs of the circuit can be separated anatomically (macroreentry), such as in Wolff–Parkinson–White syndrome, or contained at a single location (microreentry), such as the AV node in AV nodal reentry tachycardia.

Reentrant mechanisms are usually triggered by premature complexes that happen to occur while one limb is still refractory and the other is able to be depolarized. In patients with the appropriate electrical substrate, states of catecholamine excess provide conditions that are ripe for reentry by exaggerating the differences in the electrical properties of conductive tissue and increasing the frequency of premature

complexes. It is not unusual for cancer patients to present with reentrant supraventricular tachycardia for the first time after major surgery or during intensive chemotherapy.

ECG features include a regular, narrow-complex tachycardia, with occasional exceptions as noted above. Differential diagnosis of narrow-complex tachycardia also includes sinus tachycardia, atrial tachycardia, atrial flutter, and atrial fibrillation. Distinguishing types of reentrant tachycardias can usually be accomplished by careful scrutiny of the surface ECG (see below), but sometimes intracardiac electrophysiologic studies are needed to confirm the correct diagnosis.

Atrioventricular nodal reentrant tachycardia (AVNRT) is the most common cause of paroxysmal supraventricular tachycardia. The reentry circuit occurs within or in the proximity of the AV node. Ventricular rates fall between 150 and 250 bpm. Retrograde P waves are usually buried in the QRS complex and thus may not be readily apparent.

Atrioventricular reentry tachycardia (AVRT) involves a macroreentrant circuit with AV conduction occurring at a site distant from the AV node. This bypass tract usually can conduct only in a retrograde fashion, such that the ECG will look normal when the patient is in normal sinus rhythm (i.e., the bypass tract is concealed). When anterograde AV conduction is possible through the bypass tract, ventricular pre-excitation is evident during normal sinus rhythm, and the phenomenon is termed *Wolff–Parkinson–White* pattern. Retrograde P waves occur just after the QRS complex.

Wolff–Parkinson–White syndrome deserves a bit more consideration here because of two unique features. Because anterograde conduction down the bypass tract is possible, reentrant circuits occurring in this manner result in QRS complexes that are broad and bizarre, and this wide-complex tachycardia can be confused with ventricular tachycardia (VT). Furthermore, when atrial fibrillation occurs in the context of Wolff–Parkinson–White syndrome, anterograde conduction through the bypass tract can lead to an unusually rapid ventricular response, which may be poorly tolerated and which can rapidly degenerate into ventricular arrhythmias and sudden death. AV nodal blocking agents such as digoxin and beta-blockers will not slow the ventricular response in this case and paradoxically can increase the rate by shortening the refractory period of the bypass tract tissue and are thus contraindicated. Lidocaine, procainamide, intravenous (IV) amiodarone, and electrical cardioversion are preferred in this situation, and any of these therapeutic modalities is suitable for use in cancer patients.

Several cases of Wolff–Parkinson–White syndrome have been described in pediatric patients with tuberous sclerosis and associated cardiac rhabdomyomas.[20,21] If these neoplasms are well enough differentiated to retain the conductive properties of cardiac myocytes, and if they are so positioned to bridge normal atrial and ventricular tissue, preexcitation and reentry tachycardia can occur. Although there was initially some debate over whether the rhabdomyomas were the actual source of preexcitation, there has been subsequent correlation between tumor location on imaging and accessory pathway localization on electrophysiologic study.[22] Cure has been achieved in such cases either by tumor resection or radiofrequency ablation of the pathway, but spontaneous regression can also occur.

Treatment of an ongoing symptomatic episode of reentry tachycardia consists of slowing or blocking conduction through the AV node by vagal maneuvers such as Valsalva or by IV adenosine, given as an initial bolus of 6 mg followed by 12 mg if necessary. Since most reentrant circuits involve the AV node, these methods are successful in terminating the arrhythmia in the vast majority of cases. Other medications that affect AV nodal conduction, such as beta-blockers, verapamil, or diltiazem, can also be effective in terminating reentrant rhythms but are considered second-line agents because of their longer half-lives and propensity to cause hypotension. Acutely ill patients with hemodynamic compromise are more appropriately treated with adenosine or electrical cardioversion. Prevention of recurrent arrhythmias can usually be achieved with beta-blockers or nondihydropyridine calcium channel blockers. Alternatively, or for medically refractory cases, catheter-based radiofrequency ablation can offer a cure rate of greater than 90%. Such modalities are not contraindicated in cancer patients even with advanced malignancy if their life expectancy is greater than 3 months.

■ Multifocal Atrial Tachycardia

Multifocal atrial tachycardia (MAT) is defined by an atrial rate of greater than 100 bpm and P waves of at least three differing morphologies with the absence of a dominant pacemaker (Figure 9-1). The differential diagnosis includes sinus tachycardia with frequent APCs and atrial fibrillation, although all three of these rhythm disturbances fall along the spectrum of increased atrial excitability and are related mechanistically. Indeed, MAT often degenerates into atrial fibrillation. The distinction between MAT and atrial fibrillation is important, however, because the treatments, discussed below, differ significantly. MAT is typically irregular and has 1:1 ventricular conduction with usual rates between 100 and 130 bpm.

MAT is classically associated with acute respiratory failure and chronic obstructive lung disease and is especially common among patients with progressive lung cancer. MAT is often triggered by increases in right atrial pressures, such as occurs in the perioperative period following lung resection. MAT has also been associated with congestive heart failure and the use of theophylline. Treatment consists of rate control with beta-blockers or nondihydropyridine calcium channel blockers and management of the underlying disease. Cardiac glycosides, such as digoxin, are contraindicated because they often increase the atrial rate. Beta-blockers, although effective, must be used with caution in patients with underlying lung disease, especially when a significant bronchospastic component is present. Other antiarrhythmics are notably ineffective. Because MAT does not involve a reentry circuit, electrical cardioversion is ineffective. Thus, MAT can be difficult to manage and, when present, usually confers a poor overall prognosis.

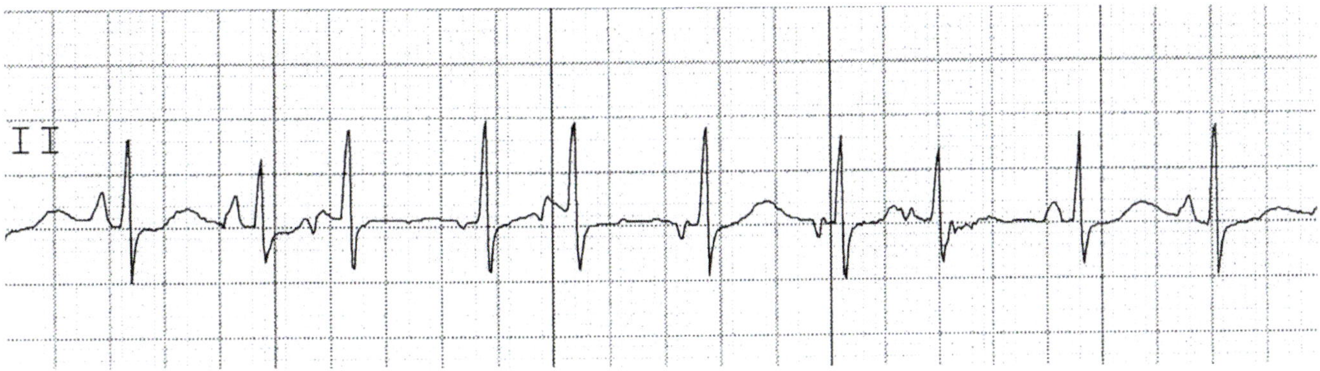

FIGURE 9-1 Multifocal atrial tachycardia on a 12-lead electrocardiogram.

Ectopic Atrial Tachycardia

Ectopic atrial tachycardia presents with a regular atrial rate of 100 to 220 beats per minute and a P-wave morphology that differs from P waves originating from the sinus node. AV block can occur and, when present, suggests digoxin toxicity. A case of ectopic atrial tachycardia caused by a right atrial leiomyosarcoma has been reported,[23] as has a case linked to ifosfamide.[24] AV nodal blocking agents can slow ventricular response but do nothing to terminate the rhythm. Treatment includes correction of electrolyte disturbances and withdrawal of toxic proarrhythmic agents, such as digoxin, although, occasionally, catheter ablation techniques or specific antiarrhythmic medications are necessary.

Atrial Flutter and Fibrillation

Atrial flutter and fibrillation are rhythms that lie on a spectrum of atrial electrical and mechanical disarray. They share several clinical aspects and treatment strategies and, in fact, overlap mechanistically more than is usually recognized. Therefore, it is most useful to consider them together. As discussed above, both of these arrhythmias are seen frequently in cancer patients. Mechanically, the dysrhythmic atria become essentially nonfunctional, both during the arrhythmia and temporarily after conversion back to normal sinus rhythm. This leads to stasis of blood in the atria and predisposes the patient to the development of intracardiac thrombi and associated systemic embolization. By far the most common site of thrombus formation is the left atrial appendage.[25]

On the ECG, typical atrial flutter is characterized by regular atrial activity (F waves) at approximately 300 bpm. The waves are asymmetric, often leading to a "saw-toothed" pattern, which is usually best demonstrated in lead II. There is generally some block at the level of the AV node; the most common conduction ratios are 2:1 and 4:1, although other conduction ratios are not infrequently seen. Ventricular response can be regular (i.e., with fixed 2:1 block) or irregular (i.e., with variable block). RR intervals will generally be some multiple of the flutter cycle length, which is typically 200 milliseconds. When a fixed conduction ratio of 2:1 exists, the ventricular rate is approximately 150 bpm. In this situation, typical flutter waves can be obscured, and distinguishing flutter from paroxysmal supraventricular tachycardia (PSVT) or even sinus tachycardia can be challenging. If careful inspection of the 12-lead ECG does not allow definitive diagnosis, administration of adenosine while the patient is being observed with continuous ECG monitoring may be undertaken.

Although adenosine will not usually terminate atrial flutter, increasing block at the AV node will allow the underlying atrial rhythm to become apparent. As discussed above, most PSVTs will terminate with adenosine.

Atrial fibrillation is usually easily recognized on ECG as an irregularly irregular rhythm with a baseline of unorganized atrial activity. The ventricular rate is widely variable, depending mostly on AV nodal conduction properties.

The clinical presentation of atrial fibrillation and flutter covers a broad range of possibilities in cancer patients, as it does in the normal population. Arrhythmia can be found incidentally on physical examination of an asymptomatic patient or can present as acute, life-threatening hemodynamic instability. When present, symptoms are usually related to either the heart rate, loss of AV synchrony, or thromboembolic complications. Paroxysmal arrhythmias typically presents with episodic palpitations and dyspnea. If the ventricular rate is fast enough or if underlying coronary disease is present, chest pain can ensue, along with ischemic ECG changes and elevated levels or serum cardiac markers owing to a myocardial oxygen supply and demand mismatch. Hemodynamically significant hypotension can lead to lightheadedness or syncope. If patients have any predisposition to left ventricular systolic or diastolic dysfunction, decreased left ventricular filling time and loss of the atrial contribution to filling can lead to congestive heart failure. Because of their predisposition to thromboembolic disease, cancer patients are more likely than the general population to present with these phenomena. Because most intracardiac thrombi related to atrial fibrillation and flutter originate from the left atrial appendage, stroke and systemic embolization are seen. Sometimes mental status changes or failure to thrive are the only symptoms of this arrhythmia in the older patient or those with more advanced stages of their malignancy.

The most important risk factor for the development of atrial fibrillation or flutter is intrinsic cardiac disease. Conditions that increase atrial size, contribute to elevated atrial pressures, or cause direct inflammation of the atrial structures (such as pericarditis) are especially likely to result in atrial dysrhythmia. Other risk factors include age, hypertension, lung disease, thyrotoxicosis, surgery, and other states with increased catecholamine levels. Atrial fibrillation is especially common in cancer patients. When de novo fibrillation or flutter develops in the patient with malignancy, a workup for secondary causes is crucial, regardless of whether intrinsic cardiac disease is present. Pulmonary embolus, acute or chronic pericarditis, and infection should always remain in the differential diagnosis.

Thyrotoxicosis and other metabolic derangements should also be ruled in or out in all patients. As noted above, atrial fibrillation should be anticipated in the perioperative setting, especially in patients undergoing lung resection.

Treatment of atrial fibrillation and flutter can be divided into three distinct therapeutic goals: (1) control of the ventricular rate, (2) rhythm control, and (3) prevention of thromboembolic complications. These are considered separately below.

Control of the ventricular rate is carried out with agents that slow conduction through the AV node, including β-blockers, calcium channel blockers, and digoxin. First-line agents for the acutely ill patient include the short-acting preparations of beta-blockers or diltiazem, but care must be taken to avoid systemic hypotension. In patients who present with hypotension, these agents are not recommended, and other treatment strategies should be considered (i.e., cardioversion). Digoxin has the advantage of slowing AV conduction without causing hypotension, but it may take several hours to achieve therapeutic levels, and digoxin is generally less effective than other agents. Stable patients with normal blood pressure can usually be controlled with longer-acting beta-blockers, diltiazem, or verapamil. In patients with frequent symptomatic paroxysmal events, rate-controlling agents are usually continued during sinus rhythm to prevent excessive tachycardia when the arrhythmia occurs. In these situations, a balance is sought that avoids marked sinus bradycardia on the one hand while controlling the ventricular response to the arrhythmia on the other. In some patients, this balance cannot be achieved without the aid of a permanent pacemaker, which is frequently indicated for this form of tachycardia–bradycardia syndrome.

Before discussing rhythm control, it is worth noting that the reestablishment of sinus rhythm is not necessarily a goal of treatment. Some patients tolerate chronic atrial fibrillation extraordinarily well. Successful conversion and maintenance of sinus rhythm becomes less likely in the setting of prolonged chronic arrhythmia, previous failed attempts at conversion, or predisposing structural heart disease. Thus, before blindly embarking on a strategy of maintaining sinus rhythm, one must take into account variables such as the case-specific risks, the level of medical necessity, and the likelihood of success. Furthermore, the results of recent trials suggest that rhythm control offers no mortality benefit over rate control with anticoagulation.[26]

Conversion of atrial fibrillation and flutter to normal sinus rhythm can be spontaneous or can be achieved with electrical shock or antiarrhythmic medications. For the acutely unstable patient, emergent synchronized DC cardioversion should be performed per Advanced Cardiac Life Support (ACLS) protocols.[27] Short-acting general anesthetic agents should be administered to all conscious patients prior to electrical cardioversion. For elective cardioversion, strategies are tailored to minimize the risk of thromboembolism. Because thrombi in the left atrial appendage can be dislodged at the time of or in the weeks following cardioversion, ruling out, preventing, or treating this entity is of utmost importance prior to elective cardioversion (see below). Success rates generally exceed 80%, with treatment failure more likely in patients with long-standing chronic atrial fibrillation and structural abnormalities of the atria. Chemical cardioversion with amiodarone can be pursued in the non-emergent setting, and short courses do not expose patients to the multiple organ toxicities of chronic administration. It should also be mentioned that treatment of any predisposing conditions will help facilitate cardioversion and maintenance of normal sinus rhythm afterward. Maintenance of normal sinus rhythm can be furthered with antiarrhythmic medications or catheter ablation procedures. Antiarrhythmic medications can carry significant toxicities and can be proarrhythmic, and thus are generally administered only under the guidance of a cardiologist.

Thromboembolic sequelae remain a significant source of morbidity and mortality in patients with atrial fibrillation and flutter. Although evidence is emerging that selected patients are at low enough risk of embolic events to forego systemic anticoagulation despite their arrhythmia,[28] cancer patients are less likely to be in this category owing to such factors as their advanced age, hypercoagulable state, or multisystem comorbid illness. Although some patients will carry contraindications to systemic anticoagulation, it should at least be considered in all patients with atrial fibrillation or flutter and coexisting active malignancy. Unfortunately, cancer patients also carry a higher risk of bleeding complications from chronic anticoagulation. Guidelines generally recommend the CHA_2DS_2-VASc score in the estimation of the risk for thromboembolism in patients with non-valvular atrial fibrillation along with the HAS-BLED risk score to estimate risk of major bleeding with anti-coagulation therapy.[29] However, these risk scores have not been sufficiently validated in patients with cancer.[30] Recent, large, nation-wide data sets have shown some conflicting results and therefore, some caution needs to be exercised while using these scores in cancer patients to define risk for stroke or systemic embolism.[31,32]

Full anticoagulation with warfarin to achieve an international normalized ratio of 2 to 3 or with enoxaparin is recommended for episodes of arrhythmia that last greater than 48 hours. Caution must be used when attempting to determine the timing of arrhythmia onset from a patient's history because studies correlating symptoms with dysrhythmia on Holter monitoring have found history to be an unreliable determinant of the duration of the disturbance. If atrial fibrillation or flutter is known or suspected to have been present for more than 48 hours, anticoagulation should be continued for at least 4 weeks after restoration of normal sinus rhythm. Because the mechanical function of the atria does not return to normal immediately after conversion, the risk of thrombus formation paradoxically increases during this time period. If the patient experiences frequent recurrences of paroxysmal arrhythmia or if the underlying risk factors are expected to progress over time, anticoagulation should be continued indefinitely. In patients who are deemed to be poor candidates for anticoagulation with warfarin, aspirin (325 mg daily) should be offered.

Non-vitamin K antagonist oral anticoagulants (NOACs) which includes the direct thrombin inhibitor dabigatran and the factor Xa inhibitors rivaroxaban, apixaban and edoxaban are attractive and suitable alternatives to warfarin for stroke prevention in AF.[33] However, the experience of their use in patients with malignancy is limited. The only randomized control trial specifically evaluating NOACs in patients with malignancy is in the setting of secondary prevention of venous thromboembolic disease (VTE) in the HOKUSAI-VTE Cancer study.[34] Edoxaban was noninferior as compared to dalteparin with respect to the composite outcome of recurrent VTE and major bleeding; however, major bleeding itself occurred more frequently in patients treated with edoxaban, especially in patients with gastrointestinal malignancies.

Much of the efforts to use NOACs in patients with malignancy and atrial fibrillation is thus inferred from this trial as well as the original trials validating the use of these NOACs.[33] However, most of the NOAC atrial fibrillation trials excluded patients with active malignancies. The ARISTOTLE trial did include these patients, and a sub-group analysis of 1236 patients with either a remote or active history of cancer showed the superior efficacy and safety of apixaban as compared to warfarin for preventing strokes/systemic embolism in these patients, results that are similar to those without a history of cancer.[35] Similarly, a single center registry of patients with malignancy receiving Rivaroxaban for Atrial Fibrillation showed low rates of cumulative 1-year incidence of stroke (1.4%) and major bleeding (1.2%),[36] rates which are comparable to the original ROCKET-AF study.[37]

In general, the European Heart Rhythm Association recommends a team approach while defining anti-coagulation therapy for patients with malignancy and atrial fibrillation.[33] This approach includes taking into account the stroke/systemic embolism risk, the bleeding risk, especially in the context of the specific malignancy and treatment received, patient preference, drug interactions (CYP3A4 and/or Pg-P interaction) and need for adjustment based on specific patient factors like thrombocytopenia or renal dysfunction.

With elective cardioversion, a standard regimen would include documented therapeutic anticoagulation for 3 weeks prior to conversion and continued for at least 4 weeks afterward. An alternative strategy that has been shown to be safe and effective is to undergo imaging for left atrial thrombi with transesophageal echocardiography immediately prior to cardioversion.[38] If no thrombi are seen, cardioversion is performed while anticoagulated, with subsequent anticoagulation for 4 weeks. If a left atrial thrombus is seen, a period of anticoagulation followed by reimaging to confirm resolution prior to cardioversion is the usual course. It should be reemphasized that cancer patients have several nontraditional risk factors for stroke in the setting of atrial fibrillation. Given the results of the AFFIRM trial[26] and others that show higher stroke rates after discontinuation of warfarin, indefinite anticoagulation should be strongly considered in patients with cancer and atrial fibrillation, even when sinus rhythm can be restored and traditional risk factors are absent.

VENTRICULAR ARRHYTHMIAS

Ventricular arrhythmias encompass disturbances initiated by ectopic beats originating from the ventricles and reentrant rhythms involving ventricular pathways. Such disturbances are manifested by wide QRS complexes. Ventricular tachycardia (VT) is defined as three or more ventricular extrasystoles in succession at a rate greater than 120 bpm. Runs of ventricular beats between 60 and 120 bpm are referred to as accelerated idioventricular rhythm. VT may be self-terminating but is described as "sustained" if it lasts longer than 30 seconds or results in hemodynamic collapse. VT is described as "monomorphic" when the QRS complexes have the same general appearance and "polymorphic" if there is wide beat-to-beat variation in QRS morphology.

In general, ventricular arrhythmias are considered far more serious than their supraventricular counterparts because rapid or disorganized ventricular activity dramatically compromises cardiac output and can result in sudden cardiac death. Efforts to rapidly treat such cases of hemodynamically unstable ventricular arrhythmias have led to the increase in the availability of defibrillators in public places.[39] Cancer patients have an increased likelihood of such disturbances; often they have underlying heart disease, and they have the additional risk factors of exposure to stressful and potentially cardiotoxic anticancer treatments, increased use of a wide variety of medicines that may be proarrhythmic, and a high likelihood of hormonal and metabolic abnormalities that further the initiation and propagation of ventricular dysrhythmia.

Although more than 80% of wide-complex tachycardias will be of ventricular origin, supraventricular tachycardia with aberrant intraventricular conduction remains in the differential diagnosis. Underlying structural heart disease strongly favors the diagnosis of ventricular arrhythmia. Several criteria have been proposed to help distinguish whether a given ECG tracing favors ventricular or supraventricular tachycardia with aberrant conduction.[40] In general, AV dissociation, capture or fusion beats, QRS duration > 140 milliseconds, extreme QRS axis, and concordance of the QRS complexes across the precordial leads all favor VT. The definitive diagnosis sometimes requires intracardiac electrophysiologic testing.

Ventricular Premature Complexes

VPCs are the most common form of ventricular arrhythmia. They are often present in healthy patients with structurally normal hearts and thus do not always represent a worrisome underlying pathophysiology. Ventricular ectopy increases with the multiple physiologic stresses that are encountered in cancer patients. VPCs are also more common in patients with heart disease and can be associated with an increased risk of malignant ventricular rhythms.[41] They may be asymptomatic, discovered incidentally on physical examination, while a patient is on inpatient telemetry monitoring, or during long-term ambulatory ECG monitoring (i.e., Holter monitoring). VPCs may also be associated with symptoms of palpitations and, when in repetitive patterns associated with a slow effective ventricular rate, occasional lightheadedness. Historically, VPCs were considered dangerous and were widely treated, but studies have subsequently shown that zealous suppression proved considerably more dangerous than the arrhythmia itself.[42,43] VPCs do not require specific treatment, except in rare cases in which the symptoms are significant enough to warrant suppression. Beta-blockers usually suffice in these instances and do not carry the proarrhythmic tendencies of other antiarrhythmics.

Ventricular Tachycardia

VT is characterized by a wide-complex tachycardia originating from the ventricular tissue. As noted above, VT can be sustained or non-sustained, monomorphic or polymorphic, and related to primary or secondary etiologies. *Torsades de pointes* comprises a unique subgroup of VT with different risk factors, ECG manifestations, and treatment considerations and is discussed separately. VT is usually initiated by a VPC that occurs during the vulnerable period of the cardiac cycle.

Predisposing risk factors for the development of VT include, first and foremost, structural heart disease. In the general population, acute or chronic ischemic heart disease and various types of nonischemic cardiomyopathy are the most common causes. In the cancer patient, there are several primary causes of this dysrhythmia, including primary and metastatic cardiac tumors,[44] coronary vasospasm (i.e., during 5-fluorouracil or capecitabine administration), and anthracycline-related cardiomyopathy. In hospitalized patients, central venous catheters and devices that enter the right ventricle can also trigger VT.[45] Secondary causes include severe alkalosis, hypokalemia (adrenal tumors), hypomagnesemia, thyrotoxicosis, pheochromocytoma, and mediator release associated with the carcinoid syndrome.

Specific cardiac tumors that have been frequently associated with VT include lymphomas, rhabdomyomas, fibromas, and lipomas.[46–49] Cases involving hamartoma, vascular tumors, and metastatic disease have also been described.[50–52] A case of positional VT related to esophageal carcinoma has also been reported, notable for the lack of pericardial invasion on pathologic examination.[53] Fortunately, such manifestations of local tumor effects are unusual.

Chemotherapeutic medications have also been implicated as possible causes of ventricular arrhythmias. VT has been reported as an early manifestation of toxicity following administration of anthracyclines.[54] VT is more common after the development of cardiomyopathy after cumulative exposure to anthracyclines.[55] Interleukin-2 and alemtuzumab have also been associated with VT.[56,57] Ibrutinib, a Bruton's tyrosine kinase (BTK) inhibitor has been shown to be associated with polymorphic ventricular tachycardia, without prolonging the QT interval.[58,59] Miscellaneous causes of ventricular arrhythmia in the cancer patient include surgical manipulation of adrenal tumors, including non–catecholamine-secreting tumors[60]; a case of ventricular arrhythmias related to deployment of an esophageal stent for malignant dysphagia has also been reported.[61]

Immune checkpoint inhibitors (ICI) are novel form of cancer immunotherapy which help the adaptive immune system preferentially target cancer cells. These have been associated with myocarditis in small case series.[62,63] A recent review of their use in a multicenter retrospective and prospective study indicated that myocarditis may be more common than is appreciated with ICI and is associated with risk for major adverse cardiac events (MACE), including ventricular arrhythmias and sudden cardiac death.[64] Furthermore, utilization of combination ICI therapy actually increases risk of myocarditis and subsequent MACE.[62] In patients with early recognition of this syndrome, high dose steroid therapy was found to be effective to prevent MACE; however, the utility of a variety of immunosuppressive therapies including intravenous immunoglobin, mycophenolate, anti-thymocyte globulin and infliximab remains undetermined.[64] Further research is needed in this area as the use of this promising class of medicines is likely to the grow in the coming years.[65]

Symptoms during VT depend mostly on ventricular rate and the duration of the arrhythmia, although the underlying cardiac substrate plays a role as well. Non-sustained VT can be asymptomatic or can present with palpitations, chest pain, dyspnea, or presyncope. Sustained VT can present with any of these symptoms but frequently results in hemodynamic collapse with either syncope or sudden cardiac death. Sustained VT can degenerate into ventricular fibrillation and is more likely to do so at faster rates.

The initial therapeutic approach to VT should begin with considerations of both urgency and causality. In the unstable patient, emergent restoration of sinus rhythm is required. The standard treatment algorithms for VT and ventricular fibrillation as recommended in the ACLS protocols should be followed,[27] with an emphasis on delivering the first electrical shock as soon as possible after the arrhythmia is discovered because the prognosis worsens rapidly with each passing minute during cardiopulmonary arrest. Even conscious patients with VT and symptoms such as chest pain or severe dyspnea are at high risk of the development of VF, and urgent cardioversion under conscious sedation should be considered. For hemodynamically stable VT without evidence of cardiac ischemia or heart failure, an approach involving chemical cardioversion and reversal of any predisposing conditions is reasonable. Acute suppression of ventricular arrhythmias can be carried out with IV agents, including amiodarone, lidocaine, beta-blockers, and procainamide. Acute cardiac ischemia must be considered in any patient with new-onset VT, even when other possible etiologies are present. Abnormalities in serum electrolyte concentrations should be sought and corrected. Serum potassium and magnesium should be kept above 4.0 mEq/L and 2.0 mg/dL, respectively. Echocardiography can help evaluate for any structural heart disease. Further workup and treatment can be tailored to the individual patient based on the underlying malignancy and treatments thereof. If recurrent ventricular arrhythmias are a problem, longer-term suppression with oral agents such as beta-blockers, amiodarone, or mexiletine may be indicated.

Other than antiarrhythmic medications, secondary prevention of ventricular arrhythmias can involve treatment of the underlying malignancy, catheter-based radiofrequency ablation, or an implantable defibrillator. In cases of VT as a primary arrhythmia caused by intracardiac masses, treatment of the tumor either with surgery (i.e., for rhabdomyoma, lipoma, or hamartoma)[47,49,50,66] or with chemotherapy and/or radiation (i.e., for lymphoma)[46,67] has resulted in cure of the arrhythmia. Likewise, secondary ventricular arrhythmias caused by biologically active metabolites from tumors such as pheochromocytoma have been ameliorated following surgical resection.[68,69] When a single anatomic focus is suspected as the etiology of VT, such as an ischemic scar, referral to an electrophysiologist for radiofrequency ablation may be appropriate. The use of implantable defibrillators in the cancer patient is discussed separately below.

■ Ventricular Fibrillation

Ventricular fibrillation is characterized by chaotic, low-voltage electrical activity on ECG. Mechanically, there is likewise no organized activity; therefore, this is a non-perfusing rhythm. Complete hemodynamic collapse uniformly results, and death is imminent unless electrical activity is restored within a few minutes either spontaneously or by electrical cardioversion. The risk factors for ventricular fibrillation are the same as for VT, except that sustained very rapid tachycardias, including VT, can degenerate into ventricular fibrillation if coronary perfusion is compromised or metabolic abnormalities such as profound hypoxia exist. Treatment is also similar to that of VT, with resuscitation as per ACLS protocols[27] and correction of the underlying predisposing conditions when possible. Unfortunately, resuscitation efforts have a lower likelihood of success in cancer patients compared with the general population.

■ Torsades de Pointes

Torsades de pointes is a distinctive subset of polymorphic VT associated with a prolonged QT interval, which may be congenital or acquired. *Torsades de pointes* literally means twisting of points (referring to beat-to-beat changes of the QRS axis) and is thus characterized by a gradual change in the amplitude and twisting of the QRS complexes around the isoelectric line (Figure 9-2).[70] Although this rhythm characteristically terminates spontaneously, it frequently recurs and may degenerate into sustained VT and ventricular fibrillation and is therefore potentially lethal. Rate is typically 200 to 250 bpm. In most but not all cases, *torsades de pointes* is initiated by a characteristic sequence of a long RR interval followed by a short RR interval, with premature depolarization interrupting the preceding repolarization.[71] *Torsades de pointes* can rarely occur in cases with a normal QT interval.[72]

The QT interval is measured from beginning of the QRS complex to the return of the T wave to the isoelectric baseline. It is measured in the ECG lead that gives the longest duration. Because the QT interval varies with heart rate, a corrected QT interval (QTc) is used to define normal values: QTc = QT interval divided by the square root of the RR interval expressed in seconds. Normal values for the QT interval also depend on sex. Criteria for normal, borderline, and prolonged QTc are depicted in Table 9-2.[73] A QTc interval > 500 milliseconds in men or women has been shown to be clearly associated with an increased risk of *torsades de pointes* and is considered dangerous.[74] In addition to the absolute value of the QTc interval, an increase of 60 milliseconds above baseline for an individual patient is generally considered also to represent an increased risk.[73]

Hence, prolongation of the QT interval to longer than 500 milliseconds during drug therapy should prompt a critical reevaluation of the risks and benefits of that therapy and consideration of therapeutic alternatives, in concert with a search for underlying predisposing factors, such as hypokalemia or drug interactions.

Risk factors for *torsades de pointes* include any agent or mechanism that prolongs the QT interval (Table 9-3).[70,75] Congenital forms of long QT syndrome exist, and the molecular mechanisms have been elucidated, but are not discussed further here. In cancer patients, acquired long QT syndrome is not an infrequent occurrence and is most commonly associated with drug administration, but a combination of multiorgan system disease, malnutrition, electrolyte abnormalities, and polypharmacy makes this group particularly susceptible. Those cancer patients with coexisting or malignancy-related cardiac disease are at even higher risk.

A list of medications that can prolong the QT interval is shown in Table 9-4.[76] Among the worst offenders are certain cardiac antiarrhythmics (especially class IC and class III agents), which affect ion channels in the heart as their primary mechanism. Several chemotherapy agents are well known to prolong the QT interval.[77] Among them, arsenic trioxide has been most closely associated with *torsades de pointes*, but other medications such as tamoxifen,[76] doxorubicin,[78] 5-fluorouracil[79] and combretastatin A-4[80] can also prolong the QT interval. Also considered to have "possible risk of *torsades*" are lapatinib, nilotinib and sunitinib.[76] Other classes of medications that have been implicated in *torsades de pointes* include various antimicrobial agents, psychiatric medications, and antiemetics, all of which are used frequently in the cancer patient. In one study, about 16% of patients with cancer in a palliative care unit were found to have a prolonged QT interval.[81] The potential to prolong the QT interval and develop *torsades de pointes* is not limited to prescribed medications but is also extended to over-the-counter medications, such as cesium chloride,

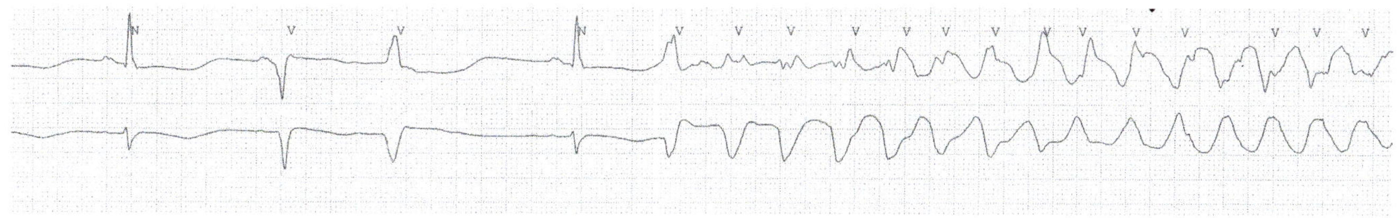

FIGURE 9-2   *Torsades de pointes* associated with acquired long QT syndrome.

TABLE 9-2   Normal and abnormal values for corrected QT interval (QTc) in milliseconds

	ADULT MALES	ADULT FEMALES
Normal	< 430	< 450
Borderline	431–450	451–470
Prolonged	> 450	> 470

Source: Adapted from Committee for Proprietary Medicinal Products, 1997.[73]

Table 9-3 Causes of long QT syndrome

Congenital long QT syndromes (adrenergic dependent)
Jervell and Lange-Nielsen syndrome
Romano-Ward syndrome
Acquired long QT syndromes
Drugs: see Table 9-4
Electrolyte abnormalities: hypokalemia, hypomagnesemia, hypocalcemia
Endocrine disorders: hypothyroidism, hyperparathyroidism, pheochromocytoma, hyperaldosteronism
Cardiac conditions: myocardial ischemia, myocardial infarction, myocarditis, bradyarrhythmia, complete atrioventricular block
Intracranial disorders: subarachnoid hemorrhage, thalamic hematoma, cerebrovascular accident, encephalitis, head injury
Nutritional disorders: anorexia nervosa, starvation, liquid protein diets, gastroplasty and ileojejunal bypass, celiac disease

Source: Adapted from Viskin S, 1999[70] and Khan IA, 2003.[75]

Table 9-4 Drugs associated with known risk of *Torsades de Pointes*

Aclarubicin[a]
Amiodarone
Anagrelide
Arsenic trioxide
Azithromycin
Chloroquine
Chlorpromazine
Cilostazol
Ciprofloxacin
Citalopram
Clarithromycin
Cocaine
Disopyramide
Dofetilide
Domperidone[a]
Donepezil
Dronedarone
Droperidol
Erythromycin
Escitalopram
Flecainide
Fluconazole
Halofantrine[a]
Haloperidol
Ibogaine[a]
Ibutilide
Levofloxacin
Levomepromazine[a]
Levosulpiride[a]
Methadone
Moxifloxacin
Ondansetron
Oxaliplatin
Papaverine
Pentamidine
Pimozide
Procainamide
Propofol
Quinidine
Roxithromycin[a]
Sevoflurane
Sotalol
Sulpiride[a]
Sultopride[a]
Terlipressin[a]
Terodiline[a]
Thioridazine
Vandetanib

Source: Adapted from www.CredibleMeds.org, 2018.[76]
[a]Available outside of the U.S. market.

which is commonly used as an alternative therapy for various types of malignancies and which also has been associated with *torsades de pointes*.[82]

After initiation of a medication that affects the QT interval, a prolongation of the QTc interval of more than 25% from the baseline or a QTc interval longer than 500 milliseconds increases the risk of precipitating drug-induced *torsades de pointes*, regardless of the specific agent.[83,84] One exception is amiodarone, which routinely prolongs the QT interval to more than 500 milliseconds but rarely causes *torsades de pointes*.[85] Overall, more than 90% of drug-induced *torsades de pointes* occurs when the QTc interval exceeds 500 milliseconds.[86]

Because of individual variability, it is often difficult to predict the QT response to a patient's medications.[87] However, a number of risk factors for the development of drug-induced *torsades de pointes* have been recognized. These include congenital long QT syndromes, female gender, electrolyte abnormalities such as hypokalemia and hypomagnesemia, diuretic use, bradycardia, cardiac hypertrophy, congestive heart failure, renal and liver insufficiency, coadministration of drugs blocking P-450 isoenzyme CYP3A4, and baseline ECG abnormalities.[86]

In clinical practice, physicians prescribing noncardiac medications that prolong the QT interval face a challenging dilemma because although the odds of unintentionally provoking arrhythmias relating to long QT syndrome with noncardiac drugs are small, the risk of sudden unexpected death remains. Most clinicians follow the serial QT interval and electrolytes and minimize concurrent offending agents. While prescribing any agents that prolong the QT interval, it is important to look at the age, sex, and associated conditions because almost all patients in whom *torsades de pointes* develops in association with the use of noncardiac drugs have at least one additional risk factor, and 72% have two risk factors, which can be easily identified before administration of the culprit drug is initiated.[88]

The second question that physicians face is to how long one should follow these patients. Short term follow up may not be sufficient, as only 18% of these patients develop arrhythmias within 72 hours of the onset of oral therapy; 42% of arrhythmias occurred between 3 and 30 days, and 40% occurred more than 1 month after the onset of oral therapy.[88] Elderly women, persons with advanced heart disease, patients receiving other drugs that prolong the QT interval directly or indirectly (e.g., diuretics that cause hypokalemia), patients with a family history of sudden death, and patients with a complex medical regimen are all at increased risk. Certain drugs frequently interfere with hepatic metabolism and thus should be a cause for special concern; examples include erythromycin, clarithromycin, ketoconazole, itraconazole, amiodarone, and many antidepressants and antiretroviral agents.[89]

If therapy with a drug that has QT interval–prolonging potential is started, patients should be warned to report promptly any symptoms, such as new palpitations and near-syncope or syncope, as well as concurrent conditions or therapies that can cause hypokalemia (e.g., gastroenteritis or the addition of a diuretic to the patient's regimen). Routine ECG examination during treatment to detect asymptomatic prolongation of the QT interval may be considered in such high-risk situations, and in some instances, the offending agent can be replaced. Specific monitoring guidelines exist for arsenic trioxide.[90]

Treatment of *torsades de pointes* differs from that of VT or ventricular fibrillation in general; its unique mechanism allows for some specific targeted interventions. The usual strategies for acute management of *torsades de pointes* include defibrillation, magnesium, and increasing heart rate. These and other strategies are discussed briefly.

Magnesium is the drug of choice for suppressing ectopic beats and terminating *torsades de pointes*, even in patients with normal magnesium levels.[91] Magnesium can be given in a dose of 2 g IV initially over 30 to 60 seconds, which then can be repeated twice at 5- to 15-minute intervals.[70] Rapidly infused magnesium can be followed by a continuous infusion. Magnesium therapy does not affect the QTc interval and is not effective in the long-term management of this syndrome.

Acceleration of the heart rate can also be effective in treating recurrent *torsades de pointes* and may be achieved by using beta1-adrenergic agonists, such as isoproterenol, or with overdrive electrical pacing. Isoproterenol can be considered when *torsades de pointes* is caused by acquired long QT syndrome, there is underlying bradycardia, *torsades de pointes* is pause dependent, and cardiac pacing cannot be started immediately.[70] It should be avoided in patients with hypertension and ischemic heart disease. It should be administered as a continuous IV infusion to keep the heart rate faster than 90 bpm until overdrive pacing can be started. It should be emphasized that the therapeutic window of isoproterenol is very narrow, and its administration can often provoke arrhythmias even more severe than the initial indication.

Temporary cardiac pacing can also be effective in terminating *torsades de pointes* by increasing the heart rate, shortening the QT interval, and suppressing ectopy. Initially, a higher heart rate (100–140 bpm) may be needed to prevent *torsades de pointes*. Once the arrhythmia has been controlled, the pacing rate should be decreased to the lowest rate that prevents ventricular ectopy.

Long term treatment of acquired long QT syndrome usually is not required because the QT interval returns to normal once the inciting factor or predisposing condition has been corrected. Future administration of agents that prolong the QT interval should be avoided. In those patients in whom bradycardia, pause, or AV block was the precipitating event, a permanent pacemaker can be considered. In the absence of structural heart disease, acquired long QT syndrome is usually reversible and thus carries a good prognosis.

BRADYARRHYTHMIAS

Bradyarrhythmias generally fall under one of two mechanistic categories: disease intrinsic to the conduction system of the heart (i.e., primary dysrhythmia) and reflex-mediated disease (secondary). Both are important causes of symptoms in cancer patients and are considered below.

The conduction system of the heart can be interrupted at all levels by primary and metastatic tumors or by infiltrative processes such as amyloidosis. Among the most common sites of involvement are the sinus node, the AV node, and the infranodal conduction bundles; disruption at any of these sites may lead to significant bradycardia.

■ Sinus Node Dysfunction

Sinus node dysfunction encompasses a number of arrhythmias caused by abnormalities of this structure, including sinus bradycardia, sinus arrest, sinoatrial exit block, and the tachycardia-bradycardia syndrome. When these entities are associated with symptoms such as dizziness, fatigue, mental status changes, heart failure, or syncope, the sick sinus syndrome is said to exist. The sinus node undergoes gradual degenerative changes, and sinus node dysfunction is thus found more frequently in the elderly population. Among the specific tumors associated with sick sinus syndrome are cardiac involvement by lymphoma,[92] rhabdomyoma,[93] and other right atrial mass lesions. Radiation and infiltrative disease such as amyloidosis can also involve the sinus node.

Sinus bradycardia is defined by a heart rate less than 60 bpm, with each QRS complex preceded by a P wave of normal morphology. When symptoms of presyncope or syncope are present and if they can be correlated to the bradycardia, evaluation and treatment are warranted. The sinus node can be affected by increased vagal tone, metabolic abnormalities, drugs, or direct alteration of the sinus node. In cancer patients, sinus bradycardia has been associated with several antineoplastic medications, such as cisplatin, paclitaxel, irinotecan, mitoxatrone, octreotide, and thalidomide. Ethanol injection for hepatocellular carcinoma often causes sinus bradycardia and AV block but rarely results in significant symptomatology.[94] Pheochromocytoma can cause

bradycardia in approximately 10% of cases as a reflex response to the episodic hypertension.[95] One case of sinoatrial block temporally related epirubicin administration has been reported[96]; if a causal relationship exists, it is very rare.

Treatment of sinus bradycardia is rarely indicated. If the symptoms necessitate treatment, however, acute treatment involves atropine, ephedrine, theophylline, or temporary pacing. Removal of offending agents should be carried out when reasonable, but major restructuring of anticancer treatment plans is not usually required. Long-term treatment includes a permanent pacemaker, but, again, only when symptoms are present and attributable to the bradycardia is this indicated and only if the underlying cause is not likely to be reversible.

Tachycardia-bradycardia syndrome is a common form of sinus node dysfunction. Paroxysms of atrial fibrillation or flutter are interspersed with sinus arrest or sinus bradycardia, with junctional or ventricular escape beats possible. The most common scenario is a transient symptomatic bradycardia immediately following spontaneous conversion of an atrial tachyarrhythmia. AV nodal blocking agents used to control heart rate during the tachyarrhythmia invariably worsen the severity of the bradyarrhythmic episodes, making treatment without a permanent pacemaker quite challenging. Since the risk factors include age and the presence of atrial fibrillation or flutter, this entity is found coincidentally more often in cancer patients. Chest radiation has also been implicated as a rare cause of tachycardia-bradycardia syndrome, presumably related to direct damage to the sinus node.[97]

■ AV Block

AV block describes an abnormal conduction between the atria and the ventricles. In addition to block at the AV node proper, lesions can occur distally along the conduction system at the His bundle or the bundle branches.

In first-degree AV block, conduction between the atria and ventricles is delayed, but all impulses are conducted. The ECG manifestation is a prolongation of the PR interval. The lesion is usually located at the AV node, and the normal narrow-complex QRS is then preserved. The slight dyssynchrony of the atrial and ventricular contractions is rarely enough to cause symptoms. The rhythm is benign, and no treatment is warranted.

Second-degree AV block is characterized by intermittent nonconducted beats. These dropped beats can be seemingly random or can occur in regular patterns, resulting in grouped beating. Second-degree AV block is divided into two subgroups, Mobitz type I and type II, which have important clinical distinctions. Mobitz type I is also known as Wenckebach phenomenon. In type I block, the AV node is unable to process the impulses presented to it, resulting in progressive prolongation of the PR interval and dropped beats. In type II block, the PR interval remains constant prior to the dropped beat. Because type I block is usually located within the AV node, the QRS complexes are often narrow. Type II block is almost always more distal, occurring in the His-Purkinje system, and is often associated with a bundle branch block and hence a wide QRS complex. Type I AV block is considered benign and does not usually progress to complete heart block. Treatment with a pacemaker is generally not indicated. Type II block, on the other hand, is associated with progression to advanced AV block, potentially resulting in syncope or sudden death. A permanent pacemaker is therefore warranted. When a fixed 2:1 block exists, it is impossible to distinguish type I and II block from the surface ECG, although the QRS interval duration can be suggestive.

Third-degree AV block, also known as complete heart block, occurs when none of the atrial impulses are able to conduct to the ventricles. The rate of the escape mechanism is dependent on the level of the block, with more distal disease associated with slower escape rhythms. AV dissociation is present. If the escape rhythm is fast enough, patients can occasionally be asymptomatic, but most patients present with profound fatigue, decreased exercise capacity, congestive heart failure, lightheadedness, syncope, or sudden cardiac death. Acute treatment includes a temporary pacemaker, although medications such as atropine may be used temporarily. Isoproterenol, under extremely careful monitoring, can also be effective for short periods of time. A permanent pacemaker is almost uniformly indicated for the acquired forms of third-degree heart block.

AV block is a common cause of arrhythmia in cancer patients. Intracardiac tumors, especially lymphoma, are frequently associated with AV block. Primary cystic tumors of the AV nodal region itself have been described[98,99] and are not surprisingly associated with AV block. Treatment of cardiac tumors with chemotherapy or surgery can result in recovery of normal cardiac conduction. Pheochromocytoma[100] and thymoma[101] have included AV block as part of their systemic manifestations. High-dose chemotherapy and stem cell transplantation can also induce AV block,[54] presumably through increased vagal tone. Individual chemotherapy agents associated with transient AV block include paclitaxel[77] and octreotide.[102] Amongst newer therapies, the immune

checkpoint inhibitors (ICI) have been associated with brady-arrhythmias, ranging from asymptomatic PR prolongation to the development of complete heart block which frequently requires cardiac pacing.[64] Of note, in our institutional experience, due to the significant myocardial inflammation associated with ICI, transvenous right ventricular pacing may be associated with failure to capture or capture at higher thresholds and thus, may present some unique challenges to delivering pacing in this population.

▪ Reflex-Mediated Bradycardia

In addition to the intrinsic pacemakers of the cardiac conduction system, heart rate is influenced by sympathetic and parasympathetic tone. As discussed above, increased catecholamine states can lead to sinus tachycardia and various atrial and ventricular tachyarrhythmias. This is achieved not only through circulating factors but also via activation of the sympathetic cardiac nerves. Conversely, parasympathetic activity via the vagus nerve will slow the heart rate by decreasing the automaticity of the pacemaker cells. In pathologic states, excess vagal tone can lead to inappropriate sinus bradycardia or sinus arrest and result in symptoms. Parasympathetic tone also decreases the conduction velocity throughout the cardiac conduction system. This is especially evident at the AV node; thus, AV block is another potential manifestation of a pathologic increase in vagal tone. In addition to affecting heart rate and cardiac conduction velocity, vagal tone also reduces systemic blood pressure.

The vagus nerve serves as the efferent limb of several different reflex arcs that involve the heart. One of the best known and clinically most important of such reflexes involves the carotid sinus baroreceptors. These receptors, located at the bifurcation of the common carotid arteries, respond to stretching of the tissue, which usually occurs in the setting of increased blood pressure. Afferent fibers contained in the glossopharyngeal nerve arrive at the dorsal vagal nucleus in the medulla, where the vagus nerve is activated, reducing heart rate and blood pressure. In carotid sinus hypersensitivity, inappropriate triggering of the baroreceptors results in symptomatic bradycardia, hypotension, or both.

Cancer patients can suffer from carotid sinus hypersensitivity when masses impinge on this structure or any other component of the reflex arc. Bradycardia-related syncope is sometimes the presenting symptom of neck masses. More commonly, however, bradyarrhythmias complicate surgical resection or other manipulation of the tumor, including radiation.[103] Carotid sinus hypersensitivity has been

TABLE 9-5 Recommendations for CIED management of patients undergoing radiation therapy

RECOMMENDATIONS:
• Avoid placing CIEDs in the field of therapy
• Inform patients of possible device malfunction prior to administration of RT
• Review manufacturer recommendations for CIED exposure to radiation
• Estimate radiation dose to the CIED; avoid neutron producing or high energy (>10 MV) photon beams
• Avoid cumulative dose of >10 Gy, consider device repositioning if risks acceptable.
• Furthermore, absorbed dose to PPM should be limited to ≤ 2 Gy, and ≤ 0.5-1 Gy to ICDs
• Consider telemetry and pulse oximetry at least for the first session. These should be considered for each session in high risk patients (with >10 Gy cumulative dose).
• Consider placing magnet during RT for ICDs to suspend tachycardia therapies.
• Depending on risk (cumulative RT dose, patient dependency, rhythm abnormalities seen), individualized schedules should be made for device interrogation after the therapy. Consideration should be given for device interrogation within 24 hours for high risk patients.
• Use of shielding to protect should be discussed with Radiation Oncology, with the caveat that it was not effective in some trials, though is still recommended by some device manufacturers.

CIED, Cardiac implantable Electronic devices; Gy, Gray; ICD, Implantable cardiac defibrillator; MV, megavolts; PPM, permanent pacemaker; RT, radiation therapy.

associated with a variety of mass lesions in this area, including carcinomas of the head and neck, lymphomas, neurofibromatosis, carotid body tumors, and metastatic disease (usually to the cervical lymph nodes). Less commonly, other components of the reflex arc have been implicated, such as involvement of the glossopharyngeal nerve, medulla, and vagus nerve itself.[103]

A variation of carotid sinus hypersensitivity is the Cushing reflex. In response to head trauma, neurosurgery, or a generalized increase in intracranial pressure, systemic blood pressure is increased to maintain cerebral perfusion pressure. This increase in blood pressure can then result in reflex bradycardia via activation of the carotid sinus or other baroreceptors. Any intracranial mass or resection thereof can result in bradycardia. A similar physiology is involved with the oculocardiac reflex, as illustrated by a case of an orbital mass presenting with bradycardia.[104] Corticosteroids given in the perioperative setting have been shown to reduce the incidence of bradycardia and hemodynamic instability associated with neurosurgery.[105]

Separate from the carotid sinus pathway is the trigeminocardiac reflex, in which stimulation of the trigeminal nerve can result in hypotension and bradycardia. The efferent limb is again mediated by the vagus nerve. Several cases of intraoperative bradycardia or asystole have been reported involving resection of tumors associated with the trigeminal nerve.[106,107]

Lastly, although not technically a reflex, is the abnormal stimulation of the vagus nerve by seizure activity. Intracranial neoplasms often present with seizure activity, and specific areas localized to the temporal lobes can result in ictal bradyarrhythmias.[108,109]

Reflex-mediated bradycardias should be considered in the differential diagnosis of syncope in the cancer patient. Even when a strong suspicion for vagally mediated syncope is present, careful evaluation is needed to determine whether symptoms are due to the cardioinhibitory or vasodepressor component of the reflex because the treatments are different. In the acute setting, atropine or sympathomimetics can reverse vagally induced bradycardia. Preventive measures such as temporary pacing or glucocorticoid administration can be taken prior to surgery when a high risk of bradycardia is thought to exist. Treatment of the underlying cause can be curative. In some instances, if a clear causal relationship exists between bradycardia and syncope and if the cause is not reversible, permanent pacing is indicated. Atrial pacing alone is not appropriate for this indication because reflex bradycardia can involve some degree of AV block as well. It should be emphasized that these reflexes also produce hypotension, and correction of the heart rate alone with a pacemaker may not eliminate syncopal symptoms if a substantial vasodepressor component exists.

CARDIAC IMPLANTABLE ELECTRONIC DEVICES

Cardiac Implantable Electronic Devices (CIEDs), which include permanent pacemakers (PPMs), Implantable Cardiac Defibrillators (ICDs) and Cardiac

Resynchronization Therapy devices without or with defibrillation (CRT-P/CRT-D) are used to treat several rhythm disorders. Implantable cardiac defibrillators (ICDs) are used for primary and secondary prevention of ventricular arrhythmias in a variety of settings. Given studies that have shown a mortality benefit of ICDs as primary prevention in patients with ischemic and non-ischemic cardiomyopathies[110,111] and the expanded indications for ICD placement under the Centers for Medicare and Medicaid Services, we are currently experiencing an explosion in the numbers of devices being used. Formal recommendations regarding the indications for these devices can be found among the American Heart Association–American College of Cardiology guidelines and are not reviewed here.[112] ICDs have been used successfully to prevent recurrent ventricular arrhythmias in patients with cardiac tumors, such as rhabdomyoma or lipoma.[47,52] Although, in general, the same guidelines apply to CIED use in cancer patients, a few additional comments should be made.

First, studies involving ICDs for primary arrhythmia prevention in cardiomyopathy failed to show a mortality benefit for those patients in class IV congestive heart failure. One of the reasons for this was felt to be the extremely poor overall prognosis in this population, who are just as likely to die from congestive heart failure and comorbid conditions as they are from arrhythmia. This line of reasoning can be applied to patients with malignancies; even if patients are otherwise candidates for ICD therapy, a life expectancy of less than 1 year owing to their malignancy makes them unlikely to achieve a mortality benefit from such a device. Even when life expectancy exceeds 1 year, but the patient still carries a terminal diagnosis, ICDs cannot be expected to significantly affect quality-adjusted life years and thus are rarely offered to such patients in practice. These considerations, however, can be revisited for CRT-P devices. Second, several cancer treatments can cause reduced left ventricular function that is reversible.[113] Although it may be appropriate to consider ICD therapy in someone with severe progressive left ventricular dysfunction several years after anthracycline therapy, caution must be undertaken when dealing with potentially reversible decreases in left ventricular function. Third, ICD placement can interfere with the diagnosis and treatment of malignancy and vice versa. The inability to undergo magnetic resonance imaging studies is particularly relevant in this population. Special precautions with respect to electrocautery need to be undertaken during surgery in patients with devices. Lastly, patients with ICDs who progress to the terminal phase of their malignancies should have their device therapies inactivated as they enter comfort care.[114]

Radiation therapy can damage CIEDs, particularly beyond a certain cumulative dose; especially if the device is in the direct radiation field.[115–117] Common CIEDs failure described in literature can range from a temporary change in the sensing thresholds or pacing rates to rare permanent damage, battery depletion or loss of capture for the device.[118] Most patients; however, tolerate radiation therapy well with transient device dysfunction detected only in a minority of patients, especially with neutron producing radiation therapy.[119,120] Recommendations and guidelines vary for radiation therapy delivery in patients with CIEDs[119–124] and these are summarized in Table 9-5. Furthermore, previous chest radiation can pose challenging access issues if an ICD is later required.

REFERENCES

1. Chung MK, Martin DO, Sprecher D, et al. C-reactive protein elevation in patients with atrial arrhythmias: inflammatory mechanisms and persistence of atrial fibrillation. *Circulation*. 2001;104(24):2886–2891.
2. Guzzetti S, Costantino G, Fundarò C. Systemic inflammation, atrial fibrillation, and cancer. *Circulation*. 2002;106(9):e40; author reply e40.
3. Hidalgo JD, Krone R, Rich MW, et al. Supraventricular tachyarrhythmias after hematopoietic stem cell transplantation: incidence, risk factors and outcomes. *Bone Marrow Transplant*. 2004;34(7):615–619.
4. Alexandre J, Moslehi JJ, Bersell KR, Funck-Brentano C, Roden DM, Salem J-E. Anticancer drug-induced cardiac rhythm disorders: current knowledge and basic underlying mechanisms. *Pharmacol Ther*. 2018;189:89–103.
5. Thorp BC, Badoux X. Atrial fibrillation as a complication of ibrutinib therapy: clinical features and challenges of management. *Leuk Lymphoma*. 2018;59(2):311–320.
6. Dimopoulos MA, Tedeschi A, Trotman J, et al. Phase 3 Trial of Ibrutinib plus Rituximab in Waldenström's Macroglobulinemia. *N Engl J Med*. 2018;378(25):2399–2410.
7. Thompson PA, Lévy V, Tam CS, et al. Atrial fibrillation in CLL patients treated with ibrutinib. An international retrospective study. *Br J Haematol*. 2016;175(3):462–466.
8. Singla A, Hogan WJ, Ansell SM, et al. Incidence of supraventricular arrhythmias during autologous peripheral blood stem cell transplantation. *Biol Blood Marrow Transplant*. 2013;19(8):1233–1237.
9. Jhingran A, Eifel PJ. Perioperative and postoperative complications of intracavitary radiation for FIGO stage I-III carcinoma of the cervix. *Int J Radiat Oncol Biol Phys*. 2000;46(5):1177–1183.
10. Shalaby AA, Rhee J, McBride D, Kart B. Mediastinal carcinoma invading the left inferior pulmonary vein and presenting as refractory atrial arrhythmia. *Pacing Clin Electrophysiol*. 2002;25(8):1280–1281.
11. Hancock EW. Atrial flutter in a man with mediastinal cancer. *Hosp Pract (1995)*. 1996;31(1):15–16, 20.

12. Murthy SC, Law S, Whooley BP, Alexandrou A, Chu K-M, Wong J. Atrial fibrillation after esophagectomy is a marker for postoperative morbidity and mortality. *J Thorac Cardiovasc Surg*. 2003;126(4):1162–1167.

13. Sekine Y, Kesler KA, Behnia M, Brooks-Brunn J, Sekine E, Brown JW. COPD may increase the incidence of refractory supraventricular arrhythmias following pulmonary resection for non-small cell lung cancer. *Chest*. 2001;120(6):1783–1790.

14. Amar D, Roistacher N, Burt ME, et al. Effects of diltiazem versus digoxin on dysrhythmias and cardiac function after pneumonectomy. *Ann Thorac Surg*. 1997;63(5):1374–1381; discussion 1381–1382.

15. Joo JB, DeBord JR, Montgomery CE, et al. Perioperative factors as predictors of operative mortality and morbidity in pneumonectomy. *Am Surg*. 2001;67(4):318–321; discussion 321–322.

16. Cardinale D, Martinoni A, Cipolla CM, et al. Atrial fibrillation after operation for lung cancer: clinical and prognostic significance. *Ann Thorac Surg*. 1999;68(5): 1827–1831.

17. Barbetakis N, Vassiliadis M. Is amiodarone a safe antiarrhythmic to use in supraventricular tachyarrhythmias after lung cancer surgery? *BMC Surg*. 2004;4:7.

18. Ciriaco P, Mazzone P, Canneto B, Zannini P. Supraventricular arrhythmia following lung resection for non-small cell lung cancer and its treatment with amiodarone. *Eur J Cardiothorac Surg*. 2000;18(1):12–16.

19. Handschin AE, Lardinois D, Schneiter D, Bloch K, Weder W. Acute amiodarone-induced pulmonary toxicity following lung resection. *Respiration*. 2003;70(3):310–312.

20. Wu CT, Chen MR, Hou SH. Neonatal tuberous sclerosis with cardiac rhabdomyomas presenting as fetal supraventricular tachycardia. *Jpn Heart J*. 1997;38(1):133–137.

21. Bosi G, Lintermans JP, Pellegrino PA, Svaluto-Moreolo G, Vliers A. The natural history of cardiac rhabdomyoma with and without tuberous sclerosis. *Acta Paediatr*. 1996;85(8):928–931.

22. Van Hare GF, Phoon CK, Munkenbeck F, Patel CR, Fink DL, Silverman NH. Electrophysiologic study and radiofrequency ablation in patients with intracardiac tumors and accessory pathways: is the tumor the pathway? *J Cardiovasc Electrophysiol*. 1996;7(12):1204–1210.

23. Gehrmann J, Kehl HG, Diallo R, Debus V, Vogt J. Cardiac leiomyosarcoma of the right atrium in a teenager: unusual manifestation with a lifetime history of atrial ectopic tachycardia. *Pacing Clin Electrophysiol*. 2001;24(7):1161–1164.

24. Müller L, Kramm CM, Lawrenz W, Schmidt KG, Wessalowski R. Recurrent atrial ectopic tachycardia following chemotherapy with ifosfamide. *Pediatr Hematol Oncol*. 2004;21(4):307–311.

25. Isbell DC, Dent JM. The role of transesophageal echocardiography in atrial fibrillation. *Cardiol Clin*. 2004;22(1):113–126, ix.

26. Wyse DG, Waldo AL, DiMarco JP, et al. A comparison of rate control and rhythm control in patients with atrial fibrillation. *N Engl J Med*. 2002;347(23):1825–1833.

27. Link MS, Berkow LC, Kudenchuk PJ, et al. Part 7: adult advanced cardiovascular life support: 2015 American Heart Association guidelines update for cardiopulmonary resuscitation and emergency cardiovascular care. *Circulation*. 2015;132(18 suppl. 2):S444–S4464.

28. The SPAF III Writing Committee for the Stroke Prevention in Atrial Fibrillation Investigators. Patients with nonvalvular atrial fibrillation at low risk of stroke during treatment with aspirin: Stroke Prevention in Atrial Fibrillation III Study. The SPAF III Writing Committee for the Stroke Prevention in Atrial Fibrillation Investigators. *JAMA*. 1998;279(16):1273–1277.

29. January CT, Wann LS, Alpert JS, et al. 2014 AHA/ACC/ HRS guideline for the management of patients with atrial fibrillation: a report of the American College of Cardiology/American Heart Association Task Force on practice guidelines and the Heart Rhythm Society. *J Am Coll Cardiol*. 2014;64(21):e1–e76.

30. Zamorano JL, Lancellotti P, Rodriguez Muñoz D, et al. 2016 ESC Position Paper on cancer treatments and cardiovascular toxicity developed under the auspices of the ESC Committee for Practice Guidelines: The Task Force for cancer treatments and cardiovascular toxicity of the European Society of Cardiology (ESC). *Eur Heart J*. 2016;37(36):2768–2801.

31. D'Souza M, Carlson N, Fosbøl E, et al. CHA2DS2-VASc score and risk of thromboembolism and bleeding in patients with atrial fibrillation and recent cancer. *Eur J Prev Cardiol*. 2018;25(6):651–658.

32. Hu W-S, Lin C-L. Impact of atrial fibrillation on the development of ischemic stroke among cancer patients classified by CHA2DS2-VASc score-a nationwide cohort study. *Oncotarget*. 2018;9(7):7623–7630.

33. Steffel J, Verhamme P, Potpara TS, et al. The 2018 European Heart Rhythm Association Practical Guide on the use of non-vitamin K antagonist oral anticoagulants in patients with atrial fibrillation. *Eur Heart J*. 2018;39(16):1330–1393.

34. Raskob GE, van Es N, Verhamme P, et al. Edoxaban for the treatment of cancer-associated venous thromboembolism. *N Engl J Med*. 2018;378(7):615–624.

35. Melloni C, Dunning A, Granger CB, et al. Efficacy and safety of apixaban versus warfarin in patients with atrial fibrillation and a history of cancer: insights from the ARISTOTLE trial. *Am J Med*. 2017;130(12):1440–1448.e1.

36. Laube ES, Yu A, Gupta D, et al. Rivaroxaban for stroke prevention in patients with nonvalvular atrial fibrillation and active cancer. *Am J Cardiol*. 2017;120(2):213–217.

37. Bansilal S, Bloomgarden Z, Halperin JL, et al. Efficacy and safety of rivaroxaban in patients with diabetes and nonvalvular atrial fibrillation: the Rivaroxaban Once-daily, Oral, Direct Factor Xa Inhibition Compared with Vitamin K Antagonism for Prevention of Stroke and Embolism Trial in Atrial Fibrillation (ROCKET AF Trial). *Am Heart J*. 2015;170(4):675–682.e8.

38. Klein AL, Grimm RA, Murray RD, et al. Use of transesophageal echocardiography to guide cardioversion in patients with atrial fibrillation. *N Engl J Med*. 2001;344(19):1411–1420.

39. Caffrey SL, Willoughby PJ, Pepe PE, Becker LB. Public use of automated external defibrillators. *N Engl J Med*. 2002;347(16):1242–1247.

40. Brugada P, Brugada J, Mont L, Smeets J, Andries EW. A new approach to the differential diagnosis of a regular tachycardia with a wide QRS complex. *Circulation*. 1991;83(5):1649–1659.

41. Cairns JA, Connolly SJ, Roberts R, Gent M. Randomised trial of outcome after myocardial infarction in patients with frequent or repetitive ventricular premature depolarisations: CAMIAT. Canadian Amiodarone Myocardial Infarction Arrhythmia Trial Investigators. *Lancet*. 1997;349(9053):675–682.

42. Echt DS, Liebson PR, Mitchell LB, et al. Mortality and morbidity in patients receiving encainide, flecainide, or placebo. The Cardiac Arrhythmia Suppression Trial. *N Engl J Med*. 1991;324(12):781–788.

43. Buxton AE, Lee KL, Fisher JD, Josephson ME, Prystowsky EN, Hafley G. A randomized study of the prevention of sudden death in patients with coronary artery disease. Multicenter Unsustained Tachycardia Trial Investigators. *N Engl J Med*. 1999;341(25):1882–1890.

44. Hogarth AJ, Bebb OJ, Graham LN. A case of malignant arrhythmia. *Heart*. 2012;98(20):1539.

45. Ray S, Stacey R, Imrie M, Filshie J. A review of 560 Hickman catheter insertions. *Anaesthesia*. 1996;51(10): 981–985.

46. Manojkumar R, Sharma A, Grover A. Secondary lymphoma of the heart presenting as recurrent syncope. *Indian Heart J*. 2001;53(2):221–223.

47. Chen HM, Chiu CC, Lee CS, Lai WD, Lin YT. Intractable ventricular tachycardia in a patient with left ventricular epicardial lipoma. *J Formos Med Assoc*. 2001;100(5):339–342.

48. Khan A, Dewhurst N. Use of sympathomimetic nasal spray in association with cardiac fibroma: an unusual cause of ventricular tachycardia. *Br J Clin Pract*. 1997;51(3):192–193.

49. Enbergs A, Borggrefe M, Kurlemann G, et al. Ventricular tachycardia caused by cardiac rhabdomyoma in a young adult with tuberous sclerosis. *Am Heart J*. 1996;132(6):1263–1265.

50. Greenberg HM, Aretz HT. Case records of the Massachusetts General Hospital. Weekly clinicopathological exercises. Case 31-1999. A 33-year-old man with wide-complex tachycardia and a left ventricular mass. *N Engl J Med*. 1999;341(16):1217–1224.

51. Leak D. Amiodarone for control of recurrent ventricular tachycardia secondary to cardiac metastasis. *Tex Heart Inst J*. 1998;25(3):198–200.

52. Thøgersen AM, Helvind M, Jensen T, Andersen JH, Jacobsen JR, Chen X. Implantable cardioverter defibrillator in a 4-month-old infant with cardiac arrest associated with a vascular heart tumor. *Pacing Clin Electrophysiol*. 2001;24(11):1699–1700.

53. Gautam PL, Kathuria S, Sood D, Kaul TJK. Recurrent positional ventricular tachycardia in a patient with carcinoma of the oesophagus. *Anaesthesia*. 2003; 58(1):98.

54. Ando M, Yokozawa T, Sawada J, et al. Cardiac conduction abnormalities in patients with breast cancer undergoing high-dose chemotherapy and stem cell transplantation. *Bone Marrow Transplant*. 2000;25(2):185–189.

55. Gupta M, Thaler HT, Friedman D, Steinherz L. Presence of prolonged dispersion of qt intervals in late survivors of childhood anthracycline therapy. *Pediatr Hematol Oncol*. 2002;19(8):533–542.

56. Lenihan DJ, Alencar AJ, Yang D, Kurzrock R, Keating MJ, Duvic M. Cardiac toxicity of alemtuzumab in patients with mycosis fungoides/Sézary syndrome. *Blood*. 2004;104(3):655–658.

57. Oleksowicz L, Escott P, Leichman GC, Spangenthal E. Sustained ventricular tachycardia and its successful prophylaxis during high-dose bolus interleukin-2 therapy for metastatic renal cell carcinoma. *Am J Clin Oncol*. 2000;23(1):34–36.

58. Tomcsányi J, Nényei Z, Mátrai Z, Bózsik B. Ibrutinib, an approved tyrosine kinase inhibitor as a potential cause of recurrent polymorphic ventricular tachycardia. *JACC Clin Electrophysiol*. 2016;2(7):847–849.

59. Beyer A, Ganti B, Majkrzak A, Theyyunni N. A perfect storm: tyrosine kinase inhibitor-associated polymorphic ventricular tachycardia. *J Emerg Med*. 2017;52(4):e123–e127.

60. Cheong MA, Kim YC, Park HK, et al. Paroxysmal tachycardia and hypertension with or without ventricular fibrillation during laparoscopic adrenalectomy: two case reports in patients with noncatecholamine-secreting adrenocortical adenomas. *J Laparoendosc Adv Surg Tech A*. 1999;9(3):277–281.

61. Khan HA, Ahmad I, Ahmed W. Ventricular fibrillation after insertion of a self-expanding metallic stent for malignant dysphagia. *Am J Gastroenterol*. 2000;95(3):827.

62. Johnson DB, Balko JM, Compton ML, et al. Fulminant myocarditis with combination immune checkpoint blockade. *N Engl J Med*. 2016;375(18):1749–1755.

63. Reddy N, Moudgil R, Lopez-Mattei JC, et al. Progressive and reversible conduction disease with checkpoint inhibitors. *Can J Cardiol*. 2017;33(10):1335.e13–1335.e15.

64. Mahmood SS, Fradley MG, Cohen JV, et al. Myocarditis in patients treated with immune checkpoint inhibitors. *J Am Coll Cardiol*. 2018;71(16):1755–1764.

65. Andrews A. Treating with checkpoint inhibitors-figure $1 million per patient. *Am Health Drug Benefits*. 2015;8(Spec Issue):9.

66. Krasuski RA, Hesselson AB, Landolfo KP, Ellington KJ, Bashore TM. Cardiac rhabdomyoma in an adult patient presenting with ventricular arrhythmia. *Chest*. 2000;118(4):1217–1221.

67. Miyashita T, Miyazawa I, Kawaguchi T, et al. A case of primary cardiac B cell lymphoma associated with ventricular tachycardia, successfully treated with systemic chemotherapy and radiotherapy: a long-term survival case. *Jpn Circ J*. 2000;64(2):135–138.

68. Li W-M, Huang C-H, Su C-M, Chai C-Y, Wu W-J, Chou Y-H. Extra-adrenal pheochromocytoma presenting with life-threatening ventricular tachycardia: a case report. *Kaohsiung J Med Sci*. 2004;20(12):612–615.

69. Petit T, de Lagausie P, Maintenant J, Magnier S, Nivoche Y, Aigrain Y. Thoracic pheochromocytoma revealed by ventricular tachycardia. Clinical case and review of the literature. *Eur J Pediatr Surg*. 2000;10(2):142–144.

70. Viskin S. Long QT syndromes and torsade de pointes. *Lancet*. 1999;354(9190):1625–1633.

71. Kay GN, Plumb VJ, Arciniegas JG, Henthorn RW, Waldo AL. Torsade de pointes: the long-short initiating sequence and other clinical features: observations in 32 patients. *J Am Coll Cardiol*. 1983;2(5):806–817.

72. Leenhardt A, Glaser E, Burguera M, Nürnberg M, Maison-Blanche P, Coumel P. Short-coupled variant of torsade de pointes. A new electrocardiographic entity in the spectrum of idiopathic ventricular tachyarrhythmias. *Circulation*. 1994;89(1):206–215.

73. Committee for Proprietary Medicinal Products. Points to consider: the assessment of the potential for QT interval prolongation by non-cardiovascular medicinal products. *CPMP/986/96 1997*

74. Priori SG, Schwartz PJ, Napolitano C, et al. Risk stratification in the long-QT syndrome. *N Engl J Med*. 2003;348(19):1866–1874.

75. Khan IA. Clinical and therapeutic aspects of congenital and acquired long QT syndrome. *Am J Med*. 2002;112(1):58–66.

76. Woosley R, Heise C, Romero K. www.CredibleMeds.org/research-scientists/, QTdrugs List [Internet]. AZCERT, Inc.; [cited 2018 Jun 20]. *https://crediblemeds.org/*

77. Yeh ETH, Tong AT, Lenihan DJ, et al. Cardiovascular complications of cancer therapy: diagnosis, pathogenesis, and management. *Circulation*. 2004;109(25):3122–3131.

78. Ferrari S, Figus E, Cagnano R, Iantorno D, Bacci G. The role of corrected QT interval in the cardiologic follow-up of young patients treated with Adriamycin. *J Chemother*. 1996;8(3):232–236.

79. Oztop I, Gencer M, Okan T, et al. Evaluation of cardiotoxicity of a combined bolus plus infusional 5-fluorouracil/folinic acid treatment by echocardiography, plasma troponin I level, QT interval and dispersion in patients with gastrointestinal system cancers. *Jpn J Clin Oncol*. 2004;34(5):262–268.

80. Cooney MM, Radivoyevitch T, Dowlati A, et al. Cardiovascular safety profile of combretastatin a4 phosphate in a single-dose phase I study in patients with advanced cancer. *Clin Cancer Res*. 2004;10(1 pt 1): 96–100.

81. Walker G, Wilcock A, Carey AM, Manderson C, Weller R, Crosby V. Prolongation of the QT interval in palliative care patients. *J Pain Symptom Manage*. 2003;26(3):855–859.

82. Saliba W, Erdogan O, Niebauer M. Polymorphic ventricular tachycardia in a woman taking cesium chloride. *Pacing Clin Electrophysiol*. 2001;24(4 pt 1):515–517.

83. Bednar MM, Harrigan EP, Ruskin JN. Torsades de pointes associated with nonantiarrhythmic drugs and observations on gender and QTc. *Am J Cardiol*. 2002;89(11):1316–1319.

84. Makkar RR, Fromm BS, Steinman RT, Meissner MD, Lehmann MH. Female gender as a risk factor for torsades de pointes associated with cardiovascular drugs. *JAMA*. 1993;270(21):2590–2597.

85. Lazzara R. Amiodarone and torsade de pointes. *Ann Intern Med*. 1989;111(7):549–551.

86. Gowda RM, Khan IA, Wilbur SL, Vasavada BC, Sacchi TJ. Torsade de pointes: the clinical considerations. *Int J Cardiol*. 2004;96(1):1–6.

87. Roden DM. Drug-induced prolongation of the QT interval. *N Engl J Med*. 2004;350(10):1013–1022.

88. Zeltser D, Justo D, Halkin A, Prokhorov V, Heller K, Viskin S. Torsade de pointes due to noncardiac drugs: most patients have easily identifiable risk factors. *Medicine (Baltimore)*. 2003;82(4):282–290.

89. Abernethy DR, Flockhart DA. Molecular basis of cardiovascular drug metabolism: implications for predicting clinically important drug interactions. *Circulation*. 2000;101(14):1749–1753.

90. US Food and Drug Administration. *Trisenox - Label [Internet]*. 2018. https://www.accessdata.fda.gov/drugsatfda_docs/label/2018/021248s015lbledt.pdf

91. Tzivoni D, Banai S, Schuger C, et al. Treatment of torsade de pointes with magnesium sulfate. *Circulation*. 1988;77(2):392–397.

92. Suzuki T, Ishibashi S, Qin X, et al. Sick sinus syndrome in association with malignant lymphoma. *Eur Heart J*. 1996;17(6):968.

93. Cowley CG, Tani LY, Judd VE, Shaddy RE. Sinus node dysfunction in tuberous sclerosis. *Pediatr Cardiol*. 1996;17(1):51–52.

94. Ferlitsch A, Kreil A, Bauer E, et al. Bradycardia and sinus arrest during percutaneous ethanol injection therapy for hepatocellular carcinoma. *Eur J Clin Invest*. 2004;34(3):218–223.

95. Schürmeyer TH, Engeroff B, Dralle H, von zur Mühlen A. Cardiological effects of catecholamine-secreting tumours. *Eur J Clin Invest*. 1997;27(3):189–195.

96. Okamoto T, Ogata J, Minami K. Sino-atrial block during anesthesia in a patient with breast cancer being treated with the anticancer drug epirubicin. *Anesth Analg*. 2003;97(1):19–20, table of contents.

97. Watanabe T, Okazaki O, Izumo K, Michihata T, Katagiri T, Harumi K. Brady-tachycardia syndrome after radiotherapy for lung cancer. Assessment by computed tomography and carbon-11 methionine positron emission tomography. *Jpn Heart J*. 1999;40(5):677–681.

98. Paniagua JR, Sadaba JR, Davidson LA, Munsch CM. Cystic tumour of the atrioventricular nodal region: report of a case successfully treated with surgery. *Heart*. 2000;83(4):E6.

99. Declich P, Sironi M, Isimbaldi G, Bana R. Atrioventricular nodal tumor associated with polyendocrine anomalies. *Pathol Res Pract*. 1996;192(1):54–59; discussion 60–61.

100. Paschalis-Purtak K, Puciłowska B, Prejbisz A, Januszewicz A. Cardiac arrests, atrioventricular block, and pheochromocytoma. *Am J Hypertens*. 2004;17(6): 544–545.

101. Pentz WH. Advanced heart block as a manifestation of a paraneoplastic syndrome from malignant thymoma. *Chest*. 1999;116(4):1135–1136.

102. Dilger JA, Rho EH, Que FG, Sprung J. Octreotide-induced bradycardia and heart block during surgical resection of a carcinoid tumor. *Anesth Analg*. 2004;98(2):318–320, table of contents.

103. Hong AM, Pressley L, Stevens GN. Carotid sinus syndrome secondary to head and neck malignancy: case

report and literature review. *Clin Oncol (R Coll Radiol).* 2000;12(6):409–412.

104. Westerling D, Blohmé J, Stigmar G. Orbital mass in a child causing somnolence, nausea and bradycardia. *Can J Anaesth.* 1998;45(8):777–780.

105. Mursch K, Buhre W, Behnke-Mursch J, Markakis E. Peroperative cardiovascular stability during brainstem surgery. The use of high-dose methylprednisolone compared to dexamethasone. A retrospective analysis. *Acta Anaesthesiol Scand.* 2000;44(4):378–382.

106. Schaller B, Probst R, Strebel S, Gratzl O. Trigeminocardiac reflex during surgery in the cerebellopontine angle. *J Neurosurg.* 1999;90(2):215–220.

107. Bauer DF, Youkilis A, Schenck C, Turner CR, Thompson BG. The falcine trigeminocardiac reflex: case report and review of the literature. *Surg Neurol.* 2005;63(2):143–148.

108. van der Sluijs BM, Renier WO, Kappelle AC. Brain tumour as a rare cause of cardiac syncope. *J Neurooncol.* 2004;67(1–2):241–244.

109. Kahane P, Di Leo M, Hoffmann D, Munari C. Ictal bradycardia in a patient with a hypothalamic hamartoma: a stereo-EEG study. *Epilepsia.* 1999;40(4):522–527.

110. Moss AJ, Zareba W, Hall WJ, et al. Prophylactic implantation of a defibrillator in patients with myocardial infarction and reduced ejection fraction. *N Engl J Med.* 2002;346(12):877–883.

111. Bardy GH, Lee KL, Mark DB, et al. Amiodarone or an implantable cardioverter-defibrillator for congestive heart failure. *N Engl J Med.* 2005;352(3):225–237.

112. Epstein AE, DiMarco JP, Ellenbogen KA, et al. ACC/AHA/HRS 2008 Guidelines for Device-Based Therapy of Cardiac Rhythm Abnormalities: a report of the American College of Cardiology/American Heart Association Task Force on Practice Guidelines (Writing Committee to Revise the ACC/AHA/NASPE 2002 Guideline Update for Implantation of Cardiac Pacemakers and Antiarrhythmia Devices) developed in collaboration with the American Association for Thoracic Surgery and Society of Thoracic Surgeons. *J Am Coll Cardiol.* 2008;51(21):e1–e62.

113. Ewer MS, Lippman SM. Type II chemotherapy-related cardiac dysfunction: time to recognize a new entity. *J Clin Oncol.* 2005;23(13):2900–2902.

114. Lampert R, Hayes DL, Annas GJ, et al. HRS Expert Consensus Statement on the Management of Cardiovascular Implantable Electronic Devices (CIEDs) in patients nearing end of life or requesting withdrawal of therapy. *Heart Rhythm.* 2010;7(7):1008–1026.

115. John J, Kaye GC. Shock coil failure secondary to external irradiation in a patient with implantable cardioverter defibrillator. *Pacing Clin Electrophysiol.* 2004;27(5):690–691.

116. Lloyd Jones S, Mason RA. Laser surgery in a patient with Romano-Ward (long QT) syndrome and an automatic implantable cardioverter defibrillator. *Anaesthesia.* 2000;55(4):362–366.

117. Gomez DR, Poenisch F, Pinnix CC, et al. Malfunctions of implantable cardiac devices in patients receiving proton beam therapy: incidence and predictors. *Int J Radiat Oncol Biol Phys.* 2013;87(3):570–575.

118. Viganego F, Singh R, Fradley MG. Arrhythmias and other electrophysiology issues in cancer patients receiving chemotherapy or radiation. *Curr Cardiol Rep.* 2016;18(6):52.

119. Brambatti M, Mathew R, Strang B, et al. Management of patients with implantable cardioverter-defibrillators and pacemakers who require radiation therapy. *Heart Rhythm.* 2015;12(10):2148–2154.

120. Grant JD, Jensen GL, Tang C, et al. Radiotherapy-induced malfunction in contemporary cardiovascular implantable electronic devices: clinical incidence and predictors. *JAMA Oncol.* 2015;1(5):624–632.

121. Hurkmans CW, Knegjens JL, Oei BS, et al. Management of radiation oncology patients with a pacemaker or ICD: a new comprehensive practical guideline in The Netherlands. *Radiat Oncol.* 2012;7:198.

122. Crossley GH, Poole JE, Rozner MA, et al. The Heart Rhythm Society (HRS)/American Society of Anesthesiologists (ASA) Expert Consensus Statement on the perioperative management of patients with implantable defibrillators, pacemakers and arrhythmia monitors: facilities and patient management this document was developed as a joint project with the American Society of Anesthesiologists (ASA), and in collaboration with the American Heart Association (AHA), and the Society of Thoracic Surgeons (STS). *Heart Rhythm.* 2011;8(7):1114–1154.

123. Makkar A, Prisciandaro J, Agarwal S, et al. Effect of radiation therapy on permanent pacemaker and implantable cardioverter-defibrillator function. *Heart Rhythm.* 2012;9(12):1964–1968.

124. Marbach JR, Sontag MR, Van Dyk J, Wolbarst AB. Management of radiation oncology patients with implanted cardiac pacemakers: report of AAPM Task Group No. 34. American Association of Physicists in Medicine. *Med Phys.* 1994;21(1):85–90.

10 Cardiac Ultrasonography, Doppler Imaging, and Related Techniques for Cancer Patients

Jose Banchs ■ *Thomas H. Marwick*

LEFT VENTRICULAR ASSESSMENT WITH TWO-DIMENSIONAL ECHOCARDIOGRAPHY

■ Left Ventricular Dimensions

The use of two-dimensional (2D) echocardiography can yield information about the size of the cardiac chambers, the wall thickness, the left ventricular ejection fraction (LVEF), and regional function. In our laboratories, the protocol for 2D echocardiography follows the recommendations of the American Society of Echocardiography (ASE) guidelines for chamber quantification.[1] We obtain measurements of septal and posterior wall thickness and LV internal dimensions (LVID) by using M-mode and 2D echocardiography. LVID in diastole (LVIDd), LVID in systole (LVIDs), and wall thickness are measured at the LV minor axis, approximately at the tips of the mitral valve leaflet. We conventionally obtain these measurements from the 2D parasternal long-axis view and complement them with motion mode (M-mode) images. M-mode echocardiography yields excellent temporal resolution, but measurements may be erroneous if the absence of an appropriate imaging window leads to off-axis imaging.

■ Calculation of Ejection Fraction and Assessment of Regional Function

The biplane method of disks (modified Simpson rule) is the most commonly used 2D method for evaluating ejection fraction, and the one recommended for routine clinical use by the most recent ASE guidelines. The principle underlying this method is that the total LV volume is calculated by adding the volumes from a column of 20 elliptical disks drawn over the ventricular cavity space. The height of each disk is calculated as a fraction of the LV long axis. The LV long axis used is the longer of the two lengths from the 2- and 4-chamber views (Figure 10-1). The cross-sectional area of the disk is based on the two diameters obtained from the 2- and 4-chamber views. When two adequate orthogonal views are not available, a single plane can be used; the area of the disk is then assumed to be circular. The main limitation of this method is the inability to image the true apex of the heart in most cases, and the geometrical assumptions used in the model, which make it particularly problematic when the ventricles are asymmetric, when there is regional dysfunction, or when the ventricles are aneurysmal.

The LVEF is calculated as follows:

$$EF = 100 \times (end-diastolic\ volume - end-systolic\ volume) \div end-diastolic\ volume$$

LVEF as calculated by echocardiography with quantitative methods, such as the method of discs, correlates well with the LVEF calculations obtained from radionuclide or contrast ventriculography.[2,3] Echocardiography can also provide information about the size and the global and regional function of the right ventricle, which are associated with long-term survival for patients with heart failure and valvular heart disease.

Another important aspect of 2D echocardiography is that it allows evaluation of regional wall motion. We assess regional function by visually evaluating endocardial motion and wall thickening of each of the 17 segments in the parasternal long- and short-axis views, as well as in the apical axis views. We then integrate this information to determine whether the regional dysfunction follows a coronary artery territory, as is the case in ischemic heart disease, or whether the regional dysfunction does not follow the distribution of a coronary artery or arteries, as is the case in Tako-tsubo cardiomyopathy, which may be found among cancer patients.Regional systolic function is of vital importance in detecting cardiotoxicity, because the distribution of dysfunction may be regional (resembling myocarditis), not necessarily global.

■ Left Ventricular Mass

It is important to obtain accurate measurements of LV mass during the initial examination and follow-up of patients at risk of cardiotoxicity. The recommended

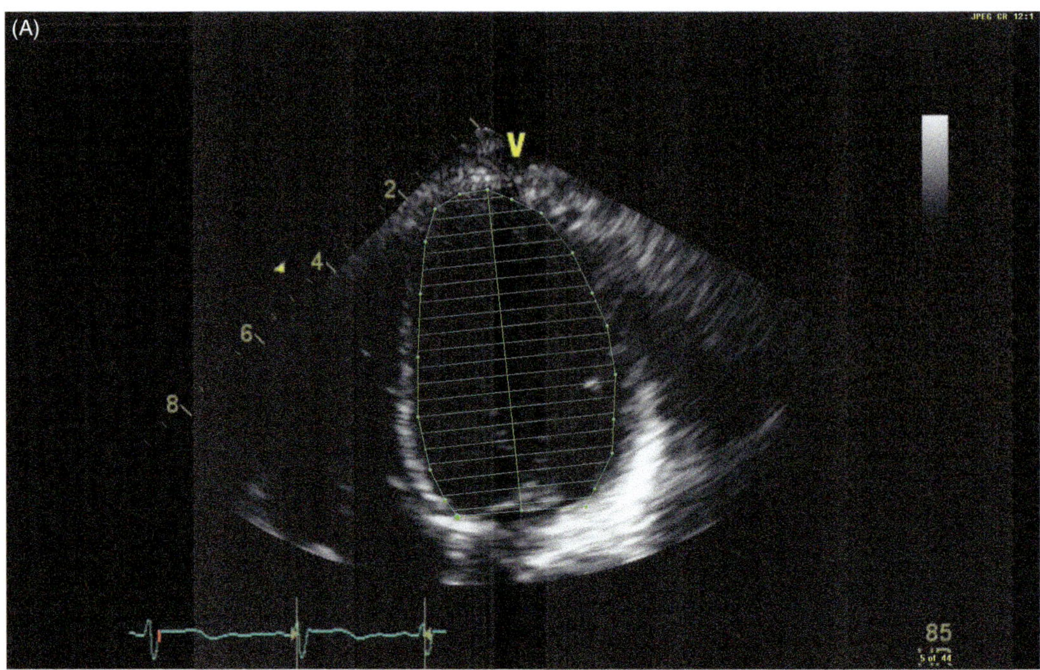

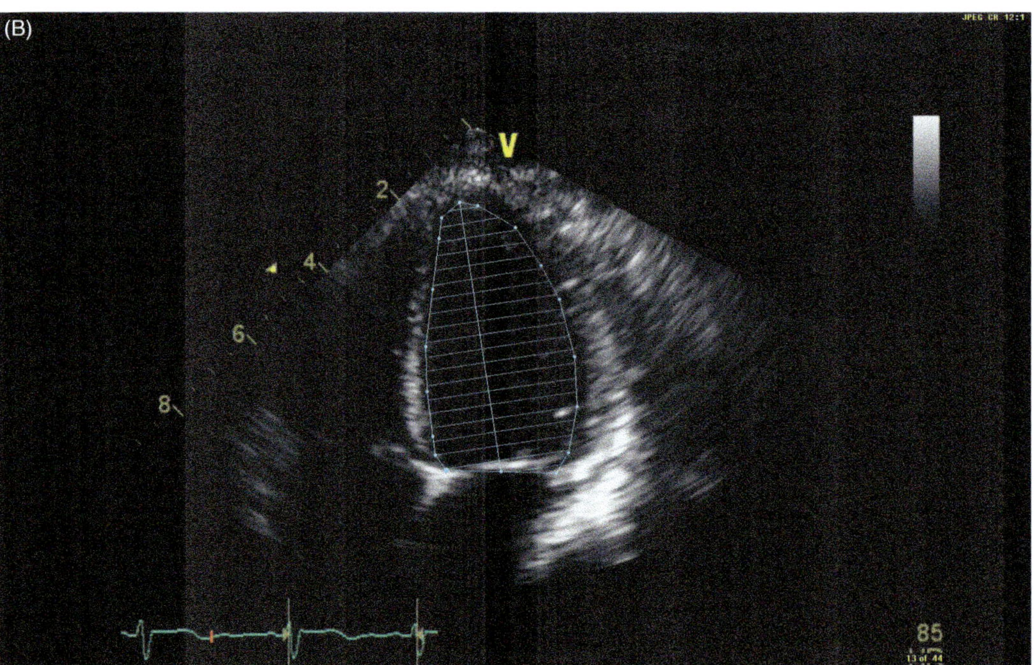

FIGURE 10-1 Example of endocardial tracing using the method of disks from the apical 4-chamber cardiac view of a young patient. (A) End-diastolic volume frame. (B) End-systolic volume frame.

formula for estimating LV mass from LV linear dimensions, and the one that is used in our laboratories, is based on a model of the LV as a prolate ellipse:

$$LV\ mass = 0.8 \times [1.04(LVIDd + PWTd + SWTd)^3 - (LVIDd)^3] + 0.6\ g$$

where LVIDd is left ventricular internal diameter at the end of diastole; PWTd is posterior wall thickness at the end of diastole; and SWTd is septal wall thickness at the end of diastole. This formula is appropriate only for patients with no serious distortions of LV geometry, and, because cubing of the linear measurements is required, small errors in these measurements will be greatly magnified.

Another important calculation is the assessment of relative wall thickness (RWT) with the following formula:

$$RWT = (2 \times PWTd) \div LVIDd$$

This formula allows categorization of an increase in LV mass as either concentric (RWT ≥ 0.42) or eccentric (RWT ≤ 0.42) hypertrophy and also allows identification of concentric remodeling (normal LV mass with increased RWT). Patients with normal LV mass have either concentric remodeling (normal LV mass with increased RWT ≥ 0.42) or normal geometry (RWT ≤ 0.42) and normal LV mass. Patients with increased LV mass have either concentric (RWT ≥ 0.42) or eccentric (RWT ≤ 0.42) hypertrophy.

■ Other Information

The 2D echocardiography signal also permits observations about the intensity and pattern of the reflected echo signal from the LV myocardium. Cardiac amyloidosis should be considered especially for patients with multiple myeloma. Amyloidosis may be appreciated as an infiltrative form of cardiomyopathy, characterized by symmetrical thickening of the left and right ventricles, with an abnormal speckled appearance of the myocardium. These patients exhibit normal LV chamber size, normal systolic function until the disease is at an advanced stage, bi-atrial enlargement, and pericardial effusions (Figure 10-2).

LEFT VENTRICULAR ASSESSMENT WITH DOPPLER ECHOCARDIOGRAPHY

Doppler echocardiography evaluates changes in the frequency with which red blood cells move within the cardiac chambers or valves. Doppler calculations allow an accurate calculation of stroke volume, cardiac output, valvular stenosis, and regurgitation, as well as an evaluation of diastolic function and congenital shunts.

■ Stroke Volume and Cardiac Output

It is possible to calculate the stroke volume with Doppler echocardiography. Flow (Q) is the product of the cross-sectional area of the orifice (CSA) and the time velocity integral (TVI) across the orifice, as in the following equation:

$$Q = \text{stroke volume} = CSA \times TVI$$

Cardiac output can then be calculated by multiplying stroke volume by heart rate. Stroke volume and cardiac output are most commonly calculated from measurements of the LV outflow tract. The stroke volume obtained from this orifice is usually the most accurate because the LV outflow tract most closely resembles a circle. Validation studies have shown an excellent correlation between cardiac output derived from the ventricular outflow Doppler method and cardiac output measured by thermodilution.[4]

Doppler echocardiography can also be used to estimate the right ventricular systolic pressure (RVSP) noninvasively. RVSP is calculated with the modified Bernoulli equation:

$$\text{Pressure gradient} = 4V^2$$

where V stands for velocity of the tricuspid regurgitant jet. Therefore, RVSP can be estimated as follows:

$$RVSP = 4V^2 + RAP$$

where RAP is right atrial pressure calculated on the basis of the size and collapsibility of the inferior vena cava (IVC).

■ Assessment of Diastolic Function

In our laboratories we evaluate diastolic function according to the most recent ASE recommendations.[5] We obtain Doppler measurements of mitral inflow and pulmonic vein inflow as seen in an apical 4-chamber cardiac view. We record mitral inflow (peak E wave, A wave velocities, E/A ratio, and E deceleration time [DT] in milliseconds) and annular tissue Doppler velocities (cm/sec). We also report left atrial volumes indexed to body surface area by using the biplane method of disks (modified Simpson rule). For grading purposes, in our laboratory we follow the grading system proposed by the recent ASE document.[5] These recommendations describe stages of LV diastolic function: grade I (impaired early LV relaxation pattern), grade II (pseudonormalization), and grade III (restrictive filling), as determined on the basis of a majority of physiologic signals, and also recognizing the new possibility of an indeterminate pattern.

We routinely report the medial, lateral, and average tissue Doppler velocities. These measurements are particularly attractive for several reasons; Doppler tissue imaging (DTI) waveforms are obtainable from nearly all patients, regardless of image quality; the measurements are known to correlate well with invasive LA measurements[6,7]; they are reproducible and relatively load-independent; they help determine the presence of pseudonormalization phenomena[8]; and, finally, DTI has also been reported to be useful in the evaluation of pericardial constriction,[9] which is often a pathologic condition of concern for cancer patients.

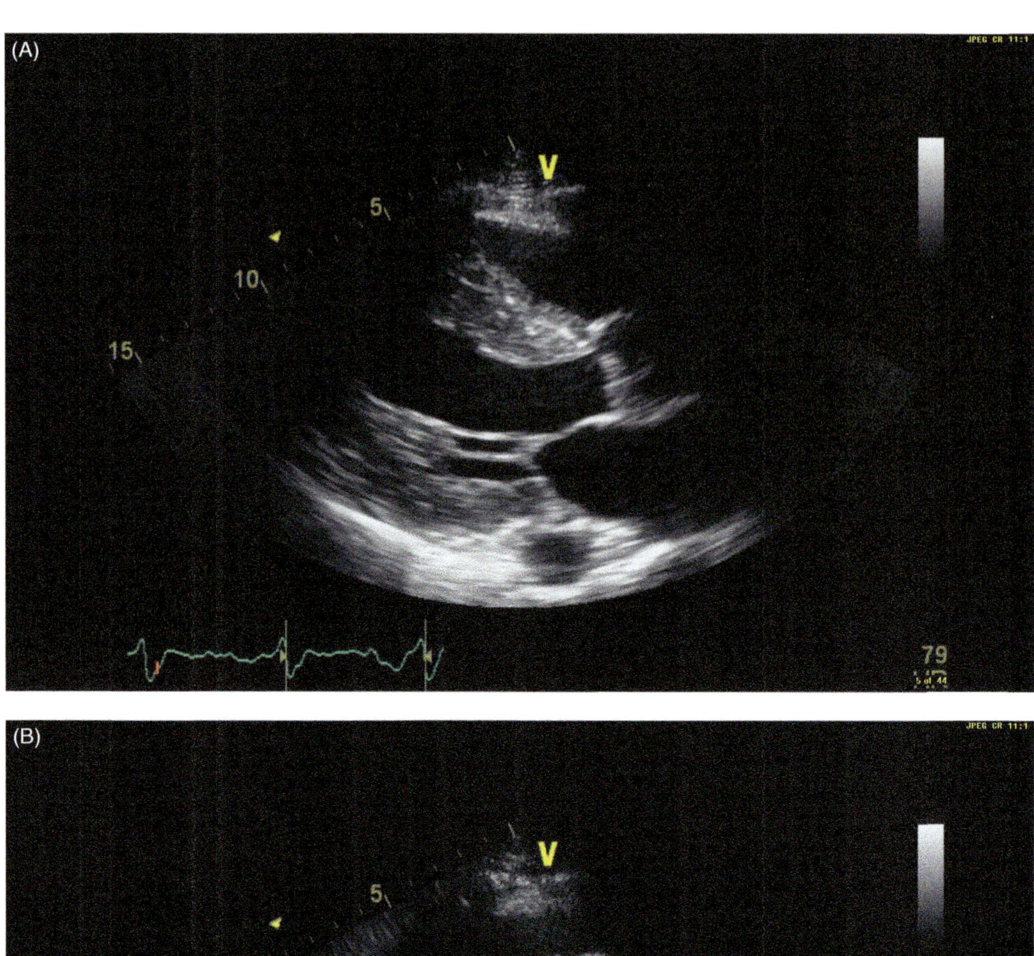

FIGURE 10-2 Classic example of amyloid heart disease as shown by echocardiography. (A) Parasternal long-axis view. (B) Parasternal short-axis views. Note the extent of wall thickening and the speckled pattern of the left ventricle.

Once mitral flow and annular velocities with time intervals have been obtained, several ratios can be calculated. These include the E/A ratio and the ratio of mitral peak early filling velocity (E) to tissue Doppler early mitral annular (E′) velocity, or E/E′. The latter ratio is the most frequently used for estimating LV filling pressures.[6,7]

Diastolic Function and Detection of Cardiotoxicity

Measurements of diastolic function by Doppler echocardiography may be a marker for the early detection of toxicity. One study found that the isovolumetric relaxation time was significantly prolonged (from 66 ± 18 to

84 ± 24 ms; $P < 0.05$) after a cumulative doxorubicin dose of 100 to 120 mg/m². Ain increase of more than 37% in volumetric relaxation time was 78% (7 of 9) sensitive and 88% (15 of 17) specific for predicting the ultimate development of doxorubicin-induced systolic dysfunction[10]; however, the results regarding the value of diastolic dysfunction as an indicator of this diagnosis are contradictory. Because of the influence of hypertension and other risk factors on diastolic function, this signal is certainly nonspecific.

The myocardial performance (Tei) index is another important Doppler-derived tool (Figure 10-3).[11,12] This index expresses the ratio of the sum of the isovolumetric contraction time and the isovolumetric relaxation time divided by the ejection time. This formula combines systolic and diastolic myocardial performance without geometrical assumptions and correlates well with the results of invasive measurements. The normal value of this index is 0.39 ± 0.05; higher values indicate worse systolic and worse diastolic function. The value is appealing for use with cancer patients, because it appears to be independent of heart rate, mean arterial pressure, and degree of mitral regurgitation. It has also been found to be sensitive and accurate in detecting subclinical cardiotoxicity associated with anthracycline therapy.[13] Studies using the Tei index show that this index is better than the ejection fraction in detecting anthracycline-induced deterioration in LV function among adults: it detects this deterioration earlier in the course of treatment and

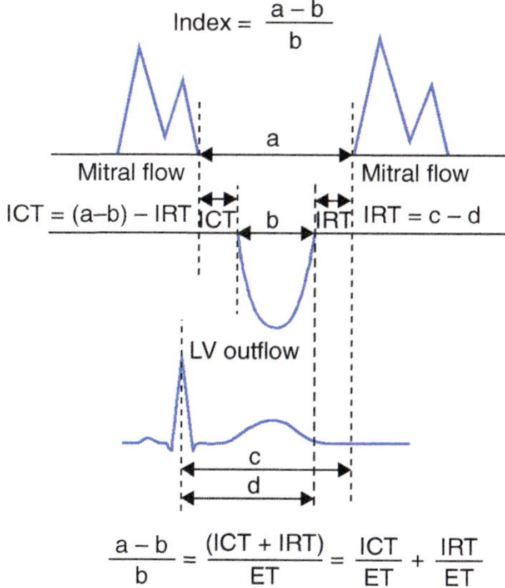

FIGURE 10-3   Tei index diagram and formula for calculation.[12] (Reproduced with permission from the *Journal of the American Society of Echocardiography.*) ET, ejection time; ICT, isovolumic contraction time; IRT, isovolumic relaxation time; LV, left ventricle.

is more likely to detect statistically significant differences.[14] The same group of researchers has also found that low-dose anthracycline chemotherapy regimens exert a differential effect on LV and RV function, causing a significant negative impact on LV function but sparing RV function.[15]

LV ASSESSMENT WITH 3-DIMENSIONAL ECHOCARDIOGRAPHY

The feasibility of real-time 3-dimensional echocardiography (RT3DE) is based on new matrix-array transducers. This imaging method improves and expands the diagnostic capabilities of cardiac ultrasound.[16] The recent position statement of the ASE provides guidelines for appropriate application of this technique, based on the currently available published reports. The document recommends the clinical application of RT3DE for the accurate calculation of LV volumes and function, the evaluation of valvular heart disease, and the assessment of the patients with congenital heart disease.[16]

Three acquisition modes are used with RT3DE: wide-angle or full-volume acquisition (pyramidal data set of 90 degrees × 90 degrees), live 3D or narrow-angle acquisition (pyramidal data set of 50 degrees × 30 degrees), and 3D zoom (smaller, magnified pyramidal data set of 30 degrees × 30 degrees).[16] The full-volume acquisition (wide-angle) requires a trade-off between temporal and spatial resolution. Electrocardiographic (ECG) gating enables merging 2 to 4 narrower pyramidal scans obtained over 2 to 4 consecutive beats. A wide-angle imaging can be obtained with single-beat full-volume acquisitions but at the sacrifice of spatial and temporal resolution. Full-volume acquisitions can be obtained from the parasternal, apical 4-chamber, and subcostal acoustic windows.

A complete 3D examination includes evaluation of ejection fraction, valvular structure and function, and hemodynamics.[16] Imaging with narrow angles (live 3D) can be used if high resolution is desired.

LEFT VENTRICULAR CHAMBER MEASUREMENT AND ACCURATE ESTIMATION OF EJECTION FRACTION

RT3DE avoids the geometric assumptions and consequences of foreshortening that limit the calculation of LV volumes with 2D echocardiography. The ability to capture a full-volume acquisition of the LV allows for accurate identification of the true apex of the heart. An algorithm based on the detection of the endocardial

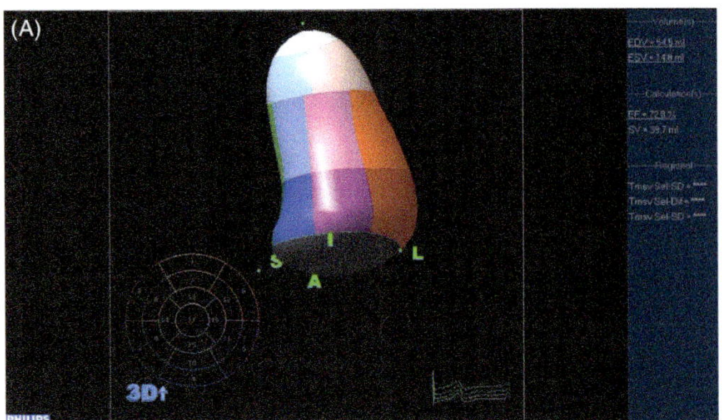

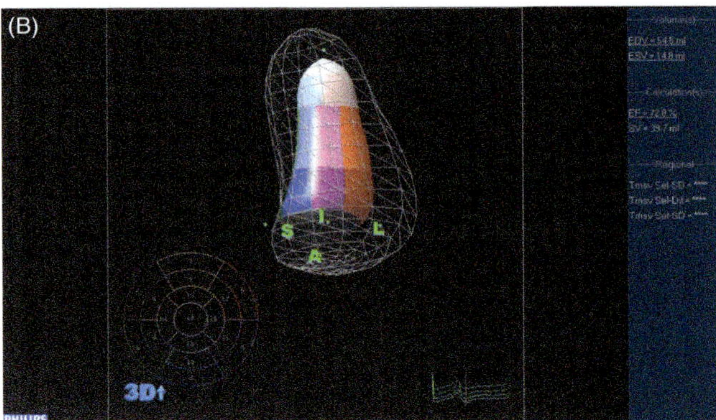

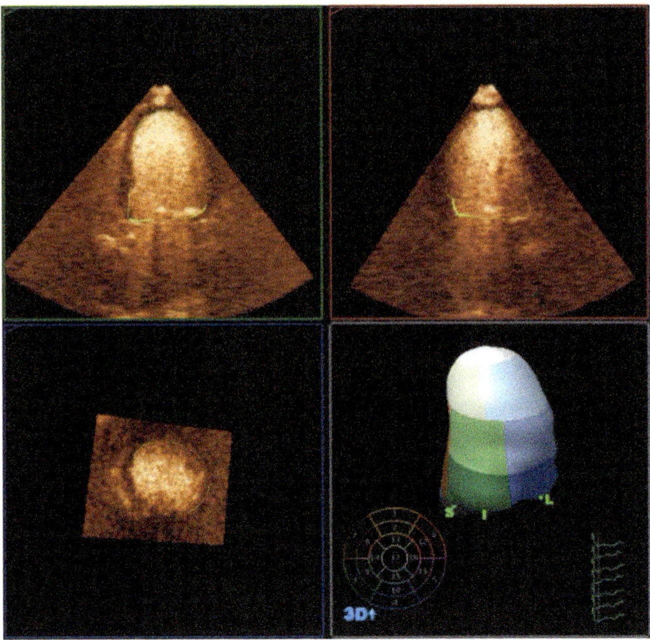

FIGURE 10-5   Calculation of three-dimensional (3D) ejection fraction from images obtained by echocardiography with enhancement.

FIGURE 10-4   Evaluation of ejection fraction as shown by three-dimensional (3D) echocardiography. (A) End-diastolic volume. (B) End-systolic volume.

border then allows for direct quantification of LV volumes, without multiplane tracing or geometric modeling (Figure 10-4). Jacobs and colleagues compared 2D and 3D echocardiography against cardiac magnetic resonance imaging (CMRI) in their ability to accurately calculate end diastolic volume (EDV), end systolic volume (ESV), and EF. RT3DE measurements of the LV correlate well with CMRI values (ESV, $r = 0.96$; ESV, $r = 0.97$, and EF, $r = 0.93$).[17] Importantly, the limits of agreement were wider for volumes and ejection fraction when 2D transthoracic echocardiography (TTE) was used instead of RT3DE,[17] such that 2D EF can be potentially miscalculated by approximately 10 points. In contrast, calculating LV volume and EF with RT3DE is a fast, accurate, and reproducible method, superior to the conventional 2D methods. The small negative biases associated with the calculation of volumes and EF by RT3DE rather than CMRI can be reduced by taking care to include endocardial trabeculations within the LV cavity.[18]

More recently, contrast has been used to enhance RT3DE images. Contrast enhancement has been found not only to improve the accuracy and reproducibility of LV volume measurements when image quality is poor but also to enhance the assessment of regional wall motion from RT3DE datasets. The

authors found that, when selective dual triggering is used to minimize bubble destruction by ultrasound energy, contrast enhancement renders RT3DE-based analysis of regional LV function more accurate than CMRI methods and increases its reproducibility to levels similar to those noted with images of optimal quality (Figure 10-5).[19]

The accurate calculation of volumes and EF is an essential part of the initial and follow-up evaluations of patients being treated with cardiotoxic regimens. At our institution, the administration of anthracyclines is discontinued if patients exhibit a symptomatic drop of more than 5% to an EF lower than 55%, or an asymptomatic drop of more than 10% to an EF lower than 55%. Miscalculating the EF by 2DTTE can lead oncologists to discontinue an anthracycline-based regimen because of concerns about toxicity, even though no toxicity exists and the indications of toxicity are caused simply by a mistake in the calculation as the result of the inherent limitations of the technology used.

LV ASSESSMENT WITH STRAIN IMAGING

Two-dimensional strain (2DS) imaging is a semi-automated and quantitative technique that provides a multidimensional evaluation of myocardial mechanics.[20] The technique is based on conventionally acquired gray-scale images, and the measurement is derived from frame-by-frame tracking of individual speckles throughout the cardiac cycle. Unlike the preceding tissue-Doppler approach, 2DS imaging does not suffer from angle dependency and is easier to calculate.

2DS imaging can be used to calculate the EF with the following formula:

$$EF = -4.35 * (GLS + 3.9)^{21}$$

where GLS stands for global longitudinal strain.

However, the use of this method to calculate EF misses the point that the greatest strength of this technique is the identification of subclinical dysfunction. The most practically useful aspects relate to measurement of longitudinal and circumferential motion, with the signals from radial and rotational motion being primarily of research interest. The most robust parameter is GLS, which represents the average longitudinal deformation from the apical 4-chamber, 2-chamber, and long-axis views. Normal peak longitudinal strain ranges from –16% to –20% (Figures 10-6 and 10-7).[22-24]

This technique is prognostically powerful. Studies comparing GLS to EF and wall motion score index (WMSI) have shown that GLS may be a better superior predictor of outcome than either of the other variables.

The advent of this technology has generated much interest in its use as a tool in the recognition of subclinical or preclinical LV dysfunction. A recently published study[25] with participation from our center, sought to evaluate whether sensitive echocardiographic measurements and biomarkers could predict later cardiac dysfunction in 43 chemotherapy-treated patients. LVEF, peak systolic myocardial longitudinal and radial strain, echocardiographic markers of diastolic function, N-terminal pro-brain natriuretic peptide (NT-proBNP) concentrations, and cardiac troponin I (cTnI) concentrations were measured. Cardiotoxicity developed in 9 patients (21%), 1 at 3 months and 8 at 6 months. The decrease in longitudinal strain from baseline to 3 months and a detectable troponin concentration at 3 months were independent predictors of the development of cardiotoxicity at 6 months. LVEF, diastolic function variables, and NT-proBNP concentrations did not predict cardiotoxicity. This and other studies have emphasized that changes in the peak longitudinal strain predict the development of later cardiotoxicity among patients treated with anthracyclines and trastuzumab. The evaluation of this novel variable may be useful in determining which chemotherapy-treated patients may benefit from alternative therapies, thereby decreasing the incidence of cardiotoxicity and its associated morbidity and mortality (Figure 10-8).

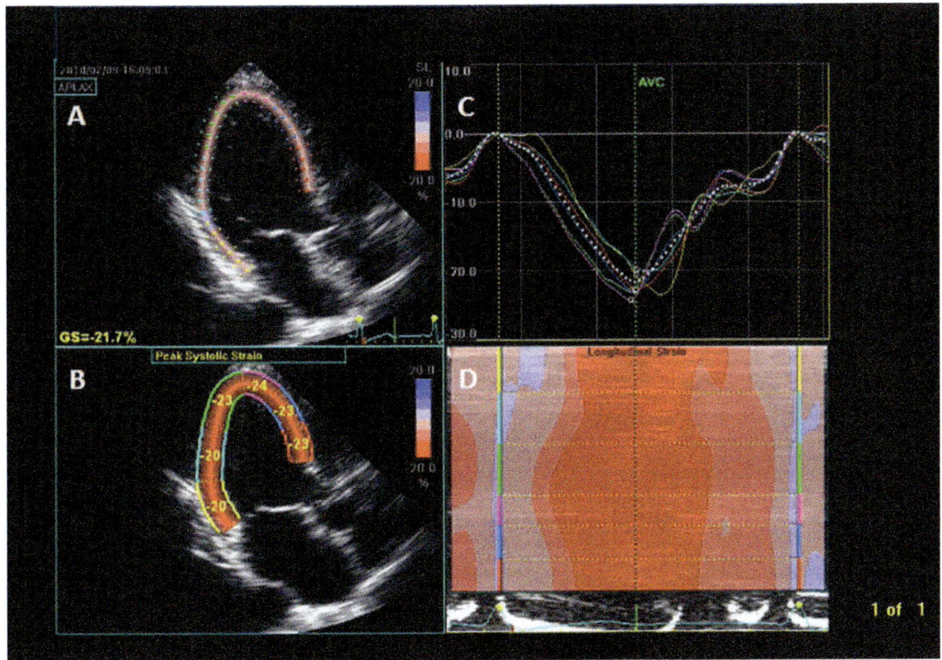

FIGURE 10-6   Two-dimensional (2D) echocardiography–based strain analysis (speckle tracking) of an apical long-axis view of a normal left ventricle. The left upper panel (A) shows the tracking of the various segments. The left lower panel (B) shows the global peak longitudinal strain for this view, as well the strain values for the individual segments. The right upper panel (C) illustrates the times to peak longitudinal strain of the segments, in reference to aortic valve opening (yellow dotted line) and aortic valve closure (green dotted line). The right lower panel (D) shows a color display of the strain of the segments throughout the cardiac cycle.

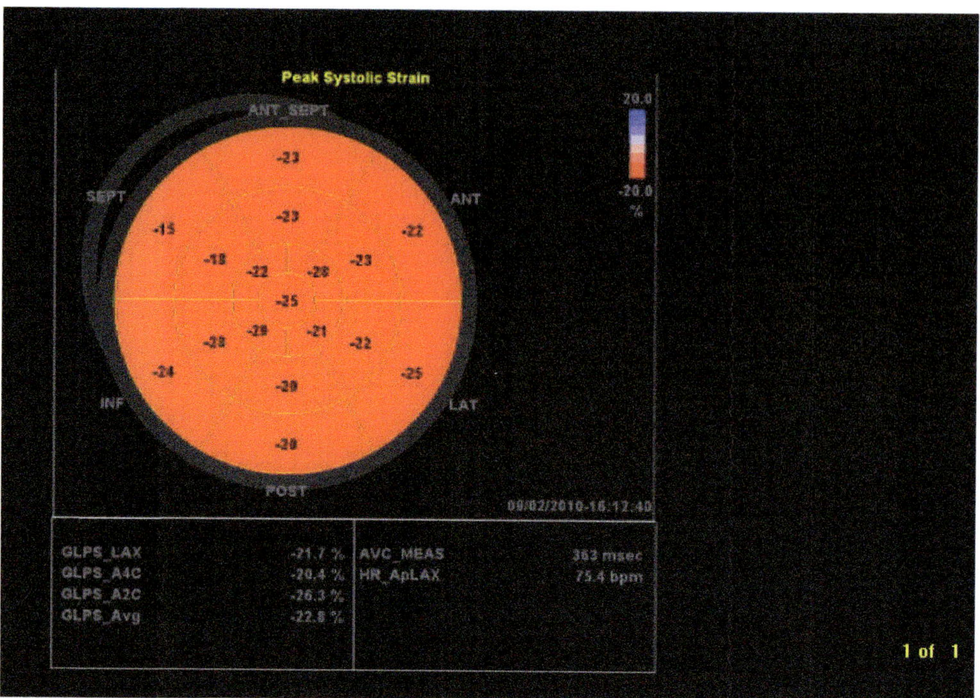

FIGURE 10-7 Polar map of two-dimensional (2D)-based strain values of a normal patient.

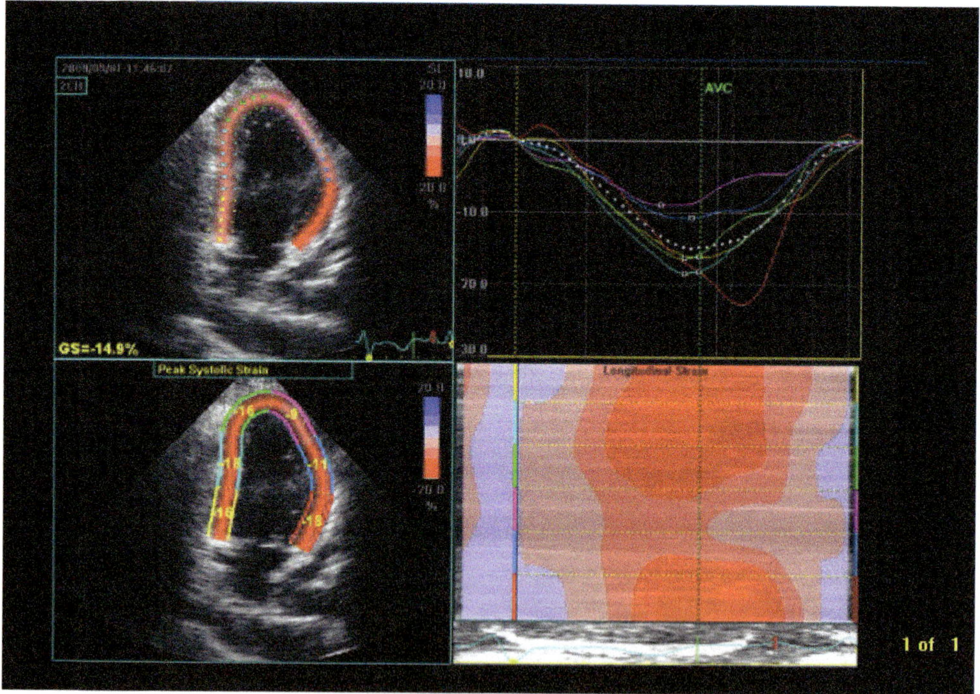

FIGURE 10-8 Abnormal two-dimensional (2D)-based strain values of a patient undergoing anthracycline-based chemotherapy apical 2-chamber view. The mean peak longitudinal strain for this view is abnormal (-14.9%). The individual strain values for the mid- and apical anterior wall segments are also abnormal.

PERICARDIAL DISEASE

■ Pericardial Effusion

The most common form of pericardial disease encountered at our institution is pericardial effusion with or without evidence of hemodynamic compromise. The management of pericardial disease largely depends on the size of the effusion, its hemodynamic compromise, the presence of neoplastic disease in the pericardial space, and the risk of recurrence; however, attempts have recently been made to establish guidelines for the management of the spectrum of pericardial disease.[26,27]

The pericardium consists of two sacs; an inner and an outer. The inner, serous, or visceral pericardium is composed of serosa, a monolayer of mesothelial cells that covers the coronary vessels. The outer, more fibrous (parietal) pericardium is composed of fibrocollagenous tissue and elastic fibers.

We classify pericardial effusions on the basis of the maximum diameter of fluid seen at the end of diastole. We classify a pericardial effusion as small if its diameter is less than 1 cm, moderate if its diameter is 1 to 2 cm, and large if its diameter is more than 2 cm. An effusion is called circumferential when all conventional views show that it surrounds the heart. An effusion is classified as loculated if there is visual evidence of an isolated pocket of fluid. We commonly find such fluid when fibrous adhesions are present between the pericardial layers adhering the visceral and parietal layers of the pericardium.

■ Cardiac Tamponade

Cardiac tamponade is defined as a hemodynamic abnormality produced by the accumulation of pericardial fluid that exerts sufficient pericardial pressure to impair the diastolic filling of the ventricles.

Although the diagnosis of cardiac tamponade is a clinical one, it is usually confirmed by echocardiography, with close attention to 2D echocardiographic and Doppler variables obtained with a respirometer. In our laboratory, the two main diagnostic criteria are the presence of early diastolic RV collapse and the documentation of a clinically significant variation (> 25%) in MV inflow with respiration. Diastolic RV collapse can be well documented either with subcostal views showing the RV in a longitudinal profile or with the parasternal long-axis view. M-mode can be used to accurately time the events.

Pericardiocentesis is the treatment of choice for circumferential large pericardial effusions with demonstrated evidence of hemodynamic compromise (Figure 10-9).[27] This procedure is most commonly performed via a subxiphoid approach under echocardiographic guidance. Alternatively, it can be performed via the apical approach. The procedure is performed in our noninvasive laboratory or at the bedside in the intensive care unit. Pericardiocentesis is safe when performed by trained personnel. When a loculated effusion is diagnosed, patients are referred to Interventional Radiology for CT-guided pericardiocentesis. In cases of recurrent effusions, we consult cardiothoracic surgery for the placement of a pericardial window.

If at the time of the initial diagnosis of the pericardial effusion the risk of recurrence is considered high because of the oncologic diagnosis, we consider injecting sclerosing agents. The use of these agents has been documented in published reports for the past two decades.[28] The agent used at our institution is N,N',N''-triethylenethiophosphoramide (thiotepa). Thiotepa is a synthetic antitumor agent that has an indication for controlling intracavitary effusions secondary to diffuse or localized neoplastic diseases of various serosal cavities.[28] Thiotepa for injection is an ethylenimine-type compound that is available and supplied as a nonpyrogenic, sterile lyophilized powder for intravenous, intracavitary, or intravesical administration in a 15-mg vial. Our protocol uses 15 mg of thiotepa followed by 150 mg of hydrocortisone. These drugs are injected after the effusion has been completely drained; the drain is then clamped for 48 hours to allow the drug to take effect. Repeat injections have been used for a total dose of 45 mg of thiotepa. No procedure-related complications or adverse effects have been reported with thiotepa, and the incidence of recurrent effusion is less than 10%.[28]

■ Constrictive Pericarditis

Constrictive pericarditis occurs when the fibrotic pericardium impairs normal diastolic filling. Usually, 2D echocardiography shows thickening of the pericardium; however, the pericardium can be of normal thickness in as many as 20% of the cases. The thickened pericardium is not necessarily seen circumferentially and can be patchy. Pericardial constriction is typically chronic, but a transient variant has been recently reported. This transient form of constrictive pericarditis has been reported to occur in 10%–20% of cases during the resolution of pericardial inflammation.[29]

Another important consideration is effusive-constrictive pericarditis. This clinical syndrome is characterized by concurrent pericardial effusion and pericardial constriction, and constrictive

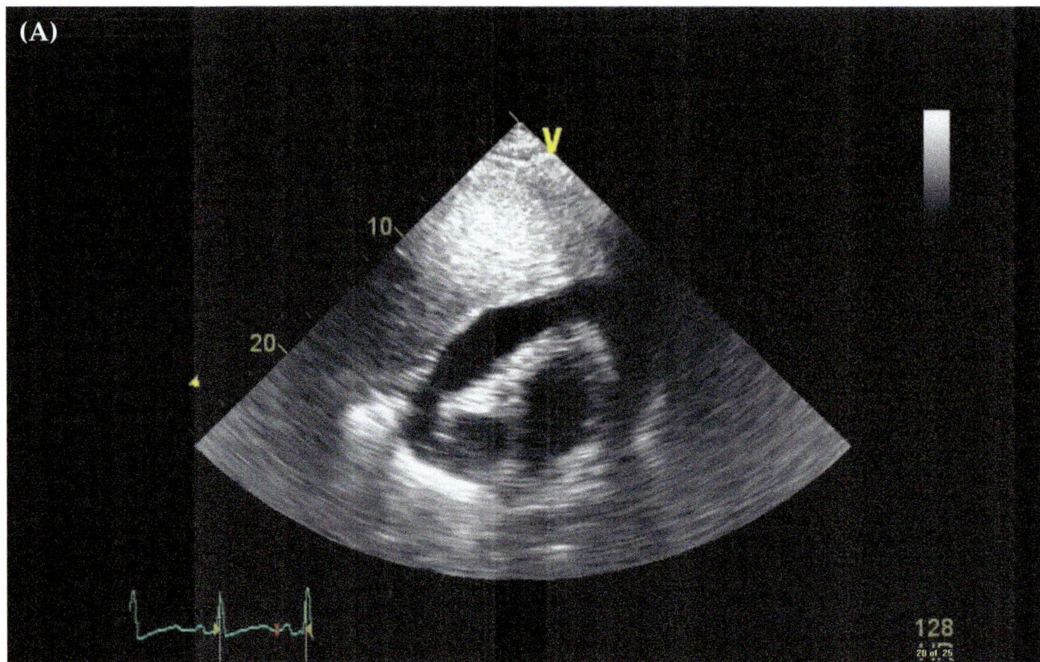

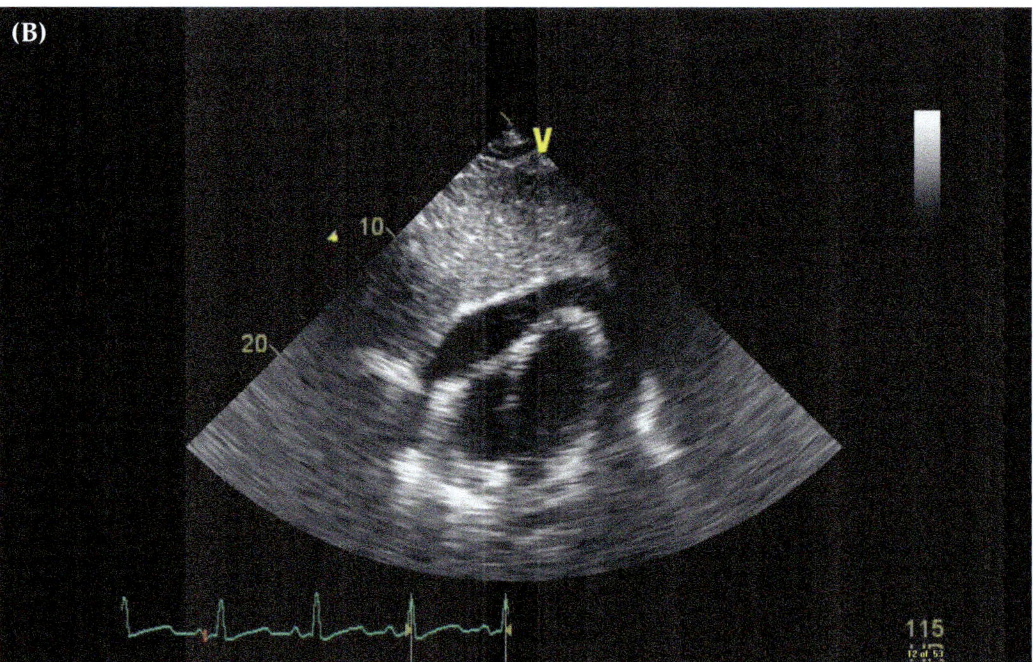

FIGURE 10-9 (A) Example of a large, circumferential pericardial effusion shown by echocardiography. Note the early, almost complete diastolic collapse of the right ventricle (RV). (B) Ultrasound-guided pericardiocentesis. Note the injection of agitated saline for confirmation of adequate location.

hemodynamics persists after the drainage of the pericardial effusion. In effusive-constrictive pericarditis, the visceral layer of the pericardium, rather than the parietal layer, constricts the heart. This is a rare condition; however, effective recognition is important because pericardiectomy is indicated for management.

ECHOCARDIOGRAPHIC ASSESSMENT OF INTRACARDIAC MASSES

Echocardiography is the method of choice for diagnosis and evaluation of prognosis of cardiac masses, whether they are thrombi, vegetation, or tumors.[30] This assessment begins with a thorough description of the location of the mass and its relationship to adjacent structures. Masses can be either intracardiac or extracardiac. The description should include the location and mechanism of implantation of the mass, (i.e., a pedunculated mass attached to the apical segment of the inferior wall through a long stalk), or the route of access of the mass to the heart (superior, inferior vena cava, or pulmonary veins) if the mass is not primarily attached to the heart (Figure 10-10). The characterization of the shape, the longest dimensions, and, ideally, the volume of the mass is essential. Maximum diameter measurements obtained via 2D echocardiography are routinely used to determine the size of the mass. The size of an intracardiac mass has important clinical relevance as a predictor of embolic events, congestive heart failure, and death, and as an efficacy assessment after treatment (anticoagulation, antibiotics, and chemotherapy.[31]

Additionally, a description of the hemodynamic consequences of the mass should also be reported. The echocardiographer should then integrate all of the available information to generate a differential diagnosis. Once all of this information has been obtained, a decision can be made as to the most appropriate treatment for the patient. The complete echocardiographic evaluation of a cardiac mass is summarized in Box 10-1.

The differential diagnosis of intracardiac masses includes tumors (benign, malignant, or metastatic), normal structures or their variants, embryonic remnants, thrombi, masses associated with cardiomyopathy (apical hypertrophic cardiomyopathy, noncompaction cardiomyopathy, and hypereosinophilic syndrome), masses, and complications associated with device implantation (Box 10-1). Primary tumors are much less common than metastatic tumors in the heart, occurring in at least 7 of every 10,000 persons.[32] Benign primary cardiac tumors occur more frequently than malignant ones. The most common cardiac tumor is the myxoma. A large single-institution series of primary cardiac tumors at the University of Minnesota found that 42% were cardiac myxomas and 16% were malignant tumors (sarcomas).[33]

Echocardiography is the most frequently used imaging modality in the assessment of intracardiac masses. Historically, this evaluation was based on the analysis of 2D slices of the heart; the information obtained from orthogonal tomographic planes from several acoustic windows was used to mentally reconstruct a model of the 3D appearance of the mass and its spatial orientation to adjacent structures.

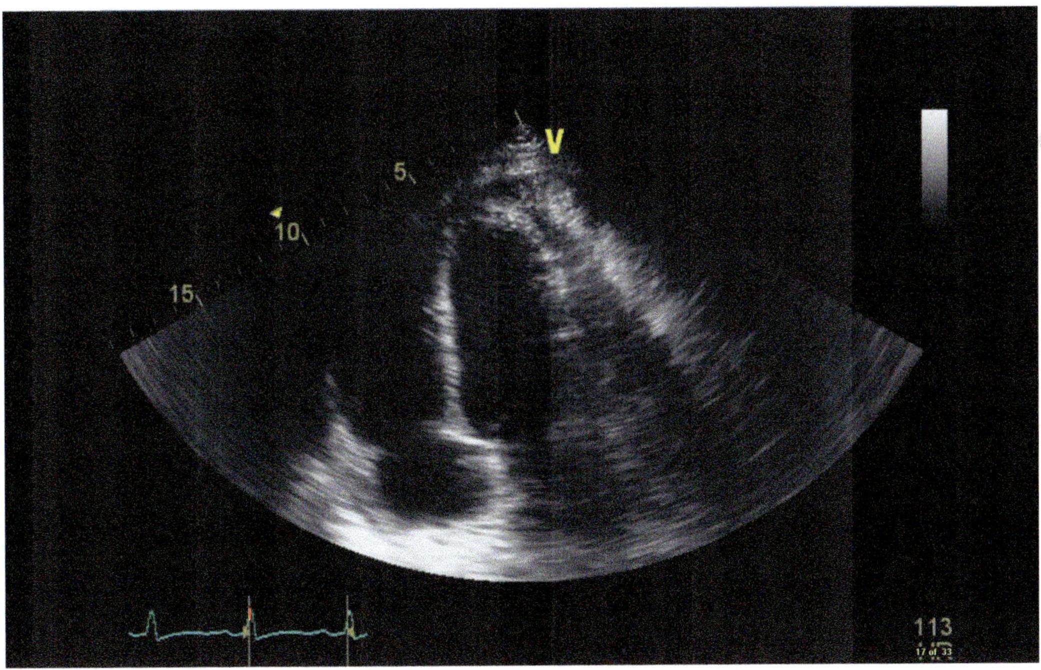

FIGURE 10-10   Apical 4-chamber view of a patient with a primary cardiac sarcoma. The tumor originates from the inferolateral and anterolateral walls of the left ventricle. A large pleural effusion is seen, with large amounts of echodense material floating in the space.

BOX 10-1   Echocardiographic evaluation of cardiac masses

1. Characterization of the mass
   a. Location: intracardiac or extracardiac
   b. Relationship with adjacent structures
   c. Site and mechanism of implantation
   d. Route of access to the heart
   e. Shape, size, and volume
   f. Hemodynamic consequences

2. Differential diagnosisa
   a. Benign
      1. Embryonic remnants
      2. Normal variants (false chords, heavy trabeculations, accessory papillary muscles)
      3. Thrombi (mural or associated with catheter or other devices)
      4. Benign cardiac tumors
      5. Cardiomyopathy (apical hypertrophic cardiomyopathy, noncompaction cardio-myopathy)
      6. Vegetations
   b. Malignant
      1. Primary
      2. Metastatic

3. Accurate estimation of left ventricular volumes and ejection fraction
4. Therapeutic decision making

REAL-TIME THREE-DIMENSIONAL ECHOCARDIOGRAPHY IN THE ASSESSMENT OF CARDIAC TUMORS

Although the ASE does not include the evaluation of cardiac masses as part of the proposed applications in its position paper, we consider RT3DE extremely useful in assessing cardiac masses. At our institution, the evaluation of a cardiac mass via transthoracic RT3DE includes, at a minimum, a full-volume acquisition in the parasternal long axis and in the apical 4-chamber views. If the mass in question is located in the right atrium, full-volume acquisition, live 3D, and subcostal images are obtained from the right modified inflow. Live 3D images of the right parasternal and supraclavicular windows have been used in the echocardiographic assessment of thrombus in the innominate vein and the superior vena cava.[34]

Once a 3D data set has been acquired, it can be sliced and cropped in many different ways. Images can also be manipulated to provide views and planes and to align structures in ways that were previously impossible with 2D imaging. This feature is particularly useful in a workflow situation in which the images captured by a sonographer are later interpreted by the physician when the patient is no longer available to provide additional images. The availability of the full-volume acquisition allows echocardiographers to slice and crop the heart as they would have done if they were directly imaging the patient (Figure 10-11A and 11B). In most cases, the full-volume loop allows good visualization of location, shape, attaching interface, and relationship to adjacent structures of cardiac masses.

Emphasis should also be placed on evaluating the composition of the cardiac mass (Figure 10-12). For patients with myxomas and hemangiomas, 3D imaging appears to be superior to 2DTTE in assessing left atrial tumors because of the unique ability of live RT3DE to systematically section and view the contents of an intracardiac mass. Left atrial (LA) myxomas can

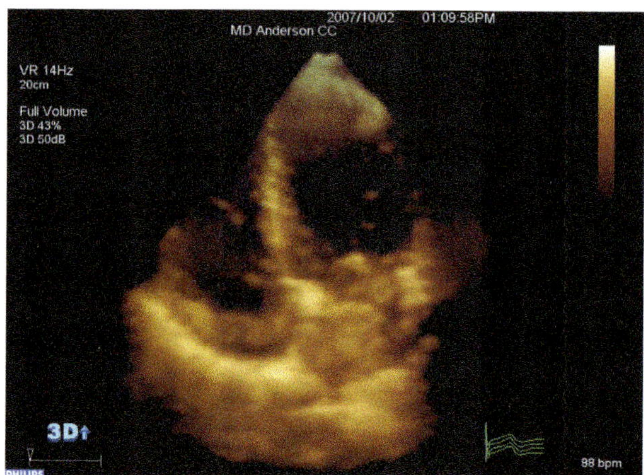

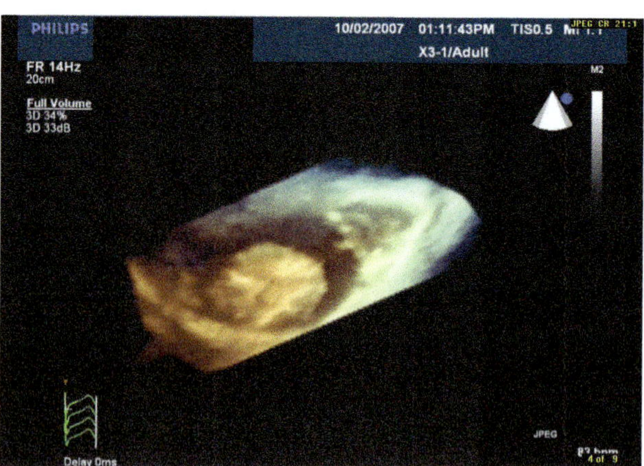

FIGURE 10-11 Full-volume acquisition image (A) and cropped image (B) obtained from a patient with recurrent metastatic osteosarcoma. The mass enters the right atrium from the right upper pulmonary vein.

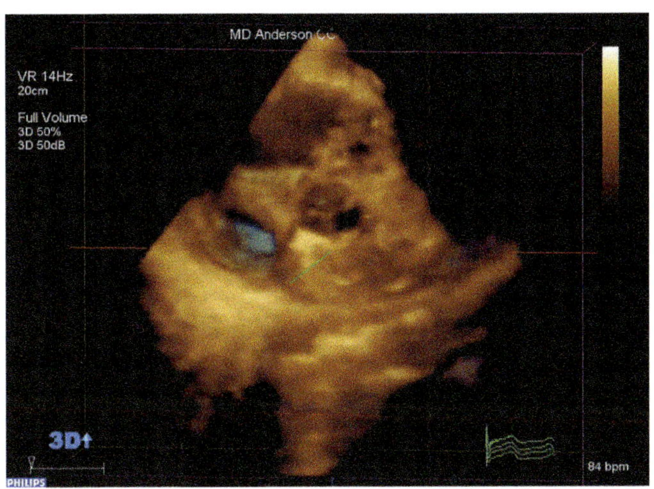

FIGURE 10-12 Full-volume acquisition image obtained from the short-axis view of a patient with metastatic osteosarcoma. The mass was not surgically resectable due to extensive aortic root involvement.

be confidently diagnosed by noting isolated echolucent areas consistent with hemorrhage or necrosis in the tumor mass. In contrast, RT3DE images of hemangiomas show much more extensive and closely packed echo-lucency with little solid tissue.[35] Overall, RT3DE provides a more comprehensive assessment of the inner structure of the mass, an assessment that correlates better with pathologic findings (necrosis, hemorrhage, cystic areas, or fibrotic bands).[30,36]

Because most masses are irregularly shaped, accurately imaging them or selecting the largest diameter can be difficult. Nanda and colleagues reported that 2D measurements obtained from a transthoracic or a transesophageal study underestimate the true maximal diameter of irregularly shaped structures.[37] In the case of cardiac masses, this underestimation can lead to a misrepresentation of the patient's prognosis. RT3DE images the entire volume of a mass, allowing for accurate measurements in multiple planes. Asch and associates reported that, as compared to RT3DE, 2D transthoracic images lead to consistent underestimation of the maximal diameter by 24.6% ($P < 0.001$) and 2D transesophageal images, by 19.8% ($P = 0.01$). In addition, RT3DE allows more rapid determination of measurements with excellent intraobserver and interobserver variability (better than with 2D echocardiography).

We suggest that RT3DE may be the technique of choice for the noninvasive evaluation of the size of intracardiac masses.[31]

Normal cardiac structures (moderator band or false cords) or their variants (accessory papillary muscles) can be confused with cardiac masses on 2DTTE images. In such cases, we find it very useful to obtain a full-volume acquisition so that we can understand the 3D relationship of the structure. This is particularly a problem in the right atrium, because the differential diagnosis includes a normal structure (prominent IVC ridge or crista terminalis), embryonic remnants (prominent Eustachian valve or Chiari network), thrombus, tumor, or tumor-thrombus arising from the IVC.[38-40] The ability to use the live 3D mode to see these 3D structures in motion has allowed us in many instances to properly diagnose these conditions without the need for more invasive testing, such as TEE.

REAL-TIME THREE-DIMENSIONAL TRANSESOPHAGEAL ECHOCARDIOGRAPHY IN THE ASSESSMENT OF CARDIAC TUMORS

Recent advances in ultrasound transducer technology have allowed the miniaturization of matrix array transducers to produce a real-time 3D matrix array transesophageal echocardiogram (3D-MTEE).[41] If clinical questions are not successfully answered by transthoracic RT3DE, 3D-MTEE is performed. In addition to the images obtained according to our laboratory protocol, a full-volume acquisition view of the LV is obtained. Depending on the location of the mass in question, 3D zoom images are obtained from the mitral valve (MV), the tricuspid valve (TV), the left atrial appendage (LAA), the left upper pulmonary vein (LUPV), and the interatrial septum (IAS). A full-volume acquisition and live 3D imaging in the bicaval view are useful in the characterization of masses in the superior vena cava (SVC), the IVC, and the right atrium.

One of the biggest limitations of 2D echocardiography in the assessment of cardiac masses is the possibility of "missing" the mass during the evaluation. As mentioned above, orthogonal planes are used to evaluate these masses, and if a mass happens to be located in an area between the imaging planes, it will not become apparent during the examination. One advantage of 3D-MTEE is that is allowed us to visualize the full volume of 3D structures with unparalleled anatomic detail.

Muller and co-workers evaluating the value of 3D-MTEE as an adjunct to conventional 2D imaging in the preoperative evaluation of cardiac masses. In 37% of patients, 3D-MTEE revealed one or more items of additional information regarding type and site of attachment, surface features, and spatial relationship to surrounding structures. These researchers estimate that for at least 18% of all intra-cardiac masses 3D-MTEE can be expected to deliver supplementary information. For 6 of their patients, the additional findings led to decisions deviating from those made on the basis of 2DTEE. The authors concluded that the information revealed by 3D imaging facilitates therapeutic decision making, especially the choice of the optimal surgical access before the removal of the intracardiac mass.[42] Sugeng and associates showed that 3D-MTEE may become one of the modalities of choice to assess the MV during preoperative planning of MV surgery, including the resection of tumors from the valve.[21,31,37,41–46] Likewise, in the assessment of tumors of the aortic valve (papillary fibroelastomas), Le Tourneau and colleagues reported that the use of live 3D-MTTE improved their operative planning.[47] In addition, 3D-MTEE has been used to assess neoplasms of the pulmonic valve.[48]

ECHOCARDIOGRAPHIC ASSESSMENT OF CARDIAC THROMBI

Cardiac thrombi are most frequently seen in the apex, the left atrial appendage, and the right atrium or SVC. The evaluation of cardiac masses at the apex can be extremely challenging when only orthogonal planes are used, and RT3DE has the benefit of showing the structure and function of the true apex of the heart. With live 3D TTE, thrombi can be easily viewed from all sides. In addition, by cropping the 3D images sequentially in transverse (horizontal and short-axis), longitudinal (vertical or long-axis), frontal, and oblique planes, the degree and extent of lysis within the thrombus, which represents an integral part of the clot-resolution process, can be comprehensively assessed in sequential studies.[49] In addition, the administration of ultrasound contrast provides the opportunity to carefully crop the ventricle from apex to base, fully confirming or ruling out the presence of an apical thrombus.

■ Evaluation of the Left Atrium

The LA is the most important location for the formation of thrombi in many cardiovascular conditions. Most of these clots occur in the LAA, a structure ranging from 1.2 to 4.5 cm in length; its shape and location allows for stasis of blood in atrial fibrillation, mitral stenosis, and other conditions with low cardiac output, particularly states with poor LV function or enlargement of the LA. In 80% of the general population, the LAA may contain 1 to 4 lobes, with pectinate muscles larger than 1 mm in diameter.[50] Traditionally, it has been difficult to visualize by 2D TTE, the accuracy of 2D TEE and 3D TTE combined is comparable to that of 2D TEE in evaluating the LA and the LAA for thrombus. In some patients, 2DTEE but not 3DTTE may lead to the misdiagnosis of pectinate musculature as thrombus.[51]

Patients with cancer and atrial fibrillation are at risk of stroke but may also have absolute contraindications to treatment with warfarin. For such patients, LAA occlusion devices may be a novel treatment option. Recent studies have shown that the use of 3D-MTEE for the visualization and quantitative assessment of the LAA orifice is feasible and that it yields results that correlate well with those of 64-slice cardiac CT.[43]

■ Evaluation of the Left Ventricle

Noncompaction cardiomyopathy results from the failure of myocardial development during embryogenesis. A maximal end-systolic ratio of noncompacted cardiomyopathy to compacted cardiomyopathy of more than 2 is considered diagnostic (Figure 10-13).[52] RT3DE supplements 2DTTE in yielding a definitive diagnosis of clots coexisting with trabeculations in the

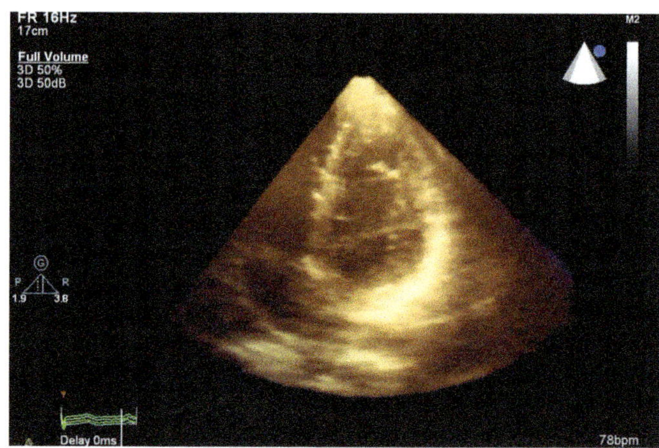

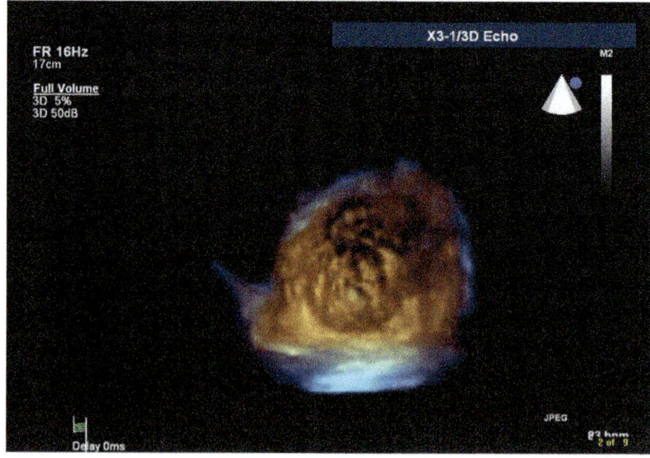

FIGURE 10-13 Cropped images acquired by 3D full-volume echocardiography of a person with the diagnosis of non-compaction cardiomyopathy. The image shows the spongiform appearance of the left ventricular (LV) apex, with numerous trabecula.

LV. RT3DE best demonstrates the mobility of clots and the presence of central echolucencies consistent with clot lysis, and it also allows confident differentiation of clots from adjacent trabeculations. Contrast can further assist in the definition of the trabeculations and the recesses in noncompaction cardiomyopathy.

In cases of hypereosinophilic syndrome, both ventricles of the heart are often involved, with mural endocardial thickening of the inflow portions and apices of the ventricles. Echocardiography commonly demonstrates localized thickening of the posterobasal LV wall, with absent or markedly limited motion of the posterior leaflet of the MV. The apex may be obliterated by thrombus. RT3DE is very useful in the evaluation of patients with hypereosinophilic syndrome, because the obliteration of the apex (Figure 10-14), the thickening of the posterobasal wall, and the limited motion of the LV wall can be easily demonstrated by cropping the full-volume acquisition images. Contrast may be helpful in defining the obliteration of the apex in patients with hypereosinophilic syndrome.

■ Evaluation of Masses and Complications Associated with Devices

Thrombi or vegetations can occur as a complication of the implantation of catheters or pacemakers. Among oncology patients, a common cause of thrombus formation in the RA is the presence of a catheter whose tip is far beyond the junction of the SVC and the RA. The jet of fluid then hits the wall of the RA, denuding the endothelium and provoking the formation of a thrombus in that location. Live RT3DE (especially 3D zoom) is useful

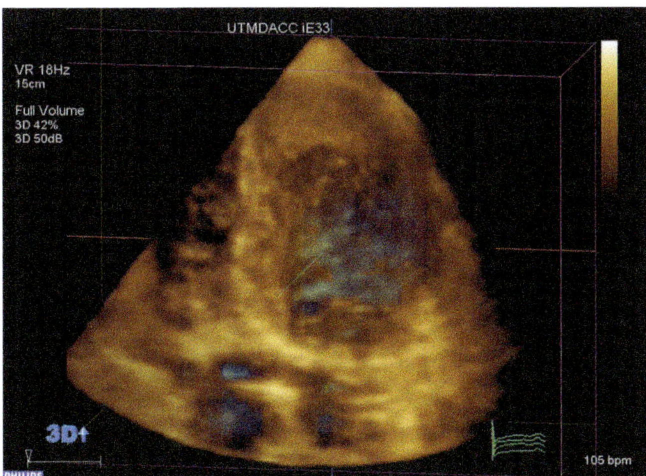

FIGURE 10-14 Full-volume 3D echocardiography images acquired from an apical 4-chamber cardiac view of patient with hypereosinophilic syndrome.

for evaluating these cardiac masses. Anticoagulation and repositioning of the catheter are essential.

RT3DE can also be used to diagnose complications associated with the placement of pacemakers. Daher and colleagues reported the use of full-volume acquisition to demonstrate a pacemaker lead perforation of the interventricular septum with the pacer tip in the LV.[53]

CONCLUSION

This chapter has discussed the standard protocols used for the echocardiographic examination of the cancer patient. The improvement in the quality of conventional echocardiographic modalities and the introduction of new ones have established echocardiography as the modality of choice for imaging the heart of the cancer patient. Echocardiography allows a comprehensive evaluation of the structure and function of the heart. When compared with other modalities, echocardiography has obvious advantages: it is noninvasive, radiation-free, cost-effective, portable, and reliable. These benefits are likely to be augmented by increases in miniaturization, increases in automation, and reductions in cost.

REFERENCES

1. Lang RM, Bierig M, Devereux RB, et al. Recommendations for chamber quantification: a report from the American Society of Echocardiography's Guidelines and Standards Committee and the Chamber Quantification Writing Group, developed in conjunction with the European Association of Echocardiography, a branch of the European Society of Cardiology. *J Am Soc Echocardiogr*. 2005;18(12):1440–1463. doi:10.1016/j.echo.2005.10.005 [published Online first: 2005/12/27]

2. Mohan HK, Livieratos L, Gallagher S, et al. Comparison of myocardial gated single photon emission computerised tomography, planar radionuclide ventriculography and echocardiography in evaluating left ventricular ejection fraction, wall thickening and wall motion. *Int J Clin Pract*. 2004;58(12):1120–1126. [published Online first: 2005/01/14]

3. Folland ED, Parisi AF, Moynihan PF, et al. Assessment of left ventricular ejection fraction and volumes by real-time, two-dimensional echocardiography. A comparison of cineangiographic and radionuclide techniques. *Circulation*. 1979;60(4):760–766. [published Online first: 1979/10/01]

4. Lewis JF, Kuo LC, Nelson JG, et al. Pulsed Doppler echocardiographic determination of stroke volume and cardiac output: clinical validation of two new methods using the apical window. *Circulation*. 1984;70(3): 425–431. [published Online first: 1984/09/01]

5. Nagueh SF, Smiseth OA, Appleton CP, et al. Recommendations for the evaluation of left ventricular diastolic function by echocardiography: an update from the American Society of Echocardiography and the European Association of Cardiovascular Imaging. *J Am Soc Echocardiogr*. 2016;29(4):277–314. doi:10.1016/j.echo.2016.01.011 [published Online first: 2016/04/03]

6. Nagueh SF, Middleton KJ, Kopelen HA, et al. Doppler tissue imaging: a noninvasive technique for evaluation of left ventricular relaxation and estimation of filling pressures. *J Am Coll Cardiol*. 1997;30(6):1527–1533. [published Online first: 1997/11/15]

7. Ommen SR, Nishimura RA, Appleton CP, et al. Clinical utility of Doppler echocardiography and tissue Doppler imaging in the estimation of left ventricular filling pressures: A comparative simultaneous Doppler-catheterization study. *Circulation*. 2000;102(15):1788–1794. [published Online first: 2000/10/12]

8. Sohn DW, Chai IH, Lee DJ, et al. Assessment of mitral annulus velocity by Doppler tissue imaging in the evaluation of left ventricular diastolic function. *J Am Coll Cardiol*. 1997;30(2):474–480. [published Online first: 1997/08/01]

9. Stoddard MF, Seeger J, Liddell NE, et al. Prolongation of isovolumetric relaxation time as assessed by Doppler echocardiography predicts doxorubicin-induced systolic dysfunction in humans. *J Am Coll Cardiol*. 1992;20(1): 62–69. [published Online first: 1992/07/01]

10. McCall R, Stoodley PW, Richards DA, et al. Restrictive cardiomyopathy versus constrictive pericarditis: making the distinction using tissue Doppler imaging. *Eur J Echocardiogr*. 2008;9(4):591–594. doi:10.1093/ejechocard/jen112 [published Online first: 2008/05/21]

11. Tei C, Ling LH, Hodge DO, et al. New index of combined systolic and diastolic myocardial performance: a simple and reproducible measure of cardiac function—a study in normals and dilated cardiomyopathy. *J Cardiol*. 1995;26(6):357–366. [published Online first: 1995/12/01]

12. Tei C, Nishimura RA, Seward JB, et al. Noninvasive Doppler-derived myocardial performance index: correlation with simultaneous measurements of cardiac catheterization measurements. *J Am Soc Echocardiogr*. 1997;10(2):169–178. [published Online first: 1997/03/01]

13. Ishii M, Tsutsumi T, Himeno W, et al. Sequential evaluation of left ventricular myocardial performance in children after anthracycline therapy. *Am J Cardiol*. 2000;86(11):1279–1281, A9. [published Online first: 2000/11/25]

14. Belham M, Kruger A, Mepham S, et al. Monitoring left ventricular function in adults receiving anthracycline-containing chemotherapy. *Eur J Heart Fail*. 2007;9(4):409–414.doi:10.1016/j.ejheart.2006.09.007[published Online first: 2006/10/28]

15. Belham M, Kruger A, Pritchard C. The Tei index identifies a differential effect on left and right ventricular function with low-dose anthracycline chemotherapy. *J Am Soc Echocardiogr*. 2006;19(2):206–210. doi:10.1016/j.echo.2005.08.018 [published Online first: 2006/02/04]

16. Hung J, Lang R, Flachskampf F, et al. 3D echocardiography: a review of the current status and future directions. *J Am Soc Echocardiogr*. 2007;20(3):213–233. doi:10.1016/j.echo.2007.01.010 [published Online first: 2007/03/06]

17. Jacobs LD, Salgo IS, Goonewardena S, et al. Rapid online quantification of left ventricular volume from real-time three-dimensional echocardiographic data. *Eur Heart J*. 2006;27(4):460–468. doi:10.1093/eurheartj/ehi666 [published Online first: 2005/12/02]

18. Mor-Avi V, Sugeng L, Lang RM. Real-time 3-dimensional echocardiography: an integral component of the routine echocardiographic examination in adult patients? *Circulation*. 2009;119(2):314–329. doi:10.1161/CIRCULATIONAHA.107.751354 [published Online first: 2009/01/21]

19. Corsi C, Coon P, Goonewardena S, et al. Quantification of regional left ventricular wall motion from real-time 3-dimensional echocardiography in patients with poor acoustic windows: effects of contrast enhancement tested against cardiac magnetic resonance. *J Am Soc Echocardiogr*. 2006;19(7):886–893. doi:10.1016/j.echo.2006.02.010 [published Online first: 2006/07/11]

20. Cho GY, Marwick TH, Kim HS, et al. Global 2-dimensional strain as a new prognosticator in patients with heart failure. *J Am Coll Cardiol*. 2009;54(7):618–624. doi:10.1016/j.jacc.2009.04.061 [published Online first: 2009/08/08]

21. Zamorano J, Cordeiro P, Sugeng L, et al. Real-time three-dimensional echocardiography for rheumatic mitral valve stenosis evaluation: an accurate and novel approach. *J Am Coll Cardiol*. 2004;43(11):2091–2096. doi:10.1016/j.jacc.2004.01.046 [published Online first: 2004/06/03]

22. Sun JP, Popovic ZB, Greenberg NL, et al. Noninvasive quantification of regional myocardial function using Doppler-derived velocity, displacement, strain rate, and strain in healthy volunteers: effects of aging. *J Am Soc Echocardiogr*. 2004;17(2):132–138. doi:10.1016/j.echo.2003.10.001 [published Online first: 2004/01/31]

23. Edvardsen T, Gerber BL, Garot J, et al. Quantitative assessment of intrinsic regional myocardial deformation by Doppler strain rate echocardiography in humans: validation against three-dimensional tagged magnetic resonance imaging. *Circulation*. 2002;106(1):50–56. [published Online first: 2002/07/03]

24. Kowalski M, Kukulski T, Jamal F, et al. Can natural strain and strain rate quantify regional myocardial deformation? A study in healthy subjects. *Ultrasound Med Biol*. 2001;27(8):1087–1097. [published Online first: 2001/08/31]

25. Sawaya H, Sebag IA, Plana JC, et al. Early detection and prediction of cardiotoxicity in chemotherapy-treated patients. *Am J Cardiol*. 2011;107(9):1375–1380. doi:10.1016/j.amjcard.2011.01.006 [published Online first: 2011/03/05]

26. Shabetai R. Corticosteroids for recurrent pericarditis: on the road to evidence-based medicine. *Circulation*. 2008

;118(6):612–613. doi:10.1161/CIRCULATIONAHA.108. 795567 [published Online first: 2008/08/06]

27. Maisch B, Seferovic PM, Ristic AD, et al. Guidelines on the diagnosis and management of pericardial diseases executive summary; The Task force on the diagnosis and management of pericardial diseases of the European society of cardiology. *Eur Heart J.* 2004;25(7):587–610. doi:10.1016/j.ehj.2004.02.002 [published Online first: 2004/05/04]

28. Martinoni A, Cipolla CM, Cardinale D, et al. Long-term results of intrapericardial chemotherapeutic treatment of malignant pericardial effusions with thiotepa. *Chest.* 2004;126(5):1412–1416. doi:10.1378/chest.126.5.1412 [published Online first: 2004/11/13]

29. Haley JH, Tajik AJ, Danielson GK, et al. Transient constrictive pericarditis: causes and natural history. *J Am Coll Cardiol.* 2004;43(2):271–275. [published Online first: 2004/01/23]

30. Suwanjutah T, Singh H, Plaisance BR, et al. Live/ real time three-dimensional transthoracic echocardiographic findings in primary left atrial leiomyosarcoma. *Echocardiography.* 2008;25(3):337–339. doi:10.1111/j.1540-8175.2007.00573.x [published Online first: 2008/03/01]

31. Asch FM, Bieganski SP, Panza JA, et al. Real-time 3-dimensional echocardiography evaluation of intracardiac masses. *Echocardiography.* 2006;23(3):218–224. doi:10.1111/j.1540-8175.2006.00196.x [published Online first: 2006/03/10]

32. Reynen K. Cardiac myxomas. *N Engl J Med.* 1995;333(24): 1610–1617. doi:10.1056/NEJM199512143332407 [published Online first: 1995/12/14]

33. Molina JE, Edwards JE, Ward HB. Primary cardiac tumors: experience at the University of Minnesota. *Thorac Cardiovasc Surg.* 1990;38(suppl 2):183–191. doi:10.1055/s-2007-1014064 [published Online first: 1990/08/01]

34. Upendram S, Nanda NC, Vengala S, et al. Live three-dimensional transthoracic echocardiographic assessment of thrombus in the innominate veins and superior vena cava utilizing right parasternal and supraclavicular approaches. *Echocardiography.* 2005;22(5):445–449. doi:10.1111/j.1540-8175.2005.50023.x [published Online first: 2005/05/20]

35. Mehmood F, Nanda NC, Vengala S, et al. Live three-dimensional transthoracic echocardiographic assessment of left atrial tumors. *Echocardiography.* 2005;22(2): 137–143. doi:10.1111/j.0742-2822.2005.03088.x [published Online first: 2005/02/08]

36. Pothineni KR, Nanda NC, Burri MV, et al. Live/real time three-dimensional transthoracic echocardiographic description of chordoma metastatic to the heart. *Echocardiography.* 2008;25(4):440–442. doi:10.1111/j.1540-8175.2008.00639.x [published Online first: 2008/03/28]

37. Nanda CN, Abd-El RSM, Gajendra K, et al. Incremental value of three-dimensional echocardiography over transesophageal multiplane two-dimensional echocardiography in qualitative and quantitative assessment of cardiac masses and defects. *Echocardiography.* 1995;12(6): 619–628. doi:doi:10.1111/j.1540-8175.1995.tb00854.x

38. Pothineni KR, Nanda NC, Burri MV, et al. Live/real time three-dimensional transthoracic echocardiographic visualization of Chiari network. *Echocardiography.* 2007;24(9):995–997. doi:10.1111/j.1540-8175.2007.00503.x [published Online first: 2007/09/27]

39. McKay T, Thomas L. Prominent crista terminalis and Eustachian ridge in the right atrium: two dimensional (2D) and three dimensional (3D) imaging. *Eur J Echocardiogr.* 2007;8(4):288–291. doi:10.1016/j.euje. 2006.03.006 [published Online first: 2006/04/20]

40. Roldan FJ, Vargas-Barron J, Vazquez-Antona C, et al. Three-dimensional transesophageal echocardiography of the atrial septal defects. *Cardiovasc Ultrasound.* 2008;6:38. doi:10.1186/1476-7120-6-38 [published Online first: 2008/07/22]

41. Sugeng L, Shernan SK, Salgo IS, et al. Live 3-dimensional transesophageal echocardiography initial experience using the fully-sampled matrix array probe. *J Am Coll Cardiol.* 2008;52(6):446–449. doi:10.1016/j. jacc.2008.04.038 [published Online first: 2008/08/02]

42. Muller S, Feuchtner G, Bonatti J, et al. Value of transesophageal 3D echocardiography as an adjunct to conventional 2D imaging in preoperative evaluation of cardiac masses. *Echocardiography.* 2008;25(6):624–631. [published Online first: 2008/07/25]

43. Stewart JA, Silimperi D, Harris P, et al. Echocardiographic documentation of vegetative lesions in infective endocarditis: clinical implications. *Circulation.* 1980;61(2): 374–380. [published Online first: 1980/02/01]

44. Zamorano J, Perez de Isla L, Sugeng L, et al. Noninvasive assessment of mitral valve area during percutaneous balloon mitral valvuloplasty: role of real-time 3D echocardiography. *Eur Heart J.* 2004;25(23):2086–2091. doi:10.1016/j.ehj.2004.09.041 [published Online first: 2004/12/02]

45. Monaghan MJ. Role of real time 3D echocardiography in evaluating the left ventricle. *Heart.* 2006;92(1):131–136. doi:10.1136/hrt.2004.058388 [published Online first: 2005/12/21]

46. Handke M, Schochlin A, Schafer DM, et al. Myxoma of the mitral valve: diagnosis by 2-dimensional and 3-dimensional echocardiography. *J Am Soc Echocardiogr.* 1999;12(9):773–776. [published Online first: 1999/09/08]

47. Le Tourneau T, Pouwels S, Gal B, et al. Assessment of papillary fibroelastomas with live three-dimensional transthoracic echocardiography. *Echocardiography.* 2008;25(5):489–495. doi:10.1111/j.1540-8175.2008.00631.x [published Online first: 2008/03/18]

48. Singh A, Miller AP, Nanda NC, et al. Papillary fibroelastoma of the pulmonary valve: assessment by live/ real time three-dimensional transthoracic echocardiography. *Echocardiography.* 2006;23(10):880–883. doi:10.1111/j.1540-8175.2006.00336.x [published Online first: 2006/10/31]

49. Sinha A, Nanda NC, Khanna D, et al. Morphological assessment of left ventricular thrombus by live three-dimensional transthoracic echocardiography. *Echocardiography.* 2004;21(7):649–655. doi:10.1111/j.0742-2822.2004.04062.x [published Online first: 2004/10/19]

50. Veinot JP, Harrity PJ, Gentile F, et al. Anatomy of the normal left atrial appendage: a quantitative study of age-related changes in 500 autopsy hearts: implications for echocardiographic examination. *Circulation*. 1997;96(9):3112–3115. [published Online first: 1997/12/31]

51. Karakus G, Kodali V, Inamdar V, et al. Comparative assessment of left atrial appendage by transesophageal and combined two- and three-dimensional transthoracic echocardiography. *Echocardiography*. 2008;25(8):918–924. doi:10.1111/j.1540-8175.2008.00758.x [published Online first: 2008/11/07]

52. Jenni R, Oechslin E, Schneider J, et al. Echocardiographic and pathoanatomical characteristics of isolated left ventricular non-compaction: a step towards classification as a distinct cardiomyopathy. *Heart*. 2001;86(6):666–671. [published Online first: 2001/11/17]

53. Daher IN, Saeed M, Schwarz ER, et al. Live three-dimensional echocardiography in diagnosis of interventricular septal perforation by pacemaker lead. *Echocardiography*. 2006;23(5):428–429. doi:10.1111/j.1540-8175.2006.00231.x [published Online first: 2006/05/12]

Ali Agha ▪ *Purvi Parwani* ▪ *Juan C. Lopez-Mattei*

INTRODUCTION

Proper identification and characterization of cardiac masses is an important aspect for the health care team evaluating a new or recurrent intracardiac abnormality suspicious of malignancy. For most intra-cavitary structures, transthoracic echocardiography (TTE) and/ or transesophageal echocardiography (TEE) will provide sufficient information to determine the type of cardiac mass. The differential diagnosis includes: benign or malignant tumor, thrombus or artifact (see also Chapters 10 and 14). Proper identification of the cardiac mass is essential, as this will guide clinical management. We will not discuss benign primary cardiac tumors in this chapter, as the diagnosis of cardiac myxomas has been addressed in other chapters of this volume as well as in other resources.[1] Myxomas often are managed in high-volume cardiovascular care centers, and afflicted patients often may not require cardio-oncologic care.

ETIOLOGY

There are multiple potential etiologies of a cardiac mass. Most importantly, a clinician must differentiate between whether the mass is a tumor or thrombus, as this guides therapeutic decision-making and interventions; while a thrombus may require that the patient receive anticoagulation, a cardiac tumor may require open biopsy to determine a specific tumor type, resection, and further oncologic intervention.

If malignancy is identified, it is important to determine if this is primary or secondary malignancy. In the case of a secondary malignancy, one may need to identify the primary tissue type. Characteristics of the malignancy will guide the timing of treatment. For example, some patients may benefit from concurrent chemotherapy and resection while others may benefit from chemotherapy followed by subsequent surgery that may be influenced by the response to initial treatment.

The incidence of primary malignant cardiac tumors is quite low, representing less than 1% of all cardiac tumors. Of the primary cardiac tumors, approximately one-quarter are malignant. Three-quarters of these malignant tumors are sarcomas (see Figure 11-1).[2] Notwithstanding the rarity of these tumors, it is important to recognize that the prognosis of patients with primary cardiac malignancy remains poor, with a mean survival of approximately 26 months.[3]

Secondary cardiac malignancy is far more common than primary, and are seen regularly in tertiary cancer centers.[4] Identifying the origin of the cardiac mass can be challenging, as cancers can invade the heart by either contiguous spread (lung, esophageal, or breast cancer, thoracic lymphomas, etc.) or intravascular spread (renal, uterine, colon, hepatic cancer, etc.). The natural history of malignant melanoma may

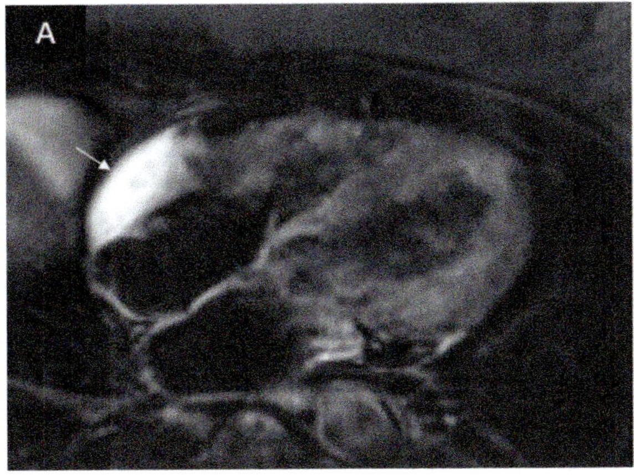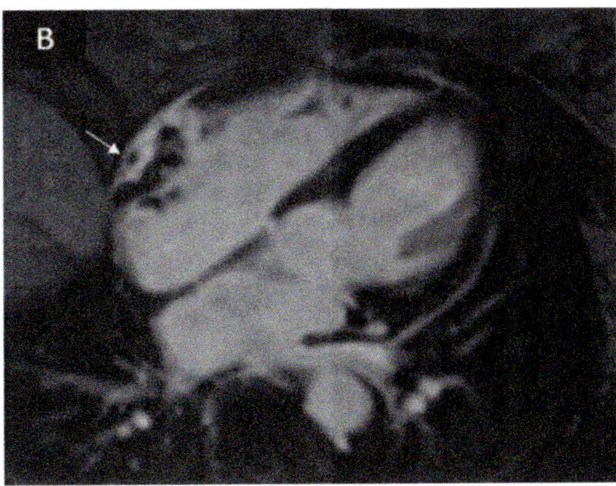

FIGURE 11-1 Cardiac MRI example of a primary cardiac angiosarcoma: This is an example of a cardiac angiosarcoma located in the right atrium (white arrows). In T2 weighted imaging with fat saturation (A), high signal within the mass can be appreciated. In late gadolinum enhancement image (B) borders are predominantly enhancing, with a central non-enhancing core.

ultimately involve spread to both the heart and the pericardium.[5]

As noted above, thrombus formation should be considered in the differential diagnosis of any cardiac mass. Many cancer patients have central lines in place for the administration of their chemotherapy, increasing the incidence of thrombus formation. Chemotherapy related contractile dysfunction and cardiomyopathy is an additional predisposing factor in thrombus formation. Similarly the hypercoagulable state associated with malignancy furthers the formation of intra-cardiac thrombi.

Although TTE is a useful tool to identify cardiac masses, it may sometimes produce artifacts that falsely appear to represent cardiac masses. Mirroring and "side lobes" may mimic masses, in addition to normal anatomic variants including Eustachian valves, Chiari networks, and lipomatous hypertrophy of the interatrial septum.[6] In cases of possible artifact on TTE, a TEE is typically recommended as an additional imaging study.

ECHOCARDIOGRAPHY

Echocardiography is usually the initial test for evaluation of a suspected cardiac mass. It is widely available for most patients. A standardized approach is required for echocardiographic evaluation of an echogenic structure inside a cardiac chamber that is not an evident artifact or a likely thrombus, according to imaging features and clinical context, as follows[7]:

■ General Location within the Heart

Location is an important aspect of determining the identity of the cardiac mass. Supporting evidence of thrombus is: (1) in TEE, a rounded echogenic structure at the left atrial appendage in a patient with atrial fibrillation; (2) in TTE, echogenicity in an akinetic apex in a patient post-myocardial infarction (post-MI). In these cases, the clinical context and findings are usually sufficient to allow for a confident diagnosis of thrombus. However, if a mass has an atypical location for a thrombus (i.e., a mass not associated with hypokinesis or akinesis of a myocardial segment, a mass not associated to atrial arrhythmias such as atrial fibrillation or flutter, or a right-sided mass) or a mass with an invasive appearance (i.e., sessile attachments to endocardium, thickening of myocardium associated with mass attachment), further assessment is essential.

■ Proximity to Superior Vena Cava (SVC) Indwelling Catheters

In cancer patients, thrombus associated with catheter use is encountered frequently. The mechanisms may be due to hypercoagulable states, direct injury to the vessel or the right atrium during central line insertion, and/or venous stasis caused by the indwelling catheter itself.[8] Often these TTE findings need corroboration through TEE. Three-dimensional (3D) TEE acquisition often helps in clarifying the relationship of the catheter to the mass. The closer the mass is to the catheter, the higher the suspicion of thrombus.

■ Vascularization

A thrombus is an avascular structure. In echocardiography, color Doppler may help not only to assess, based on turbulence generated by the mass, but also whether there is evidence that small vessels are feeding the mass;

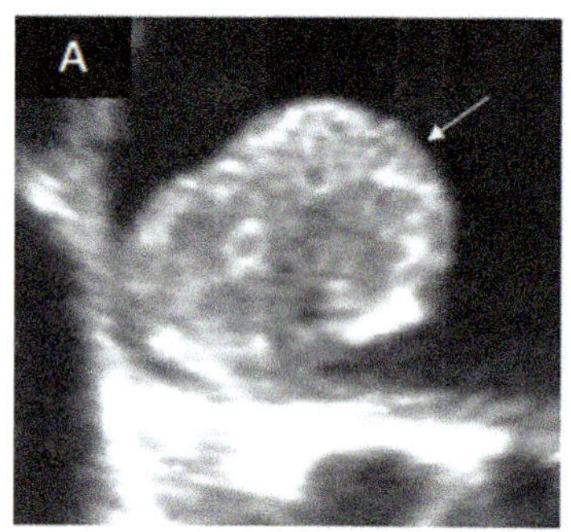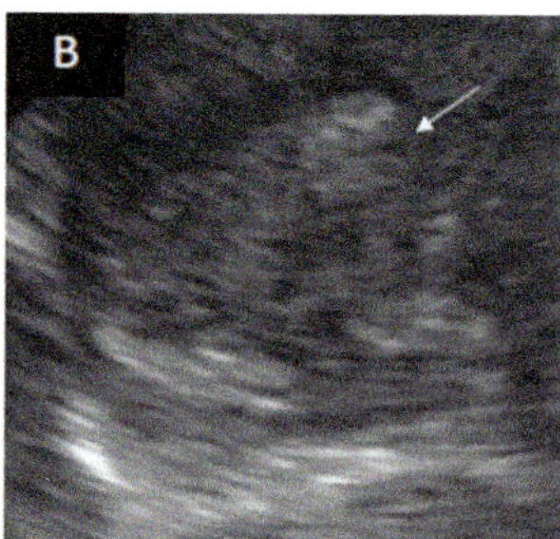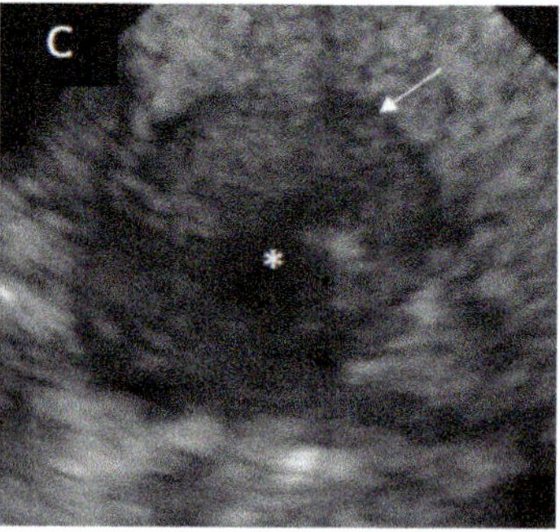

FIGURE 11-2 UEA echocardiography in a cardiac tumor. In (A), we have a 2D TEE acquisition of a mass (white arrow) in the left atrium before IV injection of an ultrasonic enhancing agent (UEA). During IV ultrasound contrast administration, as shown in (B), there seems to be significant perfusion, evidenced by the substantial enhancement that makes the mass (white arrow) difficult to distinguish from the cavity. In (C), a slight increase in mechanical index (MI) shows attenuation (due to destruction of microbubbles given high MI) at its core (*) and some of the periphery, excluding image saturation and confirming perfusion. This is consistent with tumor.

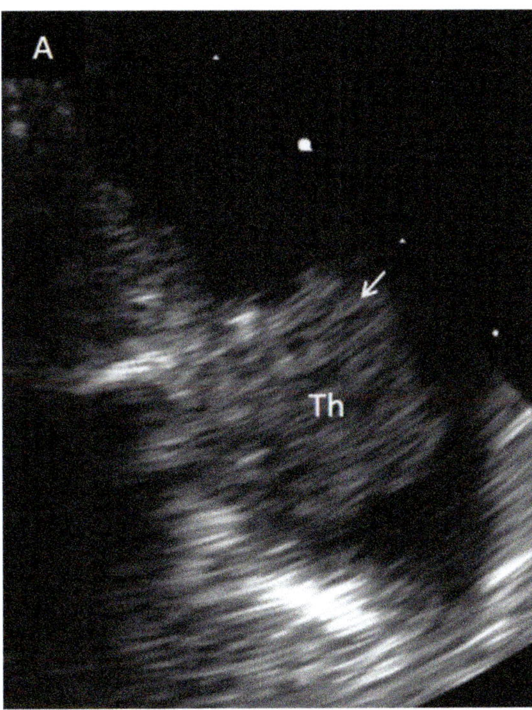
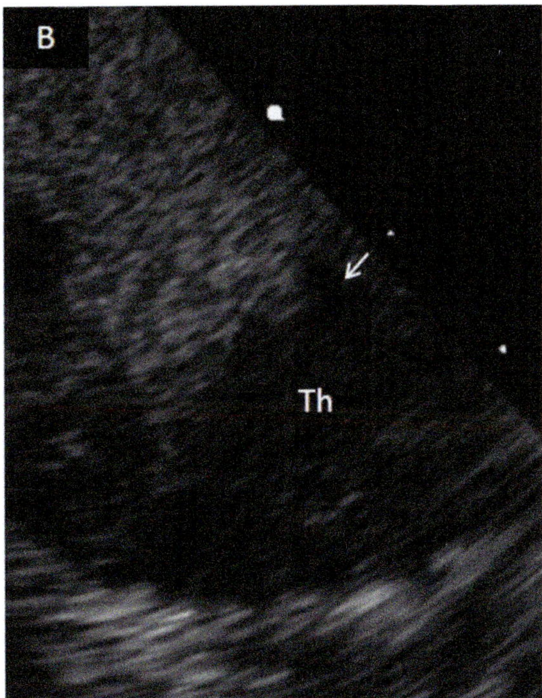

FIGURE 11-3 Contrast TEE in cardiac thrombus. In (A), there is a TEE off axis view of a mass (white arrow) in the RA before IV ultrasonic enhancing agent (UEA). In (B), during IV UEA administration, there is no perfusion because the mass (white arrow) is a thrombus. RA = right atrium, Th, thrombus.

the latter can be better visualized by TEE, due to its superior spatial resolution when compared with TTE. The use of ultrasonic enhancing agents (UEA) in echocardiography is very helpful because the presence or absence of enhancement within the mass can, in some cases, be appreciated by TTE/TEE.[9] If there is evidence of perfusion (enhancement with UEA) this is more consistent with tumor, because such enhancement suggest a vascular supply. Thrombus does not exhibit perfusion enhancement (see Figures 11-2 and 11-3).

■ Wall Motion Abnormalities

The presence of left ventricular segmental wall motion abnormalities that follow a coronary distribution suggest that a mass in the left ventricle is a thrombus. Tumor infiltration due to tethering of the myocardium can cause regional wall motion abnormalities; wall thickening might also be identified in a still ultrasound image. When the mass is a tumor in the ventricle, the ventricular systolic function is usually preserved, except when the mass causes obstruction to the outflow, leading to an increase in ventricular afterload, and ultimately, global systolic dysfunction; this is seen more commonly when tumors invade the right ventricle. Spontaneous echocardiographic contrast in relation to a mass also supports the diagnosis of thrombus.

In echocardiography, the ability to characterize tissue is limited, and the application of the backscatter technique to identify cardiac masses is not well established. When using the structured approach (described above) to determine the course of management, the characteristics of the mass encountered by echocardiography (as discussed above) need to be weighted with a determination of whether the mass has tumor versus thrombus characteristics. If the mass has characteristics of a thrombus, then anticoagulation followed by re-imaging in two months is appropriate. If follow-up imaging indicates that there is no decrease in the mass size, then other imaging modalities such as cardiac magnetic resonance imaging (MRI) may be considered.

CARDIAC MRI

Echocardiography may not be sufficient to distinguish between masses is a tumors, thrombi, or artifacts. In such instances, cardiac MRI can be very useful. The greatest benefit of cardiac MRI in the assessment of cardiac abnormalities is its ability to characterize tissue. The implementation of techniques such as first-pass perfusion and late gadolinium enhancement add important information for those evaluation intracardiac abnormalities. T1 and T2 weighted cardiac

MRI produce patterns that can distinguish tumor from thrombus, and some tumors are associated with pathognomonic findings on cardiac MRI. Contrast enhanced cardiac MRI with prolonged inversion time (TI: 600 msec) is the gold standard cardiac imaging technique to characterize thrombi (see Figures 11-4 and 11-5).[10] The standarized approach for echocardiography which was described above also applies to cardiac MRI.[7]

■ T1 and T2 Tissue Characterization

T1 (a characteristic of increasing magnetization) and T2 (decreasing magnetization) weighted imaging are useful in the characterization of cardiac masses. This evaluation is based on the precession of protons and the signal they generate in MRI. When the mass is a thrombus, the intensity of the signal, will be lower than the signal generated by the myocardium in both

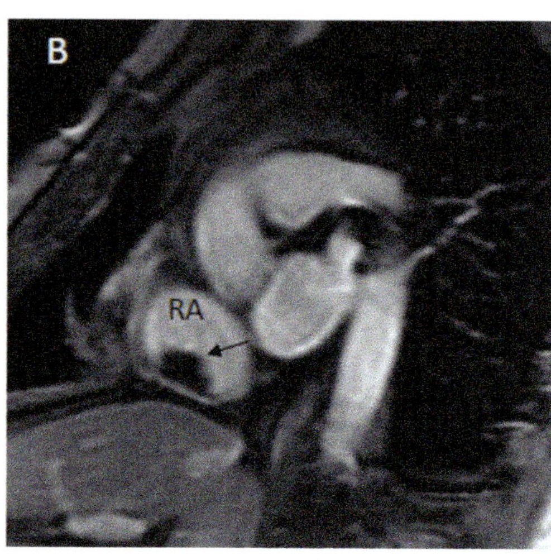

FIGURE 11-4 Cardiac MRI findings in cardiac thrombus. In (A), there is a still frame of a sagittal cine view of a mass (black arrow) in the RA. In (B), in a post-contrast acquisition with long inversion time (TI:600 msec), there is no enhancement within the mass, (black arrow), this finding supports the diagnosis of thrombus. RA, right atrium

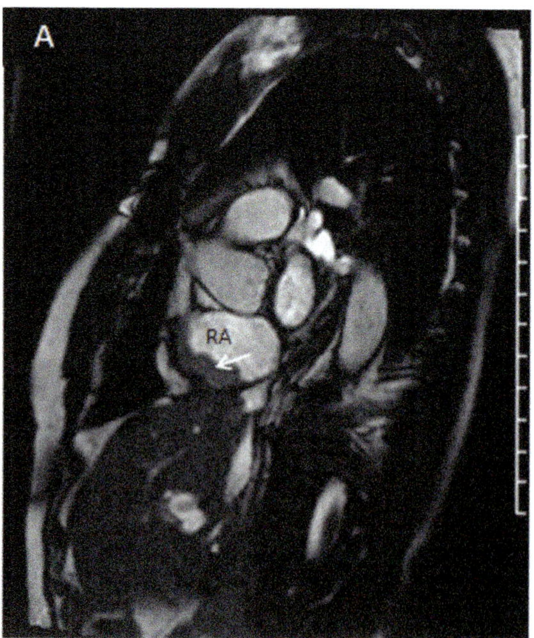
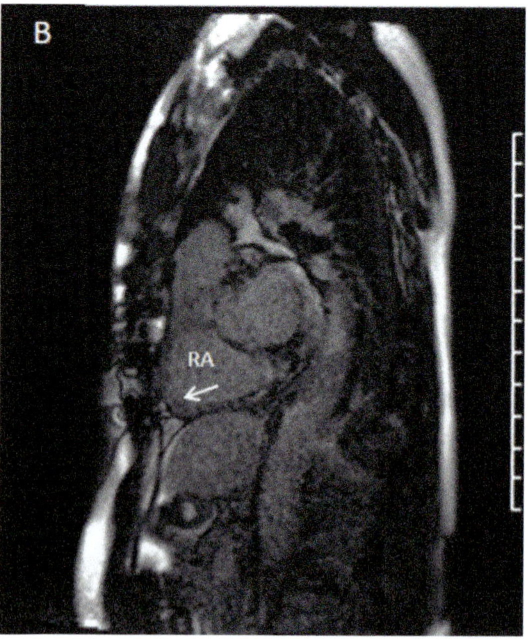

FIGURE 11-5 Cardiac MRI delayed enhancement in cardiac tumor. In (A), there is a still frame of an axial cine view of a mass (white arrow) in the RA. In (B), 10 minutes after IV administration of a gadolinium based contrast, there is delayed enhancement within the mass (increase in brightness, to the point of almost "disappearing" within the blood pool of contrast) as shown by the white arrow, this finding supports the diagnosis of tumor. RA, right atrium

T1 and T2 parameters. If the suspect mass is a tumor, generally the intensity of the signals will be similar to myocardium or is higher in both T1 and T2 weighted imaging. Among the different types of tumors, however, there could be overlap with a thrombus regarding T1 and T2 findings.

■ First-Pass Perfusion

In first-pass perfusion, image acquisition is performed during intravenous administration of a gadolinium-based contrast, focusing the view on the mass of interest. Enhancement of the mass during first-pass perfusion implies that the mass is vascularized, a finding which supports the diagnosis of tumor. If the mass is avascular in nature, enhancement will not be observed, suggesting thrombus.

■ Delayed Enhancement

This acquisition technique relies on the differential kinetics of gadolinium deposition between the intracellular and extracellular space. Usually image acquisition is performed 10 minutes after the administration of a gadolinium-based contrast. In general, enhancement is diagnostic of tumor. Inversion time (IR) is a parameter of image acquisition that describes the timing of nulling (or suppressing the signal) of different tissues after an inversion recovery pulse in MRI. If there is no enhancement and the mass nulls at a fixed inversion time of 600 msec, this is diagnostic of thrombus (Figures 11-4 and 11-5).[10]

Generally, if there is evidence of contrast uptake, the mass is a tumor. Thrombus characterization using delayed enhancement with long inversion time is a well-validated technique that has been corroborated by comparison with pathologic specimens and clinical outcomes.[10] Cardiac MRI is not a first-line technique for this type of assessment, but it increases the diagnostic certainty when needed.

CARDIAC CT

Cardiac computed tomography (CCT) has an excellent spatial resolution (<1 mm) and a larger field of view than echocardiography. While it can be used to better assess the anatomical relationship of structures, its temporal resolution is limited; if tissue characterization is performed using the Hounsfield unit scale (measurement derived from different attenuation coefficients of tissues in CT) to assess an intra-cardiac mass, there can be overlap in the units to distinguish tumor vs. thrombus. Tumor vascularization may be evident, but that is not a consistent finding. For anatomical location of a cardiac mass, cardiac CTA can be very useful.[11]

FDG PET-CT

When evaluating a cardiac tumor in patients with no history of cancer or an unidentified primary cancer, it is important to determine if it is a primary or a secondary malignancy, as the treatment recommendation will change significantly. Whole body F18 fluorodeoxyglucose positron emission tomography-computed tomography (FDG PET-CT) is useful to assess whether there is a primary malignancy that has metastasized to the heart[7]; if that is the case, the treatment usually will be systemic therapy focusing on the primary cancer lesion in the absence of mechanical compromise. If there is no suspicious peripheral metabolic activity, referral for an open biopsy or resection, if feasible, is recommended.[7]

SUMMARY

1. When TTE/TEE findings are suggestive of a cardiac mass, the standardized approach[7] (determine location, catheter proximity, level of vascularization, and presence of wall motion abnormalities) should be used to determine whether the mass has the characteristics of a tumor, a thrombus, or an artifact (see Figure 11-6).
   a. If the mass has thrombus characteristics, use of anticoagulation and follow-up imaging in two months is recommended.
   b. If differentiation is unclear, consider use of cardiac MRI as that technique remains the most promising non-invasive technique for thrombus characterization.
   c. If the mass has tumor characteristics, then consider using cardiac MRI plus whole body PET CT for further differentiation.
   d. If the cardiac MRI and PET CT findings are suggestive of primary cardiac tumor, consider open biopsy (and resection, if feasible) or percutaneous biopsy in selective cases.
   e. If the cardiac mass evaluated by cardiac MRI and PET CT indicates cardiac metastasis with a known primary tumor, then the recommendation, in most of the cases, will be to treat the underlying malignancy and perform follow-up imaging.

2. It is important to use echocardiography-based tumor and thrombus characteristics to determine what will be the downstream testing and treatment strategy.

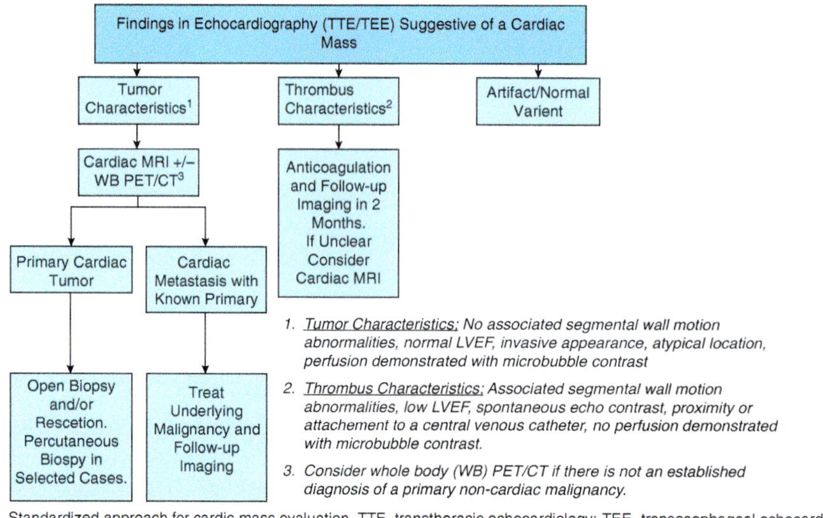

FIGURE 11-6 MD Anderson's algorithm for cardiac mass evaluation. (Reprinted by permission from Springer Nature, *Current Treatment Options in Cardiovascular Medicine* [Evaluation and management of cardiac tumors, Palaskas et al., 2018].[7])

KNOWLEDGE GAPS

1. What is the role of molecular imaging with echocardiography, cardiac MRI and cardiac PET in the non-invasive characterization of cardiac tumors?

2. What is the feasibility of using percutaneous biopsy for cardiac tumor tissue diagnosis?

3. What is the appropriate imaging interval to assess response to chemotherapy in malignant cardiac tumors?

REFERENCES

1. Butany J, Nair V, Naseemuddin A, Nair GM, Catton C, Yau T. Cardiac tumours: diagnosis and management. *The Lancet Oncol*. 2005;6(4):219–228.

2. Bisel HF, Wroblewski F, Ladue JS. Incidence and clinical manifestations of cardiac metastases. *JAMA*. 1953;153(8):712–715.

3. Yusuf SW, Bathina JD, Qureshi S, et al. Cardiac tumors in a tertiary care cancer hospital: clinical features, echocardiographic findings, treatment and outcomes. *Heart Int*. 2012;7(1):e4.

4. Lopez-Mattei J, Iliescu C, Durand JB, et al. The role of cardiac MRI in cardio-oncology. *Future Cardiol*. 2017;13(4):311–316.

5. Amano J, Nakayama J, Yoshimura Y, Ikeda U. Clinical classification of cardiovascular tumors and tumor-like lesions, and its incidences. *Gen Thorac Cardiovasc Surg*. 2013;61(8):435–447.

6. Alam M. Pitfalls in the echocardiographic diagnosis of intracardiac and extracardiac masses. *Echocardiography*. 1993;10(2):181–191.

7. Palaskas N, Thompson K, Gladish G, et al. Evaluation and management of cardiac tumors. *Curr Treat Options Cardiovasc Med*. 2018;20(4):29.

8. Verso M, Agnelli G. Venous thromboembolism associated with long-term use of central venous catheters in cancer patients. *J Clin Oncol*. 2003;21(19):3665–375.

9. Porter TR, Mulvagh SL, Abdelmoneim SS, et al. Clinical applications of ultrasonic enhancing agents in Echocardiography: 2018 American Society of Echocardiography guidelines update. *J Am Soc Echocardiogr*. 2018;31(3):241–274.

10. Weinsaft JW, Kim HW, Shah DJ, et al. Detection of left ventricular thrombus by delayed-enhancement cardiovascular magnetic resonance prevalence and markers in patients with systolic dysfunction. *J Am Coll Cardiol*. 2008;52(2):148–157.

11. Kassop D, Donovan MS, Cheezum MK, et al. Cardiac masses on cardiac CT: a review. *Curr Cardiovasc Imaging Rep*. 2014;7:9281.

12 Pericardial Disease in the Cancer Patient

Steven M. Ewer

INTRODUCTION

Cancer is among the leading causes of death in developed countries. Involvement of the heart is a frequent occurrence, as is extensively detailed in these chapters. The heart can be a site of metastatic disease, and is also vulnerable to treatment-related complications. The pericardium is of special interest to those treating patients with cancer, as it is the cardiac structure most frequently affected by tumor spread, and it is the cardiac structure most sensitive to the effects of ionizing radiation. Pericardial disease and cancer are therefore frequently intertwined.

It is estimated that approximately 9% of patients that ultimately die from their cancer have direct malignant involvement of the pericardium, and for 80% of these patients, this pericardial involvement will contribute to their death.[1] An even greater number develop pericardial disease via other mechanisms that are related to their malignancy. Likewise, 7% of patients presenting with acute pericardial disease have a neoplastic etiology,[2] and 35% of procedures performed for pericardial disease are done so on cancer patients.[3] Typically, pericardial disease presents well after the diagnosis of cancer has been established. Relevant clinical questions then include the etiology of the pericardial disease, implications for prognosis and further cancer treatment, and management approach to the pericardial disease. However, among patients that present with pericardial disease without previously known malignancy, a new diagnosis of malignancy is discovered less than 5% of cases of acute percardiditis[2] and 23% of large pericardial effusions.[4]

Malignant pericardial disease was historically considered a medical curiosity, diagnosed almost exclusively on autopsy. With the advent of improved imaging technology, earlier diagnosis became possible, but prognosis remained grim, and little could be offered to patients besides palliation. Currently, diagnosis of malignant pericardial disease is common, and a much greater number of treatments are available for the systemic and local management of their malignancy. These advances have rendered pericardial disease in the cancer patient increasingly relevant in modern medicine. Despite these accomplishments, however, quality evidence for optimizing diagnostic and therapeutic strategies for these conditions has lagged, and we are left with uncertainty as to the ideal management of this complex group of patients.

Malignancy and its treatment cause pericardial disease in a variety of ways. While primary pericardial tumors are very rare, metastases are quite common. Nearly all cancers are capable of metastasizing to the pericardium through either direct extension (i.e., lung, esophageal), retrograde lymphatic spread (i.e., lung, breast), or hematogenous seeding (i.e., melanoma, lymphoma, leukemia). Other causes of pericardial disease besides direct invasion include adjacent inflammation, interruption of lymphatic or venous drainage, infection, hypoalbuminemia, congestive heart failure, renal failure, toxicies of chemotherapeutics, and chest irradiation. It should be recognized that pericardial disease can also be idiopathic and unrelated to the underlying malignancy. The etiology of a pericardial abnormality is thus critical to the management of cancer patients, having important implications for prognosis and treatment.

Symptoms of pericardial disease are often vague and nonspecific, and can mimic disease in many other organ systems, which are often also affected by the malignancy. Diagnosis can be challenging, and treatment of existing pericardial disease does not ensure relief of symptoms. The clinician must approach these patients with a broad view of clinical medicine in order to minimize the possibility of incorrect diagnoses and inappropriate interventions. Despite these challenges, the management of such problems may be tremendously gratifying, such as the dramatic improvement upon relief of pericardial tamponade. As cancer treatments continue to improve, we will have increasing opportunity to offer our patients both quantity and quality of life through management of their pericardial disease.

After a brief discussion of normal pericardial structure and function, this chapter will examine the spectrum of primary and metastatic tumors of the pericardium, pericardial sequelae of chest radiation, and other aspects of malignancy and its treatment that affect the pericardium. We will then review the more common manifestations of pericardial disease as it pertains to the patient with diagnosed or undiagnosed malignancy.

Mechanisms, diagnosis, and treatment of these entities, including acute pericarditis, pericardial effusion, tamponade, and pericardial constriction will be discussed.

NORMAL PERICARDIAL STRUCTURE AND FUNCTION

The pericardium is a fibrous sac surrounding the heart consisting of two layers: the inner *visceral pericardium*, attached directly to the epicardial surface of the heart, and the outer *parietal pericardium*. These layers are separated by the *pericardial space*, which normally contains a small amount of serous fluid, but can greatly expand in pathologic states, holding as much as two liters. The two meet at or near the origin of the great vessels, and these attachments serve to anchor the pericardium and heart within the mediastinum.

The visceral pericardium consists of a monolayer of mesothelial cells on the surface of the epicardium. The parietal pericardium likewise has a mesothelial layer, but also contains a thicker serosa, which is made of fibrous connective tissue including collagen and elastin, and normally measures 1–3.5 mm in thickness.[5] This thickness increases with most pericardial disease states including those related to malignancy and indeed is the primary abnormality in the case of constriction. Most references to "the pericardium" as a tissue structure are understood to imply the parietal pericardium; the visceral pericardium usually is included as part of the "epicardium". While this convention has the potential for confusion, the meaning is usually clear from the context. Metastases to the pericardium, however may involve both the parietal and visceral layers.

Pericardial innervation is derived from the phrenic nerve anteriorly and the esophageal plexus posteriorly, both supplied by the vagus nerve. Myocardial innervation is supplied by the same nerves, which helps explain the similarities of anginal pain and pericardial pain when prominent pleuritic features are absent. Lymphatic drainage is to the anterior and posterior mediastinal lymph nodes, and retrograde spread through these vessels is an important source of metastatic tumor spread, especially for cases of breast and lung cancers. Lymphatic obstruction by tumor is also a mechanism of pericardial effusion.

The pericardial space normally contains up to 50 ml of fluid, which is continuously secreted by the mesothelial cells of the visceral pericardium. This plasma ultrafiltrate serves to lubricate the movements of the heart. Pericardial fluid is resorbed via lymphatics and veins. When secretion is increased as in acute pericarditis or resorption is decreased (i.e., tumor obstruction of lymphatics), fluid can accumulate abnormally in the pericardial space.

The pericardium serves many other physiologic functions in addition to lubrication of the heart. The relatively fixed volume and inherent elasticity combine to keep the pericardial sac under tension, which contributes to diastolic pressures within the heart and helps maintain the classic pressure-volume relationships of cardiac physiology. Within the pericardial space, there is a small negative pressure (~3 mmHg) that serves to augment diastolic filling.[5] Other functions include a physical tethering of the heart within the mediastinum, a barrier against infection and inflammation, participation in the cardiac autonomic reflexes, and paracrine functions (releasing mediators such as endothelin and prostacyclines). When cancer results in a diseased pericardium, any of these functions can be disrupted, often leading to complex pathophysiology.

PRIMARY TUMORS OF THE PERICARDIUM

Primary pericardial tumors (both benign and malignant) are extraordinarily rare. The reported incidence of all primary cardiac tumors range from 0.001%–0.28% in autopsy series,[6] and pericardial tumors make up only a fraction of these cases. (By comparison, incidence of pericardial metastases is approximately 2.5% in similar general autopsy series.) A list of primary tumors of the pericardium is shown in Table 12-1. Five tumor types

TABLE 12-1   Primary pericardial tumors (relative frequency)

BENIGN	MALIGNANT
Pericardial Cyst (62%)	Mesothelioma (15%)
Teratoma (11%)	Angiosarcoma (7%)
Bronchogenic Cyst	Malignant Teratoma (3%)
Dermoid	Kaposi's Sarcoma
Lipoma	Rhabdomyosarcoma
Fibroma	Fibrosarcoma
Solitary Fibrous Tumor	Synovial Sarcoma
Neuroma	Spindle Cell Sarcoma
Lymphangioma	Thymoma
Lymphangioepithelioma	Primary Cardiac Lymphoma
Hemangioma	Hodgkin Lymphoma
Neurofibroma	Malignant Nerve Sheath Tumor
Leiomyoma	Hemangioepithelioma
Hamartoma	Liposarcoma
	Pheochromocytoma

make up the vast majority of primary pericardial tumors, accompanied by a longer list of very rare entities. Benign pericardial tumors are more common than primary malignancies, and present more commonly in the pediatric population. Malignant tumors are seen more frequently after the third decade. We will briefly discuss some of the more common pericardial tumors below. The bulk of epidemiologic data regarding primary cardiac tumors comes from a series of 533 such cases by the Armed Forces Institute of Pathology,[7] and has been summarized and updated more recently.[6]

Pericardial cyst

Pericardial cysts make up the most common primary pericardial tumor. They consist of a lining of mesothelial cells surrounded by fibrous connective tissue and contain a clear, straw-colored fluid, which may communicate with the pericardial space. Pericardial cysts are usually small (less than 3 cm) but have the capacity to expand considerably, and may achieve dimensions of up to 15 cm.[6] The most common location is along the right heart border (Figure 12-1).[6] The majority of pericardial cysts are diagnosed before the age of 30. Only 1/3 of patients present with symptoms, which can include chest pain, dyspnea and arrhythmias.[5] More typically, an abnormality is seen incidentally on chest X-ray. More detailed imaging can be obtained with echocardiography, computed tomography (CT), or magnetic resonance imaging (MRI). Treatment, when necessary, consists of surgical excision, percutaneous drainage, or thorascopic drainage. Prognosis is excellent.

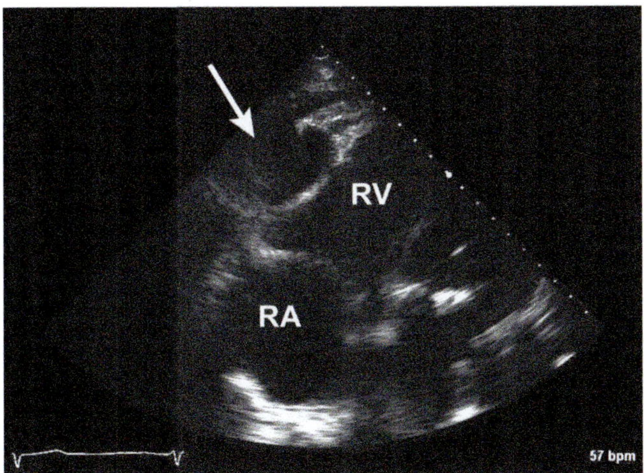

FIGURE 12-1 Off-axis echocardiographic image of a large pericardial cyst (arrow) along the right ventricular free wall. RV, right ventricle; RA, right atrium.

Teratoma

Teratomas are tumors derived from all three germ layers, and though usually benign, can carry malignant potential. Pericardial teratomas arise from the base of the pulmonary artery or aorta, which often complicates their surgical removal. Approximately 80% occur in the pediatric population,[6] typically in infancy or in utero.[8,9] There is a remarkable female-to-male preponderance. Clinical presentation can be dramatic, with compression of the right atrium or right ventricle, or tamponade from an associated pericardial effusion. Presentation includes hydrops fetalis, fetal pericardial effusion, and dyspnea, cyanosis, cardiomegaly, cardiac murmurs, and sudden cardiac death in the neonatal or pediatric patient. Treatment includes surgical excision, and a non-trivial operative mortality exists for these patients. Occasionally, fetal pericardiocentesis is also necessary.[10] After recovery from surgery, the prognosis is excellent and recurrences are uncommon. In rare cases of malignant transformation, teratomas can invade adjacent structures such as myocardium. In these unfortunate cases surgical excision is not feasible and the prognosis is poor.

Mesothelioma

Mesothelioma is the most common primary malignancy of the pericardium. It usually presents in middle age, with males affected twice as often as females.[11] It is controversial whether exposure to inhaled asbestos is a significant risk factor for pericardial mesothelioma as it is for its pleural counterpart, as several cases without any apparent asbestos exposure have been documented.[5,12] Another series however found no difference in asbestos exposure in patients with pleural versus pericardial mesothelioma,[13] implying an association. Further confounding the debate is the fact that some mesotheliomas thought to be of pericardial origin are actually derived from the pleura with local invasion into the pericardium. Some evidence implicates Simian Virus 40 as well as asbestos in the pathogenesis of mesothelioma; this virus has been found in up to 80% of patients with mesothelioma, and has been found to cause mesothelioma in animal models.[14]

Mesothelioma usually spreads uniformly throughout the pericardial space, although localized nodules can exist. Local invasion can occur to the pleura, mediastinum, mediastinal lymph nodes, and occasionally through the diaphragm to the peritoneum. Invasion to the deep myocardium is rare, in contrast with other pericardial malignancies. Distant metastases are also notably uncommon, but have been found in the brain.[15] Clinical presentation includes acute pericarditis, pericardial effusion, and constriction. Diagnosis of mesothelioma is confirmed by pathologic evaluation of the pericardial fluid or biopsy. Treatment is mainly palliative, and consists of radiation, chemotherapy, and local measures to control pericardial symptoms. Given the behavior patterns of this malignancy, surgical resection is very difficult, and operative mortality high. Prognosis is poor with or without surgery, with one series reporting a 60% 6-month mortality.[6]

■ Angiosarcoma

Angiosarcoma is the second most common primary pericardial malignancy after mesothelioma and originates in either the right atrium or pericardium in 80% of cases.[6] Patients usually present as young or middle-aged adults, and men are more susceptible than women. Unlike mesothelioma, angiosarcoma commonly invades the myocardium, and can present with intracardiac masses or valvular obstruction. Distant metastases are possible and occur in approximately 1/4 of all cases,[6] with a predilection for the central nervous system. Symptoms and clinical findings include those of acute pericarditis, pericardial effusion, congestive heart failure, arrhythmias, and constitutional symptoms. Pericardial effusions are typically hemorrhagic. Surgical resection may be possible in selected patients but treatment is generally palliative, and includes chemotherapy and radiation.

■ Other primary pericardial tumors

Pericardial lipomas resemble those found elsewhere in the body. They are slow-growing benign tumors that are asymptomatic until they begin to compress adjacent structures. Unlike teratomas, there is no significant inflammatory reaction, and effusion is usually absent. If not compressing critical structures, they can grow to giant proportions—nearly 5 kg in one case report.[16] They can be confused with pericardial cysts, in part because of their homogenous, low-density signal on various imaging modalities. Surgery is curative, and offered only when symptoms warrant intervention or diagnostic uncertainty remains. As with lipomas elsewhere, there is a low rate of malignant transformation to liposarcoma. Once resected, lipsarcomas can recur, and repeat surgery can be an effective way to manage such cases.[17,18]

Primary cardiac lymphoma is usually of B-cell origin and tends to involve both the myocardium and pericardium simultaneously (Figure 12-2). Treatment is similar to extracardiac lymphoma. Hemangiomas and lymphangiomas can occur in the pericardium, often mimicking pericardial cysts. Occasionally,

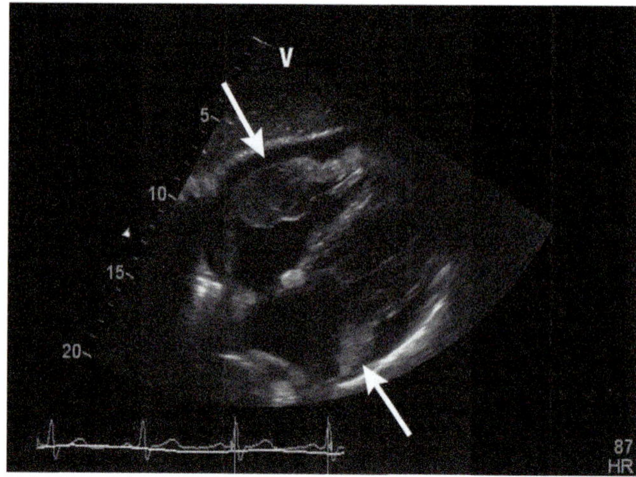

FIGURE 12-2 Subcostal echocardiographic image of a patient with primary cardiac T-cell/NK cell lymphoma. Tumor is seen in the right and left atrioventricular grooves (arrows). Note the associated pericardial effusion.

thymomas can arise from the parietal pericardium without evidence of anterior mediastinal involvement. Tumors can be benign or malignant, and do not appear to be associated with myasthenia gravis. Intrapericardial pheochromocytoma is a rare but well-documented phenomenon. Diagnosis includes measurement of active metabolites in the blood and urine, and imaging with MRI or targeted nuclear scanning. Pericardial tumors have been described in the context of neurofibromatosis 1.

METASTATIC DISEASE OF THE PERICARDIUM

Malignant pericardial disease is very common, and contributes heavily to morbidity and mortality.[1] In several large autopsy series, 10% of all patients who die of cancer have metastases to the heart, and the vast majority of these have pericardial involvement.[19] Pericardial metastases outnumber primary pericardial tumors approximately 100-fold, and thus are by far the more important clinical entities. Nearly all cancers have been found to metastasize to the pericardium, but only a handful of these are seen with any meaningful frequency. Table 12-2 lists the more common pericardial metastases with their relative frequencies.[20-22] Lung, breast, and hematologic malignancies together account for approximately 2/3 of pericardial metastases. In some series, this group accounts for 80%.[19] These numbers reflect the overall higher incidence of these malignancies. Of equal relevance is the likelihood of a given malignancy to metastasize to the pericardium. Melanoma is the most likely to do

TABLE 12-2 Metastatic disease of the pericardium (relative frequency)

| Lung Cancer (33%) |
| Breast Cancer (19%) |
| Hematologic Malignancies (13%) |
| Gastrointestinal Carcinomas (8%) |
| Melanoma (5%) |
| Prostate Cancer (4%) |
| Thyroid Cancer (4%) |
| Pancreatic Cancer (4%) |
| Gynecologic Malignancies (4%) |

so, with up to 70% of metastatic cases involving the pericardium.[19] Leukemia and lymphoma are found to involve the pericardium in approximately 33% of cases, breast cancer in 21%, and lung cancer in 19%.[1]

Cancer can metastasize to the pericardium via one of three mechanisms: direct extension, retrograde lymphatic spread, and hematogenous seeding. Direct extension is facilitated by aggressive tumor behavior and proximity to the heart. Malignancies in this category include lung cancer, esophageal cancer, and to a lesser degree breast cancer. Other members of this category are primary cardiac tumors that originate elsewhere in the heart and invade the pericardium, such as rhabdomyosarcoma and fibrosarcoma. Angiosarcoma is a unique, albeit confusing example in that it can originate in either the myocardium or pericardium and then proceed to invade adjacent structures. Lymphatic spread is probably the most common mechanism of pericardial metastasis. Careful histologic study has confirmed this mechanism in the majority of cases.[23–25] Cancers that frequently metastasize to the anterior and posterior mediastinal nodes, most notably breast and lung cancer, can reach the pericardium in this manner (Figure 12-3). Of note, breast cancer located in the inner quadrants may be more likely to cause malignant pericardial effusion.[26] Invasion and obstruction of lymphatics is also likely to be the main contributor to malignant and non-malignant pericardial effusions in this group. Leukemia, lymphoma, and melanoma most commonly seed the heart, including the pericardium, through the blood vessels (Figure 12-4). Hemorrhage often accompanies metastases in this category, contributing to the pericardial effusion. It is notable that these malignancies are the same ones that have a higher propensity to involve the pericardium.

Presentation of metastatic pericardial disease is highly variable, spanning the spectrum from incidental

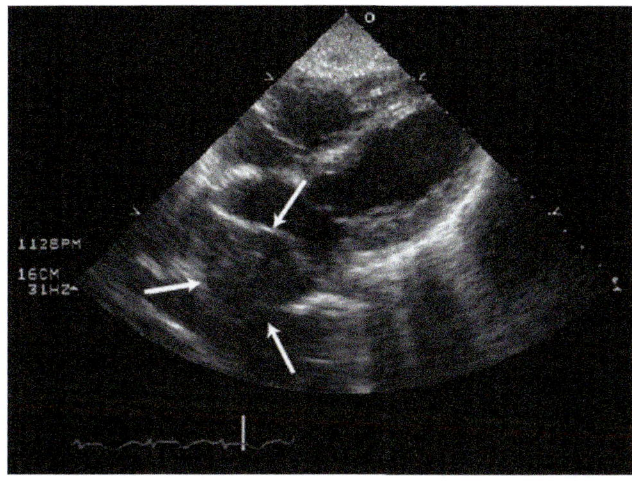

FIGURE 12-3 Parasternal long axis echocardiographic image showing a large pericardial tumor (arrows) compressing the left atrium in a patient with metastatic lung cancer.

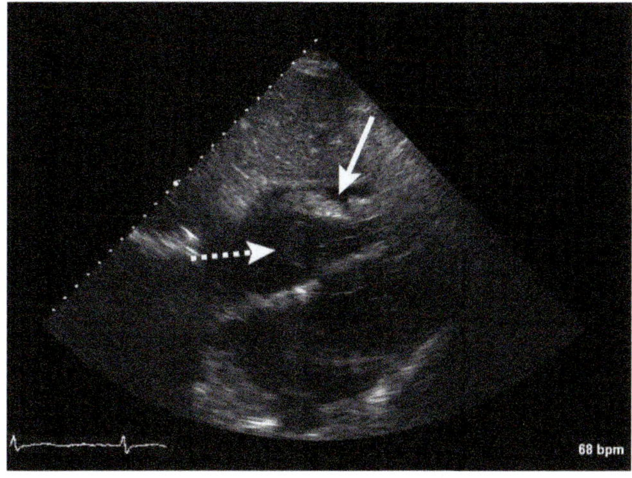

FIGURE 12-4 Subcostal echocardiographic image of a patient with post-transplant lymphoproliferative disease. Pericardial thickening and tumor infiltration are evident (arrow), in addition to a small pericardial effusion. Also present is a round tumor attached to the tricuspid valve (dotted arrow) for which tissue pathology was not available.

finding to life-threatening catastrophic event. The common pericardial syndromes, namely acute pericarditis, chronic effusion, tamponade, and constrictive disease all occur in cancer patients and will be discussed in detail below. In general, malignant pericardial disease presents more often as chronic pericardial effusions or tamponade. Case series have been published that specifically look at symptoms and signs of metastatic pericardial disease. The most frequent symptoms are dyspnea and cough, and the most common findings include tachycardia, elevated jugular venous pressure, pleural effusion and abnormal chest X-ray.[20,27] Symptoms are non-specific and can mimic other diseases, especially those involving the lungs, which frequently serve as the primary site of malignancy. Atrial arrhythmias are a common manifestation of malignant pericardial disease, and new occurrence in a cancer patient should raise suspicion for cardiac metastases. Because symptoms are relatively non-specific, the differential diagnosis in these patients is always broad and the clinician must have a high index of suspicion to detect pericardial involvement.

Transthoracic echocardiogram is the imaging modality of choice for the evaluation of pericardial disease because of its high diagnostic yield, ready availability, and non-invasive nature (Figure 12-5). Echocardiographic findings for specific entities will be discussed below. Chest X-ray may reveal cardiomegaly, pleural effusions, and mediastinal lymphadenopathy. Electrocardiography may reveal several aspects of pericardial disease, and these will also be considered below. Computed tomography (CT) and magnetic resonance imaging (MRI) can be helpful adjuncts, especially useful because of their expanded field of view, including lungs, pleura, mediastinum, and great vessels, which helps put malignant pericardial disease in a broader context (Figure 12-6). MRI can often visualize cardiac tumors with extraordinary contrast resolution.[28,29] Because melanin can bind paramagnetic metals, melanoma has unique features on MRI, giving a bright appearance on T1-weighted images in contrast to other tumors.[28] Both MRI and CT can help determine pericardial thickness if constriction is being considered.

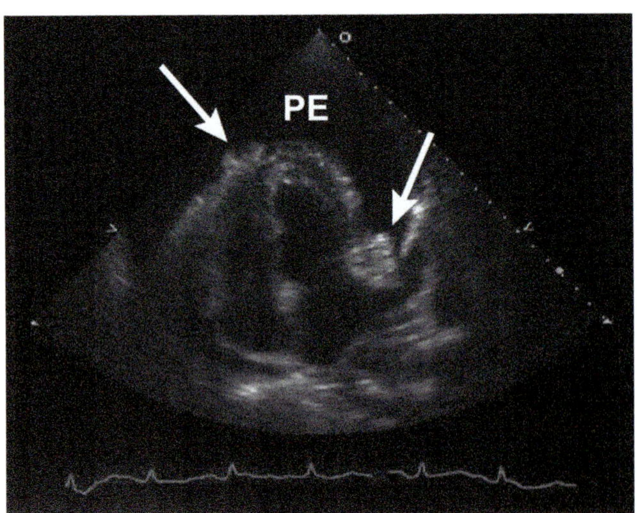

FIGURE 12-5 Apical 4-chamber view of a large malignant pericardial effusion (PE) in a patient with squamous cell carcinoma of the lung. Note visible pericardial metastases (arrows).

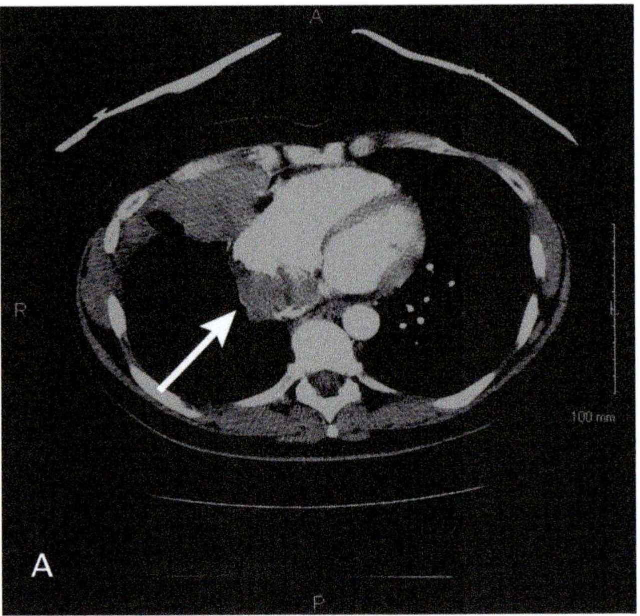

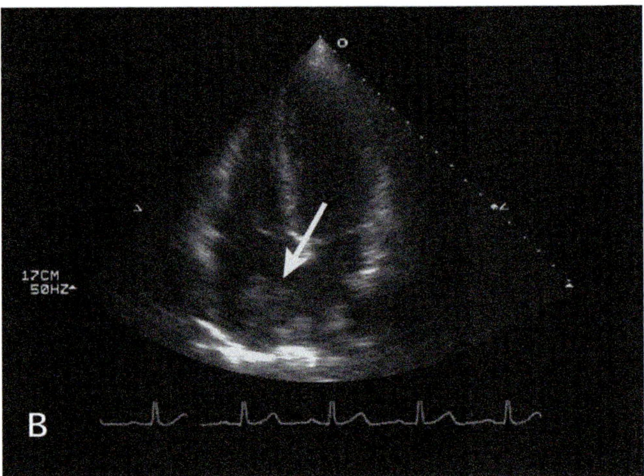

FIGURE 12-6 Leiomyosarcoma of the uterus metastatic to the pericardium. (A) CT imaging of the pericardial-based mass protruding into the right atrium (arrow). (B) Apical 4-chamber echocardiographic image of the same patient.

Pathology plays a major role in diagnosis, including cytology of pericardial fluid and tissue from surgical specimens. The finding of malignant cells in pericardial fluid or in tissue samples of parietal or visceral pericardium help establish the diagnosis of a *malignant pericardial effusion*, defined as an effusion associated with any evidence for malignant invasion of the pericardium. Not all pericardial effusions in a patient with cancer are necessarily malignant (see below). The reported sensitivity of cytology from pericardial effusions ranges around 80%–90% in most studies, and the specificity approaches 100%.[1,12] False-negatives have been attributed to either very low cell counts or large amounts of obscuring blood.

Sensitivity of cytology is lower in certain malignancies, namely leukemia and lymphoma.[12]

Diagnostic yield for malignant pericardial disease can be enhanced with biopsy. Percutaneous biopsy of the parietal pericardium or intrapericardial tumors has been shown to be feasible,[30,31] but surgery is the more typical method of obtaining tissue samples. Through a surgical approach, specimens can be obtained from both the visceral and parietal pericardium. This can be facilitated by pericardioscopy, which can directly visualize tumors protruding into the pericardial space. Pericardial biopsy without direct visualization is less sensitive than cytology because of sampling error.[32] When both cytology and pericardioscopy-guided biopsy are used, sensitivity is maximized. Fluid analysis is usually adequate to establish the diagnosis, but if cytology findings are benign and clinical suspicion for malignant effusion remains high, more rigorous investigation may be warranted.

Tumor markers are beginning to make progress in characterizing serous effusions related to malignancy.[33] In particular, carcinoembryonic antigen (CEA) levels are elevated in the pericardial fluid of patients with malignant effusions due to many different cancers.[34,35] Although case series have been small, results have been promising. DNA ploidy analysis by flow cytometry has been investigated as an additional means of diagnosing malignant pericardial effusions. Exclusively diploid DNA is associated with benign pathology, and aneuploid or tetraploid with positive cytology.[36–38] Immunocytochemistry has shown promise not only in diagnosing malignancy, but also helping to distinguish among various forms. For example, fluid Ber-EP4 positivity was 95% sensitive for carcinoma, but was not seen in any cases of mesothelioma or in benign effusions.[39] In the future, tumor-specific markers may be available for use in evaluating pericardial effusions of unclear origin in the cancer patient.

Treatment of malignant pericardial disease involves both local control of the pericardial disease and if appropriate, systemic treatment for the underlying malignancy. Palliation is usually the goal, since the overall prognosis generally poor. Tumor type and aggressiveness must be taken into account. As with any treatment in oncology, quality and quantity of life must both be considered when choosing a therapeutic strategy. In general, the more definitive procedures carry a higher risk of morbidity and mortality, and less burdensome strategies are sometimes more prudent. Specific interventions are discussed below. Good communication between the cardiologist, oncologist, primary care physician, patient and family is useful in arriving at an appropriate treatment strategy that can optimize outcomes for the patient.

NON-MALIGNANT PERICARDIAL DISEASE IN CANCER PATIENTS

It has been estimated that nearly 2/3 of patients with malignancy who present with pericardial disease do not have direct pathologic invasion of the pericardium by the tumor.[3] Radiation pericarditis and opportunistic infections are examples of indirect effects of malignancy. In some instances pericardial disease is completely unrelated to the malignancy. We will discuss some of the non-malignant but malignancy-related conditions here.

■ Radiation-induced pericardial disease

It has been well established that radiation fields that include the heart are associated with cardiac sequelae. This topic is more extensively covered in Chapter 7 (Effects of Radiation Therapy on the Cardiovascular System), and only aspects related to pericardial disease are discussed here. The pericardium is the most radiosensitive of the cardiac structures.[6] Radiation-related pericardial disease depends mostly on radiation dose, volume of the heart exposed, and specific techniques used, but other factors play a role, including age at the time of exposure (younger patients are at higher risk) and even genetic susceptibility.[40] The mechanism of pericardial damage from radiation is thought to consist of microvascular destruction (including lymphatics) and apoptosis from direct cellular injury.[41] Inflammation from necrosis of tumor cells and hypersensitivity reactions may also play a role.[6] Over time, pericardial thickening, fibrosis and effusion can develop. Although pathologic changes can be found in many patients exposed to radiation, symptoms occur in a relatively small minority.

The most common malignancies treated with chest radiation and thus associated with cardiac disease are lung cancer, breast cancer, and lymphoma. Other relevant malignancies are esophageal and thyroid cancer, and those treated with total body radiation. Radiation doses typically associated with cardiac disease in adults start around 25 Gy (2500 Rads), with disease quite common at doses above 40 Gy. One study found acute pericarditis in over 30% of patients who received greater than 40 Gy to the heart.[6] Incidence of cardiac sequelae also increases when more than 50% of the volume of the heart is contained in the radiation field.[42] Two large cohorts of survivors of childhood cancer suggest significant risk with radiation doses smaller than previously reported, down to 5–15 Gy.[43,44]

The exact incidence of radiation-related pericardial disease is difficult to discern because of the potentially long delay between radiation exposure and the development of late pericardial disease.

Furthermore, improvements in radiation techniques over the last 30 years have led to remarkable reductions in the incidence of disease, making older epidemiologic studies somewhat obsolete. One study examined the burden of cardiac radiation in all patients with pericardial disease and found radiation to be the cause in 7.3%. This was further broken down, and radiation was implicated in 11% of cases of constriction, 7.5% of pericardial effusion, and 9.1% of acute pericarditis.[21]

Hodgkin lymphoma carries the highest incidence of radiation-related cardiac disease, attributable to disease prevalence, rate of cure, younger patient population, and anatomic considerations. The relative risk of fatal cardiac events has been reported as high as 7.2 after treatment.[45,46] In one study of 48 long-term Hodgkin survivors with an average of 14 year follow-up and a median dose of 40 Gy, all patients studied were found to have pericardial thickening, and one was found to have constriction.[47] An autopsy study of young patients who received over 35 Gy to the heart found pericardial thickening in 15 of 16 cases, and clinical evidence of tamponade was present in 5 cases prior to death.[48] In the largest cohort to date of patients with mediastinal radiation for Hodgkin lymphoma, 2.2% of 590 patients developed clinical pericardial disease.[49]

Breast cancer is typically treated with tangential radiation fields, such that no more than 2 cm of lung or chest wall tissue is involved. Respiratory gating with breath-holding techniques can further reduce cardiac radiation.[50] The heart is nearly completely shielded during radiation of right-sided breast cancer, and is minimized with modern techniques for left-sided disease. Significant cardiac toxicities of radiation for breast cancer are fairly uncommon, including pericardial disease. One study found no increase in cardiac mortality when comparing patients with left and right-sided breast cancer treated with radiation and followed for 12 years.[51]

Chemoradiation for esophageal cancer is associated with a 5-fold increase in pericardial disease compared with a matched cohort treated with surgery alone.[52] Proximity to the heart readily explains this phenomenon, and radiation dose to the heart is the strongest predictor of pericardial disease in this group.[53] Radiation therapy for lung cancer is usually palliative, and usually administered only to active macroscopic lesions. Extent of heart involvement thus is highly dependent on location of disease. The heart can be fairly effectively shielded during left hilar radiation. Prognosis is generally very poor in this group of patients, so manifestations of late pericardial disease are uncommon. Acute pericarditis is possible, but infrequent.

Clinical manifestations of radiation-induced pericardial disease are highly variable, and include acute pericarditis, chronic pericardial effusion, and (non-calcific) pericardial constriction. Patients can present acutely during their treatment, sub-acutely weeks or months later, or as late as decades after radiation exposure. The peak incidence of pericardial sequelae occurs 5–9 months after radiation exposure,[42] but all patients are indefinitely susceptible, with incidence increasing with the duration of follow-up.[5] Interestingly, acute disease does not seem to predispose a higher risk of late chronic disease.[42] Another known complication of radiation is the development of secondary malignancies. These can arise from virtually any tissue exposed to the radiation, including the pericardium in very rare instances. Cases involving "primary" pericardial lymphoma,[54] pericardial angiosarcoma,[55] and pericardial mesothelioma[56] have been described, occurring years after radiation therapy to the chest for the initial malignancy.

Chemotherapy-related pericardial disease

Several anti-cancer agents have been implicated in pericardial disease,[57] and are summarized in Table 12-3. The incidence of chemotherapy-related pericardial disease is rare, and the mechanisms are generally poorly understood. Nonetheless, this phenomenon is important to include in the differential diagnosis of pericardial conditions in the cancer patient. Chemotherapy-related pericardial disease is usually self-limited, and may be treated with anti-inflammatory drugs and removal of the offending agent when practical. In very rare cases,

TABLE 12-3 Anticancer drugs associated with pericardial disease

MEDICATION	COMMENT
Cytarabine	Pericarditis, Effusion
Cyclophosphamide	Pericarditis
Ifosfamide	Pericarditis
Anthracyclines	Myopericarditis
Sargramostim	Effusion, Constriction
Busulfan	Effusion, Fibrosis
Cisplatin	Pericarditis
Methotrexate	Pericarditis, Effusion
Imatinib	Effusion
All-*trans* Retinoic Acid	Effusion (Retinoic Acid Syndrome)

pericardiocentesis may be necessary to treat tamponade or as a diagnostic intervention to help rule out malignant effusion or infection.

Anthracyclines can cause myopericarditis as a manifestation of their early cardiotoxicity. These effects are not related to cumulative dose, but a relationship with later cardiac dysfunction has been suggested. Pericarditis alone should not be considered sufficient grounds for aborting an anthracycline-containing chemotherapeutic regimen in patients who are otherwise stable.[58]

All-*trans* retinoic acid is used for induction and maintenance of remission in patients with acute promyelocytic leukemia. A major toxicity of this agent is retinoic acid syndrome, which consists of fever, weight gain, interstitial pulmonary infiltrates, pleural and pericardial effusions, hypotension, and acute renal failure. It is seen during induction in approximately 25% of cases, but not observed during maintenance therapy. Pleural and pericardial manifestations can occur in up to 1/3 of patients with the syndrome.[59] The mechanism involves the differentiation and extravasation of leukemic cells into affected organs, which causes a brisk inflammatory response and capillary leak. Mortality ranges from 5%–30%, but cause of death is not usually related directly to the pericardial effusion.[59] Treatment involves early recognition and administration of corticosteroids. Development of retinoic acid syndrome does not preclude further treatment with this agent, but prophylactic steroids and close monitoring are required.

◼ Infection-related pericardial disease

Of all recognized causes of pericardial disease, infections make up the largest category. A long list of potential pathogens exist, including viruses, bacteria, rickettsia, fungi, and parasites.[5] Cancer patients are uniquely susceptible because of immunosuppression, multi-system organ disease, and loss of tissue integrity (Figure 12-7). Frequent hospitalizations and long-term intravascular access catheters add to the infectious burden. Thus, infections should routinely be included in the differential diagnosis of malignant pericardial disease. During any pericardial drainage procedure, samples should always be collected for cell count, Gram stain, and culture, with additional microbiologic studies obtained if indicated. Because treatment is usually curative, correct diagnosis is essential.

Cancer or complications of its treatment can lead to suppurative infections of the pericardium via fistula formation. Given the close proximity of the esophagus to the heart, esophageal cancers can

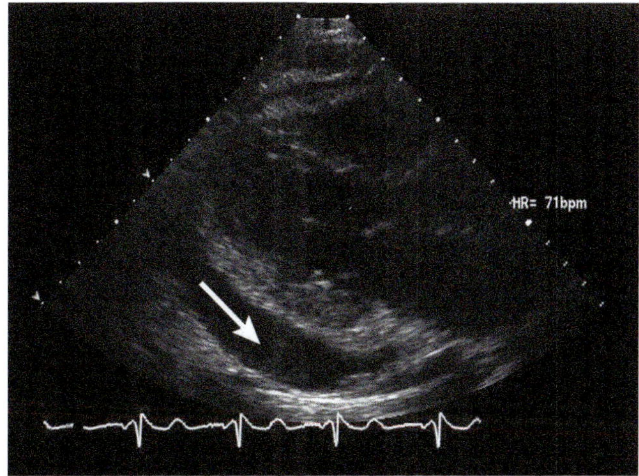

FIGURE 12-7 Parasternal long axis echocardiographic image in a patient with lymphoma and purulent pericarditis. Note the inflammatory stranding within the pericardial space (arrow). Cultures of the fluid grew coagulase-negative Staphylococcus aureus.

invade locally and create esophago-pericardial fistulas with resulting purulent pericarditis.[60–62] Metallic stents placed into the esophagus for obstructing tumor can also lead to fistula formation.[63] Gastric cancer has likewise created fistulas to the pericardium in rare cases.[64]

Tuberculous pericarditis is relevant in the cancer patient because of this organism's predilection for immunocompromised hosts and the elderly, and because clinical features can often mimic malignant disease. Although *Myocbacterium tuberculosis* can present with the entire spectrum of pericardial syndromes, the most common presentation is chronic effusive pericarditis, which can progress to calcific constrictive disease. Chronic fevers and cachexia are frequent. Pulmonary infection need not be present.[5] Diagnosis requires a high index of suspicion.

Human immunodeficiency virus (HIV) is associated with both malignancies and pericardial disease and is thus of special interest. HIV can lead to pericardial disease via direct effects, secondary infections and malignancies.[65] Prior to the use of highly active antiretroviral therapy (HAART), the incidence of pericardial effusion was 11% per year and conferred a poor prognosis.[66] Typical pericardial effusions are small, asymptomatic and sterile, but tamponade and constrictive disease are possible. Secondary pericardial infections include typical and atypical mycobacteria and fungi. HIV-related malignancies such as primary cardiac lymphoma, metastatic lymphoma, and Kaposi's sarcoma have all been known to involve the pericardium.

PERICARDIAL SYNDROMES IN THE CANCER PATIENT

Pericardial disease in the cancer patient presents with an array of clinical syndromes, including acute pericarditis, pericardial effusion, cardiac tamponade and constriction. Although some degree of overlap is frequently seen in actual practice, it is helpful to organize one's approach to pericardial disease within this framework. Presentation and management of these entities will be discussed, with emphasis on their relevance in cancer patients.

■ Acute pericarditis

Acute pericarditis is a chest pain syndrome caused by inflammation of the pericardium and surrounding structures. A component of myocarditis is frequently present and accounts for some of the clinical features; the term "myopericarditis" may be more accurate. A pericardial effusion may or may not be present. Idiopathic and viral etiologies make up the majority of cases. Many of the less common causes are associated with well-established diagnoses or obvious clinical scenarios. The causes of acute pericarditis are summarized in Table 12-4.

In the general population, acute pericarditis is rarely the first presentation of a malignancy. In one series, of 387 patients with acute pericarditis without tamponade,[9] (2.3%) were ultimately found to have occult malignancy as the cause.[2] Features that favored malignancy include a large associated effusion and the lack of response to anti-inflammatory medications. Of

TABLE 12-4   Causes of acute pericarditis

Idiopathic
Viral (Coxackie, Echovirus, Influenza, HIV)
Tuberculosis
Lyme Disease
Other Infections (Bacterial, Fungal, Parasitic)
Collagen Vascular Disease
Drug Reactions
Hypothyroidism
Myocardial Infarction
Post-Pericardiotomy
Renal Disease
Malignancy
Radiation
Trauma

malignancies that present with acute pericarditis as the first manifestation, almost all are primary lung cancers. In the patient with known malignancy, idiopathic and viral etiologies are still the most likely, but the possibility of malignant pericarditis must obviously be carefully considered. In addition to the clinical clues mentioned above, a reasonable search for other metastatic disease is helpful, as the pericardium is very seldom the only site of metastatic spread. Radiation, chemotherapy, renal failure and infection are possible etiologies, given the appropriate setting.

Acute pericarditis presents with chest pain, fever, dyspnea and cough. The chest pain is classically located over the left precordium, sharp in quality, and demonstrates positional and pleuritic features. Alternately, the pain can mimic myocardial ischemia with a dull pressure-like quality and radiation to the jaw, left shoulder and arm, probably a manifestation of myocardial involvement. Onset can be abrupt. Rapid shallow breathing or splinting are commonly present with pleuritic pain, and can be confused with true dyspnea. Physical exam findings of acute pericarditis can include low-grade fever, tachycardia, and a pericardial rub. Rubs are characteristically transient and are often positional, and may not be heard at all. Thus, while the presence of a pericardial rub is specific for pericarditis, it is not a very sensitive finding.

Electrocardiographic findings of acute pericarditis are generated by the superficial myocarditis that is generally present. Diffuse ST elevation reflects a current of injury, but in a non-coronary distribution (Figure 12-8). This is often accompanied by PR depression. When present, these findings are diagnostic, but many patients will not demonstrate classic ECG features. Echocardiography is used to detect an associated pericardial effusion, and can also reveal pericardial pathology such as metastatic disease. Other findings include markers of systemic inflammation, including elevated C-reactive protein, erythrocyte sedimentation rate and leukocyte counts. Serum cardiac markers such as CK-MB and troponin can be mildly elevated, reflecting some degree of associated myocarditis.

Differential diagnosis of acute pericarditis includes acute myocardial ischemia, pulmonary embolism, pneumonia and metastatic disease to the ribs, among others. Prompt establishment of the correct diagnosis is crucial given the high acuity of some of these entities. Also, anticoagulation is relatively contraindicated in acute pericarditis due to the risk of developing a hemorrhagic effusion. Management of acute pericarditis consists of non-steroidal anti-inflammatory drugs and colchicine.[67,68] Corticosteroids may be needed for refractory cases but are generally avoided given their substantial side-effect profile and possible increased likelihood of recurrence.

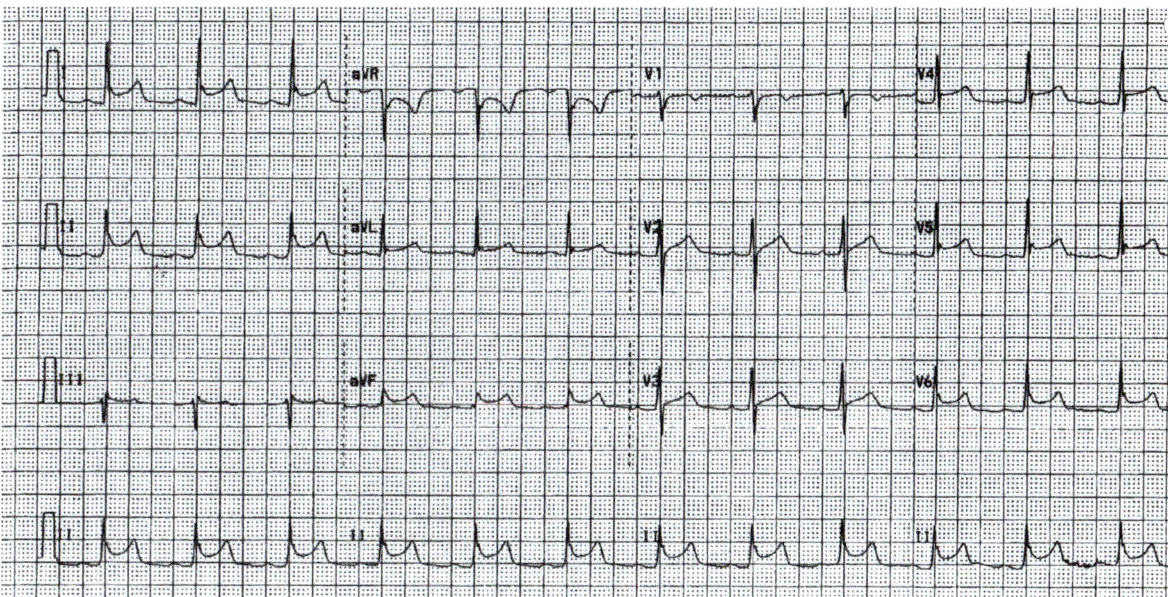

FIGURE 12-8 Electrocardiogram from a patient with multiple myeloma and acute pericarditis. Diffuse ST elevation in a non-coronary distribution is evident.

Even in the cancer patient, acute pericarditis without effusion that responds rapidly and completely to therapy is unlikely to represent malignant disease, and an exhaustive search for pathologic evidence of pericardial invasion is not usually warranted. Features that render malignant pericarditis more likely include recurrent or refractory symptoms, the presence of a pericardial effusion, and other evidence of widespread metastatic disease. Pericardial masses on echocardiography are highly suggestive of malignant involvement. As noted above, when radiation or chemotherapy are the likely causes of pericarditis, the physician can usually continue these treatments after initial symptoms have resolved with the administration of anti-inflammatory drugs.

■ Pericardial effusion

Pericardial effusions are commonly encountered in cancer patients. Clinical presentation is widely variable and potential etiologies are numerous. Unlike acute "dry" pericarditis, which is less likely to be directly related to malignancy, a pericardial effusion in a patient with cancer is always of concern, and often a poor prognostic sign (associated with a 27% 1-year survival in one study).[69] Because malignant invasion of the pericardium occurs frequently, all patients with pericardial effusion need to be carefully evaluated. It should be noted, however, that up to 2/3 of cancer patients who develop pericardial effusions do so through mechanisms other than malignant invasion of the pericardium (Figure 12-9).[3] In the general population, large

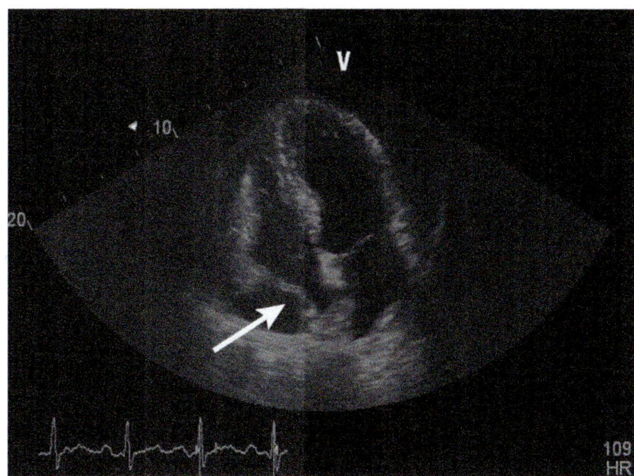

FIGURE 12-9 Apical 4-chamber view of a large malignant pericardial effusion in a patient with synchronous lung and esophageal cancer. Note systolic notching of the right atrium (arrow), suggesting hemodynamic compromise. The recurrent effusion was non-malignant, with repeatedly negative cytology.

pericardial effusions are usually associated with an obvious non-malignant etiology. When a significant effusion is discovered unexpectedly however, and especially when clinical features of inflammation are absent, the likelihood of finding malignancy is significantly increased. Cytology can discover previously unrecognized malignancy in 3%–8% of symptomatic pericardial effusions.[70,71] Among patients that present with large pericardial effusion without previously known malignancy, a new diagnosis of malignancy is discovered in up to 23% of cases.[4]

Pericardial effusions usually result from increased production or decreased resorption of pericardial fluid. Alternately, foreign material such as blood, lymph, pus, or tumor can fill the pericardial space. The pericardial space has even been found to be a site of extramedullary hematopoiesis in cases of chronic myeloid leukemia,[72,73] and amyloid accumulation in multiple myeloma.[74] Thus, the nature of the pericardial fluid provides clues as to its origin. Any cause of acute pericarditis (see Table 12-4) including malignant invasion, radiation, and chemotherapy agents can lead to an effusion due to increased production of an inflammatory exudate. Diseases that alter the hydrostatic balance between serum and tissue such as heart failure, renal failure or hypoalbuminemia can result in effusions as well. Decreased resorption occurs when pericardial lymphatics or veins are obstructed by tumor or fibrinous inflammatory debris. When malignancy invades and disrupts the normal tissue integrity, hemorrhagic effusions can result.

Pericardial effusions are often asymptomatic, discovered as incidental findings on chest X-ray or CT scan. Other presentations include acute or chronic pericarditis, cough, dyspnea and reduced functional capacity. Symptoms are related less to the size of the effusion, but rather to intrapericardial pressure, a feature that depends on rapidity of fluid accumulation and distensibility of the pericardium. In the absence of acute pericarditis or frank tamponade, physical exam findings may be absent. Decreased intensity of heart sounds is neither sensitive nor specific. The ECG may show non-specific findings; decreased QRS voltage can sometimes help to raise suspicion of pericardial effusion, but is also seen with other conditions such as a left-sided pleural effusion and obesity. If pericardial effusion is suspected or discovered on cardiac imaging, echocardiography is the test of choice for confirmation of the diagnosis and assessment of its hemodynamic significance. In addition to determining the size and location of the effusion, other features such as fibrinous stranding, loculations, and adhesions may also be evident. Tumors from metastatic disease can sometimes be seen on either the parietal or visceral pericardial surfaces (Figure 12-10).

For diagnostic or therapeutic purposes, pericardial fluid can be drained percutaneously and the fluid analyzed. The European Society of Cardiology has issued guidelines regarding indications for pericardiocentesis.[3] Class I indications include cardiac tamponade, symptomatic moderate-to-large effusions not responsive to medical therapy and suspicion for

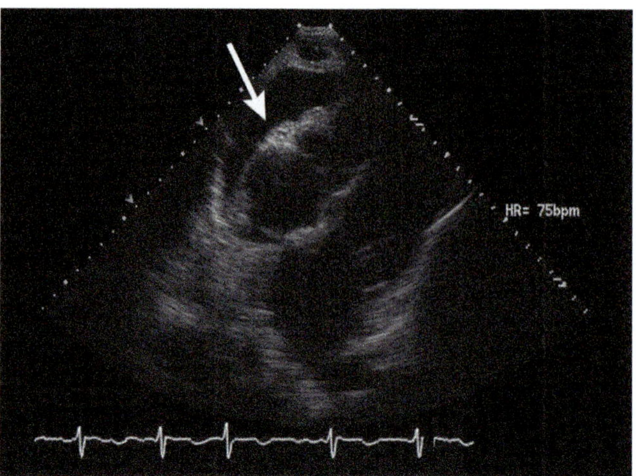

FIGURE 12-10 Subcostal echocardiographic image of a patient with esophageal cancer, pericarditis and malignant effusion. Note pericardial metastases (arrow).

unknown bacterial or neoplastic etiology. Thus in a cancer patient with a suspected malignant pericardial effusion, a relatively low threshold exists for drainage as long as it is safe to do so. Findings that favor malignant effusion are larger size, recurrent or refractory effusions, unclear etiology, widespread metastatic disease elsewhere, and lack of inflammatory features such as chest pain and fever.

Gross features of pericardial fluid such as color and consistency at the time of pericardial drainage can provide useful information. Pus, chylous effusion, and frank hemorrhage are easily recognized. Increasing levels of inflammation will render the fluid turbid with cells and fibrinous debris, which also increase the viscosity. Analysis of pericardial fluid should include cell count, leukocyte differential, Gram stain, culture, and cytology to rule out infection and malignancy; additional studies may also be indicated depending on the clinical scenario. Some authors suggest that a bloody effusion with a protein level > 3 mg/dL is highly suggestive of malignancy.[19] Chemistries such as lactate dehydrogenase, glucose and protein levels are unlikely to yield additional diagnostic information. Malignant pericardial effusion, if diagnosed, carries a poor prognosis, but since up to 2/3 of such patients will have a non-malignant and treatable etiology, the distinction is of utmost importance.

Treatment of pericardial effusions in the cancer patient includes managing the underlying cause when appropriate. Acute inflammation, infection, hypothyroidism, heart failure, renal failure, etc. can all be managed medically, and favorable outcomes with regards to the pericardial disease can be expected. When a chemotherapeutic agent or chest radiation is the culprit, conservative management is usually adequate, and treatment strategy need not usually be altered significantly. Malignant effusions are managed with a combination of local measures and systemic anti-tumor therapy if indicated. Chest radiation for pericardial metastases can help control aggressive disease as well.

If the pericardial effusion warrants intervention for diagnostic or therapeutic drainage, percutaneous pericardiocentesis with extended catheter drainage is emerging as the initial treatment strategy of choice (Figure 12-11). A recent series of 212 patients who underwent pericardiocentesis with extended drainage demonstrated 99% procedural success rate, a 2% rate of serious complications and a 10%–14% rate of recurrent effusion.[75] Compared with isolated pericardiocentesis, extended catheter drainage decreases the rate of recurrent effusion from 38% to 12%, and is thus an important component of this procedure.[76] Optimal duration of catheter drainage appeared to be 3–5 days, which minimized both the recurrence rate as well as the infectious risks associated with longer duration of catheter use.[75] If pericardiocentesis with extended catheter drainage fails, a variety of percutaneous and minor surgical approaches can provide additional treatment options.

In some centers intrapericardial administration of sclerosing agents or anti-tumor agents through the drainage catheter is used to help manage recurrent malignant effusions. Several small series have been published with encouraging results. Sclerosis with tetracycline analogues provides control of malignant pericardial disease in 90% of patients,[77–79] preventing recurrent effusion and alleviating symptoms. Significant side effects including pain with administration, fever, and atrial arrhythmias are less common with newer agents such as minocycline. Intrapericardial chemotherapy has also shown promise for local control of malignant disease. This mode of delivery allows for higher drug concentrations than can be obtained with systemic therapy.[80] Agents that have studied for intrapericardial delivery include cisplatin,[32,81–83] mitoxantrone,[84,85] 5-fluorouracil,[86] thiotepa[87] and bleomycin.[88]

Subxiphoid pericardiotomy is a minimally-invasive surgical procedure that can be performed under local anesthesia. It allows for direct visualization as well as thorascopic examination. A pleuropericardial window can also be created via the subxiphoid approach. Fluid and tissue specimens can be obtained for diagnostic purposes. In a retrospective review comparing surgical pericardiotomy to perciardiocentesis with extended drainage, surgical pericardiotomy had a similar rate of recurrent effusion, but a higher rate of complications.[89] Pericardioperitoneal shunt is an

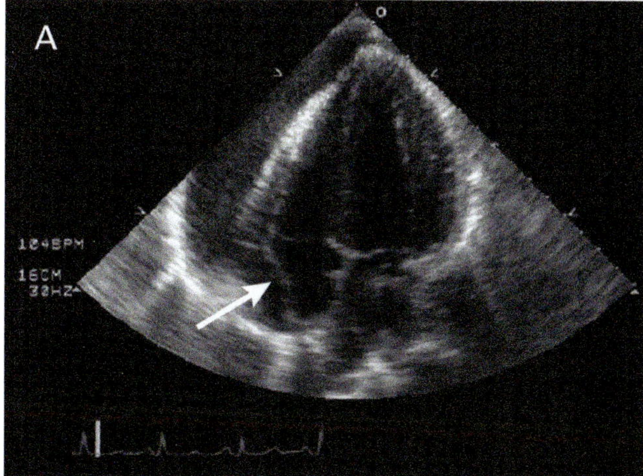

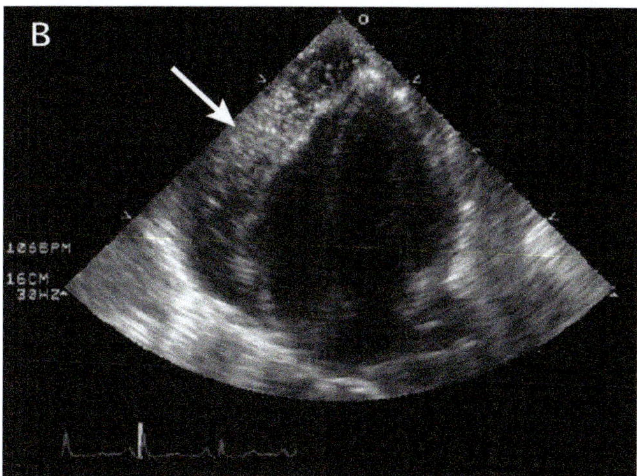

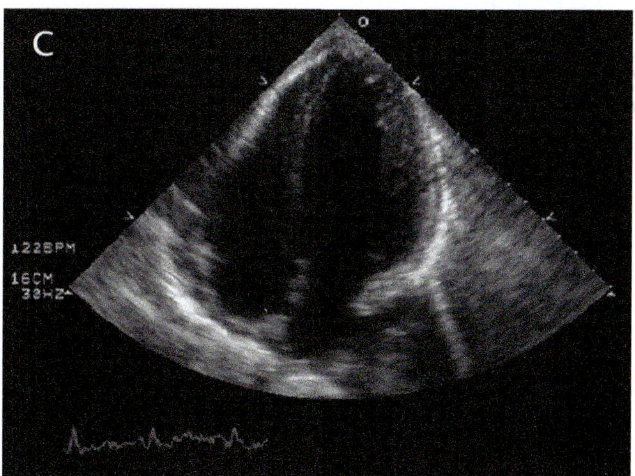

FIGURE 12-11 Echocardiography-guided pericardiocentesis (apical 4-chamber views). (A) A large effusion is present with systolic notching of the right atrium (arrow). (B) Agitated saline (arrow) has been injected into the pericardial space to confirm proper location of the needle. (C) After drainage, the effusion is no longer evident and all four cardiac chambers have re-expanded.

alternative drainage procedure that is likewise minimally invasive and can be done under local anesthesia. It is technically simpler than subxiphoid pericardiotomy and has been associated with shorter recovery times.[90] Catheter-based pericardiotomy, using a balloon across the pericardium that can be inflated to disrupt the pericardium and allow drainage, has been developed but is now less often performed, given the success of subxiphoid pericardiotomy. More definitive surgical management of malignant pericardial disease requires partial or complete pericardiectomy. This requires general anesthesia for anterior thoracotomy or sternotomy, and is associated with significant morbidity and mortality. In most patients with malignant pericardial effusions, prognosis is limited and less invasive strategies are preferred.

■ Cardiac tamponade

Cardiac tamponade exists when the pericardial space contains fluid under sufficient pressure to interfere with cardiac filling, resulting in decreased cardiac output and the inability to sustain vital functions. Malignant pericardial disease is the most frequent cause of cardiac tamponade in the general population. Furthermore, among the various pericardial syndromes, tamponade is the most likely to be associated with malignancy.[1] Cardiac tamponade can be the first presentation of malignancy; in one series of consecutive patients with tamponade and no prior diagnosis of cancer, 9 of 52 patients (17%) were ultimately diagnosed with malignant effusions.[2] More typically, tamponade will develop in patients with a previous diagnosis of cancer. Any malignancy that spreads to the pericardium is capable of causing pericardial tamponade. Despite the close association between tamponade and malignant pericardial disease, non-malignant pericardial disease can also lead to tamponade. A broad differential diagnosis should be considered, even in a patient with known malignancy.

Symptoms of tamponade initially consist of increasing dyspnea. Anxiety, cough, and severe weakness are other common symptoms. The chest discomfort of pericarditis is often absent. Overt tamponade can present as cardiogenic shock or pulseless electrical activity requiring immediate intervention. Physical examination characteristically demonstrates hypotension, tachycardia, distant heart sounds and jugular venous distention; jugular venous pulsations demonstrate a prominent *x* descent. The pulse is characteristically weak, and may show an exaggerated decrease during inspiration, known as *pulsus paradoxus.* This finding is a manifestation of the interdependence of the right and left cardiac chambers; a preferential filling of the right ventricle during inspiration must be at the expense of left ventricular filling due to the limitations imposed by the pressurized effusion. An abnormal pulsus paradoxus is defined as a >10 mmHg drop in systolic blood pressure with normal inspiration. It may also be appreciated by palpating the radial pulse, which can disappear during inspiration in frank tamponade.

Cardiac tamponade is confirmed with diagnostic studies. The chest radiograph shows an enlarged cardiac silhouette with a sac-like configuration. The electrocardiogram may show electrical alternans (beat-to-beat alternation of the QRS voltage), caused by swinging of the heart within the effusion. The most useful non-invasive test is echocardiography, which not only demonstrates the size and location of the pericardial effusion, but several hemodynamic findings suggestive of tamponade as well. One of the early findings is notching of the right atrium during systole, as this chamber typically has the lowest pressures (Figure 12-12A). As tamponade progresses, right ventricular compression during diastole may be evident (Figure 12-12B). In all patients with frank tamponade, the inferior vena cava is dilated and fails to collapse with inspiration, correlating with elevated central venous pressure. Doppler echocardiography reveals exaggerated respiratory variation of the left-sided forward flow velocities, an equivalent hemodynamic finding to pulsus paradoxus (Figure 12-12C). Cardiac tamponade progresses along a continuum, and not all of the above echocardiographic findings may be present in individual patients. Furthermore, care must be taken not to attempt to predict the pace of progression based on echocardiography alone; it is impossible to tell the rate of fluid accumulation and the distensibility of the pericardium. Cardiac tamponade is ultimately a clinical diagnosis, with echocardiography serving a confirmatory role.

Tamponade constitutes a medical emergency, as hemodynamic collapse and death may be imminent. Expedient drainage, usually via pericardiocentesis, often provides dramatic symptomatic improvement. Temporizing measures while drainage is being arranged include IV volume resuscitation to prevent right-sided chamber collapse and if necessary, hemodynamic support with phenylephrine. In cases in which hemodynamic collapse does not appear imminent, consideration can be given to some of the other methods of pericardial drainage discussed above as appropriate. Any therapeutic strategy for tamponade must be instituted without delay however, as small increases in pericardial fluid volume are associated with large increases in intrapericardial pressure; rapid progression can occur without warning and may be fatal.

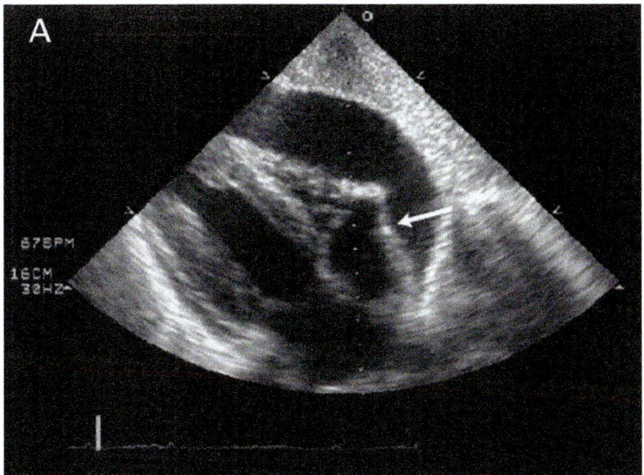

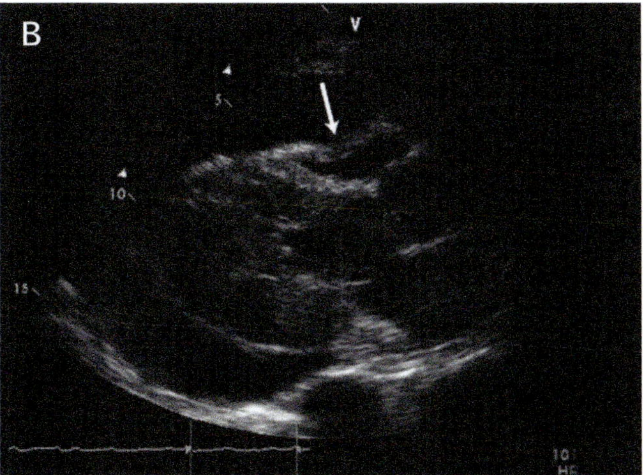

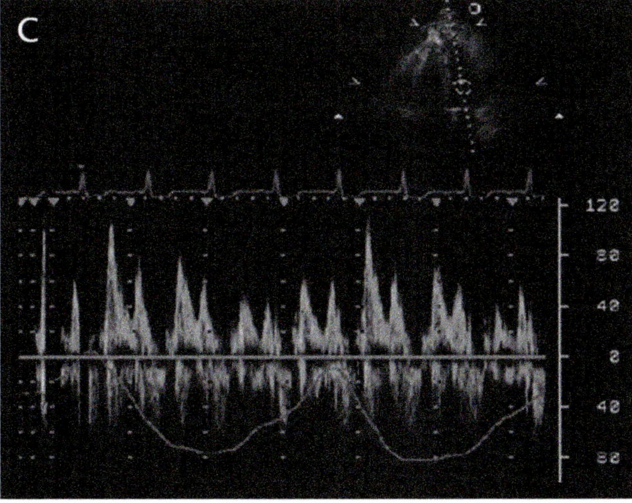

FIGURE 12-12 Echocardiographic features of tamponade. (A) Non-traditional 4-chamber view showing a large pericardial effusion and systolic notching of the right atrium (arrow). (B) Diastolic compression of the right ventricle (arrow). (C) Pulse-wave Doppler across the mitral valve showing marked respiratory variation of the inflow velocities.

■ Pericardial constriction

Pericardial constriction occurs when abnormal pericardial tissue creates a rigid shell that compresses the heart and interferes with normal chamber filling. It causes a syndrome seemingly similar to congestive heart failure, but right and left ventricular systolic function are preserved, and important differences exist in the pathophysiology. Constriction usually results from a fibrous or calcific response to chronic pericardial inflammation. In the general population, most cases of pericardial constriction are idiopathic or follow cases of pericarditis which are themselves idiopathic.[21] Of the known causes, infection, post-cardiac surgery, and chest radiation are the most common. Tuberculous pericarditis was formerly the most common etiology of constriction, but its incidence has decreased in industrialized nations. Any cause of acute or chronic pericardial disease however can lead to subsequent constriction.

In the cancer patient, chest radiation is the most common etiology of constrictive disease. Other possible causes include any pericardial disease that results in a hemorrhagic effusion, as blood typically produces a brisk inflammatory response. Malignant pericardial disease (especially from breast or lung cancer) can lead to constriction, but this is not a common entity, likely because malignant effusions are not especially inflammatory and overall prognosis tends to be poor. Complete encasement of the heart by solid tumor in the pericardium can also be clinically indistinguishable from constriction.[91]

Pericardial constriction can result from pathologic changes to the parietal pericardium, visceral pericardium, or both. These changes primarily include fibrotic thickening and chronic lymphocytic inflammation, with gross calcification present in less than 1/3 of cases.[21] Pericardial thickening is usually symmetric and completely encases the heart, but other patterns are possible including loculated or band-like pathology. At its maximum thickness, the parietal pericardium ranged from 1–17 mm with a mean of 4 mm in a series of patients with constriction.[21] Interestingly, 4% of cases were categorized as having normal pericardial thickness.

Effusive-constrictive disease is a related condition, which includes features of constriction as well as an effusion. It can be seen with malignant pericardial invasion or radiation. Patients typically present with tamponade, and features of constriction become apparent after pericardiocentesis. The visceral as opposed to parietal pericardium is the primary site of pathology.

The pathophysiology of pericardial constriction involves impaired right and left ventricular filling and ventricular interdependence, which is caused by the externally imposed volume limit. Any increased filling in the right heart must be at the expense of left-sided filling, and vice versa. Diastolic pressures in all four cardiac chambers are nearly equalized as well as significantly elevated. Hemodynamic findings with respiratory variation are a key diagnostic feature of constriction, with characteristic patterns during catheterization and echocardiography that are unique to constriction.

Symptoms of constriction arise from elevation of either left- or right-sided filling pressures. Gradually worsening weakness, fatigue, and dyspnea on exertion are prominent, but highly non-specific in the cancer patient. Lower extremity edema, abdominal congestion, and ascites are common, and are often confused with liver failure or myocardial disease.

Physical exam findings mimic those seen in right-sided heart failure, with elevated jugular venous pressure, hepatomegaly (sometimes pulsatile), and peripheral edema. Jugular venous pulsations reveal prominent x and y descents and Kussmaul's sign (failure of the central venous pressure to decrease with inspiration). An S3 may be present, in this setting referred to as a pericardial knock, and is due to early rapid ventricular filling.

MRI and CT can define pericardial anatomy fairly well and are both more accurate at determining pericardial thickness than echocardiography. They can also show dilation of the superior and inferior vena cavae. Diagnosis of constriction really requires the hemodynamic data available from echocardiography or catheterization, however.

Echocardiography can reveal several aspects of pericardial constriction, but the findings can be subtle, and the interpreting cardiologist must have a reasonable index of suspicion to make the diagnosis. Pericardial anatomy can be visible, but image quality is often limited by the high echogenicity of the pericardium, especially when calcification is present. Increased pericardial thickness can sometimes be measured (Figure 12-13A), but this is not a consistent finding and is better evaluated by CT or MRI. The inferior vena cava is dilated and fails to compress with respiration. The interventricular septum can show a characteristic "bounce" corresponding to the rapid ventricular filling in early diastole. An M-mode through the posterior wall of the left ventricle sometimes shows separate densities corresponding to parietal and visceral pericardium that are adherent to the posterior wall and move with the myocardium, a phenomenon known as "tram-tracking" (Figure 12-13B).

Doppler examination of mitral inflow reveals a restrictive filling pattern of severe diastolic

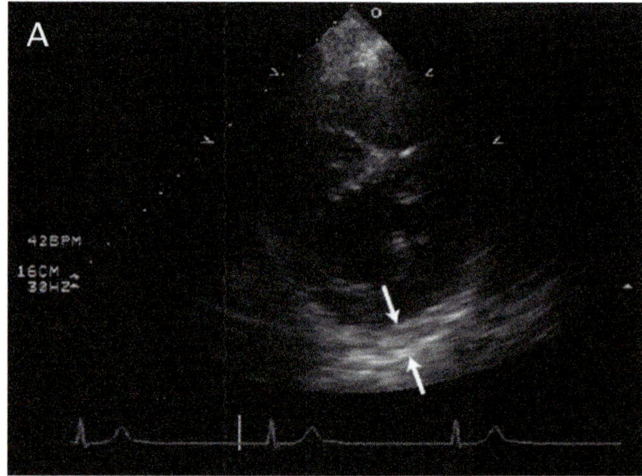

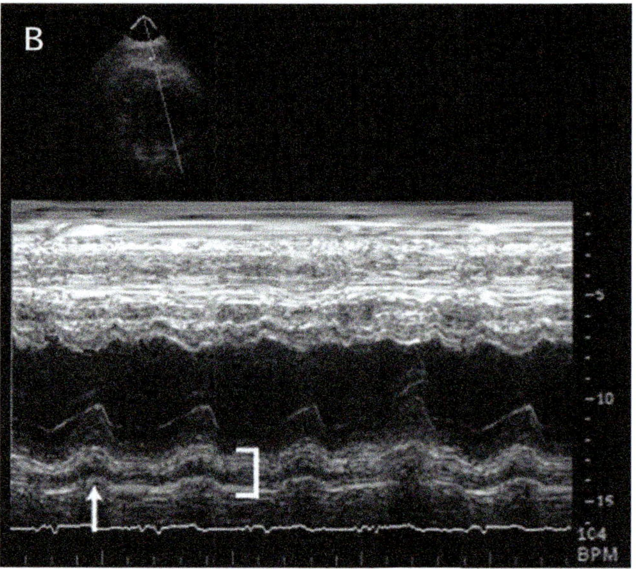

FIGURE 12-13 Echocardiographic features of pericardial constriction. (A) Parasternal short axis view demonstrating marked thickening and echogenicity of the posterior pericardium (arrows). (B) M-mode through the left ventricle demonstrating pericardial thickening (bracket) and adherent pericardium moving with the left ventricle (arrow).

dysfunction, including E wave >> A wave velocities and very rapid deceleration time. Unlike restrictive cardiomyopathy however, tissue Doppler measurements of the mitral annulus remain normal or are increased. Ventricular interdependence is the most specific finding, and is demonstrated by exaggerated changes to the forward flow velocities with respiration. Left-sided velocities peak during expiration whereas right-sided velocities peak during inspiration.

Hemodynamic measurements during cardiac catheterization play a confirmatory role. Elevation and equalization of diastolic pressures is seen. Left

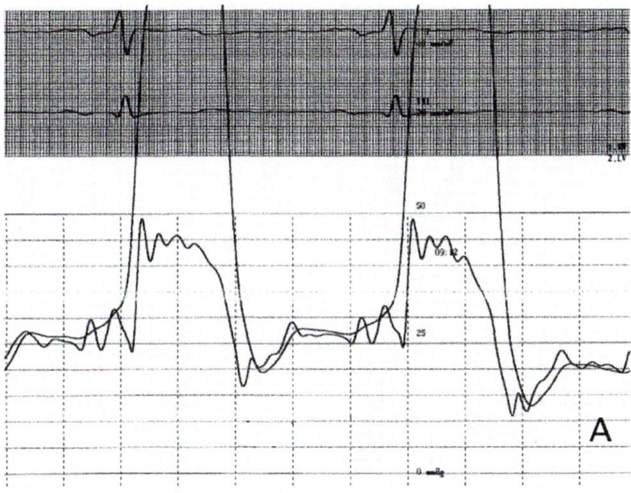

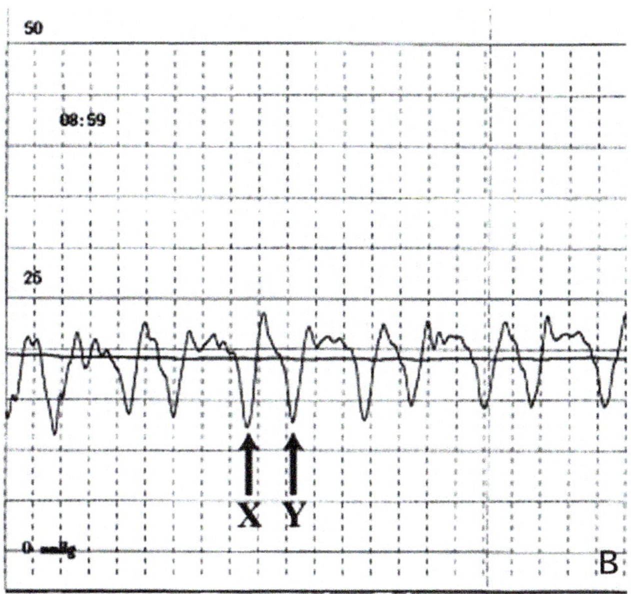

FIGURE 12-14 Catheter-based hemodynamic features of pericardial constriction. (A) Simultaneous pressures from the right and left ventricle showing elevation and equalization of pressures in diastole, as well as the characteristic "dip-and-plateau." (B) Right atrial pressure tracing showing elevated mean right atrial pressure (19 mmHg) and prominent *x* and *y* descents (labeled).

and right ventricles both show a characteristic diastolic pressure tracing—"dip and plateau"—which reflects rapid early filling followed by abrupt cessation of filling due to a rigid unexpandable heart (Figure 12-14A). Right atrial pressure tracings demonstrate the prominent *x* and *y* descents (Figure 12-14B) and Kussmaul's sign. Simultaneous right atrial and pulmonary capillary wedge tracings can demonstrate ventricular interdependence with one rising while the other falls.

In practice, diagnosis of pericardial constriction is not straightforward, as many of the above findings can also be seen with tamponade, restrictive cardiomyopathy, or right ventricular failure. The findings that are most specific for constriction are often the hardest to measure. Furthermore, combinations of these entities exist, such as in effusive-constrictive disease or the combined restriction and constriction that frequently occurs after chest irradiation. Sometimes endomyocardial biopsy is used to help rule out a myopathic process if surgical intervention for constriction is being considered. Diagnosis requires a high index of suspicion in the appropriate clinical setting, and multiple diagnostic tests are usually required to establish the diagnosis of pericardial constriction.

Treatment of pericardial constriction is surgical, and complete pericardiectomy is required, usually through a median sternotomy approach. Surgery is typically long and technically challenging due to adherent fibrotic debris, and can be complicated by severe bleeding, myocardial damage, arrhythmias, and hypotension. Overall operative mortality is 6%–12%, and is even higher (21%) in the case of radiation disease.[3] If coexisting myocardial fibrosis is present, the results after pericardiectomy are poor. Good outcomes rely on careful patient selection, and it is the rare patient with metastatic cancer who is able to tolerate such a procedure.

REFERENCES

1. Wilding G, Green HL, Longo DL, Urba WJ. Tumors of the heart and pericardium. *Cancer Treat Rev.* 1988;15(3):165–181.
2. Imazio M, Demichelis B, Parrini I, et al. Relation of acute pericardial disease to malignancy. *Am J Cardiol.* 2005;95(11):1393–1394.
3. Adler Y, Charron P, Imazio M, et al; European Society of Cardiology (ESC). 2015 ESC Guidelines for the diagnosis and management of pericardial diseases: the task force for the diagnosis and management of pericardial diseases of the European Society of Cardiology (ESC). Endorsed by: the European Association for Cardio-Thoracic Surgery (EACTS). *Eur Heart J.* 2015;36(42):2921–2964.
4. Corey GR, Campbell PT, Van Trigt P, et al. Etiology of large pericardial effusions. *Am J Med.* 1993;95(2):209–213.
5. Spodick DH. *The Pericardium: A Comprehensive Textbook.* New York, NY: Marcel Dekker, Inc.; 1997.
6. McAllister HA Jr, Hall RJ, Cooley DA. Tumors of the heart and pericardium. *Curr Probl Cardiol.* 1999;24(2):57–116.
7. McAllister HA Jr, Fenoglio JJ Jr. Tumors of the cardiovascular system. In *Atlas of Tumor Pathology, Series 2.* J Rosai,

LH Sobin, Eds. Washington, DC: Armed Forces Institute of Pathology; 1978, pp. 20-25.

8. Roy N, Blurton DJ, Azakie A, Karl TR. Immature intrapericardial teratoma in a newborn with elevated alpha-fetoprotein. *Ann Thorac Surg*. 2004;78(1):e6-e8.

9. Ragupathy R, Nemeth L, Kumaran V, Rajamani G, Krishnamoothy P. Successful surgical management of a prenatally diagnosed intrapericardial teratoma. *Pediatr Surg Int*. 2003;19(11):737–739.

10. Tollens M, Grab D, Lang D, Hess J, Oberhoffer R. Pericardial teratoma: prenatal diagnosis and course. *Fetal Diagn Ther*. 2003;18(6):432–436.

11. Thomason R, Schlegel W, Lucca M, Cummings S, Lee S. Primary malignant mesothelioma of the pericardium. Case report and literature review. *Tex Heart Inst J*. 1994;21(2):170–174.

12. Hancock EW. Neoplastic pericardial disease. *Cardiol Clin*. 1990;8(4):673–682.

13. Murai Y. Malignant mesothelioma in Japan: analysis of registered autopsy cases. *Arch Environ Health*. 2001;56(1):84–88.

14. Carbone M, Rizzo P, Pass H. Simian virus 40: the link with human malignant mesothelioma is well established. *Anticancer Res*. 2000;20(2A):875–877.

15. Bohn U, Gonzalez JL, Martin LM, Casado A, Diaz-Rubio E, Aragoncillo P. Meningeal and brain metastases in primary malignant pericardial mesothelioma. *Ann Oncol*. 1994;5(7):660–661.

16. Lang-Lazdunski L, Oroudji M, Pansard Y, Vissuzaine C, Hvass U. Successful resection of giant intrapericardial lipoma. *Ann Thorac Surg*. 1994;58(1):238–240.

17. Noji T, Morikawa T, Kaji M, Ohtake S, Katoh H. Successful resection of a recurrent mediastinal liposarcoma invading the pericardium: report of a case. *Surg Today*. 2004;34(5):450–452.

18. Kendall SW, Williams EA, Hunt JB, Petch MC, Wells FC, Milstein BB. Recurrent primary liposarcoma of the pericardium: management by repeated resections. *Ann Thorac Surg*. 1993;56(3):560–562.

19. Kralstein J, Frishman W. Malignant pericardial diseases: diagnosis and treatment. *Am Heart J*. 1987;113(3):785–790.

20. MacGee W. Metastatic and invasive tumours involving the heart in a geriatric population: a necropsy study. *Virchows Arch A Pathol Anat Histopathol*. 1991;419(3):183–189.

21. Oh KY, Shimizu M, Edwards WD, Tazelaar HD, Danielson GK. Surgical pathology of the parietal pericardium: a study of 344 cases (1993-1999). *Cardiovasc Pathol*. 2001;10(4):157–168.

22. Abraham KP, Reddy V, Gattuso P. Neoplasms metastatic to the heart: review of 3314 consecutive autopsies. *Am J Cardiovasc Pathol*. 1990;3(3):195–198.

23. Kline IK. Cardiac lymphatic involvement by metastatic tumor. *Cancer*. 1972;29(3):799–808.

24. Williams PL, Warwick R. *Gray's Anatomy*. 36th ed. Edinburgh: Churchill Livingstone; 1980.

25. Rouvière H. *Anatomie des lymphatiques de l'homme*. Paris: Masson; 1981

26. Pokieser W, Cassik P, Fischer G, Vesely M, Ulrich W, Peters-Engl C. Malignant pleural and pericardial effusion in invasive breast cancer: impact of the site of the primary tumor. *Breast Cancer Res Treat*. 2004;83(2):139–142.

27. Thurber DL, Edwards JE, Achor RW. Secondary malignant tumors of the pericardium. *Circulation*. 1962;26:228–241.

28. Chiles C, Woodard PK, Gutierrez FR, Link KM. Metastatic involvement of the heart and pericardium: CT and MR imaging. *Radiographics*. 2001;21(2):439–449.

29. Grizzard JD, Ang GB. Magnetic resonance imaging of pericardial disease and cardiac masses. *Cardiol Clin*. 2007;25(1):111–140, vi

30. Ziskind AA, Rodriguez S, Lemmon C, Burstein S. Percutaneous pericardial biopsy as an adjunctive technique for the diagnosis of pericardial disease. *Am J Cardiol*. 1994;74(3):288–291.

31. Gupta K, Mathur VS. Diagnosis of pericardial disease using percutaneous biopsy: case report and literature review. *Tex Heart Inst J*. 2003;30(2):130–133.

32. Maisch B, Pankuweit S, Brilla C, et al. Intrapericardial treatment of inflammatory and neoplastic pericarditis guided by pericardioscopy and epicardial biopsy—results from a pilot study. *Clin Cardiol*. 1999;22(1 suppl 1):I17–I22.

33. Pomjanski N, Grote HJ, Doganay P, Schmiemann V, Buckstegge B, Böcking A. Immunocytochemical identification of carcinomas of unknown primary in serous effusions. *Diagn Cytopathol*. 2005;33(5):309–315.

34. Szturmowicz M, Tomkowski W, Fijalkowska A, et al. Diagnostic utility of CYFRA 21-1 and CEA assays in pericardial fluid for the recognition of neoplastic pericarditis. *Int J Biol Markers*. 2005;20(1):43–49.

35. Tatsuta M, Yamamura H, Yamamoto R, Ichii M, Iishi H, Noguchi S. Carcinoembryonic antigens in the pericardial fluid of patients with malignant pericarditis. *Oncology*. 1984;41(5):328–330.

36. Bardales RH, Stanley MW, Schaefer RF, Liblit RL, Owens RB, Suhrland MJ. Secondary pericardial malignancies: a critical appraisal of the role of cytology, pericardial biopsy, and DNA ploidy analysis. *Am J Clin Pathol*. 1996;106(1):29–34.

37. Decker D, Stratmann H, Springer W, Schwering H, Varnai N, Bollmann R. Benign and malignant cells in effusions: diagnostic value of image DNA cytometry in comparison to cytological analysis. *Pathol Res Pract*. 1998;194(11):791–795.

38. Fischler DF, Wongbunnate S, Johnston DA, Katz RL. DNA content by image analysis. An accurate discriminator of malignancy in pericardial effusions. *Anal Quant Cytol Histol*. 1994;16(3):167–173.

39. Motherby H, Kube M, Friedrichs N, et al. Immunocytochemistry and DNA-image cytometry in diagnostic effusion cytology I. Prevalence of markers in tumour cell positive and negative smears. *Anal Cell Pathol*. 1999;19(1):7–20.

40. Janjan NA, Strom, E, Perkins, G, et. al. Effects of radiation on the heart. In: Ewer MS, Yeh E, eds. *Cancer and the Heart*. Hamilton, Ontario: BC Decker Inc.; 2006.

41. Stone RM, Bridges, KR, Libby, P. Hematological-oncological disorders and the cardiovascular

system. In: Braunwald E, Zipes DP, Libby P, eds. *Heart Disease: A Textbook of Cardiovascular Medicine*. 6th ed. Philadelphia, PA: W.B. Saunders Company; 2001, pp. 2223-2243.

42. Spodick DH. Pericardial diseases. In: Braunwald E, Zipes DP, Libby P, eds. *Heart Disease: A Textbook of Cardiovascular Medicine*. 6th ed. Philadelphia, PA: W.B. Saunders Company; 2001:1823-1876.

43. Mulrooney DA, Yeazel MW, Kawashima T, et al. Cardiac outcomes in a cohort of adult survivors of childhood and adolescent cancer: retrospective analysis of the Childhood Cancer Survivor Study cohort. *BMJ*. 2009;339:b4606.

44. Tukenova M, Giobout C, Oberlin O, et al. Role of cancer treatment in long-term overall and cardiovascular mortality after childhood cancer. *J Clin Oncol*. 2010;28(8):1308–1315.

45. Ewer MS, Ewer SM, Suter T. Cardiac complications. In: Bast RC, Croce CM, Hait WN, et al., eds. *Holland-Frei Cancer Medicine*. 9th ed. Hoboken, NJ: John Wiley & Sons, Inc.; 2017.

46. Adams MJ, Hardenbergh PH, Constine LS, Lipschultz SE. Radiation-associated cardiovascular disease. *Crit Rev Oncol Hematol*. 2003;45(1):55–75.

47. Adams MJ, Lipsitz SR, Colan SD, et al. Cardiovascular status in long-term survivors of Hodgkin's disease treated with chest radiotherapy. *J Clin Oncol*. 2004;22(15):3139–3148.

48. Brosius FC 3rd, Waller BF, Roberts WC. Radiation heart disease. Analysis of 16 young (aged 15 to 33 years) necropsy patients who received over 3,500 rads to the heart. *Am J Med*. 1981;70(3):519–530.

49. Tarbell NJ, Thompson L, Mauch P. Thoracic irradiation in Hodgkin's disease: disease control and long-term complications. *Int J Radiat Oncol Biol Phys*. 1990;18(2):275–281.

50. Pedersen AN, Korreman S, Nyström H, Specht L. Breathing adapted radiotherapy of breast cancer: reduction of cardiac and pulmonary doses using voluntary inspiration breath-hold. *Radiother Oncol*. 2004;72(1):53–60.

51. Nixon AJ, Manola J, Gelman R, et al. No long-term increase in cardiac-related mortality after breast-conserving surgery and radiation therapy using modern techniques. *J Clin Oncol*. 1998;16(4): 1374–1379.

52. Murthy SC, Rozas MS, Adelstein DJ, et al. Induction chemoradiotherapy increases pleural and pericardial complications after esophagectomy for cancer. *J Thorac Oncol*. 2009;4(3):395–403.

53. Wei X, Liu HH, Tucker SL, et al. Risk factors for pericardial effusion in inoperable esophageal cancer patients treated with definitive chemoradiation therapy. *Int J Radiat Oncol Biol Phys*. 2008;70(3):707–714.

54. Yukiiri K, Mizushige K, Ueda T, Kohno M. Second primary cardiac B-cell lymphoma after radiation therapy and chemotherapy—a case report. *Angiology*. 2001;52(8):563–565.

55. Killion MJ, Brodovsky HS, Schwarting R. Pericardial angiosarcoma after mediastinal irradiation for seminoma. A case report and a review of the literature. *Cancer*. 1996;78(4):912–917.

56. Velissaris TJ, Tang AT, Millward-Sadler GH, Morgan JM, Tsang GM. Pericardial mesothelioma following mantle field radiotherapy. *J Cardiovasc Surg (Torino)*. 2001;42(3):425–427.

57. Yeh ET, Tong AT, Lenihan DJ, et al. Cardiovascular complications of cancer therapy: diagnosis, pathogenesis, and management. *Circulation*. 2004;109(25): 3122–3131.

58. Ewer MS, Benjamin RS. Doxorubicin cardiotoxicity: clinical aspects, recognition, monitoring, treatment, and prevention. In: Ewer MS, Yeh E, eds. *Cancer and the Heart*. Hamilton, Ontario: BC Decker Inc.; 2006, pp. 9-32.

59. Tallman MS, Andersen JW, Schiffer CA, et al. Clinical description of 44 patients with acute promyelocytic leukemia who developed the retinoic acid syndrome. *Blood*. 2000;95(1):90–95.

60. Touati GD, Carmi D, Nzomvuama A, Marticho P. Purulent pericarditis caused by malignant oesophago-pericardial fistula. *Eur J Cardiothorac Surg*. 2003;24(5): 847–849.

61. Kaufman J, Thongsuwan N, Stern E, Karmy-Jones R. Esophageal-pericardial fistula with purulent pericarditis secondary to esophageal carcinoma presenting with tamponade. *Ann Thorac Surg*. 2003;75(1) :288–289.

62. Luthi F, Groebli Y, Newton A, Kaeser P. Cardiac and pericardial fistulae associated with esophageal or gastric neoplasms: a literature review. *Int Surg*. 2003;88(4):188–193.

63. Dennert B, Ramirez FC, Sanowski RA. Pericardioesophageal fistula associated with metallic stent placement. *Gastrointest Endosc*. 1997;45(1):82–84.

64. Chinnaiyan KM, Ali MI, Gunaratnam NT. Gastric cancer presenting as gastropericardial fistula in a patient with familial adenomatous polyposis syndrome. *J Clin Gastroenterol*. 2004;38(3):298.

65. Hsue PY, Waters DD. What a cardiologist needs to know about patients with human immunodeficiency virus infection. *Circulation*. 2005;112(25):3947–3957.

66. Heidenreich PA, Eisenberg MJ, Kee LL, et al. Pericardial effusion in AIDS. Incidence and survival. *Circulation*. 1995;92(11):3229–3234.

67. Imazio M, Bobbio M, Cecchi E, et al. Colchicine in addition to conventional therapy for acute pericarditis: results of the COlchicine for acute PEricarditis (COPE) trial. *Circulation*. 2005;112(13):2012–2016.

68. Imazio M, Bobbio M, Cecchi E, et al. Colchicine as first-choice therapy for recurrent pericarditis: results of the CORE (COlchicine for REcurrent pericarditis) trial. *Arch Intern Med*. 2005;165(17):1987–1991.

69. Dequanter D, Lothaire P, Berghmans T, Sculier JP. Severe pericardial effusion in patients with concurrent malignancy: a retrospective analysis of prognostic factors influencing survival. *Ann Surg Oncol*. 2008;15(11):3268–3271.

70. Wiener HG, Kristensen IB, Haubek A, Kristensen B, Baandrup U. The diagnostic value of pericardial

cytology. An analysis of 95 cases. *Acta Cytol.* 1991; 35(2):149–153.

71. Ben-Horin S, Bank I, Guetta V, Livneh A. Large symptomatic pericardial effusion as the presentation of unrecognized cancer: a study in 173 consecutive patients undergoing pericardiocentesis. *Medicine (Baltimore).* 2006;85(1):49–53.

72. Bradford CR, Smith SR, Wallis JP. Pericardial extramedullary haemopoiesis in chronic myelomonocytic leukaemia. *J Clin Pathol.* 1993;46(7):674–675.

73. Shih LY, Lin FC, Kuo TT. Cutaneous and pericardial extramedullary hematopoiesis with cardiac tamponade in chronic myeloid leukemia. *Am J Clin Pathol.* 1988;89(5):693–697.

74. Kornberg A, Rapoport M, Yona R, Kaufman S. Amyloidosis of the pericardium in multiple myeloma: an unusual cause of bloody pericardial effusion. *Isr J Med Sci.* 1993;29(12):794–797.

75. El Haddad D, Iliescu C, Yusuf SW, et al. Outcomes of cancer patients undergoing percutaneous pericardiocentesis for pericardial effusion. *J Am Coll Cardiol.* 2015;66(10):1119–1128.

76. Virk SA, Chandrakumar D, Villanueva C, Wolfenden H, Liou K, Cao C. Systematic review of percutaneous interventions for malignant pericardial effusion. *Heart.* 2015;101(20):1619–1626.

77. Celermajer DS, Boyer MJ, Bailey BP, Tattersall MH. Pericardiocentesis for symptomatic malignant pericardial effusion: a study of 36 patients. *Med J Aust.* 1991;154(1):19–22.

78. Grau JJ, Estapé J, Palombo H, et al. Intracavitary oxytetracycline in malignant pericardial tamponade. *Oncology.* 1992;49(6):489–491.

79. Maher EA, Shepherd FA, Todd TJ. Pericardial sclerosis as the primary management of malignant pericardial effusion and cardiac tamponade. *J Thorac Cardiovasc Surg.* 1996;112(3):637–643.

80. Lerner-Tung MB, Chang AY, Ong LS, Kreiser D. Pharmacokinetics of intrapericardial administration of 5-fluorouracil. *Cancer Chemother Pharmacol.* 1997;40(4):318–320.

81. Fiorentino MV, Daniele O, Morandi P, et al. Intrapericardial instillation of platin in malignant pericardial effusion. *Cancer.* 1988;62(9):1904–1906.

82. Tomkowski W, Szturmowicz M, Fijalkowska A, Filipecki S, Figura-Chojak E. Intrapericardial cisplatin for the management of patients with large malignant pericardial effusion. *J Cancer Res Clin Oncol.* 1994;120(7):434–436.

83. Tondini M, Rocco G, Bianchi C, Severi C, Corbellini D. Intracavitary cisplatin (CDDP) in the treatment of metastatic pericardial involvement from breast and lung cancer. *Monaldi Arch Chest Dis.* 1995;50(2):86–88.

84. Kuhn K, Purea H, Selbach J, Westerhausen M. Treatment with locally applied mitoxantrone. *Acta Med Austriaca.* 1989;16(3-4):87–90.

85. Musch E, Gremmler B, Nitsch J, Rieger J, Malek M, Chrissafidou A. Intrapericardial instillation of mitoxantrone in palliative therapy of malignant pericardial effusion. *Onkologie.* 2003;26(2):135–139.

86. Morere JF, Delanian S, Boaziz C, Breau JL, Israel L. Intracavitary 5-fluoro-uracil (5-FU) in combination with systemic chemotherapy. *Acta Med Austriaca.* 1989;16(3-4):74–75.

87. Martinoni A, Cipolla CM, Cardinale D, et al. Long-term results of intrapericardial chemotherapeutic treatment of malignant pericardial effusions with thiotepa. *Chest.* 2004;126(5):1412–1416.

88. Kunitoh H, Tamura T, Shibata T, et al. A randomised trial of intrapericardial bleomycin for malignant pericardial effusion with lung cancer (NCOG9811). *Br J Cancer.* 2009;100(3):464–469.

89. Patel N, Rafique AM, Eshaghian S, et al. Retrospective comparison of outcomes, diagnostic valvue, and complications of percutaneous prolonged drainage versus surgical pericardiotomy of pericardial effusion associated with malignancy. *Am J Cardiol.* 2013;112(8): 1235–1239.

90. Wang N, Feikes JR, Mogensen T, Vyhmeister EE, Bailey LL. Pericardioperitoneal shunt: an alternative treatment for malignant pericardial effusion. *Ann Thorac Surg.* 1994;57(2):289–292.

91. Ako J, Eto M, Kim S, et al. Pericardial constriction due to malignant lymphoma. *Jpn Heart J.* 2000;41(5): 673–679.

13 Arterial and Venous Thromboembolic Diseases in Cancer Patients

Elie Mouhayar

INTRODUCTION

The association between malignancy and thromboembolic diseases is well established in the literature. In fact, both arterial and venous thromboembolic events related to cancer and cancer therapies are common and are known to be a leading cause of morbidity and mortality in this patient population.[1] Patients with underlying malignancy have added increased risks for thromboembolism related to the inherent thrombophilia associated with their cancer and its therapy. The clinical presentation and management vary based on the venous and arterial bed and the organ involved; clinical spectrum includes upper and lower extremities deep vein thrombosis and pulmonary embolism, stroke, myocardial infarction, visceral and limb ischemia. These events often require long-term antiplatelet and/or anticoagulation with associated increase in bleeding and recurrence events. These patients have in general a worse prognosis than patients with cancer who did not experience thromboembolic events and their survival is particularly poor when the diagnosis of cancer is concurrent with the thromboembolic event.[2]

PREVALENCE

Venous thromboembolism (VTE) is particularly common in cancer patients. VTE can be the presenting first manifestation of an occult malignancy and 10% of patients with idiopathic VTE develop cancer within 2 years.[3] On the other hand and among all patients with VTE, 20% have underlying active malignancy.[4] Among hospitalized cancer patients, the cumulative incidence of deep venous thrombosis (DVT) has been reported at 4.6%.[5] The true incidence of subclinical DVT is believed to be much higher since up to 50% of cancer patients were found to have evidence of DVT at autopsy.[6] Compared to controls, patients with active malignancy have a higher risk of first and recurrent VTE, as well as higher bleeding risks while on anticoagulants.[2]

Unlike VTE, there have been very few epidemiologic studies looking at incidence of arterial ischemic events in cancer patients. Most of the demographic data available, comes from Khorana and his group from the University of Rochester. Looking at two large, separate cohorts of patients with cancer, they reported an incidence of 1.5%–3.1% of arterial ischemic events.[7] The most common being cardiac and less than 0.5% involved limb ischemia. This rate is much higher when looking at specific cancer population, like patients with myeoproloferative disorders or hematologic malignancies with secondary amyloidosis.[8,9] It is also much more common with specific cancer therapies like radiation therapy or certain chemotherapeutic agents.

MECHANISMS AND PATHOPHYSIOLOGY

In addition to the usual causes and the traditional risk factors typically associated with acute vascular syndromes in the general population, patients with underlying malignancy have added increased risks for venous and arterial thrombotic events related to the inherent thrombophilia associated with their cancer and its therapy. A summary of potential causes of vascular events in patients with malignancy is listed in Table 13-1. From clinical perspective, it is useful to divide these cancer related etiologies into two broad categories; the first category includes a mechanistic classification and the second group includes more specific cancer etiologies.

■ Specific Mechanisms

Hypercoagulability: Multifactorial mechanisms have been implicated in the pathogenesis of hypercoagulability and thrombosis in the setting of underlying cancer: This includes local and systemic activation of the coagulation cascade, thrombocytosis, factors C and S depletion, increased fibrinogen levels and fibrinolytic inhibition.[10–12] On the other hand, endothelial

TABLE 13-1   Etiology

CAUSES OF ARTERIAL ISCHEMIC EVENTS IN NON-CANCER PATIENTS		CAUSES OF ARTERIAL ISCHEMIC EVENTS IN PATIENTS WITH MALIGNANCY, HEMATOLOGIC DISORDERS OR CANCER THERAPY
Thrombotic	**Embolic**	
Atherosclerosis	Aneurysms (aortic, carotid, popliteal)	Multiple Myeloma
Shock/Low flow state	Paradoxic emboli	Myeloproliferative disorders
Heparin-Induced thrombocytopenia	Aortic arch atherosclerosis	Leukemia
Thrombophilia	Valvular prosthesis	Neurofibromatosis
Antiphospholipid syndrome	Infective endocarditis	Cardiac Tumors
Antithrombin deficiency	Mitral stenosis	Phlegmasia syndrome
Protein C and S deficiency	Acute Myocardial infarction	DIC
	Atrial fibrillation	Therapy (chemotherapy, radiotherapy, supportive therapy)

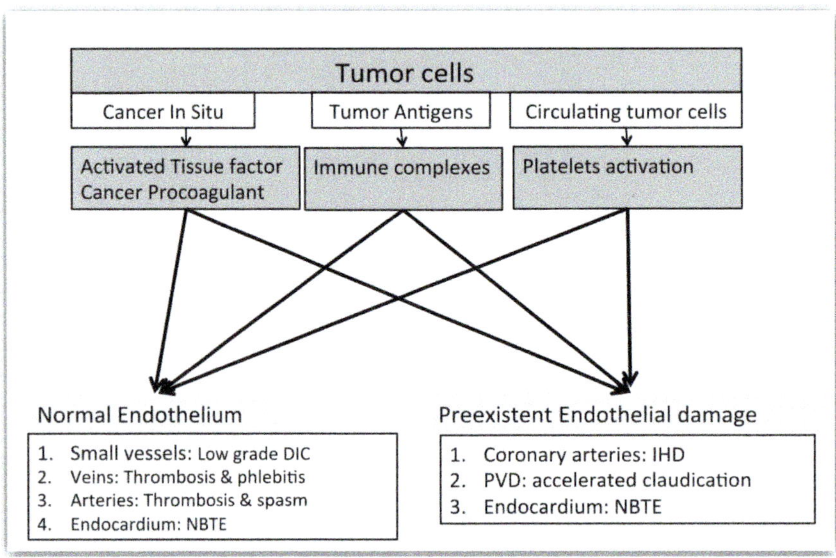

FIGURE 13-1   Circulating and in-situ cancer cells can enhance activity of tissue and activates platelets. These mediators can then set off coagulation in previously damaged or even healthy vessels. The end result is cancer enhanced thrombosis. (Adapted from Naschitz et al., *Cancer*, 69(1992), 2712–2720.)

damage triggered by cancer cells mediated vessel injury or iatrogenic mechanisms (vessel catheterization, surgery and chemotherapeutic agents), has also been suggested as a major cause leading to excessive thrombosis[13]: As shown in Figure 13-1, cancer cells—circulating and in-situ—can enhance activity of tissue factor and other cancer procoagulant factors in addition to activating platelets. These mediators can then set off coagulation in previously damaged vessels like the coronary arteries or peripheral arteries and/or even previously healthy vessels. The end result is cancer enhanced thrombosis, which manifest as (1) low grade disseminated intravascular coagulation; (2) venous thrombophlebitis; (3) arterial thrombosis; (4) accelerated ischemic cardiac and peripheral vascular disease; (5) Nonbacterial thrombotic endocarditis (NBTE) (Figure 13-2).

Paraneoplastic syndrome: Another subgroup of cancer patients with hypercoagulable condition present with digital ischemia with no evidence of large vessel involvement (Figure 13-3). Mechanism is suspected to be related to antigen mediated antibody complexes from tumor cells with capillary deposition. This paraneoplastic syndrome is usually very hard to treat and patient symptoms do not respond to usual vascular therapy till the cancer is fully controlled.[14]

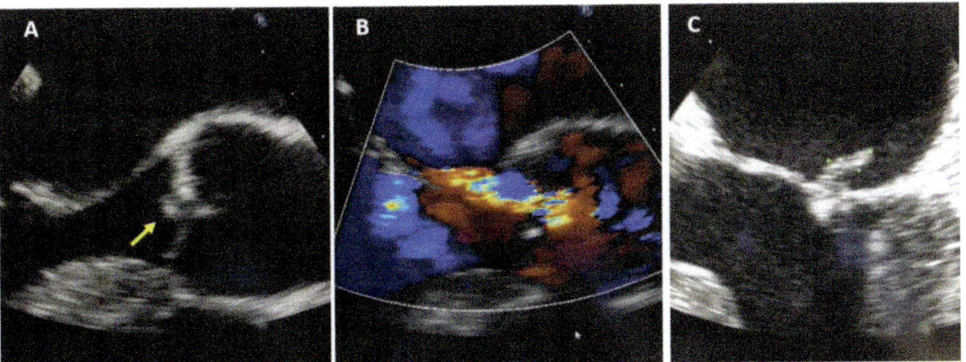

FIGURE 13-2   Sixty six year old patient with pancreatic cancer presents with stroke. His transesophageal echocardiogram showed evidence of aortic (A) and mitral (C) valves vegetation with severe secondary aortic regurgitations. He was diagnosed with non-bacterial thrombotic endocarditis based on the abnormal valves leaflets morphology shown above in the absence of fever and negative blood cultures.

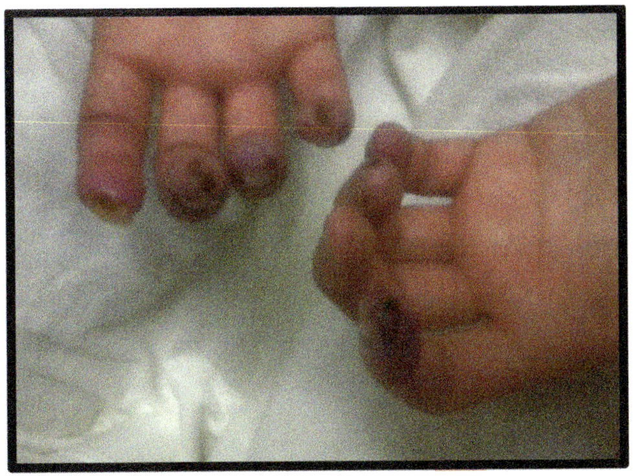

FIGURE 13-3   Digital ischemia in a 54 year old male with small cell lung cancer and digital ischemia.

Other mechanisms: The presence of underlying atherosclerotic disease by itself constitutes an additional risk factor for increased incidence in ischemic events related to cancer therapy. Jurado and Thompson reported a 2–5 times increase in coronary artery thrombosis risk in patients with known coronary artery disease undergoing radiation therapy.[15] Other reported unique mechanisms for arterial ischemic events include include tumor embolization, vessel wall invasion by tumor and paradoxical embolization. Often, a specific cause is never identified. In our cohort of 74 patients[16] with acute arterial limb ischemia, 24 confirmed pathology samples were available. The majority of patients (67%) had thrombus and 21% had associated underlying significant atherosclerotic disease. Tumor invasion of the artery was observed in two cases and only one patient with leukemia had leukemic cell aggregates (Figure 13-4). On the venous side, a relatively common trigger of upper extremity, superior vena cava and even right atrial thrombosis include catheter mediated vessel or right atrial wall injury (Figure 13-5).

■ Thrombotic Events Associated with Specific Malignancies

Myeloproliferative disorders: Myeloproliferative disorders (MPDs), such as polycythemia vera (PV) and essential thrombocythemia (ET) are associated with vascular events characterized by microcirculatory disregulation and thrombosis in various central and peripheral terminal venous and arterial beds leading to a plethora of symptoms including auditory and visual, intractable headaches, Reynaud's phenomenon, ischemic strokes, acute coronary syndrome, mesenteric and limb venous thrombosis.[17,18] The incidence of thrombosis upon diagnosis with PV and ET has been reported between 9.7 and 38.6% in various studies, with 64%–96.7% of these being arterial events.[8] Also reported is the tendency for these events to manifest 5–6 years before the diagnosis of MPD. The pathogenesis of thrombsis in MPDs is related to red blood cells increased adhesiveness, erythrocytosis, thrombocytosis, leucocytosis, and enhanced platelet activation.[8] Primary prevention of thrombosis in MPD patients involves the use of Aspirin which significantly lowers the composite cardiovascular risk in this population. Patients with platelet counts greater than 600,000 and symptomatic patients benefit from cell reduction therapy like Hydroxyurea , Interferon alfa, Anagrelide and/or phlebotomy.[19]

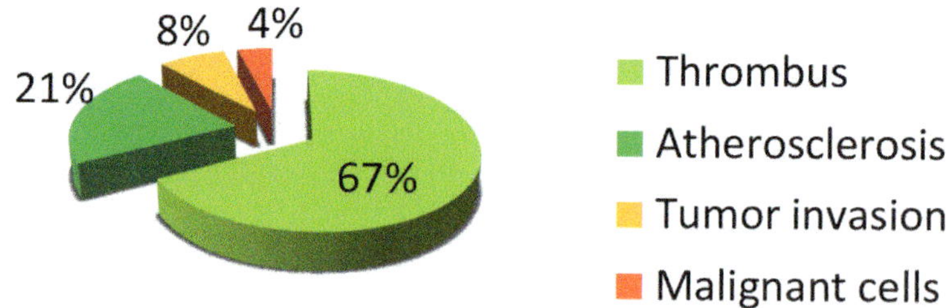

FIGURE 13-4 Mechanism of arterial thrombosis in cancer patients. (Adapted from Mouhayar et al., *Vasc Med*, 19(2014), 112–117.)

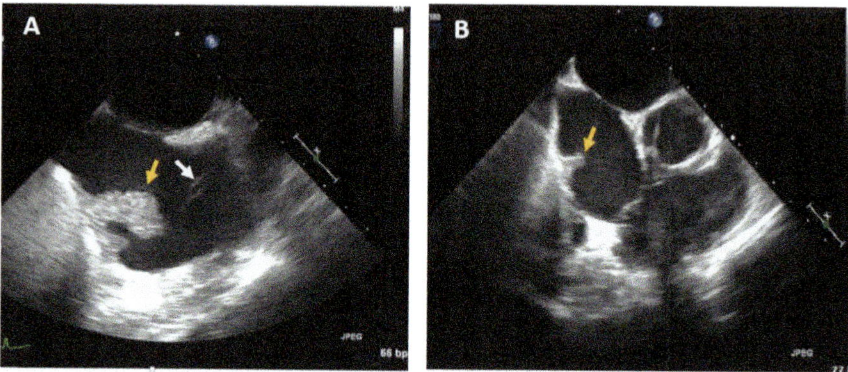

FIGURE 13-5 (A) Catheter (white arrow) mediate clot (yellow arrow) formation within the right atrium as seen by TEE. (B) Follow up TEE study showed almost complete resolution of the clot following catheter removal and three months of full anticoagulation.

Acute Leukemia: Although hemorrhage is the typically described complication in acute leukemia, venous and arterial ischemic thrombotic events can occur as well. De Stefano et al. reported a 1.4% incidence of thrombosis at presentation in acute lymphoblastic leukemia and 9.6% in acute promyelocytic leukemia, with an increase to 10.6% with L-asparaginase treatment.[20] More than half of the thromboses in this study were reported as the presenting manifestation, with 80% VTEs and 20% arterial ischemic events. Thrombotic mechanisms in acute leukemia include increased blast cell secretion of tumor necrosis factor alpha (TNFα) and interleukin-1 beta (IL-1β) leading to enhanced expression of endothelial tissue factor[21], thrombomodulin down-regulation and adhesion molecule up-regulation.[22] Other suspected mechanisms include increased fractional volume of leukocytes and reduced cell deformability.[23,24] Options for management include leukapheresis and urgent chemotherapy whereas revascularization is sometimes needed for large artery occlusion.

Cardiac Amyloidosis: Primary amyloidosis, particularly AL type has been associated with both venous and also intracardiac thrombosis (Figure 13-6). These patients are at high risk for arterial thromboembolic events despite preserved left ventricular ejection fraction

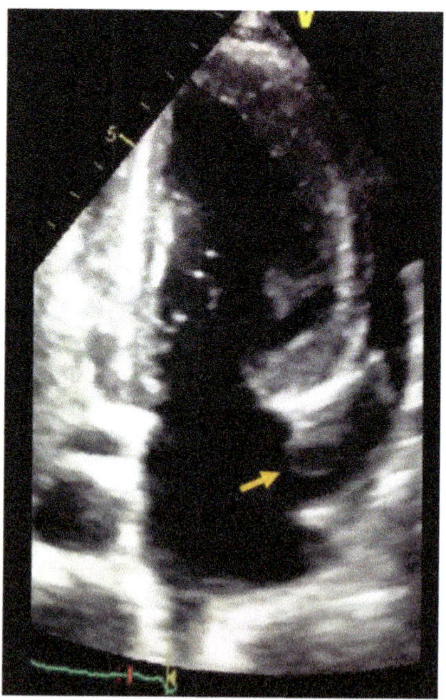

FIGURE 13-6 Two chambers view by transthoracic echocardiogram showing large left atrial appendage clot (arrow) in a patient with amyloid heart disease. Clot formation occurred despite absence of any evidence of atrial fibrillation.

TABLE 13-2 Chemotherapeutic Agents Associated with Arterial Ischemic events

Cisplatin
L-Asparaginase
Fluorouracil
Gemcitabine
Capecitabine

Angiogenesis inhibitors:
   Thalidomide
   Bevacizumab
   Sunitinib
   Sorafenib
   Ponatinib

and absence of cardiac arrhythmias, with an incidence ranging from 26% to 33%.[9,25] Arterial thromboembolism related mortality of 26% in one study.[9] A variety of mechanistic etiologies have been proposed for this phenomenon including endothelial dysfunction and myocardial damage,[26] direct myocardial toxic effect,[27] left ventricular diastolic dysfunction and stasis, atrial systolic failure and hypercoagulability.[28] In managing these patients the benefit of prophylactic anticoagulation needs to be balanced against the risk of hemorrhage from amyloid deposited fragile blood vessels.[29]

■ Thrombotic Events Associated with Specific Cancer Therapies

Chemotherapy: Although chemotherapeutic agents are now considered an independent risk factor for thrombosis in cancer patients, the true incidence of vascular events secondary to chemotherapy remains largely unknown, with most available data generated from case reports. The mechanisms of chemotherapy related thrombosis include endogenous procoagulant–anticoagulant mismatch,[30,31] accentuated tumor and endothelial cell death, and cytokine release leading to increased expression of tissue factor[32,33] enhanced endothelial cell reactivity to platelets and induced expression of macrophage-monocyte tissue factor.[34] Certain chemotherapeutic agents are known to have a stronger association with arterial ischemic events due to specific pathophysiological mechanisms. These drugs can be divided into two categories (Table 13-2): First category includes several standard chemotherapeutic agents like L-Asparaginase, Cisplatin, 5-Fluorouracil, Capecitabine, and Gemcitabine. In a study by De Stefano et al. the incidence of thrombosis in a population with acute lymphoblastic leukemia was shown to increase from 1.4% to 10.6% with L-asparaginase treatment.[20] Cisplatin, a central component of several Cisplatin-based chemotherapeutic regimens, is known to induce thrombosis by causing endothelial damage,[34] increasing monocyte tissue factor activity and platelet activation with a reported 12%–17.6%[35] incidence of thrombosis, including strokes, recurrent peripheral arterial events and aortic thrombosis.[36] 5-Fluorouracil on the other hand leads to decrease in protein C and increase in fibrinopeptide A levels, endothelial damage and even endothelial independent vasoconstriction via protein kinase C.[37] Gemcitabine has been associated with vascular events ranging from systemic capillary leaks, thrombotic microangiopathy, VTE and digital ischemia.[38] Despite the presence of several case reports in the literature on this subject, the exact incidence of vascular events with Gemcitabine remains largely unknown. (Figure 13-7).

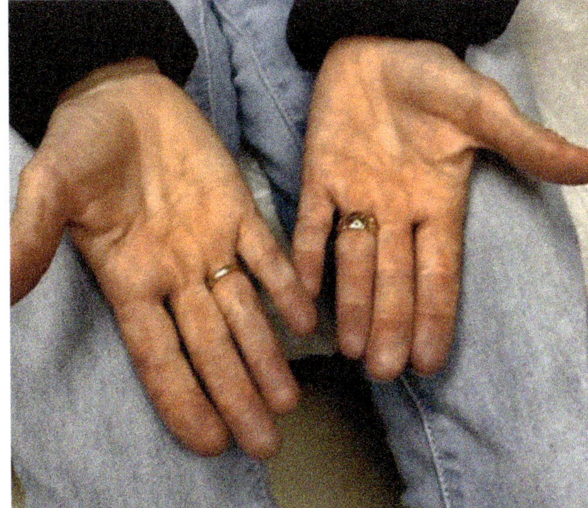

RIGHT PRESSURES & DBI		
Brachial	141	
Thumb	112	0.79
Index	81	0.57
Middle	34	0.24
Ring	33	0.23
Little	85	0.60

LEFT PRESSURES & DBI		
Brachial	140	
Thumb	107	0.76
Index	23	0.16
Middle	45	0.32
Ring	21	0.15
Little	65	0.46

FIGURE 13-7 68-year-old patient with pancreatic cancer and digital pain and discoloration within 2 weeks of starting gemcitabine. Digital ischemia was confirmed based on an abnormal PPG study with severely diminished digital pressures and digital-brachial indices involving several fingers in both hands.

The second category of cancer drugs associated with vascular thromboembolism includes the group of angiogenesis inhibitors like thalidomide and several targeted therapy drugs also known as the vascular signaling pathway inhibitors drugs or VSPI. These include Bevacizumab and several tyrosine kinase inhibitors (TKIs) like sunitinib, sorafenib, axitinib, pazopanib and also ponatinib. Thalidomide and lenalidomide are both associated with a risk for venous and also arterial thrombosis due to their anti-angiogenetic and anti-cyclo-oxygenase action and also immune stimulation and modulation of adhesion molecules.[39,40] Venous thromboembolism with these drugs is especially common in those receiving concomitant therapy with dexamethosne: lenalidomide for example in combination with high-dose dexamethasone is associated with VTE rates of 26%–67% in patients with newly diagnosed multiple myeloma.[41] In contrast, the risk of VTE is significantly reduced to 12% with low-dose dexamethasone. In the relapsed/refractory setting, the risk of VTE in patients treated with lenalidomide plus high-dose dexamethasone is 11%–15%.[42] The increased risks for arterial ischemia in these patients was evaluated by Libourel et al. In their prospective cohort study of 195 patients with multiple myeloma, 11 patients developed arterial ischemic event over a period of 522 patient-years (5.6%).[43] Interestingly, several of these patients developed arterial thrombosis while receiving anticoagulation therapy: four were receiving vitamin K antagonist and 2 were on DVT prophylaxis dose of low molecular weight heparin.

Bevacizumab, a vascular endothelial growth factor (VEGF) inhibitor, has been linked to serious vascular thrombotic events[44,45] through mechanisms such as endothelial damage, exposure of subendothelial collagen, reduction of endothelial renewal capacity, tissue factor activation and over expression of proinflammatory cyclooxygenase-2 and E-selectin genes.[46–48] In their population of patients receiving concurrent bevacizumab and chemotherapy, Scappaticci et al. reported the absolute rate of arterial events as 5.5 events per 100-person years.[49] Pereg and Lisher reported the efficacy of low-dose Aspirin in preventing cardiovascular complications in patients 65 years of age or older who had a prior history of thromboembolic events and were currently receiving Bevacizumab.[44] The mechanism of vascular toxicities associated with TKIs is not well understood and is suspected to be partially mediated by nitric oxide inhibition versus accelerated atherosclerosis and possible interference with platelets function. In a met-analysis by Choueiri et al. the incidence of arterial ischemia was reported at 4% with 3 fold increase in risk in those patient being treated with sunitinib or sorafenib.[50] Arterial ischemia with

Ponatinib has been reported to be greater than 20% leading to the implementation of major restrictions on indications and monitoring by the FDA.[51]

Other cancer therapies:

1. Erythropoetin (EPO): EPO use in cancer patients is associated with an increased risk for thromboembolic events, especially when used in combination with chemotherapy with rates ranging from 13% to 27% in various studies.[52,53] Some studies have indicated a role of altered protein C and S levels, factor VIII, and vWF secondary to EPO in the pathogenesis of arterial and venous thrombotic events,[54] while others point to increased level of C-reactive protein, nitric oxide and thrombin activatable fibrinolytic inhibitor as the causative factors for EPO-related thrombosis.[55]

2. Hormonal therapy: The use of certain adjuvant hormonal therapy in patients with positive-receptor breast cancer has been linked to a slight increased risk of arterial ischemia including peripheral vascular events.[56] These events were especially reported with certain aromatase inhibitors (i.e., letrozole, anastrozole) when compared to the selective estrogen-receptor modulator tamoxifen.[57] The relative beneficial effect of Tamoxifen on the lipid profile can partially explain this difference in some cardiovascular endpoints. Clinical monitoring and adequate management of the usual cardiovascular risk factors is recommended to allow initiation and continuation of these drugs due to their large survival benefit in breast cancer patients compared to the relative low incidence of cardiovascular complications.

3. Blood and blood component transfusion: A retrospective analysis of a cohort of 70,542 cancer patients, reported an arterial ischemic events rate of 5.2% in the patients that received RBC transfusions versus 3.1% for the non-transfused patients. Both RBC and platelet transfusion were found to be predictors of arterial ischemic events.[58] Various mechanisms have been proposed for transfusion induced thrombosis that include: increase in circulating RBC mass and consequent vascular stasis; vasoconstriction due to nitric oxide depleted RBCs[59]; delivery of increased amount of redox-active iron leading to oxidative stress; and inadvertent delivery of pro-thrombotic agents such as activated platelets and platelet microparticles.[60,61]

4. Radiation therapy is a well-known to accelerate atherosclerosis and lead to arterial occlusive disease. The risk of arterial ischemic events depends on the radiation dose, technique, extent of vasculature exposed and type of cancer.[15] Radiation causes oxidative stress leading to endothelial damage, activation of the coagulation cascade leading to fibrin deposition, accelerated transforming growth factor beta mediated transformation of fibroblasts to fibrocytes, and accelerated atherosclerosis—all of which predispose patients to thrombosis.[62,63] Primary prevention in patients with documented atherosclerosis following radiation therapy includes diet and lifestyle modifications to lower traditional atherosclerotic risk factors and optimal management of diabetes, hypertension, and dyslipidemia.[64] Lifelong antiplatelet therapy along with statin therapy are recommended for pharmacologic management, chosen for their anti-inflammatory and anti-thrombotic effects on the irradiated endothelium.[65] Radiation induced scarring makes surgical intervention difficult; hence percutaneous angioplasty with or without stenting is becoming the preferred revascularization method with encouraging results for radiation induced renal, iliac, and femoral symptomatic obstructive arterial disease[64] (Figure 13-8).

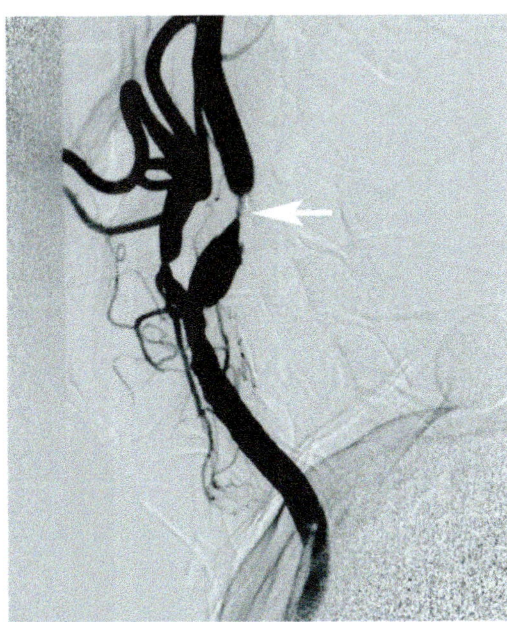

FIGURE 13-8   Critical left internal carotid artery stenosis in a 55-year-old patient presenting with transient ischemic attack 15 years after radiation therapy for Hodgkin's lymphoma. No recurrent events following medical therapy and carotid stenting.

MANAGEMENT

The management strategy varies depending on the patient clinical scenario, the type of cancer and cancer therapy and also on the site and vascular bed involved. There are specific clinical scenarios where primary prevention is indicated for the prevention of both arterial and venous events. The short and the long-term management plans should be tailored to the patients' clinical condition, the cancer type and the presence or absence of reversible etiology.

■ Prophylaxis

Primary preventive strategies for the prevention of arterial events include lifelong antiplatelet therapy and statins for radiation-induced and known underlying atherosclerotic disease; aspirin and/or hydroxyurea for myeloproliferative disorders[66]; and use of aspirin for patients with a history of prior cardiovascular events or who are over 65 and receiving Bevacizumab.[44]

When it comes to the more common venous events, the recommendations related to VTE prophylaxis are more complex and differ between the ambulatory and the inpatient settings. In fact, routine VTE prophylaxis using LMWH is strongly recommended for inpatients admitted for acute medical illness and surgery. Post-operative prophylaxis for up to 4 weeks is also recommended for those undergoing abdominal and pelvic surgeries.[67]

On the other hand, routine thromboprophylaxis is not recommended for ambulatory patients. Despite the increased risks of VTE in cancer patients in general, the individual patients' risks vary significantly based on the malignancy and also multiple host clinical factors. Several risk stratification models have been used in trials assessing role of thromboprophylaxis in the ambulatory cancer patients setting. The most validated VTE predictive model is the one proposed by Khorana et al.[68] Using simple patient clinical data with assigned risk scores, these patients are divided into a high risk, an intermediate and a low risk group. While the high risk score patients may potentially benefit from prophylaxis with LMWH, the current available data[69] does not support thromboprophylaxis in ambulatory setting based on the high number of patients needed to treat to prevent a single VTE event (NNT=60). One exception to this ambulatory setting rule is related to patients with multiple myeloma receiving immunomodulatory therapy and steroids. In fact, patients receiving lenalidomide or thalidomide in combination with dexamethasone are at significantly higher risk for VTE and outpatient prophylaxis with

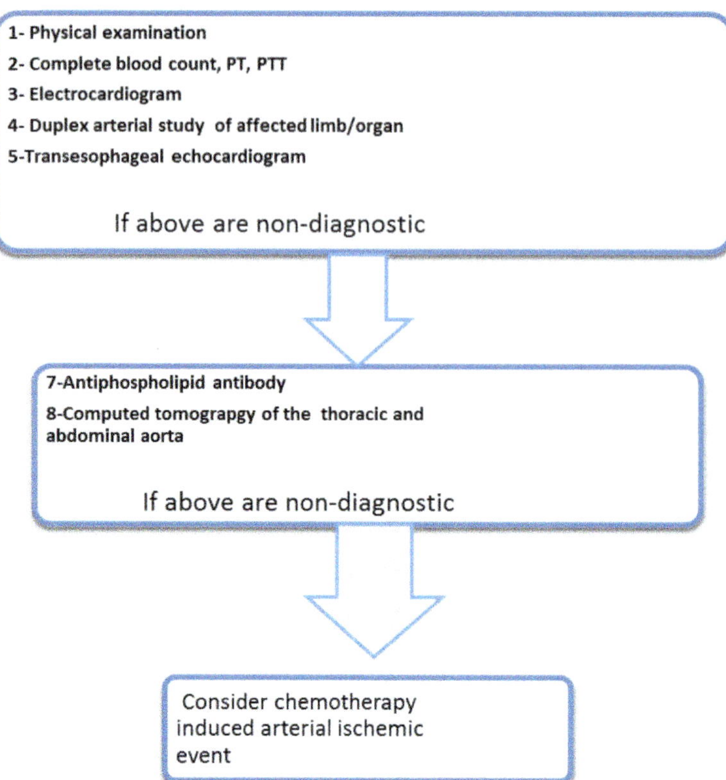

FIGURE 13-9   Suggested diagnostic evaluation chart.

LMWH in this group of patient, was associated with a significant reduction in symptomatic VTE when compared with warfarin (RR 0.33, 95% CI 0.14–0.83). Aspirin also appear to be effective since the difference between LMWH and aspirin was not statistically significant (RR 0.51, 95% CI 0.22–1.17).[69]

■ Management of Acute Arterial Ischemic Events

For patients with malignancy presenting with acute arterial ischemic events, the standard evaluation should include a complete physical exam, complete blood count, basic metabolic panel, coagulation profile and electrocardiography to identify arrhythmia (Figure 13-9). Echocardiography is indicated to evaluate a potential cardiac source of embolism. Given the high incidence of NBTE in this patient population, a low threshold for performing transesophageal echocardiogram (TEE) is justified. If these studies are unremarkable, computed tomographic angiography of the chest and abdominal aorta may be necessary (Figure 13-10). In the setting of a suspected central nervous system embolic event or an affecting the upper extremities carotid or upper limb duplex imaging study should be performed. TEE, transcranial Doppler (TCD), or agitated saline contrast echocardiography can be performed to excluding an intra-cardiac shunt in the presence of a suspected paradoxical embolism. If a thrombotic arterial event is suspected, further testing to exclude the presence of anti-phospholipid antibody or tumor-induced blood vessel compression may become necessary. If the aforementioned testing is non-diagnostic, chemotherapy-induced arterial ischemic events should be suspected. In non-cancer patients, it is unclear if extensive screening for occult malignancy is justified in patients who present with an idiopathic arterial ischemic events. Oktar et al. recommended a moderate screening strategy utilizing basic laboratory testing, chest X-ray, and abdominopelvic ultrasonography to search for occult cancer in patients presenting with idiopathic VTE and a more extensive screening strategy in patients with high risk features for malignancy, such as thrombosis in unusual sites.[70] El Sakka et al.[71] recommended screening with a chest X-ray based on findings from their study, in which lung cancer was the predominant malignancy in patients presenting with critical leg ischemia; Treatment of the acute arterial events varies by type of organ involved (cardiac, central nervous system, limb or bowel

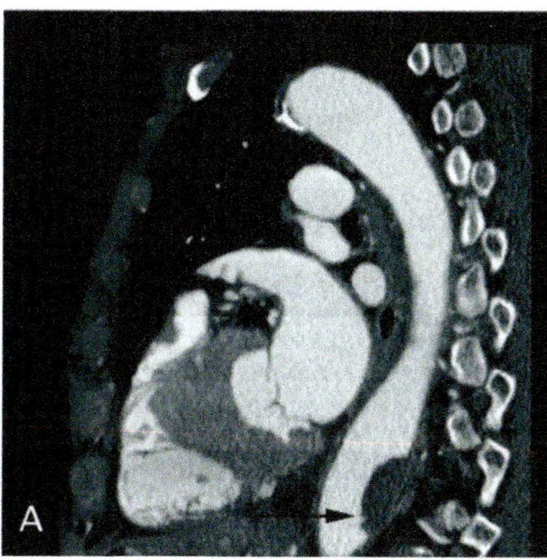

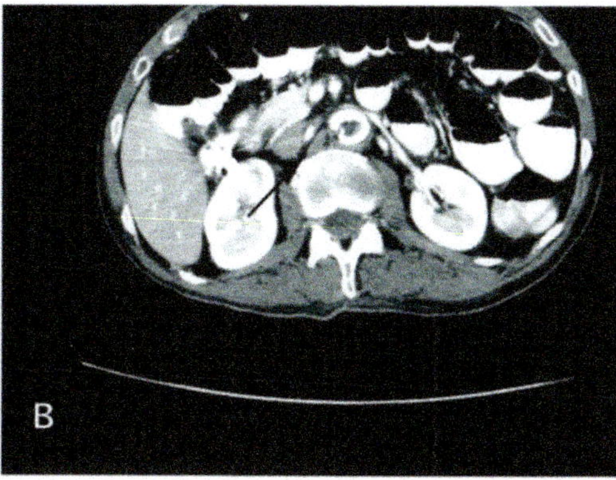

FIGURE 13-10 62 year old patient with bladder cancer. Incidental finding of a sessile thrombus involving his abdominal aorta wall on CT-Scan study of the abdomen and pelvis (A) saggital section; (B) coronal section. He subsequently developed acute left lower limb ischemia necessitating embolectomy.

ischemia) and is aimed towards reversing ischemia and minimizing organ damage followed by long-term therapy and secondary prevention. The decision to use medical therapy versus surgical or percutaneous approach for revascularization should be determined by the general condition of the patient and availability of local expertise. Management of these patients is often a challenge based on their bleeding risks especially in the setting of associated thrombocytopenia. While acute coronary intervention has been shown to be reasonably safe in these patients[72] there is a significant concern related to the need for dual antiplatelets therapy for extended period of time. Drug-eluting coronary stents pose a special problem in this setting and should be avoided. We typically recommend using bare metal stents since many of these patients will end up receiving more chemotherapy and/or surgery for the management of their cancer. The type of long-term

anticoagulation recommended for secondary prevention, depends on the underlying mechanism and etiology: Table 13-3 summarizes some of the therapeutic interventions for arterial ischemic events observed in the setting of malignancy or hematologic disorders.

■ Management of Venous Thromboembolic Events

Cancer patients often face the challenge of having multiple comorbidities which can impact the choice and the dosing of pharmacologic anticoagulants. This include, for example, the complexity related to inherent hypercoagulable state, the higher than usual bleeding risk during thrombocytopenia, the complexity of drug-drug interactions between anticoagulants and several chemotherapies. Indications for VTE prophylaxis and treatment of acute VTE events in these patients are aimed at decreasing DVT occurrence, preventing extension into pulmonary embolism, and minimizing VTE recurrence. The duration of therapy and the choice of pharmacologic approach for such therapy are sometimes different compared to those with no underlying cancer.

In general, patients presenting with VTE are typically risk stratified into low, intermediate or high risk categories depending on the presence or absence of pulmonary embolism and its secondary hemodynamic effects.

Outpatient anticoagulation for 3 to 6 months is typically used for simple DVT or low risk VTE with normal hemodynamics. The American College of Chest Physicians (ACCP) recommend treating cancer related uncomplicated VTEs with full anticoagulation for 3 months[73] while the medical Society of Clinical Oncology (ASCO) specify in their 2013 guidelines[74] that initial VTE therapy should be for 6 months.

The armamentarium of anticoagulation therapy for DVT in the general population include warfarin, low molecular weight heparin, fondaparinux, and the direct oral anticoagulants (DOACs). In patients with malignancy, LMWH is the long-term anticoagulant of choice for the management of VTE based on its safety and efficacy and also its superiority in reducing recurrence VTE rate compared to other agents. Warfarin and fondaparinux are both associated with similar bleeding risks as LMWH but both are associated with higher recurrence rate.[75] Other advantages of LMWH compared to warfarin include the more predictable response and standardized dosing with less drug-drug interaction.

As for the newer oral anticoagulation agents, expert panels continue to recommend against the use

TABLE 13-3 Therapeutic interventions of potential benefit for arterial ischemic events in cancer patients

ARTERIAL ISCHEMIC EVENTS ASSOCIATED WITH	TREATMENT OPTIONS
Acute Leukemia	-Chemotherapy and Leukapheresis -Surgical thromboembolectomy
Radiation therapy	-Antiplatelet therapy -Statin therapy -Percutaneous angioplasty with or without stenting -Surgery
Paradoxical embolization	-Systemic anticoagulation -PFO closure for recurrent events
Myeloproliferative disorders	-Aspirin (For primary and secondary prevention) -Cell Reduction therapy (i.e., Phlebotomy, Hydroxyurea, Anagrelide, Interferon alpha)
Cardiac Amyloidosis	-Systemic anticoagulation
Bevacizumab	-Aspirin (For primary prevention in patients over 65 years age or with a history of cardiovascular events)
NBTE	-Systemic anticoagulation

NBTE, Non-bacterial thrombotic endocarditis; PFO, Patent foramen ovale.

of these drugs in patients with cancer. In fact, The National Comprehensive Cancer Network (NCCN) guidelines recommend against using DOACs in cancer patients[74] based on the limited data regarding their safety in patients with active malignancy. Other Reasons to avoid use of these drugs in the cancer population include the lack of convincing efficacy data in this subgroup of patients in addition to the lack of reversal agents' availability, the limited options for standardized testing for monitoring and, more importantly, the unpredictable and complicated drug-drug interactions with chemotherapy agents.

Limited clinical data suggest similar efficacy between DOACs and warfarin in cancer patients with VTE. The scarce safety and effectiveness outcome data in cancer patients were derived mainly from limited observational studies and from several small subgroup analysis studies obtained from large clinical trials that mainly included non-cancer[76–78] and typically excluded patients undergoing active chemotherapy. These studies have the usual inherent limitations of meta-analysis related to the difference and the heterogeneity of trial protocols like baseline patients' clinical characteristics and the pre-defined outcomes and complications. Moreover, there are several clinical and metabolic features in cancer patients that can alter the DOACs pharmacodynamics with secondary unpredictable clinical response to these drugs: These features include altered renal and hepatic functions, cancer cachexia and malnutrition, coagulopathy and thrombocytopenia and more importantly the unpredicted response caused by

drug-drug interaction with cancer therapies. In fact, data about the combined use of chemotherapeutic agents and DOACs is rare. DOACS interact with CYP3A4 and P-glycoprotein, making them theoretically susceptible to plasma concentrations' fluctuations when taken with inhibitors or inducers of these enzymes. Several categories of chemotherapeutic agents, including antimitotic microtubule inhibitors, tyrosine kinase inhibitors and immune-modulating agents are known substrates to either or both of CYP3A4 and P-glycoprotein.[79–80] Theoretically, these types of pharmacodynamics drug-drug interactions can lead to attenuation of the DOACs effects, increasing the risk of thrombosis, or exacerbation of their anticoagulation effects leading to an increase in bleeding risks. The current NCCN guidelines recommend against the use of DOACs in patients with active cancer.[74] These recommendations are based mainly on the many reasons listed above and will likely hold until more safety data is available. There are currently multiple randomized and also observational ongoing trials investigating the safety and efficacy of these drugs in cancer patients (clinicaltrials.gov: NCT 02048865, NCT 02073682, NCT 01708850, and NCT 01727427) that will hopefully further clarify the role of these drugs in managing cancer patients. Until a better understanding of bleeding risks related to DOACs' pharmacodynamics interaction with chemotherapy and a better evidence of clinical safety are both available, vigilance and caution are recommended when using DOACs in cancer patients. In particular when combined with drugs that strongly interact with CYP3A4 or P-glycoprotein.

Duration of Therapy and Other Special Clinical Scenarios

1. *Duration of therapy:* The American College of Chest Physicians (ACCP) recommend treating cancer related uncomplicated VTEs with full anticoagulation for 3 months[73] while the medical Society of Clinical Oncology (ASCO) recommend low molecular weight heparin (LMWH) for a total of 6. Treatment beyond 3–6 month is a debatable approach: The current ASCO guidelines[74] and expert panels recommend anticoagulation beyond 6 months should be considered for selected patients who are at high risk for recurrent VTE, such as those with metastatic disease or actively undergoing chemotherapy. Patients with evidence of recurrent VTE should be assessed for compliance and be considered for alternate anticoagulation regimen or be considered for any increase in their LMWH dose by 25%.[81]

2. *Incidental venous thromboembolism*, including pulmonary emboli, should be treated similarly and for the same duration as symptomatic VTEs.

3. *Upper extremity DVT* is often related to indwelling venous catheters. Management recommendations from the ACCP[73] include recommending removal of the offending catheter only if it is no longer needed or if it is occluded. Otherwise, these catheters should be preserved during chemotherapy and anticoagulation should be initiated and continued as long as catheter is being used and followed by a minimum of 3 months of anti-coagulation after its removal. *Catheter related right atrial clot* is also a secondary complication and usually related to mechanical injury by deeply inserted central venous catheter. It is typically managed by retrieving the catheter tip by about 3–5 centimeters and full anticoagulation for 3 months.

4. *Thrombocytopenia and VTEs*: In the common clinical scenarios of cancer- or chemotherapy-induced severe thrombocytopenia, platelet transfusions is sometimes used to allow anticoagulation. Based on experts' opinion, full therapeutic anticoagulation with LMWH should be used if the platelet count can be maintained above 50×10^9/L. For platelet counts between 20 and 50×10^9/L, 50% reduction in LMWH is recommended with close clinical monitoring for bleeding. For platelet count below 20×10^9/L, anticoagulation should be avoided.[82]

5. *Pulmonary embolism*: The treatment of high risk patients who are hemodynamically unstable on initial presentation with PE, is to proceed with reperfusion therapy (systemic thrombolytics, catheter directed thrombolysis or surgery). Those who are hemodynamically stable are typically treated with anticoagulation for 6 months. It has been shown, however, that 31% of normotensive patients have evidence of right

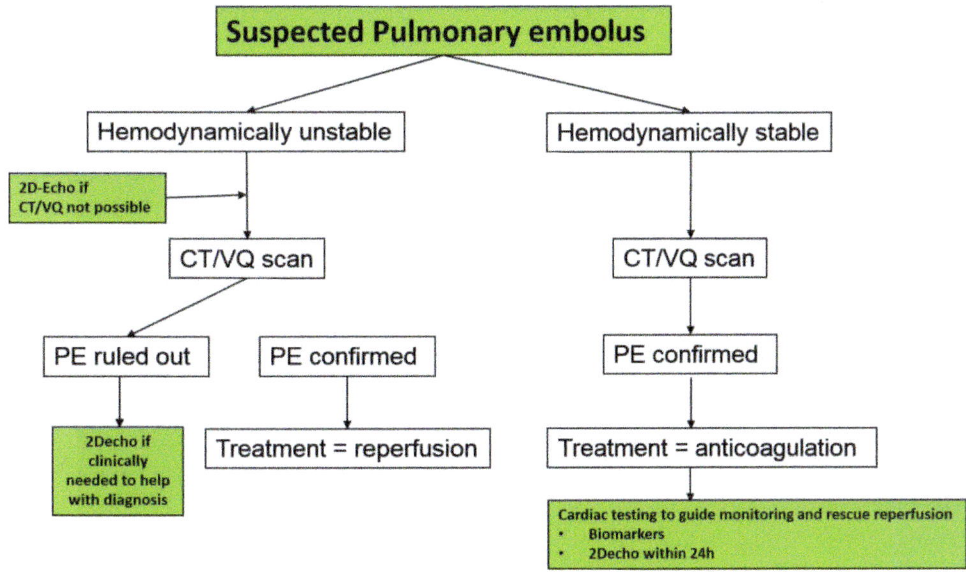

FIGURE 13-11 Timing and indication for cardiac testing for risk stratification in patients with suspected acute pulmonary embolism.

ventricular dysfunction leading to late clinical deterioration with 10% shock at 48h and 5% related death.[83] There is no individual clinical, imaging or laboratory test findings that has been shown to accurately predict worsening outcome that is considered high enough to justify primary reperfusion in normotensive patients with VTE. Current risk assessment strategies using echocardiography and cardiac biomarkers in acute PE concentrate on identification of patients who appear to be stable at presentation but have impending right ventricular failure and high risk of subsequent shock or death. Cardiac testing in this subgroup of patients is becoming a well-recognized tool to help further risk stratify these patients (low versus intermediate-risk) and can guide clinical monitoring in order to establish rescue reperfusion in those with delayed hemodynamic instability and shock that was not present initially on presentation.[73,84] Figure 13-11 below shows a proposed and suggested algorithm related to the timing and indication of cardiac testing in patients with suspected PE.

OUTCOME

Appropriate prevention and treatment of cancer-associated thrombosis is vital to reduce its burden on patients with malignancy. Data related to cancer patients' outcomes following thromboembolic events is limited and mostly based on retrospective analysis of small cohort studies or data registry. Despite these limitations, these studies findings are consistent with the message of worsening outcome when these events occur.

In order to assess the significance and outcome of these events, Khorana et al. prospectively followed more than 4000 cancer patients receiving active chemotherapy and reported that thromboembolic complications competed with infectious diseases as the second most common cause of death in these patients (1). They also observed a higher rates of death from arterial events compared to venous events. Patients with VTE have in general a worse prognosis than patients with cancer who did not experience thromboembolic events and their survival is particularly poor when the diagnosis of cancer is concurrent with the thromboembolic event.[2] As for the arterial ischemic events, several recent studies found and reported that an aggressive approach for the treatment thromboembolic events in cancer patients, including even complex surgeries for life threatening arterial events do not appear to be associated with a prohibitively high mortality rate.[16,85] Conservative management as the main therapeutic modality is not justified in these

circumstances. Except in extreme cases of terminal cancer where palliative care is a reasonable option, selection of treatment modality, in our opinion, should follow the established standard of care.[16,85]

SUMMARY

Venous and arterial thromboembolic diseases are common source of serious morbidities and are considered the third most common cause of mortality in cancer patients after cancer itself and infection. Patients with certain malignancies are at significantly increased risks for these vascular events due to the inherent thrombophilia associated with these cancers and cancer therapies. In general, the clinical presentation vary based on the venous or arterial bed and organs involved. Management is often a challenge due to the presence of several clinical factors that can impact the choice and dosing of antiplatelets and anticoagulants in managing these patients. These challenges also include the higher than usual bleeding risks in these patients (low platelets, brain metastasis, the need for procedures and surgeries) in addition to the complexity of drug-drug interaction between anticoagulants and several chemotherapeutic agents. Long-term cancer patients' outcomes are often impacted by these thromboembolic events and include longer hospitalizations and shorter lifespan. In daily clinical practice, a good understanding of the nuances surrounding management of these complex patients is critical for improved outcome and it is our believe that a multidisciplinary approach between oncologist and other medical specialists (cardiology, vascular surgery, interventional radiology) is essential in the management of these patients aiming for optimal outcome.

REFERENCES

1. Khorana AA, Francis CW, Culakova E, Kuderer NM, Lyman GH. Thromboembolism is a leading cause of death in cancer patients receiving outpatient chemotherapy. *J Thromb Haemost*. 2007;5(3):632–634.
2. Sorensen HT, Mellemkjaer L, Olsen JH, Baron JA. Prognosis of cancers associated with venous thromboembolism. *N Engl J Med*. 2000;343(25):1846–1850.
3. Murchison JT, Wylie L, Stockton DL. Excess risk of cancer in patients with primary venous thromboembolism: a national, population-based cohort study. *Br J Cancer*. 2004;91(1):92–95.
4. Imberti D, Agnelli G, Ageno W, et al. Clinical characteristics and management of cancer-associated acute venous thromboembolism: findings from the MASTER Registry. *Haematologica*. 2008;93(2):273–278.
5. Khorana AA, Francis CW, Culakova E, Kuderer NM, Lyman GH. Frequency, risk factors, and trends for

venous thromboembolism among hospitalized cancer patients. *Cancer*. 2007;110(10):2339–2346.

6. Johnson MJ, Sproule MW, Paul J. The prevalence and associated variables of deep venous thrombosis in patients with advanced cancer. *Clin Oncol (R Coll Radiol)*. 1999;11(2):105–110.

7. Khorana AA, Francis CW, Culakova E, Fisher RI, Kuderer NM, Lyman GH. Thromboembolism in hospitalized neutropenic cancer patients. *J Clin Oncol*. 2006;24(3):484–490.

8. Landolfi R, Di Gennaro L, Falanga A. Thrombosis in myeloproliferative disorders: pathogenetic facts and speculation. *Leukemia*. 2008;22(11):2020–2028.

9. Feng D, Edwards WD, Oh JK, et al. Intracardiac thrombosis and embolism in patients with cardiac amyloidosis. *Circulation*. 2007;116(21):2420–2426.

10. Javid M, Magee TR, Galland RB. Arterial thrombosis associated with malignant disease. *Eur J Vasc Endovasc Surg*. 2008;35(1):84–87.

11. Kwaan HC, Parmar S, Wang J. Pathogenesis of increased risk of thrombosis in cancer. *Semin Thromb Hemost*. 2003;29(3):283–290.

12. Lee AY, Levine MN. The thrombophilic state induced by therapeutic agents in the cancer patient. *Semin Thromb Hemost*. 1999;25(2):137–145.

13. Naschitz JE, Yeshurun D, Abrahamson J. Arterial occlusive disease in occult cancer. *Am Heart J*. 1992;124(3):738–745.

14. Chow SF, McKenna CH. Ovarian cancer and gangrene of the digits: case report and review of the literature. *Mayo Clin Proc*. 1996;71(3):253–258.

15. Jurado JA, Bashir R, Burket MW. Radiation-induced peripheral artery disease. *Catheter Cardiovasc Interv*. 2008;72(4):563–568.

16. Mouhayar E, Tayar J, Fasulo M, et al. Outcome of acute limb ischemia in cancer patients. *Vasc Med*. 2014;19(2):112–117.

17. Rossi C, Randi ML, Zerbinati P, Rinaldi V, Girolami A. Acute coronary disease in essential thrombocythemia and polycythemia vera. *J Intern Med*. 1998;244(1):49–53.

18. Marchioli R, Finazzi G, Landolfi R, et al. Vascular and neoplastic risk in a large cohort of patients with polycythemia vera. *J Clin Oncol*. 2005;23(10):2224–2232.

19. Harrison CN, Campbell PJ, Buck G, et al. Hydroxyurea compared with anagrelide in high-risk essential thrombocythemia. *N Engl J Med*. 2005;353(1):33–45.

20. De Stefano V, Sora F, Rossi E, et al. The risk of thrombosis in patients with acute leukemia: occurrence of thrombosis at diagnosis and during treatment. *J Thromb Haemost*. 2005;3(9):1985–1992.

21. Bombeli T, Karsan A, Tait JF, Harlan JM. Apoptotic vascular endothelial cells become procoagulant. *Blood*. 1997;89(7):2429–2442.

22. Romer LH, McLean NV, Yan HC, Daise M, Sun J, DeLisser HM. IFN-gamma and TNF-alpha induce redistribution of PECAM-1 (CD31) on human endothelial cells. *J Immunol*. 1995;154(12):6582–6592.

23. Fass R, Haddad M, Zaizov R, et al. Recurrent peripheral arterial occlusion by leukemic cells sedimentation

in acute promyelocytic leukemia. *J Pediatr Surg*. 1992;27(5):665–667.

24. Posacioglu H, Apaydin AZ, Buyukkececi F, Soydan S, Durmaz . Recurrent peripheral arterial occlusion in acute promyelocytic leukemia. *EJVES Extra*. 2003;6(5):100–102.

25. Roberts WC, Waller BF. Cardiac amyloidosis causing cardiac dysfunction: analysis of 54 necropsy patients. *Am J Cardiol*. 1983;52(1):137–146.

26. Berghoff M, Kathpal M, Khan F, Skinner M, Falk R, Freeman R. Endothelial dysfunction precedes C-fiber abnormalities in primary (AL) amyloidosis. *Ann Neurol*. 2003;53(6):725–730.

27. Liao R, Jain M, Teller P, et al. Infusion of light chains from patients with cardiac amyloidosis causes diastolic dysfunction in isolated mouse hearts. *Circulation*. 2001;104(14):1594–1597.

28. Browne RS, Schneiderman H, Kayani N, Radford MJ, Hager WD. Amyloid heart disease manifested by systemic arterial thromboemboli. *Chest*. 1992;102(1):304–307.

29. Yood RA, Skinner M, Rubinow A, Talarico L, Cohen AS. Bleeding manifestations in 100 patients with amyloidosis. *JAMA*. 1983;249(10):1322–1324.

30. Rogers JS, 2nd, Murgo AJ, Fontana JA, Raich PC. Chemotherapy for breast cancer decreases plasma protein C and protein S. *J Clin Oncol*. 1988;6(2):276–281.

31. Mannucci PM, Bettega D, Chantarangkul V, Tripodi A, Sacchini V, Veronesi U. Effect of tamoxifen on measurements of hemostasis in healthy women. *Arch Intern Med*. 1996;156(16):1806–1810.

32. Greeno EW, Bach RR, Moldow CF. Apoptosis is associated with increased cell surface tissue factor procoagulant activity. *Lab Invest*. 1996;75(2):281–289.

33. Wang J, Weiss I, Svoboda K, Kwaan HC. Thrombogenic role of cells undergoing apoptosis. *Br J Haematol*. 2001;115(2):382–391.

34. Walsh J, Wheeler HR, Geczy CL. Modulation of tissue factor on human monocytes by cisplatin and adriamycin. *Br J Haematol*. 1992;81(4):480–488.

35. Numico G, Garrone O, Dongiovanni V, et al. Prospective evaluation of major vascular events in patients with nonsmall cell lung carcinoma treated with cisplatin and gemcitabine. *Cancer*. 2005;103(5):994–999.

36. Grenader T, Shavit L, Ospovat I, Gutfeld O, Peretz T. Aortic occlusion in patients treated with Cisplatin-based chemotherapy. *Mt Sinai J Med*. 2006;73(5):810–812.

37. Alter P, Herzum M, Soufi M, Schaefer JR, Maisch B. Cardiotoxicity of 5-fluorouracil. *Cardiovasc Hematol Agents Med Chem*. 2006;4(1):1–5.

38. Dasanu CA. Gemcitabine: vascular toxicity and prothrombotic potential. *Expert Opin Drug Saf*. 2008;7(6):703–716.

39. Fanelli M, Sarmiento R, Gattuso D, et al. Thalidomide: a new anticancer drug? *Expert Opin Investig Drugs*. 2003;12(7):1211–1225.

40. Baz R, Li L, Kottke-Marchant K, et al. The role of aspirin in the prevention of thrombotic complications of thalidomide and anthracycline-based

chemotherapy for multiple myeloma. *Mayo Clin Proc.* 2005;80(12):1568–1574.

41. Rajkumar SV, Jacobus S, Callander NS, et al. Lenalidomide plus high-dose dexamethasone versus lenalidomide plus low-dose dexamethasone as initial therapy for newly diagnosed multiple myeloma: an open-label randomised controlled trial. *Lancet Oncol.* 2010;11(1):29–37.

42. Weber DM, Chen C, Niesvizky R, et al. Lenalidomide plus dexamethasone for relapsed multiple myeloma in North America. *N Engl J Med.* 2007;357(21):2133–2142.

43. Libourel EJ, Sonneveld P, van der Holt B, de Maat MP, Leebeek FW. High incidence of arterial thrombosis in young patients treated for multiple myeloma: results of a prospective cohort study. *Blood.* 2010;116(1):22–26.

44. Pereg D, Lishner M. Bevacizumab treatment for cancer patients with cardiovascular disease: a double edged sword? *Eur Heart J.* 2008;29(19):2325–2326.

45. Grivas AA, Trafalis DT, Athanassiou AE. Implication of bevacizumab in fatal arterial thromboembolic incidents. *J BUON.* 2009;14(1):115–117.

46. Yoon S, Schmassmann-Suhijar D, Zuber M, Konietzny P, Schmassmann A. Chemotherapy with bevacizumab, irinotecan, 5-fluorouracil and leucovorin (IFL) associated with a large, embolizing thrombus in the thoracic aorta. *Ann Oncol.* 2006;17(12):1851–1852.

47. Ferrara N. Vascular endothelial growth factor: basic science and clinical progress. *Endocr Rev.* 2004;25(4):581–611.

48. Kilickap S, Abali H, Celik I. Bevacizumab, bleeding, thrombosis, and warfarin. *J Clin Oncol.* 2003;21(18):3542; author reply 3.

49. Scappaticci FA, Skillings JR, Holden SN, et al. Arterial thromboembolic events in patients with metastatic carcinoma treated with chemotherapy and bevacizumab. *J Natl Cancer Inst.* 2007;99(16):1232–1239.

50. Choueiri TK, Schutz FA, Je Y, Rosenberg JE, Bellmunt J. Risk of arterial thromboembolic events with sunitinib and sorafenib: a systematic review and meta-analysis of clinical trials. *J Clin Oncol.* 2010;28(13):2280–2285.

51. Bair SM, Choueiri TK, Moslehi J. Cardiovascular complications associated with novel angiogenesis inhibitors: emerging evidence and evolving perspectives. *Trends Cardiovasc Med.* 2013;23(4):104–113.

52. Dusenbery KE, McGuire WA, Holt PJ, et al. Erythropoietin increases hemoglobin during radiation therapy for cervical cancer. *Int J Radiat Oncol Biol Phys.* 1994;29(5):1079–1084.

53. Gladding PA, Webster MW, Kay P. Late drug-eluting stent thrombosis and erythropoietin: cause and effect? *Heart Lung Circ.* 2007;16(4):305–307.

54. Haddad TC, Greeno EW. Chemotherapy-induced thrombosis. *Thromb Res.* 2006;118(5):555–568.

55. Tobu M, Iqbal O, Fareed D, et al. Erythropoietin-induced thrombosis as a result of increased inflammation and thrombin activatable fibrinolytic inhibitor. *Clin Appl Thromb Hemost.* 2004;10(3):225–232.

56. Mouridsen H, Keshaviah A, Coates AS, et al. Cardiovascular adverse events during adjuvant endocrine therapy for early breast cancer using letrozole or tamoxifen: safety analysis of BIG 1-98 trial. *J Clin Oncol.* 2007;25(36):5715–5722.

57. Ewer MS, Gluck S. A woman's heart: the impact of adjuvant endocrine therapy on cardiovascular health. *Cancer.* 2009;115(9):1813–1826.

58. Khorana AA, Francis CW, Blumberg N, Culakova E, Refaai MA, Lyman GH. Blood transfusions, thrombosis, and mortality in hospitalized patients with cancer. *Arch Intern Med.* 2008;168(21):2377–2381.

59. Reynolds JD, Ahearn GS, Angelo M, Zhang J, Cobb F, Stamler JS. S-nitrosohemoglobin deficiency: a mechanism for loss of physiological activity in banked blood. *Proc Natl Acad Sci USA.* 2007;104(43):17058–17062.

60. Blumberg N, Gettings KF, Turner C, Heal JM, Phipps RP. An association of soluble CD40 ligand (CD154) with adverse reactions to platelet transfusions. *Transfusion.* 2006;46(10):1813–1821.

61. Khan SY, Kelher MR, Heal JM, et al. Soluble CD40 ligand accumulates in stored blood components, primes neutrophils through CD40, and is a potential cofactor in the development of transfusion-related acute lung injury. *Blood.* 2006;108(7):2455–2462.

62. Burger A, Loffler H, Bamberg M, Rodemann HP. Molecular and cellular basis of radiation fibrosis. *Int J Radiat Biol.* 1998;73(4):401–408.

63. Riley PA. Free radicals in biology: oxidative stress and the effects of ionizing radiation. *Int J Radiat Biol.* 1994;65(1):27–33.

64. Jurado J, Thompson PD. Prevention of coronary artery disease in cancer patients. *Pediatr Blood Cancer.* 2005;44(7):620–624.

65. Gaugler MH, Vereycken-Holler V, Squiban C, Vandamme M, Vozenin-Brotons MC, Benderitter M. Pravastatin limits endothelial activation after irradiation and decreases the resulting inflammatory and thrombotic responses. *Radiat Res.* 2005;163(5):479–487.

66. Landolfi R, Marchioli R, Kutti J, et al. Efficacy and safety of low-dose aspirin in polycythemia vera. *N Engl J Med.* 2004;350(2):114–124.

67. Khorana AA, Carrier M, Garcia DA, Lee AY. Guidance for the prevention and treatment of cancer-associated venous thromboembolism. *J Thromb Thrombolysis.* 2016;41(1):81–91.

68. Khorana AA, Kuderer NM, Culakova E, Lyman GH, Francis CW. Development and validation of a predictive model for chemotherapy-associated thrombosis. *Blood.* 2008;111(10):4902–4907.

69. Di Nisio M, Porreca E, Ferrante N, Otten HM, Cuccurullo F, Rutjes AW. Primary prophylaxis for venous thromboembolism in ambulatory cancer patients receiving chemotherapy. *Cochrane Database Syst Rev.* 2012;12:CD008500.

70. Oktar GL, Ergul EG, Kiziltepe U. Occult malignancy in patients with venous thromboembolism:

risk indicators and a diagnostic screening strategy. *Phlebology*. 2007;22(2):75–79.

71. El Sakka K, Gambhir RP, Halawa M, Chong P, Rashid H. Association of malignant disease with critical leg ischaemia. *Br J Surg*. 2005;92(12):1498–1501.

72. Iliescu C, Durand JB, Kroll M. Cardiovascular interventions in thrombocytopenic cancer patients. *Tex Heart Inst J*. 2011;38(3):259–260.

73. Kearon C, Akl EA, Ornelas J, et al. Antithrombotic therapy for VTE disease: CHEST guideline and expert panel report. *Chest*. 2016;149(2):315–352.

74. Lyman GH, Bohlke K, Khorana AA, et al. Venous thromboembolism prophylaxis and treatment in patients with cancer: american society of clinical oncology clinical practice guideline update 2014. *J Clin Oncol*. 2015;33(6):654–646.

75. Lee AY, Levine MN, Baker RI, et al. Low-molecular-weight heparin versus a coumarin for the prevention of recurrent venous thromboembolism in patients with cancer. *N Engl J Med*. 2003;349(2):146–153.

76. Prins MH, Lensing AW, Brighton TA, et al. Oral rivaroxaban versus enoxaparin with vitamin K antagonist for the treatment of symptomatic venous thromboembolism in patients with cancer (EINSTEIN-DVT and EINSTEIN-PE): a pooled subgroup analysis of two randomised controlled trials. *Lancet Haematol*. 2014;1(1):e37–e46.

77. Vedovati MC, Germini F, Agnelli G, Becattini C. Direct oral anticoagulants in patients with VTE and cancer: a systematic review and meta-analysis. *Chest*. 2015;147(2):475–483.

78. Schulman S, Kakkar AK, Goldhaber SZ, et al. Treatment of acute venous thromboembolism with dabigatran or warfarin and pooled analysis. *Circulation*. 2014;129(7):764–772.

79. Gnoth MJ, Buetehorn U, Muenster U, Schwarz T, Sandmann S. In vitro and in vivo P-glycoprotein transport characteristics of rivaroxaban. *J Pharmacol Exp Ther*. 2011;338(1):372–380.

80. Harvey RD, Morgan ET. Cancer, inflammation, and therapy: effects on cytochrome p450-mediated drug metabolism and implications for novel immunotherapeutic agents. *Clin Pharmacol Ther*. 2014;96(4):449–457.

81. Carrier M, Le Gal G, Cho R, Tierney S, Rodger M, Lee AY. Dose escalation of low molecular weight heparin to manage recurrent venous thromboembolic events despite systemic anticoagulation in cancer patients. *J Thromb Haemost*. 2009;7(5):760–765.

82. Lee AY, Peterson EA. Treatment of cancer-associated thrombosis. *Blood*. 2013;122(14):2310–2317.

83. Grifoni S, Olivotto I, Cecchini P, et al. Short-term clinical outcome of patients with acute pulmonary embolism, normal blood pressure, and echocardiographic right ventricular dysfunction. *Circulation*. 2000;101(24):2817–2822.

84. Konstantinides SV, Torbicki A, Agnelli G, et al. 2014 ESC guidelines on the diagnosis and management of acute pulmonary embolism. *Eur Heart J*. 2014;35(43):3033–3069, 69a-69k.

85. Nicolajsen CW, Dickenson MH, Budtz-Lilly J, Eldrup N. Frequency of cancer in patients operated on for acute peripheral arterial thrombosis and the impact on prognosis. *J Vasc Surg*. 2015;62(6):1598–1606.

14 Cardiac Tumors

Daniel Perry ■ *Monika Leja* ■ *Scott Schuetze* ■ *Shanda H. Blackmon* ■ *Michael J. Reardon*

INTRODUCTION

Although cardiac masses are rare, malignant tumors typically have a less than one year survival without intervention. Retrospective reviews of cardiac surgeries have revealed the incidence of primary cardiac tumors to be 0.3%[1,2] to 0.7%.[3] Clinical series from busy cardiac centers such as the Methodist DeBakey Heart Center,[4] Stanford University,[5] and the Texas Heart Institute[6] covering over 20 years, each only report 85, 42, and 114 patients, respectively, with primary cardiac tumors treated surgically. In these series, about 72% of tumors were benign and 28% were malignant, with sarcomas comprising 75% of the malignant tumors. Because cardiac neoplasms are rare, the data on the true prevalence of cardiac tumors is scant and the incidence will likely increase as the routine use of imaging modalities such as echocardiography (Echo), cardiac computed tomography (CCT), and cardiac magnetic resonance imaging (CMR) increases[7] as well as data capture among various medical centers.

Cardiac neoplasms can be divided into primary tumors arising from the heart and secondary tumors that have metastasized to the heart. Metastatic tumors to the heart are a much more common entity than primary cardiac tumors[8] with 10%–20% of patients dying from disseminated cancer also having metastatic involvement of the heart and pericardium.[9–12] Of these, primary cardiac tumors are three times more likely to be benign than malignant[3,10] (Table 14-1). A final category of cardiac tumors of interest is the direct extension of infradiaphragmatic tumors, which can occur with almost any cell type but occurs in 4% to 10% of renal cell tumors,[13–15] typically extending into the vena cava and right atrium.

Management of cardiac tumors is a complex decision based on malignant potential, location, thromboembolic potential, and resection potential. A discussion of the chemotherapeutic, and surgical evolution of care follows. For most malignant cardiac tumors, surgical excision after systemic chemotherapy remains the best treatment for malignant cardiac tumors when possible if distant metastatic control can be achieved, as well as a negative margin. There are isolated exceptions to this rule such as cardiac lymphoma, which may need chemotherapy only. The principal problem with surgical resection of primary cardiac tumors has been the tumor's extensive involvement of cardiac structures, which makes access difficult. Complete resection is

TABLE 14-1 Tumors and cysts of the heart and pericardium

TYPE	NUMBER	%
Benign		
Myxoma	130	24.4
Lipoma	45	8.4
Papillary fibroelastoma	42	7.9
Rhabdomyoma	36	6.8
Fibroma	17	3.2
Hemangioma	15	2.8
Teratoma	14	2.6
Mesothelioma of the atrioventricular node	12	2.3
Granular cell tumor	3	
Neurofibroma	3	
Lymphangioma	2	
Subtotal	**319**	**59.8**
Pericardial cyst	82	15.4
Bronchogenic cyst	7	1.3
Subtotal	**89**	**16.7**
Malignant		
Angiosarcoma	39	7.3
Rhabdomyosarcoma	26	4.9
Mesothelioma	19	3.6
Fibrosarcoma	14	2.6
Malignant lymphoma	7	1.3
Extraskeletal osteosarcoma	5	
Neurogenic sarcoma	4	
Malignant teratoma	4	
Thymoma	4	
Leiomyosarcoma	1	
Liposarcoma	1	
Synovial sarcoma	1	
Subtotal	**125**	**23.5**
Total	**533**	**100.0**

often a technical challenge with newer techniques such as left sided autotransplantation providing a novel approach. Metastatic disease remains the challenge in malignant disease, and a systemic approach is necessary.

SURGICAL HISTORICAL PERSPECTIVE

Cardiac tumors have always aroused the interest of cardiac surgeons because of the grave consequences inherent in their untreated natural history. There have been several advances in the surgical history leading to the development of advanced procedures such as autotransplantation and complicated reconstructions of the heart. The first case of primary cardiac neoplasm was described by Realdo Colomnus in 1562.[16] The classification system used today originates from Yater who reported nine cases of cardiac tumors in 1931,[17] all postmortem cases. It remained for Barnes and colleagues in 1934 to make the first clinical antemortem diagnosis of a primary cardiac tumor, a sarcoma, from an electrocardiogram and a lymph node biopsy.[18] The surgical treatment of cardiac tumors began in 1938, when Beck successfully removed an intrapericardial cystic teratoma that extended to the right ventricle.[19] Maurer successfully excised the first primary cardiac tumor of the heart, an epicardial lipoma external to the left ventricle, in 1951.[19] However, no real surgical progress in the excision of cardiac tumors was made until the introduction of cardiopulmonary bypass (CPB) by John Gibbon in 1953, who used the principles

established by Michael E. DeBakey's roller pump to create artificial blood flow, allowing a controlled and reproducible access to the interior chambers of the heart.[20] This was followed shortly afterward by the successful excision of a left atrial myxoma using CPB by Crafoord in 1954.[21] The first successful right ventricular myxoma excision was achieved in 1960, showing that tumors of all cardiac chambers could be excised.[22]

A second major event, which impacted the diagnosis and surgical treatment of cardiac tumors, was the introduction of echocardiography allowing a noninvasive method to view the interior and exterior of the heart (Figure 14-1). The first echocardiographic diagnosis of a cardiac tumor was made in 1968, and this tumor was later successfully excised.[23] Cardiac MRI is now used frequently, as it can provide non-invasive, high-resolution images of the heart, which is useful in differentiating tumor from thrombus as well as evaluating the degree of myocardial involvement. Operations for myxoma are now routinely performed in multiple centers with minimal morbidity and mortality.[24,25]

Primary malignant tumors of the heart remain a surgical challenge owing to the technical difficulties of major cardiac resections and the aggressive biological nature of these tumors, but new methods with minimal morbidity and mortality are developing.[25–27] Despite these difficulties, survival has been shown to improve with surgical resection and neoadjuvant chemotherapy,[28–30] and novel approaches allowing a more complete tumor resection, such as cardiac autotransplantation, have been introduced.[28,31] Cardiac

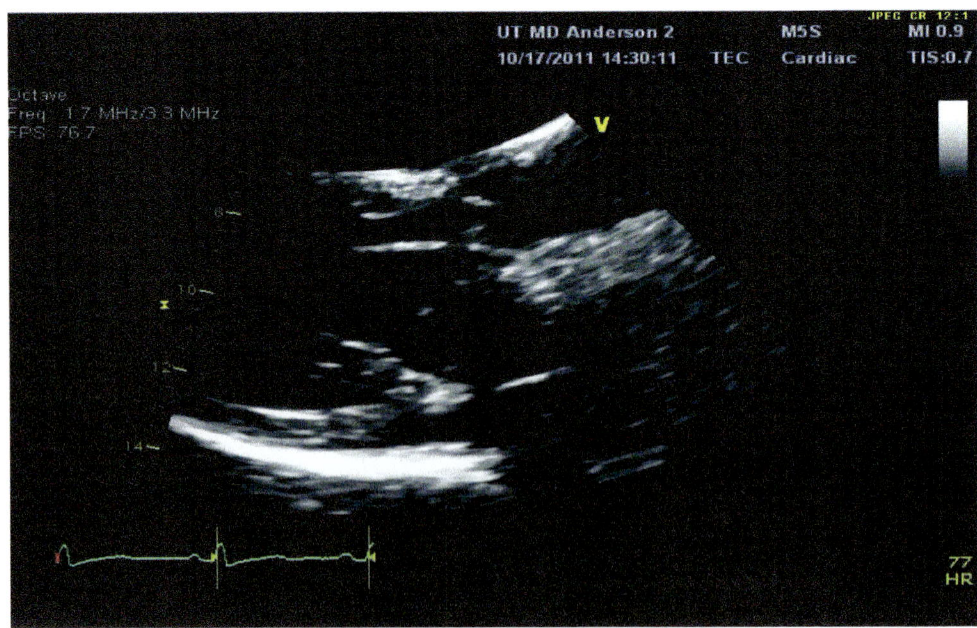

FIGURE 14-1   Transthoracic echocardiogram of a left atrial leiomyosarcoma.

autotransplantation was introduced by Reardon et al. in 1998 to manage the technical dificulties of large left atrial primary sarcomas. This involved complete cardiac explantation, ex vivo tumor resection, and cardiac reconstruction.[26] This approach combined with aggressive neoadjuvant systemic chemotherapy is the best chance at curative option or survival benefit for left sided malignant tumors except for lymphoma. Right sided primary malignant tumors also behave in a similar fashion with extensive resection involving up to 30% of the RV free wall and possible tricuspid valve replacement with biological valve.

CLINICAL PRESENTATION

Cardiac tumors cause signs and symptoms based on tumor location, size, adherent clot formation, and tissue type. These can be further classified into constitutional, cardiac, obstructive, and thromboembolic events.[32] Predominant constitutional symptoms include fever, fatigue, malaise, and weight loss.[33] These are especially evident in cardiac myxomas and may be associated with an increase in cytokine release, such as IL 6, that has been noted with these tumors.[34] One of the most common symptoms in adults includes dyspnea while the most frequent symptom in children was hypoxia.[24] Dyspnea can be related to position if the tumor is in some way obstructing the atrio-ventricular valves, and can worsen when the patient is lying flat.[35] However, dyspnea can be a result of other cardiac manifestations such as congestive heart failure (CHF) and thromboembolic disease. Chest pain may occur and is more common with malignant and pericardial tumors. Angiosarcomas are known to invade the coronary arterial system and cause myocardial infarction, and can also lead to coronary steal.[36] Constitutional symptoms are diffuse and have also included more rare symptoms such as night sweats, polymyositis, hepatic dysfunction, and Raynaud's phenomenon.[34,37]

Arrhythmias are also associated with cardiac tumors. Diverse ECG abnormalities have been noted including sinus tachycardia, supraventricular tachycardia, atrial fibrillation or flutter,[38] or ST segment changes.[37,39] Heart block from infiltration of the AV node and sick sinus syndrome has been reported.[40] Mesotheliomas can replace the AV node causing AV block or sudden cardiac death.[41,42] Ventricular tachycardia[43] has also been seen with one report even detailing the rapid onset of death following such an arrhythmia as the tumor infiltrated the conduction system.[44]

Obstructive symptoms occur from mechanical obstruction of the tumor on the structures of the heart such as valves, pulmonary veins, etc. These include hypotension, syncope, dyspnea,[45–47] and edema.

Other symptoms may include hemoptysis or cough.[37] Obscure presentations can include epistaxis[48] or positional cyanosis.[49] The positional cyanosis was seen in a pedunculated tumor that protruded through the tricuspid valve, causing intermittent obstruction with diversion of blood through a patent foramen ovale. This significant shunting of blood from right to left resulted in cyanosis. Portal vein thrombosis and subsequent Budd–Chiari syndrome secondary to a right atrial tumor have also been reported.[50] The mass effect of an intracavitary tumor can obstruct the transfer of blood through the cardiac chambers or can interfere with normal coaptation of cardiac valvular structures. Congestive heart failure can occur, especially if the tumor invades the myocardium and impairs ventricular contraction or if it obstructs the valve, essentially creating valvular stenosis which has been seen in both the mitral and tricuspid positions.[34,35]

Embolic symptoms are a common phenomena associated with cardiac malignancy.[34] Reports include systemic embolization of tumor fragments causing stroke. Peripheral arterial occlusion for left-sided tumors and pulmonary hypertension for right-sided tumors are frequently seen. Angina and myocardial infarction can also occur from tumor embolus. Systemic emboli from left-sided heart lesions are much more frequently seen than pulmonary tumor emboli from right-sided heart lesions, possibly because these are easier to diagnose. No current recommendations have been proposed for anticoagulation with cardiac tumors. Anticoagulation needs to be tailored to the patient's clinical presentation and degree of thrombus on the tumor with mobility of the tumor raising concern for thromboembolic potential. Another difficult problem clinicians face with embolic presentation of the tumor includes the further timing of resection and bypass immediately following the stroke. Intervention too soon can result in hemorrhage into the brain while intervention later may allow more emboli to shower, patient condition to worsen, and the resection to become more complex.

Cardiac tamponade, hemopericardium, and pericardial rub are an early and frequent manifestation of the disease but cause symptoms only 10% of the time in affected patients with cytology frequently not showing malignant cells.[51] Malignancies which are commonly associated with metastasis to the heart include leukemia, lung, breast, sarcoma, and melanoma, although many other cancers can result in cardiac metastasis.

Pinede et al. described that up to one-third of their patients with left atrial myxoma had non-specific laboratory abnormalities including anemia and elevated ESR, serum C-reactive protein, or globulin level. Anemia was usually normochromic or hypochromic. Hemolytic anemia does occur with mechanical destruction of erythrocytes by the tumor.[34] The tumor itself may be causing a systemic inflammatory and immune response. High levels of IL-6 were found in patients with left atrial myxomas before resection, which returned to normal after resection.[52]

Children have distinctively different presentations than adults who present with cardiac tumors with wide and varied symptoms. However, dyspnea, seizure, cardiac murmur, and cyanosis were prominent in a small series of patients evaluated by Wang and colleagues.[53] The most common cardiac tumor in children is rhabdomyoma.[3] Stiller and colleagues and Bertolini and colleagues both reviewed their institution's experience, finding over 41 pediatric tumors in all. Based on their retrospective reviews, they advocated intervening surgically for benign cardiac tumors only when obstructive or life-threatening symptoms arose.[54,55] Complete resection was not the mainstay of treatment, but instead myocardial function and anatomic preservation for future survival was key. Since many of the benign tumors regressed, relief from hemodynamic compromise was the goal of resection. Fetal diagnosis has also been made, allowing the physician to develop a plan of care prenatally.[55] Most of these patients have families with tuberous sclerosis[56–58] who were in screening programs.

■ Diagnosis

Because the signs and symptoms are nonspecific, diagnosis of cardiac tumors requires a high degree of clinical suspicion and some form of imaging technique. The diagnosis may be presumed by chest radiography reflecting the changes seen within the cardiac chambers as a tumor occupies more and more space. Specifically, these changes may be cardiomegaly, pleural effusion, pulmonary nodules, or an altered right atrial silhouette.[37] Occasionally, tumor calcification may be identified,[59] occurring most commonly in right atrial tumors. Similarly, the electrocardiogram may reflect electrical changes within the heart from a tumor. Arrhythmias are common as the tumor enlarges, but specific electrical abnormalities are not reliably diagnostic on their own.

As mentioned in the surgical history, echocardiography is the most important diagnostic modality used today for cardiac tumors. This technology has not only become so advanced as to reveal the mass, it can also often help determine the implantation site and discriminate between vegetation, thrombi, and tumor (Figure 14-2).[60] Echocardiography is both noninvasive and readily available and can be repeated in the operating room at the time of surgery. Any echocardiogram with evidence of a right atrial mass, not consistent with

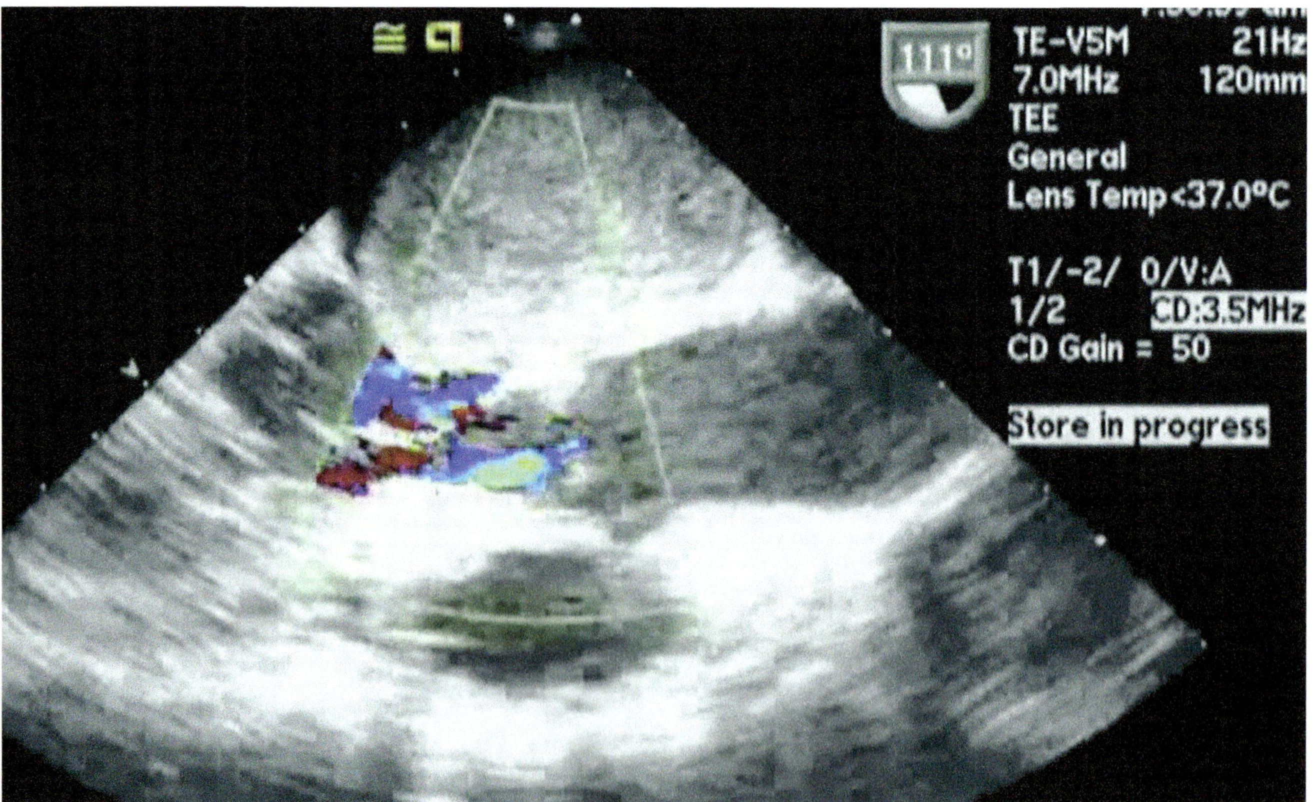

FIGURE 14-2 Echocardiogram of a left atrial myxoma.

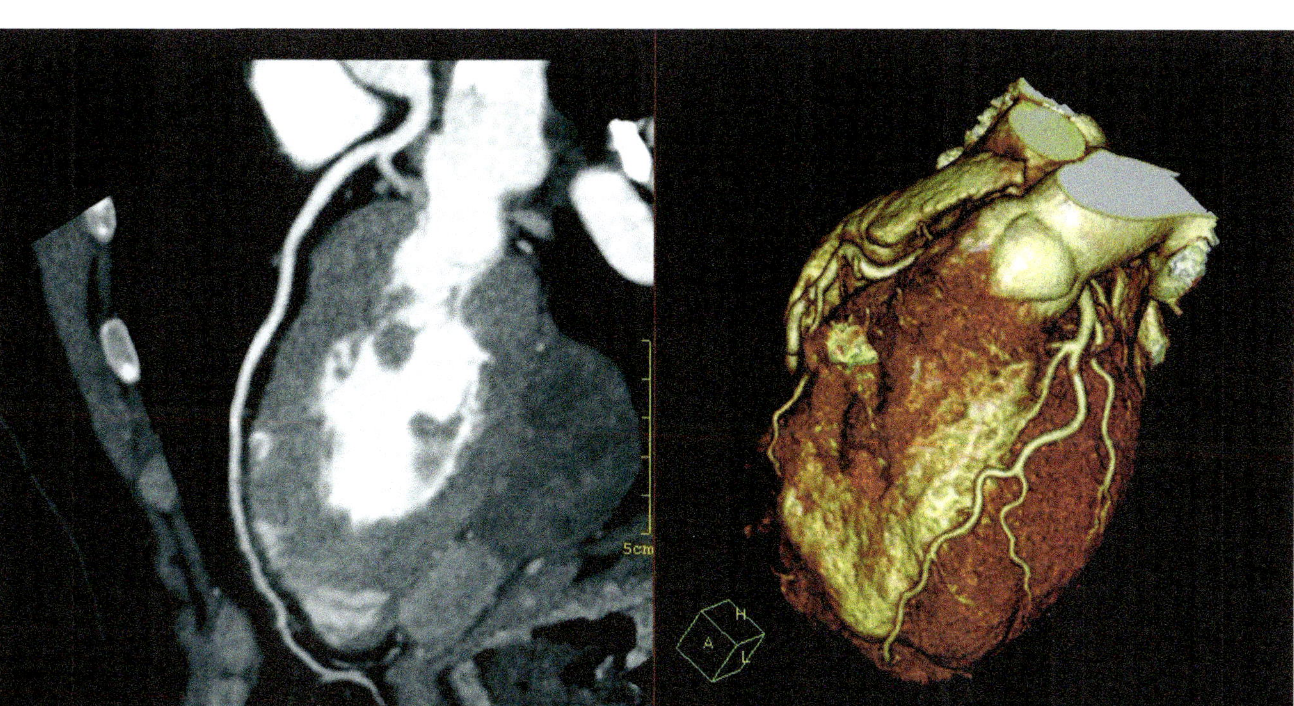

FIGURE 14-3   Image of right ventricular tumor with cardiac computed tomographic scan.

thrombus material, in association with a pericardial effusion, should be highly suspicious of a primary cardiac malignancy and warrant further investigation.

Although echocardiography is the most common evaluation for cardiac tumors, magnetic resonance imaging (MRI) and computed tomography (CT) can give a more complete view of mediastinal, lung parenchymal, and pleural structures and are complementary imaging modalities. All cardiac tumors should likely be imaged with cardiac MRI as can easily help differentiate between tumor and thrombus, myxoma versus malignant and becomes essential when planning a surgical resection for complicated tumors to assess myocardial invasion. Solid, fatty, or liquid tumors are easily identified by either CT or MRI.[61] MRI is superior to echocardiography in delineating the intra- and extracardiac extension of cardiac tumors and, unlike CT, does not require iodinated contrast if concomitant renal dysfunction. Magnetic resonance angiography can also aid in determining invasion and differentiating tumor from adjacent vascular structures (Figures 14-3 and 14-4).[62] Cine MRI mode is used to visualize heart motion, blood flow, and intracavitary signal intensities.

Multimodality imaging of cardiac tumors with echo, MRI, and/or CT will likely become accepted as a standard of care as each modality offers different but additional information to tumor diagnosis and follow up. Currently, transthoracic echocardiography remains the screening modality of choice. However, cardiac MR

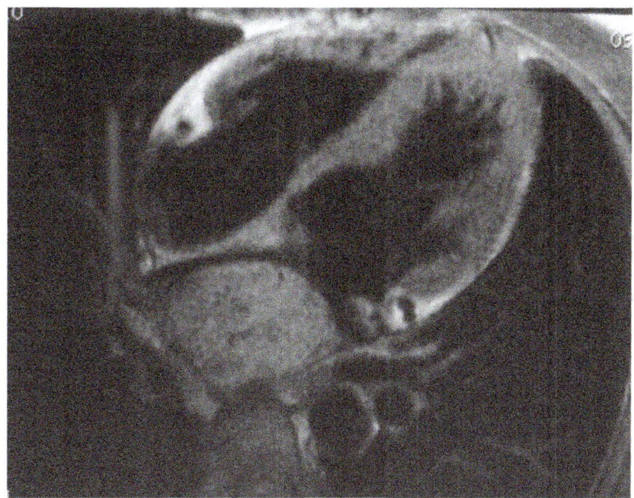

FIGURE 14-4   Magnetic resonance image of a large left atrial paraganglioma.

and CT both are essential in the staging and identification of cardiac masses. Cardiac magnetic resonance imaging offers more detailed information than echo on tumor extent, hemorrhage and necrosis, vascularity, and invasion of adjacent structures. By showing perfusion, it may assist the practitioner by helping differentiate between tumor and thrombus, which are often very difficult by echo but can be accomplished by gadolinium enhancement with CMR. Gadolinium enhancement occurs when one tissue has a higher affinity or vascularity as compared to another. Thrombus remains dark with gadolinium but cardiac tumors tend to enhance.[63,64] Tl, T2, and proton density images of CMR can be used for tissue characterization to differentiate between benign and malignant lesions, although this can be quite difficult and pathology should be the final determinant.[64] All cardiac tumors should likely have a baseline cardiac MRI. Cardiac CT can also be complimentary by showing a noninvasive means of visualizing coronary involvement by the tumor prior to surgery, as well as pericardial involvement.

Cardiac catheterization and angiography are often very helpful in determining the diagnosis. However, catheter manipulation and contrast injection can also cause dislodgment of tumor fragments. Because of this, trans-septal puncture of the left atrium should be approached with care. Angiography may be especially helpful in determining the difference between a coronary aneurysm and tumor[65] or determining the involvement of coronary arterial branches, which may directly supply the tumor, especially angiosarcomas (Figure 14-5). This tumor may be identified as a filling defect when dye is injected into the cardiac chamber.[37] Endomyocardial biopsy has also been performed, with a 50% false-negative rate.[37] Right atrial biopsy has been done safely and, if possible, should be recommended with transesophageal echocardiographic guidance. The risk of thromboembolism from catheter manipulation can be assessed by cardiac MRI prior to procedure. If significant thrombus is present on the surface of the tumor, would likely shy away from a right sided catheter biopsy and attempt open excision. There is no evidence that biopsy of a cardiac tumor causes seeding of the tumor. If anything, it will allow for a more rapid diagnosis than open excisional biopsy. However, tumor diagnosis, if possible is essential as outcomes are improved with neoadjuvant chemotherapy prior to surgery.[66]

Pericardiocentesis has been described as an adjunctive tool to diagnose malignant cells within the pericardial space or as a palliative tool to temporize patients who present with pericardial tamponade from rapid tumor growth.[67,68] Pericardial windows can be created to relieve constant effusions in patients who are not deemed operable. Pericardiocentesis may not be diagnostic and has been shown to have a negative cytology from effusions from malignant primary tumors.[69]

A final diagnostic tool is aspiration or surgical removal of contents from peripheral emboli that have showered from the primary tumor. These emboli can help lead to the tissue of origin and help the physician plan the order of treatment. If metastatic disease is present, we recommend biopsy of distal metastases prior to cardiac biopsy if hemodynamically stable from the cardiac mass. Resection of the cardiac mass is complex, and often the last place to secure a diagnosis when other sites can be reached.

As imaging of the chest and heart increases with all modalities, more cardiac masses will likely be incidentally diagnosed. The future of imaging cardiac tumors will become more challenged as to diagnosis and evaluating tumors from new perspectives. An exciting arena will be the advance of molecular imaging of cardiac tumors for correct diagnosis and to determine negative margins and early metastasis to distant organs. After surgery, distant metastasis is a major contributor to the prognosis of the patient with clean margins associated with a longer disease-free period with majority of the patients dying from metastatic disease rather than primary tumor. Current modalities are effective at gross imaging, but it will become important to view these tumors at a molecular level at the time of diagnosis and surveillance.

SURGICAL TREATMENT

The surgical approach to the patient with a primary malignant or complex benign cardiac tumor can be quite complicated. Surgical excision remains the best treatment when possible. Although advances in surgical technique have allowed an increasing number of these tumors to be resected, the average cardiac surgeon will encounter a cardiac tumor only in 1 of every 500 cases, and most of these will be simple primary myxomas. Anatomic evaluation in the preoperative setting is crucial to planning the operation. Even with the imaging detail available today, attachment and invasion may not be appreciated until the interior chambers of the heart are examined. The following is a general description of several operative techniques used when excising cardiac tumors. This approach can

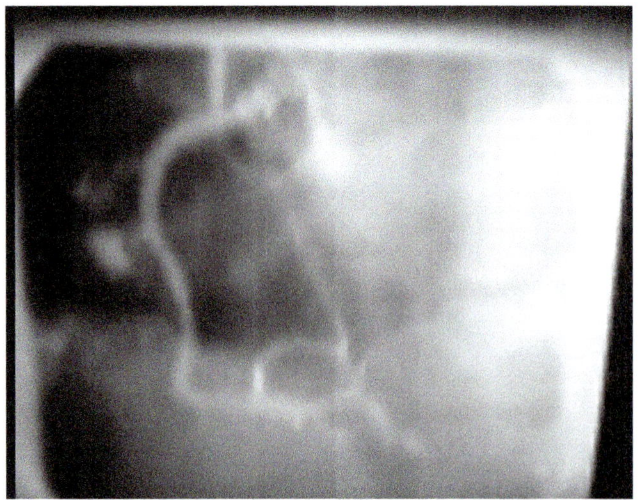

FIGURE 14-5 Right heart catheterization with tumor blush.

be divided by anatomy, including left- versus right-sided tumors, atrial versus ventricular tumors, right ventricular outflow tract tumors, atrial extension of infradiaphragmatic tumors, and special considerations regarding the histologic type of tumor. Minimally invasive strategies are also discussed in this section.

ANATOMIC APPROACHES

Since the location of the tumor is a main pathophysiologic factor, each approach is divided into anatomic sections. The second most important physiologic factor is size and extent of invasion into the myocardium, and for those tumors that are too large to resect through conventional approaches, alternatives are discussed, including radical resections of tumors and reconstruction. As for all of the following approaches in which a sternotomy is performed, the patient is prepared and draped in a sterile fashion for all cardiac tumors from the neck to the legs, making the groins easily accessible and the saphenous vein available in the event it is needed. The traditional median sternotomy is used unless otherwise described, and median pericardiotomy, potentially opening both pleural spaces and systemically heparinizing, is employed. When excising intracardiac tumors, CPB has two main uses: it allows visualization of the interior chambers of the heart while maintaining systemic blood flow, and it may also prevent embolization of tumor fragments into the lungs as the tumor is manipulated. The aortic cross-clamp prevents systemic embolization during dissection as well.[6]

RIGHT ATRIAL TUMOR RESECTION

All right sided tumors, other than those that are clearly simple benign tumors, require a tissue diagnosis prior to resection if possible. This is to eliminate those tumors that do not need surgery, like lymphoma, and to allow neoadjuvant therapy to shrink the tumor if sarcoma.

Right atrial tumors require bicaval cannulation. The most common primary malignant tumor reported in the right atrium is angiosarcoma. Intraoperative transesophageal echocardiography (TEE) is especially important during placement of cannulas to ensure that tumor thrombi are not dislodged.

Right atrial tumors are approached using a standard full sternotomy. Either vena cava may be cannulated directly, or right atrial appendage with guidance into the superior vena cava may be employed (Figure 14-6). Cannulation of the right atrial appendage rarely works for right atrial masses, and the most common technique used is direct superior vena caval cannulation. When atrial or caval cannulation is not possible without causing tumor dislodgment, jugular,

innominate, or femoral cannulation is another option. It is more typical to have difficulty with low-lying tumors that preclude inferior vena caval cannulation, and in this instance, femoral vein cannulation provides adequate venous drainage of the lower half of the body.

After the patient has been placed on CPB, the aorta is cross-clamped and the patient is given 10 cc/kg of antegrade cold blood cardioplegia. Prior to atriotomy, the cavae should be snared to minimize the amount of blood in the field. The right atrium may be opened from the superior vena cava to the inferior vena cava, but, again, it is important not to incise the tumor during atriotomy. The temperature is allowed to drift down, but systemic hypothermia is not a goal in these more easily resected tumors. Most right atrial sarcomas originate in the lateral right atrial wall. They tend to be extensive and infiltrative and may extend to involve the right coronary artery and tricuspid valve. Excision should include a rim of normal tissue and a full-thickness portion of the wall if possible. Prior to reconstruction, a tour of the available chambers of

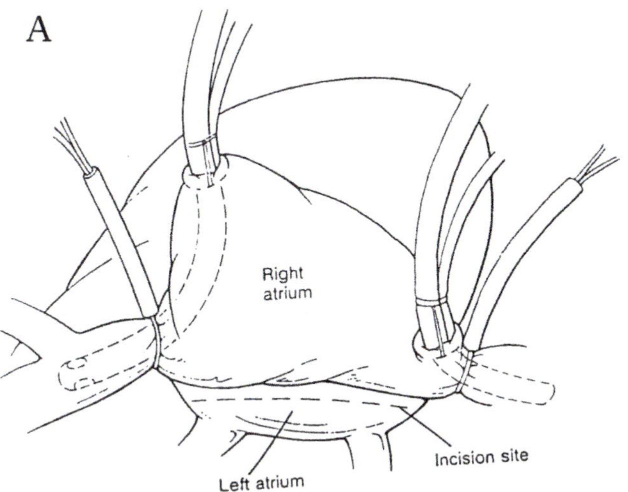

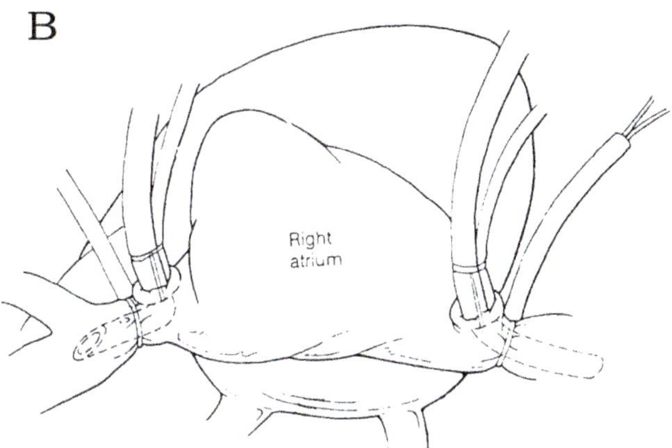

FIGURE 14-6 (A) Standard venous cannulation of the superior vena cava through the right atrial appendage and, (B) superior vena cava cannulation.

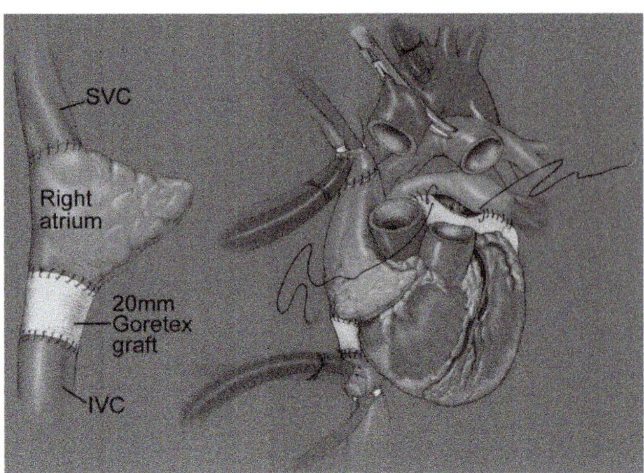

FIGURE 14-7 Reconstruction of the inferior vena cava after the tumor has been excised.

the heart can help identify any additional implants or fragments that may have been left behind.

Reconstruction options are depicted in Figure 14-7, which illustrates the reconstruction of the inferior vena cava after the tumor has been excised. The right atrium or septum may be reconstructed using pericardium or expanded polytetra-fluoroethylene. Prior to decannulation, TEE should be used again to look for any additional fragments or tumor implants. It becomes important to record in both the operative note and the TEE record any unusual anatomic features that may become suspect at later follow-up TEE. For example, if a pledgeted suture or rim of patch is visible on the postoperative TEE, notation at the time of surgery may prevent this abnormality from mistakenly being diagnosed as a recurrence. Benign right atrial tumors are approached in much the same way but tend to originate from the interatrial septum and be far less extensive.

Many complex right atrial tumors may also involve the tricuspid valve and extend into the ventricle (Figure 14-8). Right atrial tumors may also originate from an infradiaphragmatic source. Please see infradiaphragmatic tumor section following this for discussion.

LEFT ATRIAL TUMOR RESECTION

The left atrium is the most common tumor site within the heart, with myxomas being the most common benign type and malignant fibrous histiocytoma being the most common malignant type. Delay in treatment is not recommended owing to the risk of embolization and obstruction being much higher with faster-growing tumors. For left atrial tumors that are clearly myxoma, a right thoracotomy approach or even robotic resection is reasonable. For large tumors or those with a likelihood of malignancy then sternotomy is best. Care is taken not to cause dislodgment

of tumor fragments while placing the patient on CPB and dissecting around the heart. Pericardial stay sutures are placed low in the pericardium on the right to rotate the heart to the left and increase exposure of the left atrium (Figure 14-9). Extensive mobilization of the superior vena cava will also improve left atrial exposure. The inferior vena caval–right atrial junction is also dissected to free the inferior vena cava.

The interatrial groove[70] is dissected, and the left atrium is entered on its most rightward anterior surface, leaving a 5 to 10 mm rim of tissue for closure. The incision line should be just anterior to the right-sided pulmonary veins (Figure 14-10) and should be carried onto the lateral left atrium posterior to the superior and inferior venae cavae. The surgeon must carefully incise the wall of the left atrium, making sure not to incise the tumor lying underneath. If the tumor is noted to be extending from the septum, it is important to excise a rim of normal tissue around the insertion of the tumor to decrease the likelihood of recurrence. Occasionally, it may be necessary to incise both atria to completely visualize the septum and facilitate closure. The septum may be over sewn or recreated with a Dacron or pericardial patch (Figure 14-11). As usual, a vent is used to evacuate the air from the cardiac chambers, and decannulation and closing the chest are routine. Inspection of all chambers of the heart for additional tumor fragments prior to closure of the suture lines is performed.

LEFT VENTRICULAR TUMOR RESECTION

Left ventricular tumors can be approached via three main techniques. Our preferred approach is through the atrioventricular valve, but transaortic valvular and ventricular incisions have also been described.[71] There are some reports of no recurrence after partial wall excision of benign ventricular tumors, but because malignant tumors have a much higher propensity to recur and the exact pathology of the tumor is often not known at the time of resection, complete excision, when feasible, is recommended. Accessing the ventricle, then, becomes even more important as the surgeon attempts to access as much of the ventricle as possible. This atrioventricular valvular approach may make accessing the tumor through the valve possible without disruption of any additional anatomic structures. Again, one must inspect the entire ventricle for additional tumor fragments. Cardiotomy suction should be limited during tumor manipulation because distant implants have been reported in the literature.[61,72] Occasionally, ventricular tumors may be aggressive enough to invade valvular structures and require valve repair, as well as complete excision and replacement. Ventricular tumors may also require large resections of the entire thickness of the ventricular wall, and these can be closed with a

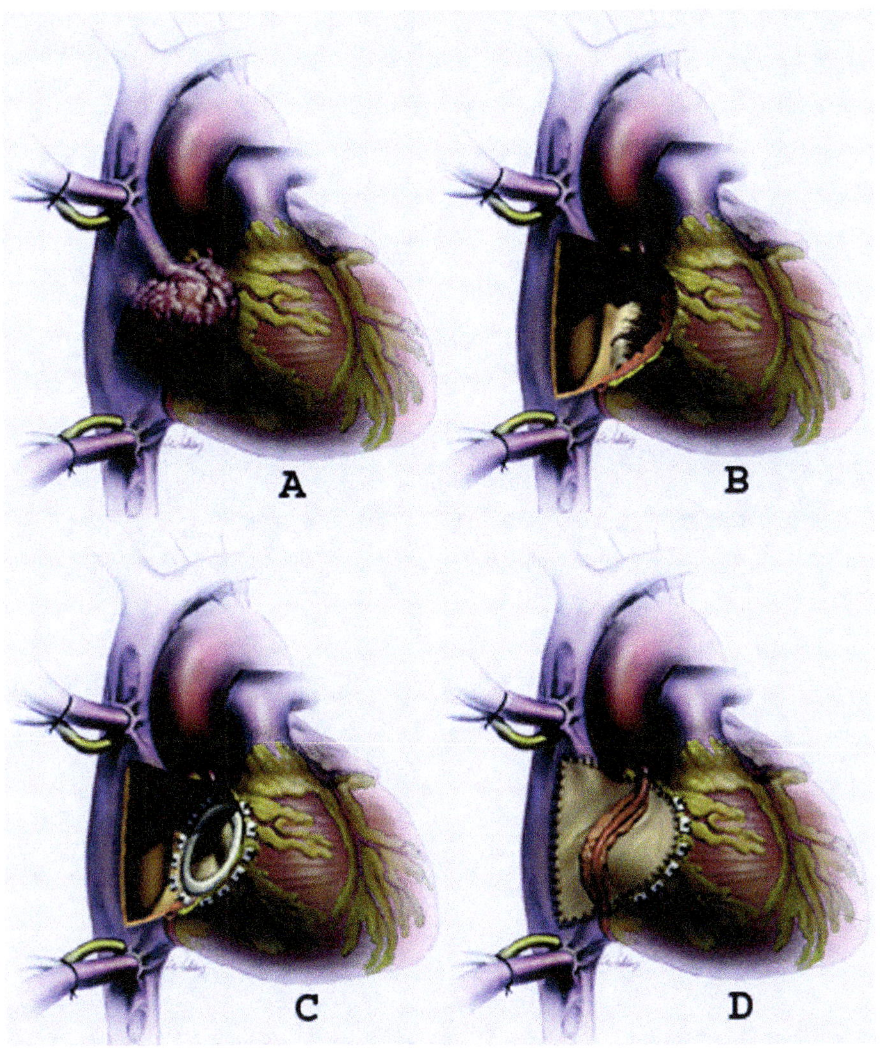

FIGURE 14-8   Right atrial angiosarcoma involving the right coronary artery and tricuspid valve with reconstruction.

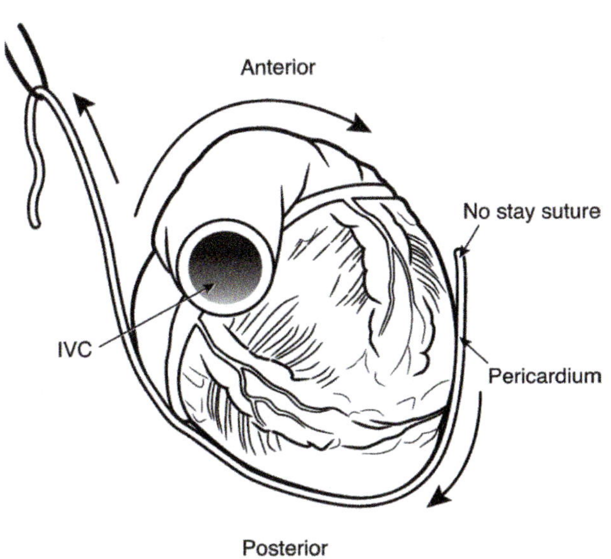

FIGURE 14-9   Rotation of the heart with pericardial stay sutures.

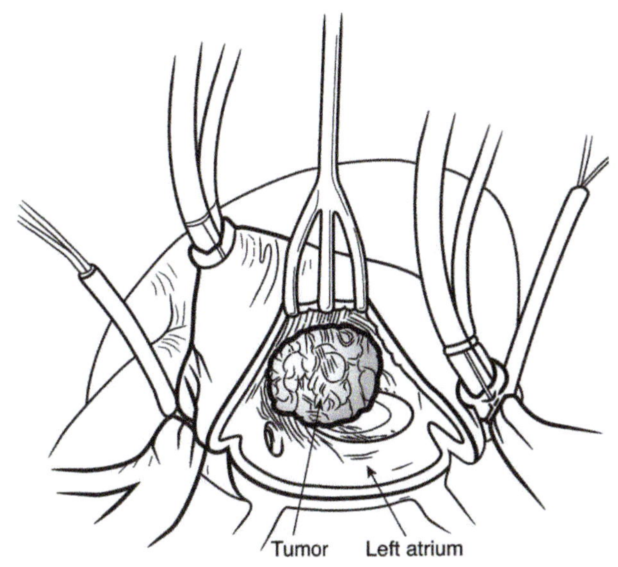

FIGURE 14-10   Left atriotomy incision opened with subsequent exposure of tumor.

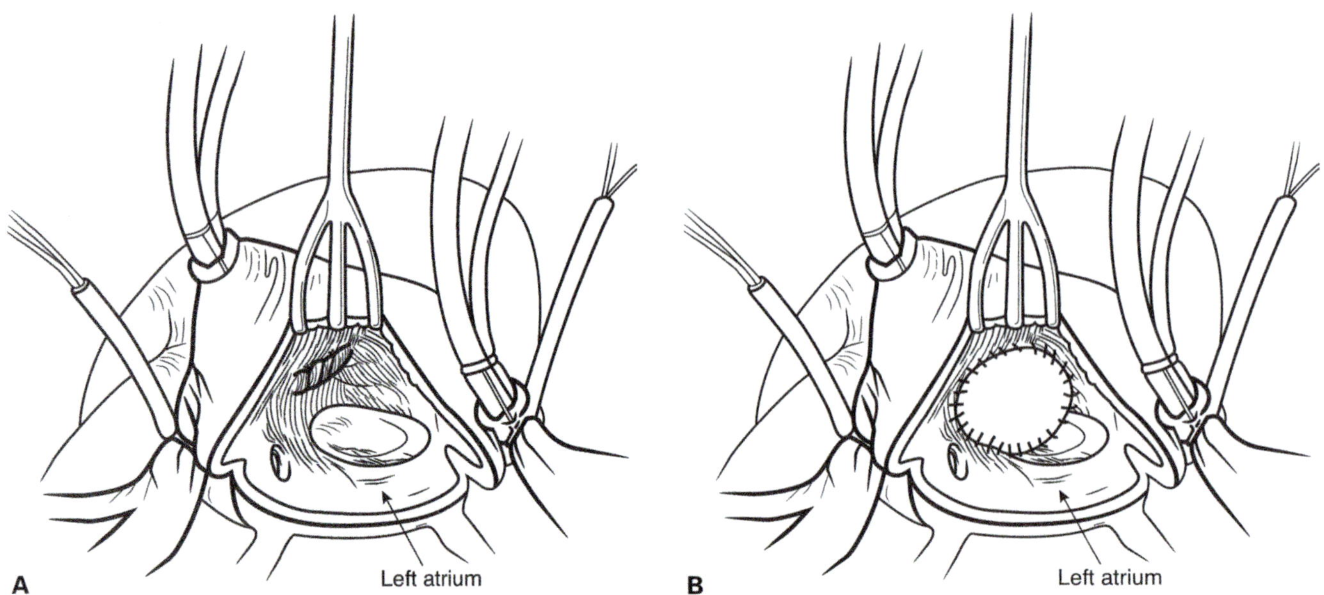

FIGURE 14-11   (A) Oversewn septal resection; (B) patch closure of septum.

large patch and reinforcement, such as the Dor technique. Others are too large for such reconstruction, and the patch may be left exposed (Figure 14-12).

The left atrial approach to ventricular tumors can include an annular incision on the anterior leaflet of the mitral valve. This allows the chordal structures to be displaced downward and out of the way for visualization. Right ventricular tumors may be approached in the same manner through the tricuspid valve, or by direct ventriculotomy. For unresectable ventricular tumors, total artificial heart implantation has been used.[73]

CARDIAC AUTOTRANSPLANTATION

Some left-sided atrial tumors may be so large that they may not be excised via the conventional method, and newer, more innovative techniques have been employed for such situations (Figure 14-13).[6,28,29,31] Sarcomas can arise from the anterior surface of the left atrium, and a complete resection with adequate reconstruction necessitates better exposure than traditional methods can afford (Figure 14-14). Derivations of myxomas include giant left atrial myxomas, which can involve the orifices of the pulmonary veins.[26] The cardiac autotransplantation technique involves complete cardiac excision, ex vivo tumor removal with cardiac reconstruction, and cardiac reimplantation. Our institution has reported 35 cases in the literature, most being performed for complex left-sided primary cardiac tumors.[74]

The first half of cardiac surgery is much like that of a simple left atrial tumor. The pulmonary artery catheter is placed high in the superior vena cava, where it will not interfere with the autotransplantation. The TEE probe is placed prior to draping and is most helpful when weaning the patient from CPB, watching for wall motion abnormalities, assessing the heart's response to volume loading, and ensuring that all of the air has been removed. Several modifications to the standard resection for orthotopic cardiac transplantation have been employed because the resected heart will later be reimplanted, often after some type of reconstruction to one or more chambers has been made. The traditional median sternotomy, as stated in the beginning of the chapter, is employed. The distal segments of the ascending aorta and superior and inferior venae cavae are all cannulated for CPB. Two concentric purse-string Tevdec sutures are used to secure the aortic cannula. A 4-0 purse-string suture is used to secure both caval cannulas, with pledgets used only for the inferior vena cava cannulation site. An alternative to inferior vena cava cannulation is femoral vein cannulation, which has been successfully performed in 3 of the 12 cases reported by Reardon.[68] The inferior vena cava is mobilized from its attachment to the diaphragm. A posterolateral right atrial cannulation for the inferior vena cava cannula may be used, and the superior vena cava is typically directly cannulated. We use small, 24F caval cannulae and active venous assist suction to concomitantly assist in exposure and venous drainage, respectively. Caval snares are used to prevent leakage of blood into the incised atrium. The superior vena cava is mobilized from its pericardial attachments and from the right pulmonary artery.

After institution of CPB, the aorta is separated from the pulmonary artery and cross-clamped close to the arterial cannula. Mobilization is the key to success in excision of the heart. Both the superior and inferior venae cavae are extensively mobilized. Antegrade

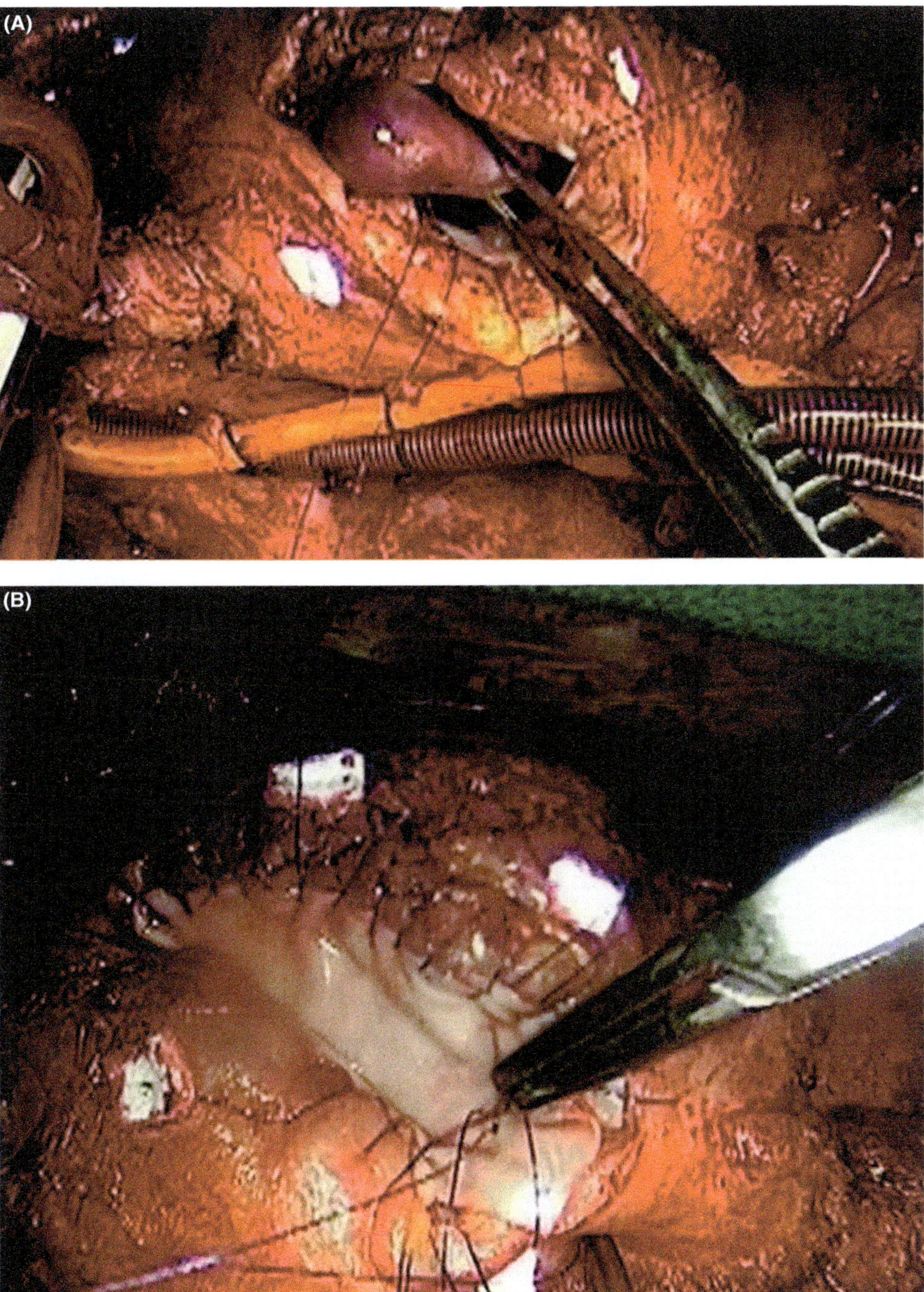

FIGURE 14-12 (A) Right ventricle with tumor excision; (B) right ventricle with patch closure.

cold blood cardioplegia is given at 10 cc/kg. The temperature is allowed to drift down, and time cooling is only employed when circulatory arrest is anticipated. Sondergaard's groove is mobilized. This should be relatively easy because the only true connection of the atria is at the fossa ovalis. The left atrium is incised anterior to the right pulmonary veins and extended along its superior most aspect. The incision may be extended in a medial direction parallel to the right pulmonary artery to provide additional exposure. The left

atrial tumor is inspected, and the decision is made to either use the standard approach for left atrial tumors or to proceed with cardiac autotransplantation.

If cardiac autotransplantation is planned, the superior and inferior venae cavae are transected, leaving enough of a cuff proximal to the cannula to sew to during reimplantation. It is important to stress that caval cannulation needs to be far enough away from the atrium to allow division and then enough tissue space for reconnection. We find that the inferior vena

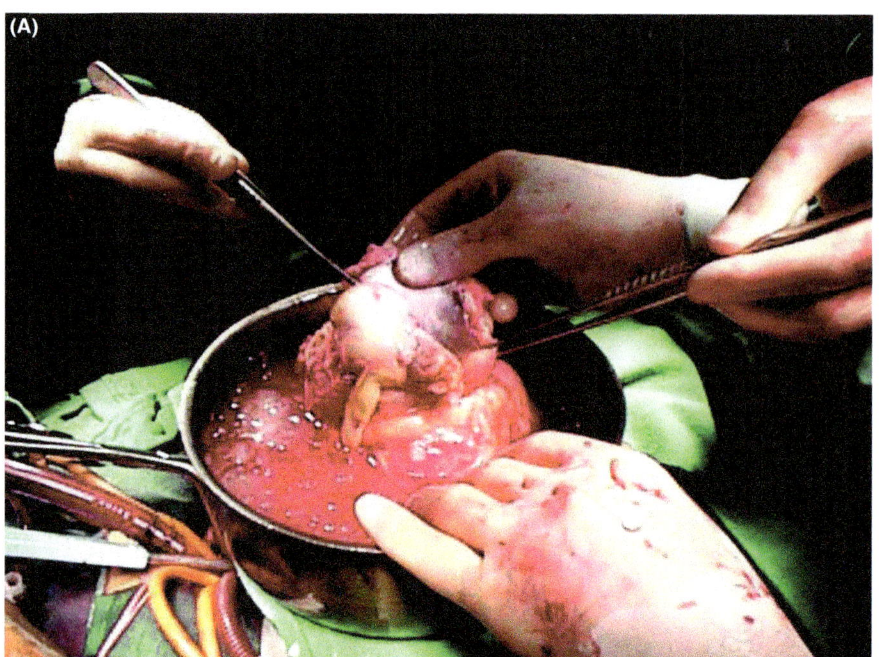

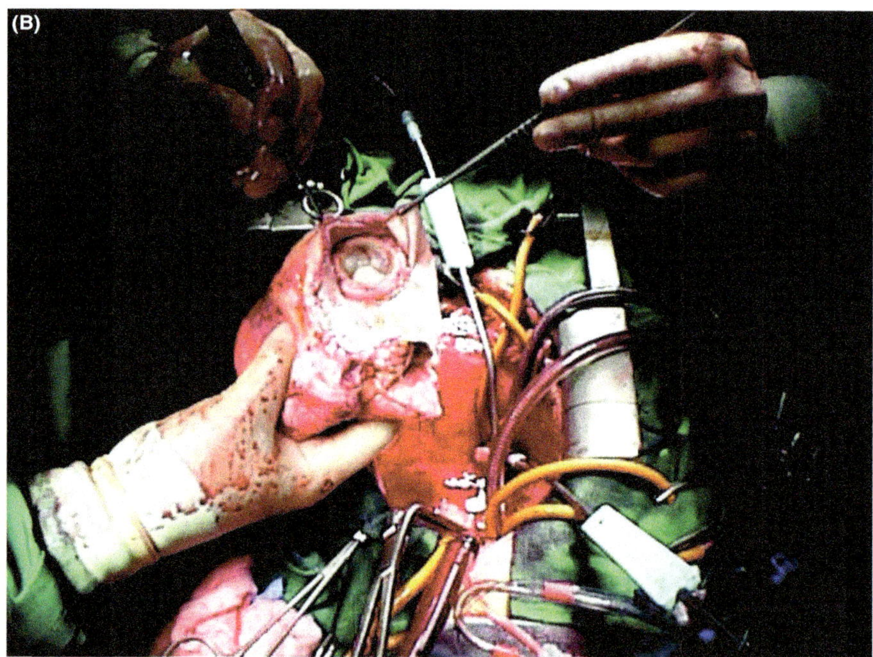

FIGURE 14-13 (A) Explanted heart as seen during autotransplantation; (B) reconstructed heart with MVR and pericardial replacement of anterior left atrial wall.

cava tends to shrink back the most after transection. The aorta is divided proximal to the clamp, 1 cm distal to the sinotubular junction. Prior to division of the pulmonary artery, a suture or pen mark can be made to secure alignment for reimplantation. Following this, the pulmonary artery is divided 3 mm proximal to the bifurcation. At this point, the only thing holding the heart in place is the left atrium. The left atrial incision should run parallel and posterior to the atrio-

ventricular groove anteriorly and continue parallel to the coronary sinus. Unlike the standard orthotopic heart transplantation technique, in which the incision transects the coronary sinus, the incision should be halfway between the mitral valve and the left pulmonary veins, taking care to avoid the coronary sinus, which runs along the posterior portion of the mitral valve (Figure 14-15). The incision is continued to the left side of the atrium, between the left atrial

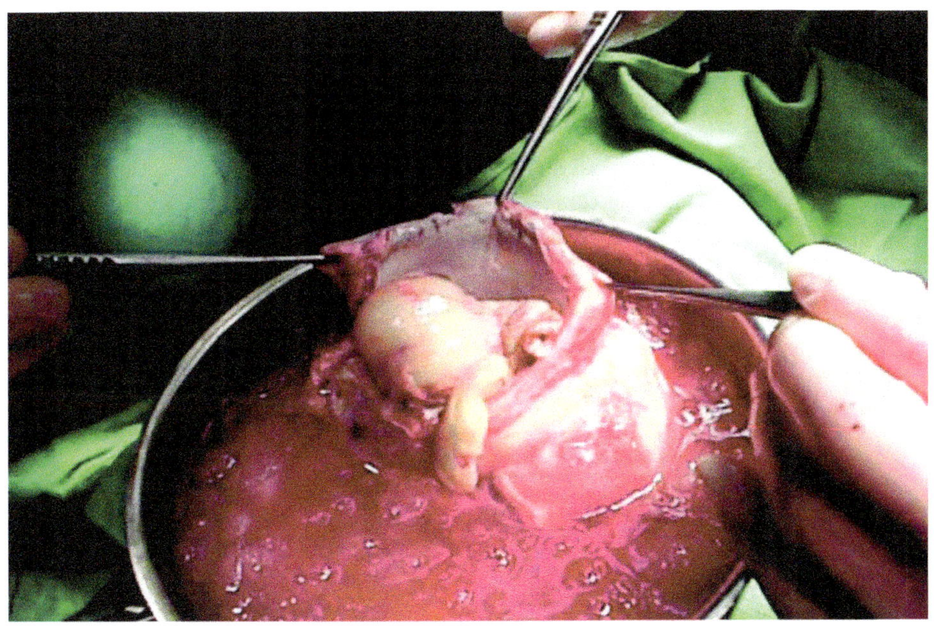

FIGURE 14-14 Ex vivo heart showing large sarcoma arising from the anterior left atrial wall.

appendage and the pulmonary vein (Figure 14-16). Creating an incision too close to the pulmonary vein may result in a very small cuff of pulmonary vein, limiting optimal reimplantation. These cardiectomy modifications must allow for planned reimplantation of the heart and a minimal amount of distortion as the ends are transected and sewn back together.

Once the heart is removed, a cuff of the left posterior aspect of the atrial wall and pulmonary veins should be left behind. Any mediastinal lymph nodes may be resected at this time for staging. The left atrial tumor is resected (Figure 14-17), and often a complex reconstruction is necessary (Figure 14-18). Some of these reconstructions may include such procedures

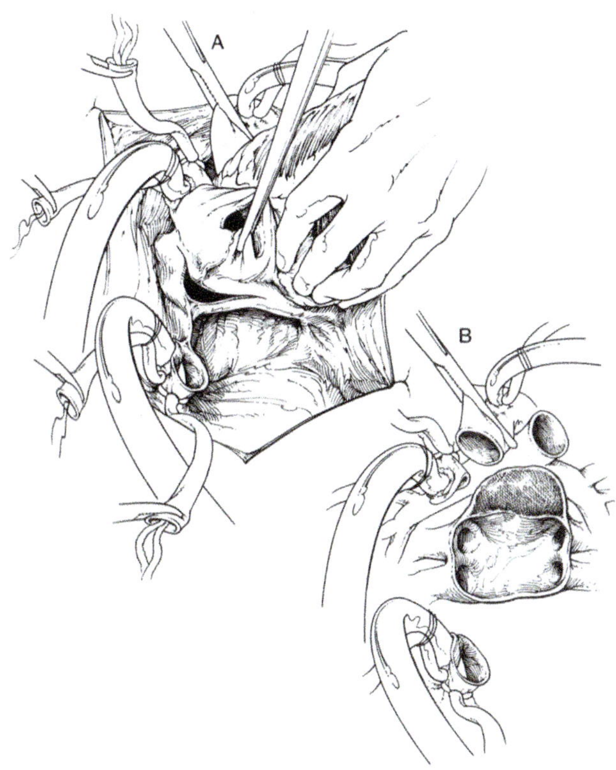

FIGURE 14-15 Left atrial incision for explantation of the heart.

FIGURE 14-16 Explantation of the heart for exposure of extensive left atrial sarcoma.

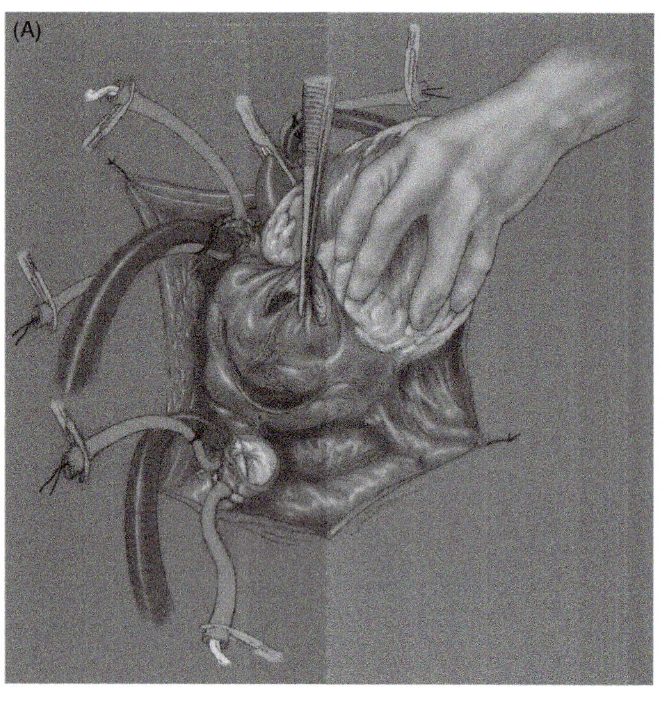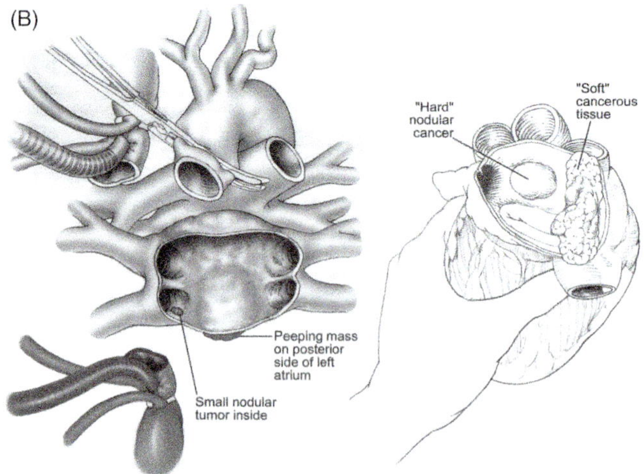

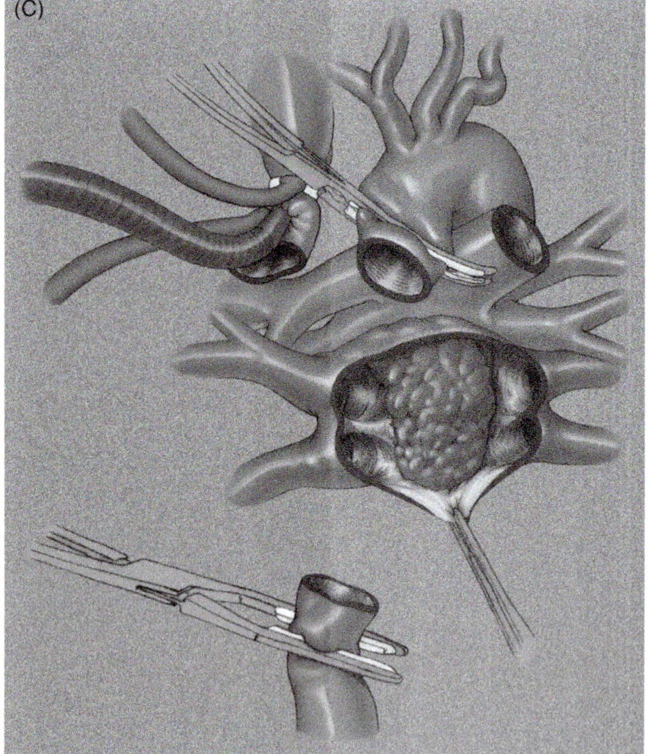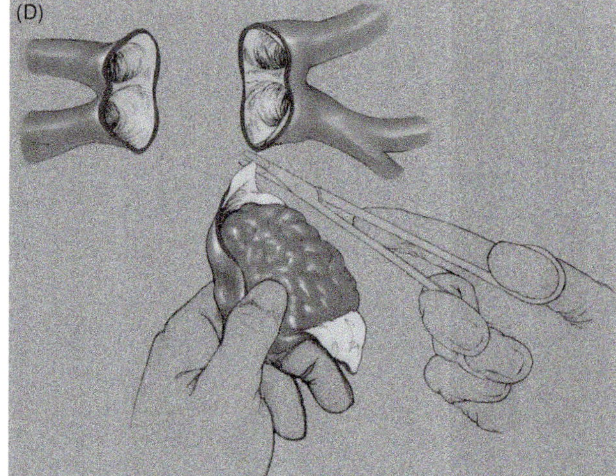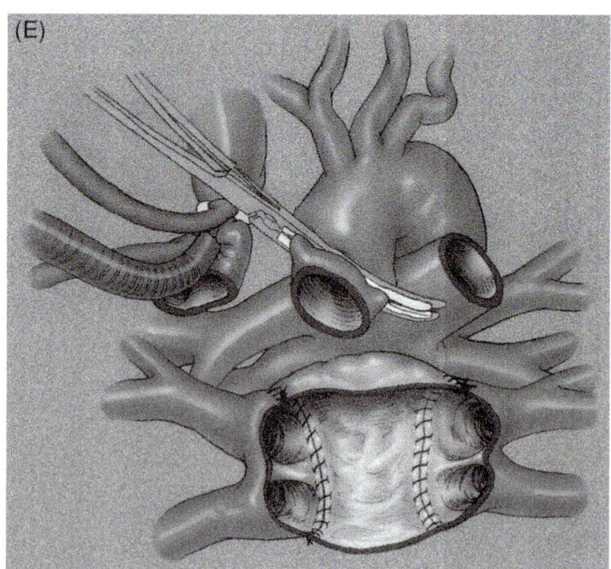

FIGURE 14-17 (A) Excision of heart during autotrans-plantation. (B) Explanted heart after excision revealing two different left atrial tumor implants. (C) Tumor resection from the back of the left atrium. (D) Excision of tumor from the left atrial wall between the pulmonary veins.(E) Repaired posterior aspect of the left atrium after tumor has been resected. *(continued)*

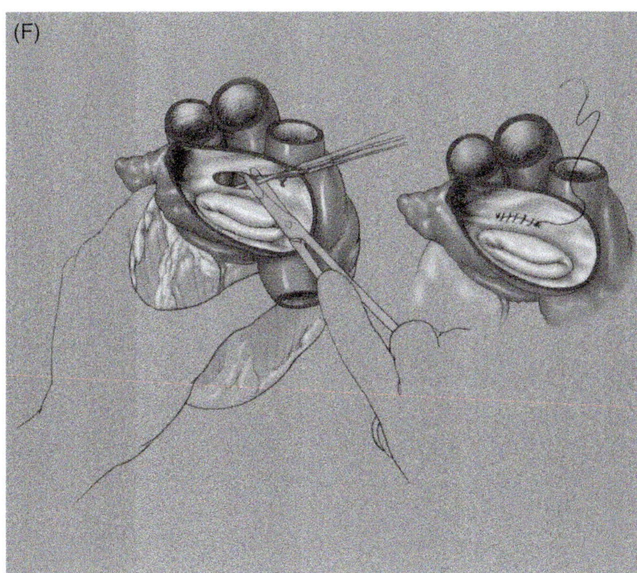

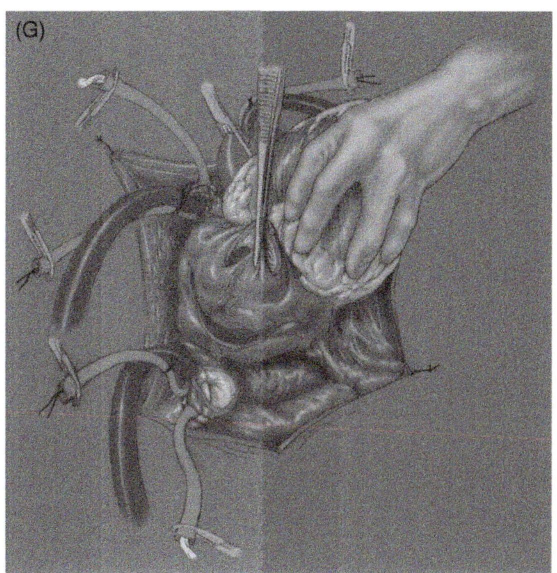

FIGURE 14-17   **(continued)** (F) Excision of tumor from anterior aspect of the left atrium and subsequent primary repair. (G) Reconstruction of the left atrium from explanted heart.

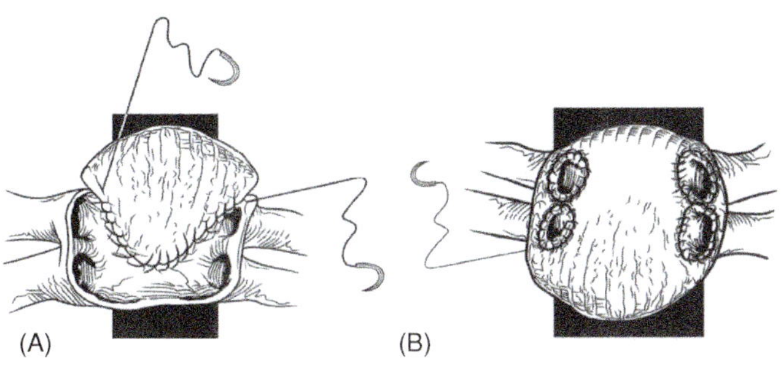

FIGURE 14-18   Reconstruction options for left atrium: (A) reconnecting intact sided pulmonary veins; (B) reconstruction for tumor involving the orifice of one or more of the pulmonary veins.

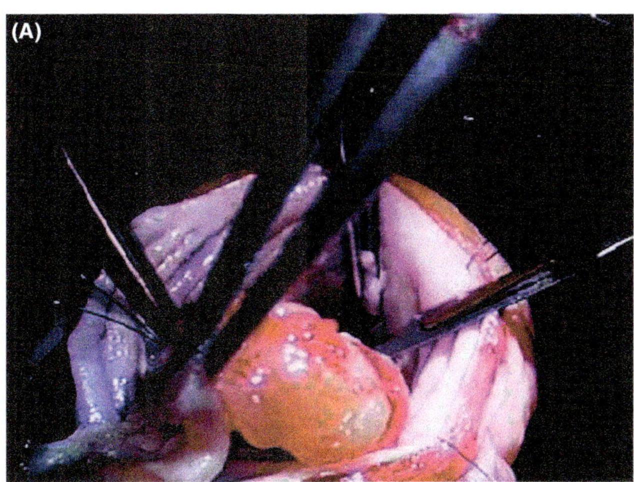

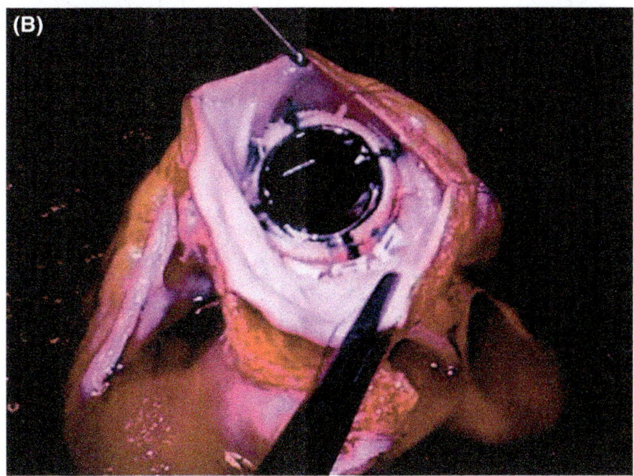

FIGURE 14-19   Left ventricular sarcoma: (A) exposure of the tumor; (B) reconstruction with mechanical valve replacement.

as mitral valve replacement or repair, ventricular septum reconstruction, inferior vena cava reconstruction, creation of a new left atrium, or concomitant pneumonectomy. Occasionally, it may become necessary to reconnect the pulmonary veins separately with tumors that involve one or more orifices. Caution is warranted as tumors approach the fibrous skeleton of the heart, especially those superior and inferior to the tricuspid valve near the aorta. Reconstruction of the left atrium is performed with pericardium, and the inferior vena cava may be reconstructed if necessary with Gore-Tex (W.L. Gore & Associates, Newark, DE) or a spiral saphenous vein graft. Most left atrial tumors can be more completely resected with the additional exposure afforded by explantation of the heart. Ventricular tumors may require excision of involved valvular structures that are also involved, complicating reconstruction (Figure 14-19). Tissue valves have the benefit of avoiding warfarin therapy, which may make management of patients receiving adjuvant chemotherapy difficult.

A the coronary arteries with either antegrade or retrograde cold blood cardioplegia can be employed to identify any injury to the explanted heart. It will be much easier to make any repairs at this time because the heart may be rotated at will. Valve replacement and most of the reconstruction may also be performed at this time. An incision may be made through the pulmonary veins to create an enlarged cuff for the anastomosis.

Once the heart has been reconstructed and repaired (Figure 14-20), the left atrial anastomosis is performed first with a 48 inch-long 4-0 polypropylene suture. Care must be taken not to narrow the venae cavae or the pulmonary veins. The most difficult repair so far has been the inferior vena cava, which can be difficult to reach, given the deep placement within the pericardium and the obstruction of view from the heart. A 48-inch double-armed 4-0 polypropylene suture is used for the running anastomosis of left atrial cuff edges. Care must be taken to align the venae cavae such that the

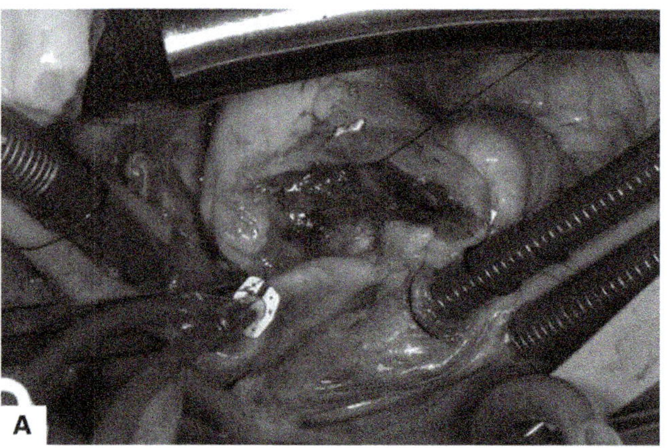

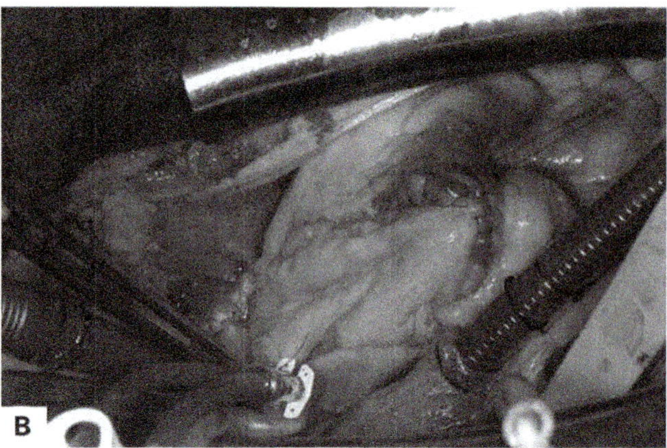

FIGURE 14-20 RVOT tumor (A) excised and (B) with reconstruction.

right atrium anastomosis is not under tension. The suture line is begun at the left atrial appendage and continued toward the right side of the patient. This allows the operator to sew toward herself.

A left ventricular vent is placed in the right superior pulmonary vein and positioned through the mitral valve into the left ventricle for de-airing. The right atrium is closed with a 5-0 RB needled polypropylene for each bicava anastomosis, with care being taken not to damage the sinoatrial node near the superior vena cava anastomosis. The pulmonary artery and aorta are reimplanted with running 4-0 polypropylene sutures. Remember that the pulmonary artery has been marked for realignment, and the suture line may be left untied for a period of time to allow air to escape from the right side of the heart as it fills with blood. The vent is temporarily occluded to distend the heart and fill the aorta during the completion of the suture line. De-airing maneuvers are employed with TEE, used to confirm the displacement of such air. If the patient has been cooled, he or she is rewarmed at this time. Temporary pacing wires are always used, and tube thoracostomy is employed for drainage of the pleural space if they are entered. A mediastinal chest tube is also placed, and a Dacron mesh is used to create a pericardial space and prevent cardiac herniation in the event of a right or left concomitant pneumonectomy.

It is common to have pump times exceeding 200 minutes with a cross-clamp time of more than 2 hours. Inotropic support is commonly used in these patients as they are being weaned from CPB. Two hundred milliliters of warm blood cardioplegia are given just prior to declamping. The umbilical tapes are removed from around the cavae.

Unique postoperative issues may relate mainly with bradycardia because the vagal innervation to the heart has been interrupted. Some critics of this technique argue for partial ex situ removal of cardiac neoplasms.[75] This technique involves transection of the inferior vena cava with a concomitant left atrial incision. This technique does not involve transection of the aorta, superior vena cava, or pulmonary artery. The procedure has been performed with the heart fibrillating and aorta cross-clamped for only 85 minutes by Kallenbach and Haverich.[75] This simpler method may be used in certain cases in which the tumor can be exposed in such a manner. Although orthotopic heart transplantation has been performed for primary malignant cardiac tumors,[76] it is both expensive and poorly available, and immunosuppression may adversely affect outcomes in patients who may later receive chemotherapy; therefore, we do not recommend it.

Right Ventricular Outflow Tract and Pulmonary Artery Tumor Resection

Tumors involving the right ventricular outflow tract have conventionally been determined to be unresectable until now. Our first case of a pulmonary valve homograft replacement of the right ventricular outflow tract was performed at the Methodist DeBakey Heart Center in 2004 (Figure 14-20). This included similar techniques of pulmonary artery root resection and implantation of homograft as described by Chambers and colleagues and Conklin and Reardon.[77,78] Particular hazards of resecting the pulmonary root include avoiding the left main coronary artery as it courses behind the pulmonary artery root, and especially the first septal perforator. The largest pulmonary artery homograft from the donor closest to that person's age should be chosen. This particular case was a resection of a pulmonary artery angiosarcoma that involved the main pulmonary artery trunk and pulmonic valve (Figure 14-21). A right pneumonectomy was performed, as well as pulmonary trunk and valve resection (Figure 14-22). If sections of the pulmonary artery have to be resected and reconstructed, pericardium, Gore-Tex or Dacron may be used as a patch or conduit.

Extension of Infradiaphragmatic Tumors

Right atrial tumors may also originate from an infradiaphragmatic source. The most frequent source of these tumors is renal cell carcinomas with caval extension of a tumor thrombosis. Although these do not typically involve the myocardium, they can occupy the right atrium (4%–10% of cases[13–15]) and, less frequently, the right ventricle and require CPB for their safe removal. If a complete resection can be performed, the 5-year survival rate can reach 64%.[79]

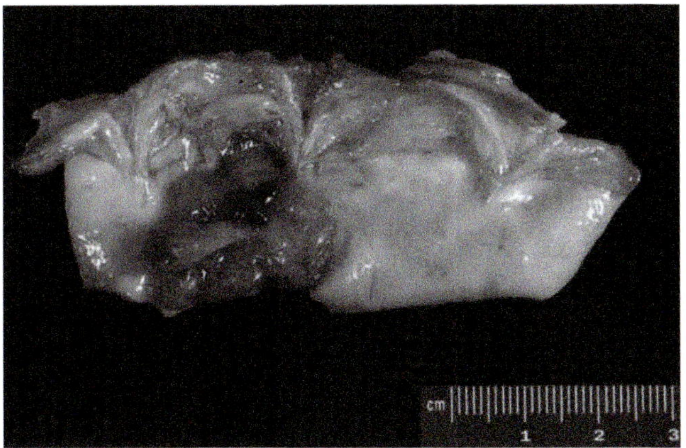

FIGURE 14-21 Pulmonary valve with involved tumor.

The preoperative evaluation involves a CT scan of the abdomen and chest with bone scintigraphy. The cephalic extent of the tumor can also be preoperatively defined by TEE or MRI. Those cases classified as level III (suprahepatic) or level IV (into the atrium) will undergo preoperative percutaneous renal artery embolization.[80] A period of 48 to 72 hours is usually taken prior to surgery to allow the tissue planes and edema to develop. Embolization can cause retraction of the tumor caudally and aid in the endarterectomy dissection, thus facilitating tumor removal.[80]

In the operating room, TEE is used throughout the procedure monitoring for tumor migration or embolization during mobilization of the kidney. The abdomen is first exposed to ensure that the tumor is resectable. In our experience, resection of the intracaval tumor is greatly facilitated by first mobilizing the kidney. If the tumor distends the cava significantly and is firmly seated within the cava, the renal vein can be transected and the kidney removed. If there is concern that division of the renal vein will allow propagation of the tumor, then the kidney is left in situ. The liver is completely mobilized, and the suprahepatic cava is freed from the diaphragmatic attachments and both phrenic veins are divided. If the cephalad limit of the tumor is at the cavoatrial junction, then the diaphragmatic incision can be extended anteriorly from the inferior vena cava, allowing access to the pericardium without sternotomy. However, for more cephalad extension, a formal sternotomy is required. Rarely, venovenous bypass can be used to permit adequate dissection and mobilization for tumor removal. In many instances, the tumor can be manipulated inferiorly into the region of the hepatic veins, the cavoatrial junction clamped, and the tumor removed without CPB.[81] If the tumor is too bulky or extends too deeply into the atrium, CPB will be required. The superior vena cava and aorta are cannulated, and CPB is initiated. The distal inferior vena cava in the abdomen and the contralateral renal vein are clamped, along with a Pringle maneuver. A low atriotomy extending onto the suprahepatic cava is performed without cardiac arrest. The tumor is transected below the hepatic veins and removed. The atriotomy is closed, and a clamp is placed at the cavoatrial junction. The patient is weaned from CPB while the liver is rotated into the right upper quadrant, exposing the intrahepatic cava. A lateral venotomy is performed here to remove the rest of the thrombus. The venotomy is extended to incorporate the renal vein ostia. Repair of the venotomy is begun cephalad, and, when

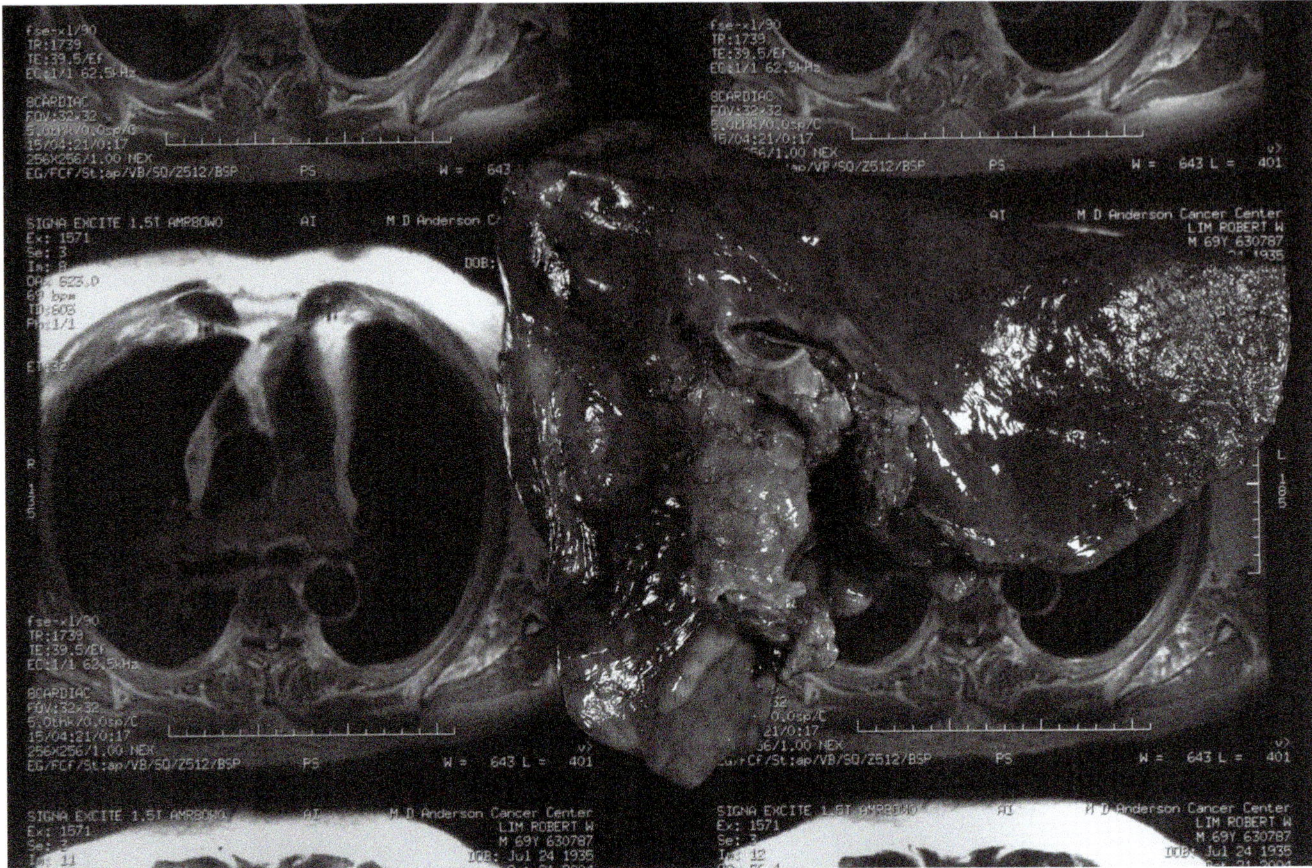

FIGURE 14-22   Gross specimen with underlying image of computed tomographic scan appearance.

possible, a clamp is placed along the infrahepatic cava, allowing the Pringle and the cavoatrial clamp to be removed. If there is significant bland thrombus in the pelvic veins, then a Greenfield filter is inserted into the inferior vena cava prior to completing the repair of the venotomy.

Over 15 years of experience with these tumors from The University of Texas MD Anderson Cancer Center was reviewed in 2002, including 96 patients with 8% of the tumors at level III and 15% at level IV. Their overall surgical 5-year survival rate was 35%. This review and others have found that the level of tumor thrombus propagation was not a predictor of overall survival.[80–83] For this reason, radical surgical excision has been advocated and remains the gold standard for treatment.

■ Minimally Invasive Approaches

Some surgeons have described resecting these cardiac tumors via a less invasive method.[84–87] Incomplete surgical resection of a malignant cardiac tumor is associated with a poor prognosis and overall no benefit to the patient. Because each cardiac tumor should be treated as if it were malignant, minimally invasive approaches are limited with respect to an exit portal for the tumor. These minimally invasive approaches are more acceptable for benign rather than malignant tumors. However, there have been instances where what was thought to be a benign tumor was malignant on final pathology. We advocate making a smaller skin incision, which is about 12 cm in length, and complete sternotomy underneath. Raising skin flaps may also aid in mobilizing tissue to allow the retractor to expose the heart.

■ Pathologic Features Affecting Surgical Approach

Sarcomas are the most common form of malignant disease of the heart, comprising 75% of these tumors. Cardiac sarcomas, or other tumors in the heart, may interfere with function and necessitate removal for cure or palliation. There is also the possibility that a mural thrombus may be mistaken for tumor; thus, the initial approach for these patients is similar to that of the cardiac tumor patient. In general, certain benign tumors or cysts may be mistaken for malignant tumors,[88] and myxomas are even known to recur;

therefore, it is always prudent to treat each tumor as if it were malignant to reduce such a recurrence. Showered thrombotic emboli may occasionally mimic metastatic involvement.[89] Clinical features that may increase the suspicion of malignant disease are evidence of metastatic disease, rapid growth of tumor size, a hemorrhagic pericardial effusion, location of the tumor on the right side of the heart or on the atrial free wall, an intramural location, an intracavitary location, or extension into the pulmonary veins.

As stated earlier, cardiac tumors can be divided into primary and secondary. Primary cardiac tumors can further be categorized as benign or malignant. Benign cardiac tumors include: thrombus, myxoma, rhabdomyoma, fibroma, lipoma, lipomatous hypertrophy of the interatrial septum, papillary fibroelastoma, teratoma, and hemangioma. Thymoma, paraganglioma, pheochromocytoma, and mesothelioma of the atrioventricular node are considered benign, but have malignant potential. Seventy-five percent of malignant cardiac tumors are sarcomas, which include angiosarcoma, undifferentiated pleomorphic sarcoma, rhabdomyosarcoma, fibrosarcoma, myxosarcoma, liposarcoma, leiomyosarcoma, extraskeletal osteosarcoma, chondrosarcoma, and other variants. Plasmacytoma, malignant schwannoma, and lymphoma make up the remaining portion of malignant cardiac tumors. Secondary cardiac tumors are either from direct extension from the infradiaphragmatic region or metastases and are 30 times more likely than a primary malignant cardiac tumor.

PRIMARY BENIGN TUMORS

Almost half of benign heart tumors are myxomas.[90] Some benign heart tumors can undergo malignant transformation, thus excision is likely the best option and can also prevent emboli.[91] Myxomas are generally pedunculated with a short 1 to 2 cm based attachment to the endocardial septum, usually in the left atrium close to the fossa ovalis (Figure 14-23), have endothelium-lined crevices and clefts, have a predilection for the atria, are often gelatinous or mucoid, can have areas of hemorrhage, are likely to produce emboli, are very friable, and can frequently masquerade as many other more common cardiovascular and systemic diseases.[92] Because of their friability, it is important to remove fragments by irrigation to avoid seeding myxomatous material within the heart and pericardium. Partial excision may be warranted in selected cases. The distribution of these tumors is as follows: 74.5% from the left atrium, 18.1% from the right atrium, 3.7% from the right ventricle, and

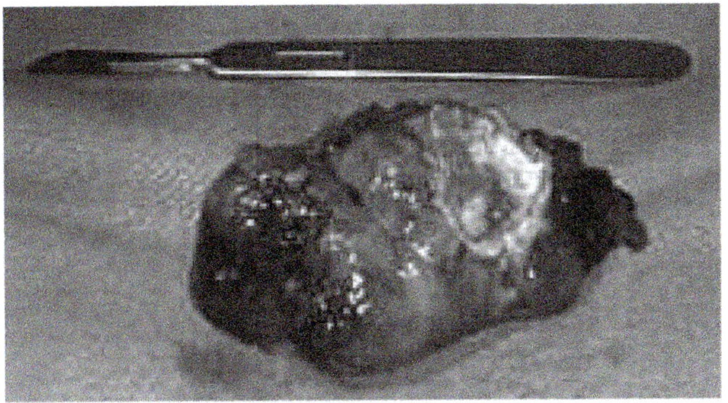

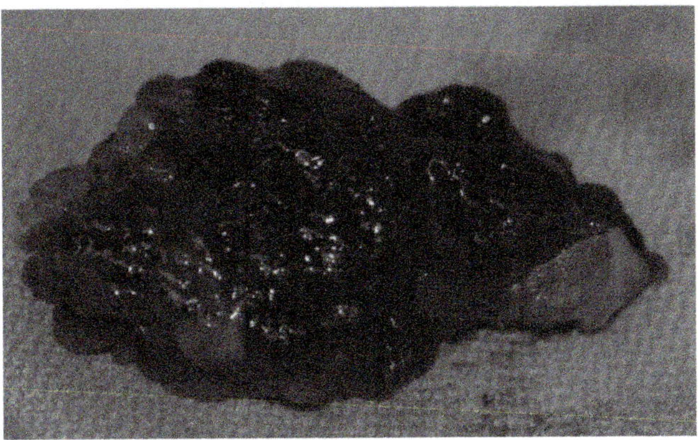

FIGURE 14-23 Two photographs of myxomatous tumors.

3.7% from the left ventricle.[90] Extensive local invasion has been noted. There are many reports of local recurrences, but distant metastases have been noted, with independent growth at these separate sites. They can be infected or multifocal.[56,93–95] They usually arise from the region of the limbus of the fossa ovalis. Right atrial myxomas tend to have a broader attachment to the septal wall or septum, requiring a broader septal resection. Atypical myxomas can occur on the left atrial appendage and even the chordae of the mitral valve.[90] Surgical resection cures the patient in more than 95% of cases.

In a clinical series, as many as 80% to 90% of patients who have rhabdomyomas tend also to have tuberous sclerosis or a family history.[56,93,95] They are probably the same as hamartomas, Purkinje cell tumors, glycogenic tumors, and histiocytoid cardiomyopathy.[96] These are benign yellow-gray tumors that invariably occur in the cardiac ventricles or atrioventricular valves.[94] Rhabdomyomas are the most common primary cardiac tumors in children and can be multiple. Fetal diagnosis can be made. In infants with incessant ventricular tachycardia,[6] the only gross finding may be a grayish white discoloration of the endocardium at the site identified by electrophysiologic mapping. These tumors are frequently determined to be unresectable at operation and thus are frequently observed and tend to regress.[56,58] The only indication for surgery in patients with biopsy-proven rhabdomyoma is when the tumor is causing life-threatening symptoms.[97] Cooley resected 21 rhabdomyomas, with 18 of the 21 patients being cured of their dysrhythmia after resection.[6] Unresected tumors should be followed by serial echocardiography.

Fibromas grossly resemble uterine leiomyomatomatas, with a whorled appearance on cut section, compressing surrounding structures as they grow. They may also be categorized as hamartomas. They almost exclusively occur or originate within the left ventricle more than the right ventricle or ventricular septum,[98] often arising within the myocardium.[6,97,99] The tumor can often be easily separated from the surrounding myocardium. Tumor calcification can be seen on chest radiography, leading to a diagnostic evaluation. Most are diagnosed in infancy, and they are the second most common childhood cardiac tumor; untreated cases can eventually obstruct ventricular inflow or outflow. A case report by Waller and colleagues discussed single ventricular palliation for a large fibroma in an infant who later received a successful cardiac transplantation. Today, autotransplantation with reconstruction should be considered in tumors that grow too large for complete resection otherwise, unless a reconstruction was not possible or allowances for growth could not be secured. The Batista principles have also been described in the resection of such fibromas by Zidere and colleagues.[100] More than 5- to 17-year survival durations have been reported.[6,101] Jamieson and colleagues successfully treated a left ventricular fibroma in 1981 with orthotopic heart transplantation.[102]

Lipomas are encapsulated tumors that are composed of mature fat cells. They can arise from epicardial or pericardial fat and may be quite large. Intramyocardial tumors are usually quite small. Many of these are discovered at the time of operation, and we advise resecting these owing to the risk of emboli and obstruction. A right ventricular tumor presenting with ventricular tachycardia was successfully resected by Schrepfer and colleagues.[43] Masses with lipomatous hypertrophy of the interatrial septum are usually observed[103] and if resected tend not to require CPB because they can usually be separated from the intra-atrial groove. Incidental lipomatous hypertrophy of the interatrial septum found on echo may be observed without resection.

Papillary fibroelastomas are usually small tumors but have a predilection for valve leaflets, especially the mitral or tricuspid valves.[104] They have characteristic papillary fronds with a central core of dense connective tissue sometimes lined by hyperplastic endocardial tissue (Figure 14-24). Papillary fibroelastomas can be multicentric. The Texas Heart Institute documented 14 patients diagnosed with cardiac papillary fibroelastoma from 1992 to 2014, all of whom had their lesions surgically excised, with no 30-day deaths.[105]

Mesothelioma of the atrioventricular node is also called a cardiac conduction tumor. Grossly, this tumor appears to be poorly circumscribed and can be multicystic in nature. It is reported to usually be below

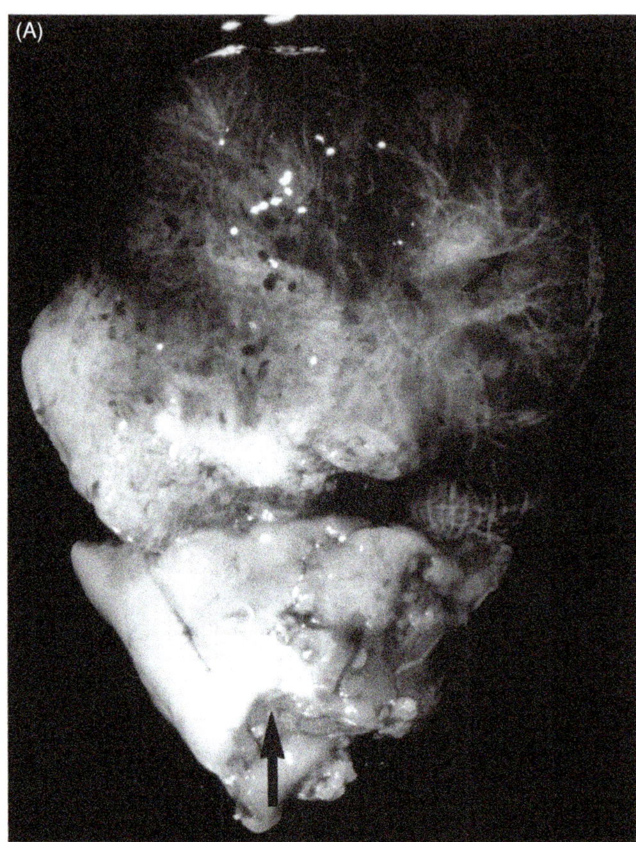

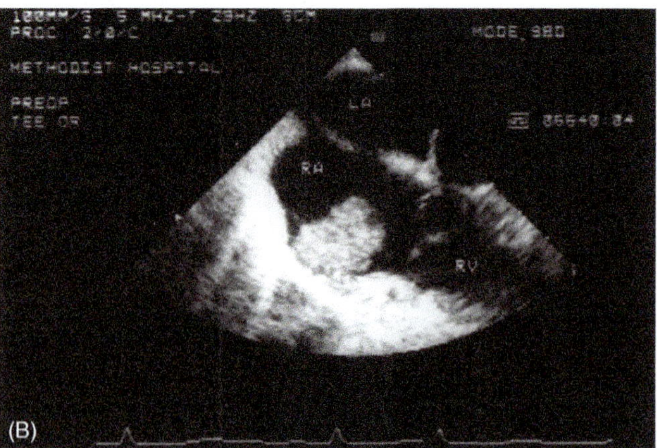

FIGURE 14-24 (A) Fibroelastoma. (B) echocardiographic image of fibroelastoma of the right atrium and ventricle.

15 mm in diameter and located in the atrial septum superior to the septal leaflet of the tricuspid valve in the vicinity of the atrioventricular node. Because of this tumor's propensity to cause ventricular arrhythmias and heart block, it was called the "smallest tumor to cause sudden death" by Wolf and Bing.[106] Interestingly, this tumor has never been diagnosed antemortem.[107] If the diagnosis is suspected but not proven, palliative treatment should include defibrillation or ablation, as well as pacing, because previous reports of pacing have only failed to prevent sudden death.[90,107,108] Young adults with complete heart block should be evaluated for this type of tumor.

Pheochromocytomas are potentially lethal functioning chromaffin tumors of the sympathetic nervous system that occur rarely within the pericardium and on the surface of the heart. These are soft fleshy tumors that can be flattened between the surface of the heart and pericardium. Severe and sometimes episodic hypertension is noted in this disease. These patients have elevated levels of urinary catecholamines and can be localized by CT scan or[109] I metaiodobenzylguanidine. Widespread metastases have been reported. Prior to surgical resection, it is important to employ alpha blockade and then beta blockade when necessary. An alpha-adrenergic blocker is given 10 to 14 days preoperatively, followed by beta-adrenergic blockade two to three days preoperatively if needed. Beta blockade should never be given first due to the risk of unopposed alpha stimulation and further blood pressure elevations. Reports of this tumor suggest that it is often intimately involved with vascular structures such as the coronary arteries and the aorta. The tumor has to be resected from its attachments and should not be enucleated.

Other benign tumors include paragangliomas (Figure 14-25), neurilemmomas, teratomas, and hemiangiomas. Paragangliomas are predominantly located in the posterior mediastinum if they are intrathoracic. These tumors are of endocrine origin and may secrete catecholamines, causing their presentation to be much like that of a pheochromocytoma. Neurilemmoma has been described infiltrating the portal vein, and successful reconstruction has been described, including reconstruction of the right atrium, left atrium, and septum. There have been only about 10 cases reported in the literature. The majority of teratomas are in young patients and in the right atrium. Twenty percent of these are malignant. These tumors more commonly arise from the anterior mediastinum.[110] Hemangiomas comprise 1% to 2% of benign neoplasms. Successful excision from the tricuspid valve and left atrium have been described,[86,111] and right ventricular recurrence has also been discussed.[112] These tumors can also arise from major vessels, including the coronary arteries.[113] Most are diagnosed at autopsy, but early diagnosis is associated with prolonged survival of up to 26 years.[6] Primary malignant tumors are more likely to invade surrounding structures and produce chest pain, effusions, or obstruction owing to their rapid growth.

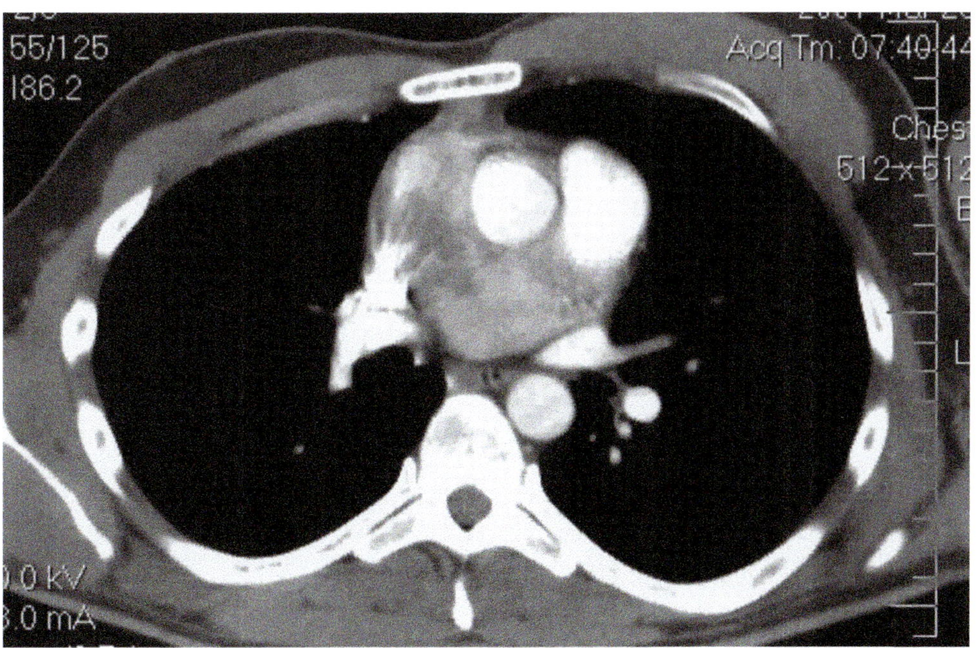

FIGURE 14-25 Paraganglioma.

PRIMARY MALIGNANT TUMORS

Sarcomas are the main type of primary malignant tumor found within the heart. Although the division of sarcomas into several subclassifications has been made easier with the advent of antibody labeling and newer immunohistochemical techniques,[114] this differentiation does not appear to be clinically prognostic. Primary cardiac sarcomas have an extremely poor prognosis due to difficulty in complete resection, advanced disease at diagnosis, and high prevalence of brain metastases. The overall survival of resected cardiac sarcomas is reported to be less than 11 months.[97,115] Neoadjuvant therapy to achieve cytoreduction prior to excision of non-life-threatening tumors has been performed with some success.[116] A recent study by Abu Saleh et al suggests that neoadjuvant chemotherapy followed by radical surgery is a safe and effective strategy in patients with right-side heart sarcoma, and that this treatment multimodality enhances successful negative margin resection that translates into improved patient survival.[66] It is well documented that sarcomas show rapid growth, local invasion, and distant metastasis (Figure 14-26).[117] The surgeon should treat each of these tumors in a similar manner, but particular features are discussed in the following section such that their behavior may influence approach. In a review of the Houston Methodist Hospital cardiac tumor database, 95 patients with primary cardiac sarcoma underwent surgical excision with a postoperative 1-year mortality of 35%.[118] Patients with radically resected sarcomas tend to die from metastatic disease rather than local recurrence,[31,119] thus, surgical resection is typically considered palliative. The most important part of a preoperative evaluation for primary malignant tumors of the heart is imaging (usually CT scan to include lungs, and MRI and/or echocardiography) to evaluate the extent of disease and determine resectability. Survival correlates with the completeness of resection and tumor grade in patients diagnosed with localized sarcoma.[30,97] Median survival in patients who underwent complete resection was 24 months versus 10 months in all other patients. Cardiac transplantation and cardiac autotransplantation have been successfully performed to obtain complete local control. Other patients may benefit from incomplete resection to palliate obstructive symptoms or heart failure.

Angiosarcomas, the most common type of malignant sarcoma in the heart, has a predilection for the right heart (80%) and are twice as common in men.[90] They are the most common form of malignant heart tumor,[90] tend to be bulky and aggressively invade adjacent structures,[31] often present with obstruction or right-sided heart failure, and can be multifocal.[31] Spontaneous rupture into the pericardium has been described with eventual cardiac tamponade and death.[120] Ninety percent of patients die within 9 to 12 months of diagnosis if their tumor is not resected, and metastasis is a greater problem than recurrence. Sixty-six percent to 89% of tumors will metastasize, most often to the lung, liver, or brain.[121] Rettmar's review of over 108 cases of primary cardiac angiosarcomas revealed the mean age at presentation to be 40 years and the survival time after the onset of symptoms to be 6.7 months. If the patients had their tumor resected, survival seemed to increase to 8 months.[117] It is difficult to say whether these patients were being compared with later-stage non-operative candidates and if surgical margins were free of tumor.

Other types of tumors that are malignant include undifferentiated pleomorphic sarcomas, leiomyosarcomas, liposarcomas, plasmacytoma, myxosarcoma, extraskeletal osteosarcoma, chondrosarcoma, carcinosarcoma, and malignant schwannoma. Undifferentiated pleomorphic sarcoma (malignant fibrous histiocytoma in older literature) usually occurs in the left atrium, and mimics myxoma.[122] It is commonly incompletely excised owing to being mistaken for a myxoma. Many of the above-mentioned tumors have the characteristic behavior that their extracardiac counterparts possess. Metastases to brain is common.

Malignant mesothelioma is a rare tumor of the pericardial mesothelial cells. Exposure to asbestos can be associated with this disease but is rarer than with the pleural mesothelioma. Nodules of firm white tissue are often identified. There are no data to indicate that resection improves overall survival. Chemotherapy provides minimal benefit in this disease, however new immunotherapy agents are being studied.

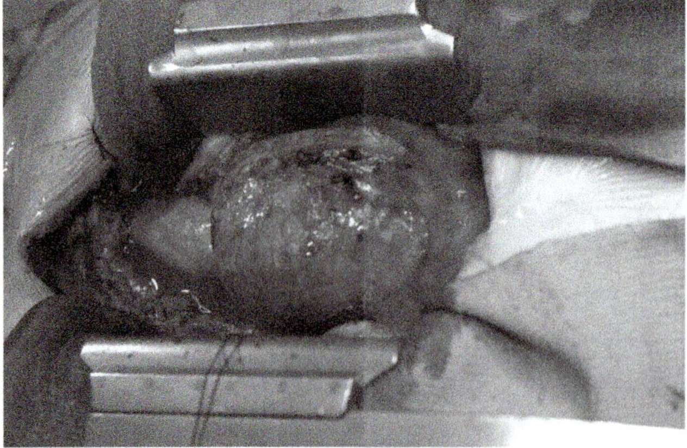

FIGURE 14-26 Appearance of angiosarcoma after dissection with open chest.

Lymphoma has been known to invade the conduction system[38,44] or into other heart structures, such as the interatrial septum.[123] There are many reports of either complete or debulking successful resections with prolonged survival,[109,124] but there are also reports of prolonged survival with chemotherapy alone.[125] Other patients have had the tumor resected but have died from perioperative complications, such as disseminated intravascular coagulation leading to hemopericardium.[126] Chemotherapy alone is likely the best choice.

Leukemia has also been noted in the cardiac chambers, including predominantly right ventricular wall lesions.[127,128] Most of these patients are treated with chemotherapy, and their tumors tended to regress.[127,128]

SECONDARY CARDIAC TUMORS

This classification includes both tumors arising from the infradiaphragmatic region and metastatic tumors. These are 20 to 30 times more frequent than primary cardiac tumors.[90] Although the approach is completely different, it is important to note that these can be from multiple primary tissue origins and anatomic locations as well.

Tumors arising from the infradiaphragmatic region can be of renal, hepatocellular,[129–131] uterine,[132,133] or testicular in origin. One of the tumors of hepatocellular origin included tumor extending into the right atrium with a significant thrombus below the tumor lying in the hepatic veins and inferior vena cava.[130] Another hepatocellular carcinoma was initially diagnosed as thrombus until it was later found to extend into the heart.[129] Distinguishing the difference between these may be done with either CT or MRI.[131] Reports of treatment include resections such as simple infradiaphragmatic removal to circulatory arrest.[134]

Metastatic cardiac tumors can be from any primary tumor, most frequently from lung cancer, breast cancer, melanoma,[40,135] and leukemia,[41,136] but can also arise from carcinoid tumor,[137] non-Hodgkin's lymphoma,[41,138] renal cell carcinoma,[80] cervical carcinoma,[40] hepatocellular,[139] rectal adenocarcinoma,[140] testicular germ cell tumors,[141] and sarcoma.[142] These are predominantly located in the right atrium and occasionally in the right ventricle. Therapy is palliative here, although there has been some success with resection of isolated metastases. Autopsy reviews have found up to 20% to 30% of patients with advanced cancer having metastatic disease in the heart.[90] One report described extension of cervical carcinoma metastasis from the right ventricle into the right ventricular outflow tract.[90] A case of high-grade pleomorphic sarcoma metastatic to the heart was described by authors from the Texas

Heart Institute with complete successful reconstruction of the heart, including the right ventricle and mitral valve replacement.[143] Metastatic tumors in the heart were also found to be the most common cause of pericardial tamponade.[144]

RECURRENCE

The degree of complete resection seems to be the main factor affecting recurrence of tumor. A left atrial myxoma diagnosed during evaluation of repeated embolic events recurred 5 months after resection in the right ventricular outflow tract and another myxoma recurred 14 years later in the left atrium and left ventricle concomitantly.[145] The recurrence rate of myxoma that was completely excised was between 1%[146] and 4.7%[147] in two large studies, although there are many reports of no recurrences.[53,148–152]

Some patients have a predilection for tumor recurrence. About 5% of patients with cardiac myxoma have a family history of the disorder, Carney's syndrome, and in this group, the tumor is most likely to recur after surgery. Carney's syndrome consists of myxomas, spotty pigmentation, and endocrine overactivity. These patients tend to be in their twenties, are more likely to have tumors in other areas than the left atrium, occasionally have bilateral tumors, and are more likely to develop recurrences.[153] In these patients, it is important to explore all of the chambers of the heart when feasible and to especially perform a complete preoperative evaluation to locate any additional myxomas.

DISCUSSION

When a diagnosis of a cardiac tumor has been made, it is imperative to first determine if the mass is benign or malignant, and if malignant, is it primary or metastatic disease to the heart. Following the appropriate evaluation, if the patient is an otherwise operative candidate, primary malignant tumors should almost always be excised after appropriate neoadjuvant chemotherapy if complete resection with negative margins is able to be achieved, with lymphoma being the primary exception to resection. Because both malignant and benign tumors can cause obstructive symptoms, irreversible heart failure, or death and the etiology of the tumor is often not known prior to resection, each tumor should be treated as if it were malignant and should be excised completely. Some tumors that were initially thought to be benign can later be diagnosed as malignant. There is also an argument for incomplete resection of benign tumors involving conductive tissue or valves or the fibrous skeleton of the heart, but each case must be weighed against the specific risk-benefit ratio.

The aggressive biologic nature of these tumors makes treatment complex and difficult, but advances and refinement in surgical technique have provided some hope for these patients. The principal problem with surgical resection of primary cardiac tumors has been extensive involvement of cardiac structures by the tumor with difficult access to the tumor limiting adequate resection. As surgical techniques advance, these obstacles may be overcome. The Autotransplant Program for cardiac tumors became available at Methodist DeBakey Heart Center, Houston, TX in 1998. Reardon et al.[25,26] demonstrated the benefit of resection of both right and left atrial sarcomas. In a retrospective review of 57 patients who underwent extensive resection of the right atrium for sarcoma with bovine pericardial reconstruction, the 30-day mortality was 14%, with a survival benefit shown for the tumors with negative surgical margins (median survival 27 months vs. 4 months) and a significantly higher overall 5-year survival rate (36% vs. 0%; p = 0.0003) than patients with positive surgical margins. In a series of 35 autotransplants from 1998 through 2013 for complex left-sided otherwise unresectable cardiac tumors by traditional methods, overall 30-day, 1-year, and 2-year procedural survival was 85%, 59%, and 44%, respectively, with one patient survival beyond 5 years and 6 months and a median survival of 36 months.[74] These data are supported by other retrospective reviews such as Truong, et al which reviewed 16 patients in the British Columbia Center between 1990 and 1996 showing complete surgical resection in patients with no metastatic disease experienced improved survival (25 month medial survival versus 6 months).[154] Similar data were also found in a small 16 patient series by Mayer et al. showing survival benefit for patients receiving both surgery and chemotherapy in patients with localized and resectable disease.[155] Mayo Clinic reviewed their data over a 32-year period and found 34 patients who had undergone resection of cardiac sarcoma.[156] Median survival time of 12 months was extended to 17 months with a negative margin. This group also showed that angiosarcoma had a shorter survival than the other forms of cardiac sarcoma.[156] These data emphasize the importance of complete surgical Improvement in systemic treatment is essential as patients continue to later die from metastatic disease.

The role of adjuvant therapy in soft tissue sarcomas is evolving and improving. Putnam and colleagues demonstrated no significant difference in the survival of patients with primary malignant sarcomas of the heart who underwent surgical intervention alone compared with those who had adjuvant postoperative chemotherapy, however this study was underpowered to show a real benefit.[30] However, several studies have advocated combined therapy,[157–160] especially in patients with extracardiac metastases.[136] Chemotherapy agents often used as systemic treatment in sarcoma are doxorubicin, and ifosfamide with response rates >20% in metastatic disease.[161] Doxorubicin and olaratumab are newer combinations for treatment of locally advanced or metastatic soft tissue sarcoma resulting in objective response in 15%–20% of cases. However, the use of adjuvant chemotherapy in localized disease is controversial and has not always provided evidence of improved outcome. In the series by Reardon, there was an observation that early deaths after resection occurred in patients who refused chemotherapy.[27] More recently published work by Reardon et al. also reflect patients receiving neoadjuvant chemotherapy had a higher likelihood of a negative margin resection in right sided cardiac tumors and the median survival of patients who had negative margin resection was 53.5 months compared with 9.5 months for a positive margin resection. Neoadjuvant chemotherapy led to a doubling of survival (20 versus 9.5 months).[66]

New therapy for sarcoma is emerging. Weekly paclitaxel has been used for metastatic angiosarcoma with a tumor control rate of 70%. The primary tumors were not however cardiac.[162,163] The Sarcoma Meta-Analysis Collaboration was an analysis of 1568 patients from 14 trials of doxorubicin based therapy. It showed evidence that adjuvant doxorubicin based chemotherapy improved time to local and distant recurrence and overall recurrence-free survival with a trend towards improved overall survival in sarcoma patients, especially in sarcomas of the extremities. Whether this data can be applied to cardiac sarcomas is yet to be defined.[164] Chemotherapy targets will likely change as the role of antiangiogenesis drugs advances with VEGF inhibitors and immune targeted therapies.[165,166] Radiation therapy is limited owing to the risk of cardiotoxicity in the heart and generally excluding most surgical treatments after radiation.

The role of factors such as genetics in predicting sarcoma response to chemotherapy is still to be determined.

Gene therapy and the current availability of microarray analysis will likely play a larger role in the study and treatment of primary cardiac tumors.[167] The genetics of sarcoma are complicated and may involve random complex alterations as in undifferentiated pleomorphic sarcoma, leiomyosarcoma and osteosarcoma, or recurrent genetic alterations as in myxoid liposarcoma and synovial sarcoma. One recurrent translocation involving chromosomes 12 and 15 (12;15) (p13q25), which combines a transcription factor with a tyrosine kinase receptor, occurs in a subset of congenital fibrosarcomas.[168] There have been at least 19 specific translocations associated with specific sarcoma subtypes.[169] Translocations disrupt genes located at chromosomal break-points creating chimeric genes which may be translated into fusion proteins.[169] Chromosomal translocations that have been associated with the formation of fusion proteins are found in the Ewing family of tumors,[170,171] alveolar rhabdomyosarcomas,[172,173] and synovial sarcomas,[174,175] among others. Gene models may also be used as predictors of chemoresistance as was shown in pediatric osteosarcomas by Man et al.[176] Cytogenetics of sarcoma will likely also become an important adjunct to diagnosis, classification, and treatment and may make choosing the correct therapy easier as many sarcomas present as poorly differentiated tumors lacking clear phenotypic features.[168,177]

Surgery is still the mainstay of treatment in soft tissue sarcomas of the abdomen and extremities.[161,178] Large randomized trials of cardiac tumors have not been performed owing to the rarity of this disease. Good outcomes have been reported with complete surgical resection and often radical cardiac reconstruction with a median survival reported as high as 25 months,[4,157] Since the completeness of resection correlates with survival,[97,115] more radical approaches to cardiac tumors seem warranted.[25,28,31,179,180] Survival in autotransplanted patients appears to exceed that of patients receiving standard resections.[25] The recent advances in cardiac surgery and technology make the treatment of cardiac tumors both exciting and promising, as evidenced by a recent case report detailing the use of total artificial heart implantation following resection of a right ventricular angiosarcoma,[73] suggesting that complete excision of both ventricles and total cardiac replacement may be an option in carefully selected patients with primary cardiac sarcoma with extensive ventricular involvement. Future studies are needed to determine the best mode of therapy for such patients.

In today's environment of safer cardiac surgery with protective hypothermia and cardioplegia, complete and radical resection with pre-operative neo-adjuvant chemotherapy is the best option for most malignant cardiac tumors in carefully selected patients. Multidisciplinary cooperation between cardiology, oncology, radiology, pathology and surgery is essential. As such, many of these more complicated resections and reconstructions should be performed only in centers where this level of care can be offered. Heart centers with experience in complex cardiac reconstruction and transplantation and oncology centers with experience treating rare tumors should be considered when treating this unique group of patients.

Research into cardiac tumors is necessary. Although a rare, but fatal disease, it offers invaluable information into the nature of sarcoma and the physiology of the heart. Future directions for cardiac tumor patients will likely be varied, including complete excision of the heart and pericardium, with temporary implantation of an artificial heart or assist device. Cardiac resection will likely be accompanied by tailored genetic therapy and personalized chemotherapy. The patient would be able to receive adjuvant chemotherapy with such agents as doxorubicin without the concern for myocardial toxicity. Outcome studies of cardiac surgery need to be developed to better improve surgical technique and appropriate timing of systemic therapeutic agents must be explored. Also, a major weakness of therapy is the ability to image microscopic disease, with metastatic disease being the primary reason patients die from their cardiac tumors. There is evidence already that tumor-free margins provide longer survival in cardiac resections. As molecular imaging becomes more advanced, the ability to detect disease will become much more sophisticated with the possibility of improved outcomes and ability for targeted therapy. The optimal use of multimodality treatment with chemotherapy, radiation, and surgery of primary cardiac tumors can improve patient survival and is evolving. Success likely lies in a more biological targeted approach to treatment with better detection of microscopic disease.

REFERENCES

1. Holley DG, Martin GR, Brenner JI, et al. Diagnosis and management of fetal cardiac tumors: a multicenter experience and review of published reports. *J Am Coll Cardiol*. 1995;26(2):516–520.
2. Roberts WC. Primary and secondary neoplasms of the heart. *Am J Cardiol*. 1997;80(5):671–682.
3. Yu K, et al. Epidemiological and pathological characteristics of cardiac tumors: a clinical study of 242 cases. *Interact Cardiovasc Thorac Surg*. 2007;6(5):636–639.
4. Bakaeen FG, et al. Surgical outcome in 85 patients with primary cardiac tumors. *Am J Surg*. 2003;186(6):641–647; discussion 647.
5. Dein JR, et al. Primary cardiac neoplasms. Early and late results of surgical treatment in 42 patients. *J Thorac Cardiovasc Surg*. 1987;93(4):502–511.
6. Cooley DA. Surgical treatment of cardiac neoplasms: 32-year experience. *Thorac Cardiovasc Surg*. 1990;38(suppl 2):176–182.
7. Perchinsky MJ, Lichtenstein SV, Tyers GF. Primary cardiac tumors: forty years' experience with 71 patients. *Cancer*. 1997;79(9):1809–1815.

8. Bisel HF, Wroblewski F, Ladue JS. Incidence and clinical manifestations of cardiac metastases. *J Am Med Assoc.* 1953;153(8):712–715.

9. Hanfling SM. Metastatic cancer to the heart. Review of the literature and report of 127 cases. *Circulation.* 1960;22:474–483.

10. Hoey ET, et al. MRI and CT appearances of cardiac tumours in adults. *Clin Radiol.* 2009;64(12):1214–1230.

11. Reynen K. Cardiac myxomas. *N Engl J Med.* 1995;333 (24):1610–1617.

12. Smith C. Tumors of the heart. *Arch Pathol Lab Med.* 1986;110(5):371–374.

13. Fine G. Neoplasms of the pericardium and heart. In: Gould S, ed. *Pathology of the Heart and Blood Vessels.* Springfield, IL: Charles C. Thomas; 1968:851–883.

14. Marshall VF, et al. Surgery for renal cell carcinoma in the vena cava. *J Urol.* 1970;103(4):414–420.

15. Nesbitt JC, et al. Surgical management of renal cell carcinoma with inferior vena cava tumor thrombus. *Ann Thorac Surg.* 1997;63(6):1592–1600.

16. Columbus M. *De Re Anatomica.* Venice: N Bevilacque; 1559:14.

17. Yater W. Tumors of the heart and pericardium: pathology, symptomatology and report of nince cases. *Arch Intern Med.* 1931;48(4):627–666.

18. Barnes A, Beaver D, Snell AM. Primary sarcoma of the heart: report of a case with electrocardiographic and pathological studies. *Am Heart J.* 1934;9(4):480–91.

19. Beck CS. An intrapericardial teratoma and a tumor of the heart: both removed operatively. *Ann Surg.* 1942;116(2):161–174.

20. Gibbon JH Jr. The development of the heart-lung apparatus. *Am J Surg.* 1978;135(5):608–619.

21. Crafoord C. Panel discussion of late results of mitral commissurotomy. Paper presented at: *Henry Ford Hospital International Symposium on Cardiovascular Surgery.* 1955:202–203.

22. Gerbode F, Kerth WJ, Hill JD. Surgical management of tumors of the heart. *Surgery.* 1967;61(1):94–101.

23. Schattenberg TT. Echocardiographic diagnosis of left atrial myxoma. *Mayo Clin Proc.* 1968;43(9):620–627.

24. Piazza N, et al. Primary cardiac tumours: eighteen years of surgical experience on 21 patients. *Can J Cardiol.* 2004;20(14):1443–1448.

25. Reardon MJ, et al. Cardiac autotransplant for surgical treatment of a malignant neoplasm. *Ann Thorac Surg.* 1999;67(6):1793–1795.

26. Reardon MJ, et al. Cardiac autotransplantation for primary cardiac tumors. *Ann Thorac Surg.* 2006;82(2): 645–650.

27. Reardon MJ, Walkes JC, Benjamin R. Therapy insight: malignant primary cardiac tumors. *Nat Clin Pract Cardiovasc Med.* 2006;3(10):548–553.

28. Cooley DA, et al. Human cardiac explantation and autotransplantation: application in a patient with a large cardiac pheochromocytoma. *Tex Heart Inst J.* 1985;12(2):171–176.

29. Mery GM, et al. A combined modality approach to recurrent cardiac sarcoma resulting in a prolonged remission: a case report. *Chest.* 2003;123(5):1766–1768.

30. Putnam JB Jr, et al. Primary cardiac sarcomas. *Ann Thorac Surg.* 1991;51(6):906–910.

31. Hoffmeier A, Schmid C, Scheld HH. Reply: "Ex situ resection of primary cardiac tumors". *Thorac Cardiovasc Surg* 2003; 51: 293–294. *Thorac Cardiovasc Surg.* 2004;52(2):125.

32. Butany J, et al. Cardiac tumours: diagnosis and management. *Lancet Oncol.* 2005;6(4):219–228.

33. Debourdeau P, et al. [Malignant cardiac tumors]. *Bull Cancer.* 2004;91(suppl 3):136–146.

34. Pinede L, Duhaut P, Loire R. Clinical presentation of left atrial cardiac myxoma. A series of 112 consecutive cases. *Medicine.* 2001;80(3):159–172.

35. Thung KH, et al. Cardiac tumor masquerading as obstructive sleep apnea syndrome. *Interact Cardiovasc Thorac Surg.* 2008;7(2):358–359.

36. Glancy DL, Morales JB Jr, Roberts WC. Angiosarcoma of the heart. *Am J Cardiol.* 1968;21(3):413–419.

37. Rettmar K, et al. Primary angiosarcoma of the heart. Report of a case and review of the literature. *Jpn Heart J.* 1993;34(5):667–683.

38. Hayes D Jr, Liles DK, Sorrell VL. An unusual cause of new-onset atrial flutter: primary cardiac lymphoma. *South Med J.* 2003;96(8):799–802.

39. Molina JE, Edwards JE, Ward HB. Primary cardiac tumors: experience at the University of Minnesota. *Thorac Cardiovasc Surg.* 1990;38(suppl 2):183–191.

40. Marti G, et al. [Cardiac metastases of malignant melanoma mimicking sick sinus syndrome]. *Rev Esp Cardiol.* 2004;57(6):589–591.

41. Strauss WE, Asinger RW, Hodges M. Mesothelioma of the AV node: potential utility of pacing. *Pacing Clin Electrophysiol.* 1988;11(9):1296–1298.

42. Thorgeirsson G, Liebman J. Mesothelioma of the AV node. *Pediatr Cardiol.* 1983;4(3):219–223.

43. Schrepfer S, et al. Successful resection of a symptomatic right ventricular lipoma. *Ann Thorac Surg.* 2003;76(4):1305–1307.

44. Ottaviani G, et al. Sudden death due to lymphomatous infiltration of the cardiac conduction system. *Cardiovasc Pathol.* 2003;12(2):77–81.

45. Aoyagi S, et al. Right atrial myxoma in a patient presenting with syncope. *Kurume Med J.* 2004;51(1):91–93.

46. Bassi D, et al. Primary cardiac precursor B lymphoblastic lymphoma in a child: a case report and review of the literature. *Cardiovasc Pathol.* 2004;13(2):116–119.

47. Fuzellier JF, et al. [Fibroelastoma of the tricuspid valve presenting with syncope]. *Arch Mal Coeur Vaiss.* 2004;97(1):67–69.

48. Pego-Fernandes PM, et al. Right atrial lipoma. *Arq Bras Cardiol.* 2003;80(1):97–99, 94–96.

49. Levitas A, et al. Positional cyanosis in infants: an unusual presentation of right-sided cardiac masses. *Cardiol Young.* 2004;14(1):46–49.

50. Anagnostopoulos GK, et al. Budd-Chiari syndrome and portal vein thrombosis due to right atrial myxoma. *Ann Thorac Surg.* 2004;78(1):333–334.

51. Weinberg BA, Conces DJ Jr, Waller BF. Cardiac manifestations of noncardiac tumors. Part I: Direct effects. *Clin Cardiol.* 1989;12(5):289–296.

52. Seguin JR, et al. Interleukin 6 production by cardiac myxomas may explain constitutional symptoms. *J Thorac Cardiovasc Surg*. 1992;103(3):599–600.

53. Wang JN, et al. Cardiac tumor in infants and children. *Acta Paediatr Taiwan*. July-Aug, 2003;44(4):215–9.

54. Bortolotti U, et al. Surgical excision of intracardiac myxomas: a 20-year follow-up. *Ann Thorac Surg*. 1990;49(3):449–453.

55. Stiller B, et al. Primary cardiac tumours: when is surgery necessary? *Eur J Cardiothorac Surg*. 2001;20(5):1002–1006.

56. Paladini D, et al. Prenatal ultrasound diagnosis of Nager syndrome. *Ultrasound Obstet Gynecol*. 2003;21(2):195–197.

57. Beghetti M, et al. Pediatric primary benign cardiac tumors: a 15-year review. *Am Heart J*. 1997;134(6):1107–1114.

58. Borges AC, et al. Preoperative two- and three-dimensional transesophageal echocardiographic assessment of heart tumors. *Ann Thorac Surg*. 1996;61(4): 1163–1167.

59. Smythe WR, et al. Antisense therapy for malignant mesothelioma with oligonucleotides targeting the bcl-xl gene product. *J Thorac Cardiovasc Surg*. 2002;123(6): 1191–1198.

60. Mikhail P, et al. An incidental calcified right atrial mass. *Can J Cardiol*. 2003;19(13):1551–1553.

61. Daniel WG, Mugge A. Transesophageal echocardiography. *N Engl J Med*. 1995;332(19):1268–1279.

62. Attum AA, et al. Malignant clinical behavior of cardiac myxomas and "myxoid imitators". *Ann Thorac Surg*. 1987;44(2):217–222.

63. Gilkeson RC, Chiles C. MR evaluation of cardiac and pericardial malignancy. *Magn Reson Imaging Clin N Am*. 2003;11(1):173–186, viii.

64. Sparrow PJ, et al. MR imaging of cardiac tumors. *Radiographics*. 2005;25(5):1255–1276.

65. Thakrar A, et al. Multimodality cardiac imaging for the noninvasive characterization of intracardiac neoplasms. *Int J Cardiol*. 2009;132(2):e74–e76.

66. Anfinsen OG, et al. Coronary artery aneurysms mimicking cardiac tumor. *Eur J Echocardiogr*. 2004;5(4):308–312.

67. Abu Saleh WK, et al. Improved outcomes with the evolution of a neoadjuvant chemotherapy approach to right heart sarcoma. *Ann Thorac Surg*. 2017;104(1):90–96.

68. Gidlewski J, Petrie JP. Pericardiocentesis and principles of echocardiographic imaging in the patient with cardiac neoplasia. *Clin Tech Small Anim Pract*. 2003;18(2):131–134.

69. Kamiya H, et al. Surgical treatment of primary cardiac tumors: 28 years' experience in Kanazawa University Hospital. *Jpn Circ J*. 2001;65(4):315–319.

70. Fortmann T. [Hemorrhagic nonspecific pericardial effusion as an initial symptom of angiosarcoma of the right heart]. *Z Kardiol*. 2004;93(10):807–812.

71. Larbalestier RI, Chard RB, Cohn LH. Optimal approach to the mitral valve: dissection of the interatrial groove. *Ann Thorac Surg*. 1992;54(6):1186–1188.

72. Bortolotti U, et al. Right ventricular myxoma: review of the literature and report of two patients. *Ann Thorac Surg*. 1982;33(3):277–284.

73. Read RC, et al. The malignant potentiality of left atrial myxoma. *J Thorac Cardiovasc Surg*. 1974;68(6):857–868.

74. Bruckner BA, et al. Total artificial heart implantation after excision of right ventricular angiosarcoma. *Tex Heart Inst J*. 2016;43(3):252–254.

75. Ramlawi B, et al. Autotransplantation for the resection of complex left heart tumors. *Ann Thorac Surg*. 2014;98(3):863–868.

76. Kallenbach K, Haverich A. Explantation of the heart for resection of primary cardiac tumors can be avoided by partial ex situ heart surgery. *Thorac Cardiovasc Surg*. 2003;51(5):293–294.

77. Goldstein DJ, et al. Experience with heart transplantation for cardiac tumors. *J Heart Lung Transplant*. 1995;14(2):382–386.

78. Chambers JC, et al. Pulmonary autograft procedure for aortic valve disease: long-term results of the pioneer series. *Circulation*. 1997;96(7):2206–2214.

79. Conklin LD, Reardon MJ. Autotransplantation of the heart for primary cardiac malignancy: development and surgical technique. *Tex Heart Inst J*. 2002;29(2):105–108; discussion 108.

80. Swierzewski, DJ, Swierzewski MJ, Libertino JA. Radical nephrectomy in patients with renal cell carcinoma with venous, vena caval, and atrial extension. *Am J Surg*. 1994;168(2):205–209.

81. Sweeney P, et al. Surgical management of renal cell carcinoma associated with complex inferior vena caval thrombi. *Urol Oncol*. 2003;21(5):327–333.

82. Hatcher PA, et al. Surgical management and prognosis of renal cell carcinoma invading the vena cava. *J Urol*. 1991;145(1):20–23; discussion 23–24.

83. Libertino JA, Zinman L, Watkins E Jr. Long-term results of resection of renal cell cancer with extension into inferior vena cava. *J Urol*. 1987;137(1):21–24.

84. Neves RJ, Zincke H. Surgical treatment of renal cancer with vena cava extension. *Br J Urol*. 1987;59(5):390–395.

85. Gulbins H, et al. Minimally invasive extirpation of a left-ventricular myxoma. *Thorac Cardiovasc Surg*. 1999;47(2):129–130.

86. Ko PJ, et al. Video-assisted minimal access in excision of left atrial myxoma. *Ann Thorac Surg*. 1998;66(4): 1301–1305.

87. Lapenna E, et al. Cavernous hemangioma of the tricuspid valve: minimally invasive surgical resection. *Ann Thorac Surg*. 2003;76(6):2097–2099.

88. Ravikumar E, et al. Minimal access approach for surgical management of cardiac tumors. *Ann Thorac Surg*. 2000;70(3):1077–1079.

89. Prasad A, Callahan MJ, Malouf JF. Acquired right atrial blood cyst: a hitherto unrecognized complication of cardiac operation. *J Am Soc Echocardiogr*. 2003;16(4):377–378.

90. Gosse P, et al. Myxoma of the mitral valve diagnosed by echocardiography. *Am Heart J*. 1986;111(4):803–805.

91. McAllister H. *Tumors of the Cardiovascular System*. Washington, DC: Armed Forces Institute of Pathology; 1978.

92. Eckhardt BP, et al. Giant cardiac myxoma with malignant transformed glandular structures. *Eur Radiol*. 2003;13(9):2099–2102.

93. Teja K, Gibson RS, Nolan SP. Atrial extension of mitral annular calcification mimicking intracardiac tumor. *Clin Cardiol*. 1987;10(9):546–548.

94. Bosi G, et al. The natural history of cardiac rhabdomyoma with and without tuberous sclerosis. *Acta Paediatr.* 1996;85(8):928–931.

95. Parsons AM, Detterbeck FC. Multifocal right atrial myxoma and pulmonary embolism. *Ann Thorac Surg.* 2003;75(4):1323–1324.

96. Visrutaratna P, Sivasomboon C, Oranratanachai K. Clinics in diagnostic imaging (78). Cardiac rhabdomyoma in tuberous sclerosis. *Singapore Med J.* 2002;43(10):541–546.

97. Jacob B, et al. Unexpected infant death attributable to cardiac tumor or cardiomyopathy. Immunohistochemical and electron microscopical findings in three cases. *Z Rechtsmed.* 1990;103(5):335–343.

98. Burke AP, Virmani R. Cardiac rhabdomyoma: a clinicopathologic study. *Mod Pathol.* 1991;4(1):70–74.

99. Cho JM, et al. Surgical resection of ventricular cardiac fibromas: early and late results. *Ann Thorac Surg.* 2003;76(6):1929–1934.

100. Bapat VN, et al. Right-ventricular fibroma presenting as tricuspid stenosis–a case report. *Thorac Cardiovasc Surg.* 1996;44(3):152–154.

101. Zidere V, Lubaua I, Lacis A. Giant fibroma of the right ventricle. *Cardiol Young.* 2002;12(6):584–586.

102. Williams DB, et al. Cardiac fibroma: long-term survival after excision. *J Thorac Cardiovasc Surg.* 1982;84(2):230–236.

103. Jamieson SW, et al. Operative treatment of an unresectable tumor of the left ventricle. *J Thorac Cardiovasc Surg.* 1981;81(5):797–799.

104. Nadra I, et al. Lipomatous hypertrophy of the interatrial septum: a commonly misdiagnosed mass often leading to unnecessary cardiac surgery. *Heart.* 2004;90(12):e66.

105. Targa L, et al. [Papillary fibroelastoma of the septal leaflet of the tricuspid valve. Report of a case and review of the literature]. *Ital Heart J Suppl.* 2003;4(10):862–865.

106. Abu Saleh WK, et al. Cardiac papillary fibroelastoma: single-institution experience with 14 surgical patients. *Tex Heart Inst J.* 2016;43(2):148–151.

107. Wolf PL, Bing R. The smallest tumor which causes sudden death. *JAMA.* 1965;194(6):674–675.

108. Nishida K, Kamijima G, Nagayama T. Mesothelioma of the atrioventricular node. *Br Heart J.* 1985;53(4):468–470.

109. Lewman LV, Demany MA, Zimmerman HA. Congenital tumor of atrioventricular node with complete heart block and sudden death. Mesothelioma or lymphangioendothelioma of atrioventricular node. *Am J Cardiol.* 1972;29(4):554–557.

110. Igawa T, et al. Surgical resection of malignant lymphoma in the right atrium after systemic chemotherapy. *Intern Med.* 2003;42(4):336–339.

111. Cox JN, et al. Teratoma of the heart. A case report and review of the literature. *Virchows Arch A Pathol Anat Histopathol.* 1983;402(2):163–174.

112. Abu Saleh WK, et al. Case report: a rare case of left atrial hemangioma: surgical resection and reconstruction. *Methodist Debakey Cardiovasc J.* 2016;12(1):51–4.

113. Colli A, et al. Recurrence of a right ventricular hemangioma. *J Thorac Cardiovasc Surg.* 2003;126(3):881–883.

114. Weston CF, et al. Cardiac haemangioma associated with a facial port-wine stain and recurrent atrial tachycardia. *Eur Heart J.* 1988;9(6):668–671.

115. Donsbeck AV, et al. Primary cardiac sarcomas: an immunohistochemical and grading study with long-term follow-up of 24 cases. *Histopathology.* 1999;34(4):295–304.

116. Fyfe AI, et al. Leiomyosarcoma of the left atrium: case report and review of the literature. *Can J Cardiol.* 1991;7(4):193–196.

117. Lajos P, et al. Spindle cell sarcoma of the pericardium: a case report. *J Card Surg.* 2004;19(2):139–141.

118. Janigan DT, Husain A, Robinson NA. Cardiac angiosarcomas. A review and a case report. *Cancer.* 1986;57(4):852–859.

119. Ramlawi B, et al. Surgical treatment of primary cardiac sarcomas: review of a single-institution experience. *Ann Thorac Surg.* 2016;101(2):698–702.

120. Mahdhaoui A, et al. [Right atrium angiosarcoma disclosed by alveolar hemorrhage]. *Rev Med Suisse Romande.* 2004;124(2):115–116.

121. Corso RB, et al. Spontaneous rupture of a right atrial angiosarcoma and cardiac tamponade. *Arq Bras Cardiol.* 2003;81(6):611–613, 608–610.

122. Thomas CR Jr, et al. Primary malignant cardiac tumors: update 1992. *Med Pediatr Oncol.* 1992;20(6):519–531.

123. Korbmacher B, et al. Malignant fibrous histiocytoma of the heart—case report of a rare left-atrial tumor. *Thorac Cardiovasc Surg.* 1992;40(5):303–307.

124. Anghel G, et al. Primary cardiac lymphoma: report of two cases occurring in immunocompetent subjects. *Leuk Lymphoma.* 2004;45(4):781–788.

125. Gowda RM, Khan IA. Clinical perspectives of primary cardiac lymphoma. *Angiology.* 2003;54(5):599–604.

126. Boccardi L, Pino PG. [Primary lymphoma of the right atrium: a case report]. *Ital Heart J Suppl.* 2004;5(6):487–491.

127. Ricchi A, et al. Asymptomatic cardiac lymphoma in a hepatitis C virus-positive thalassemic patient. *Ital Heart J.* 2004;5(4):302–304.

128. Barbaric D, et al. It is ALL in the heart: a patient with acute lymphoblastic leukemia and cardiac infiltration at time of diagnosis. *Leuk Lymphoma.* 2002;43(12):2417–2419.

129. Potenza L, et al. Cardiac involvement in malignancies. Case 2. Right ventricular lesion as presenting feature of acute promyelocytic leukemia. *J Clin Oncol.* 2004;22(13):2742–2744.

130. Carnero Fernandez M, et al. [Massive venous thrombosis with cardiac invasion as primary manifestation of hepatocarcinoma]. *An Med Interna.* 2003;20(10):537–539.

131. Kubota H, et al. Surgical treatment of malignant tumors of the right heart. *Jpn Heart J.* 2002;43(3):263–271.

132. Lazaros G, et al. Growth of hepatocellular carcinoma into the right atrium. A case of antemortem diagnosis with magnetic resonance imaging of the heart. *Acta Cardiol.* 2003;58(6):563–565.

133. Fujiwara K, et al. Successful one-stage surgical removal of intravenous uterine leiomyomatosis with right heart xtension. *Jpn J Thorac Cardiovasc Surg.* 2003;51(9):462–465.

134. Jerez Anera M, Delange Segura L, Carmona Aurioles J. [Uterine leiomyoma with cardiac extension: anesthetic management]. *Rev Esp Anestesiol Reanim.* 2004;51(1):40–43.

135. Horvath G, et al. [Surgical treatment of malignant renal tumors invading the inferior vena cava and right atrium]. *Magy Seb.* 2003;56(6):239–241.

136. Messner G, et al. Surgical management of metastatic melanoma to the ventricle. *Tex Heart Inst J.* 2003;30(3):218–220.

137. Loffler H, Grille W. Classification of malignant cardiac tumors with respect to oncological treatment. *Thorac Cardiovasc Surg.* 1990;38(suppl 2):173–175.

138. Collins HA, Collins IS. Clinical experience with cardiac myxoma. *Ann Thorac Surg.* 1972;13(5):450–457.

139. Zuo XY, Xu SY. [A case of non-Hodgkin's lymphomas metastasize to the cardiac right atrium]. *Hunan Yi Ke Da Xue Xue Bao.* 2002;27(2):175.

140. Masci G, et al. Metastasis of hepatocellular carcinoma to the heart: a case report and review of the literature. *Tumori.* 2004;90(3):345–347.

141. Koizumi J, et al. Solitary cardiac metastasis of rectal adenocarcinoma. *Jpn J Thorac Cardiovasc Surg.* 2003;51(7):330–332.

142. Stefka J, et al. Sarcomatoid intracardiac metastasis of a testicular germ cell tumor closely resembling primary cardiac sarcoma. *Hum Pathol.* 2003;34(10):1074–1077.

143. Shafique QS, Rajesh CM, Rakesh SN. Cardiac metastases of osteosarcoma. *J Coll Physicians Surg Pak.* 2004;14(7):430–432.

144. Harting MT, et al. Sarcoma metastatic to the right ventricle: surgical intervention followed by prolonged survival. *Tex Heart Inst J.* 2004;31(1):93–95.

145. Markiewicz W, et al. Echocardiographic detection of pericardial effusion and pericardial thickening in malignant lymphoma. *Radiology.* 1977;123(1):161–164.

146. Hermans K, et al. Four cardiac myxomas diagnosed three times in one patient. *Eur J Echocardiogr.* 2003;4(4):336–338.

147. McCarthy PM, et al. The significance of multiple, recurrent, and "complex" cardiac myxomas. *J Thorac Cardiovasc Surg.* 1986;91(3):389–396.

148. Castells E, et al. Cardiac myxomas: surgical treatment, long-term results and recurrence. *J Cardiovasc Surg (Torino).* 1993;34(1):49–53.

149. Evans BJ, Haw MP. Surgical clearance of invasive cardiac leiomyosarcoma with concomitant pneumonectomy. *Eur J Cardiothorac Surg.* 2003;24(5):843–846.

150. Hanson EC, et al. The surgical treatment of atrial myxomas. Clinical experience and late results in 33 patients. *J Thorac Cardiovasc Surg.* 1985;89(2):298–303.

151. Livi U, et al. Cardiac myxomas: results of 14 years' experience. *Thorac Cardiovasc Surg.* 1984;32(3):143–147.

152. Richardson JV, et al. Surgical treatment of atrial myxomas: early and late results of 11 operations and review of the literature. *Ann Thorac Surg.* 1979;28(4):354–358.

153. Semb BK, et al. Angiographic and echocardiographic observations in surgical patients with atrial myxoma. *Cardiovasc Intervent Radiol.* 1985;8(3):119–126.

154. Carney JA, et al. The complex of myxomas, spotty pigmentation, and endocrine overactivity. *Medicine (Baltimore).* 1985;64(4):270–283.

155. Truong PT, et al. Treatment and outcomes in adult patients with primary cardiac sarcoma: the British Columbia Cancer Agency experience. *Ann Surg Oncol.* 2009;16(12):3358–3365.

156. Mayer F, et al. Primary malignant sarcomas of the heart and great vessels in adult patients–a single-center experience. *Oncologist.* 2007;12(9):1134–1142.

157. Simpson L, et al. Malignant primary cardiac tumors: review of a single institution experience. *Cancer.* 2008;112(11):2440–2446.

158. Babatasi G, et al. Leiomyosarcoma of the pulmonary veins extending into the left atrium or left atrial leiomyosarcoma: multimodality therapy. *J Thorac Cardiovasc Surg.* 1998;116(4):665–667.

159. Percy RF, et al. Prolonged survival in a patient with primary angiosarcoma of the heart. *Am Heart J.* 1987;113(5):1228–1230.

160. Pessotto R, et al. Primary cardiac leiomyosarcoma: seven-year survival with combined surgical and adjuvant therapy. *Int J Cardiol.* 1997;60(1):91–94.

161. Rhomberg W, Grass M. [Angiosarcoma of the right atrium: local control via low radiation doses and razoxane. A case report]. *Strahlenther Onkol.* 1999;175(3):102–104.

162. Cormier JN, Pollock RE. Soft tissue sarcomas. *CA Cancer J Clin.* 2004;54(2):94–109.

163. Fata F, et al. Paclitaxel in the treatment of patients with angiosarcoma of the scalp or face. *Cancer.* 1999;86(10):2034–2037.

164. Penel N, et al. Phase II trial of weekly paclitaxel for unresectable angiosarcoma: the ANGIOTAX Study. *J Clin Oncol.* 2008;26(32):5269–5274.

165. Sarcoma Meta-analysis Collaboration (SMAC). Adjuvant chemotherapy for localised resectable soft tissue sarcoma in adults. *Cochrane Database Syst Rev.* 2000;(2):CD001419.

166. Fernandez PM, Rickles FR. Tissue factor and angiogenesis in cancer. *Curr Opin Hematol.* 2002;9(5):401–406.

167. Ganjoo K, Jacobs C. Antiangiogenesis agents in the treatment of soft tissue sarcomas. *Cancer.* 2010;116(5):1177–1183.

168. Quackenbush J. Microarray analysis and tumor classification. *N Engl J Med.* 2006;354(23):2463–2472.

169. Graadt van Roggen JF, et al. Diagnostic and prognostic implications of the unfolding molecular biology of bone and soft tissue tumours. *J Clin Pathol.* 1999;52(7):481–489.

170. Tomescu O, Barr FG. Chromosomal translocations in sarcomas: prospects for therapy. *Trends Mol Med.* 2001;7(12):554–559.

171. Ginsberg JP, et al. EWS-FLI1 and EWS-ERG gene fusions are associated with similar clinical phenotypes in Ewing's sarcoma. *J Clin Oncol.* 1999;17(6):1809–1814.

172. Zucman J, et al. EWS and ATF-1 gene fusion induced by t(12;22) translocation in malignant melanoma of soft parts. *Nat Genet.* 1993;4(4):341–345.

173. Kelly KM, et al. Common and variant gene fusions predict distinct clinical phenotypes in rhabdomyosarcoma. *J Clin Oncol*. 1997;15(5):1831–1836.

174. Sorensen PH, et al. PAX3-FKHR and PAX7-FKHR gene fusions are prognostic indicators in alveolar rhabdomyosarcoma: a report from the children's oncology group. *J Clin Oncol*. 2002;20(11):2672–2679.

175. Guillou L, et al. Histologic grade, but not SYT-SSX fusion type, is an important prognostic factor in patients with synovial sarcoma: a multicenter, retrospective analysis. *J Clin Oncol*. 2004;22(20):4040–4050.

176. Ladanyi M, et al. Impact of SYT-SSX fusion type on the clinical behavior of synovial sarcoma: a multi-institutional retrospective study of 243 patients. *Cancer Res*. 2002;62(1):135–140.

177. Man TK, et al. Expression profiles of osteosarcoma that can predict response to chemotherapy. *Cancer Res*. 2005;65(18):8142–8150.

178. Momand J, Zambetti GP. Mdm-2: "big brother" of p53. *J Cell Biochem*. 1997;64(3):343–352.

179. Hueman MT, et al. Management of extremity soft tissue sarcomas. *Surg Clin North Am*. 2008;88(3):539–557, vi.

180. Murphy MC, et al. Surgical treatment of cardiac tumors: a 25-year experience. *Ann Thorac Surg*. 1990;49(4):612–617; discussion 617–618.

181. Wippermann J, et al. Redo- extirpation of a cardiac leiomyosarcoma to avoid transplantation. *Thorac Cardiovasc Surg*. 2002;50(1):62–63.

Saamir A. Hassan

INTRODUCTION

Carcinoid disease is caused by rare neuroendocrine tumors that most commonly arise from the gastrointestinal (GI) tract but may also originate in the lungs or, more rarely, in other organs. The most common locations of GI carcinoids are the appendix and the terminal ileum. The most malignant carcinoid tumors arise in the ileum and metastasize to produce the well-described clinical picture of carcinoid syndrome. Patients with carcinoid syndrome present with vasomotor changes, hypermotility of the GI tract, hypotension, and bronchospasm; ultimately, changes in cardiac valves add to the clinical picture seen in patients with advanced or late-stage carcinoid disease.

Carcinoid heart disease is the initial presentation of carcinoid disease in as many as 20% of patients and occurs in more than 50% of patients with carcinoid syndrome.[1,2] Carcinoid heart disease usually involves the right-sided structures of the heart. Less frequently, but more commonly in patients with primary carcinoid in the lung, left-sided valvular involvement is evident. Although carcinoid heart disease is rare, it can lead to substantial morbidity and mortality.

ETIOLOGY AND PATHOPHYSIOLOGY

The incidence of carcinoid tumors is 1 or 2 cases per 100,000 population. The sites most commonly affected by carcinoid tumors are the GI tract (73.7%) and the bronchopulmonary system (25.1%). Within the GI tract, the small bowel (28.7%), appendix (18.9%), and rectum (12.6%) are the most common sites of involvement.[3] Invasive or metastatic carcinoid tumors can manifest themselves in cardiac structures because of the release of vasoactive substances such as serotonin, bradykinin, tachykinins, prostaglandins, and histamine.

The characteristic finding of carcinoid heart disease is plaque-like deposits of fibrous tissue. These carcinoid plaques are composed of smooth muscle cells, myofibroblasts, extracellular matrix, and an overlying endothelial layer. The fibrous deposits may involve the tricuspid valve, the pulmonary valve, the cardiac chambers, the pulmonary artery, the vena cava, and the coronary sinus.[2,3] The fibrous reaction occurs most commonly on the endocardium of the valvular cusps, but it can also involve the subvalvular apparatus and the papillary muscles. These fibrous deposits can lead to stenosis or regurgitation of the valve, although regurgitation is more common. The ventricular aspects of the tricuspid valve and the arterial aspects of the pulmonary valve are generally affected.[4] Right-sided carcinoid heart disease is most common because of inactivation of humoral substances by the lung. However, left-sided involvement is seen in 5%–10% of cases and is usually associated with a right-to-left intracardiac shunt, extensive liver metastases, or bronchial carcinoid.[1,2,5,6]

Although the cause of this fibrous plaque formation is not entirely clear, animal studies have implicated serotonin and bradykinin in its development.[7] Alterations in the metabolism of serotonin, its associated receptors, and a transporter gene have been proposed as mechanisms of serotonin-induced carcinoid heart disease.[8,9] Furthermore, indirect evidence indicating that serotonin levels are higher in patients with known carcinoid heart disease than in patients without carcinoid heart disease points to the role of high serotonin levels as an important contributor to the development of carcinoid heart disease.[10–12]

CLINICAL PRESENTATION AND DIAGNOSIS

The symptoms of carcinoid heart disease usually manifest themselves in patients in the fifth through seventh decades of life. Because the clinical manifestations are often subtle early in the course of the disease, a high index of suspicion is necessary for the diagnosis of carcinoid heart disease. In addition, a time lag of 2 to 5 years can exist between the onset of symptoms and the confirmation of the diagnosis.[13–15] Patients usually present with fatigue and shortness of breath. As the disease progresses, right-sided heart failure with edema, ascites, and dyspnea ensues.

Cardiac physical examination often detects murmurs caused by tricuspid regurgitation and pulmonary valve stenosis; initially the murmurs may be soft, but they generally progress and become harsher over time. Jugular venous pressure is usually elevated, and a right ventricular impulse is palpable. Indications of advanced disease are peripheral edema, ascites, and hepatomegaly due to right ventricular failure. In 30%–50% of cases the results of electrocardiography are normal; in other cases, these results may show low voltage, nonspecific ST segment changes, and, commonly, sinus tachycardia. A right bundle branch block may also be seen.[1,16] Chest radiographs can demonstrate cardiomegaly, prominent right-sided cardiac chambers, and mild pulmonary congestion.

A key tool for diagnosing carcinoid heart disease is the measurement of urinary excretion of 5-hydroxyindoleacetic acid (5-HIAA) over 24 hours. Metastatic carcinoid tumors take up tryptophan and, though a biochemical pathway (Figure 15-1), metabolize it to serotonin. Serotonin is later broken down into 5-HIAA, which is excreted almost exclusively in the urine; therefore, patients with carcinoid heart disease exhibit elevated levels of 5-HIAA. In one series of patients with carcinoid heart disease, the mean 24-hour urinary excretion of 5-HIAA was more than 10-fold higher than the reference value.[15,16]

A study from the Mayo Clinic showed that urinary excretion of 5-HIAA may also predict the progression of carcinoid heart disease. In that study, which involved 71 patients, a cardiac score was used to evaluate the progression and severity of disease. Patients with an increase of more than 25% in the cardiac score exhibited significantly higher levels of urinary excretion of 5-HIAA.[13]

Echocardiography plays an important role in the detection of carcinoid heart disease. In addition, because the extent of cardiac involvement is the main predictor of clinical outcomes for patients with the carcinoid syndrome, echocardiography can also quantify the extent of disease and document the progression of valvular lesions. As noted above, carcinoid heart disease usually involves the tricuspid and pulmonary valves. Cardiac ultrasonography can often show thickening, retraction, and, sometimes, immobility of the tricuspid valve leaflets, abnormalities that lead to tricuspid regurgitation. Moderate to severe tricuspid regurgitation may be seen in as many as 90% of patients with carcinoid heart disease; tricuspid stenosis is less common (Figures 15-2 and 15-3).[1] The continuous Doppler profile of tricuspid regurgitation shows a characteristic dagger-shaped spectrum with early peak pressure and rapid decline (Figure 15-4). Often, the pulmonary valve is also involved, and this involvement leads to immobility of the pulmonic valve cusps, valve regurgitation, and, less commonly, stenosis.[17]

In the largest reported series of 74 carcinoid patients with comprehensive echocardiographic data, the following spectrum of structural heart disease was noted: all patients had tricuspid valve regurgitation, and moderate to severe regurgitation was present in 90% of cases. Pulmonary valve regurgitation was present in 81% of patients, and pulmonary valve stenosis was present in 53%. Left-sided valve involvement was seen in 7% of patients, and a small pericardial effusion was seen in 14%.[1] The combination of severe tricuspid valve regurgitation and pulmonary valve stenosis may be particularly problematic because the stenotic right ventricular outflow valve exacerbates the degree of tricuspid regurgitation, thereby furthering right-heart failure.[17]

Cardiac magnetic resonance imaging (MRI) is of additional value in carcinoid heart disease because it improves diagnostic accuracy when echocardiographic image quality is suboptimal (Figure 15-5).[18] Cardiac MRI also allows velocity-encoded phase contrast sequences that can quantify the degree of dysfunction, whether it be regurgitation or stenosis, of the tricuspid and pulmonary valves.[19] Furthermore, fibrotic carcinoid

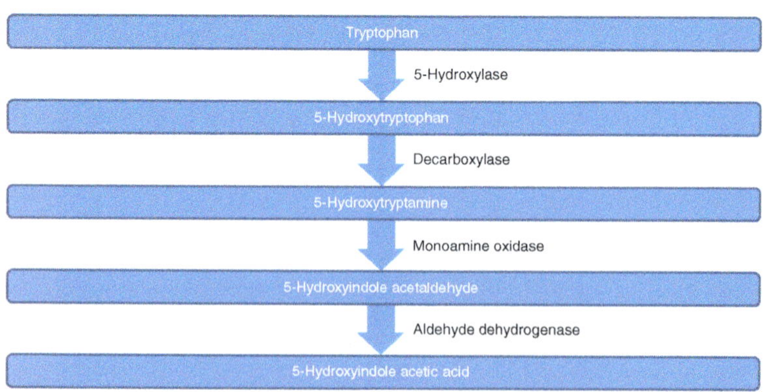

FIGURE 15-1 Biochemical pathway of the synthesis and degradation of serotonin (5-hydroxytryptamine).

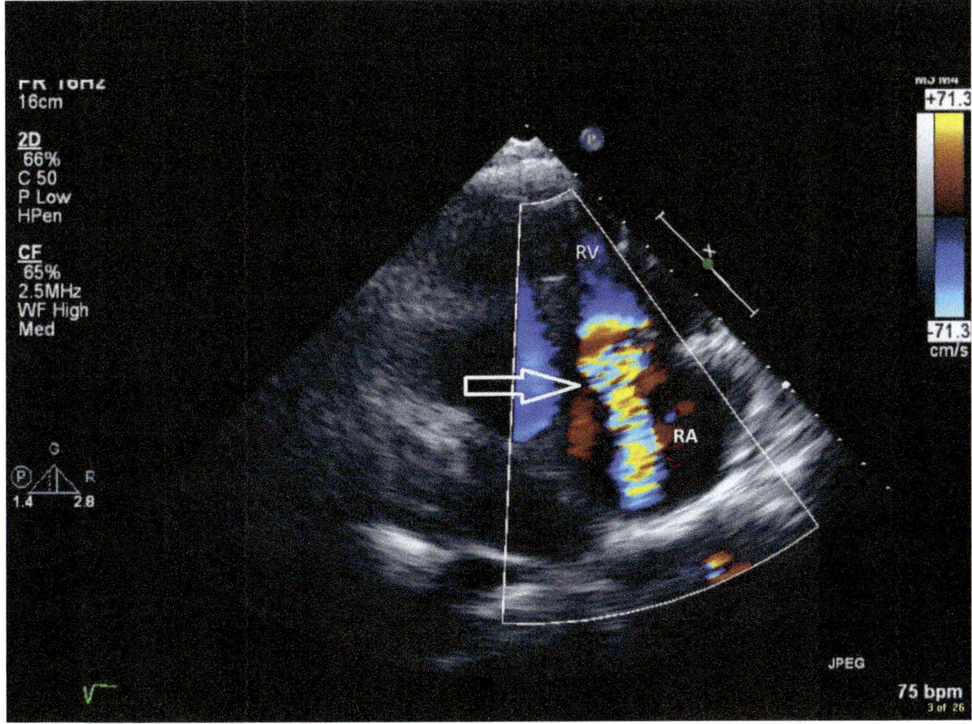

FIGURE 15-2 Transthoracic echocardiogram from a modified right-ventricular inflow view, showing thickened, fixed, non-coapting tricuspid valve leaflets (arrow). RA, right atrium; RV, right ventricle.

FIGURE 15-3 Transthoracic echocardiogram from a modified right-ventricular inflow view, showing color flow Doppler imaging of severe tricuspid valve regurgitation (Arrow). RA, right atrium; RV, right ventricle.

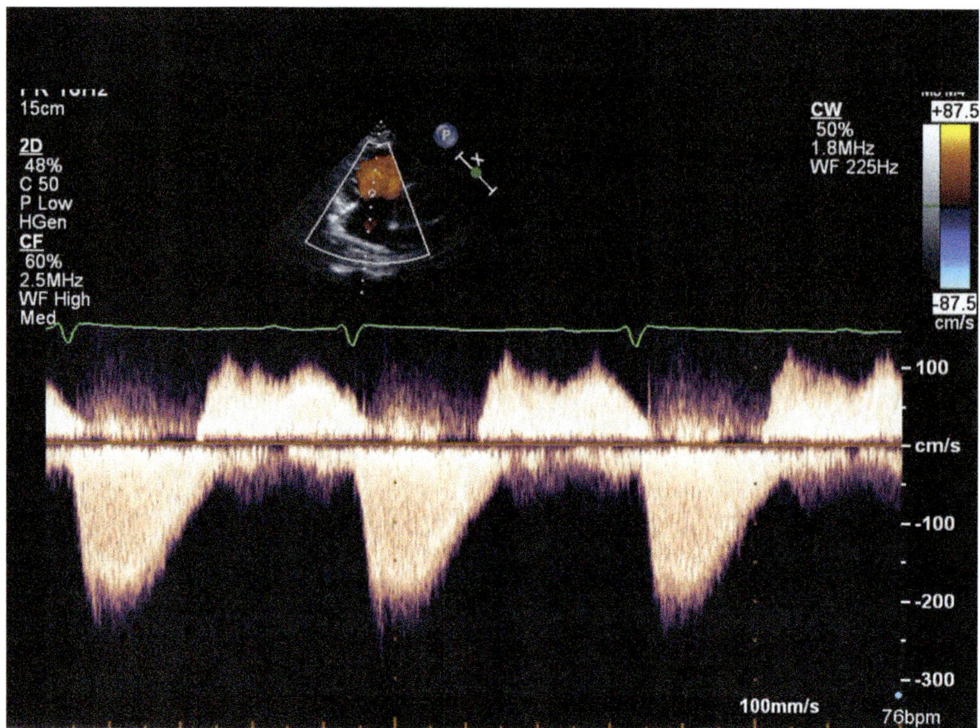

FIGURE 15-4 Continuous flow Doppler image of severe tricuspid regurgitation, showing the characteristic dagger shape with early peak pressure and rapid decline.

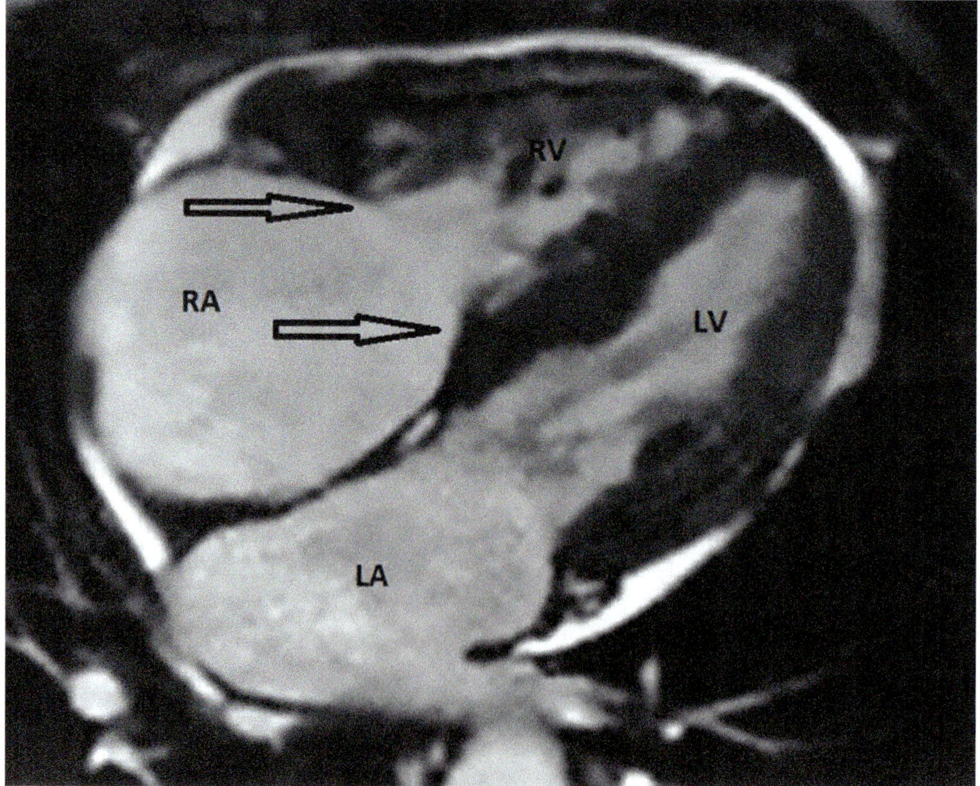

FIGURE 15-5 Cardiac magnetic resonance image showing a four-chamber view with non-coaptation of the tricuspid valve leaflets (arrows) during systole. RA, right atrium; RV, right ventricle; LA, left atrium; LV, left ventricle.

plaques can be detected by cardiac MRI using delayed-enhancement imaging with gadolinium. Late enhancement and thickening can be seen in the valve leaflets, the annulus, and the endocardium of the right ventricle and the right ventricular outflow tract.[20]

MANAGEMENT

The overall prognosis for patients with advanced disease is poor; most patients die in less than one year as the result of progressive right-sided heart failure.[21] Treatment goals are limited to palliation and symptom management.

Somatostatin analogs have been used to provide symptomatic relief for patients with carcinoid disease. Octreotide, an eight-amino-acid peptide, binds to somatostatin receptors and directly reduces the levels of the vasoactive peptides that are responsible for some of the symptoms of carcinoid syndrome. Approximately 70% of patients obtain some relief from symptoms of diarrhea and flushing, along with a concomitant decrease in levels of 5-HIAA in urine and serum. However, treatment with somatostatin analogs does not appear to affect valve disease. Although such therapy causes substantial declines in 5-HIAA levels, existing valvular disease does not regress.[1,3,12] In the rare circumstance that carcinoid heart disease is caused by an ovarian carcinoid tumor without liver metastases, surgical procedures, although they are curative with regard to the primary tumor, do not lead to regression of cardiac lesions.[22]

Medical therapy for heart failure is usually limited to the administration of diuretics. A regimen of salt and water restriction, careful monitoring of fluid balance, the use of compression stockings, and treatment of heart failure with loop diuretics is often used. Although diuretics improve the degree of edema, they may increase the patient's level of fatigue and can adversely affect blood pressure by reducing left-sided cardiac output.

Valve surgery is the only definitive treatment for carcinoid heart disease and should be considered for patients with symptomatic but controlled metastatic carcinoid syndrome. Furthermore, surgery should be performed early after the onset of cardiac symptoms, because delay can worsen right-sided heart failure and increase the risks associated with surgery. Patients with progressive fatigue, worsening exercise capability, and declining right ventricular function in the presence of controlled metastatic disease should be evaluated for valve surgery.

Tricuspid valve replacement is the surgical procedure of choice; however, the choice of valve prosthesis requires thoughtful discussion and careful patient selection. Mechanical prostheses are believed to be durable and unaffected by vasoactive substances, but they require the administration of anticoagulants, which may increase the risk of bleeding for patients with extensive liver disease.[17,21] The risk of thrombosis with mechanical tricuspid valves is approximately 4% per year for all patients.[23] In contrast, bioprosthetic valves do not require the administration of anticoagulants but are susceptible to premature degeneration among patients with carcinoid heart disease. It is believed that bioprosthetic valve dysfunction may be caused by thrombosis, carcinoid plaque deposition, or accelerated degeneration.[24,25] Pulmonary valve replacement and valvectomy have also been used to treat patients with pulmonary valve carcinoid disease, and, although available data are limited, a small study found that pulmonary valve replacement may be the method of choice because it reduces the risk of adverse right-heart dilation after the surgical procedure.[26]

Special consideration should be given to patients who have hepatic carcinoid disease and require surgery. Patients with severe carcinoid heart disease are not candidates for hepatic surgery because of the risk of hepatic hemorrhage induced by elevated right-sided pressures; therefore, cardiac surgical intervention can be considered for this group of patients even though they exhibit minimal cardiac symptoms.[27]

Because anesthesia can precipitate carcinoid storm among patients with carcinoid syndrome, these patients require treatment with an intravenous bolus or a continuous infusion of a somatostatin, which reduces the risk of this complication during the perioperative period. Patients with carcinoid storm exhibit profound changes in blood pressure, as well as arrhythmias, bronchoconstriction, confusion, and flushing. Treatment with antihistamines can reduce flushing and bronchospasm, and treatment with corticosteroids can reduce the production of bradykinin.[17,28–30]

PROGNOSIS OF PATIENTS WITH CARCINOID HEART DISEASE

Valve surgery may increase patients' longevity and quality of life; however, studies have found that the operative mortality rate is high (35%–63%) because of postoperative bleeding and heart failure and because of difficulty in weaning patients from cardiopulmonary bypass.[14,21,31] Other studies have found that survival times are longer for patients undergoing valve replacement surgery than for those treated with medical therapy. Operative outcome is improving as the result of better patient selection and earlier surgical intervention before the onset of advanced or symptomatic cardiac decompensation.[32]

REFERENCES

1. Pellikka PA, Tajik AJ, Khandheria BK, et al. Carcinoid heart disease. Clinical and echocardiographic spectrum in 74 patients. *Circulation*. 1993;87(4):1188–1196.
2. Lundin L, Norheim I, Landelius J, Oberg K, Theodorsson-Norheim E. Carcinoid heart disease: relationship of circulating vasoactive substances to ultrasound-detectable cardiac abnormalities. *Circulation*. 1988;77(2):264–269.
3. Modlin IM, Sandor A. An analysis of 8305 cases of carcinoid tumors. *Cancer*. 1997;79:813–829.
4. Pandya UH, Pellikka PA, Enriquez-Sarano M, Edwards WE, Schaff HV, Connolly HM. Metastatic carcinoid tumor to the heart: echocardiographic-pathologic study of 11 patients. *J Am Coll Cardiol*. 2002;40(7):1328–1332.
5. Schweizer W, Gloor F, Von Bertrab R, Dubach UC. Carcinoid heart disease with left-sided lesions. *Circulation*. 1964;29:253–257.
6. Strickman NE, Rossi PA, Massumkhani GA, Hall RJ. Carcinoid heart disease: a clinical pathologic, and therapeutic update. *Curr Prob Cardiol*. 1982;6(11):1–42.
7. Spatz M. Pathogenetic studies of experimentally induced heart lesions and their relation to the carcinoid syndrome. *Lab Invest*. 1964;13:288–300.
8. Chaowalit N, Connolly HM, Schaff HV, Webb MJ, Pellikka PA. Carcinoid heart disease associated with primary ovarian carcinoid tumor. *Am J Cardiol*. 2004;93(10):1314–1315.
9. Roth BL. Drugs and valvular heart disease. *N Engl J Med*. 2007;356(1):6–9.
10. Simula DV, Edwards WD, Tazelaar HD, Connolly HM, Schaff HV. Surgical pathology of carcinoid heart disease: a study of 139 valves from 75 patients spanning 20 years. *Mayo Clin Proc*. 2002;77(2):139–147.
11. Robiolio PA, Rigolin VH, Wilson JS, et al. Carcinoid heart disease. Correlation of high serotonin levels with valvular abnormalities detected by cardiac catheterization and echocardiography. *Circulation*. 1995;92(4):790–795.
12. Denney WD, Kemp WE Jr, Anthony LB, Oates JA, Byrd BF 3rd. Echocardiographic and biochemical evaluation of the development and progression of carcinoid heart disease. *J Am Coll Cardiol*. 1998;32(4):1017–1022.
13. Zuetenhorst JM, Bonfrer JM, Korse CM, Bakker R, van Tinteren H, Taal BG. Carcinoid heart disease: the role of urinary 5-hydroxyindoleacetic acid excretion and plasma levels of atrial natriuretic peptide, transforming growth factor-beta and fibroblast growth factor. *Cancer*. 2003;97(7):1609–1615.
14. Connolly HM, Schaff HV, Mullany CJ, Rubin J, Abel MD, Pellikka PA. Surgical management of left-sided carcinoid heart disease. *Circulation*. 2001;104(12 suppl 1):I36–I40.
15. Møller JE, Connolly HM, Rubin J, Seward JB, Modesto K, Pellikka PA. Factors associated with the progression of carcinoid heart disease. *N Engl J Med*. 2003;348(11):1005–1015.
16. Westberg G, Wängberg H, Ahlman C, Bergh CH, Beckman-Suurküla M, Caidahl K. Prediction of prognosis by echocardiography in patients with midgut carcinoid syndrome. *Br J Surg*. 2001;88(6):865–872.
17. Fox DJ, Khattar RS. Carcinoid heart disease: presentation, diagnosis, and management. *Heart*. 2004;90(10):1224–1228.
18. Bastarrika G, Cao MG, Cano D, Barba J, de Buruaga JD. Magnetic resonance imaging diagnosis of carcinoid heart disease. *J Comput Assist Tomogr*. 2005;29(6):756–759.
19. Sandmann H, Pakkal M, Steeds R. Cardiovascular magnetic resonance imaging in the assessment of carcinoid heart disease. *Clin Radiol*. 2009;64(8):761–766.
20. Moerman VM, Dewilde D, Hermans K. Carcinoid heart disease: typical findings on echocardiography and cardiac magnetic resonance. *Acta Cardiol*. 2012;67(2):245–258.
21. Connolly HM, Nishimura RA, Smith HC, Pellikka PA, Mullany CJ, Kvols LK. Outcome of cardiac surgery for carcinoid heart disease. *J Am Coll Cardiol*. 1995;25(2):410–416.
22. Robboy SJ, Norris HJ, Scully RE. Insular carcinoid primary in the ovary. A clinicopathologic analysis of 48 cases. *Cancer*. 1975;36(2):404–418.
23. Thorburn CW, Morgan JJ, Shanahan MX, Chang VP. Long-term results of tricuspid valve replacement and the problem of prosthetic valve thrombosis. *Am J Cardiol*. 1983;51(7):1128–1132.
24. Ridker PM, Chertow GM, Karlson EW, Neish AS, Schoen FJ. Bioprosthetic tricuspid valve stenosis associated with extensive plaque deposition in carcinoid heart disease. *Am Heart J*. 1991;121(6 pt 1):1835–1838.
25. Pislaru SV, Hussain I, Pellikka PA, et al. Misconceptions, diagnostic challenges and treatment opportunities in bioprosthetic valve thrombosis: lessons from a case series. *Eur J Cardiothorac Surg*. 2015;47(4):725–732.
26. Connolly HM, Schaff HV, Mullany CJ, Abel MD, Pellikka PA. Carcinoid heart disease: impact of pulmonary valve replacement in right ventricular function and remodeling. *Circulation*. 2002;106(12 suppl 1):I51–I56.
27. McDonald ML, Nagorney DM, Connolly HM, Nishimura RA, Schaff HV. Carcinoid heart disease and carcinoid syndrome: successful surgical treatment. *Ann Thorac Surg*. 1999;67(2):537–539.
28. Mason RA, Steane PA. Carcinoid syndrome: its relevance to the anaesthetist. *Anaesthesia*. 1976;31(2):228–242.
29. Vaughan DJ, Brunner MD. Anesthesia for patients with carcinoid syndrome. *Int Anesthesiol Clin*. 1997;35(4):129–142.
30. Weingarten TN, Abel MD, Connolly HM, Schroeder DR, Schaff HV. Intraoperative management of patients with carcinoid heart disease having valvular surgery: a review of one hundred consecutive cases. *Anesth Analg*. 2007;105(5):1192–1199.
31. Robiolio PA, Rigolin VH, Harrison JK, et al. Predictors of outcome of tricuspid valve replacement in carcinoid heart disease. *Am J Cardiol*. 1995;75(7):485–488.
32. Møller JE, Pellikka PA, Bernheim AM, Schaff HV, Rubin J, Connolly HM. Prognosis of carcinoid heart disease: analysis of 200 cases over two decades. *Circulation*. 2005;112(21):3320–3327.

16 Cardiac Monitoring During Clinical Trials

Nicolas Palaskas ▪ *Michael Ewer*

INTRODUCTION

Every year there is continued innovation and production of new cancer therapeutic drugs.[1] Personalized medicine and improved genomics has led to a shift in development of more targeted therapies for a variety of cancers. Five new cancer therapeutic drugs were added by the U.S. Food and Drug Administration (FDA) in 2016 alone, which adds to a list of over 200 approved therapies.[1] These drugs are clearly effective as evidenced by the 15.5 million cancer survivors in 2016 which is expected to increase to 20.3 million over the next decade.[1] Various cardiotoxicities from cancer therapeutics have been described beginning with doxorubicin induced cardiomyopathy almost a half century ago.[2] As cancer survivorship has increased, the early and late cardiotoxicity of cancer therapeutics has been increasingly recognized as an important knowledge gap that needs to be addressed. In 2013, the National Cancer Institute (NCI) and the National Heart, Lung, and Blood Institute (NHLBI) came together to discuss the state of cancer treatment related cardiotoxicity in a two day workshop in Bethesda, Maryland.[3] Various cardiotoxicities, that include cardiomyopathy but extend to many more cardiac conditions, have been realized as side effects from the introduction of newer cancer drugs. With the realization of cardiotoxicity playing a crucial role in long term survivorship, clinical trials of cancer therapeutics have changed to better evaluate cardiac side effects. In this chapter we present the evolution of defining cardiotoxicity and focus on cardiomyopathy monitoring in various clinical trials.

DEFINING CARDIOTOXICITY

To better identify and study cardiotoxicity, one of the first steps, as recommended by the 2013 NCI-NHLBI workshop, was to implement a uniform grading of cardiac toxicities.[3] Oncologic trials often use a standardized reporting of toxicities including cardiac and non-cardiac events. In 1983, the NCI developed the common toxicity criteria (CTC) which through many new versions and editions has now become the common terminology criteria for adverse events (CTCAE). Each new version of the CTCAE introduces more specific definitions, severity criteria, and modifies adverse event nomenclature. Currently, the CTCAE just introduced version 5.0 in April 2018. Each toxicity is graded for severity scaled from 1 to 5: grade 1–mild, grade 2–moderate, grade 3–severe, grade 4–life-threatening or disabling, and grade 5–death. Of note, previous CTCAE versions did not include grade 5–death which was added on the 4th version. Also, previous versions of the CTCAE split cardiac toxicities into two sections; "cardiac arrhythmia" and "cardiac general." Newer versions have included definitions of each toxicity and lumped all cardiac toxicities into one section, "cardiac disorders." Examples of such definitions include "heart failure" with the definition listed as "a disorder characterized by the inability of the heart to pump blood at an adequate volume to meet tissue metabolic requirements, or, the ability to do so only at an elevation in the filling pressure." (Table 16-1). Also there is "left ventricular systolic dysfunction" with the definition being "a disorder characterized by failure of the left ventricle to produce adequate output." (Table 16-1). With the introduction of CTCAE version 5.0 there were significant changes in the definition of "left ventricular systolic dysfunction." Per CTCAE version 4.03 it was defined as "a disorder characterized by failure of the left ventricle to produce adequate output despite an increase in distending pressure and in end-diastolic volume. Clinical manifestations may include dyspnea, orthopnea, and other signs and symptoms of pulmonary congestion and edema" (Table 16-1). While more specific definitions of cardiac toxicities are being made, how cardiotoxicity is monitored is still variable and difficult to define in practice and current clinical trials. Under the category "investigations" the adverse event listed as "ejection fraction decrease" lists rather arbitrary cut-offs for left ventricular ejection fraction as below:

Grade 1–None

Grade 2–Resting ejection fraction 40%–50%; 10%–19% drop from baseline

Grade 3–Resting ejection fraction 20%–39%; ≥ 20% drop from baseline

Grade 4–Resting ejection fraction <20%

Grade 5–None

TABLE 16-1　　CCTCAE cardiac disorders

CTCAE VERSION 5.0						
Adverse Event	**Definition and Grades**					
Heart Failure	Definition: A disorder characterized by the inability of the heart to pump blood at an adequate volume to meet tissue metabolic requirements, or, the ability to do so only at an elevation in the filling pressure.					
	Grade	1	2	3	4	5
		Asymptomatic with laboratory (e.g., BNP [B-Natriuretic Peptide]) or cardiac imaging abnormalities	Symptoms with moderate activity or exertion	Symptoms at rest or with minimal activity or exertion; hospitalization; new onset of symptoms	Life-threatening consequences; urgent intervention indicated (e.g., continuous IV therapy or mechanical hemodynamic support)	Death
Left ventricular systolic dysfunction	Definition: A disorder characterized by failure of the left ventricle to produce adequate output.					
	Grade	1	2	3	4	5
		-	-	Symptomatic due to drop in ejection fraction responsive to intervention	Refractory or poorly controlled heart failure due to drop in ejection fraction; intervention such as ventricular assist device, intravenous vasopressor support, or heart transplant indicated	Death
CTCAE VERSION 4.03						
Adverse Event	**Definition and Grades**					
Heart Failure	Definition: A disorder characterized by the inability of the heart to pump blood at an adequate volume to meet tissue metabolic requirements, or, the ability to do so only at an elevation in the filling pressure.					
	Grade	1	2	3	4	5

(continued)

CTCAE VERSION 5.0					
Adverse Event	**Definition and Grades**				
		Asymptomatic with laboratory (e.g., BNP [B-Natriuretic Peptide]) or cardiac imaging abnormalities	Symptoms with mild to moderate activity or exertion	Severe with symptoms at rest or with minimal activity or exertion; intervention indicated	Life-threatening consequences; urgent intervention indicated (e.g., continuous IV therapy or mechanical hemodynamic support)	Death
Left ventricular systolic dysfunction	Definition: A disorder characterized by failure of the left ventricle to produce adequate output despite an increase in distending pressure and in end-diastolic volume. Clinical manifestations may include dyspnea, orthopnea, and other signs and symptoms of pulmonary congestion and edema.				
	Grade	1	2	3	4	5
		-	-	Symptomatic due to drop in ejection fraction responsive to intervention	Refractory or poorly controlled heart failure due to drop in ejection fraction; intervention such as ventricular assist device, intravenous vasopressor support, or heart transplant indicated	Death

The most specific description of cardiomyopathy was formulated by the Cardiac Review and Evaluation Committee (CREC) supervising trastuzumab clinical trials, who defined drug-associated cardiotoxicity as one or more of the following: 1) cardiomyopathy characterized by a decrease in left ventricular ejection fraction (LVEF) globally or due to regional changes in interventricular septum contraction; 2) symptoms associated with heart failure (HF); 3) signs associated with HF, such as S3 gallop, tachycardia, or both; 4) decline in initial left ventricular ejection fraction (LVEF) of at least 5% to less than 55% with signs and symptoms of heart failure or asymptomatic decrease in LVEF of at least 10% to less than 55%.[4] This is similar but not identical to the American Society of Echocardiography (ASE) expert consensus statement by Plana et al. that defined chemotherapeutic related cardiac dysfunction (CTRCD) as a decrease in LVEF by 10% or to below LVEF 53%.[5] Neither the American Society of Clinical Oncology (ASCO) clinical practice guidelines (CPG) or the European Society of Medical Oncology (ESMO) CPG define a specific LVEF cutoff for asymptomatic left ventricular dysfunction or chemotherapy related cardiac dysfunction.[6,7] Both CPG mention the variability of definitions used in clinical trials and that there is no consensus definition to date.[6,7]

In addition to clinical heart failure and asymptomatic left ventricular dysfunction, another common cardiotoxicity of cancer therapeutics is hypertension. Tyrosine kinase inhibitors (TKI) are the most common newer chemotherapeutic associated with hypertension.[8] For example, in four phase II and III clinical trials of sunitinib, hypertension was the most common side effect.[9–13] The CTCAE version 5 classification of hypertension is listed under "vascular disorders" and not "cardiac disorders". The definition of hypertension per CTCAE is "A disorder characterized by a pathological increase in blood pressure" with grades 1-5 (Table 16-2):

Grade 1–Adult: Systolic BP 120–139 mm Hg or diastolic BP 80–89 mm Hg Pediatric: Systolic/diastolic BP >90th percentile but < 95th percentile

Grade 2–Adult: Systolic BP 140–159 mm Hg or diastolic BP 90–99 mm Hg if previously WNL; change in baseline medical intervention indicated; recurrent or persistent (≥24 hrs.); symptomatic increase by >20 mm Hg (diastolic) or to >140/90 mm Hg; monotherapy indicated initiated Pediatric and adolescent: Recurrent or persistent (≥24 hrs) BP >ULN;

TABLE 16-2 CTCAE vascular disorders

CTCAE VERSION 5.0					
Adverse Event	**Definition and Grades**				
Hypertension	Definition: A disorder characterized by a pathological increase in blood pressure.				
	Grade	1	2	3	4	5
		Adult: Systolic BP 120 - 139 mm Hg or diastolic BP 80 - 89 mm Hg; Pediatric: Systolic/ diastolic BP >90th percentile but< 95th percentile; Adolescent: BP ≥120/80 even if < 95th percentile	Adult: Systolic BP 140 - 159 mm Hg or diastolic BP 90 - 99 mm Hg if previously WNL; change in baseline medical intervention indicated; recurrent or persistent (>=24 hrs); symptomatic increase by >20 mm Hg (diastolic) or to >140/90 mm Hg; monotherapy indicated initiated; Pediatric and adolescent: Recurrent or persistent (>=24 hrs) BP >ULN; monotherapy indicated; systolic and /or diastolic BP between the 95th percentile and 5 mmHg above the 99th percentile; Adolescent: Systolic between 130-139 or diastolic between 80-89 even if < 95th percentile	Adult: Systolic BP >=160 mm Hg or diastolic BP >=100 mm Hg; medical intervention indicated; more than one drug or more intensive therapy than previously used indicated; Pediatric and adolescent: Systolic and/ or diastolic > 5 mmHg above the 99th percentile	Adult and Pediatric: Life-threatening consequences (e.g., malignant hypertension, transient or permanent neurologic deficit, hypertensive crisis); urgent intervention indicated	Death

monotherapy indicated; systolic and /or diastolic BP between the 95th percentile and 5 mmHg above the 99th percentile Adolescent: Systolic between 130–139 or diastolic between 80–89 even if < 95th percentile Adolescent: BP ≥120/80 even if < 95th percentile

Grade 3–Adult: Systolic BP ≥ 160 mm Hg or diastolic BP ≥ 100 mm Hg; medical intervention indicated; more than one drug or more intensive therapy than previously used indicated; Pediatric and adolescent: Systolic and/or diastolic > 5 mmHg above the 99th percentile

Grade 4–Adult: Life-threatening consequences (e.g., malignant hypertension, transient or permanent neurologic deficit, hypertensive crisis); urgent intervention indicated.

Grade 5–Adult and Pediatric: Death.

The diagnosis and measurement of blood pressure by non-invasive blood pressure cuff monitoring is much simpler and easier to define than cardiomyopathy or heart failure. The impact of the recent release of new hypertension guidelines by the American College of Cardiology (ACC) and American Heart Association (AHA) has yet to be seen in the determination of cardiac side effects and treatment indications.[14] These new guidelines set definitions of hypertension lower than the previous 140/90 mmHg but treatment indications are largely unchanged.[14]

Another common major cardiac adverse event that is closely monitored in clinical trials is drug effects on myocardial cell repolarization that results in QT prolongation, usually reported as a value corrected for heart rate using one of several formulae for correction. The most common of these are the Bazett and the more commonly used Fridericia formulae. Many drugs cause QT/QTc prolongation most commonly seen in antimicrobials and psychiatric medications. The risk of ventricular arrhythmias, particularly *torsades de pointes* that can degenerate into ventricular fibrillation, is the concern with QT/QTc prolongation. Commonly used thresholds for discontinuing the study medication are QTc>500msec or an increase of >60msec. The FDA recommends most new pharmaceuticals have a thorough QT/QTc study performed in which ECG monitoring of QT/QTc is the main focus. Cancer therapeutic agents are typically not studied in this manner because healthy young volunteers cannot receive cancer therapeutics. Also, cancer patients are on multiple medicines resulting in possible drug interactions contributing to QT/QTc prolongation. A common symptom of cancer or its treatment is nausea and vomiting for which antiemetics are used; these agents are known to cause QT/QTc prolongation independently. This confounds the results of studying QT/QTc prolongation in new cancer therapeutic trials. It may result in the over-reporting of repolarization effects of cancer drugs. Defining QT/QTc prolongation is also simpler than defining cardiomyopathy with clear numerical cutoffs for grades of toxicity as seen in Table 16-3. Also for this cardiac adverse event, the CTCAE lists it under the category "Investigations," not "cardiac disorders," and it is labeled "Electrocardiogram QT corrected interval prolonged" (Table 16-3). The only controversy regarding QT/QTc prolongation would be which of the several corrected calculations is used. There are several proposed methods for correcting QT interval for heart rate but there is no consensus on which should be used in cancer patients. The Fridericia formula mentioned above is more commonly used in cancer patients.

Defining each cardiotoxicity is an ever-evolving process. With each new version of the CTCAE more specific criteria and definitions are provided. Newer studies are becoming more standardized in their classification and reporting of adverse events. This is partly due to the increased emphasis on long-term cardiovascular health with increasing cancer survivorship.

FDA APPROVAL PROCESS

The vast majority of developing drugs never make it to the market or even to be tested in humans due to toxicities that are first seen during animal testing. All drugs must be tested in animals prior to administration to humans. Once the drug is determined to be safe and effective in laboratory and animal research then it is tested in humans sequentially in phase I, II, and III clinical trials. Phase I clinical trials focus on the safety of a particular drug with regards to the dose, frequency, duration, and side effects. Phase II clinical trials, while still addressing safety, also shift to better assess the effectiveness of the drug, usually comparing the standard treatment to the new drug or in addition to the new drug. If the cancer therapeutic continues to perform well in phase II trials, then phase III trials begin in which the focus is on whether the new agent is more effective and/or has fewer side effects than the current best known treatment. The inherent cytotoxicity of cancer therapeutics and the morbidity and mortality of cancer allows for accepting a higher threshold of toxicity for limited benefit when evaluating cancer drugs.

TABLE 16-3   CTCAE investigations

CTCAE VERSION 5.0					
Adverse Event	**Definition and Grades**				
Ejection Fraction Decreased	Definition: The percentage computed when the amount of blood ejected during a ventricular contraction of the heart is compared to the amount that was present prior to the contraction.				
	Grade	1	2	3	4	5
		-	Resting ejection fraction (EF) 50%–40%; 10%–19% drop from baseline	Resting ejection fraction (EF) 39%–20%; >=20% drop from baseline	Resting ejection fraction (EF) <20%	-
Electrocardiogram QT corrected interval prolonged	Definition: A finding of a cardiac dysrhythmia characterized by an abnormally long corrected QT interval.				
	Grade	1	2	3	4	5
	-	Average QTc 450–480 ms	Average QTc 481–500 ms	Average QTc >= 501 ms; >60 ms change from baseline	Torsade de pointes; polymorphic ventricular tachycardia; signs/ symptoms of serious arrhythmia	-

After completing clinical trials, the drug manufacturers then present the data on effectiveness and toxicity to the FDA. Specifically, the FDA's Center for Drug Evaluation and Research (CDER) evaluates new drugs before they can be brought to market and sold to the consumer. Based on the available clinical trials, CDER determines if the benefits outweigh the risks of the new drug in the intended patient population for whom it was developed. The FDA also considers the current available treatments and the severity of the illness for which the drug was made. Included in the final FDA-approved drug label, is also information for mitigating the toxicities or risks of the drug. The benefits of this process are to provide accurate and third-party independent information to patients and prescribers to guide appropriate use of the new therapy.[15]

In 1992, the FDA implemented the Accelerated Approval process for expedited introduction of new drugs to the market. This is usually used for serious conditions in which there is an unmet medical need as in the late 1980s and early 1990s with the HIV/AIDS epidemic. With "Accelerated Approval" the drug only needs to show improvement in an intermediate outcome that is likely to result in an overall clinical benefit in traditional endpoints such as mortality. Even after the drug is approved through this process it still needs to be further studied to ultimately prove that benefits in the intermediate outcome result in overall traditional endpoint benefit. These continued trials are referred to as Phase IV clinical trials. If the resultant clinical benefit is not found to be met then the drug approval can be terminated. Many new cancer therapeutics have been approved through the "Accelerated Approval" process by showing that a new drug can shrink the tumor size (intermediate outcome) which is reasonably likely to predict an improvement in survival. Also with new cancer therapeutics, the FDA has several drug development designations that can expedite approval, including Fast Track, Breakthrough Therapy, and Priority Review. The details of which are outside the scope of this chapter. In addition, cancer therapeutics are evaluated by the Oncologic Drug Advisory Committee (ODAC) which consists of 13 voting members in the various fields of oncology. One of the 13 voting members is a technically qualified member for consumer interests who is recommended by consumer-oriented organizations.[15]

PHASE I CLINICAL TRIALS

Phase I clinical trials are conducted in a small number of patients and are the first performed in humans receiving newly developed drugs. Novel agents must first show efficacy in animal studies prior to their use in humans. Normally, phase I trials are conducted on healthy young volunteers with no preexisting comorbidities but in oncologic novel agents this is often not the case. Chemotherapeutics are usually tested in patients with metastatic advanced cancer and numerous comorbidities therefore the tolerance of side effects is higher than other classes of drugs. Cancer patients enrolled in phase I trials have often already been treated with several established chemotherapeutics and radiation placing them at higher risk for cumulative toxicities. This may also result in difficulty determining which agent actually caused the toxicity. Often in phase I trials of trastuzumab, patients that developed cardiomyopathy were thought to be secondary to previous use of anthracyclines.[16] Trastuzumab was not expected to cause cardiotoxicity therefore initial phase I trials were not designed to closely monitor for cardiac side effects.

Left ventricular dysfunction and congestive heart failure were not expected complications of both doxorubicin and trastuzumab. Therefore close monitoring of left ventricular function was not performed in phase I trials for either. With doxorubicin, initial phase I trials suggested possible signals of cardiotoxicity although subsequent phase II trials did not plan for regular cardiac assessment. It wasn't until after retrospective reviews of phase II and phase III trials specifically focusing on cardiotoxicity that cardiomyopathy was appreciated as a cardiac adverse event of both doxorubicin and trastuzumab. See Chapters 3 and 4.

Currently, immune checkpoint inhibitors are the most recent cancer therapeutic class of medications to be introduced to the market. Phase I trial of these medications did not show increased cardiac side effects but cardiac monitoring again was not clearly defined in many of these trials. In contrast to doxorubicin and trastuzumab, many but not all of the checkpoint inhibitor initial phase I trials used strict LVEF cutoff, usually >50%, for inclusion into the trials. Again phase I

trials have limitations in detecting signals of cardiotoxicity especially if the toxicity event rate is low given the small number of patients in phase I trials. There are retrospective studies showing that myocarditis and decreased left ventricular systolic function are being found with check-point inhibitors as their use has increased in the "real-world" population after FDA approval.[17] To some extent, this follows a similar path of elucidation of cardiotoxicities that was seen with doxorubicin and trastuzumab.

One of the focuses of phase I trials is monitoring for life-threatening arrhythmias. Key to this measure is monitoring of the QT/QTc interval, of which prolongation may lead to *torsades de pointes*. As mentioned above, the correction formula used differs depending on trial and institution. Several QT corrections exist, each with its own bias and limitation depending on heart rate. Typically the QTc is averaged on at least two electrocardiograms prior to each drug administration. Most clinical trials have QTc interval cut-offs for trial eligibility and for cessation of the trial drug or modification of the dose. Resting ECGs which are a 6 second snapshot of the electrical function of the heart are not designed to detect paroxysmal arrhythmias but often phase I trials include close and rigorous clinical follow up and supervision. Upon the development of any symptoms such as palpitations or dizziness further workup with ECG and possible holter monitoring can detect these arrhythmias. The main purpose of ECG monitoring is to detect potentially fatal arrhythmias that would halt drug development.

Besides toxicity monitoring, classically phase I trials in oncology attempt to define what is referred to as the maximum tolerated dose (MTD). Typically oncology drugs have had significant cytotoxicity leading to bone marrow suppression and thus limiting the dose tolerated. With the advent of targeted therapy, bone marrow suppression is much less of a problem and cardiac toxicities are being found to be a limiting factor. The initial phase I trials of trastuzumab monitored the serum concentration and based on the effective serum concentration further phase II and phase III trials dosed trastuzumab accordingly.[18]

PHASE II CLINICAL TRIALS

After sufficient phase I trials have showed a favorable safety profile for novel anticancer agents, phase II trials are designed to further look at the safety and shift some of the focus to the efficacy of the novel agent. Phase II trials are still conducted on small numbers of patients, usually less than 100, as is performed in phase I trials. Patients entering phase II trials also similarly to phase I have already received several chemotherapeutic agents and have advanced metastatic cancer. The efficacy endpoint measured can vary from mortality to disease progression or response to treatment. It may be difficult to detect a marginal benefit in such a small population with already advanced disease. The same holds true to detecting cardiotoxicity especially if the true incidence of the cardiotoxicity is low for the investigational chemotherapeutic. Partly this is due to a high background rate of cardiac comorbidities that may mask the increase in trial drug induced toxicity. The detection of cardiotoxicity in phase II trials is difficult and often lags behind that of the detection performed later in drug development.

Unfortunately, as will be discussed later, both doxorubicin and trastuzumab clinical trials initially were not designed with rigorous cardiac monitoring or cardiac inclusion and exclusion criteria.[4,19] The cardiac toxicities were only realized after retrospective review of phase II trials for both of these cancer therapeutics.[4] In the case of trastuzumab, it was only after these retrospective reviews that the cardiotoxicity of trastuzumab was realized to be due to the concomitant administration with doxorubicin.[20]

The initial trials of trastuzumab for adjuvant chemotherapy were the first to implement stringent cardiac inclusion and exclusion criteria. These initial trials of trastuzumab in the adjuvant setting also employed rigorous cardiac monitoring with serial cardiac exams, assessment of LV function, and ECG monitoring.[21–24] Since the development of oncologic clinical trials for trastuzumab in the adjuvant setting, strict criteria for inclusion patients based on normal LV function assessment prior to enrollment have become the standard. This has resulted in oncologic clinical trials being less representative of the "real world" population.

Unfortunately, with the expansion to many sites and smaller oncology practices there is a loss of control or standardization of processes. Despite standardized definitions of cardiotoxicity listed in the CTCAE, reporting may differ between sites in a multi-center study. There are practice and cultural differences between sites that may influence how reporting and classification of adverse events are recorded. While having many sites recruit patients at the same time may provide a more timely signal of efficacy of a study drug, it may at the same time result in delayed reporting of toxicities. Toxicities in phase III studies are reported to a central location which may lead to delays between reporting and recognition of significant increases in toxicity.

As mentioned earlier, oncologic patients enrolled in clinical trials have often exhausted all other currently approved therapeutic options. In the case of phase III trials of trastuzumab in metastatic breast cancer, this resulted in many of the cardiac toxicities at the time being attributed to prior use of anthracyclines. It was not until the H0648 g phase III trial showed several cases of congestive heart failure that trastuzumab cardiotoxicity was suspected and the cardiac review and evaluation committee (CREC) was created.[20] As mentioned earlier, trials with trastuzumab in the adjuvant setting implemented some of the strictest cardiac monitoring criteria. For example, the HERA trial, a phase III trial, introduced some of the strictest cardiac monitoring that has been seen in any oncologic clinical trial which included a full physical exam, ECG, cardiac questionnaire, and LV function assessment with MUGA performed at baseline, 3, 6, 12, 18, 24, 30, 36, and 60 months.[23] The need for this extensive monitoring is being questioned; in some instances of metastatic HER2 positive breast cancer, trastuzumab has been given for periods in excess of 10 years.

PHASE III CLINICAL TRIALS

Phase III clinical trials shift the focus to efficacy of drugs, especially in novel cancer therapeutics where it may take high patient numbers to detect small improvements in efficacy. To achieve higher patient numbers in a timely manner phase III studies are often multi-center or even international cooperative groups that allow for increased and more efficient patient recruitment. The involvement of many centers limits biases that may come from single center studies and more accurately reflects "real-world" practice. Often smaller oncology practices, as opposed to only large tertiary referral centers, recruit patients for phase III trials. This allows for patients with more comorbidities and more representative of the general population.

PHASE IV CLINICAL TRIALS

After completion of several phase II and III trials, drugs are submitted for FDA approval as discussed above. Even after a drug is presented to the market with FDA approval pharmaceutical companies must continue to obtain safety data and sometimes even in formal trials. These trials after approval of a drug are considered to be Phase IV clinical trials. The number of patients receiving a chemotherapeutic after approval substantially increases and at times it is not until this phase that cardiotoxicities are appreciated. This may be due to the incidence of cardiotoxicity being relatively low compared to a high incidence of cardiac conditions in the general population. In this scenario it requires vastly increased numbers of patients receiving a drug to detect an increase in cardiac toxicities. It is for this reason that ongoing safety monitoring is critical after drugs are introduced to the general population. It is in these Phase IV studies that a drug most closely reflects that of the "real-world" practice.

Immune checkpoint inhibitors (ICI) are some of the latest chemotherapeutic agents introduced to the market. They work by blocking tumor cells' ability to evade the immune system, specifically T cells. With this activation of the immune system, ICI may have off target immune related adverse events (IRAE) such as rashes, colitis, and even myocarditis. The initial reports from Bristol-Myers Squibb on incidence of myocarditis in patients being treated with the ICI nivolumab, ipilimumab, or both was only 0.09%.[25] Post-marketing data is just starting to reveal that this number may actually be higher. Mahmood et al. found the prevalence of myocarditis to be 1.14% when retrospectively evaluating data from an 8 site multicenter registry.[17] More importantly, as often seen in Phase IV trials, the clinical relevance of adverse events is better appreciated. In Mahmood et al.'s review almost half of the patients who developed myocarditis had a major adverse cardiovascular event, and in some instances death.[17] This underscores the importance of continued safety monitoring after drug approval.

ASSESSMENT OF LVEF AND CHF

Congestive heart failure is defined by a clinical syndrome of dyspnea, orthopnea, paroxysmal nocturnal dyspnea, and lower extremity edema. Patients with congestive heart failure may have systolic left ventricular dysfunction or diastolic dysfunction. A retrospective analysis of several phase II trials of anthracyclines by Von Hoff et al. in 1979 is one of the most cited studies regarding cardiotoxicity of anthracyclines.[2] This was the first study that clearly showed the dose dependent nature of doxorubicin induced cardiomyopathy.[2] It should be noted that the presence of cardiomyopathy in this retrospective review was defined as "clinical signs and symptoms of congestive heart failure believed to be secondary to doxorubicin by the clinical investigator caring for the patient."[2] This highlights one of the criticisms in determining cardiotoxicity in that there is not a uniform definition of cancer therapeutic induced cardiotoxicity. There is clinical heart failure and subclinical cardiomyopathy/LV dysfunction that need to both be considered when evaluating toxicity. In addition, the modality for determining cardiac function differs between many phase I, II, and III trials including echocardiography, multi-gated

acquisition (MUGA), and cardiac magnetic resonance imaging (cMRI). Even within echocardiography, classically left ventricular ejection fraction (LVEF) has been the standard for systolic function evaluation but trials use various cut-offs for what defines a significant decrease in LVEF ranging from 5% to 20%.[26] Also the definition of what a normal cutoff for ejection fraction varies from 45% to 55%.[5,21–24] Newer echocardiographic techniques such as strain imaging, particularly global longitudinal strain, ventricular-arterial coupling, and even diastolic parameters have shown promise in predicting subsequent cardiotoxicity as measured by the traditional LVEF, but have not yet been universally included in the evaluation of cancer patients.[5,27,28] Therefore, if a patient develops diastolic dysfunction or reductions in strain, should the patient be classified as having a cardiotoxic event secondary to the cancer drug? The NCI's CTCAE is not nearly specific enough to differentiate between all of these factors. CTCAE lists both "heart failure" and "left ventricular dysfunction" as cardiotoxicity adverse events. Going by the classic definition, "heart failure" should include the clinical constellation of symptoms orthopnea, paroxysmal nocturnal dyspnea, and lower extremity edema but does not differentiate whether there is systolic dysfunction or diastolic dysfunction (now termed heart failure with reduced ejection fraction (HFrEF) and heart failure with preserved ejection fraction (HFpEF) respectively). Left ventricular dysfunction also does not differentiate between diastolic or systolic dysfunction and does not clarify how one should be monitoring systolic function and by which imaging modality. In general practice, echocardiography with assessment of left ventricular systolic function has become the imaging modality of choice due to its relatively low cost, no ionizing radiation exposure, and portability. Some studies have shown MUGA is more reproducible in terms of LVEF but the aforementioned benefits of echocardiography outweigh the relatively higher inter-observer variability in LVEF assessment.[29] High cost and lack of portability/availability of cMRI limits the widespread use of this imaging modality for general surveillance.

DOXORUBICIN CARDIOTOXICITY MONITORING IN CLINICAL TRIALS (SEE ALSO CHAPTER 3)

In the 1970s, initial phase I clinical trials for doxorubicin were designed with electrocardiogram monitoring and monitoring for clinical heart failure given the expected possibility of cardiotoxicity seen in the closely related chemical, daunorubicin, which had been used especially in pediatric patients with observed cardiotoxicities.[30] The initial phase I clinical trial of Adriamycin performed at MD Anderson Cancer Center monitored electrocardiograms every 3 weeks.[30] Acute ECG changes were observed in 4 patients but resolved with discontinuation of the drug.[30] More concerning were 6 cases of severe congestive heart failure in which 2 patients died out of a total of 67 patients receiving doxorubicin.[30] Despite cardiotoxicity being observed, early studies were listing the major triad of toxicity from doxorubicin being alopecia, mucositis, and bone marrow suppression.[31] In the mid-1970s, retrospective analysis of phase I, II, and III studies of doxorubicin were what brought cardiotoxicity and specifically congestive heart failure to the forefront in consideration of major dose-limiting toxicity.[2,31] The only cardiac monitoring performed in the phase I, II, and III trials of the time were periodic electrocardiograms (usually every 3 weeks) and clinical exams for heart failure.[2] Most of the studies note that by the time congestive heart failure was present it was already too late and most patients progressed to hypotension and subsequent death.[2] At the same time, the transient ECG abnormalities seen in these clinical trials were usually reversible and did not result in clinical congestive heart failure.[30] Soon after the realization that once clinical heart failure presented, it was too late for intervention, different modalities for detecting subsequent heart failure began to be employed and incorporated to monitoring during clinical trials. Initially there was promise in detecting ECG voltage decrease and subsequent heart failure.[32,33] Also noted were declines in left ventricular systolic function noted on both echocardiography and equilibrium radionuclide angiography.[34,35] Initially the problem with this decline in left ventricular systolic function was that it was subclinical and not necessarily all patients who had a decline in LVEF by these measurements would go on to develop clinical heart failure. This caused concern that premature cessation of doxorubicin may be occurring. Nuclear studies then came into favor and cardiac monitoring during clinical trials was performed by multi-gated acquisition (MUGA) studies.[35] Echocardiography technology improved and now with 2D and 3D imaging, echocardiography has become the favorable test. Its low cost, portability, and lack of radiation make it ideal for monitoring during clinical trials. There are some patients who have poor acoustic windows and uninterpretable echocardiograms for which increasing use in cardiac MRI has made this a viable option for monitoring during clinical trials. The lack of ionizing radiation is the benefit cardiac MRI has over MUGA but it is more costly and less portable with availability limited to large medical centers. Despite the known cardiotoxicity and potentially fatal congestive heart failure from doxorubicin, a paucity of oncologic clinical trials have cardiotoxicity as a primary or secondary end point.[36] Verma et al. in 2011 found that only 1% (46 out of 3482) of clinical trials for breast cancer had cardiac primary or secondary endpoints.[36]

The dose and the schedule of administration of doxorubicin is known to have an effect on its cardiotoxicity.[2] Doxorubicin began to be studied in the adjuvant setting of breast cancer treatment with higher doses at shorter intervals or so called "dose-dense" therapy. The reasoning for this dosing adjustment was its improved cancer outcomes due to human cancer cell Gompertzian kinetics.[37] The CALBG 9741 trial was one of the first to randomize patients to the new dose-dense therapy compared to the conventional three week scheduling.[38] Due to the elevated doses at shorter intervals there was speculation of increased cardiotoxicity. Some studies revealed dose dense scheduling had half the cardiomyopathy compared to conventional dosing[38,39] although long-term cardiac safety of dose dense anthracycline therapy cannot be predicted from early ejection fraction data.[40] Dose dense scheduling in addition to subsequent therapy including trastuzumab has also been studied. The monitoring of LVEF in these trials is typically at baseline, 2 months (after completion of dose dense doxorubicin, and then varying frequencies between 2–18 months while on subsequent therapy.[41] As opposed to conventional doxorubicin followed by subsequent trastuzumab trials, those patient's that developed an asymptomatic drop in LVEF at the 2 month monitoring post dose dense doxorubicin were not precluded from continuing therapy. These patients did not have increased clinical cardiotoxicity.[41]

The results of how LVEF was measured in these trials has led to various recommended LVEF monitoring schedules in clinical practice that is beyond the scope of this chapter. Generally, at least a baseline LVEF assessment and follow up assessment after completing therapy are recommended. Various clinical factors may influence more frequent or less frequent monitoring which is controversial and there is no clear consensus.

TRASTUZUMAB CARDIOTOXICITY MONITORING IN CLINICAL TRIALS (SEE ALSO CHAPTER 4)

The initial trials for trastuzumab were for metastatic breast cancer and were performed in patients who had received several other chemotherapeutics and had multiple comorbidities. Initial phase I trials of trastuzumab had cardiomyopathy events but these were often attributed to previous use of anthracyclines therefore the initial subsequent phase II and phase III trials did not design monitoring of left ventricular function into their monitoring schedule.[4,42] Once again, upon retrospective review of phase II and III clinical trials, the cardiac adverse events were realized in trastuzumab trials.[20] This is what led to the development of the CREC mentioned above. Also, this led to the frequent monitoring of LVEF in clinical practice and the eventual realization trastuzumab induced asymptomatic reversible decline in LVEF.[43]

In the early 2000s, trastuzumab was beginning to be tested in the adjuvant setting for potential micrometastases after surgical resection. This patient population is different from the typical patient population of oncologic clinical trials. These patients do not have a large burden of cancer and have not received multiple chemotherapies in the past. Also, they are potentially cured of their malignancy therefore the threshold for acceptable toxicity is lower. This eventually led to some of the most stringent cardiac eligibility criteria and cardiac exclusion criteria upon the design of trastuzumab for adjuvant therapy trials as opposed to the trastuzumab for metastatic breast cancer trials. The landmark studies for adjuvant trastuzumab are the National Surgical Adjuvant Breast and Bowel Project (NSABP) B-31, North Central Cancer Treatment Group N9831, Breast Cancer International Research Group 006 (BCIRG), Herceptin Adjuvant Trial Study (HERA), and Finland Herceptin Study Investigators (FinHer).[21-23,44,45] All had strict LVEF inclusion cut-offs ranging from 50% to 55% with BCIRG stating the cut-off was per the lower limit of normal set by the institution performing the monitoring (Table 16-4). All of the studies also excluded patients with any history of congestive heart failure. Each study also had long lists of cardiac exclusions including varying definitions of coronary artery disease, hypertension, and conduction abnormalities. The HERA trial even excluded patients that had received cumulative anthracycline doses above 360 mg/m2 for doxorubicin or 720 mg/m2 for epirubicin. The frequency of cardiac monitoring increased substantially compared to prior oncologic clinical trials. The B31 and N9831 trials had patients assess LVEF before entry, after completion of doxorubicin, and then at 6,9,12, and 18 months. It should also

TABLE 16-4 Cardiac inclusion criteria in adjuvant trastuzumab studies

	STUDY				
	NSABP B-31	**HERA**	**FinHer**	**BCIRG 006**	**N9831**
LVEF cut-off	LVEF > 50%	LVEF > 55% (after doxorubicin before randomization to trastuzumab)	LVEF > 50%	LVEF > lower limit of normal for institution	LVEF > 50%
Cardiac monitoring schedule	LVEF assessment at baseline, after completion of doxorubicin, and 6, 9, 18 months after randomization. LVEF assessed by **MUGA**.	Cardiac questionnaire, physical exam, 12-lead ECG, assessment of LVEF by **echocardiography or MUGA** at baseline, 3, 6,12, 18, 24, 30,36, and 60 months after randomization	LVEF assessment by **echocardiography or MUGA** at baseline, after last FEC cycle, and 12, 36 months after therapy	LVEF assessed 7 times over 48 months. Decline in LVEF defined as a decrease in LVEF by 10% on 2 occasions or at final assessment. **Modality or interval of LVEF assessment not specified.**	LVEF assessment at baseline, after completion of doxorubicin, and 6, 9, 18 months after randomization. LVEF assessed by **MUGA or echocardiography**

be noted that patients were not randomized to receive trastuzumab until after LVEF had been assessed following completion of doxorubicin. Therefore, about 7% of patients were determined to be ineligible for trastuzumab and never proceeded with the trial. This may suggest that patients selected for these clinical trials had more cardiac reserve. This may be why the limit of 4% increase in cardiotoxicity that was set as the cutoff for early termination of the trials was never met. Again, the most rigorous cardiac monitoring was performed in the HERA trial with every visit at baseline, 3, 6, 12, 18, 24, 30, 36, and 60 months consisting of a cardiac questionnaire, physical exam, 12-lead ECG, and assessment of LVEF by echocardiography or MUGA. All of the trials measured LVEF by either MUGA, Echocardiogram, or both for which the specifics are listed in the table (Table 16-4).

Often trastuzumab associated decline in LVEF is asymptomatic and of unknown clinical significance. Many patients will not go on to develop congestive heart failure and many will have reversal to normal LVEF even tolerating re-initiation of trastuzumab.[43] Therefore, as with doxorubicin, it is unclear how often to monitor LVEF and how or when to intervene medically. There is no consensus among the different medical societies and the practice varies among institutions.

CONCLUSION

Oncologic clinical trials continue to develop and study new chemotherapeutics with increasing efficacy and cancer survivorship. These novel therapeutics add to the efficacy of older therapies and allow for more time to recognize potential cardiac side effects. Clinical trials are essential for determining these adverse events and defining the risks and benefits from newer therapies. Cardiotoxicity has become a point of emphasis given the significant morbidity and mortality associated with cardiac disease. Congestive heart failure has a mortality comparable to and at times worse than that of cancer. This is why monitoring of cardiac function and for symptoms of heart failure has become a challenge that is assessed throughout the drug development process. Oncology clinical trials are unique in the differentiation of metastatic disease trials and adjuvant therapy trials. The acceptable tolerance of cardiotoxicity in metastatic disease is higher than due to the risk of no cancer therapy in these patients. In contrast, adjuvant chemotherapeutic studies have strictly changed their criteria for including and excluding patients with rigorous cardiac monitoring due to a lower tolerance of cardiac side effects. The emphasis for both has been on earlier detection of asymptomatic cardiac disease. Unfortunately the clinical significance of asymptomatic cardiac disease is unknown and needs further study. Also when to stop chemotherapeutics or how to treat asymptomatic cardiac disease is challenging and needs to be addressed in clinical trials. This will allow translation of practices in clinical trials to clinical practice and overall improved cardiovascular health of the cancer patient.

REFERENCES

1. American Society of Clinical Oncology. The State of Cancer Care in America, 2017: A report by the American Society of Clinical Oncology. *J Oncol pract.* 2017;13(4):e353–e394. doi:10.1200/jop.2016.020743 [published Online first: 2017/03/23]
2. Von Hoff DD, Layard MW, Basa P, et al. Risk factors for doxorubicin-induced congestive heart failure. *Ann Intern med.* 1979;91(5):710–717. [published Online first: 1979/11/01]
3. Shelburne N, Adhikari B, Brell J, et al. Cancer treatment-related cardiotoxicity: current state of knowledge and future research priorities. *J Natl Cancer Inst.* 2014;106(9):1–3. doi:10.1093/jnci/dju232 [published Online first: 2014/09/12]
4. Seidman A, Hudis C, Pierri MK, et al. Cardiac dysfunction in the trastuzumab clinical trials experience. *J Clin Oncol.* 2002;20(5):1215–1221. doi:10.1200/jco.2002.20.5.1215 [published Online first: 2002/03/01]
5. Plana JC, Galderisi M, Barac A, et al. Expert consensus for multimodality imaging evaluation of adult patients during and after cancer therapy: a report from the American Society of Echocardiography and the European Association of Cardiovascular Imaging. *J Am Soc Echocardiogr.* 2014;27(9):911–939. doi:10.1016/j.echo.2014.07.012 [published Online first: 2014/08/31]
6. Armenian SH, Lacchetti C, Barac A, et al. Prevention and monitoring of cardiac dysfunction in survivors of adult cancers: American society of clinical oncology clinical practice guideline. *J Clin Oncol.* 2017;35(8):893–911. doi:10.1200/jco.2016.70.5400 [published Online first: 2016/12/06]
7. Curigliano G, Cardinale D, Suter T, et al. Cardiovascular toxicity induced by chemotherapy, targeted agents and radiotherapy: ESMO Clinical Practice Guidelines. *Ann Oncol.* 2012;23(suppl 7):vii155–vii166. doi:10.1093/annonc/mds293 [published Online first: 2012/11/20]
8. Zhu X, Stergiopoulos K, Wu S. Risk of hypertension and renal dysfunction with an angiogenesis inhibitor sunitinib: systematic review and meta-analysis. *Acta Oncol (Stockholm, Sweden).* 2009;48(1):9–17. doi:10.1080/02841860802314720 [published Online first: 2008/08/30]
9. Motzer RJ, Michaelson MD, Redman BG, et al. Activity of SU11248, a multitargeted inhibitor of vascular endothelial growth factor receptor and platelet-derived growth factor receptor, in patients with metastatic renal cell carcinoma. *J Clin Oncol.* 2006;24(1):16–24. doi:10.1200/jco.2005.02.2574 [published Online first: 2005/12/07]

10. Motzer RJ, Hutson TE, Tomczak P, et al. Sunitinib versus Interferon alfa in metastatic renal-cell carcinoma. *N Engl J Med*. 2007;356(2):115–124. doi:10.1056/NEJMoa065044

11. Motzer RJ, Rini BI, Bukowski RM, et al. Sunitinib in patients with metastatic renal cell carcinoma. *JAMA*. 2006;295(21):2516–2524. doi:10.1001/jama.295.21.2516 [published Online first: 2006/06/08]

12. Demetri GD, van Oosterom AT, Garrett CR, et al. Efficacy and safety of sunitinib in patients with advanced gastrointestinal stromal tumour after failure of imatinib: a randomised controlled trial. *Lancet*. 2006;368(9544):1329–1338. doi: 10.1016/S0140-6736(06)69446-4

13. Ewer MS, Suter TM, Lenihan DJ, et al. Cardiovascular events among 1090 cancer patients treated with sunitinib, interferon, or placebo: a comprehensive adjudicated database analysis demonstrating clinically meaningful reversibility of cardiac events. *Eur J Cancer* 2014;50(12):2162–2170. doi:10.1016/j.ejca.2014.05.013

14. Whelton PK, Carey RM, Aronow WS, et al. 2017 ACC/AHA/AAPA/ABC/ACPM/AGS/APhA/ASH/ASPC/NMA/PCNA guideline for the prevention, detection, evaluation, and management of high blood pressure in adults. *J Am Coll Cardiol*. 2018;71(19):2199-2269.

15. U.S. Food & Drug Administration. Accelerated approval program. *https://www.fda.gov*. Updated April 1, 2018. Accessed 03/28/2018.

16. Esteva FJ, Valero V, Booser D, et al. Phase II study of weekly docetaxel and trastuzumab for patients with HER-2–overexpressing metastatic breast cancer. *J Clin Oncol*. 2002;20(7):1800–1808. doi:10.1200/JCO.2002.07.058

17. Mahmood SS, Fradley MG, Cohen JV, et al. Myocarditis in patients treated with immune checkpoint inhibitors. *J Am Coll Cardiol*. 2018;71(16):1755-1764. doi:10.1016/j.jacc.2018.02.037 [published Online first: 2018/03/24]

18. Baselga J. Phase I and II clinical trials of trastuzumab. *Ann Oncol*. 2001;12(suppl 1):S49–S55. doi:10.1093/annonc/12.suppl_1.S49

19. Marty M, Cognetti F, Maraninchi D, et al. Randomized Phase II trial of the efficacy and safety of trastuzumab combined with docetaxel in patients with human epidermal growth factor receptor 2–positive metastatic breast cancer administered as first-line treatment: the M77001 study group. *J Clin Oncol*. 2005;23(19):4265–4274. doi:10.1200/JCO.2005.04.173

20. Slamon DJ, Leyland-Jones B, Shak S, et al. Use of chemotherapy plus a monoclonal antibody against HER2 for metastatic breast cancer that overexpresses HER2. *N Engl J Med*. 2001;344(11):783–792. doi:10.1056/NEJM200103153441101

21. Romond EH, Perez EA, Bryant J, et al. Trastuzumab plus adjuvant chemotherapy for operable HER2-positive breast cancer. *N Engl J Med*. 2005;353(16):1673–1684. doi:10.1056/NEJMoa052122

22. Tan-Chiu E, Yothers G, Romond E, et al. Assessment of cardiac dysfunction in a randomized trial comparing doxorubicin and cyclophosphamide followed by paclitaxel, with or without trastuzumab as adjuvant therapy in node-positive, human epidermal growth factor receptor 2-overexpressing breast cancer: NSABP B-31.

23. Piccart-Gebhart MJ, Procter M, Leyland-Jones B, et al. Trastuzumab after adjuvant chemotherapy in HER2-positive breast cancer. *N Engl J Med*. 2005;353(16):1659–1672. doi:10.1056/NEJMoa052306

24. Perez EA, Rodeheffer R. Clinical cardiac tolerability of trastuzumab. *J Clin Oncol*. 2004;22(2):322–329. doi:10.1200/jco.2004.01.120 [published Online first: 2004/01/15]

25. Johnson DB, Balko JM, Compton ML, et al. Fulminant myocarditis with combination immune checkpoint blockade. *N Engl J Med*. 2016;375(18):1749–1755. doi:10.1056/NEJMoa1609214 [published Online first: 2016/11/03]

26. Swain SM, Whaley FS, Ewer MS. Congestive heart failure in patients treated with doxorubicin: a retrospective analysis of three trials. *Cancer*. 2003;97(11):2869–2879. doi:10.1002/cncr.11407 [published Online first: 2003/05/27]

27. Narayan HK, French B, Khan AM, et al. Noninvasive measures of ventricular-arterial coupling and circumferential strain predict cancer therapeutics–related cardiac dysfunction. *JACC Cardiovasc Imaging*. 2016;9(10):1131–1141. doi:10.1016/j.jcmg.2015.11.024

28. Nagiub M, Nixon JV, Kontos MC. Ability of nonstrain diastolic parameters to predict doxorubicin-induced cardiomyopathy: a systematic review with meta-analysis. *Cardiol Rev*. 2018;26(1):29–34. doi:10.1097/crd.0000000000000161 [published Online first: 2017/10/19]

29. Bellenger NG, Burgess MI, Ray SG, et al. Comparison of left ventricular ejection fraction and volumes in heart failure by echocardiography, radionuclide ventriculography and cardiovascular magnetic resonance; are they interchangeable? *Eur Heart J*. 2000;21(16):1387–1396. doi:10.1053/euhj.2000.2011 [published Online first: 2000/08/23]

30. Middleman E, Luce J, Frei E. Clinical trials with adriamycin. *Cancer*. 1971;28(4):844–850. doi:10.1002/1097-0142(1971)28:4<844::AID-CNCR2820280407>3.0.CO;2-9

31. Lefrak EA, Pitha J, Rosenheim S, et al. A clinicopathologic analysis of adriamycin cardiotoxicity. *Cancer*. 1973;32(2):302–314. [published Online first: 1973/08/01]

32. Minow RA, Benjamin RS, Lee ET, et al. Adriamycin cardiomyopathy—risk factors. *Cancer*. 1977;39(4):1397–1402. doi:10.1002/1097-0142(197704)39:4<1397::AID-CNCR2820390407>3.0.CO;2-U

33. Ali MK, Buzdar AU, Ewer MS, et al. Noninvasive cardiac evaluation of patients receiving adriamycin-containing adjuvant chemotherapy (FAC) for stage II or III breast cancer. *J Surg Oncol*. 1983;23(3):212–216. [published Online first: 1983/07/01]

34. Lenzhofer R, Dudczak R, Gumhold G, et al. Noninvasive methods for the early detection of doxorubicin-induced cardiomyopathy. *J Cancer Res Clin Oncol*. 1983;106(2):136–142. doi:10.1007/BF00395392

35. Mitani I, Jain D, Joska TM, et al. Doxorubicin cardiotoxicity: prevention of congestive heart failure with serial

cardiac function monitoring with equilibrium radionu-clide angiocardiography in the current era. *J Nucl Cardiol.* 2003;10(2):132–139. doi:10.1067/mnc.2003.7 [published Online first: 2003/04/04]

36. Verma S, Ewer MS. Is cardiotoxicity being adequately assessed in current trials of cytotoxic and targeted agents in breast cancer? *Ann Oncol.* 2011;22(5):1011–1018. doi:10.1093/annonc/mdq607

37. Norton L. A Gompertzian model of human breast cancer growth. *Cancer Res.* 1988;48(24 pt 1):7067–7071. [published Online first: 1988/12/15]

38. Citron ML, Berry DA, Cirrincione C, et al. Randomized trial of dose-dense versus conventionally scheduled and sequential versus concurrent combination chemotherapy as postoperative adjuvant treatment of node-positive primary breast cancer: first report of inter-group trial C9741/cancer and leukemia group B trial 9741. *J Clin Oncol.* 2003;21(8):1431–1439. doi:10.1200/JCO.2003.09.081

39. Hudis C, Dang C. The development of dose-dense adju-vantchemotherapy.*BreastJ.*2015;21(1):42–51.doi:10.1111/tbj.12364 [published Online first: 2014/12/23]

40. Ewer MS, Ewer SM. Long-term cardiac safety of dose-dense anthracycline therapy cannot be pre-dicted from early ejection fraction data. *J Clin Oncol.* 2009;27(36):6073–6075. doi:10.1200/jco.2009.25.5091 [published Online first: 2009/11/11]

41. Morris PG, Dickler M, McArthur HL, et al. Dose-dense adjuvant Doxorubicin and cyclophosphamide is not associated with frequent short-term changes in left ven-tricular ejection fraction. *J Clin Oncol.* 2009;27(36):6117–6123. doi:10.1200/jco.2008.20.2952 [published Online first: 2009/11/11]

42. Baselga J, Tripathy D, Mendelsohn J, et al. Phase II study of weekly intravenous recombinant human-ized anti-p185HER2 monoclonal antibody in patients with HER2/neu-overexpressing metastatic breast cancer. *J Clin Oncol.* 1996;14(3):737–744. doi:10.1200/jco.1996.14.3.737 [published Online first: 1996/03/01]

43. Ewer MS, Vooletich MT, Durand JB, et al. Reversibility of trastuzumab-related cardiotoxicity: new insights based on clinical course and response to medical treat-ment. *J Clin Oncol.* 2005 Nov 1;23(31):7820–7826.

44. Slamon D, Eiermann W, Robert N, et al. Adjuvant tras-tuzumab in HER2-positive breast cancer. *N Engl J Med.* 2011;365(14):1273–1283. doi:10.1056/NEJMoa0910383

45. Joensuu H, Kellokumpu-Lehtinen PL, Bono P, et al. Adjuvant docetaxel or vinorelbine with or without tras-tuzumab for breast cancer. *N Engl J Med.* 2006;354(8):809–820. doi:10.1056/NEJMoa053028

17 Cardiovascular Toxicity of Antiangiogenic Therapy: Mechanisms and Management

Divyanshu Mohananey ■ *Rohit Kumar* ■ *Tochi M. Okwuosa*

INTRODUCTION

The process of forming new blood vessels is termed angiogenesis; that of forming new lymphatic vessels, lymphangiogenesis.[1] This growth of the vascular network is important for the metastatic spread of cancer tissue. In the 1970s, Judah Folkman[2] first noted that tumor cells induce angiogenesis of surrounding endothelial cells, and that solid tumors are very much dependent on sprouting angiogenesis for growth (beyond 2–3 mm in size) and survival.[2,3] At that time, neovascularization and angiogenesis were believed to be dependent on tumor angiogenesis factor (TAF), because newly formed capillaries disappear once TAF is withdrawn.

The first proangiogenic molecule to be discovered was fibroblast growth factor (FGF), followed by vascular endothelial growth factor (VEGF) and the VEGF family.[4] VEGF is specific to endothelial cells, is expressed in the vast majority of tumors such that blocking its activity inhibits experimental tumor growth in vivo, and functions as a potent pro-survival factor for endothelial cells in newly formed vessels. This process depends on 3 main points: first, VEGF is a primary requirement for sprouting angiogenesis; second, most (but not all) solid tumors overexpress VEGF; and third, VEGF inhibition has been shown to suppress tumor growth in animal models. Better understanding of this process has led to the development of numerous therapies that target angiogenesis, particularly VEGF.[4–8]

The initial assumption was that VEGF-targeted therapies would be free of toxicity. However, these agents are associated with a number of adverse events, including cardiovascular effects such as hypertension (often severe), cardiomyopathy, thromboembolic events, proteinuria, and hemorrhage, and non-cardiovascular effects such as impaired wound healing, gastrointestinal perforation, and reversible posterior leukoencephalopathy.[3,9] These adverse effects sometimes necessitate treatment breaks, reduction of drug dosage, or complete cessation of drug administration, even though some of the cardiovascular effects, such as hypertension, are predictive markers of drug efficacy. Here we discuss the details of the cardiovascular toxicity of these agents, their mechanisms of action, and preventive and management strategies.

MEANING OF TUMOR ANGIOGENESIS AND MAJOR ANGIOGENIC MODULATORS

The proliferation and metastatic spread of cancer cells depend on the supply of oxygen and nutrients and on the removal of waste products. As such, new growth in the vascular network (angiogenesis and lymphangiogenesis) is important.[1,3,7] Angiogenesis is regulated by more than a dozen proteins identified as angiogenic activator and inhibitor molecules, with varying levels of expression that determine the aggressiveness of tumor cells. The process of angiogenesis is regulated predominantly by the VEGF family and their receptors.

Five VEGF ligands (VEGF-A, VEGF-B, VEGF-C, VEGF-D, and VEGF-E) and placental growth factor (PlGF) specifically bind to three separate but structurally related tyrosine kinase receptors (Figure 17-1): VEGFR-1 (Flt-1), mainly involved in hematopoietic cell development; VEGFR-2 (Flk-1/KDR), crucial for vascular endothelial cell development; and VEGFR-3 (Flt-4), crucial for lymphatic endothelial cell development.[3,7,10] VEGFR-1 classically binds to homodimers of VEGF-A, VEGF-B, and PlGF, whereas VEGFR-2 binds to VEGF-A, VEGF-E, VEGF-C, and VEGF-D.[10,11] VEGFR-3 binds to VEGF-C and stimulates blood vessel tips; it also binds to PlGF. VEGF-A, also referred to as VEGF, is the main component and stimulates angiogenesis through VEGFR-2 activity.[7] Figure 17-1 shows the VEGF receptors and the ligands to which they bind.

Other angiogenic processes are the FGF superfamily and their receptors, the angiopoietin/TIE signaling system, and the NOTCH and WNT signaling pathways. The PDGF and TGF-β families contribute to vascular maturation and differentiation, whereas

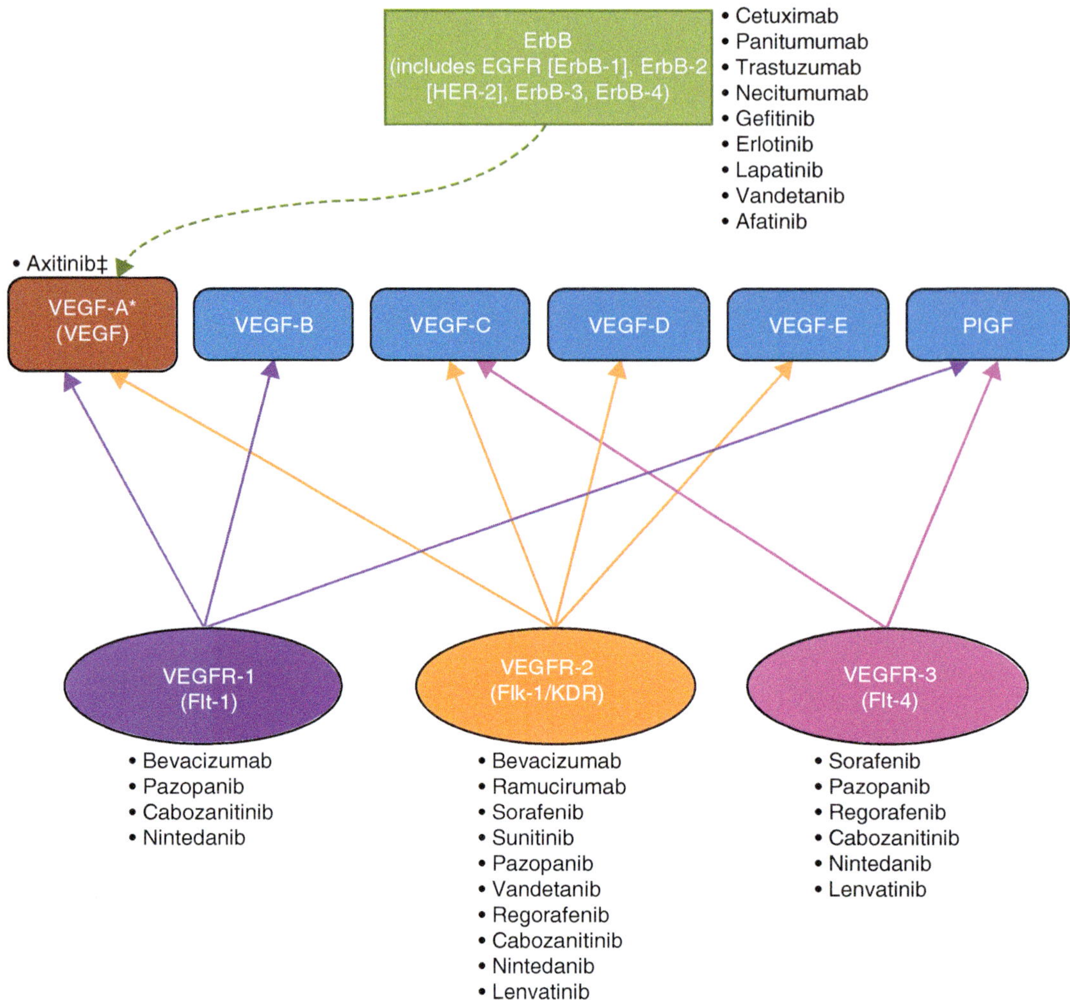

FIGURE 17-1 Receptors and ligands associated with VEGF, VEGF receptor, and specific drug therapies. VEGF, vascular endothelial growth factor; VEGFR, vascular endothelial growth factor receptor; PlGF, placental growth factor. * VEGF-A (also known as VEGF) is the main component. † Bullet points indicate antiangiogenic agents that act on the specified receptor or ligand. ‡ Inhibits the VEGF proangiogenic cytokines.

integrins and proteases, junctional molecules, chemokines, and G-protein–coupled receptors are involved in the regulation of angiogenesis.[5,7,12]

Another set of proteins with both direct and indirect effects on angiogenesis is the ErbB family of tyrosine kinase receptors, which has 4 members: epidermal growth factor receptor (EGFR; ErbB1), ErbB2 (also known as HER-2), ErbB3, and ErbB4 (Figure 17-1).[13] This family of receptors indirectly regulates the production of angiogenic factors (including VEGF, IL-8, and basic FGF [bFGF]) in tumor cells and may also directly affect tumor growth via tumor-associated endothelial cells.[13,14] Consequently, treatment with anti-EGFR or anti-ErbB2 agents significantly reduces the synthesis of these proteins by cancer cells.

MAIN CLASSES OF ANTIANGIOGENIC AGENTS

Angiogenesis may be inhibited directly or indirectly. Direct endogenous inhibitors of angiogenesis include angiostatin, endostatin, arrestin, canstatin, and tumstatin. These are fragments released upon proteolysis of distinct extracellular matrix molecules; they prevent vascular endothelial cells from proliferating and migrating in response to a spectrum of angiogenesis inducers, including VEGF, bFGF, IL-8, and PDGF.[15,16] On the other hand, indirect inhibitors of angiogenesis prevent the expression or block the activity of proangiogenic proteins.[17] For example, bevacizumab, a monoclonal antibody, neutralizes VEGF after its secretion from tumor cells; sunitinib, a multiple-receptor TKI, blocks the endothelial cell receptors (VEGFR1, VEGFR2, and VEGFR3), preventing their response to the secreted VEGF; and gefitinib, an EGFR-TKI, blocks the expression of many proangiogenic factors by tumors.[17,18]

There are 2 main classes of antiangiogenic agents: monoclonal antibodies and small-molecule TKIs, both of which are associated with clinically significant cardiovascular adverse events (Table 17-1).

■ Monoclonal Antibodies Directed Against VEGF

Bevacizumab ■ The first angiogenesis inhibitor to gain approval from the US FDA, bevacizumab (Avastin), is a humanized monoclonal antibody that binds to biologically active forms of VEGF-A and prevents its interaction with VEGF receptors (particularly VEGFR-1 and VEGFR-2).[19] Thus, it inhibits endothelial cell proliferation and angiogenesis. Bevacizumab has been approved for the treatment of metastasized colorectal cancer; recurrent or metastasized cervical cancer not amenable to chemotherapy; recurrent, metastasized, or locally advanced NSCLC not amenable to surgical excision; glioblastoma not amenable to chemotherapy; metastasized renal cell carcinoma; recurrent ovarian epithelial, fallopian tube, and primary peritoneal cancers; and cancers that are platinum resistant.[12,16,19,20] For metastatic breast cancer, bevacizumab was initially granted an accelerated FDA approval, which was later withdrawn because of a lack of evidence of improvement in disease-related symptoms or in the overall survival rate.[21,22]

Bevacizumab is associated with some cardiovascular adverse events, including hypertension that can be severe (grade 3)[23,24]; ATEs leading to cerebral infarction, stroke, MI, TIA, angina, and other ATEs; VTEs[25,26]; proteinuria[23,24]; and peripheral edema.[27] Less often, bevacizumab could also lead to cardiomyopathy with systolic LV dysfunction.[28]

Monoclonal antibodies ■ Trastuzumab is a monoclonal antibody that targets the HER-2 receptor and is approved for treatment of HER-2–positive breast cancer or metastatic adenocarcinoma of the stomach or gastroesophageal junction (GEJ).[29] Unlike anthracyclines, which are associated with type I irreversible myocyte destruction and cardiac dysfunction, trastuzumab is associated with cardiotoxicity that is not dose-related and leads to reversible ErbB2 signaling–mediated type II cardiac dysfunction without

ultrastructural changes.[30,31] The incidence of trastuzumab-associated cardiac dysfunction is about 5%–10%, with 2%–3% incidence of clinical heart failure. However, when used in combination with doxorubicin, trastuzumab is associated with a more than 7-fold higher risk of heart failure.[32]

Other monoclonal antibodies approved by the FDA for cancer treatment as of January 2016 are cetuximab and panitumumab. Both drugs inhibit angiogenesis via EGFR.

Recombinant monoclonal antibodies ■ **Ramucirumab** is a fully humanized monoclonal antibody that selectively inhibits human VEGFR-2 with much greater affinity than its natural ligands.[10,33] Ramucirumab has now been approved by the FDA for use with the combination of FOLFIRI to treat metastatic colorectal cancer; in combination with docetaxel for platinum-resistant metastatic NSCLC; in combination with paclitaxel for gastric or GEJ carcinoma; and as monotherapy for patients with advanced or metastatic gastric cancer or GEJ carcinoma for whom first-line chemotherapy has failed.[11,34,35] Cardiovascular adverse effects of ramucirumab include hypertension, arterial thrombosis (MI, cardiac arrest, cerebrovascular accident, cerebral ischemia), and proteinuria.[36]

Necitumumab is a recombinant monoclonal antibody directed against EGFR; it was approved by the FDA in November 2015 for the treatment of advanced (metastatic) squamous non–small cell lung cancer.[37] Noted adverse cardiovascular events associated with this agent include ATEs and VTEs (Table 17-1).[38]

VEGF decoy receptor ■ **Aflibercept**, also known as VEGF trap, is a human recombinant fusion protein that functions as a decoy receptor to bind VEGF-A and VEGF-B, as well as PIGF.[39] Its unique mechanism of action led investigators to speculate that it may be more universally efficacious in tumors that are dependent on pathologic angiogenesis for their growth. However, despite encouraging results from preclinical studies, aflibercept has not proved to be efficacious against various types of tumors in most later-phase clinical studies. Currently, the only FDA-approved indication for the use of aflibercept is in combination with 5-FU, leucovorin, and irinotecan for those patients with metastatic colorectal cancer previously treated with an oxaliplatin-containing chemotherapy regimen.[39] The cardiovascular adverse effects of aflibercept include hypertension, proteinuria, increased creatinine levels, VTEs, and ATEs.[40]

TABLE 17-1 FDA-approved[a] antiangiogenic inhibitors for human cancer treatment and major cardiovascular adverse events

CLASS	ANTIANGIOGENIC AGENT (TRADE NAMES)	MAJOR CARDIOVASCULAR ADVERSE EVENTS
Monoclonal Antibodies[b]	Bevacizumab (Avastin) Cetuximab (Erbitux) Panitumumab (Vectibix)	• Hypertension (56%; grades 3/4, 19%)[b] • ATEs: stroke, MI, TIA, angina, and other (~ 6%) • VTEs (~ 12%) • Proteinuria (up to 38%) • Peripheral edema • Cardiomyopathy with systolic LV dysfunction (~ 4%)
Recombinant Monoclonal Antibody	Ramucirumab (Cyramza) Necitumumab (Portrazza)	• Hypertension (ram, 16%; grades 3/4, 8%) • ATEs: MI, cardiac arrest, CVA, and cerebral ischemia (ram, 2%; nec, 5%) • Proteinuria (ram, 29.7%) • VTE (nec, 9%; grades 3/4, 5%)
VEGF Decoy Receptor (VEGF trap)	Aflibercept (Zaltrap)	• Hypertension (41%; grades 3/4, 19%) • Proteinuria (62%; grades 3/4, 8%) • Creatinine level increased (23%) • VTEs (9%) • ATEs (3%; grades 3/4, 2%)
Small-Molecule TKIs[c]	Gefitinib (Iressa) Erlotinib (Tarceva) Sorafenib (Nexavar)[d] Sunitinib (Sutent) Lapatinib (Tykerb) Pazopanib (Votrient) Vandetanib (Caprelsa) Axitinib (Inlyta) Regorafenib (Stivarga) Cabozantinib (Cometriq) Nintedanib (Ofev) Lenvatinib (Lenvima)	• Hypertension (9%–80%; grades 3/4, 9%–41.8%) • ATEs (1%–11%; grades 3/4, 1%–8%) • VTEs (1%–14%; grades 3/4, 3%–9%) • Cardiomyopathy/heart failure (4.7%–28%) • QTc prolongation[e] • Proteinuria (2.3%–36%; all grades)

FDA, U.S. Food and Drug Administration; ATE, arterial thromboembolism; MI, myocardial infarction; TIA, transient ischemic attack; VTE, venous thromboembolism; LV, left ventricular; ram, ramucirumab; nec, necitumumab; CVA, cerebrovascular accident; VEGF, vascular endothelial growth factor; TKI, tyrosine kinase inhibitor; QTc, corrected Q-T interval.

[a] As of January 2016

[b] Noted adverse events are for bevacizumab. Cetuximab and panitumumab are relatively newer agents; risk of ischemic heart disease (IHD) is 2% with cetuximab,[155] and risk of pulmonary embolism (PE) is 1% with panitumumab.[156]

[c] Rates of cardiovascular adverse events vary extensively, depending on the agent.

[d] Dual protein kinase inhibitor

[e] Noted mainly with vandetanib (8%); minimal (< 1%) risk of torsades de pointes with any of the agents

SMALL-MOLECULE TYROSINE KINASE INHIBITORS

A number of cancers are refractory to treatment with VEGF inhibitors; the extent of this resistance depends on the type of cancer and the type of VEGF blocker and differs between micrometastatic and macrometastatic disease.[41] These cancers could be intrinsically refractory, never showing any response to treatment, or could be refractory throughout the course of treatment.[7] Several mechanisms have been put forward to explain this phenomenon.[3,42] Thus, the single-pathway VEGF inhibitors discussed above are rarely used as monotherapy in the treatment of cancers but rather as adjunctive treatment with cytotoxic chemotherapy.

Because of their recognized important role in cell signaling, kinases have been one of the most intensively pursued areas of advancement in drug development within the last decade. Kinases catalyze the transfer of the gamma-phosphate group of adenosine triphosphate onto a substrate and thereby mediate most signal transduction; they also regulate a number of cellular activities, including proliferation, survival, apoptosis, metabolism, transcription, differentiation, and a variety of other cellular processes.[43] Unlike the single-pathway VEGF inhibitors discussed above, small-molecule TKIs are designed to inhibit VEGF receptor signaling pathways and, as such, exhibit single-agent activity.[3] They are therefore often used as monotherapy in the treatment of cancer.

Until 2012, an average of approximately 1 kinase per year was approved by the FDA. These rapid advances quickly led to FDA approval of more than 15 kinases between 2012 and 2015, an unparalleled progress in the history of pharmaceutical research.[44,45] As such, the development of small-molecule TKIs is one of the most pursued areas of drug discovery. Several multitargeted TKIs that block signaling pathways, such as VEGFR, FGFR, PDGFR, EGFR, Raf kinases, and c-Kit, play an important role in angiogenesis and have been approved for the treatment of various cancers.[7,12,44,45]

Imatinib is a reversible non–receptor tyrosine kinase inhibitor (NRTKI) against the BCR-Abl fusion protein. Developed in the 1990s, it was the first approved kinase inhibitor (in 2001), a revolutionary success for the treatment of CML,[44–46] and an important step toward targeted therapy. In CML particularly, the efficacy of imatinib is unparalleled, with rates of complete hematologic response approaching 100% among patients in the chronic phase.[47] Imatinib is also approved for the treatment of gastrointestinal stromal tumor (GIST) and Philadelphia chromosome–positive acute lymphoblastic leukemia. The success observed with imatinib therapy led to the investigation of multi-targeted TKIs.[12] Fluid retention and edema (including pericardial effusion), circulatory collapse, and hypotension appear to be the main cardiovascular adverse effects of imatinib.[47] Severe heart failure and LV dysfunction have been reported occasionally with this drug, particularly among patients with comorbid conditions, cardiovascular risk factors, or both.[48]

Other BCR-Abl inhibitors most recently approved by the FDA for treating various cancers are dasatinib, nilotinib, bosutinib, and ponatinib.[44,45]

Sorafenib is an oral inhibitor of the activity of VEGFR-1, VEGFR-2, VEGFR-3, PDGFR-β, B-Raf, and Raf-1 tyrosine kinase. It has received FDA approval for the treatment of patients with unresectable hepatocellular carcinoma and advanced renal cell carcinoma.[49,50]

Sunitinib targets the activity of multiple tyrosine kinases: VEGFR-1, VEGFR-2, VEGFR-3, PDGFR-β, PDGFR-α, c-Kit, colony-stimulating factor 1 receptor (CSF-1R), Flt-3, and RET. It is FDA-approved for treating advanced (metastatic) renal cell carcinoma and GIST among patients whose disease has progressed or who cannot tolerate treatment with imatinib.[49,50,12] As of July 2015, 28 TKIs had been approved for the treatment of various cancers in various stages.[44,45]

SPECIFIC CARDIOVASCULAR ADVERSE EVENTS ASSOCIATED WITH ANTIANGIOGENIC AGENTS

As noted in Table 17-1, antiangiogenic agents (including VEGF and VEGF signaling pathway inhibitors [VSPis]) are associated with a myriad of adverse cardiovascular events, which could lead to clinically significant comorbidities and even mortality. Here we discuss these cardiovascular adverse effects and their management.

■ Hypertension

Hypertension is the best-documented "class" of adverse effects associated with antiangiogenic agents that affect the VEGF pathways (VSPis). The incidence of hypertension (Table 17-2) is reported to be 9%–80% overall, and 9%–41.8% for high grade hypertension (FDA approved: up to 19%),[51,52] and is more commonly associated with direct VEGF pathway inhibitors than with EGFR inhibitors. Its incidence appears to be dose related and increases with combination VSPi therapy, although the exact mechanism of hypertension still remains elusive.[53,54]

TABLE 17-2   Incidence of hypertension[a] with various FDA-approved angiogenesis inhibitors[b]

		ALL-GRADE HYPERTENSION	≥ CTCAE GRADE 3 HYPERTENSION[c]
Small-Molecule TKIs	Gefitinib	NR	NR
	Erlotinib	NR	NR
	Sorafenib	40.6%	9.7%
	Sunitinib	41%	15%
	Lapatinib	NR	NR
	Pazopanib	80%	38%
	Vandetanib	32%	9%
	Axitinib	49%	13.7%
	Regorafenib	49%	23.4%
	Cabozantinib	37%	15%
	Nintedanib	3.5%	0.6%
	Lenvatinib	67.8%	41.8%

FDA, U.S. Food and Drug Administration; TKI, tyrosine kinase inhibitor; CTCAE, Common Terminology Criteria for Adverse Events; NR, not reported.
[a] Noted particularly for the direct vascular endothelial growth factor (VEGF) pathway inhibitors (VSPi) but not for the epidermal growth factor receptor (EGFR) inhibitors
[b] Percentages obtained from Phase 3 studies of the various agents
[c] Various CTCAE versions may have been used for individual studies

Activation of the VSP pathway triggers multiple downstream signaling cascades, and several mechanisms of VSPi-induced hypertension have been proposed. One suggested mechanism is the stimulation of nitric oxide (NO) production by VEGF: VSPis decrease NO levels, and this decrease leads to systemic vasoconstriction and BP elevation.[55] Other factors contributing to hypertension may be endothelial injury, capillary rarefaction increasing the afterload, increased levels of vasoconstrictive endothelin-1, oxidative stress, and peripheral resistance.[56,57]

VSPi-induced hypertension is classified according to the CTCAE; v4.0)[58] as Grade 1, prehypertension (SBP 120-139 mmHg or DBP 80-89 mmHg); Grade 2, Stage 1 (SBP 140-159 mmHg or DBP 90-99 mmHg or an increase in DBP >20 mmHg from baseline for >24 hours); Grade 3, Stage 2 (SBP ≥160 mmHg or DBP ≥100 mmHg); Grade 4, life-threatening consequences; and Grade 5, death.

Association with antitumor efficacy ■ Because VSPi-induced hypertension is a mechanism-based dose-dependent toxicity, it is proposed to be a biomarker of antitumor efficacy. The rationale is that the mechanism by which VSPi elevates blood pressure is believed to be same as the mechanism by which it exerts its antitumor effects.[59,60] No randomized trials have been designed to validate hypertension as a predictive biomarker for treatment efficacy, and the data from existing trials have yielded conflicting results.[61] A trial of AVF2107 (irinotecan, 5-FU, and leucovorin with bevacizumab or placebo) for patients with colorectal cancer found that patients in whom hypertension developed (increase in SBP >20 mmHg or increase in DBP >10 mmHg within 60 days of treatment) had better progression-free survival (PFS) rates (hazard ratio [HR], 0.55; P = 0.0008) and OS rates (HR, 0.43; P < 0.0001) than those with no hypertension.[62] In contrast, the NO16966 trial (FOLFOX or capecitabine plus oxaliplatin [XELOX] with or without bevacizumab) found no significant benefit in PFS or OS rates.[63]

For breast cancer, the E2100 trial[64] found that the OS times were longer for patients in whom grade 3 or 4 hypertension developed (median length of OS, 38.7 months) than for those with no hypertension (median length of OS, 25.3 months; P = 0.002), but no statistically significant benefit was found in either the AVADO or the RIBBON-1 trial.[65,66] Similarly, data from a trial of bevacizumab for non–squamous cell lung carcinoma and renal cell carcinoma have failed to show a consistent correlation between hypertension and outcome.[67,68] On the other hand, data from sunitinib trials have shown a consistent correlation of hypertension with PFS and OS.[68,69] It is noteworthy that most of the data are from retrospective analyses of studies with a single study arm, and these trials were not designed to determine the role of hypertension as a biomarker of response to VSPis. Currently, there is a need for prospective trials that can establish the predictive value of hypertension as biomarker of VSPi efficacy.

Risk factors for development of VSPi-induced hypertension ■ The risk factors that predispose patients to VSPi-induced hypertension have not yet been established by prospective studies. Some retrospective studies have linked preexisting hypertension, age 60 years or older, and BMI ≥ 25 mg/kg^2 or higher to hypertension caused by these drugs, with the risk ranging from 31% for patients with none of these risk factors to 62% for patients with all three.[70] In particular, the incidence of hypertension is higher among patients who are being treated with combination VSPi therapy.[71] Furthermore, few studies have reported a genetic predisposition to hypertension among VSPi-treated patients.[64,72]

The National Cancer Institute (NCI) guidelines stratify the risk of cerebrovascular disease (CVD; low = 0, high = 1, and higher = ≥ 2) on the basis of the following factors: SBP 160 mmHg or higher or DBP 100 mmHg or higher, diabetes, history of CVD, established or subclinical renal disease, and subclinical organ damaged as documented by ECG, echocardiogram, or carotid ultrasound. In addition, patients with 3 or more of the following risk factors were categorized as having 1 major risk factor: smoking, age (men >55 years, women >65 years), dyslipidemia (total cholesterol >190 mg/dL or LDL >130 mg/dL or TG >150 mg/dL or HDL <40 mg/dL for men and <46 mg/dL for women), abdominal obesity (male >40 in and female >35 in), fasting plasma glucose concentration (>100 mg/dL), or family history of premature (first-degree male relative age <55 y or first-degree female relative <65 y) CVD.[52] On the basis of these classifications, we recommend the implementation of more-aggressive risk-reduction interventions and close monitoring for the high-risk and higher-risk groups, targeting the modifiable risk factors as indicated.

Pretreatment assessment ■ Some level of blood pressure elevation should be anticipated for all patients who are to receive VSPi therapy. The initial assessment should include establishing a baseline blood pressure (measured on 2 different occasions) and extensively evaluating patients for cardiovascular risk factors. Furthermore, lifestyle interventions, such as the Dietary Approaches to Stop Hypertension (DASH) diet or a low-salt diet, aerobic exercise, limited alcohol intake, and weight loss, should be implemented before VSPi therapy is initiated, and treatment for hypertension should be continued throughout the duration of therapy. Similarly, pharmacological treatment should be initiated for patients whose blood pressures above target before initiation of VSPi therapy. To this end, shorter-acting antihypertensive medications with closer follow-up may be more suitable so that any delays in VSPi therapy can be avoided.

It may not be necessary to delay the initiation of VSPi therapy if the blood pressure is not at target, as long as it is not elevated to levels that are more likely associated with acute complications. As long as the patient and the physician have established an adequate plan, dose titration aimed at achieving target blood pressure levels can be achieved while the patient is receiving VSPi therapy. If the patient is already taking antihypertensive medications, the importance of adherence and regular follow up should be explained, and treatment with a single antihypertensive medication should be initiated and titrated to the maximum tolerated dose on the basis of blood pressure before a second medication is added.[52,73,74]

According to the Investigational Drug Steering Committee of the NCI,[52] the following facts should be taken into account when antihypertensive medications are selected for VSPi-induced hypertension: 1) cancer and cancer therapeutic–specific cautions and contraindications, 2) compelling considerations for preferring a specific agent in the general medical setting, 3) cautions and contraindications for avoiding a specific agent in the general medical setting, and 4) time available to titrate the dose to goal effect. Patients who exhibit an increase in DBP of more than 20 mmHg above baseline may not always cross the 140/90 mmHg threshold for hypertension. It is recommended that antihypertensive treatment be initiated so that the DBP can be maintained within 20 mmHg of baseline.

Because of the acuity of blood pressure elevation during VSPi therapy, the long-term consequences of hypertension that have been determined by studies in the general population may not be the same as those for patients with VSPi-induced hypertension. Nonetheless, for various reasons adequate control is still recommended for patients receiving VSPi therapy. First, hypertension may lead to interruption or discontinuation of VSPi therapy, which can cause tumor growth and/or resistance. Second, VSPi-induced hypertension may lead to a life-threatening hypertensive crisis.[75–77] Third, good control of hypertension may allow the administration of maximum effective VSPi dose for an adequate time period. Finally, hypertension management may improve overall survival rates.[78]

Monitoring ▪ Specific guidelines for blood pressure monitoring in patients receiving VSPi therapy have not yet been established. VSPi-induced hypertension develops acutely within hours to days after initiation of treatment.[62,79] As such, pretreatment assessment with standardized blood pressure measurement on at least two separate occasions during the clinic visit is recommended. In addition, frequent blood pressure monitoring with both clinic and home measurements should be undertaken, especially during the first cycle of chemotherapy when most of the blood pressure elevation is expected to occur. Furthermore, during therapy it is necessary to obtain in-office blood pressure measurements at least weekly for the first 6 weeks and then every 2 to 3 weeks for the duration of treatment.[52,80,74] Of note, for more potent VSPi agents such as axitinib, more frequent blood pressure monitoring may be helpful. If implemented appropriately, home blood pressure measurements can be a valuable tool for effective monitoring. One of the suggested home blood pressure monitoring schedules is 3 ambulatory measurements (the mean of three morning and night readings obtained at 5-min intervals for 3 days/week).[81]

Most VSPi regimens include drug holiday periods, which increase the risk of hypotensive episodes among patients already taking anti-hypertensive agents due to use of these drugs.[74,82] Consequently, close monitoring and appropriate dose reduction based on blood pressures should continue during this period. Following discontinuation of treatment, blood pressure may return to baseline within weeks or months, depending on the half-life of the VSPi. Therefore, monitoring should continue for a few months after completion of therapy.[52]

Management ▪ Owing to lack of standardized guidelines for management of VSPi-induced hypertension, we recommend that these patients be managed as for patients without cancer (Figure 17-2). According to recent results of the SPRINT trial, a target SBP level lower than 120 mmHg among patients at high risk of cardiovascular events but without diabetes is associated with lower rates of major cardiovascular events and death than a target SBP lower than 140 mmHg.[83] The NCI recommendations have not been updated since 2010, and are consistent with JNC-7 guidelines. With this study and these guidelines in mind, and because the primary goal is to decrease short-term morbidity associated with elevated blood pressures among patients treated with these agents, we recommend that the target blood pressure levels for patients receiving VSPi therapy should range between 120/80 mmHg and 140/90 mmHg, with the

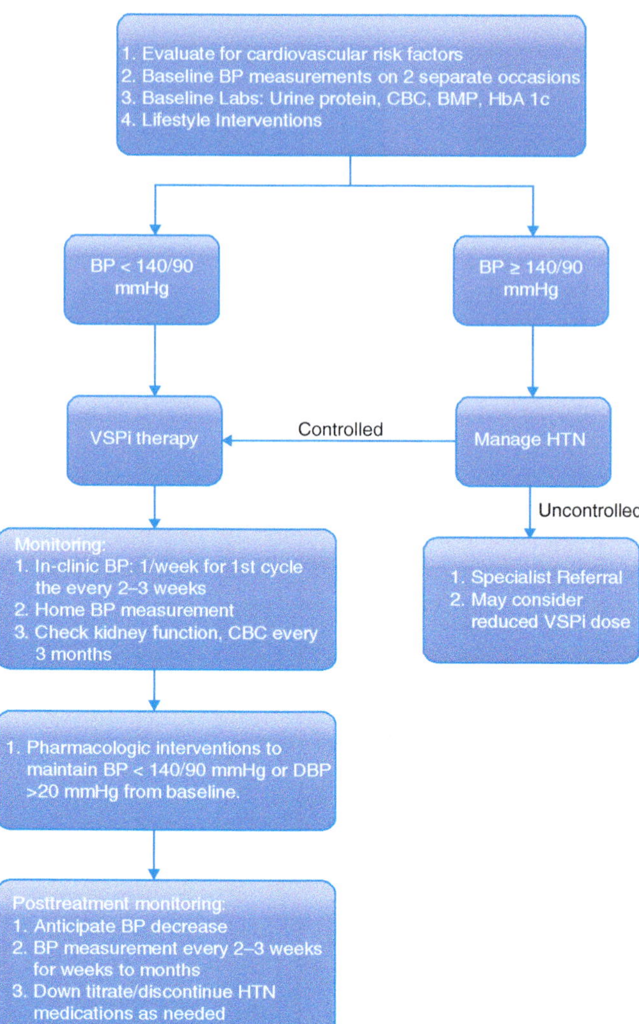

FIGURE 17-2 Algorithm for blood pressure management for patients taking antiangiogenic cancer drugs. BP, blood pressure; CBC, complete blood count; BMP, basic metabolic panel; HbA1c, hemoglobin A1c; VSPi, vascular endothelial growth factor (VEGF) signaling pathway inhibitor; HTN, hypertension; DBP, diastolic blood pressure.

exact goal dependent on comorbid conditions such as heart failure or cardiomyopathy, diabetes, CAD, renal disease, etc.

There is a lack of controlled studies suggesting any specific medication for management of VSPi-induced hypertension but the choice should be individualized on the basis of patients' comorbid conditions and general contraindications. The first-line antihypertensive medication is usually dihydropyridine CCBs (e.g., amlodipine) and hydrochlorothiazide. Adequate BP control with CCBs has been achieved in a few retrospective studies.[84,85] Non-dihydropyridine CCBs, e.g., verapamil or diltiazem should be avoided because they inhibit cytochrome P450 which can increase the plasma levels of sorafenib or sunitinib to dangerous levels.[86] ACE inhibitors/ARBs may be more suitable in these patients due to their renal and cardioprotective actions.[82] Other options include alpha- or beta-adrenoceptor blockers, nitrates, and phosphodiesterase inhibitors. Referral to a hypertension specialist should be considered early during treatment so that unnecessary delays in cancer treatment can be avoided.

For patients with CTCAE grade 4 hypertension, all VSPi agents should be discontinued, and blood pressure should be managed according to standard medical guidelines. For VSPi agents with long half-lives, e.g., bevacizumab, blood pressure usually does not normalize readily after therapy is discontinued, and the effects of dose reduction are unknown. If CTCAE grade 3 or symptomatic hypertension develops in these patients, the VSPi therapy may be discontinued for 4 weeks with the implementation of aggressive blood pressure management interventions. Once the blood pressure is within an acceptable range, reinitiating VSPi therapy may be considered, possibly with a dose reduction. If the blood pressure remains uncontrolled, discontinuation of VSPi therapy should be considered. Depending on the half-life of the VSPi, blood pressure will return to baseline (this may take up to months with certain VSPi agents, e.g., bevacizumab), and the treating physician should anticipate the need to reduce or discontinue the antihypertensive medication.[52] Of note, hypertension associated with VSPi agents is mostly manageable with appropriate therapy, and early intervention is pivotal to minimizing further cardiovascular adverse events, such as heart failure.[74]

■ Thromboembolism

It is well established that cancer itself predisposes patients to thromboembolic events.[87] In these cases, there are considerably more data on venous thrombosis than on arterial thrombosis.[88] Although the exact mechanism is unknown, thrombosis in cancer patients is most likely due to the release of prothrombotic factors into the circulation. Moreover, the elderly population is at a higher risk of CVD, and this risk is further enhanced by chemotherapeutic agents.[89] VSPi agents are notorious for causing thromboembolic events, which are believed to be due to the interruption of VEGF-regulated signaling pathways.[90] These pathways are, in part, responsible for the repair and maintenance of endothelial cells.[89] Endothelial injury is one of the main factors in Virchow's triad, along with hypercoagulability and hemodynamic changes, which are believed to contribute to thrombosis.

In addition to cancer, which already predisposes the patient to thrombosis, hypertension, which is well established as a "class" toxic effect of VSPi agents, can cause endothelial injury; thus increasing the risk of thrombosis among patients taking these agents. This increased risk of thromboembolic events is based on meta-analyses of the major VSPi trials.[90–92] CTCAE v4.0[58] defines thromboembolic events as Grade 1, superficial venous thrombosis; Grade 2, uncomplicated deep vein thrombosis; Grade 3, venous or arterial thrombosis (e.g., uncomplicated pulmonary embolism, non-embolic cardiac mural thrombus); Grade 4, life-threatening thrombosis; and Grade 5, death.

Arterial thromboembolism ■ Among patients taking VSPi agents, the incidence of all-grade ATEs is 1%–11% and that of grade 3 or higher ATEs is 1%–8%.[51] A higher risk of ATEs has been found by several meta-analyses of VSPi trials[90–92]; these events include myocardial infarction, angina, and cerebrovascular accidents. For patients being treated with bevacizumab based chemotherapy, the overall reported incidence of ATEs leading to cerebral infarction, stroke, MI, TIA, angina, and other ATEs was 6%.[25,26] On the other hand, pooled data from 12,617 patients in 20 RCTs of various tumor types showed that the incidence of all-grade ATE was 3.3% (95% CI: 2%–5.6%) and that of high-grade ATE was 2% (95% CI: 1.7%–2.5%). For this same study, the relative risk of all-grade ATEs (RR 2.08; 95% CI: 1.28-3.40) and that of high-grade cardiac ischemia (RR 2.14; 95% CI: 1.12-4.08) were significantly higher in the bevacizumab group than in the control group. There was no statistically significant difference between the 2 groups in stroke risk, and the ATE risk was unchanged when either low-dose bevacizumab (2.5 mg/kg/week) or high-dose bevacizumab (5.0 mg/kg/week) was administered.[91]

Another meta-analysis of studies involving a total of 10,255 patients treated with oral TKIs (sorafenib and sunitinib) found that the incidence of ATE among the treatment group was 1.4% (RR 3.03; 95% CI: 1.25-7.37). For this study, the incidence of various types or grades of ATEs was not reported.[92] More recently, a meta-analysis of studies involving 38,078 patients from all eligible VSPi trials (using both FDA-approved and non–FDA-approved drugs) found a significantly higher risk of MI (RR 3.54; 95% CI: 1.61–7.80) and ATEs (RR 1.80; 95% CI: 1.24–2.59) in the population studied. Again, no significant difference was found between the 2 groups in the risk of stroke.[90] The studies reported above lead to the conclusion that the risk of MI and ATE, but not that of stroke, increases significantly with use of VSPi.

Management ■ Before the initiation of VSPi therapy, patients should be extensively assessed for cardiovascular risk factors. Modifiable CVD risk factors, such as hypertension, dyslipidemia, diabetes, smoking, low physical activity, and overweight, should be aggressively managed.[93] A history of ATE is not an absolute contraindication to VSPi therapy, but this therapy should be used with caution by patients at risk of CVD and should be avoided for patients who have experienced cardiovascular events during the preceding 6 to 12 months; this suggestion is based on the exclusion criteria of the larger trials.

No standard guidelines exist for the management of ATEs among patients being treated with VSPi agents; therefore, the management of such events should be based on standard medical practice. VSPi therapy should be discontinued for patients who experience grade 3 or higher thromboembolic events.[52,74] The association of a higher risk of hemorrhage with VSPi is not a contraindication to the use of thrombolytic or anticoagulation therapy when such therapy is medically appropriate; however, these patients should be closely monitored. After acute events have resolved, the decision to resume VSPi therapy should be based on an individualized assessment of risks and benefits.

The findings of multiple trials have led to the widespread use of aspirin for both primary and secondary prevention of arterial ischemia.[94,95] Although no controlled studies have determined that aspirin is of benefit for patients undergoing VSPi therapy, it is reasonable to initiate prophylaxis with low-dose aspirin for high-risk patients, e.g., those with previous ATEs or with high Framingham Risk Scores. Furthermore, Scappaticci et al. reported that low-dose aspirin may prevent cardiovascular events among patients taking bevacizumab who are 65 years of age or older with a history of ATEs.[25]

Venous thromboembolism ■ Several meta-analyses have failed to establish a statistically significant risk of VTEs among patients treated with VSPi compared to a control group.[96–98] The incidence of all-grade VTE was 1%–14%, and that of grade 3 or higher VTE was 3%–9%.[51] Subsequently, a meta-analysis of all eligible trials of patients treated with different VSPi showed the RRs for venous thrombosis and pulmonary embolism were not statistically significant, RRs 1.14 (95% CI 0.87–1.50) and 1.18 (95% CI 0.51–2.73), respectively.[90] Cancer itself is a risk factor for VTE, and the role of VSPi agents in exaggerating this risk is uncertain.[99]

Management ■ The NCCN guidelines do not consider VSPi therapy a risk factor for VTE. For primary prevention, all hospitalized patients should receive a prophylactic dose of either LMWHs or unfractionated heparin. In contrast the administration of VTE prophylaxis in the ambulatory setting is usually not recommended except in multiple myeloma patients.[100] Furthermore, the Khorana VTE risk assessment model for cancer patients may be used in ambulatory settings. The model uses the site of the cancer, blood cell counts, and BMI to determine a patient's risk of symptomatic VTE. A score of 3 or higher confers a 7.1% to 41% risk of symptomatic VTE, and prophylaxis may be reasonable for these patients.[100,101] Routine prophylaxis may also be considered for patients taking VSPi agents in combination with immunomodulatory agents.

If VTE develops while the patient is taking VSPi agents, the therapy should be temporarily discontinued,[51] and standard anticoagulation, preferably with LMWH, initiated.[102] In such situations, thrombolytic therapy should be administered if medically appropriate. The VSPi therapy can be reinstated once the patient's condition is stable and therapeutic anticoagulation levels have been achieved. In this case, anticoagulation should be continued as long as the patient has active malignancy and this therapy is not otherwise contraindicated.[100]

There is paucity of data recommending the use of newer oral anticoagulants for the treatment of VTE among cancer patients. Similarly, limited data support the use of aspirin in the primary or secondary prevention of VTE.

■ Left Ventricular Dysfunction and Congestive Heart Failure

Angiogenesis inhibitors are known to cause LV dysfunction and CHF (Table 17-3). The pathogenesis for this effect is still unclear, but multiple mechanisms have been suggested. These drugs inhibit the VEGF pathway, which plays an important role in vascular and myocardial homeostasis.[89,103] A study of mice with cardiac myocyte–specific VEGF gene deletion found that these mice exhibited depressed basal contractile function, thinned ventricular walls, and an abnormal response to β-adrenergic stimulation.[104] Another study using murine models with experimentally induced myocardial infarctions found that VEGF exerts a cardioprotective effect.[105] Hypertension occurs commonly among these patients and may be partly responsible for the cardiac dysfunction. Another possible mechanism is the inhibition of PDGF, the absence of which has been shown to produce heart failure in mice exposed to high vascular pressures.[106,107]

CTCAE v4.0[58] grades heart failure as Grade 1 (asymptomatic with laboratory abnormalities), Grade 2 (symptoms upon mild to moderate exertion), Grade 3

TABLE 17-3 Incidence of heart failure[a] and left ventricular dysfunction with various FDA-approved angiogenesis inhibitors

NAME OF DRUG	ALL GRADE LV DYSFUNCTION	≥ CTCAE GRADE 3 HEART FAILURE/LV DYSFUNCTION[b]	REVERSIBILITY
Bevacizumab	1.5%–6.2%	1.6%	Reversible
Cetuximab	<1%	<1%	Unknown
Panitumumab	<0.2%	0.03%	Unknown
Necitumumab	NR		
Aflibercept	NR	<0.1%	Unknown
Sunitinib	4.1%	1.5%	Variable
Sorafenib	3.4%	1.5%	Reversible
Pazopanib	6.1%	1.5%	Reversible[c]
Vandetanib	0.4%	0.4%	Unknown
Ramucirumab	0.4%–2%	<1%	Unknown
Axitinib	2.7%	1.9%	Unknown
Cediranib	5.9%	2%	Unknown
Gefitinib	NR		
Erlotinib	NR		
Lapatinib	≤0.05%	0.005%	Reversible
Regorafenib	NR		Unknown
Cabozantinib	NR		
Nintedanib	NR		
Lenvatinib	7%	2%	Unknown

FDA, U.S. Food and Drug Administration; LV, left ventricular; CTCAE, Common Terminology Criteria for Adverse Events; NR, not reported.

[a] Percentages obtained from Phase 3 studies of the various agents
[b] Various CTCAE versions may have been used for individual studies
[c] Reversibility with pazopanib occurred in only 50% of patients in this study

(severe, with symptoms at rest or with minimal activity; intervention indicated), Grade 4 (life-threating consequences; urgent intervention indicated), and Grade 5 (death).

Cardiomyopathy and heart failure associated with specific angiogenesis inhibitors ■ The risk of heart failure with reduced systolic function in association with bevacizumab therapy has been reported to be as high as 4%.[28] Indeed, several clinical trials of bevacizumab have reported the sporadic occurrence of heart failure, and a meta-analysis of 5 clinical trials found that the overall incidence of high-grade heart failure (CTCAE ≥ 3) was 1.6%.[28] There is a significant difference in the incidence of high-grade heart failure (CTCAE ≥ 3)

between high-dose (5 mg/week) and low-dose (2.5 mg/week) administration of bevacizumab. Concurrent use of taxanes, capecitabine, and anthracyclines does not significantly increase the incidence or the relative risk of heart failure.[28] However, previous use of anthracyclines may cause the LVEF to be lower at baseline. A randomized controlled trial of capecitabine in combination with bevacizumab for the treatment of metastatic breast cancer found that 50% of the patients in whom CHF or cardiomyopathy developed had a baseline LVEF lower than 50%, and all of these patients had previously been treated with anthracyclines.[108]

Sunitinib has also been associated with reductions in LVEF with an incidence of 4.1%.[109,110] Animal models have suggested that acute administration of sunitinib leads to negative chronotropy and may also cause negative inotropy.[111] However, the reported incidence of LV dysfunction varies across studies, ranging from 0% to 28%.[76,110,112] A retrospective analysis of 75 patients with imatinib-resistant metastatic GIST treated with sunitinib found a mean reduction of 5% in LVEF, with an initial 2% reduction from baseline followed by a reduction of 1%–5% per cycle in subsequent cycles of therapy.[76] It is noteworthy that heart failure is an early complication and can occur as soon as 4 days after initiation of therapy.[113] Furthermore, CAD independently predicts the development of heart failure among patients taking sunitinib.[76] For these patients, histologic examination of the myocardium shows aberrant mitochondria with a notable absence of fibrosis, edema, or inflammation.[76]

The incidence of LV dysfunction among patients taking sorafenib is 4.7%, with no noted differences between sorafenib and placebo.[114] When compared to other VEGF inhibitors, pazopanib and lenvatinib are associated with a relatively higher incidence of all grades of heart failure (pazopanib, 6.1%; lenvatinib, 7%),[115,116] whereas vandetanib and ramucirumab are associated with the lowest incidences of heart failure among drugs of this class.[115,117–119]

Management ■ Assessment of cardiac function, risk stratification, and prognosis is a challenging problem. Although noninvasive imaging is commonly used for initial screening and detection of cardiac dysfunction, its accuracy is limited with regard to risk stratification.[89] Even though an assessment of LV function is not mandatory before the initiation of therapy, it should definitely be considered. Echocardiography may be preferred because it allows evaluation of structural components of the heart in addition to EF assessment.[120] Tissue Doppler and strain echocardiography have been shown to be useful for anthracycline-induced heart failure, but their value for patients taking angiogenesis inhibitors is still unknown. These limitations in imaging may be resolved by the use of biomarkers.[89,121]

BNP can be an effective tool for detecting heart failure. To this end, a small study of 6 patients treated with sunitinib found that all patients with CHF exhibited substantial elevation of BNP and that BNP evaluation was more specific than LVEF alone for diagnosis.[113] Similarly, another study of sunitinib found that 18% of patients exhibited elevated troponin I levels. However, it is unclear whether this increase indicates myocardial injury, as has been shown for anthracyclines.[76] No evidence-based guidelines exist regarding follow-up imaging for asymptomatic patients.[120]

Heart failure is an early complication of therapy with angiogenesis inhibitors, and the odds of its development decrease with treatment duration.[113,115]

Chemotherapy can be continued regardless of a decrease in LVEF as long as the EF remains above the lower limit of normal.[89,114] When the LVEF is 40%–50%, the risks and benefits of chemotherapy should be discussed with the patient, and treatment of the LV dysfunction should be considered. If the EF decreases to less than 40%, chemotherapy should be discontinued and other alternatives should be considered. LV dysfunction should be treated in these cases.

For patients with overt CHF with NYHA II symptoms, chemotherapy can be discontinued temporarily while heart failure and hypertension are managed. For patients with NYHA III to IV symptoms, chemotherapy should be discontinued and alternatives should be considered (Figure 17-3).[89] Hypertension commonly coexists with cardiac dysfunction and should be treated effectively. Although it is still uncertain whether the hypertension associated with most of these drugs is reversible, studies of bevacizumab, sunitinib, pazopanib, and sorafenib have reported reversibility with dose modification, interruption, or discontinuation, along with management of hypertension.[89,108,113,114]

■ QTc Prolongation

Approximately 4.4% of the patients treated with angiogenesis inhibitors experience corrected Q-T (QTc) interval prolongation,[122] particularly when they are treated with the small-molecule TKIs. Cancer patients often experience electrolyte disturbances and often take medications such as antiemetics and antipsychotics, which can further increase the QTc interval.[89] It is notable that the incidence of QTc prolongation is not affected by the duration of therapy,[122] and a possible proposed mechanism for QTc prolongation is interaction with the cardiac hERG potassium channel, an interaction that results in impeded electrical flow and delayed conduction.[89,122–124] CTCAE v4.0[58] grades QTc prolongation as Grade 1 (QTc 450–480 ms), Grade 2 (QTc 481-500 ms), Grade 3 (QTc > 501 ms on at least 2 separate ECGs), and Grade 4 (QTc > 501 or > 60 ms change from baseline and torsade de pointes, polymorphic ventricular tachycardia, or signs/symptoms of serious arrhythmia.)

QTc prolongation with specific angiogenesis inhibitors for cancer treatment ■ At therapeutic concentrations, sunitinib causes a dose-dependent prolongation of the QTc interval. This prolongation is usually low grade (< 500 ms) and may be more frequent among women. A study of drug interactions with sunitinib found that the most common interaction was QTc prolongation associated with the use of domperidone or loperamide.[125] However, no high-grade arrhythmias

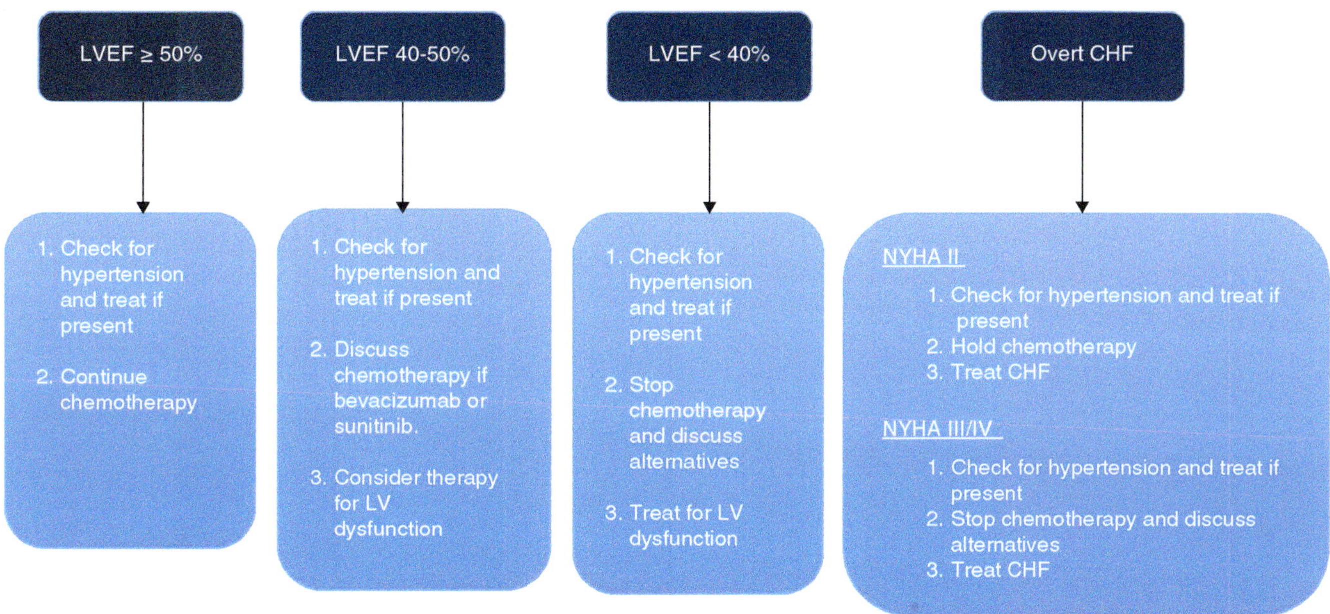

FIGURE 17-3 Management of left ventricular dysfunction and cardiomyopathy associated with angiogenesis inhibitors. LVEF, left ventricular ejection fraction; CHF, congestive heart failure; NYHA, New York Heart Association. (Adapted from Suter et al., 2013.[89])

or sudden cardiac deaths have been reported in association with sunitinib.[122,126] Similarly, pazopanib and axitinib confer a less than 1% risk of high-grade QTc prolongation with no reported cases of torsade de pointes. Unfortunately, QTc intervals were not discussed in the reports of studies of sorafenib and cediranib.[122,49,114,127]

It is remarkable that high-grade (CTCAE ≥ 3) QTc prolongation is a clinically significant adverse effect of vandetanib therapy; a trial of this therapy for metastatic medullary thyroid cancer found an incidence of 8%.[117] A subsequent meta-analysis reported the same overall incidence of QTc prolongation in association with vandetanib.[122] This effect is dose dependent: the reported incidence in association with low-dose therapy (100 mg) is 3.6%, and that in association with high-dose therapy (300 mg) is 12.2%. Nonetheless, despite this high incidence of QTc prolongation, neither study found any cases of torsade de pointes.

Risk factors and management ■ Antiangiogenic agents are associated with several risk factors for QTc prolongation (Table 17-4), such as baseline QTc prolongation, subclinical long QT syndrome, female sex, diabetes, cirrhosis, myocardial ischemia, CHF, bradycardia, atrioventricular block, electrolyte disturbances, hypothyroidism, hyperparathyroidism, hyperaldosteronism, subarachnoid hemorrhage, stroke, intracranial trauma, digitalis therapy, and rapid rate of intravenous infusion of QTc-prolonging medication(s).[128]

These factors should be identified and treated prior to initiation of chemotherapy with angiogenesis inhibitors. Cardiology evaluation should be considered before the initiation of therapy if patients have preexisting cardiac disease or are taking drugs that can potentially contribute to QTc prolongation. All patients should undergo baseline ECG, and electrolyte abnormalities should be corrected before the initiation of treatment.[129]

Of note, prophylactic drug therapy with metoprolol or diltiazem has yielded excellent results in rat models. However, the need for prophylaxis among humans is unknown.[130] Overall, it is important to watch for drug interactions that could possibly further increase the QTc interval. Important medications to consider in the setting of cancer are domperidone, ondansetron, palonosetron, granisetron, prochlorperazine, olanzapine, escitalopram, venlafaxine, sertraline, and mirtazapine.[122] ECG should be repeated 7 days after initiation of therapy and again after any dosing changes. Treatment should be stopped if monitoring shows that the QTc is lower than 500 ms.[129]

■ Proteinuria

Proteinuria is a clinically significant renal toxicity associated with the inhibition of angiogenesis. It is possible that a similar mechanism causes both proteinuria and renal disease in humans. Examination of 17 renal biopsy specimens confirmed 12 cases of

TABLE 17-4   Risk factors for drug-induced torsades de pointes

RISK FACTOR	ASPECTS
QTc prolongation on ECG	Risk is increased by baseline QTc prolongation, subclinical QTc prolongation
Sex	Female sex increases the risk of QTc prolongation
Comorbid conditions	Diabetes, cirrhosis
Intrinsic cardiac abnormalities	Myocardial ischemia, heart failure, cardiac hypertrophy, myocarditis, bradycardia, atrioventricular block
Electrolyte disturbance	Hypokalemia, hypomagnesaemia, hypocalcemia
Endocrine disorders	Hypothyroidism, hyperparathyroidism, hyperaldosteronism
CNS disorders	Subarachnoid hemorrhage, stroke, intracranial trauma
Medications	Digitalis therapy; important medications to consider in the setting of cancer include domperidone, ondansetron, palonosetron, granisetron, prochlorperazine, olanzapine, escitalopram, venlafaxine, sertraline, and mirtazapine. Of note, metoprolol or diltiazem has shown excellent results in reducing risk of torsades in the setting of QTc prolongation in rat models; data are limited in humans
Rate of infusion of anti-angiogenic medication	Rapid rate of infusion of QTc-prolonging medication increases the risk of torsades

QTc, corrected Q-T interval; ECG, electrocardiogram.

Source: Adapted from Ederhy et al., 2009.[129]

thrombotic microangiopathy; 2 cases of collapsing glomerulopathy, which were probably secondary to concurrent pamidronate therapy; and one case each of cryoglobulinemic glomerulonephritis, immune complex–associated proliferative glomerulonephritis, and sorafenib-induced interstitial nephritis.[108,131–139] CTCAE v4.0[58] classifies proteinuria as Grade 1 (1+ proteinuria; urinary protein <1 g/24 h), Grade 2 (2+ proteinuria; urinary protein 1–3.4 g/24 h), and Grade 3 (urinary protein >3.5 g/24 h). Studies using murine models showed that local reduction of VEGF production within the kidney resulted in profound thrombotic glomerular injury.[135]

Proteinuria associated with specific angiogenesis inhibitors ■ Proteinuria is a common dose-dependent adverse effect of bevacizumab treatment. The incidence of proteinuria with low-dose bevacizumab is reported to vary from 21% to 41%; its incidence with high-dose bevacizumab ranges from 22% to 63%.[140,141] However, proteinuria is usually low grade and is rarely clinically significant. A meta-analysis found that grade 3 proteinuria developed in only 1% of patients. Nonetheless, a meta-analysis of studies of bevacizumab treatment for various cancers found a consistent risk of proteinuria, even when renal cell cancer patients were excluded, a finding indicating that baseline proteinuria among patients with renal cell carcinoma is not a clinically significant confounding factor.[140] Patients among whom proteinuria develops are also more likely to have coexisting hypertension.[108] Pamidronate significantly increases the risk of proteinuria among patients taking bevacizumab.[108]

The incidence of proteinuria associated with vandetanib is approximately 10%.[142] In contrast, a study by Patel et al. found that only 2.3% of patients taking sorafenib and sunitinib experienced proteinuria. All of these patients also experienced new or exacerbated hypertension, and proteinuria preceded the development of hypertension in this study.[143] Phase II trials of axitinib found all-grade proteinuria rates of 18%–36%, and 30% of participants in a study of cediranib for ovarian cancer experienced CTCAE grade 1 or 2 proteinuria.[131,144,145]

Management ■ Given the high incidence of this adverse effect, patients should undergo urine protein/creatinine ratio testing of a second-morning void before and after receiving the drug. If a patient is hypertensive and proteinuria occurs after initiation of treatment, ACE inhibitors or ARBs should be used. In the absence of hypertension, proteinuria should be quantified and a biopsy should be performed if severe proteinuria persists. If histologic analysis shows thrombotic microangiopathy, discontinuing the causative drug should be considered.[146] Dose reduction or discontinuation has been shown to be effective in reversing proteinuria.[135,143] The role of ACE inhibitors or ARBs as prophylaxis against proteinuria among patients being treated with angiogenesis inhibitors is largely unknown.

■ Bleeding

Bleeding is commonly associated with angiogenesis inhibitors and can be classified as mild spontaneous mucocutaneous bleeding or serious tumor-related bleeding.[9] CTCAE v4.0[58] classifies colonic hemorrhage as Grade 1 (mild; no intervention needed), Grade 2 (moderate symptoms; medical intervention or minor cauterization indicated), Grade 3 (transfusion, radiological, endoscopic, or elective operative intervention indicated), Grade 4 (life-threatening consequences; urgent intervention indicated), and Grade 5 (death). The classification system for epistaxis and laryngeal bleeding is similar.

In trials of bevacizumab, mucocutaneous hemorrhage was seen in 20%–40% of patients; the most common presentation was mild epistaxis. The highest risk of bleeding is associated with tumors in the lungs and gastrointestinal tract.[9] A Phase II study of bevacizumab as therapy for non–small cell lung cancer found that 9.1% of patients experienced life-threatening pulmonary hemorrhage.[133] Squamous cell histology and baseline tumor cavitation have been reported to be independent risk factors for these patients.[147,148] On the other hand, neither central tumor location nor proximity to vascular structures has been shown to predict the risk of pulmonary hemorrhage.[148] Fatal pulmonary hemorrhage has also been reported among patients being treated with sorafenib, sunitinib, and axitinib,[149–151] whereas gastrointestinal hemorrhage is seen among patients with metastatic colorectal cancer who undergo chemotherapy with bevacizumab.[152]

Cardiovascular considerations related to bleeding risk associated with angiogenesis inhibitors ■ Angiogenesis inhibitors increase the risk of thromboembolic events, including myocardial infarction; thus, it is necessary to review the use of antiplatelet drugs and anticoagulation agents for patients taking these drugs. A meta-analysis of 5 randomized trials of bevacizumab therapy found that aspirin was protective against thromboembolic events, especially for patients with a history of such events and those older than 65 years. At the same time, aspirin users experienced only a small increase (~ 1.3-fold) in grade 3 or 4 bleeding.[25] Also, there is no reported increase in bleeding events with the use of anticoagulation therapy for patients taking bevacizumab.[63]

Although thrombocytopenia is a common complication of angiogenesis inhibitors, a small retrospective study showed that the use of aspirin by thrombocytopenic cancer patients with acute coronary syndrome significantly improved outcomes without increasing the risk of bleeding. In fact, no episodes of major gastrointestinal bleeding, intracranial bleeding, or fatal bleeding occurred among the patients in this study.[153] However, this study was not specific for angiogenesis inhibitors, which may increase the risk of bleeding beyond that posed by thrombocytopenia. Data are practically nonexistent regarding the use of dual antiplatelet therapy to treat patients taking antiangiogenic therapy, and this avenue should be explored in the future.

Because antiangiogenesis drugs have been shown to delay wound healing, current guidelines recommend temporarily stopping treatment with bevacizumab 4 weeks before surgery.[9] In a study of metastatic colorectal cancer, there was a 13% incidence of wound complications patients who underwent major surgery while taking bevacizumab had.[154] Even though no such information specific to cardiac surgery is available, we postulate that similar restrictions in the use of angiogenesis inhibitors would apply.

CONCLUSION

The dependence of solid tumors on sprouting angiogenesis for growth and survival (including metastatic spread) has led to the discovery of VEGF and VEGF-related pathways as the primary mechanism. Since the discovery of imatinib as an important step toward targeted therapy for cancer therapy and cure, and mostly owing to their effectiveness in cancer therapy, there has been an unparalleled success in the development of antiangiogenic and other agents that particularly target certain pathways in cancer growth and survival. Certain cancers can be refractory to treatment with VEGF inhibitors; therefore, the single-pathway VEGF inhibitors, such as the monoclonal antibodies, are not often used as monotherapy but are rather used as adjunctive treatment with cytotoxic chemotherapy. Consequently, multi-targeted small-molecule TKIs, which affect multiple steps in the tumor signaling pathways, have been designed to inhibit VEGF receptor signaling pathways and therefore exhibit single-agent activity.

The original assumption that VEGF-targeted therapies would be free of toxicity has not proved to be completely true. In fact, a number of toxic effects have been attributed to these agents, not the least of which is their cardiovascular toxicity, often including severe hypertension, cardiomyopathy, arterial thromboembolic events, proteinuria, hemorrhage (which makes decisions regarding the use of antiplatelet and anticoagulation agents, often used to manage CVD, challenging), and QTc prolongation with the risk of torsades de pointes. For these reasons, antiangiogenic therapies form the bulk of referrals to cardio-oncology clinics. The bulk of the challenge in managing these patients lies in a basic understanding of these agents' pathways to CVD, the expected timing of the cardiovascular disease, and an understanding of the possibility of reversal; at the same time, clinicians must remain aware of the possible need for dose adjustments of antiangiogenic therapy and the possible need for discontinuation of therapy, depending on the severity of CVD associated with these agents. Consequently, in addition to its success in cancer treatment, antiangiogenic therapy in the future will probably depend on the minimization or effective management of its associated adverse events, particularly in relation to CVD.

REFERENCES

1. Nishida N, Yano H, Nishida T, Kamura T, Kojiro M. Angiogenesis in cancer. *Vasc Health Risk Manag.* 2006;2(3):213–219.

2. Folkman J. Tumor angiogenesis: therapeutic implications. *N Engl J Med.* 1971;285(21):1182–1186.

3. Vasudev NS, Reynolds AR. Anti-angiogenic therapy for cancer: current progress, unresolved questions and future directions. *Angiogenesis.* 2014;17(3):471–494.

4. Kerbel RS. Tumor angiogenesis: past, present and the near future. *Carcinogenesis.* 2000;21(3):505–515.

5. Kerbel RS. Tumor angiogenesis. *N Engl J Med.* 2008;358(19):2039–2049.

6. Carmeliet P, De Smet F, Loges S, Mazzone M. Branching morphogenesis and antiangiogenesis candidates: tip cells lead the way. *Nat Rev Clin Oncol.* 2009;6(6):315–326.

7. Carmeliet P, Jain RK. Molecular mechanisms and clinical applications of angiogenesis. *Nature.* 2011;473(7347):298–307.

8. Olsson AK, Dimberg A, Kreuger J, Claesson-Welsh L. VEGF receptor signalling - in control of vascular function. *Nat Rev Mol Cell Biol.* 2006;7(5):359–371.

9. Chen HX, Cleck JN. Adverse effects of anticancer agents that target the VEGF pathway. *Nat Rev Clin Oncol.* 2009;6(8):465–477.

10. Aprile G, Rijavec E, Fontanella C, Rihawi K, Grossi F. Ramucirumab: preclinical research and clinical development. *Onco Targets Ther.* 2014;7:1997–2006.

11. Clarke JM, Hurwitz HI. Targeted inhibition of VEGF receptor 2: an update on ramucirumab. *Expert Opin Biol Ther.* 2013;13(8):1187–1196.

12. Al-Husein B, Abdalla M, Trepte M, Deremer DL, Somanath PR. Antiangiogenic therapy for cancer: an update. *Pharmacotherapy.* 2012;32(12):1095–1111.

13. De Luca A, Carotenuto A, Rachiglio A, et al. The role of the EGFR signaling in tumor microenvironment. *J Cell Physiol.* 2008;214(3):559–567.

14. Ciardiello F, Troiani T, Bianco R, et al. Interaction between the epidermal growth factor receptor (EGFR) and the vascular endothelial growth factor (VEGF) pathways: a rational approach for multi-target anticancer therapy. *Ann Oncol.* 2006;17(suppl 7):vii109–vii114.

15. Kerbel R, Folkman J. Clinical translation of angiogenesis inhibitors. *Nat Rev Cancer.* 2002;2(10):727–739.

16. El-Kenawi AE, El-Remessy AB. Angiogenesis inhibitors in cancer therapy: mechanistic perspective on classification and treatment rationales. *Br J Pharmacol.* 2013;170(4):712–729.

17. Folkman J. Angiogenesis: an organizing principle for drug discovery? *Nat Rev Drug Discov.* 2007;6(4):273–286.

18. Roskoski R Jr. Vascular endothelial growth factor (VEGF) signaling in tumor progression. *Crit Rev Oncol Hematol.* 2007;62(3):179–213.

19. Samant RS, Shevde LA. Recent advances in anti-angiogenic therapy of cancer. *Oncotarget.* 2011;2(3):122–134.

20. National Cancer Institute. Bevacizumab. 2016; https://www.cancer.gov/about-cancer/treatment/drugs/bevacizumab. Accessed April 5, 2019.

21. Burstein HJ. Avastin for breast cancer, 2005-2011: requiescat in pacem? *J Natl Compr Canc Netw.* 2011;9(12):1321–1323.

22. Montero AJ, Escobar M, Lopes G, Glück S, Vogel C. Bevacizumab in the treatment of metastatic breast cancer: friend or foe? *Curr Oncol Rep.* 2012;14(1):1–11.

23. Shah SR, Gressett Ussery SM, Dowell JE, Liticker J. Response to letter titled: blood pressure monitoring in patients receiving bevacizumab. *Ann Oncol.* 2013;24(4):1127–1128.

24. Shah SR, Gressett Ussery SM, Dowell JE, et al. Shorter bevacizumab infusions do not increase the incidence of proteinuria and hypertension. *Ann Oncol.* 2013;24(4):960–965.

25. Scappaticci FA, Skillings JR, Holden SN, et al. Arterial thromboembolic events in patients with metastatic carcinoma treated with chemotherapy and bevacizumab. *J Natl Cancer Inst.* 2007;99(16):1232–1239.

26. Nalluri SR, Chu D, Keresztes R, Zhu X, Wu S. Risk of venous thromboembolism with the angiogenesis inhibitor bevacizumab in cancer patients: a meta-analysis. *JAMA.* 2008;300(19):2277–2285.

27. Herbst RS, Johnson DH, Mininberg E, et al. Phase I/II trial evaluating the anti-vascular endothelial growth factor monoclonal antibody bevacizumab in combination with the HER-1/epidermal growth factor receptor tyrosine kinase inhibitor erlotinib for patients with recurrent non-small-cell lung cancer. *J Clin Oncol.* 2005;23(11):2544–2555.

28. Choueiri TK, Mayer EL, Je Y, et al. Congestive heart failure risk in patients with breast cancer treated with bevacizumab. *J Clin Oncol* 2011;29(6):632–638.

29. National Cancer Institute. Trastuzumab. 2016; https:// www.cancer.gov/about-cancer/treatment/drugs/ trastuzumab. Accessed April 5, 2019.

30. Ewer MS, Lippman SM. Type II chemotherapy-related cardiac dysfunction: time to recognize a new entity. *J Clin Oncol*. 2005;23(13):2900–2902.

31. Ewer MS, Vooletich MT, Durand JB, et al. Reversibility of trastuzumab-related cardiotoxicity: new insights based on clinical course and response to medical treatment. *J Clin Oncol*. 2005;23(31):7820–7826.

32. Bowles EJ, Wellman R, Feigelson HS, et al. Pharmacovigilance study team. Risk of heart failure in breast cancer patients after anthracycline and trastuzumab treatment: a retrospective cohort study. *J Natl Cancer Inst*. 2012;104(17):1293–1305.

33. Aprile G, Bonotto M, Ongaro E, Pozzo C, Giuliani F. Critical appraisal of ramucirumab (IMC-1121B) for cancer treatment: from benchside to clinical use. *Drugs*. 2013;73(18):2003–2015.

34. Fala L. Cyramza (Ramucirumab) approved for the treatment of advanced gastric cancer and metastatic non-small-cell lung cancer. *Am Health Drug Benefits*. 2015;8(Spec Feature):49–53.

35. National Cancer Institute. Ramucirumab. 2016; https:// www.cancer.gov/about-cancer/treatment/drugs/ ramucirumab. Accessed April 5, 2019.

36. Spratlin JL, Cohen RB, Eadens M, et al. Phase I pharmacologic and biologic study of ramucirumab (IMC-1121B), a fully human immunoglobulin G1 monoclonal antibody targeting the vascular endothelial growth factor receptor-2. *J Clin Oncol*. 2010;28(5):780–787.

37. National Cancer Institute. Necitumumab. 2016. http:// www.cancer.gov/about-cancer/treatment/drugs/necitumumab. Accessed May 30, 2016.

38. Thatcher N, Hirsch FR, Luft AV, et al. SQUIRE investigators. Necitumumab plus gemcitabine and cisplatin versus gemcitabine and cisplatin alone as first-line therapy in patients with stage IV squamous non-small-cell lung cancer (SQUIRE): an open-label, randomised, controlled phase 3 trial. *Lancet Oncol*. 2015;16(7):763–774.

39. Ciombor KK, Berlin J. Aflibercept—a decoy VEGF receptor. *Curr Oncol Rep*. 2014;16(2):368.

40. Van Cutsem E, Tabernero J, Lakomy R, et al. Addition of aflibercept to fluorouracil, leucovorin, and irinotecan improves survival in a phase III randomized trial in patients with metastatic colorectal cancer previously treated with an oxaliplatin-based regimen. *J Clin Oncol*. 2012;30(28):3499–3506.

41. Bergers G, Hanahan D. Modes of resistance to antiangiogenic therapy. *Nat Rev Cancer*. 2008;8(8):592–603.

42. Jain RK, Duda DG, Willett CG, et al. Biomarkers of response and resistance to antiangiogenic therapy. *Nat Rev Clin Oncol*. 2009;6(6):327–338.

43. Adams JA. Kinetic and catalytic mechanisms of protein kinases. *Chem Rev*. 2001;101(8):2271–2290.

44. Soria JC, Wu YL, Nakagawa K, et al. Gefitinib plus chemotherapy versus placebo plus chemotherapy in EGFR-mutation-positive non-small-cell lung cancer after progression on first-line gefitinib (IMPRESS): a phase 3 randomised trial. *Lancet Oncol*. 2015;16(8):990–998.

45. Wu P, Nielsen TE, Clausen MH. Small-molecule kinase inhibitors: an analysis of FDA-approved drugs. *Drug Discov Today*. 2016;21(1):5–10.

46. Druker BJ, Sawyers CL, Kantarjian H, et al. Activity of a specific inhibitor of the BCR-ABL tyrosine kinase in the blast crisis of chronic myeloid leukemia and acute lymphoblastic leukemia with the Philadelphia chromosome. *N Engl J Med*. 2001;344(14):1038–1042.

47. Deininger MW, O'Brien SG, Ford JM, Druker BJ. Practical management of patients with chronic myeloid leukemia receiving imatinib. *J Clin Oncol*. 2003;21(8):1637–1647.

48. Kerkelä R, Grazette L, Yacobi R, et al. Cardiotoxicity of the cancer therapeutic agent imatinib mesylate. *Nat Med*. 2006;12(8):908–916.

49. Llovet JM, Ricci S, Mazzaferro V. SHARP investigators study group. Sorafenib in advanced hepatocellular carcinoma. *N Engl J Med*. 2008;359(4):378–390.

50. Ivy SP, Wick JY, Kaufman BM. An overview of small-molecule inhibitors of VEGFR signaling. *Nat Rev Clin Oncol*. 2009;6(10):569–579.

51. Dy GK, Adjei AA. Understanding, recognizing, and managing toxicities of targeted anticancer therapies. *CA Cancer J Clin*. 2013;63(4):249–279.

52. Maitland ML, Bakris GL, Black HR, et al. Cardiovascular Toxicities Panel, convened by the Angiogenesis Task Force of the National Cancer Institute Investigational Drug Steering Committee. Initial assessment, surveillance, and management of blood pressure in patients receiving vascular endothelial growth factor signaling pathway inhibitors. *J Natl Cancer Inst*. 2010;102(9):596–604.

53. Yang JC, Haworth L, Sherry RM, et al. A randomized trial of bevacizumab, an anti-vascular endothelial growth factor antibody, for metastatic renal cancer. *N Engl J Med*. 2003;349(5):427–434.

54. Lee JM, Sarosy GA, Annunziata CM, et al. Combination therapy: intermittent sorafenib with bevacizumab yields activity and decreased toxicity. *Br J Cancer*. 2010;102(3):495–499.

55. Facemire CS, Nixon AB, Griffiths R, Hurwitz H, Coffman TM. Vascular endothelial growth factor receptor 2 controls blood pressure by regulating nitric oxide synthase expression. *Hypertension*. 2009;54(3):652–658.

56. Steeghs N, Gelderblom H, Roodt JO, et al. Hypertension and rarefaction during treatment with telatinib, a small molecule angiogenesis inhibitor. *Clin Cancer Res*. 2008;14(11):3470–3476.

57. González-Pacheco FR, Deudero JJ, Castellanos MC, et al. Mechanisms of endothelial response to oxidative aggression: protective role of autologous VEGF and induction of VEGFR2 by H_2O_2. *Am J Physiol Heart Circ Physiol*. 2006;291(3):H1395–H1401.

58. National Cancer Institute. *Common Terminology Criteria for Adverse Events (CTCAE), v4.0*. 2016. http://ctep. cancer.gov/protocolDevelopment/electronic_applications/ctc.htm. Accessed May 30, 2016.

59. Ryanne Wu R, Lindenberg PA, Slack R, Noone AM, Marshall JL, He AR. Evaluation of hypertension as a marker of bevacizumab efficacy. *J Gastrointest Cancer*. 2009;40(3–4):101–108.

60. Scartozzi M, Galizia E, Chiorrini S, et al. Arterial hypertension correlates with clinical outcome in colorectal cancer patients treated with first-line bevacizumab. *Ann Oncol*. 2009;20(2):227–230.

61. Hurwitz HI, Douglas PS, Middleton JP, et al. Analysis of early hypertension and clinical outcome with bevacizumab: results from seven phase III studies. *Oncologist*. 2013;18(3):273–280.

62. Hurwitz H, Fehrenbacher L, Novotny W, et al. Bevacizumab plus irinotecan, fluorouracil, and leucovorin for metastatic colorectal cancer. *N Engl J Med*. 2004;350(23):2335–2342.

63. Saltz LB, Clarke S, Diaz-Rubio E, et al. Bevacizumab in combination with oxaliplatin-based chemotherapy as first-line therapy in metastatic colorectal cancer: a randomized phase III study. *J Clin Oncol*. 2008;26(12):2013–2019.

64. Schneider BP, Wang M, Radovich M, et al. ECOG 2100. Association of vascular endothelial growth factor and vascular endothelial growth factor receptor-2 genetic polymorphisms with outcome in a trial of paclitaxel compared with paclitaxel plus bevacizumab in advanced breast cancer: ECOG 2100. *J Clin Oncol*. 2008;26(28):4672–4678.

65. Miles DW, Chan A, Dirix LY, et al. Phase III study of bevacizumab plus docetaxel compared with placebo plus docetaxel for the first-line treatment of human epidermal growth factor receptor 2-negative metastatic breast cancer. *J Clin Oncol*. 2010;28(20):3239–3247.

66. Robert NJ, Diéras V, Glaspy J, et al. RIBBON-1: randomized, double-blind, placebo-controlled, phase III trial of chemotherapy with or without bevacizumab for first-line treatment of human epidermal growth factor receptor 2-negative, locally recurrent or metastatic breast cancer. *J Clin Oncol*. 2011;29(10):1252–1260.

67. Dahlberg SE, Sandler AB, Brahmer JR, Schiller JH, Johnson DH. Clinical course of advanced non-small-cell lung cancer patients experiencing hypertension during treatment with bevacizumab in combination with carboplatin and paclitaxel on ECOG 4599. *J Clin Oncol*. 2010;28(6):949–954.

68. Rini BI, Cohen DP, Lu DR, et al. Hypertension as a biomarker of efficacy in patients with metastatic renal cell carcinoma treated with sunitinib. *J Natl Cancer Inst*. 2011;103(9):763–773.

69. Rixe O, Billemont B, Izzedine H. Hypertension as a predictive factor of Sunitinib activity. *Ann Oncol*. 2007;18(6):1117.

70. Hamnvik OP, Choueiri TK, Turchin A, et al. Clinical risk factors for the development of hypertension in patients treated with inhibitors of the VEGF signaling pathway. *Cancer*. 2015;121(2):311–319.

71. Langenberg MH, Witteveen PO, Roodhart J, et al. Phase I evaluation of telatinib, a VEGF receptor tyrosine kinase inhibitor, in combination with bevacizumab in subjects with advanced solid tumors. *Ann Oncol*. 2011;22(11):2508–2515.

72. Sibertin-Blanc C, Mancini J, Fabre A, et al. Vascular endothelial growth factor a c.*237C>T polymorphism is associated with bevacizumab efficacy and related hypertension in metastatic colorectal cancer. *Dig Liver Dis*. 2015;47(4):331–337.

73. Katsi V, Zerdes I, Manolakou S, et al. Anti-VEGF anticancer drugs: mind the hypertension. *Recent Adv Cardiovasc Drug Discov*. 2014;9(2):63–72.

74. Lenihan DJ, Kowey PR. Overview and management of cardiac adverse events associated with tyrosine kinase inhibitors. *Oncologist*. 2013;18(8):900–908.

75. Ozcan C, Wong SJ, Hari P. Reversible posterior leukoencephalopathy syndrome and bevacizumab. *N Engl J Med*. 2006;354(9):980–982.

76. Chu TF, Rupnick MA, Kerkela R, et al. Cardiotoxicity associated with tyrosine kinase inhibitor sunitinib. *Lancet*. 2007;370(9604):2011–2019.

77. Caro J, Morales E, Gutierrez E, Ruilope LM, Praga M. Malignant hypertension in patients treated with vascular endothelial growth factor inhibitors. *J Clin Hypertens (Greenwich)*. 2013;15(3):215–216.

78. Piccirillo JF, Tierney RM, Costas I, Grove L, Spitznagel EL Jr. Prognostic importance of comorbidity in a hospital-based cancer registry. *JAMA*. 2004;291(20):2441–2447.

79. Maitland ML, Kasza KE, Karrison T, et al. Ambulatory monitoring detects sorafenib-induced blood pressure elevations on the first day of treatment. *Clin Cancer Res*. 2009;15(19):6250–6257.

80. Wu S, Chen JJ, Kudelka A, Lu J, Zhu X. Incidence and risk of hypertension with sorafenib in patients with cancer: a systematic review and meta-analysis. *Lancet Oncol*. 2008;9(2):117–123.

81. Azizi M, Chedid A, Oudard S. Home blood-pressure monitoring in patients receiving sunitinib. *N Engl J Med*. 2008;358(1):95–97.

82. de Jesus-Gonzalez N, Robinson E, Moslehi J, Humphreys BD. Management of antiangiogenic therapy-induced hypertension. *Hypertension*. 2012;60(3):607–615.

83. SPRINT Research Group, Wright JT Jr, Williamson JD, et al. A randomized trial of intensive versus standard blood-pressure control. *N Engl J Med*. 2015;373(22):2103–2116.

84. Pande A, Lombardo J, Spangenthal E, Javle M. Hypertension secondary to anti-angiogenic therapy: experience with bevacizumab. *Anticancer Res*. 2007;27(5B):3465–3470.

85. Mir O, Coriat R, Ropert S, et al. Treatment of bevacizumab-induced hypertension by amlodipine. *Invest New Drugs*. 2012;30(2):702–707.

86. Izzedine H, Ederhy S, Goldwasser F, et al. Management of hypertension in angiogenesis inhibitor-treated patients. *Ann Oncol*. 2009;20(5):807–815.

87. Spencer FA, Emery C, Lessard D, et al. The Worcester Venous Thromboembolism study: a population-based study of the clinical epidemiology of venous thromboembolism. *J Gen Intern Med*. 2006;21(7):722–727.

88. Timp JF, Braekkan SK, Versteeg HH, Cannegieter SC. Epidemiology of cancer-associated venous thrombosis. *Blood*. 2013;122(10):1712–1723.

89. Suter TM, Ewer MS. Cancer drugs and the heart: importance and management. *Eur Heart J*. 2013;34(15):1102–1111.

90. Faruque LI, Lin M, Battistella M, et al. Systematic review of the risk of adverse outcomes associated with vascular endothelial growth factor inhibitors for the treatment of cancer. *PLOS ONE*. 2014;9(7):e101145.

91. Ranpura V, Hapani S, Chuang J, Wu S. Risk of cardiac ischemia and arterial thromboembolic events with the angiogenesis inhibitor bevacizumab in cancer patients: a meta-analysis of randomized controlled trials. *Acta Oncol*. 2010;49(3):287–297.

92. Choueiri TK, Schutz FA, Je Y, Rosenberg JE, Bellmunt J. Risk of arterial thromboembolic events with sunitinib and sorafenib: a systematic review and meta-analysis of clinical trials. *J Clin Oncol*. 2010;28(13):2280–2285.

93. Vasan RS, Sullivan LM, Wilson PW, et al. Relative importance of borderline and elevated levels of coronary heart disease risk factors. *Ann Intern Med*. 2005;142(6):393–402.

94. Hennekens CH, Dyken ML, Fuster V. Aspirin as a therapeutic agent in cardiovascular disease: a statement for healthcare professionals from the American Heart Association. *Circulation*. 1997;96(8):2751–2753.

95. Berger JS, Brown DL, Becker RC. Low-dose aspirin in patients with stable cardiovascular disease: a meta-analysis. *Am J Med*. 2008;121(1):43–49.

96. Hurwitz HI, Saltz LB, Van Cutsem E, et al. Venous thromboembolic events with chemotherapy plus bevacizumab: a pooled analysis of patients in randomized phase II and III studies. *J Clin Oncol*. 2011;29(13): 1757–1764.

97. Qi WX, Min DL, Shen Z, et al. Risk of venous thromboembolic events associated with VEGFR-TKIs: a systematic review and meta-analysis. *Int J Cancer*. 2013;132 (12):2967–2974.

98. Sonpavde G, Je Y, Schutz F, et al. Venous thromboembolic events with vascular endothelial growth factor receptor tyrosine kinase inhibitors: a systematic review and meta-analysis of randomized clinical trials. *Crit Rev Oncol Hematol*. 2013;87(1):80–89.

99. Blom JW, Doggen CJ, Osanto S, Rosendaal FR. Malignancies, prothrombotic mutations, and the risk of venous thrombosis. *JAMA*. 2005;293(6):715–722.

100. Streiff MB, Holmstrom B, Ashrani A, et al. Cancer-associated venous thromboembolic disease, Version 1.2015. *J Natl Compr Canc Netw*. 2015;13(9):1079–1095.

101. Khorana AA, Kuderer NM, Culakova E, Lyman GH. Francis CW. Development and validation of a predictive model for chemotherapy-associated thrombosis. *Blood*. 2008;111(10):4902–4907.

102. Lee AY, Levine MN, Baker RI, et al. Randomized comparison of low-molecular-weight heparin versus oral anticoagulant therapy for the prevention of recurrent venous thromboembolism in patients with cancer (CLOT) investigators. Low-molecular-weight heparin versus a coumarin for the prevention of recurrent venous thromboembolism in patients with cancer. *N Engl J Med*. 2003;349(2):146–153.

103. Chen T, Zhou G, Zhu Q, et al. Overexpression of vascular endothelial growth factor 165 (VEGF165) protects cardiomyocytes against doxorubicin-induced apoptosis. *J Chemother*. 2010;22(6):402–406.

104. Giordano FJ, Gerber HP, Williams SP, et al. A cardiac myocyte vascular endothelial growth factor paracrine pathway is required to maintain cardiac function. *Proc Natl Acad Sci USA*. 2001;98(10):5780–5785.

105. Deuse T, Peter C, Fedak PW, et al. Hepatocyte growth factor or vascular endothelial growth factor gene transfer maximizes mesenchymal stem cell-based myocardial salvage after acute myocardial infarction. *Circulation*. 2009;120(11) suppl 1:S247–S254.

106. Richards CJ, Je Y, Schutz FA, et al. Incidence and risk of congestive heart failure in patients with renal and non-renal cell carcinoma treated with sunitinib. *J Clin Oncol*. 2011;29(25):3450–3456.

107. Chintalgattu V, Ai D, Langley RR, et al. Cardiomyocyte PDGFR-beta signaling is an essential component of the mouse cardiac response to load-induced stress. *J Clin Invest*. 2010;120(2):472–484.

108. Miller KD, Chap LI, Holmes FA, et al. Randomized phase III trial of capecitabine compared with bevacizumab plus capecitabine in patients with previously treated metastatic breast cancer. *J Clin Oncol*. 2005;23(4):792–799.

109. Tocchetti CG, Gallucci G, Coppola C, et al. The emerging issue of cardiac dysfunction induced by antineoplastic angiogenesis inhibitors. *Eur J Heart Fail*. 2013;15(5):482–489.

110. Motzer RJ, Hutson TE, Tomczak P, et al. Sunitinib versus interferon alfa in metastatic renal-cell carcinoma. *N Engl J Med*. 2007;356(2):115–124.

111. Mooney L, Skinner M, Coker SJ, Currie S. Effects of acute and chronic sunitinib treatment on cardiac function and calcium/calmodulin-dependent protein kinase II. *Br J Pharmacol*. 2015;172(17):4342–4354.

112. Demetri GD, van Oosterom AT, Garrett CR, et al. Efficacy and safety of sunitinib in patients with advanced gastrointestinal stromal tumour after failure of imatinib: a randomised controlled trial. *Lancet*. 2006;368(9544):1329–1338.

113. Khakoo AY, Kassiotis CM, Tannir N, et al. Heart failure associated with sunitinib malate: a multi-targeted receptor tyrosine kinase inhibitor. *Cancer*. 2008;112(11):2500–2508.

114. Haas NB, Manola J, Ky B, et al. Effects of adjuvant sorafenib and sunitinib on cardiac function in renal cell carcinoma patients without overt metastases: results from ASSURE, ECOG 2805. *Clin Cancer Res*. 2015;21(18):4048–4054.

115. Qi WX, Shen Z, Tang LN, Yao Y. Congestive heart failure risk in cancer patients treated with vascular endothelial growth factor tyrosine kinase inhibitors: a systematic review and meta-analysis of 36 clinical trials. *Br J Clin Pharmacol*. 2014;78(4):748–762.

116. U.S. Food and Drug Administration. Lenvatinib (Lenvima). 2015. http://www.fda.gov/Drugs/

InformationOnDrugs/ApprovedDrugs/ucm434347. htm. Accessed May 30, 2016.

117. Wells SA Jr, Robinson BG, Gagel RF, et al. Vandetanib in patients with locally advanced or metastatic medullary thyroid cancer: a randomized, double-blind phase III trial. *J Clin Oncol*. 2012;30(2):134–141.

118. Wilke H, Muro K, Van Cutsem E, et al. RAINBOW study group. Ramucirumab plus paclitaxel versus placebo plus paclitaxel in patients with previously treated advanced gastric or gastro-oesophageal junction adenocarcinoma (RAINBOW): a double-blind, randomised phase 3 trial. *Lancet Oncol*. 2014;15(11):1224–1235.

119. Tabernero J, Yoshino T, Cohn AL, et al. RAISE study investigators. Ramucirumab versus placebo in combination with second-line FOLFIRI in patients with metastatic colorectal carcinoma that progressed during or after first-line therapy with bevacizumab, oxaliplatin, and a fluoropyrimidine (RAISE): a randomised, double-blind, multicentre, phase 3 study. *Lancet Oncol*. 2015;16(5):499–508.

120. Steingart RM, Bakris GL, Chen HX, et al. Management of cardiac toxicity in patients receiving vascular endothelial growth factor signaling pathway inhibitors. *Am Heart J*. 2012;163(2):156–163.

121. Tassan-Mangina S, Codorean D, Metivier M, et al. Tissue Doppler imaging and conventional echocardiography after anthracycline treatment in adults: early and late alterations of left ventricular function during a prospective study. *Eur J Echocardiogr*. 2006;7(2):141–146.

122. Ghatalia P, Je Y, Kaymakcalan MD, Sonpavde G, Choueiri TK. QTc interval prolongation with vascular endothelial growth factor receptor tyrosine kinase inhibitors. *Br J Cancer*. 2015;112(2):296–305.

123. Sanguinetti MC, Mitcheson JS. Predicting drug-hERG channel interactions that cause acquired long QT syndrome. *Trends Pharmacol Sci*. 2005;26(3):119–124.

124. Sanguinetti MC, Jiang C, Curran ME, Keating MT. A mechanistic link between an inherited and an acquired cardiac arrhythmia: HERG encodes the IKr potassium channel. *Cell*. 1995;81(2):299–307.

125. Kruse V, Somers A, Van Bortel L, De Both A, Van Belle S, Rottey S. Sunitinib for metastatic renal cell cancer patients: observational study highlighting the risk of important drug-drug interactions. *J Clin Pharm Ther*. 2014;39(3):259–265.

126. Bello CL, Mulay M, Huang X, et al. Electrocardiographic characterization of the QTc interval in patients with advanced solid tumors: pharmacokinetic- pharmacodynamic evaluation of sunitinib. *Clin Cancer Res*. 2009;15(22):7045–7052.

127. Symonds RP, Gourley C, Davidson S, et al. Cediranib combined with carboplatin and paclitaxel in patients with metastatic or recurrent cervical cancer (CIRCCa): a randomised, double-blind, placebo-controlled phase 2 trial. *Lancet Oncol*. 2015;16(15):1515–1524.

128. Zeltser D, Justo D, Halkin A, Prokhorov V, Heller K, Viskin S. Torsade de pointes due to noncardiac drugs: most patients have easily identifiable risk factors. *Medicine (Baltimore)*. 2003;82(4):282–290.

129. Ederhy S, Cohen A, Dufaitre G, et al. QT interval prolongation among patients treated with angiogenesis inhibitors. *Target Oncol*. 2009;4(2):89–97.

130. Akman T, Erbas O, Akman L, Yilmaz AU. Prevention of pazopanib-induced prolonged cardiac repolarization and proarrhythmic effects. *Arq Bras Cardiol*. 2014;103(5):403–409.

131. Izzedine H, Massard C, Spano JP, Goldwasser F, Khayat D, Soria JC. VEGF signalling inhibition-induced proteinuria: mechanisms, significance and management. *Eur J Cancer*. 2010;46(2):439–448.

132. Frangié C, Lefaucheur C, Medioni J, Jacquot C, Hill GS, Nochy D. Renal thrombotic microangiopathy caused by anti-VEGF-antibody treatment for metastatic renal-cell carcinoma. *Lancet Oncol*. 2007;8(2):177–178.

133. Johnson DH, Fehrenbacher L, Novotny WF, et al. Randomized phase II trial comparing bevacizumab plus carboplatin and paclitaxel with carboplatin and paclitaxel alone in previously untreated locally advanced or metastatic non-small-cell lung cancer. *J Clin Oncol*. 2004;22(11):2184–2191.

134. Roncone D, Satoskar A, Nadasdy T, Monk JP, Rovin BH. Proteinuria in a patient receiving anti-VEGF therapy for metastatic renal cell carcinoma. *Nat Clin Pract Nephrol*. 2007;3(5):287–293.

135. Eremina V, Jefferson JA, Kowalewska J, et al. VEGF inhibition and renal thrombotic microangiopathy. *N Engl J Med*. 2008;358(11):1129–1136.

136. Stokes MB, Erazo MC, D'Agati VD. Glomerular disease related to anti-VEGF therapy. *Kidney Int*. 2008;74(11):1487–1491.

137. Bollée G, Patey N, Cazajous G, et al. Thrombotic microangiopathy secondary to VEGF pathway inhibition by sunitinib. *Nephrol Dial Transplant*. 2009;24(2):682–685.

138. Izzedine H, Brocheriou I, Rixe O, Deray G. Interstitial nephritis in a patient taking sorafenib. *Nephrol Dial Transplant*. 2007;22(8):2411.

139. Izzedine H, Brocheriou I, Deray G, Rixe O. Thrombotic microangiopathy and anti-VEGF agents. *Nephrol Dial Transplant*. 2007;22(5):1481–1482.

140. Zhu X, Wu S, Dahut WL, Parikh CR. Risks of proteinuria and hypertension with bevacizumab, an antibody against vascular endothelial growth factor: systematic review and meta-analysis. *Am J Kidney Dis*. 2007;49(12):186–193.

141. Kappers MH, van Esch JH, Sleijfer S, Danser AH, van den Meiracker AH. Cardiovascular and renal toxicity during angiogenesis inhibition: clinical and mechanistic aspects. *J Hypertens*. 2009;27(12):2297–2309.

142. Thornton K, Kim G, Maher VE, et al. Vandetanib for the treatment of symptomatic or progressive medullary thyroid cancer in patients with unresectable locally advanced or metastatic disease: U.S. Food and Drug Administration drug approval summary. *Clin Cancer Res*. 2012;18:3722–3730.

143. Patel TV, Morgan JA, Demetri GD, et al. A preeclampsia -like syndrome characterized by reversible hypertension

and proteinuria induced by the multitargeted kinase inhibitors sunitinib and sorafenib. *J Natl Cancer Inst.* 2008;100(4):282–284.

144. Robinson ES, Matulonis UA, Ivy P, et al. Rapid development of hypertension and proteinuria with cediranib, an oral vascular endothelial growth factor receptor inhibitor. *Clin J Am Soc Nephrol.* 2010;5(3):477–483.

145. Armstrong TS, Wen PY, Gilbert MR, Schiff D. Management of treatment-associated toxicites of anti-angiogenic therapy in patients with brain tumors. *Neuro Oncol.* 2012;14(10):1203–1214.

146. Kandula P, Agarwal R. Proteinuria and hypertension with tyrosine kinase inhibitors. *Kidney Int.* 2011;80(12):1271–1277.

147. Novoty WF, Holmgren E, Griffing S, et al. Identification of squamous cell histology and central, cavitary tumores as possible risk factors for pulmonary hemorrhage in patients with advanced NSCLC receiving bevacizumab. *Proc Am Soc Clin Oncol.* 2001;19:330a. Abstract 1318.

148. Sandler AB, Schiller JH, Gray R, et al. Retrospective evaluation of the clinical and radiographic risk factors associated with severe pulmonary hemorrhage in first-line advanced, unresectable non-small-cell lung cancer treated with Carboplatin and Paclitaxel plus bevacizumab. *J Clin Oncol.* 2009;27(9):1405–1412.

149. Scagliotti G, Novello S, von Pawel J, et al. Phase III study of carboplatin and paclitaxel alone or with sorafenib in advanced non-small-cell lung cancer. *J Clin Oncol.* 2010;28(11):1835–1842.

150. Bondarenko IM, Ingrosso A, Bycott P, Kim S, Cebotaru CL. Phase II study of axitinib with doublet chemotherapy in patients with advanced squamous non-small-cell lung cancer. *BMC Cancer.* 2015;15:339.

151. Socinski MA, Novello S, Brahmer JR, et al. Multicenter, phase II trial of sunitinib in previously treated, advanced non-small-cell lung cancer. *J Clin Oncol.* 2008;26(4):650–656.

152. Kabbinavar F, Hurwitz HI, Fehrenbacher L, et al. Phase II, randomized trial comparing bevacizumab plus fluorouracil (FU)/leucovorin (LV) with FU/LV alone in patients with metastatic colorectal cancer. *J Clin Oncol.* 2003;21(1):60–65.

153. Sarkiss MG, Yusuf SW, Warneke CL, et al. Impact of aspirin therapy in cancer patients with thrombocytopenia and acute coronary syndromes. *Cancer.* 2007;109(3):621–627.

154. Scappaticci FA, Fehrenbacher L, Cartwright T, et al. Surgical wound healing complications in metastatic colorectal cancer patients treated with bevacizumab. *J Surg Oncol.* 2005;91(3):173–180.

155. Ang KK, Zhang Q, Rosenthal DI, et al. Randomized phase III trial of concurrent accelerated radiation plus cisplatin with or without cetuximab for stage III to IV head and neck carcinoma: RTOG 0522. *J Clin Oncol.* 2014;32(27):2940–2950.

156. Giusti RM, Cohen MH, Keegan P, Pazdur R. FDA review of a panitumumab (Vectibix) clinical trial for first-line treatment of metastatic colorectal cancer. *Oncologist.* 2009;14(3):284–290.

18 Heart–Lung Interactions in the Cancer Patient

Vickie R. Shannon ▪ *Saadia A. Faiz*

INTRODUCTION

The heart and lungs represent two distinct organ systems that are inextricably intertwined due to anatomic proximity and highly integrated mechanical, physiologic, and cellular mechanisms. The biological crosstalk between these two organ systems is essential to maintain body homeostasis. Under normal circumstances, the physiologic consequences of heart and lung interactions are subtle; however in disease states, derangements in one organ system may profoundly affect the performance of the other through interdependent hemodynamic, neurohumoral, and cell signaling feedback mechanisms. Thus, significant dysfunction of the heart or lungs may lead to reciprocal injury to the other organ system, resulting in structural and functional cardiorespiratory deterioration and a rapid clinical decline. The overall goal of these tightly integrated systems is the provision of an adequate oxygen supply in relation to oxygen consumption (VO_2) to the organs and tissues of the body. The balance between oxygen supply and demand is easily maintained in healthy cardiorespiratory states. Failure to meet these demands may lead to hypoxic systemic tissue injury, metabolic acidosis, and ultimately organ dysfunction and failure.

Cardiorespiratory compromise is common in the cancer setting due to the propensity for cancer therapy or the disease itself to adversely affect these two organ systems. For example, injury to the pulmonary interstitium, alveolar-capillary membrane, pleura, pulmonary circulation, or airways is a common sequelae of cancer surgery, thoracic irradiation, or pneumotoxic chemotherapeutic and immunotherapy regimens. Adult respiratory distress syndrome (ARDS), the most severe form of lung injury, may ensue, resulting in subacute or chronic erosion of the cardiopulmonary reserve. Alternatively, pulmonary embolic events resulting from thrombus, tumor, air, or fat may have acute and devastating consequences on the cardiovascular system. Tumors within the lung may exert direct effects on the heart and mediastinal structures or, alternatively, produce hormonally active substances that indirectly compromise cardiovascular function. Finally, common critical care interventions, such as positive-pressure ventilation and the institution of positive end-expiratory pressure (PEEP),

may compromise systemic blood flow, leading to cardiopulmonary collapse. Many of these pulmonary disorders appear simultaneously in the cancer setting, and patients frequently succumb to cardiac failure and respiratory failure as the end-point of a complex series of cardiopulmonary interactions. Thus, an understanding of the interactions between the circulatory and pulmonary organ systems is central to the optimal treatment of the cancer patient with lung disease.

This chapter will review some of the common mechanical and physiologic consequences of cancer and its therapy on cardiopulmonary function. Several broad areas will be emphasized, including (1) the physiologic basis for heart-lung interactions; (2) cardiac consequences of pulmonary diseases, such as COPD; (3) cancer treatment-related lung parenchymal, airway and vascular disease; (4) cancer-related disorders of ventilatory control, including the cardiovascular consequences of sleep-disordered breathing and neurologic and chest wall disorders; (5) cardiac consequences of ventilator pump failure. This review summarizes the challenges associated with identifying the pathophysiologic mechanisms of heart-lung crosstalk and provides practical algorithms for diagnosis and treatment interventions in the cancer setting.

PHYSIOLOGICAL BASIS FOR HEART-LUNG INTERACTIONS

▪ Respiration and Cardiac Function

The complex physiologic basis for heart-lung interactions requires an understanding of the effects of changes in intrathoracic pressure (ITP) and lung volumes on venous return, pulmonary vascular resistance (PVR), left ventricular (LV) ejection fraction, cardiac output, and the metabolic energy needed to create these changes. The heart is a pressure driven system within the pressure driven thorax. Therefore, changes in ITP not only effect venous return to the right ventricle (RV), but also LV afterload. ITP is decreased during spontaneous tidal inspiration due to the contraction of respiratory muscles. Contraction and descent of the diaphragmatic muscles during spontaneous inspiration result in increased intra-abdominal pressure, while ITP and right atrial pressures (RAP) are reduced, creating a pressure gradient that markedly favors systemic venous return to the right heart. As ITP decreases, intrathoracic blood volume, LV afterload, and cardiac output increase proportionately at a constant arterial pressure. Alternatively, increased ITP, as seen during positive pressure inspiration, lowers the pressure gradient for venous return by increasing RAP and decreasing LV transmural systolic pressures.

■ Ventricular Interdependence

During spontaneous inspiration, increases in RV blood flow cause septal shift into the LV lumen, decreasing LV diastolic compliance and end-diastolic volume. During expiration, blood flow entering the RV is decreased, allowing the interventricular septum to shift into the RV with augmented filling of the LV and increased LV end diastolic pressures. This phenomenon is referred to as ventricular interdependence in which the amount of blood flow into one ventricular chamber is dependent on the amount of blood flow into the other ventricle. By contrast, positive pressure ventilation (PPV) reduces biventricular volumes by compressing both ventricles onto each other, thereby minimizing ventricular interdependence. Ventricular interdependence is manifested clinically as inspiration-associated decreases in arterial pulse pressure, otherwise known as pulsus paradoxus. These hemodynamic changes are trivial under normal circumstances, but may become clinically significant with more negative ITP swings associated with vigorous ventilatory efforts. Hypovolemia, tachypnea, and increased tidal volumes also exaggerate these hemodynamic changes by delaying blood flow from the RV to the LV. In addition, pressure or volume overload of the right ventricle, as seen in cases of chronic obstructive pulmonary disease (COPD), pulmonary hypertension (PH) and atrial septal defect (ASD) may also reduce LV systolic and diastolic function due to the effect on the interventricular septum.

These physiologic concepts are particularly relevant in the understanding and management of common respiratory disorders such as COPD, pulmonary fibrosis, pulmonary vascular diseases, neuromuscular and chest wall disorders, and disorders of ventilation and ventilatory control. Each of these topics will be discussed separately.

CARDIAC CONSEQUENCES OF PULMONARY DISEASE

In the cancer setting, cardiac consequences of pulmonary disease often occur as a result of shared risk factors and / or common pathogenic mechanisms for cardiac and lung disease. Maladaptive interactions between these two pressure-driven systems may result in erosion of the cardiopulmonary reserve and cardiac failure. For example, COPD, a frequent comorbidity of lung cancer, may adversely affect cardiac function due to shared risk factors and pathogenic mechanisms, and, when severe, lead to cardiac failure as the endpoint of a complex series of cardiopulmonary interactions. Other pulmonary diseases that are common in the cancer setting, including pulmonary vascular disorders, infection-, drug- and radiation-induced lung injury, and disorders of ventilatory control, may result in severe cardiac reserve and failure.

■ Chronic Obstructive Pulmonary Disease (COPD)

Until recently, chronic obstructive pulmonary disease (COPD) was regarded as a chronic disease of the lungs and defined by its associated degree of airflow obstruction. More recent reports have redefined COPD as a chronic inflammatory condition with significant extrapulmonary manifestations.[1-3] Cigarette smoking, the major risk factor for COPD, causes diffuse inflammation of the lung parenchyma and airways and is an increasingly recognized cause of systemic cellular and humoral inflammation.[4-7] In addition, tobacco smoke-related changes in vasomotor tone, endothelial function, and increased blood concentrations of procoagulant factors also occur in COPD.[8] Inflammation and disruption of elastic fibers are common pathologic processes in both emphysema and coronary artery disease (CAD) and underlie the pathogenic mechanisms for atherosclerotic plaque development and destabilization in CAD.[9] Inflammation also plays a central role in the pathogenesis of chronic heart failure, regardless of its etiology.[10-13] Not surprisingly, COPD often coexists with chronic heart diseases, such as CAD and congestive heart failure (CHF), based on shared risk factors and mutual pathogenic mechanisms of systemic cellular and humoral inflammation. The inflammatory response in COPD may, in fact, facilitate disease progression in atherosclerosis and contribute to the higher rate of cardiovascular-related deaths in COPD.

The cardiovascular manifestations of COPD have been increasingly recognized, including cardiac dysrhythmias, left ventricular hypertrophy and atherosclerosis, myocardial infarction, pulmonary hypertension, and cor pulmonale (Table 18-1).[14-16] Contrary to the conventional paradigm that suggested that patients with COPD die from complications related to lung disease, recent studies have implicated cardiovascular disease as a major cause of death in this group of patients, particularly in patients with mild

TABLE 18-1   Cardiovascular manifestations of pulmonary disease

PULMONARY DISEASE	ASSOCIATED CARDIOVASCULAR CONDITIONS
Pulmonary hypertension	RV dysfunction Cor-pulmonale
COPD	PH with associated RV dysfunction Arrhythmias CAD Pulmonary embolism Hypoxia-related exacerbation of preexisting LV dysfunction, LV hypertrophy
Sleep-disordered breathing: Obstructive sleep apnea (OSA) Central sleep apnea (CSA)	Hypertension, CVA, CAD CHF

to moderate stages of COPD.[17] In the Lung Health Study 2, cardiovascular disease was the second leading cause of morbidity and mortality, accounting for 50% of all hospital admissions and nearly 25% of deaths among the 6000 smokers with COPD that were evaluated.[18] Subsequent studies have confirmed a 2–3 fold increased risk of cardiovascular co-morbidity, including ischemic heart disease, arrhythmias, pulmonary embolism, stroke, and heart failure, compared to those patients without COPD.[19,20] Although increased rates of atherosclerosis in patients with COPD may be attributable to tobacco use as a common risk factor, epidemiological evidence suggests that impaired lung function (as assessed by FEV1), is an independent risk factor for cardiovascular death in this group of patients.[19–21] The prevalence of airflow obstruction among patients with ischemic heart disease is also high. In a recent study, 34% of patients with angiography-proven coronary artery disease had moderate to severe airflow obstruction on spirometric testing.[22] Many of these patients did not have a prior diagnosis of COPD, suggesting that the relationship between COPD and CAD is underappreciated in the medical community.

Patients with moderate to severe COPD and associated pulmonary hypertension (PH) may have increased plasma N-terminal pro-BNP (NT-proBNP) levels due to right-sided myocardial stress. In a recent study, elevated NT-proBNP in patients with COPD was an independent predictor of one year mortality.[23] The mechanisms linking COPD and cardiovascular disease have not been completely elucidated; however, shared genetic mechanisms, and perturbations in inflammatory, neurohumoral, and oxidative responses have been implicated. Chronic inflammation has been increasingly implicated as a shared pathogenic mechanism. Lung and systemic inflammatory responses intensify during COPD exacerbations and decline with recovery. Interestingly, patients with COPD are at the highest risk for cardiovascular events, such as CAD or stroke during the first 5 days of an acute COPD exacerbation.[24] In both CAD and COPD, the production of T_H1-mediated proinflammatory cytokines contribute to local tissue injury and serve as a self-perpetuating stimulus for further immune activation. Systemic inflammatory markers such as IL1- β, IL-6, IL-8, TNF-α, MMP-9, and CRP are elevated in all stages of COPD. Interestingly, many of these markers are also increased in cardiovascular disease (Table 18-2). CRP elevations correlate with COPD exacerbations and disease severity and may have therapeutic implications.[25–38] Many of these cytokines cause the production of large amounts of potentially destructive mediators, including tissue proteases, fibrinogen, and C-reactive protein (CRP). CRP, a marker of downstream inflammation, may also promote atherogenesis.[39,40]

The recognition of chronic inflammation as a pathogenic factor in COPD and CAD has raised questions regarding the utility of anti-inflammatory strategies in the management of coexisting tobacco-related cardiopulmonary diseases. Current practice guidelines in the management of COPD, CAD, and chronic heart failure, focus primarily on the individual disease conditions, without regard for the inflammatory heart and lung interactions. However, recent investigations suggest that several well-established agents with salutatory roles in the management of cardiac diseases, such as statins, angiotensin converting enzymes (ACE) inhibitors, and angiotensin receptor blockers (ARBs) may exhibit dual cardiopulmonary protection due to

TABLE 18-2   COPD and Atherosclerosis: potential common mediators of chronic inflammation

MEDIATOR	FUNCTION	TARGET	COPD	ATHEROSCLEROSIS	REFERENCES
IL1-b	Neutrophil chemotaxis	Leukocytes	Lung inflammation;	Inflammation	Lappalainen et al.,[25] Chung,[29]
IL-8	Neutrophil chemotaxis	Leukocytes	Lung inflammation		
LTB4	Neutrophil chemotaxis	Leukocytes	Lung inflammation Tissue remodeling	Initiation/ progression of atherosclerotic plaque	Beeh,[37] Back M Cardiovasc Drugs Ther. 2009
MMP-9	Proteolysis	Extracellular matrix	Destruction of airway parenchyma leading to emphysema	Unstable atherosclerotic lesions; plaque rupture	
TGF-b	Intimal proliferation, collagen accumulation	Smooth muscle cells	Hyperinflammation; smooth muscle proliferation; peribronchial fibrosis	Hyperinflammation; smooth muscle proliferaton; accelerated atherosclerosis; intimal hyperplasia	Robertson,[30] Bobik[34]
TNF-a	Neutrophil chemotaxis	Leukocytes, vascular smooth muscle, respiratory epithelium	Lung inflammation, fibrosis and emphysema	Plaque formation; plaque rupture	Kleinbongard et al.,[26] Mukhopadhyay et al.,[27] Sun et al.[28]

their potentially beneficial effects on lung inflammation.[41] For example, in addition to their influence on systemic inflammation and cardiovascular morbidity, statins appear to have direct disease modifying effects on the airways, perhaps though their ability to reduce inflammatory markers, such as C-reactive protein (CRP).[42] Several investigations have suggested a role for statins in attenuating the annual decline in lung function, improving exercise capacity, and reducing respiratory-related urgent care, hospitalizations and deaths among patients with COPD.[43,44] Given the fact that myocardial events are highest within the first 5 days of an acute COPD exacerbation, the use of statins in preventing COPD exacerbations may reduce the rate of concomitant cardiovascular events. Although these findings are intriguing, a role for statin drugs in the management of COPD and reducing the risk of cardiovascular disease in patients with COPD has not been confirmed. These observations have,

in fact, been challenged in more recent trials[45] and require validation in larger, randomized studies. Activation of the renin-angiotensin system (RAS) has also been associated with systemic inflammation. Thus, pharmacological blockade of RAS may represent a novel therapeutic approach to patients with COPD, particularly in the setting of concomitant pulmonary hypertension.[46] In one study, reductions in total lung capacity by angiotensin II receptor blockade was seen; however, further investigations are needed to validate these findings.[47] β–blockers, which have a long history of therapeutic efficacy in the management of cardiovascular disease has been regarded as detrimental in treating patients with COPD. However, recent observational data have suggested a role for cardioselective β–blockers in reducing COPD exacerbations and mortality.[48] Anti-inflammatory medications used in the management of COPD, such as inhaled corticosteroids have been shown to significantly reduce CRP levels. As COPD and cancer—in particular lung cancer—often coexist, these types of advances have specific relevance for the cancer patient. Well-designed prospective controlled studies are needed to corroborate these findings.

Sleep-Related Breathing Disorders

Sleep ■ Sleep represents a complex, active state that is characterized by periods of rapid eye movement (REM) and non-rapid eye movement (NREM) sleep. NREM sleep is further divided into 3 stages: N1; N2; and N3 (delta or slow-wave sleep). REM sleep is predominantly a parasympathetic state that is comprised of phasic and tonic sleep. During phasic REM sleep, rapid eye movements are accompanied by bursts of sympathetic nervous system activity. The most accurate and objective measure of sleep is polysomnography (PSG), which records simultaneously several electroencephalographic (EEG) and physiologic parameters. Distinct EEG findings distinguish the stages of sleep. Each sleep cycle lasts approximately 90 to 120 minutes. Sleep onset occurs with N1 (short-lived), which progresses to N2 (50% of total sleep time), and eventually to N3 and REM sleep. The duration of REM sleep periods increases as the night progresses and accounts for 20%–25% of total sleep time in healthy middle-aged individuals.[49] Four to five sleep cycles occur during a typical night of sleep. Sleep architecture changes with age and may be disrupted by sleep disorders, medications, alcohol, underlying medical illness and/or sleep deprivation.

During normal sleep, declines in systemic blood pressure and heart rate reach a nadir during the early periods of slow-wave sleep.[50] The blood pressure may rise during REM sleep but remains lower than blood pressure elevations during awake states.[50] Intermittent hypoxia and hypercapnia may occur during sleep, owing to periods of apnea (cessation of inspiratory flow) and hypopnea (reduction in inspiratory airflow). These periods of hypoxia trigger a sympathetic response, resulting in oscillation of systemic and pulmonary pressures, heart rate, and cardiac function. Often, this event provokes sleep arousals, which may be associated with normal breathing and restoration of normal gas exchange.

In normal individuals, sleep deprivation has been reported to depress ventilatory responses to hypercapnia and hypoxia.[51,52] In patients with concomitant pulmonary and/or neuromuscular disease, sleep deprivation may have profound effects on cardiopulmonary function, including respiratory muscle endurance.[53] Prospective studies have demonstrated a reduction or absence of REM sleep in the immediate postoperative period, followed by REM rebound (an increase in the both the number of phasic events and overall REM sleep).[54,55] Although REM sleep following a period of sleep deprivation is considered restorative, reports of delirium and nightmares, along with variable heart rates, respiration and blood pressure may further disrupt sleep. REM rebound has been hypothesized to contribute to postoperative myocardial ischemia and infarction.[56,57]

There is increasing evidence to support an important role for the sleep-wake cycle in immunological functions and the homeostatic regulation of sympathetic activity. For example, IL-2 production, plasma cortisol levels, and natural killer (NK) cell responses are blunted with sleep loss. NK cells play an important role in anti-tumor immune responses and response to infectious pathogens.[58,59] In two recent prospective studies, reduced sleep duration correlated inversely with blood pressure[60] and coronary artery calcification.[61] These observations suggest a mechanism that could potentially link sleep loss with cardiovascular disorders as well as immunologic responses to infection, inflammation, and cancer biology.[59,62] Accumulating evidence also indicates that individuals who sleep fewer than four hours have increased rates of cardiovascular mortality.[63] The increasing recognition of the role of sleep disturbances on host defense and sympathetic activities has fueled interest in its potential immunologic as well as cardiovascular consequences. Optimization of sleep disorders may, thus, play a significant role in the successful treatment of a broad range of clinical diseases, including infection, cardiac disorders, and cancer.

Sleep and cancer ■ Sleep disturbances and associated symptoms of daytime hypersomnolence and fatigue are ubiquitous problems in cancer patients, which may present before, during, or after cancer therapy.[64–67] In a large cross-sectional survey of 982 cancer patients, the most prevalent complaints were fatigue (44%), leg restlessness (41%), insomnia (31%), and excessive sleepiness (28%).[68] Confounding factors, such as pain, emotional distress, anemia, nutrition, and activity level may exacerbate disturbed sleep in cancer.[66,67] In a large prospective study, Palesh and colleagues reported a 3-fold increase in symptoms of insomnia among patients undergoing chemotherapy for cancer compared to the general population.[69]

A growing body of evidence associates sleep disruption with the incidence and progression of cancer. In animal models, disruption of the circadian rhythm and sleep fragmentation has been associated with increased carcinogenesis. The suppression of Melatonin and clock genes both play a role in the sleep circadian cycle. Suppression of these two factors has been implicated in sleep disturbance and cancer pathogenesis.[70,71] Several epidemiological studies have reported that human night shift workers might be at an increased risk of cancer.[72,73] Based on animal and human studies, the Internal Agency for Research on Cancer classified shift work with circadian disruption as "probably carcinogenic."[74] Sleep duration has also been implicated in increased risk of some types of cancer, but these studies rely mostly on self-reported sleep duration and lack objective measures, such as actigraphy and PSG.[75–78]

Sleep and cardiovascular disease ■ Sleep disordered breathing (SDB) is increasingly recognized as a common co-morbidity in cardiovascular disease with important clinical implications on long-term cardiovascular outcomes. A major subgroup of SDB includes sleep apnea. The pathognomonic characteristics of sleep apnea include repeated episodes of partial (hypopnea) or complete (apnea) interruption in breathing during sleep with associated hypoxia and partial neurologic arousals (Figure 18-1).[79] The pathophysiological consequences of sleep apnea have been associated with abnormalities in lipid and glucose metabolism, systemic hypertension, stroke, and cardiovascular diseases, including myocardial ischemia, arrhythmias, and left ventricular dysfunction.[80–82]

Sleep apnea is diagnosed by PSG and may be classified as central sleep apnea (CSA), obstructive sleep apnea (OSA), or mixed. Established guidelines by the American Academy of Sleep Medicine (AASM) for the assessment of sleep apnea are based on the Apnea-Hypopnea Index (AHI) and oxygen saturation nadir during PSG. The AHI is defined as the number of apneas and hypopneas per hour of sleep. Disease severity is stratified as follows: AHI < 5, no disease; AHI 5 to <15, mild; AHI 15 to <30, moderate; and AHI ≥30, severe.[83]

CSA ■ Apneic episodes associated with CSA are triggered by instability of the respiratory control center with associated transient withdrawal of central neurological respiratory drive and cessation of respiratory effort and airflow. Oscillations in PaCO2 around the central threshold for ventilation (apneic threshold) are caused by periods of hyperventilation during sleep arousals followed by periods of hypoventilation when PaCO2 is driven below the apneic threshold. Although the proposed mechanisms for CSA and OSA are distinct, the clinical manifestations of sleep disruption, hypoxia, and partial neurologic arousals during sleep are similar. Thus, increased rates of cardiovascular disease are seen in both disorders.

CSA in heart failure is typically accompanied by Cheyne Stokes respirations and has been well studied.

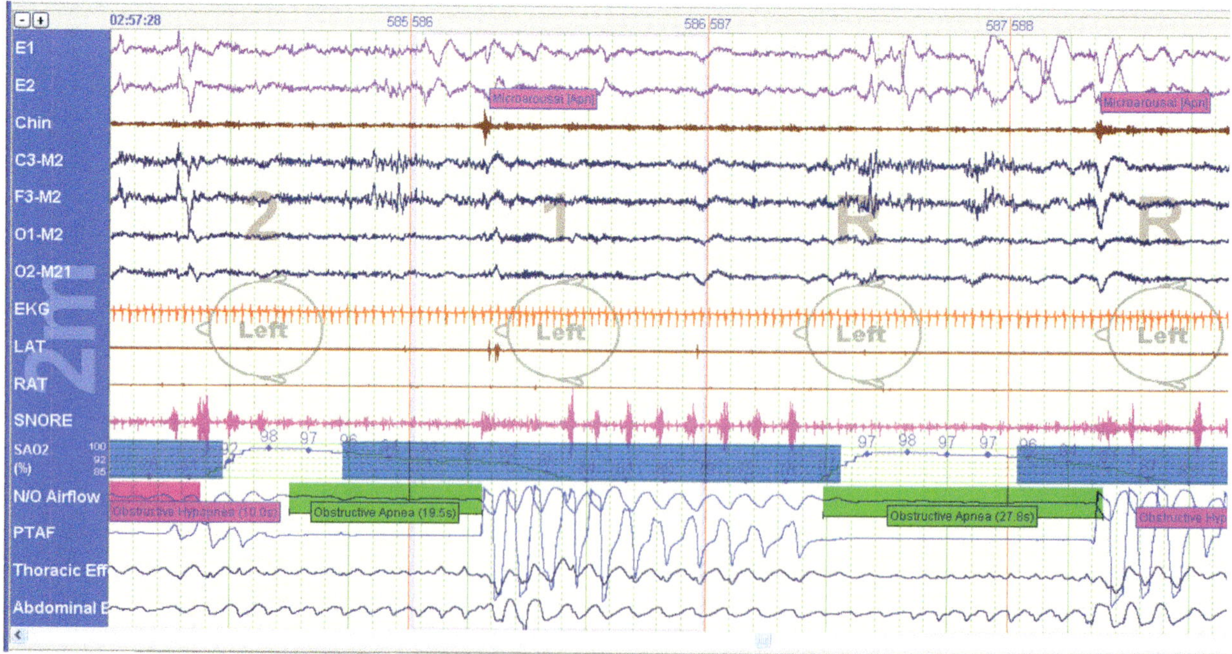

FIGURE 18-1 Standard polysomnogram displaying obstructive sleep apnea and hypopneas with repeated respiratory events with desaturations.

Approximately 35% of patients with heart failure develop CSA during the course of their illness.[2,3,84] The presence of CSA in heart failure confers increased morbidity and mortality.[2,3] Unlike OSA, optimal treatment strategies for CSA are less well defined. CSA tends to improve in parallel with successful treatment of heart failure. Therefore, medical management of heart failure is a primary focus CSA in heart failure. However, in many patients, symptoms may persist despite optimization of heart failure therapies. Other treatment options that have been offered in this setting include nocturnal oxygen supplementation, pharmacotherapies (e.g., theophylline and acetazolamide) and transvenous phrenic nerve stimulation.[85,86] Extrapolation of the results from these studies is limited by small and often nonrandomized investigations. Treatment of central sleep apnea in systolic heart failure with CPAP has been met with controversy. Early studies suggested positive effects of CPAP on sleep parameters such as AHI and nocturnal desaturation; however, improvements in hemodynamics, heart failure, and overall survival were variable, with some studies showing excess mortality among patients with CSA and CHF.[87–89] Further research is need to establish efficacy and safety in the management of CSA in heart failure.

OSA ■ In OSA, recurrent collapse of the upper airway with subsequent pharyngeal obstruction results in reduction or cessation of airflow despite ongoing respiratory effort. Airway obstruction and associated hypoxemia are eventually terminated by an arousal or entry into a lighter stage of sleep, but these cycles of desaturation continue throughout sleep. The clinical sequelae of OSA in terms of reduced quality of life, poor sleep quality, depression, reduced vigilance, and increased rates of motor vehicle accidents are well known. However, the recognition of OSA as a risk factor for cardiovascular disease is relatively new. Available data indicate that the prevalence of OSA is 2–3 fold higher among patients with cardiovascular disease compared to reference populations without heart disease.[2,3,90,91]

Several key features of OSA, namely intermittent hypoxia, hypercapnia, intrathoracic pressure swings, and sleep fragmentation, have been identified as central to the pathophysiology leading to cardiovascular consequences (Figure 18-2). Increased oxidative stress, systemic inflammation, and activation of the sympathetic nervous system have been linked to recurrent cycles of desaturation with reoxygenation in OSA. Hypoxia and sympathetic stimulation may trigger tachyarrhythmias and increased blood pressure. These derangements place increased strain on the heart, resulting in increased myocardial oxygen demand. In addition, massive negative intrathoracic pressure swings generated by ineffective respiratory efforts against a closed glottis creates a large intracardiac and extracardiac pressure differential, which

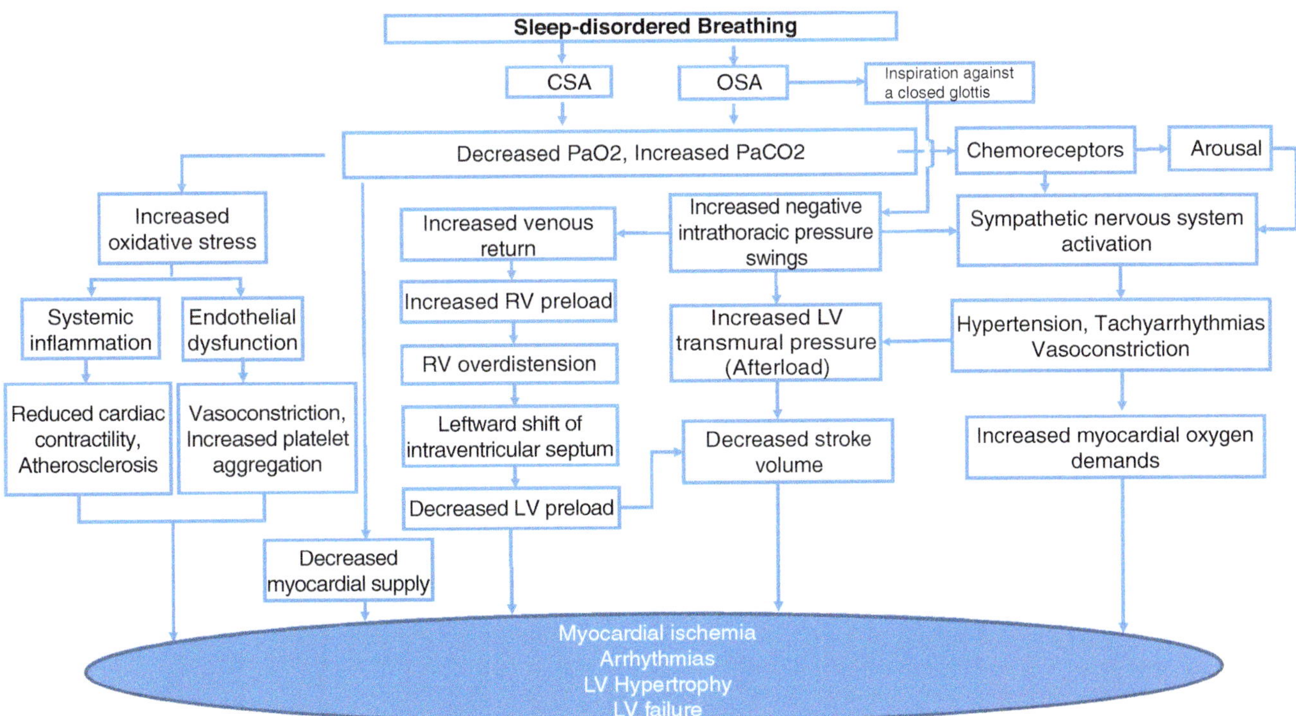

FIGURE 18-2 Proposed pathogenic features of SBD and heart disease.

leads to increased left ventricular afterload. Increased fluid return to the right ventricle due to the large negative intrathoracic pressure results in increased right ventricular preload while sympathetic discharge and hypoxia-induced pulmonary vasoconstriction at the termination of the obstructive event increase right ventricular afterload. Endothelial function, a marker of vascular function, is also impaired in patients with OSA.[92] These physiologic changes ultimately result in reduced LV function and underlie the development and/or progression of cardiovascular disease in OSA[93,94].

OSA and hypertension ■ Evidence suggesting a causal association between OSA and hypertension is compelling. The prevalence of daytime hypertension is much greater in patients with OSA. Approximately 30% of hypertensive patients have OSA.[95,96] Recurrent episodes of apneas and hypopneas during sleep result in exaggerated stimulation of vascular sympathetic activity and the release of circulating catecholamines, resulting in increased peripheral vascular resistance. Changes in intrathoracic pressures upon termination of the apneic episode cause increased cardiac output, which, in the presence of a constricted peripheral vascular bed, results in acute surges in nocturnal blood pressure. It is thought that the nocturnal increases in sympathetic vascular tone remain elevated in normoxemic conditions during the day, leading to daytime hypertension.[97] Other mechanisms that may influence the development of hypertension in patients with OSA include endothelial dysfunction and obesity-related metabolic factors, such as insulin resistance and elevated leptin levels.[98–100] PAP, the standard treatment for OSA, provides a pneumatic splint in the central airways, thus attenuating nocturnal apneas and hypopneas and reducing hypoxia-induced sympathetic activity. Long-term PAP is effective in reducing both nocturnal blood pressure surges as well as daytime hypertension. Thus, OSA should be considered in the differential diagnosis of patients with refractory hypertension, particularly those with obesity. Weight loss should be encouraged in obese patients, and bariatric surgery remains a therapeutic option for patients who fail or refuse PAP therapy.[101]

OSA and pulmonary hypertension ■ OSA may also contribute to the development of pulmonary hypertension. Endothelial damage and vascular remodeling caused by hypoxemia and apneic episodes are thought to promote the development sustained elevations in pulmonary artery pressures over time. Details of OSA-related pulmonary hypertension are discussed elsewhere in this chapter. Finally, OSA has

also been implicated in the development of stroke. The mechanism of stroke in these patients is unclear but likely relates to increased prevalence of hypertension and atherosclerosis in these patients.

OSA and heart failure ■ OSA has also been linked to the development of heart failure. Unlike CSA, which is more often associated with systolic dysfunction, OSA has been frequently linked to left ventricular diastolic dysfunction. Both conditions may coexist. As sleep progresses during the night, patients with heart failure may transition from predominantly central apneas to SDB with more obstructive features. Sleep apnea severity correlates with the degree of impairment of the left ventricular ejection fraction. In patients with mixed OSA and CSA features, substantial improvements in LVEF and function class has been documented with PAP therapy.[102]

OSA and CAD ■ OSA has also been associated with acute nocturnal ischemia and ST-segment depression. This event primarily occurs during REM sleep, which is the period of greatest oxygen desaturations and apneas. Conceivably, the REM-related hypoxemia, increased sympathetic activity, increased systemic vascular resistance, and tachycardia result in increased cardiac oxygen demand and myocardial ischemia. OSA-associated myocardial ischemia has been reported among patients with preexisting coronary artery disease as well as patients without established disease. Whether the predisposition for nocturnal ischemia in patients with OSA is directly related the process of atherogenesis or through indirect mechanisms (hypertension) is unclear.[103,104]

OSA and arrhythmias ■ Sudden cardiac death, owing to arrhythmias and myocardial infarction occurs in 46% of patients with OSA, compared to 21% of patients without this disorder.[105] The most common arrhythmias associated with OSA are sinus bradycardia and atrioventricular block (including sinus arrest and complete heart block). These bradyarrhythmias tend to be atropine-responsive and may occur in the absence of any primary disease within the cardiac conducting system.[106] An increase in vagal tone elicited by apneic or hypoxic episodes is the proposed mechanism of OSA-related bradycardia. These arrhythmias are most prominent during REM sleep and tend correlate with both apnea and hypopnea severity. Tachyarrhythmias also occur and their prevalence and severity are increased in patients with underlying cardiac disease. Both ventricular and supraventricular tachyarrhythmias have been reported. Patients with new onset atrial fibrillation should be screened for OSA.Several studies suggest higher rates of recurrence of atrial fibrillation after cardioversion among patients with untreated OSA compared to patients without OSA.[107,108]

OSA and cancer ■ The association between OSA and malignancy continues to evolve. Both intermittent hypoxia and sleep fragmentation mimic OSA. The effect of these derangements on cancer development has been studied in murine models. Almendros and colleagues demonstrated excess tumor growth, metastasis and mortality among mice with melanoma that were subjected to intermittent hypoxia versus controls.[109] Similarly, increased rates of lung carcinoma were demonstrated among male mice that were subjected to sleep fragmentation.[110] Two large observational studies have also suggested an association between malignancy and OSA among human subjects. The first study included a 22-year follow-up of a population-based cohort of 1522 patients with OSA. This investigation was the first to identify a positive relationship between the severity of OSA and mortality for all types of cancer. After adjusting for potential confounding variables, the association remained significant and persisted when patients treated with positive airway pressure therapy (PAP) were excluded.[111] The second study included 4910 patients with a median follow- up of 5 years. Both AHI and percent nocturnal desaturation below 90% ($TSat_{90}$) were used as surrogates for OSA severity in this study. A significant association was found between the incidence of cancer and severity of OSA as measured by $TSat_{90}$ after correcting for important confounding variables.[112] Both studies support an association between OSA and cancer, in which intermittent hypoxia plays a key role. Intermittent hypoxia is thought to result in oxidative stress, increased production of hypoxia-induced factor (HIF-1), and systemic inflammation. Other potential mediators in the development of malignancy may include oxidative stress, inflammation, insulin resistance and endothelial dysfunction.

OSA may complicate a variety of tumors of the head and neck region, most notably squamous cell carcinoma and sarcomas.[113] The incidence of OSA documented by polysomnography among patients with head and neck cancer varies from 8% to 92% in the published literature.[65,113,114] In contrast to obesity, which is a dominant characteristic of patients with OSA in the general population, in a study by Faiz and associates, more than half of the patients with OSA and head and neck cancer was not obese (52% with BMI < 30 kg/m²). The majority of their patients (79%) had undergone radiation therapy as part of their cancer therapy. Thus, factors other than obesity, such as architectural distortion of the proximal airway by cancer or its treatment may have played a role in the development of OSA in these patients.

Impact of CPAP on cardiovascular disease ■ Continuous positive airway pressure (CPAP) is now the standard of care in the management of patients with OSA, based on robust literature demonstrating the utility positive airway pressure in ameliorating airway obstruction in patients with this disorder. Significant improvements in daytime hypersomnolence, sleep quality, and cognitive impairments following CPAP therapy have been shown in randomized trials, particularly among patients with severe OSA (apnea-hypopnea index greater than 30). A survival benefit among CPAP users has been suggested from cohort studies; however, no large randomized studies have been performed. Among patients with OSA and cardiovascular disease, a growing body of evidence suggests improvements in cardiac function, systemic inflammatory markers (CRP, TNF-a, IL-6), biomarkers of cardiovascular disease, total cholesterol and triglyceride levels.[115] In other studies, CPAP therapy has been shown to favorably effect diurnal and nocturnal systolic and diastolic blood pressures and improve left ventricular function.[116,117] A cardioprotective benefit in terms of decreasing myocardial events, stroke, arrhythmias, and improving quality of life has also been suggested in several studies. Many of these studies were nonrandomized and insufficiently powered to establish evidence of the benefits of CPAP in cardiovascular disease and to determine its long-term benefits and safety. The most convincing evidence comes from studies demonstrating the effects of CPAP on arrhythmias. CPAP therapy significantly reduces the incidence of tachyarrhythmias and has been found to be curative in OSA-related bradyarrhythmias.[107,118] Several small studies have suggested a survival benefit among patients with OSA and cardiovascular disease; however, the quality of evidence for an improvement in mortality is, at best, weak.[119–122]

PULMONARY VASCULAR DISEASE

■ Pulmonary Thromboembolism.

Acute pulmonary embolism. ■ *Etiology* Intimal injury, venous stasis, and hypercoagulability are central to the pathogenesis of a thromboembolic disease. Each of the variables is common in the cancer setting. For example, central venous catheters, which are frequently used in cancer patients, may predispose to thrombosis formation by providing a nidus for clot formation.[123,124] Co-morbid factors, such as prolonged bed rest or major surgery that lead to venous stasis may permit an otherwise asymptomatic hypercoagulable state to become clinically manifest. Notably, risk factors for the development of thromboembolism exert their effects cumulatively and are conditioned by other co-morbid illnesses. Thus, while the patient with breast cancer and no other co-morbid illnesses has a modest risk for the development of thromboembolic disease, their risk increases substantially with the initiation of chemotherapeutic agents that have prothrombotic potential such as tamoxifen, develops treatment-related congestive heart failure, or with the development of a pathologic hip fracture.[125] These unfortunate, but all too real clinical scenarios, create important risk profiles in the cancer patient that should heighten suspicion for the diagnosis of thromboembolic events and condition the intensity of prophylactic initiatives.

Pathophysiology The consequences of massive pulmonary embolism (MPE) are usually catastrophic, resulting in acute elevations in pulmonary vascular resistance, altered right ventricular performance, severe hypoxemia, and sudden death. Preexisting cardiopulmonary disease in patients with submassive pulmonary embolism may have an equally catastrophic outcome. Mortality rates attributable to pulmonary thromboembolic phenomena range from 13.4%–24%[126–129] and may rise substantially among patients with associated hemodynamic instability.[127,130] Of those patients that succumb to PE, more than 2/3 die within the first hour of the onset of symptoms of complications related to shock. Thus, early diagnosis and treatment have a significant impact on patient outcome. In the cancer patient where comorbid illnesses may mask, mimic or simply coexist with thromboembolic disease, the diagnosis of pulmonary embolism poses an even more difficult challenge and missed diagnoses in this group of patients carry a significantly increased risk of potentially fatal consequences. Thrombus embolization typically results from migration of clot that originates in the large capacitance vessels of the pelvis and lower extremities into the central pulmonary arteries.[131,132] Other contributing sites for clot formation, including upper extremity thrombi in patients with central venous catheters and right ventricular thrombi in patients with cor pulmonale or indwelling right atrial catheters have been increasingly recognized.[124]

During the resting state, much of the tremendous, redundant, pulmonary vasculature is nonperfused. Selective recruitment of the pulmonary vasculature in response to rising cardiac outputs permits optimization of ventilation-perfusion (V/Q) balance during all phases of exercise. Vascular redundancy allows the lungs to tolerate clots that truncate significant portions (up to 50%) of the normal pulmonary circulation with little change in pulmonary hemodynamics, right heart performance or V/Q match. Massive pulmonary emboli or submassive pulmonary emboli in the setting of preexisting cardiopulmonary disease may overwhelm these compensatory mechanisms, causing a progressive rise in pulmonary vascular resistance and right ventricular afterload. The limited capacity of the RV to increase its stroke volume against acute elevations in RV afterload results in parallel increases in RV wall tension. Acute escalations in RV wall tension above 40–50 mmHg causes the right ventricle to progressively dilate and ultimately fail. This may trigger a series of hemodynamic events leading to cardiovascular collapse, including, RV dysfunction and ischemia, tricuspid regurgitation and failure of forward flow. Severe pressure elevations may also cause the opening of a patent foramen ovale. These changes may trigger intractable hypoxemia, refractory to supplemental oxygen therapy, as a consequence of the right to left intracardiac shunt. Paradoxical embolization through the patent foramen ovale may further add to the deteriorating clinical picture. Two platelet-derived chemical mediators released by the thrombus, serotonin, and bradykinin, may cause further elevations of pulmonary vascular resistance as well as pulmonary vascular redistribution and local bronchial constriction. These physiologic changes create large areas of dead space, which further aggravate V/Q imbalance and contribute to overall poor gas exchange and refractory hypoxemia. By contrast, chronic elevations in pulmonary artery systolic pressure (occurring over months to years) are better tolerated by the right ventricle, which responds over time by hypertrophy. Pulmonary embolic events most often cause abrupt rises in pulmonary artery pressures that regress to near-normal levels within 3 weeks of the acute event.[126] Among those patients that survive the initial embolic event, the recovery of PAPs and RV wall motion to normal/near normal levels is achieved in >90% of patients.[133]

Clinical presentation and evaluation Clinical evidence of pulmonary embolism is notoriously imprecise. Symptoms of unexplained hypoxemia and tachypnea, acute pleuritic chest pain, arrhythmias and hemodynamic instability, render the diagnosis intuitively obvious. However, in most cases, the presentation is sufficiently vague such that further testing is warranted. Patients may present with marked clinical symptoms but no objective signs of thrombosis. Dyspnea, the most common presenting symptom, occurs in 70%–90% of patients with angiographically proven pulmonary embolism. The symptom complex of dyspnea, pleuritic chest pain, and/or tachypnea (respiratory rate >20 breaths/minute) was noted in 97% of patients with PE.[134,135] Syncope, supraventricular arrhythmias, hypotension, and angina secondary to right ventricular ischemia presages a clinically significant clot burden and a worse prognosis. Hemoptysis is a rare complication of PE which typically occurs 12–36 hours following the embolic event and signifies pulmonary infarction. Infarction of the pulmonary vasculature requires significant compromise of two out of three of the potential sources of oxygen (airway, pulmonary and bronchial circulations). Thus, concomitant pulmonary or cardiac disease augments the risk of pulmonary infarction, which may occur in up to 20% in this group of patients. Inspection of the lower extremities for clinical evidence of deep venous thrombosis (DVT) is fruitful in less than 50% of patients. The electrocardiogram (ECG) most commonly reveals sinus tachycardia. Other tachydysrhythmias (usually atrial) are rarely seen and usually denote a large clot burden. The classic triad of an S wave in lead I, a Q wave in lead III, and a T wave in lead III ($S_1Q_3T_3$ pattern), considered pathognomic of PE, is seen in 10%–50% of cases.[136] In a recent study, this pattern was equally prevalent among patients with and without PE.[137] The electrocardiogram may also reveal changes suggestive of right heart strain, including p pulmonale (Figure 18-3A, B). This finding, as well as T wave inversion, is typically associated with massive PE with cor pulmonale. The level of hypoxemia and respiratory acidosis may vary with the clot burden and underlying cardiopulmonary reserve. Respiratory alkalosis has been reported among patients with massive pulmonary embolism and in patients with antecedent severe cardiopulmonary disease. Although radiographic findings associated with PE are nonspecific, the chest radiograph is of critical utility in excluding competing pathology. The spectrum of chest radiograph findings range from normal to studies that include hypoperfusion of the involved lung associated with enlargement of the pulmonary artery (Westermark sign), focal infiltrates, atelectasis, elevation of the ipsilateral hemidiaphragm (Figures 18-4A, B), and saddle embolus. Pleural-based, typically wedge-shaped infiltrates characteristic of pulmonary infarction may also be seen.

Rapid bedside evaluation of the unstable patient with massive PE is crucial. Among the potential markers with predictive value for the diagnosis of thromboembolic disorders, assays for D-dimer, the crossed-linked degradation product of fibrin, have been the most extensively scrutinized. D-dimer levels are virtually always elevated above 500 ng/mL in the setting of acute thrombosis. In a study by Kato and colleagues, D-dimer levels of less than 500 ng/mL were associated with a negative predictive value of 94% regardless of pretest probabilities for emboli.[138] Elevated levels of D-dimer, however, may be seen in a variety of non-thrombotic disorders, including malignancy, recent surgery, pneumonia, myocardial infarction, hemorrhage, trauma, and sepsis.[139] Furthermore, the specificity of the D-dimer assay wanes with increasing age. Hence, D-dimer assays may be of only incremental utility in the diagnostic work-up of the hospitalized, elderly patient with malignancy or other concomitant illnesses. Cardiac echocardiography with Doppler studies via the transthoracic or transesophageal routes provide indirect evidence hemodynamically significant PE. These studies are invaluable in permitting rapid bedside evaluations of the unstable patient. Echocardiography may reveal retained thrombus in the RV or pulmonary outflow tract, cor pulmonale, septal flattening with paradoxical septal motion, or a dilated right ventricle and/or right pulmonary artery (Figure 18-5). Tricuspid regurgitation is also a frequent finding in moderate to severe pulmonary hypertension. The peak velocity of the regurgitant jet across the tricuspid valve may be used to measure the pulmonary artery systolic pressure with Doppler echocardiography. Estimates of the gradient across the regurgitant tricuspid valve may be gleaned from the modified Bernoulli equation, $P = 4V^2$, where P represents the peak pressure difference between the right atrium and the right ventricle, and V is the peak velocity of the regurgitant stream. Features of acute right heart strain, indicated by right ventricular hypertrophy with widespread T wave inversion, may be seen on the electrocardiogram. Evidence of RV strain is documented in more than 40% of patients and heralds a poor outcome. In one study, mortality rates reported among patients with echocardiographic evidence of RV strain were 13-fold higher than patients with normal right ventricular findings.[130]

The diagnosis of PE is suggested by ventilation/perfusion (V/Q) scintigraphy demonstrating a high probability study and confirmed by spiral computed tomography (CT), magnetic resonance imaging (MRI), or pulmonary angiography. A high probability V/Q scan, coupled with high clinical suspicion, is usually sufficient evidence to treat. Spiral CT and MRI are established imaging modalities in the diagnostic armamentarium of PE. Clots located within the central (second to fourth order) pulmonary arteries may be identified using either of these modalities with sensitivities and specificities of greater than 80% and 90%, respectively.[140–142] Furthermore, lung windows

(A)

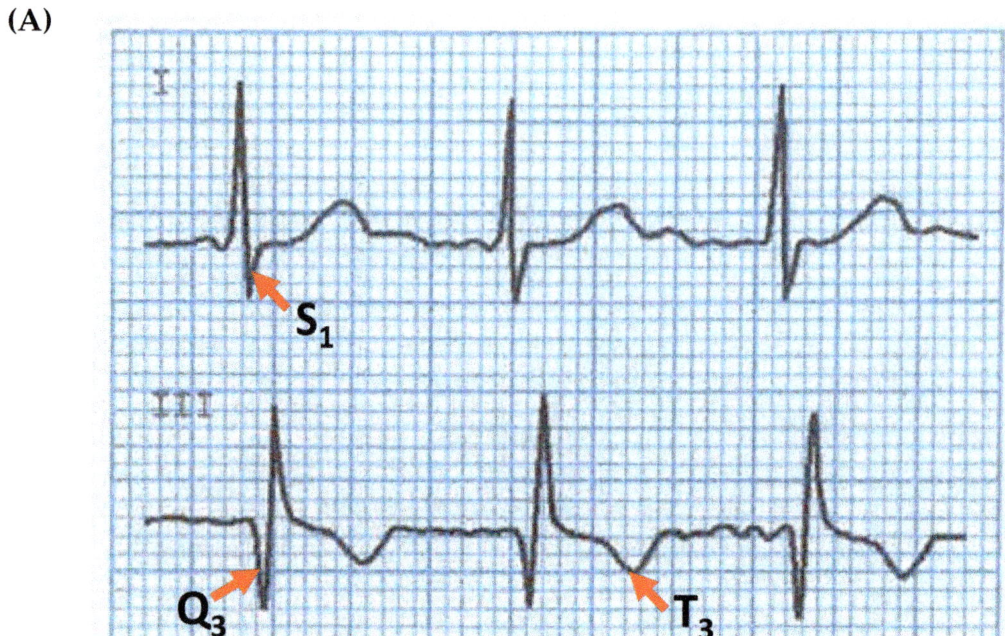

(B)

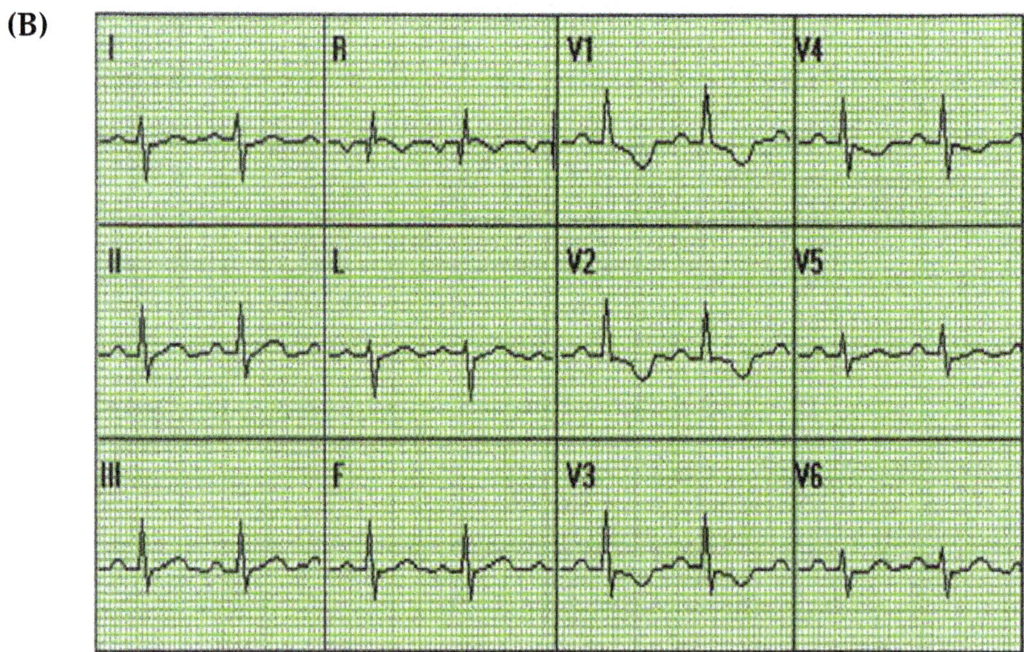

FIGURE 18-3 Electrocardiographic changes associated with pulmonary embolism (A) and right heart strain (B).

obtained during these studies offer additional information regarding competing diagnoses. Both spiral CT and MRI fail to depict clots located in the distal (subsegmental) pulmonary vasculature with any reliable degree of accuracy. Although the clinical significance of these clots has been debated, it is generally agreed that small subsegmental pulmonary emboli may presage more serious events, especially among patients with prior cardiopulmonary disease.[143,144]

Management of acute pulmonary embolism. ■ Among patients with a high clinical suspicion for PE, anticoagulation with unfractionated or fractionated heparin should be administered immediately, unless contraindicated. Treatment with one of these agents may begin even before diagnostic studies are obtained. Delays in treatment are associated with excess mortality as well as increased rates of recurrent thrombosis. Unfractionated heparin is typically bolused at 5,000

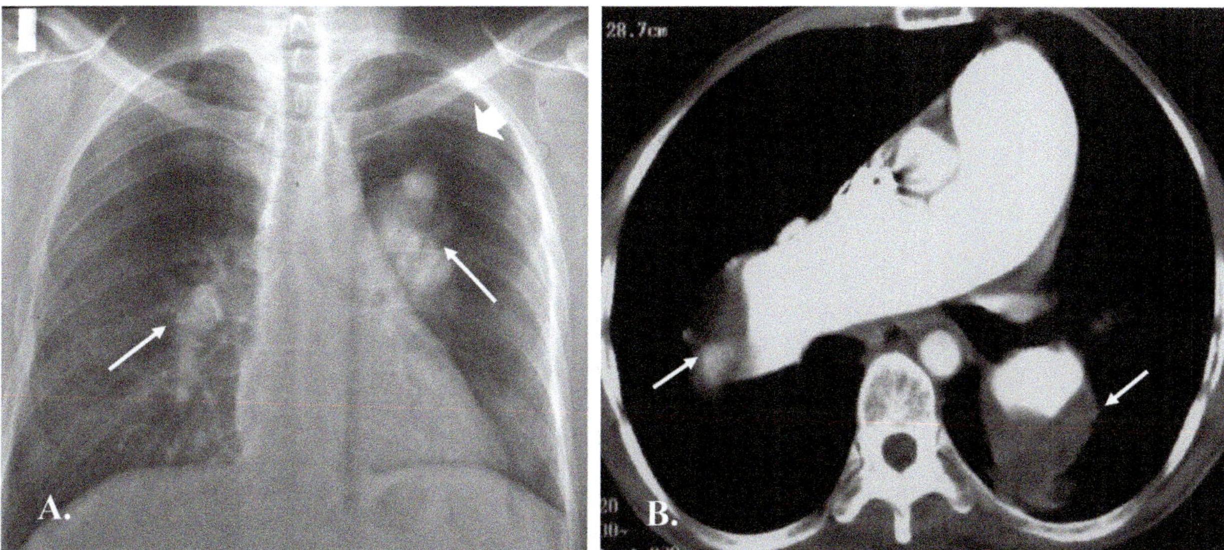

FIGURE 18-4 Chest radiograph (A) and CT angiogram (B) of large bilateral central pulmonary emboli in a 52-year-old man with renal cell carcinoma. The patient presented with an acute onset of severe shortness of breath and hypotension. Bilateral enlargement of the pulmonary arteries (arrows) is seen on the CXR with relative oligemia of the left upper lobe (arrowhead), consistent with Westermark sign is seen on the chest radiograph. Large bilateral central filling defects on the CT angiogram are indicated by arrows. Note relative elevation of the left hemidiaphragm.

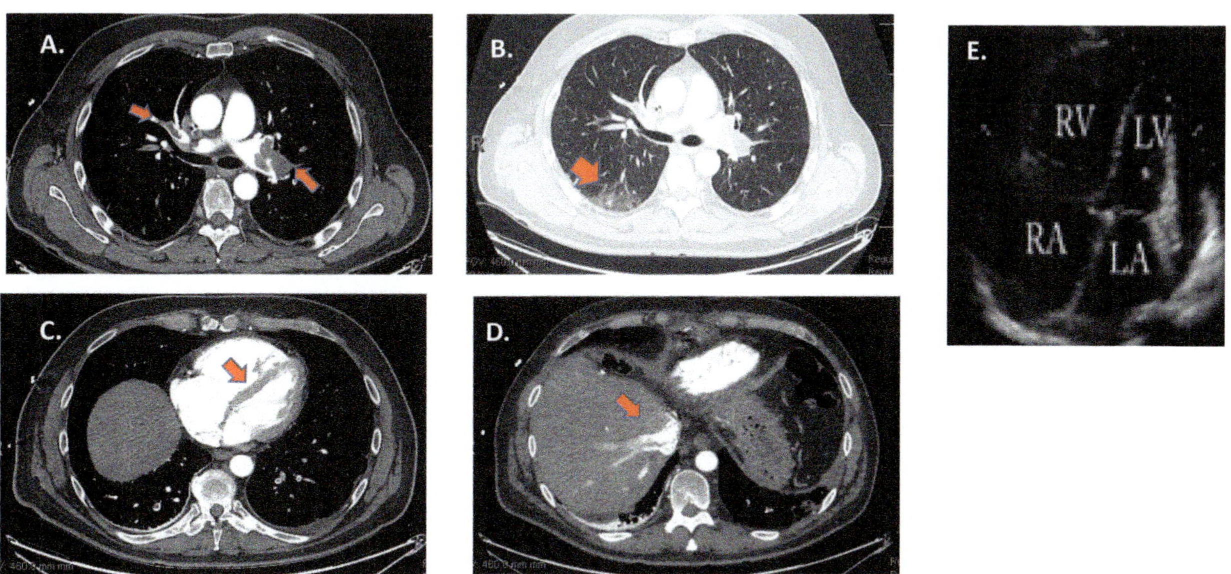

FIGURE 18-5 Saddle embolism. A 49-year-old man on panitumumab therapy for colon cancer presented with acute pleuritic chest pain, shortness of breath, hypoxemia and hypotension. A large pulmonary embolus straddles the main pulmonary arterial trunk at its bifurcation and extends into the left and right mainstem bronchi (arrows). Wedge-shaped opacities in the lower lobes, consistent with pulmonary infarction (arrow, B). Significant elevation of right sided pressures is suggested by deviation of the interventricular septum (arrow, C) and extension of contrast into the hepatic veins (arrow, D). The saddle embolism may have been precipitated by the drug, panitumumab.

to 10,000U, then given as a weight-based regimen of 18U/kg body weight/hr. A partial thromboplastin time (PTT) of 60–80 seconds or 1.5–2 times the control is a reasonable therapeutic target in most patients. Occasionally large doses of heparin are required (> 50,000 units of heparin per 24 hours), indicating heparin resistance. Unnecessary dose escalations may be avoided in these patients by monitoring the plasma heparin levels, rather than PTT. Within the first 5–10 days of an acute PE, administration of parenteral anticoagulation (unfractionated heparin, low molecular weight heparin, or fondaparinux) is indicated.[145] Overlap therapy with vitamin K antagonist is recommended. Alternatively, therapy with one of the new oral anticoagulants (dabigatran, edoxaban) may be administered as up from therapy or started 1–2 days after initiation of parenteral anticoagulant therapy.

Full anticoagulation requires depletion of both factor VII (half-life 6 hours) and thrombin (half-life 5 days). Therefore, although warfarin sodium may be added 2–3 days after therapeutic levels of PTT are achieved, heparin administration should be continued at least through the initial 5 days of warfarin therapy. Heparin prolongs the international normalized ratio (INR) by approximately 0.5. Thus, the optimal targeted initial INR of 2.0–3.0 on combined warfarin and heparin therapy may drop to 1.5–2.5 with warfarin alone.

Heparin-induced thrombocytopenia (HIT) is a potentially fatal consequence of heparin therapy. This disorder is, fortunately, rare and occurring in 1%–5% of heparin-treated patients. Both the source of heparin (decreased incidence among porcine versus bovine heparin) as well as the dose of the drug influence the occurrence of HIT. This disorder, however, has been described after intravenous line flushes and following the insertion of heparin-bonded pulmonary artery catheters. Two patterns of HIT, HIT I and HIT II, exists. HIT 1 represents a nonimmune, typically asymptomatic reduction in platelet count that most often occurs during the first day of therapy. Heparin-induced platelet clumping is felt to underlie this disorder, which commonly remits spontaneously, without interruption of therapy. HIT II, on the other hand, is felt to represent a complex autoimmune phenomenon propagated by heparin-platelet factor 4 (PF4) interactions. The heparin-PF4 complex may incite antibody formation, typically of the IgG class. Ultimately, this complex induces excessive activation of platelets and endothelial cells and intense platelet aggregation, leading to profound thrombocytopenia, massive thrombin generation, and life-threatening venous and arterial thrombotic vessel occlusion.[146–148] HIT II typically occurs 5–9 days into therapy. The diagnosis of HIT is often made on the basis of clinical findings. Laboratory evidence of HIT antibodies may be used to confirm the diagnosis. Clinical evidence of HIT, however, is sufficient to discontinue heparin therapy and initiate alternative anticoagulant treatment with agents such as danaparoid sodium, R-hirudin or argatroban. Long-term therapy with warfarin sodium is often necessary. This agent should only be initiated after effective anticoagulation has been achieved with other agents and following recovery of the platelet count and stabilization of the

patient. Although not all patients will have an anamnestic response when reexposed to heparin, re-exposition to any heparin product should be avoided.

Warfarin administration in the cancer patient can be particularly problematic. Many cancer patients are on an extensive list of medications that may interact with warfarin. The challenges of warfarin interactions with diet and concomitant drug therapy, its long half-life, and narrow therapeutic window may be particularly problematic for the cancer patient, leading to wide fluctuations in the INR and excessive bleeding or recurrent thrombosis. Disturbances in gastrointestinal absorption and hepatic function coupled with the frequent need to discontinue oral anticoagulants for invasive procedures compounds this problem. Fractionated or low molecular weight heparins (LMWH) are reasonable alternatives to Coumadin maintenance therapy and may replace unfractionated heparin in selected patients with relatively stable PE. These agents have been shown to demonstrate equivalent efficacy in this setting with the added advantages of convenient dosing and the lack of need for monitoring coagulation profiles.[149–155] Furthermore, the rapid and predictable onset of action and clearance of these agents facilitate the ease of interrupting anticoagulation coverage for invasive procedures. Lower rates of heparin-induced thrombocytopenia (HIT) and a greater degree of thrombus regression and restoration of venous patency have also been reported with LMWH administration.[156,157] In addition, the putative antineoplastic activity of these agents may confer a survival advantage among LMWH-treated patients.[158]

Although the optimal duration of anticoagulation has not been clearly defined, a minimum of 3 months of therapy is recommended after a single event, at which time the risk of bleeding versus the risk of recurrence generally offset each other.[159,160] Patients with active cancer should be treated with prolonged therapy (6–12 months) or until the cancer is in remission. Indefinite anticoagulant treatment may be appropriate for recurrent thromboembolism, neurologic disease with extremity paresis, and obesity or hematologic disorders that confer an increased risk of thromboembolism (factor V homozygous carrier, combined heterozygous carrier state for factor V Leiden, deficiencies of anti-thrombin, protein C or protein S).

Management of MPE ■ The cardinal therapeutic principles in the management of the hypoxemic, hypotensive patient with acute massive pulmonary embolism center on stabilization of cardiovascular hemodynamics, treating the current clot, and preventing clot migration while avoiding further clot formation. Hemodynamic stabilization is critical, independent of clot dynamics and considerations for thrombolysis. Unstable patients should be closely monitored, preferably in an intensive care unit setting. Judicious fluid resuscitation may augment right ventricular preload and improve both cardiac output and systemic hypotension. Right atrial pressures of 15–20 mmHg by central venous monitoring are usually sufficient to maintain adequate RV preload. Excess augmentation in preload may further distend the RV, precipitating right ventricular ischemia and further deterioration in RV function. Thus, intravenous fluids should be given judiciously, targeting RA pressures of 15–20 mmHg. Augmentation of RV contractility may be facilitated with inotropes. Although the optimal vasoactive agent has not been identified in any randomized, controlled trials, dobutamine is favored because of its inotropic properties and potent vasodilator activities on the pulmonary vascular beds. The drug may be titrated to clinical response (improved systemic blood pressure, cardiac output) from initial doses of 0.5–2 µg per kg per minute. The beneficial effects of this agent usually plateau at 15–20 µg per kg per minute. Dobutamine also possesses systemic vasodilator properties which may limit its use. In addition, the PaO2 may occasionally deteriorate following dobutamine administration, owing to increased blood flow through a fixed shunt. Norepinephrine, a potent α- and β_1-adrenoreceptor agonist, may improve systemic BP, cardiac output, peripheral vascular resistance (PVR), and RV pressures by increasing cardiac contractility and RV perfusion pressure. Norepinephrine is typically administered as a constant intravenous infusion starting at 2–4 mg per minute and titrated until the desired blood pressure is attained. Norepinephrine-dobutamine combinations may be helpful in the treatment of shock-related massive pulmonary embolism. The vasoconstrictor effects of epinephrine coupled with its β_1-mediated actions may act to improve cardiac output and reduce PVR respectively. However, the unfavorable chronotropic effects of this agent may limit its utility in this setting. Similarly, the administration of dopamine is limited in this setting because of potentially damaging tachycardia.

The utility of thrombolytic therapy in the treatment of the hemodynamically unstable patient with MPE is well established.[161–164] The critical event in the pathophysiology of acute PE is dysfunction and failure of the RV. RV dysfunction is thought to be predictive of adverse outcome.[130,163] Echocardiographic evidence of RV dysfunction and elevated serum cardiac troponin I or T levels may be used to indicate overt or impending RV failure associated with massive or submassive PE and independently predict an adverse outcome.[130,165] By accelerating clot lysis, thrombolytic agents may substantially improve RV hemodynamic

parameters.[166] By contrast, the indication and utility of thrombolysis among hemodynamically stable patients with PE-associated RV dysfunction have been sharply debated for decades. Accumulating data suggests that patients with RV dysfunction associated with hemodynamically stable PE have a mortality risk that is sufficiently high to warrant more aggressive therapy than anticoagulation alone.[165,167] In a recent study, early thrombolytic treatment of clinically stable patients is associated with an almost 50% reduction in the risk of in-hospital deaths and may confer reduced rates of clinical deterioration among hemodynamically stable patients with PE-related RV dysfunction.[164,168] The PEITHO trial compared mortality outcomes among clinically stable patients with PE-related RV dysfunction who were treated with heparin alone versus thrombolysis plus heparin. A survival benefit and improved hemodynamics were seen among the patients undergoing thrombolytic therapy. Subsequent subgroup analysis, however, suggested that the mortality benefit was based on improved hemodynamics rather than direct effects on mortality. To date, no clinical trial has been sufficiently large to convincingly demonstrate a survival advantage among patients with MPE who receive thrombolytic versus conventional heparin therapy.

Thrombolytic efficacy among the available agents urokinase, streptokinase and tissue plasminogen activator (t-PA), is roughly the same, although t-PA is infused over a shorter time period and may cause more rapid thrombolysis.[169] These drugs may be given systemically or directly into selected pulmonary arteries. More recently, direct intra-embolic infusion of low-dose thrombolytic has emerged as an alternative to systemic thrombolysis and may prove to be superior to the intravenous route of administration, with less frequent adverse effects.[170] The most devastating complication of thrombolysis is intracranial (ICH) hemorrhage. The cumulative incidence of ICH among patients treated with thrombolytic agents for MPE is considerably higher (1.9%–2.1%) than the occurrence of ICH following heparin treatment alone (0.2%).[134,161,171] Significant bleeding from other sites, including the gastrointestinal tract and venipuncture sites, occasionally occurs. In most cases, withdrawal of the lytic agent suffices to control the bleeding, as the half-life of these agents is short. Rarely, reversal of the lytic state with fresh frozen plasma, platelet transfusion, and/ or anti-fibrinolytic agents may be necessary. Surgical and/or catheter embolectomy are reasonable alternatives for patients with large, centrally-located clots and refractory systemic hypotension, echocardiographic evidence of right atrial thrombi, pulmonary artery pressures greater than 35mmHg, and contraindications to or failed thrombolytic therapy.[172] Clinician experience and available resources dictate the choice of surgical versus catheter embolectomy. Both surgical and catheter embolectomy in this setting have had anecdotal success. Individual reports have touted overall success and survival rates among patients treated with catheter embolectomy of 76% and 70%, respectively. In the setting of cardiac arrest, however, associated with MPE mortality rates following emergency embolectomy remain dismal.[173–176]

■ Pulmonary Hypertension

Definition and classification. ■ Pulmonary hypertension (PH) describes an abnormal hemodynamic state defined by a mean pulmonary arterial pressure (mPAP) greater than or equal to 25 mm Hg at rest on right heart catheterization (RHC).[177] Over the past few decades, there have been substantial advances in our understanding of both the pathophysiology and treatment for PH. The World Health Organization (WHO) groups PH into 5 major categories, based on similar pathologic and hemodynamic characteristics and management strategies.[178] The most recent revisions of this classification scheme were made in 2013 (Table 18-3).

Disorders within Group 1 include those known to cause pulmonary arterial hypertension (PAH). PAH is defined hemodynamically by the following: mPAP > 25 mm Hg, end-expiratory pulmonary artery wedge pressure (PAWP) ≤ 15 mm Hg, and pulmonary vascular resistance (PVR) > 3 Woods unit.[179] The etiologies of PAH include heritable causes, drug and toxin-induced, connective tissue diseases, HIV infection, portal hypertension, congenital heart disease, schistosomiasis and idiopathic. Pulmonary veno-occlusive disease (PVOD) and pulmonary capillary hemangiomatosis (PCH) and persistent pulmonary hypertension of the newborn (PPHN) are grouped together in PAH subcategories of 1'(PVOD, PCH) and 1''(PPHN). Other groups for PH include: pulmonary hypertension secondary to left-sided heart disease (Group 2); PH resulting in pulmonary venous hypertension (PVH); hypoxic pulmonary hypertension (Group 3); chronic thromboembolic pulmonary hypertension (CTEPH) (Group 4); and PH due to unclear and/or multifactorial causes (Group 5).

Exact estimates of the incidence of pulmonary hypertension among patients with cancer remain elusive in the published literature. Cancer-related PH has been more prominently recognized with each revised classification. This section will give a brief discussion of the current classification system for PH as it relates to the cancer patient along with new insights into its pathogenesis, prognosis, and treatment of this disease.

■ Pulmonary Hypertension: Signs and Symptoms

PH patients often present with a spectrum of subtle nonspecific symptoms, which may be difficult to dissociate from other comorbid conditions (Table 18-4). The symptoms are generally attributable to impaired oxygen transport and reduced cardiac output. Exertional

TABLE 18-3 Clinical Classification of Pulmonary Hypertension (Dana Point 2009)

GROUP 1: PAH	GROUP 2: PH OWING TO LEFT HEART DISEASE	GROUP 3: PH OWING TO LUNG DISEASES AND/OR HYPOXIA	GROUP 4: CTEPH	GROUP 5: PH WITH UNCLEAR MULTIFACTORIAL MECHANISMS

Idiopathic
Heritable
Small muscular arterioles:
  Drug-induced
  HIV
  Portal HTN,
  CHD
  CTD
Schistosomiasis
1' PVOD, PCH
	Systolic dysfunction
	Diastolic dysfunction
	Valvular Heart Disease
		COPD
		ILD
		Other pulmonary disease with mixed restrictive and obstructive pattern
		Sleep-disordered breathing
		Alveolar hypoventilation disorders
		Chronic exposure to high altitude
		Developmental abnormalities
			Unresolved clot	Hematologic disorders
				Splenectomy
				Systemic disorders
				Metabolic disorders
				Sarcoid

TABLE 18-4 Signs and symptoms of PH

SYMPTOMS	SIGNS
• Exertional Dyspnea (60%)	• Cyanosis
• Lethargy/fatigue (19%)	• Low output
• Exertional syncope/near syncope (13%, early; 33%, late)	• Venous congestion
• Exertional chest pain (7%)	• Active right ventricular impulse
• Palpitations (5%)	• Loud P2
• Peripheral edema (3%)	• High frequency TR murmur
• Anorexia (3%)	• Hi frequency diastolic PR murmur
• Abdominal pain (3%)	• Liver congestion/tenderness/hepatomegaly
• Hoarseness (2%)	• Peripheral edema
• Hemoptysis (1%–2%)	• Ascites/RUQ pain and tenderness
• Raynaud's (2%)	

dyspnea is the most frequent presenting symptom, followed by fatigue, weakness, and complaints of general exertion intolerance.[180] As the PH worsens, dyspnea at rest, chest pain, peripheral edema, abdominal distention, and syncope occur. Syncope, owing to atrial and ventricular arrhythmias, occurs in 1/3 of patients. Although the mechanism is unclear, typical angina may develop despite normal coronary arteries, and may be due to pulmonary artery stretching or right ventricular ischemia. Thus syncope and angina occur late in the course of the disease and are indicative of more severe limitations in cardiac output. These symptoms are ominous and, in 7% of patients, may presage ventricular dysrhythmias and sudden death. Other symptoms include orthopnea and paroxysmal nocturnal dyspnea which suggest elevated pulmonary venous pressure and pulmonary congestion due to sub-optimally treated left-sided heart disease. The WHO classification of functional capacity, which is an adaptation of the New York Heart Association (NYHA) system, provides a qualitative assessment of activity tolerance, and it has significant implications with regard to treatment.[180]

The physical examination may provide valuable clues to both the presence and severity of the disease. For example, the presence of an accentuated pulmonary component of the second heart sound and increased jugular "a" waves on physical examination denote high pulmonary artery and right ventricular filling pressures, respectively, and indicate the presence of severe PH. Other auscultatory findings of a tricuspid regurgitant murmur, right ventricular S_3, marked distention of the jugular veins, palpable left parasternal lift, hepatomegaly and ascites signify right ventricular dysfunction and advanced disease. Peripheral edema is also frequent in advanced disease. Findings of peripheral edema, however, are not synonymous with cor pulmonale and may instead reflect the presence of secondary hyperaldosteronism in patients with functional renal insufficiency induced by high renal vein pressures, hypercapnic acidosis and/or hypoxemia.[181,182] The electrocardiogram of a patient with moderate to severe pulmonary hypertension characteristically demonstrates evidence of right atrial enlargement and RV hypertrophy. Evidence of a prominent pulmonary trunk, RV enlargement, and pruning of peripheral pulmonary arteries on chest radiographs may also be seen with more advanced disease. Signs of right ventricular failure include right ventricular S3 gallop, marked distention of the jugular veins, pulsatile hepatomegaly, peripheral edema, and ascites. Hypotension, diminished pulse pressure, and cool extremities are particularly ominous signs that signal significantly reduced cardiac output and peripheral vasoconstriction.[180]

■ Pulmonary Hypertension: Diagnostic Evaluation

A detailed evaluation is usually needed to determine the presence of PH, the etiology and degree of functional limitation. The electrocardiogram (ECG), chest radiograph, and echocardiogram should be among the first tests in the workup, but definitive diagnosis ultimately requires an RHC.

Screening studies ■ The electrocardiogram (ECG) is not a sensitive tool for screening of PH, but may provide clues to hemodynamically significant PH. (Figure 18-6) Right ventricular hypertrophy and right axis deviation can be detected on ECG in 87% and 79% of patients, respectively.[183] Right atrial enlargement may be observed with

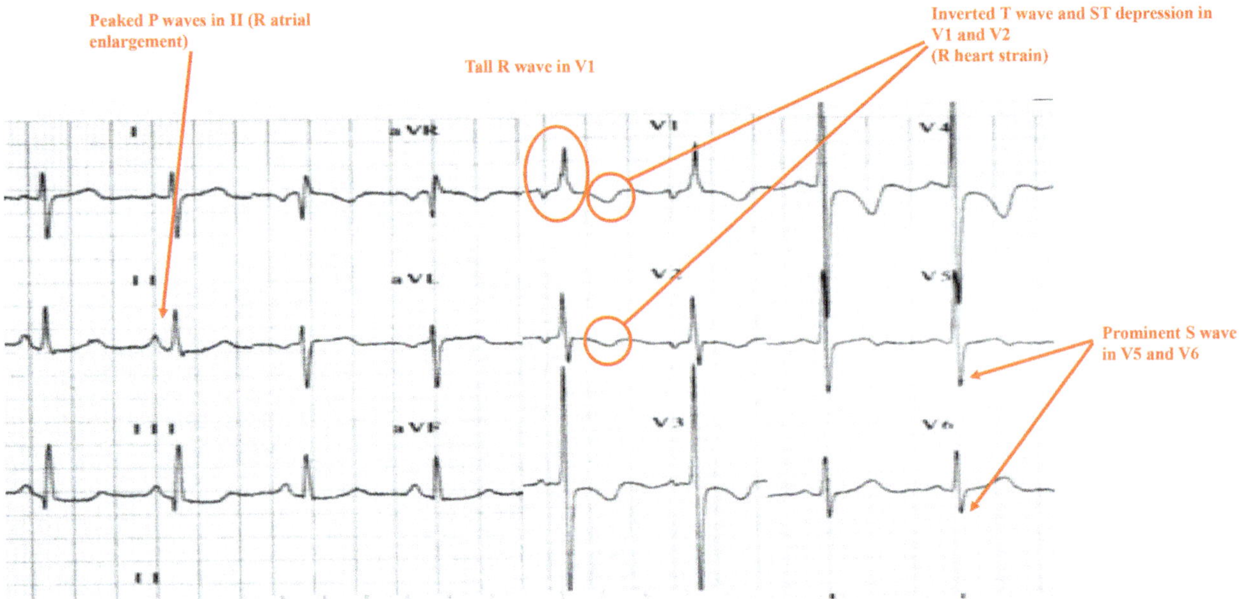

FIGURE 18-6   Typical electrocardiographic findings of PH. Right ventricular hypertrophy and R axis deviation; Peaked P waves in II suggest R atrial enlargement; Tall R wave in V1; Inverted T wave and ST depression in V1 and V2 suggest R heart strain; Prominent S wave in V5 and V6

prominent P waves in leads II, III, and/or aVF (greater than 2.5 mm). Right-sided precordial leads may display ST-T segment depression or T wave inversion. The accuracy of the chest radiograph (CXR) in detecting PH is unknown. Enlarged main and hilar pulmonary arterial shadows, attenuation of peripheral pulmonary vascular markings ("pruning"), and obscuration of the retrosternal clear space by an enlarged right ventricle are suggestive of PH (Figure 18-7). Radiographic findings of pulmonary venous congestion (associated with pulmonary venous hypertension) or lung hyperinflation (associated with chronic obstructive pulmonary disease) may also be gleaned from the chest radiograph and offer clues to the underlying diagnosis.

Standard diagnostic criteria for PH are based on transthoracic Doppler echocardiogram findings and right heart catheter-derived assessments of pulmonary artery pressures, pulmonary capillary wedge (PCW) pressures, and pulmonary vascular resistance (PVR).[180] The echocardiographic examination permits semiquantitative assessment of RV size and function, right atrial (RA) size, tricuspid regurgitant velocity for estimation of right ventricular systolic pressure (RVSP), left ventricular systolic and diastolic function, right ventricular hypertrophy and/or dilatation, left atrial size and morphologic examination of all cardiac valves. The estimation of RVSP includes RAP which is either a standardized value or an estimated value based on echocardiographic characteristics of the inferior vena cava, or the vertical height of the

jugular venous pulse on physician examination. The presence of left atrial enlargement, even in the absence of left ventricular dysfunction, should raise the possibility of left-sided heart disease that may contribute to observed pulmonary pressure elevations. In addition, intracardiac and intrapulmonary shunts may be assessed echocardiographically using bubble-contrast techniques. Thus, extrapulmonary causes of pulmonary hypertension including mitral valve disease, left ventricular dysfunction, and intracardiac shunt may be elucidated using this technique.

RHC is necessary to confirm the diagnosis or PH and accurately determine the severity of the hemodynamic derangements. This procedure permits direct and accurate measurement of RAP, pulmonary venous pressure via PCWP, PAP, mixed venous oxygen saturation, transpulmonary gradient (mean PAP-downstream pressure), and cardiac output (either by thermodilution or by using the Fick principle). It also allows for the calculation of PVR and systemic vascular resistance (SVR). The presence and/or severity of congenital or acquired left-to-right shunt may be confirmed.

Hemodynamic measurements of mean PAP exceeding 25 mm Hg at rest with a concomitant PCW of ≤ 15 mmHg and PVR > 3 Woods unit establishes the diagnosis of PAH. The National Institute of Health (NIH) registry identified 3 hemodynamic variables that correlate with an increased risk of death: increased PAP, increased RAP, and decreased cardiac index.[184]

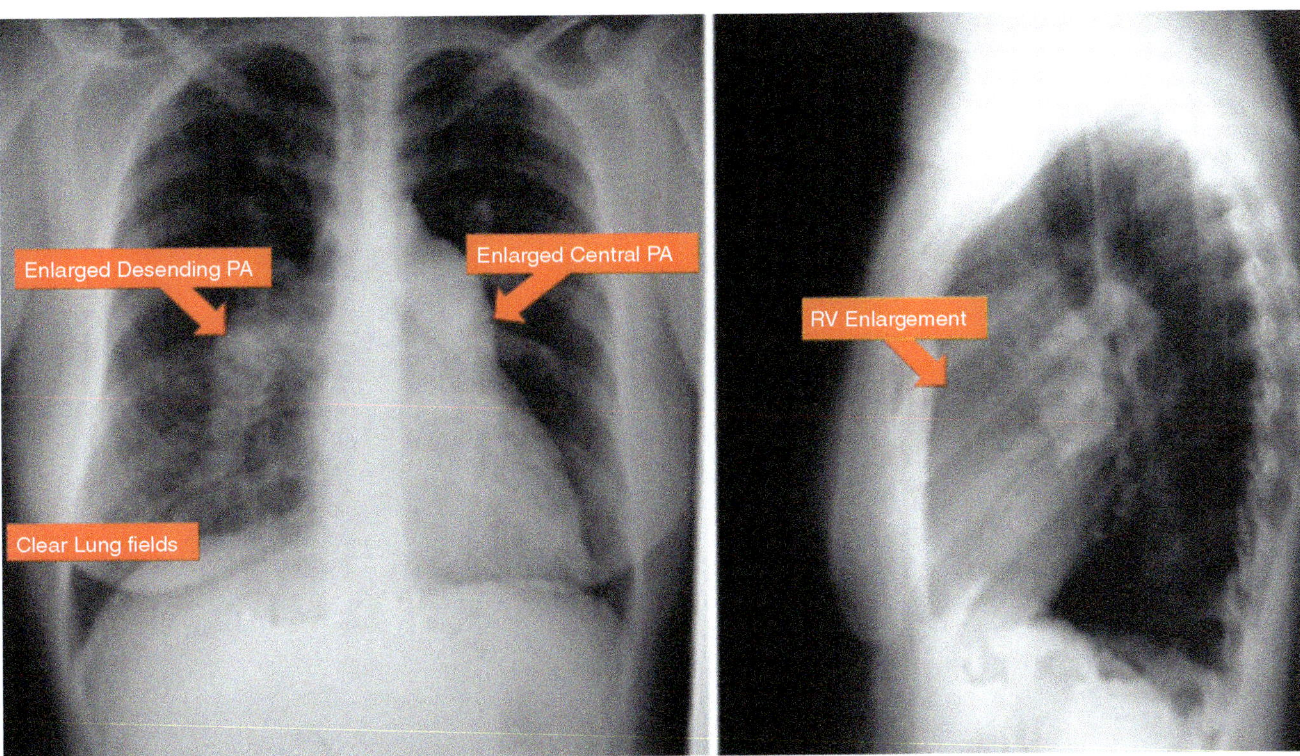

FIGURE 18-7 CXR findings of PH. Enlarged main and right hilar pulmonary arterial shadows, attenuation of peripheral pulmonary vascular markings ("pruning"), and obscuration of the retrosternal clear space by an enlarged right ventricle in the setting of clear lung fields are suggestive of PH.

A PCWP of ≥ 15 mm Hg suggests pulmonary venous hypertension. Left ventricular end diastolic pressure (LVEDP) obtained via left heart catheterization can help to confirm the PCWP and identify left-sided heart disease. Vasodilator testing is performed with inhaled nitric oxide, intravenous epoprostenol, or intravenous adenosine during the initial right heart catheterization. An acute vasodilator response, defined as a decrease in mPAP of 10 mm Hg to 40 mm Hg, with an increased or unchanged cardiac output, suggests a significant degree of reversibility. A reduction in PVR of more than 20% may also signify a positive response to vasodilator. Because of its short half-life (seconds), inhaled NO is frequently used as a screening vasodilator agent to predict the response to calcium channel blockers.[185,186] The primary goal of right heart catheterization is to identify the subset of acute responders with IPAH who could benefit from long-term monotherapy with oral calcium channel blockers.[187]

Additional studies in patients with PH ■ Laboratory studies, including liver function tests, HIV serology, thyroid function tests, complete blood count, creatinine, thyroid function studies, antinuclear antibodies, and rheumatoid factor are indicated to probe for secondary conditions associated with PH. Antinuclear antibodies may be positive at low titers in the absence of underlying collagen vascular disease.[188] If liver function tests are elevated, further evaluation with a hepatitis panel should be considered.

Pulmonary function testing with measurements of diffusing capacity of the lung for carbon monoxide (DLCO), maximum minute ventilation (MVV), total lung capacity (TLC), forced vital capacity (FVC), forced expiratory volume in 1 second (FEV1) and alveolar volume (V_A) is a sensitive, but not specific indicator of pulmonary vascular disease. These tests may help to characterize the contribution of underlying airway or parenchymal disease to the development of PH and correlate with PH severity.[189] Decreased DLCO among patients with PAH and PVH may be explained on the basis of reductions in the peripheral vascular bed coupled with muscularization and intimal thickening of smaller, more peripheral pulmonary arteries, may contribute to impaired gas transfer for carbon monoxide. In the absence of parenchymal disease, the restrictive lung defect associated with pulmonary hypertension is usually mild. Loss of normal distensibility of all lung tissues including the pulmonary vasculature and lung compression by the enlarged right heart may contribute to reduced lung volumes in some patients.

Studies to assess for PH are typically done with the patient at rest. The use of exercise echocardiography to unmask occult PH remains controversial, as no clear standardization of exercise or Doppler interrogation protocols are evident in the literature. Standard testing of functional status and the propensity to desaturate with exercise relies instead on the six-minute walk test and cardiopulmonary exercise testing (CPET). Cardiopulmonary exercise testing and the recent development of the manometer tipped catheters that permit continuous pulmonary artery pressure measurements may provide a more accurate assessment of the hemodynamic derangements in response to exercise and the impact of different treatment modalities on these changes.[190] Derangements in cardiopulmonary exercise testing, including peak O_2 uptake, anaerobic threshold, and peak O_2 pulse correlate well with abnormalities in DLCO and offer a reliable index of disease severity.[189] Nocturnal oximetry may identify patients with desaturation at night and/or underlying sleep disordered breathing. If sleep apnea is suspected, formal testing with polysomnography (PSG) should be performed.

Acute pulmonary embolism and CTEPH (Group 4) are potentially curable conditions that should be considered in all patients with unexplained PH. Evaluation for pulmonary thromboembolic disease by pulmonary radioisotope scan (ventilation/perfusion scan) or spiral computed tomography (spiral CT) is mandatory unless the underlying etiology is obvious. The ventilation-perfusion (V/Q) scan may demonstrate small, peripheral, non-segmental perfusion defects indicative of IPAH, while one or more segments of V/Q mismatch may indicate CTEPH.[180] Ventilation/perfusion defects associated with chronic thromboembolic pulmonary embolism are typically multiple, bilateral, and larger than the ventilation abnormality. A normal V/Q scan renders CTEPH unlikely. Patchy, non-segmental diffuse defects may also be seen in patients with veno-occlusive disease.[191,192] High resolution CT may be performed using spiral or electron-beam scanning (ultrafast CT) techniques. This diagnostic tool has emerged over the past decade as an important component in evaluation of the patient with suspected pulmonary embolism. High resolution CT imaging reliably depicts clot in the central (second to fourth order) pulmonary arteries, with sensitivities and specificities of greater than 80% and 90%, respectively.[140–142] In addition, the CT scan permits visualization of intrathoracic anatomy, which may be helpful in supporting or refuting the concomitant diagnoses.

Pulmonary angiography is considered the gold standard for diagnosis of CTEPH and is indicated when other investigations are inconclusive. Angiographic evidence of acute thrombi includes intravascular filling defects on two or more projections. Less consistent and nonspecific observations on angiography include vascular cut-offs, hypovascularity and vascular pruning.[134] Chronic thrombi may appear as bands or webs on angiography with associated retraction of the associated vessel wall. Rounded cutoffs of segmental vessels and irregular intimal surfaces also indicate chronicity. Five angiographic patterns associated with organized thromboembolic material during thromboendarterectomy have been identified: pouch defects; pulmonary artery webs or bands; intimal irregularities; abrupt narrowing of the major pulmonary arteries; and obstruction of lobar or segmental vessels at their origin, with complete absence of blood flow to the pulmonary segments that are normally perfused by those vessels.[193] In the past, pulmonary angiography has been regarded as a high-risk procedure, but the PIOPED investigators documented procedure-related mortality rates of less than 0.5% with procedure-related morbidity of 5%.[134] Contrast reactions, contrast-induced renal injury, and complications related to catheter insertion comprise the bulk of adverse events. An algorithm for the evaluation of PH is given in Figure 18-8.

Future screening tests ■ Magnetic resonance imaging (MRI) provides direct assessment of cardiac volumes, muscular mass, and function and is useful in the noninvasive assessment of the right heart in PH. The accuracy of MRI in detecting central clot formation is similar to that of high resolution CT. Lung windows obtained during both MRI and spiral CT offer additional information regarding competing diagnoses. In addition, MRI may delineate morphologic and functional abnormalities of lung perfusion and right heart function and offer cinematic images of the lung and lower extremity vessels without exposing the patient to ionizing radiation. Estimates of PAP and PVR with MRI may be performed with remarkable accuracy.[194] The time required for study completion is considerably longer for MRI versus high resolution CT and, thus, may not be suitable for the unstable patient with suspected pulmonary embolism. However, it is been used more frequently in the characterization of patients with PAH.[195]

Biomarkers, such as brain natriuretic peptide (BNP) and NT-proBNP, may be useful in PH patients. Elevated plasma BNP in patients with PH correlates positively with RAP, mPAP, PVR and RV mass, and inversely with cardiac index.[196,197] A recent study of 60 patient with IPAH suggested that BNP elevations also significantly correlate with decreased survival.[196]

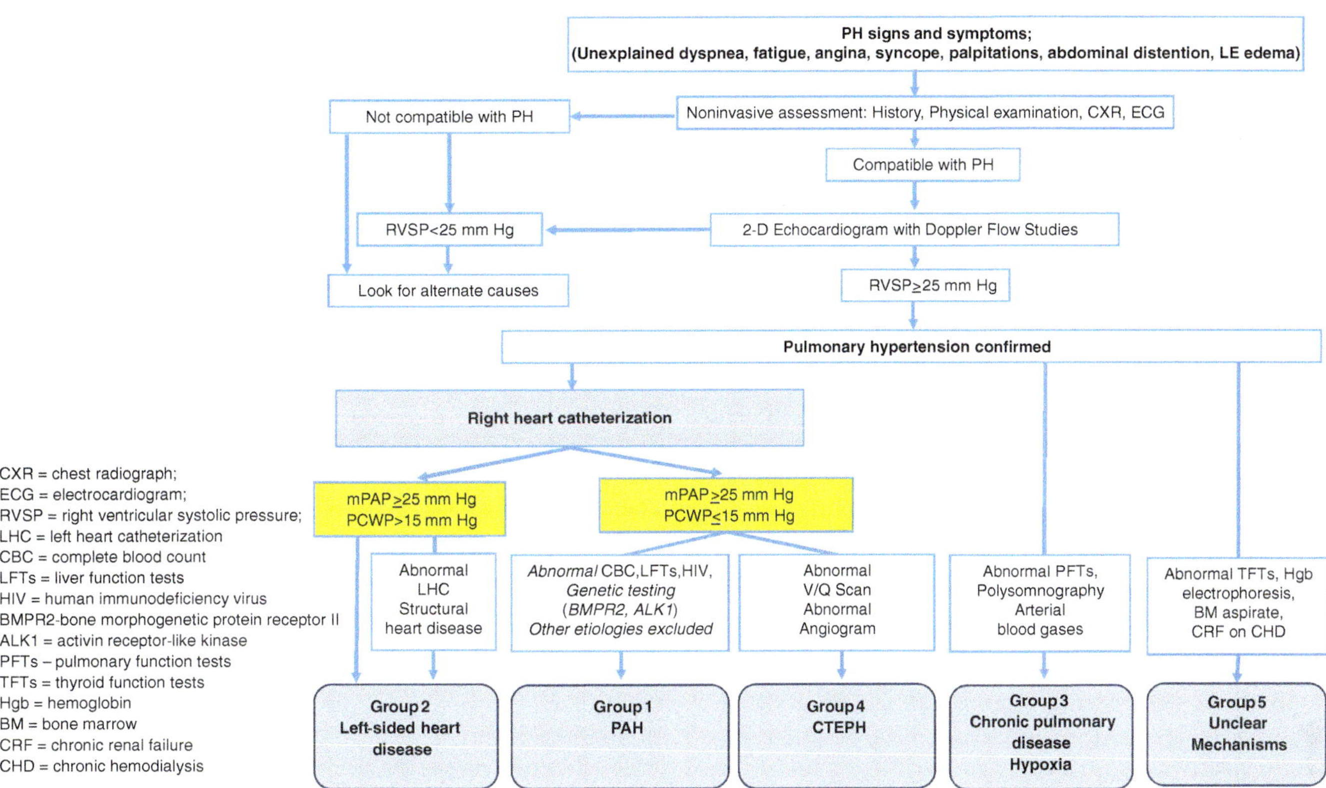

FIGURE 18-8 Algorithm for evaluation of PH.

This biomarker is not specific for PH, however, and may be elevated in other conditions, including heart failure, sepsis, pneumonia, COPD exacerbation, and pulmonary embolism. Other biomarkers, such as NT-proBNP, are also increased in patients with IPAH correlate with abnormalities in hemodynamic variables and function capacity.[198] Although the results are intriguing, biomarker assays will likely play more role in assessing the response to treatment and predicting survival and a lesser role in diagnostic testing.

■ Group 1: Pulmonary Arterial Hypertension

PAH is characterized by extensive narrowing of the pulmonary vascular bed, leading to a progressive increase in pulmonary vascular resistance, right ventricular (RV) afterload, and cardiac failure. Histologically, PAH is characterized by intimal fibrosis, increased medial thickness, pulmonary arteriolar occlusion, and plexiform lesions.[199,200] Clinical subgroups associated with the development of PAH are listed in Table 18-3. Major categories of risk factors that account for most of the reported cases of cancer-related PAH include chemotherapeutic agents, portal hypertension, and HIV infection. Dasatinib has been identified as a likely etiology for PAH. Partial clinical improvement and even

reversal of PAH after cessation of the drug has been well described.[178,201] Other chemotherapeutic agents including interferon-α and -β are classified as potential culprits resulting in PAH. Details of drug-related PAH are discussed in a separate section in this chapter.

Portopulmonary hypertension (POPH) refers to PAH in the setting of elevated pressures in the portal circulation. This form of PAH occurs in in 2%–6% of patients with portal hypertension.[178,202–204] Portal hypertension (portal pressure > 10mmHg), rather than the severity of liver disease, is the major determinant of POPH. Estimates are much higher (up to 12%) among cirrhotic patients and patients undergoing orthotopic liver transplantation.[205] The prevalence of POPH among cancer patients is unknown. Malignancy, hypercoaguability, inflammation and other conditions that compromise hepatic flow may lead to hepatic portal vein thrombosis and portal hypertension.[206,207] Portal hypertension related to splenomegaly is a well-known complication of chronic myeloproliferative diseases. A subset of patients with chronic myeloproliferative disease will develop PAH as a complication of portal hypertension and associated splenomegaly.[208] Pulmonary hypertension typically follows the development of portal hypertension by 4–7 years. While the duration of portal hypertension appears to influence the development of portopulmonary hypertension, correlations between the severity of portal hypertension and subsequent development of pulmonary hypertension have not been firmly established. The histologic changes in portopulmonary hypertension are indistinguishable from those seen in PAH. High flow associated with the hyperdynamic circulatory state and fluid overload commonly occur in advanced liver disease and may mimic PAH. Elevated PVR helps to distinguish POPH from hemodynamic changes associated with liver disease. The coexistence of pulmonary hypertension with portal hypertension worsens the overall prognosis. A mean survival of only 15 months was reported in one study, with a 50% 6-month mortality in the absence of pharmacological interventions.[209]

AIDS is associated with increased prevalence of some malignancies, including Kaposi's sarcoma, and nonHodgkin's lymphoma. The prevalence of PAH-associated HIV infection is estimated to be about 0.5%.[210] Normalization of hemodynamics and improved prognosis is seen in up to 20% of patients on PAH and HAART therapies.[211]

Over the past decade, substantial advances in the understanding of PAH pathobiology have resulted in the development of new drugs and treatment strategies with combination therapies that target multiple pathogenic pathways. Early diagnosis and the application of new treatment strategies have resulted in manageable disease in many cases with improvements in both quality of life and survival.[212] The development of PAH or pre-existing PAH prior to cancer diagnosis introduces an increased level of complexity to the management of these patients.

Pathogenesis of PAH ■ Vasoconstriction, smooth muscle cell and endothelial cell proliferation, and thrombosis are the main vascular changes in PAH. The integrity of the vascular endothelium and smooth muscle cells is tightly linked to mechanical forces, changing hemodynamics and the underlying pulmonary hormonal milieu. Rapid changes in pulmonary blood flow and shear stress result in increased release of L-arginine nitric oxide (NO), a potent selective pulmonary vasodilator, from endothelial cells.[213–215] In addition, the physiological agonists, acetylcholine and bradykinin activate endothelial cells, causing the release of NO. Available evidence suggests that basal expression of endothelial NO contributes to resting pulmonary vasorelaxation.[214–216] In addition to vasodilation, NO inhibits smooth muscle proliferation and platelet aggregation and attenuates endothelin-1 (ET-1) production.[216–218] Although the exact role of NO in the pathogenesis of pulmonary hypertension has not been full delineated, hypothetically, alterations in endothelial NO expression may contribute to pulmonary hypertension.[219,220]

This concept is strengthened by the salutary effects of inhaled NO in patients with pulmonary hypertension.[221] Decreased expression of endothelial NO and prostacyclin synthase, another potent pulmonary vasodilator with anti-platelet properties, have been noted in pulmonary arteries of patients with severe pulmonary hypertension.[219,222–224] Other endothelial-derived factors that influence pulmonary vasoreactivity include endothelin-1, thromboxane, and vascular endothelial growth factor (VEGF). Thromboxane and endothelin-1 also demonstrate potent platelet aggregation and vasoconstrictor activities, however, unlike prostacyclin and NO, levels of these substances are increased in patients with pulmonary hypertension.[225,226]; VEGF putatively exerts its effects in disease states such as pulmonary hypertension by promoting vascular cell growth, and thus may contribute to the endothelial cell clusters and plexiform lesions that characterize this disorder.[227] Altered hemostasis leading to increased thrombosis is a key factor in the development of pulmonary hypertension. Lower levels of NO and PGI_2 favor the formation of in situ thrombosis by enhancing platelet activation. In addition, the regional slowing of blood flow secondary to luminal narrowing further contributes to enhanced thrombogenicity.

A genetic component to pulmonary vasculopathy has been confirmed with the identification of a heterozygous germ line mutation in bone morphogenetic protein receptor 2 (BMPR2), a member of the TGF-beta family of proteins.[228] BMPR2 has been identified among 800% of patients with the hereditary forms of PAH and among 20% of idiopathic cases.[228,229] Rare mutations in other genes belonging to the TGF-beta super family (activin-like kinase-type 1,ALKq, endoglin, ENG; mothers against decapentaplegic, SMAD 9) have also been described.[229]

Vasoconstriction, along with vascular wall remodeling and thrombosis in situ, are three major factors that contribute to increased vascular resistance in patients with pulmonary hypertension. Vasoconstriction occurs early; proliferation of intimal and adventitial tissue follows as the disease progresses. Hypoxemia triggers a specific growth response in each cell type (endothelial cell, smooth muscle cell, and adventitial fibroblast) within the pulmonary artery wall as early as 24 hours following the hypoxic stimulus.[230] This response to hypoxia underlies the proliferative response and vascular remodeling that accompanies pulmonary hypertension.[231,232] In addition, hypoxia contributes to elevated levels of endothelin-1, a vascular endothelium peptide with potent vasoconstrictor properties.[222,232–234] An imbalance of the circulating arachidonate products, thromboxane and prostacyclin, two eicosanoids with divergent effects on vascular smooth muscle and platelet aggregation, may also play an important role in the pathogenesis of pulmonary hypertension.[235] Serotonin is a platelet- and neuroendocrine cell-derived mitogen with potent vasoconstrictor properties in the lungs. In patients with pulmonary hypertension, there is expansion of the pulmonary neuroendocrine cell population with overexpression of serotonin.[236–238] interestingly, serotonin, like hypoxemia, has profound vasodilator properties on the systemic circulation. The pathogenetic influence of serotonin in the development of dietary pulmonary hypertension is well established.[239,240] Its role in the development of other forms of pulmonary hypertension is less clear. These important observations have laid the groundwork for the development of targeted therapeutic interventions in the treatment of pathologic conditions associated with pulmonary vasculopathies.

The histopathologic changes that occur with pulmonary hypertension largely show a remarkable degree of similarity, regardless of the underlying cause or associated condition. The morphologic changes include intimal fibrosis, in situ thrombosis, fibrinoid degeneration, and medial hypertrophy of smooth muscle cells.[241] Three pathologic types of pulmonary hypertension are recognized: plexogenic, thrombotic, and veno-occlusive arteriopathy. Organized thrombi and plexiform arteriopathy were historically felt to represent pleiomorphic manifestations of one disease.[242] More recent studies, however, indicate that these patterns of vascular pathology are likely to be of clinical and prognostic significance. Plexigenic arteriopathy, the most common pathologic change, confers a worse prognosis.[241] The expansion of endothelial cell populations and disordered endothelial cell proliferation gives rise to plexiform lesions, a hallmark of both primary and some secondary forms of pulmonary hypertension that is thought to represent a form of intravascular angiogenesis. This lesion is characterized by a mass of disorganized vessels associated with smooth muscle cells, myofibroblasts, and endothelial cells, forming glomeruloid structures. These plexiform lesions modulate the release of a diverse group of growth factors and vasoactive proteins, including hypoxia-inducible factor-α (HIF-1α) and c-Src kinase, two proteins that modulate VEGF-induced production of prostacyclin and NO in the endothelial cells.[243,244] The presence of arterial thrombi distinguishes thrombogenic arteriopathy from the plexigenic form. Arterial thrombi are thought to occur as a consequence of endothelial cell injury and may appear as patchy defects on lung scintigraphy. The third histologic pattern, referred to as pulmonary veno-occlusive disease (PVOD) is characterized by intimal proliferation of the pulmonary veins rather than arteries. The distinction between PVOD and

other forms of pulmonary hypertension is important, as the use of prostacyclins and other vasodilators that are frequently used to treat other forms of pulmonary hypertension, may have catastrophic consequences in patients with PVOD.

GROUP 1: PULMONARY VENO-OCCLUSIVE DISEASE (PVOD) AND/OR PULMONARY CAPILLARY HEMANGIOMATOSIS (PCH)

PVOD and PCH are rare causes of PAH.[245] Because of specific similarities in clinical presentation, pathologic features, risk factors, and management, the new classification of PH combines PVOD and PCH into a single subcategory of PAH. Pulmonary hemosiderosis, interstitial edema and lymphatic dilatation, are prominent features of both disorders. Other histologic changes, including pulmonary arterial intimal fibrosis and medial hypertrophy are also seen in these disorders as well as in the idiopathic form of PAH. In addition, these disorders share common risk factors with PAH, including HIV, collagen vascular disease (scleroderma), and anorexigen exposure. Mutations in the BMPR2, the gene associated with idiopathic PAH, has also been isolated in patients with PVOD. Taken together, these findings suggest that PVOD, PCH, and PAH may represent different manifestations within a single disease spectrum. However, important differences in terms of clinical features, response to treatment and prognosis help to distinguish PVOD/PCH from idiopathic PAH.

Patients with PVOD/PCH frequently present with clubbing and crackles on physical examination. Ground glass opacities, septal thickening, mediastinal adenopathy, pleural effusions and reticulonodular patterns are common on chest imaging studies. Hemosiderin-laden macrophages are frequent findings on bronchoscopic examinations. Patients with PVOD/PCH tend to have lower carbon monoxide diffusing capacity and PaO2.[246,247] Importantly, treatment of PVOD/PCH patients with PAH-specific therapy may result in severe and sometimes fatal pulmonary edema. Patients with PVOD/PCH tend to have a worse prognosis than PAH, with most fatalities occurring within 2 years of the diagnosis.

PVOD has been described in cancer patients following radiation and chemotherapy (see below) and as a late sequelae of autologous and allogeneic hematopoietic stem cell transplants.[248–251] Certain malignancies, including neuroblastoma, lung cancer, multiple myeloma, leukemia, chronic myeloproliferative disease and Hodgkin lymphoma. PVOD with concomitant PCH was demonstrated in a patient with metastatic colon cancer.[249,250,252–255] The histologic hallmark of PVOD is diffuse fibrous occlusion predominantly of the postcapillary venules and small veins within the lobular septa. Medial hypertrophy of the pulmonary arteries is seen in 50% of patients with this disorder, however, arteritis and plexiform lesions are typically absent.[256,257] As the disease progresses, obliterative fibrosis and thrombosis of the affected veins occur. In PCH, proliferation of capillary channels, which may become tortuous and engorged within alveolar walls, is the dominant histologic change.

The triad of severe PAH, normal PCWP and CT findings of centrilobular ground glass opacities, septal lines and mediastinal adenopathy offer noninvasive clues to the diagnosis. Kerley B lines, a result of transudation of fluid into the interstitium and enlargement of lymphatic channels are frequent findings. Pleural effusions are commonly seen with PVOD. The pleural effusions are typically transudates and result from elevation of pulmonary capillary and visceral pleural capillary hydrostatic pressures. By contrast, pleural effusions are unusual in PAH because the high resistance vessels lie proximal to the pulmonary capillaries.[258,259] Chronic deposition of collagen fibrils within the lobular septa occurs in long-standing cases, leading to pulmonary fibrosis. Other radiographic findings include engorgement of central pulmonary arteries and patchy airspace disease. Elevations of measured PAWP may occasionally be seen, depending on the size of the involved veins, and the degree of collateral communications between the affected venous beds.[260] Interstitial edema is a prominent radiographic finding. Kerley B lines, a result of transudation of fluid into the interstitium and enlargement of lymphatic channels are frequent findings. Pleural effusions are commonly seen with PVOD. The pleural effusions are typically transudates and result from elevation of pulmonary capillary and visceral pleural capillary hydrostatic pressures. By contrast, pleural effusions are unusual in PAH because the high resistance vessels lie proximal to the pulmonary capillaries.[258,259] Chronic deposition of collagen fibrils within the lobular septa occurs in long-standing cases, leading to pulmonary fibrosis. Other radiographic findings include engorgement of central pulmonary arteries and patchy airspace disease. The diagnosis requires pathologic confirmation, although bronchoscopically obtained lung biopsies may be associated with significant bleeding and are not recommended. Findings on surgical lung biopsy specimens, including intimal fibrosis that predominantly involves the small post-capillary pulmonary veins and the absence of plexiform lesions helps to clinch the diagnosis. Although surgical lung biopsy offers the only definitive diagnosis of PVOD/PCH,

the diagnostic utility of this procedure has been questioned because of the associated increased risk of bleeding and because treatment options are very limited. A definitive diagnosis may, however, provide important prognostic information and may impact decisions regarding the considerations for lung transplantation.

Pulmonary vasodilator therapy has an established role in the treatment of PAH, its efficacy in the treatment of PVOD/PCH remains controversial. These agents may, in fact, worsen the overall cardiopulmonary status by precipitating florid and sometimes fatal pulmonary edema[256,261] Theoretically, this occurs because the vasodilator effect on the pulmonary arteries may cause a substantial drop in pulmonary arteries while resistance in the pulmonary veins remains fixed, resulting in an increased transcapillary hydrostatic pressure and fulminant pulmonary edema. Thus, vasodilator therapy in this form of pulmonary edema should be used with extreme caution. Other forms of therapy, including immunosuppressive medications with glucocorticoids and antimetabolites have been employed. Data regarding the utility of these treatment regimens are limited to small case reports and, thus, firm conclusions regarding efficacy cannot be drawn. The role of anticoagulation in the treatment of these patients remains largely unstudied. Reported one-year mortality rate of 72% yields testimony to the overall poor prognosis of patients with this disease.[262] Lung transplantation represents the sole potentially curative therapy, although cumulative experience among patients with PVOD is limited. Pulmonary transplantation remains the treatment of choice for these patients.

GROUP 2: PH OWING TO LEFT HEART DISEASE (LHD-PH)

Left-sided heart disease is probably the most common cause of PH.[246,263] In this setting, elevated pulmonary venous pressures, owing to left heart systolic dysfunction, left heart diastolic dysfunction, or valvular (usually mitral) disease led to pulmonary venous hypertension (PVH). Diastolic filling pressures are chronically elevated with LHD-PH, (as reflected in increased PCWP). Backward transmission of these pressures into the pulmonary venous system results in pulmonary venous hypertension (PVH) and vasoconstriction of the pulmonary arterial bed. The hemodynamic profile in LHD-PH includes increased PAP with an increased transpulmonary gradient (> 12 mm Hg) and a normal or near normal PVP.[264] In a small subset of patients, severe elevations in PAP occurs in association with marked increases in PVR and pulmonary diastolic pressures.[246] This phenomenon has been studied extensively in patients with mitral stenosis, and remains less characterized among patients with diastolic dysfunction. Histologic changes in PVH include thickening of the pulmonary veins and neointimal formation. These changes may be reversible with early recognition and correction of the underlying cause of PVH. Clinical signs and symptoms of PVH include dyspnea on exertion and, as the disease progresses, right sided heart failure with peripheral edema. Orthopnea and paroxysmal nocturnal dyspnea are prominent symptoms of advanced PVH, but unusual findings in early and idiopathic varieties of this disease. ECG findings of left ventricular hypertrophy may be seen, whereas in PAH right ventricular hypertrophy is more common. Echocardiography is a valuable tool in identifying systolic, diastolic and valvular abnormalities. Echocardiographic evidence of a dilated left atrium, abnormal mitral inflow pattern and LV hypertrophy or atrial fibrillation are suggestive of diastolic heart failure, which may be confirmed by documentation of elevated PCWP at right heart catheterization (RHC). Because PCWP determination is sometimes imprecise, LV end-diastolic pressure (LVEDP) measurements obtained during the procedure may provide valuable additional information. Cardiac catheterization also provides critical information regarding other hemodynamic parameters, such as pulmonary vascular resistance (PVR), right atrial pressure (RAP), transpulmonary gradient, and LVEDP. In patients with PCWP > 15, vasoreactivity testing with selective pulmonary vasodilators is not recommended.[265]

Therapy for PVD is dictated by the underlying cause. Several small studies have demonstrated a favorable response to sildenafil, a PDE5 inhibitor, when added to standard medical therapy in the treatment of in selected patients with systolic LV failure and concomitant PVH.[266,267] Although the initial data appears promising, larger controlled trials are necessary to define the safety, tolerability, and potential impact of sildenafil and other PDE5 inhibitors in this group of patients. Chronic pulmonary vasodilator therapy has not been successful in patients with mitral stenosis or diastolic dysfunction and, in fact may be dangerous.[268,269] Patients with pulmonary edema and coexisting PVH caused by severe mitral valve disease may respond to diuretic therapy while awaiting definitive surgical treatment. The approach to patients with PVH as a consequence of LV diastolic dysfunction are typically managed medically with aggressive treatment of systemic hypertension, nitrates and diuretics, although no randomized clinical trials addressing this issue is currently available.

GROUP 3: PH OWING TO LUNG DISEASES AND/OR HYPOXIA

The Group 3 disorders are characterized by alveolar hypoxia which typically occurs as a result of underlying lung disease, impaired control of breathing, or residence at high altitude.[246] Although PH is common in this group of disorders, PAP elevations are typically modest (mean PAP 20 to 35 mm Hg). Cancer and its treatment are prominent causes of hypoxic lung injury, which may be severe. The precise incidence of Group 3 PH resulting from cancer-related lung injury, however, is unknown. Hypoxic events in the cancer patient may result from a wide variety of pathologic conditions that directly and indirectly impact the lungs.

Underlying chronic obstructive pulmonary disease (COPD) often co-exists with primary bronchogenic malignancies. Pulmonary hypertension in these patients is frequently mild to moderate. Approximately 5% of patients with COPD, however, develop substantial elevations in PAP associated with severe PH (mean PAP >40 mm Hg). Severe hypoxemia, hypocapnia, and substantial reductions in diffusing capacity for carbon monoxide (DLCO) may occur despite evidence of only modest airway obstruction in this group of patients.[270] Interstitial and alveolar lung disease is also associated with mild to moderate elevations in PAP (<40 mm Hg). Injury to the lung as a consequence of radiation and/or chemotherapy, pulmonary edema, alveolar hemorrhage, atelectasis, interstitial pneumonitis, obliterative bronchiolitis, pneumonia or acute respiratory distress syndrome (ARDS) are common causes of cancer-related conditions associated with interstitial/alveolar lung disease and hypoxia with PH. Depression of host defense mechanisms by cancer as well as the treatment modalities of radiation, chemotherapy, and hematopoietic stem cell transplantation (HSCT) may trigger severe pneumonias with associated hypoxemia. Finally, sleep disordered breathing may be associated with mild pulmonary hypertension, but these patients usually have coexisting daytime hypoxemia (such as obesity hypoventilation syndrome or chronic lung disease).[271] Each of these conditions, when severe, may lead to hypoxic pulmonary arteriopathy. Thus, the cancer patient is susceptible to the development of hypoxia-associated pulmonary hypertension as an end point of a plethora of diverse insults to the lungs.

The pathologic lesion in hypoxic pulmonary arteriopathy is hyperplasia and hypertrophy of small arterioles. Plexiform lesions and neointima formation are typically absent. Although modest elevations in hypoxia-induced PH are typical, patients may present with severe hypoxia associated with profound symptoms of dyspnea. This is particularly true among patients with COPD and hypoxia-induced PH. Right heart failure may be seen in this group of patients despite only modest elevations in PAP and is thought to relate to the degree of hypoxemia, rather than PH. Additional factors, including acidemia, hypercarbia, hyperviscoscity associated with hypoxia-induced polycythemia, loss of small vessels within the pulmonary vascular bed, and compression of pulmonary vessels by the hyperinflated lungs all contribute to pulmonary hypertension and hypoxia in these patients. PH portends a poor prognosis.

Initial assessments of PH in this group of patients by echocardiogram is reasonable, although echocardiography frequently underestimates pulmonary artery pressures in this setting of COPD.[272] RHC should be pursued in patients with chronic lung disease for the following reasons: clinical worsening, progressive exercise limitation or gas exchange abnormalities are disproportionate to ventilatory impairment; severe PH is suspected by noninvasive measures; suspicion of left ventricular systolic/diastolic dysfunction; evaluation for lung transplantation. Further imaging (chest radiograph, high resolution chest tomography) and pulmonary testing may be helpful in assessing the severity of the underlying lung disease. The prognosis of PH is predicated on the severity of the underlying lung disease. Supplemental oxygen therapy and treatment strategies that focus on the underlying disease may improve overall prognosis.

Treatment should be directed towards treating the underlying pulmonary disease. Patients with chronic alveolar hypoxia should be treated with long-term oxygen therapy.[273] Positive pressure ventilation has been shown to reduce pulmonary artery systolic pressures and is the treatment of choice in patients with sleep disordered breathing.[271,274] The role of vasodilator medications has not been studied in any large, randomized trial. Caution in the use of vasodilator therapy is warranted due to the propensity of these agents to cause hypoxic vasoconstriction and worsening gas exchange. Initiation of pulmonary vasodilator therapy should be reserved for specialized centers with meticulous monitoring of patients.[275] Supplemental oxygen has been definitively shown to favorably impact survival.[273,276,277] However, improved survival has only been definitively shown in this group of patients following lung transplantation.

GROUP 4: CHRONIC THROMBOEMBOLIC PULMONARY HYPERTENSION (CTEPH)

Persistent macrovascular obstruction from unresolved pulmonary emboli may result in vasoconstriction and small vessel arteriopathy resulting in CTEPH.[278] It is estimated to occur in up to 4% of patients.[193,279–281]

Risk factors for the development of CPTEH include recurrent pulmonary embolism, younger age, large perfusion defects on scintigraphy, and idiopathic presentation of pulmonary embolism.[279,281] Subsequent pulmonary arteriopathy and in situ thrombosis may play a larger role. Histologic changes associated with CTEPH are similar to those seen in PAH.

Patients with CTEPH frequently present with unexplained dyspnea months after an acute thromboembolic event; however, no history of thromboembolic disease may be reported in 25% of patients with CTEPH.[282] Radiographic abnormalities demonstrating enlargement of central pulmonary arteries, patchy areas of hypovascularity (mosaic oligemia), and cardiomegaly may suggest the diagnosis. An echocardiogram may identify right ventricular dysfunction and elevated right ventricle systolic pressures suggestive of PH. Radionuclide ventilation/perfusion (VQ) scan is the preferred and recommended screening test for chronic thromboembolic disease in patients with PH[283] Pulmonary angiography is the gold standard for confirmation of chronic thromboembolic disease, assessment of hemodynamics and determination of operability.[278,283]

Patients with Pulmonary endarterectomy (PEA) for proximal thromboembolic disease with associated CTEHP for is potentially curative.[284] Therefore, prompt referral to a center with expertise in the management CTEPH is indicated. The feasibility of performing PEA depends on the location of the obstruction (central versus more distal pulmonary arteries), the correlation between hemodynamic findings and the degree of mechanical obstruction assessed by angiography, comorbidities, and surgical experience.[285] Patients who are not surgical candidates may benefit from balloon pulmonary angioplasty (BPA). This emerging intervention for treating segmental and subsegmental CTEPH, uses standard balloon angioplasty techniques to dilate pulmonary arteries.[286] Prospective randomized controlled trials to investigate the safety and efficacy of BPA in clinical practice are needed. Persistent PAH after PEA or in patients with inoperable disease may benefit from targeted medical therapy. Although bosentan and sildenafil have both been studied in CTEPH, only riociguat, an oral soluable guanylate cyclase stimulator, is approved for inoperable CTEPH or persistent PH after PEA in the United States and Europe.[179,283] Off-label use of other pulmonary vasodilators may be considered in specialized centers.

GROUP 5: PH WITH UNCLEAR OR MULTIFACTORIAL MECHANISMS

The final category consists of a heterogeneous group of disease processes with diverse pathologies and clinical presentations. These disorders are grouped into 4 broad categories that include hematologic disorders, systemic diseases, metabolic derangements, and other etiologies. Several of these categories are relevant to the patient with cancer and will be discussed below.

The association between PH and chronic myeloproliferative disorders (CMD) has been described in numerous reports and case series; however, many of these were based on echocardiographic data, so secondary causes were not excluded.[208,287,288] More recently, Guilipain and colleagues reported a series of 10 patients with CMD, and they described two distinct forms of PH in these patients: PAH and CTEPH.[289] Several mechanisms of PH in patients with CMD have been proposed including portal hypertension, tumor microembolism, extramedullary hematopoiesis, blood cell proliferation and enhanced angiogenesis.[208] Interestingly, indolent myeloid abnormalities such as polyclonal myelofibrosis have been described in PAH patients.[290] Murine models have also suggested an underlying myelopulmonary pathophysiologic link, for hematopoietic myeloid progenitors derived from PAH patients have resulted in endothelial injury, vascular remodeling and PAH.[291,292] A recent report describing resolution of both myelofibrosis and PAH after allogeneic hematopoietic stem cell transplantation suggests treatment of the underlying disease may be curative for PAH as well.[293] Further study is needed to determine the mechanism in this group as well as appropriate therapy.

Two of the systemic disorders that have been linked to PH, neurofibromatosis and sarcoidosis have ties to cancer.[246] Sarcoid-like reactions have been increasingly shown in a variety of hematopoietic and solid malignancies.[294,295] Both benign and malignant tumors of the nervous system are common sequelae of neurofibromatosis type 1. This autosomal-dominant disorder is occasionally complicated by systemic vasculopathy, in which lung fibrosis and/or CTEPH may play a pathogenetic role.

Among the metabolic disorders within the third group of miscellaneous diseases, derangements in thyroid function may be clinically relevant in the cancer setting. Hypothyroidism is a common sequela of certain head and neck cancers. PAH has been linked to this disorder. Pulmonary hypertension may be aggravated by hypoventilation and hypoxemia in patients with severe hypothyroid states. Alternatively, patients with PAH have a higher prevalence of both hypo- and hyperthyroid disorders. Based on these observations, it is recommended that thyroid function tests be considered in the investigation of every patient with PAH.[296,297]

Pulmonary vascular tumors, tumor emboli, fibrosing mediastinitis and metastatic carcinomas comprise the final group of disorders associated with PH. Primary tumors of the pulmonary vasculature may arise from and obstruct both the arterial and venous vascular systems. These rare tumors are often rapidly fatal.[298,299] Most cases are caused by pulmonary artery sarcomas (PAS). PAS are central tumors that mimic pulmonary thromboembolism both clinically and radiographically (Figure 18-9).[300] Dyspnea, cough, hemoptysis or chest pain are frequent presenting symptoms. Patients often present without symptom resolution despite therapeutic anticoagulation. Computed

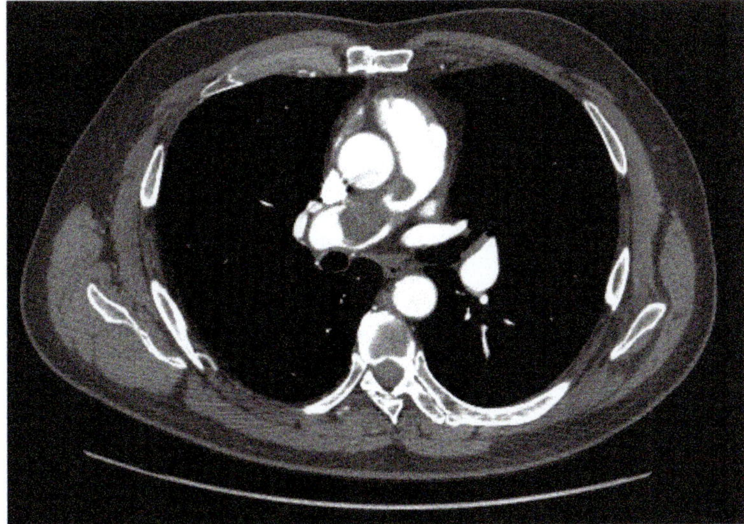

FIGURE 18-9 Pulmonary artery sarcoma mimicking pulmonary embolism. A 65-year-old man with pulmonary artery sarcoma. A large soft tumor (A) was present in the distal main pulmonary artery, extending into the right main pulmonary artery (arrow). Pulmonary artery patency was restored (B) following surgical intervention, which included endarterectomy and resection of all visualized tumor, with reconstruction of the pulmonary artery.

tomography, magnetic resonance imaging angiography (MRI-A), and fluorine-18-2-fluoro-2-deoxy-D-glucoseepositronemission tomography (FDG-PET) may assist in differentiating between tumor and thrombotic material. Heterogeneous enhancement of the filling defect on CT evaluation coupled with evidence of mediastinal invasion favors the diagnosis of PAS. Increased FDG-PET uptake, along with evidence of homogeneous mass on T1-weighted images by MRI are also helpful diagnostic clues. The therapy of choice is surgical resection combined with neoadjuvant chemotherapy may improve symptoms and extend survival, however the prognosis remains dismal, with a median survival time post-operatively of only 10 months.[301,302]

Metastatic tumor emboli are far more common etiologies of PH and typically arise from mucinous carcinomas originating in the breast, lung, stomach and colon (Figure 18-10).[303] Tumor emboli also may complicate choriocarcinomas and malignant neoplasms involving the kidneys, liver, and prostate. Ventilation perfusion scanning usually provides the greatest diagnostic utility, which may reveal multiple subsegmental mis-matched defects, whereas chest radiographs and computed tomography scans may be normal.[303] Computed tomography scans do not show proximal thombi, but they may reveal septal thickening. Diagnosis of tumor emboli may potentially be confirmed with pulmonary microvascular cytology sampling through a pulmonary artery catheter in the wedge position.[303] Estimates of a 3%–26% incidence of pulmonary tumor embolism in the medical literature are woefully inaccurate, and primarily derived from autopsy series.[304,305] Chronic pulmonary hypertension may also occur as a result of tumor thrombotic microangiopathy[306–309] This rare disorder is caused by tumor cell infiltration into the pulmonary vasculature. Adenocarcinomas involving the breast, lung, liver, stomach, kidney and choriocarcinoma are common sites of tumor origin. Histologic evidence of widespread fibrocellular intimal proliferation of small pulmonary arteries and arterioles associated with aggregates of tumor cells establishes the diagnosis, a diagnosis that is rarely made antemortem. Intimal fibrocellular proliferation leads to arterial stenosis and pulmonary arterial hypertension. PH may develop in the absence of obvious parenchymal metastases, as the small tumor cell aggregates are seldom radiographically apparent. Pulmonary hypertension due to fibrosing mediastinitis is rare, and it may present with PH owing to compression of both pulmonary arteries and veins. Most causes of fibrosing mediastinitis in the United States have been linked to *Histoplasma capsulatum* infection.[242] Rarely, fibrosing mediastinitis

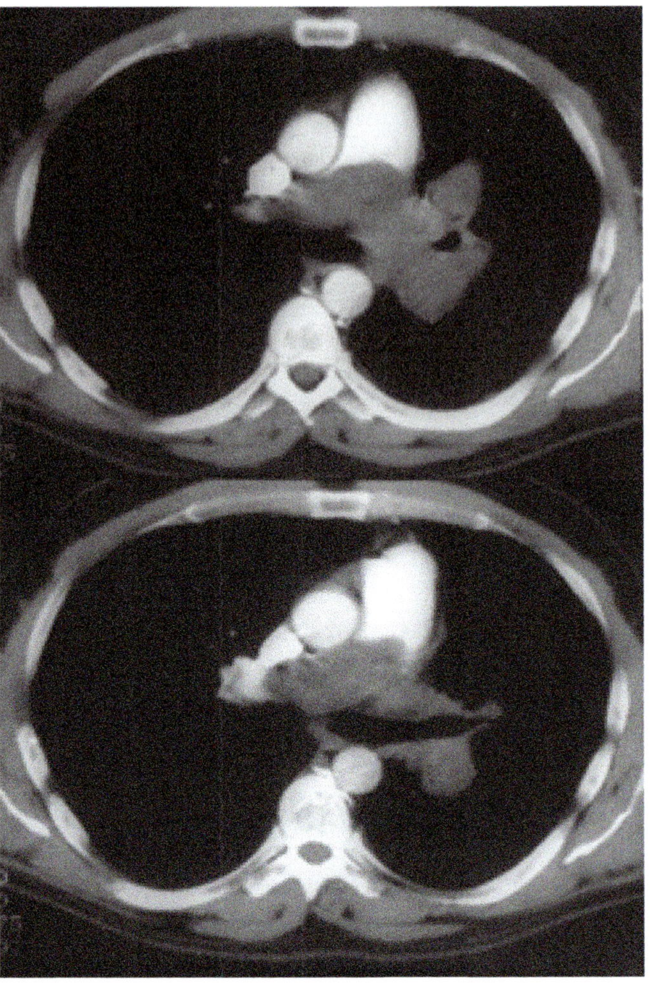

FIGURE 18-10 Metastatic tumor embolus. A 38-year-old man who presented with a 4 month history of progressive symptoms of shortness of breath. A CT angiogram showed near complete obstruction of the main pulmonary artery. Autopsy examination confirmed mucinous adenocarcinoma of the stomach with metastatic spread and obstruction of the pulmonary artery.

has also been implicated in other infections, including *Aspergillus*, *Mycobacterium tuberculosis*, *Blastomycosis*, *Mucormycosis*, and *Cryptococcosis*.[310–312] Fibrosing mediastinitis owing to radiation and Hodgkin's lymphoma have also been reported.[312,313]

■ Pulmonary Hypertension: Treatment

Over the past two decades, advancements in the understanding of PH pathogenesis and its recognition as a vasoproliferative disorder has led to a shift in the approach to treatment and has substantially broadened the therapeutic options for this disease. Only patients who demonstrate a positive response to vasodilator challenge should be considered for calcium channel blocker therapy. Close monitoring is recommended to determine both the efficacy and safety of therapy. The most frequently used short-acting vasodilators include nifedipine, diltiazem, and amlodipine. Calcium channel blocks with negative inotropic effects, such as verapamil should be avoided.[314]

The pharmacologic armamentarium used in the treatment of PH now includes a growing array of pulmonary vasodilators and agents with antiproliferative properties, in addition to the standard regimen of supplemental oxygen, and in selected cases, diuretics, digoxin, and anticoagulant therapies (Figure 18-11). Various classes of drugs are now available, including the endothelin receptor antagonists, phosphodiesterase-5 inhibitors, soluble guanylate cyclase stimulators, prostacyclin analogues and prostacyclin receptor agonists. As new pharmacologic agents emerge, the selection of the appropriate agent or combination of agents becomes more complex. The route of administration, side-effect profile, patient preference, functional status and clinical judgment all help determine the best therapy. The goal in treatment of PAH is to improve WHO functional status. Combination therapy using agents with different molecular targets may act synergistically and is advocated in patients who fail to show improvement or deteriorate with monotherapy. The goal of combination therapy should be to maximize efficacy, while minimizing toxicity. Improvement in the progression-free survival of PAH has been demonstrated in long term studies (SERAPHIN, AMBITION) with combination therapy[315]

General measures such as immunizations, psychosocial support and supervised exercise should also be considered in PH. Oxygen therapy is utilized to treat and/or prevent hypoxemia, which may cause vasoconstriction and worsening of pulmonary hypertension. Patients may be normoxemic at rest but suffer severe desaturations with exercise or sleep.

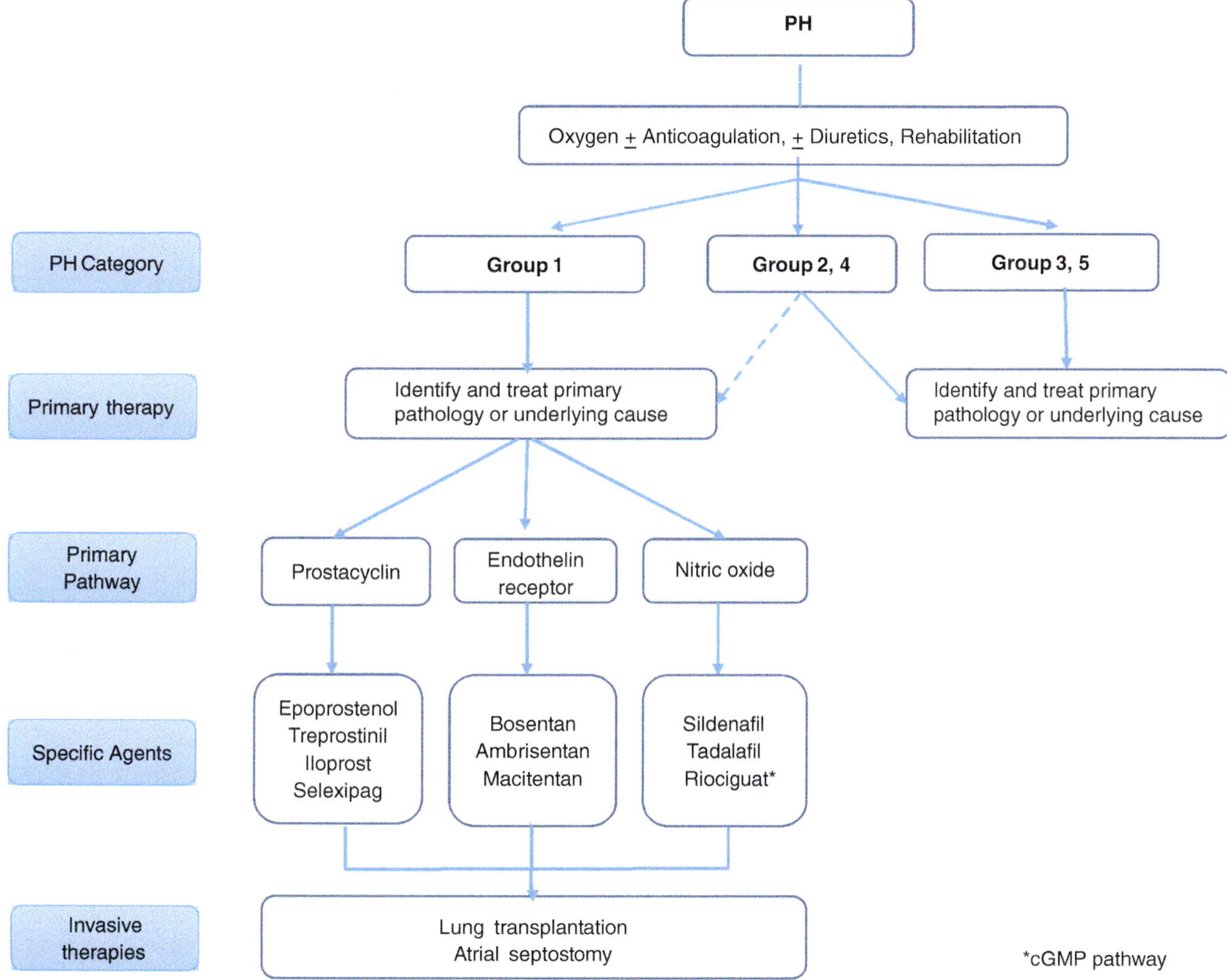

FIGURE 18-11   Algorithm for PH-specific therapy based on pathway.

Accordingly, oxygen therapy should be prescribed for patients with chronic respiratory insufficiency and arterial oxygen pressures repeatedly below 55–60 mm Hg, or for patients with major exercise-induced or sleep-associated hypoxemia. Diuretics should be administered as indicated. Improved survival has been reported with oral anticoagulation and, unless contraindicated, should be prescribed to patients with IPAH and patients with CTEPH.[316] Anticoagulation should be avoided in other forms for PH where the risk-benefit ratio may be unfavorable, such as in cancer-related thrombocytopenia.[317]

Invasive therapies ■ Interventional and surgical therapeutic options should be considered in patients with progressive functional decline and right ventricular dysfunction despite medical therapy. Atrial septostomy (AS) and transplantation (heart-lung transplantation, HLTx, and bilateral lung transplantation, BLTx) are possible options. AS effectively produces a right to left shunt, thereby decompressing the right-sided chambers and augmenting left atrial filling pressures. In so doing, RV wall tension and end diastolic pressures are reduced, RV contractility may be increased, left-sided cardiac outputs are increased, and systemic oxygen transport is improved. These hemodynamic effects are seen clinically as resolution of syncopal and precyncopal episodes, decreased systemic venous congestion, and improved exercise tolerance. Based on worldwide literature, patients undergoing AS include those with IPAH (82%), PAH associated with surgically corrected congenital heart disease (8%), collagen vascular disease (5%), distal CTEPH not amenable to surgery (3%) and miscellaneous (3%).[284] AS may be considered in patients who failed maximal medical therapy or have persistent RV failure or syncope despite medical therapy and as a bridge to transplantation.[284] Although there are no guidelines for the optimal size of the defect, a defect size of 8.5 ± 2 mm anecdotally increased cardiac output (CO) by 20% to 25%. A repeat procedure may be required if the defect closes. The optimal timing of AS is a matter of debate and experience in treating any form of PH with this procedure is very limited.[318,319]

HLTx or BLTx are both effective in treating patients with PAH. Patient selection criteria is similar to AS and includes those who failed medical therapy, patients with a functional class IV or a functional class III that is refractory to treatment. Early surgical referral for patient with IPAH, PAH related to scleroderma, PVOD, PCH, congenital right-to-left shunts or Eisenmenger syndrome is advocated.[284] Although hemodynamics are the primary determinant of

survival, functional class, exercise capacity and failure to respond to therapy all provide prognostic information. Extracorporeal support (ECLS) and ventricular assist devices may be used in critically ill patients with RV failure, but data from randomized controlled trials are lacking.

Pulmonary hypertension: Follow-up ■ Two different strategies in the follow up of PAH patients have been proposed.[320] A clinical strategy focuses on the clinical symptoms and signs and correlates these with functional status. If functional status is satisfactory (WHO functional class I and II) and there are no signs of right ventricular failure, then no change in therapy is indicated. In the goal-oriented strategy, parameters considered prognostically relevant are identified and therapy is escalated until these goals are met or significant toxicities occur. Treatment goals in the goal-oriented strategy typically include improvement of functional class to class I or II, improvement in the 6 minute walk distance to 380 m or more, a peak oxygen uptake of more than 10.4 mL/kg/minute, a maximum systolic blood pressure greater than 120 mm Hg during cardiopulmonary exercise test, or a decrease in BNP level to less than 180 pg/mL.[196,321] Close follow up every 3 to 6 months is indicated with both approaches.

DRUG-INDUCED LUNG DISEASE

Significant advancements in cancer treatment strategies over the past 2 decades, including the rapidly growing class of novel immunomodulating and molecular targeted therapies, the development of novel therapeutic agents within the class of conventional chemotherapies and the growth of complex multi-agent and multimodality regimens, have expanded cancer treatment options and contributed to improved cancer outcomes. With these advancements, organ-specific toxicities have been increasingly recognized. The lungs are particularly susceptible to injury due to drug toxicity, which may manifest as stereotyped histopathologic injury patterns involving the airways, lung parenchyma, pleura, mediastinum, and pulmonary circulation. The enhanced susceptibility of the lungs to drug-induced lung injury (DILI) has not been fully elucidated, but is felt to be due to the lung's large surface area and the propensity for higher accumulation of some drugs within the lungs versus other tissues. In addition, bioactivation and biotransformation of some drugs occur within the lung, which may lead to reactive metabolite formation, oxidative stress, and subsequent cell injury. Hypersensitivity pneumonitis caused by T-cell specific, immune-mediated mechanisms and phospholipid deposition within lung cells are additional proposed mechanisms.[322–324]

Lung injury patterns may differ in frequency, intensity, duration of pulmonary damage, and timing relative to drug exposure depending on the therapeutic class of the drug. The spectrum of lung injury patterns and clinical syndromes following conventional chemotherapeutic agents, immune checkpoint inhibitor therapies and molecular targeted agents are listed in Tables 18-5 and 18-6. While all patterns of pulmonary injury may be seen following exposure to conventional chemotherapies, molecular targeted drugs and immune modulating agents, vasculopathies, infusion reactions, pneumonitis, and pleural effusions are more common following targeted therapies. Pneumonitis and sarcoid-like reactions have been most often described following exposure to immune modulating agents. Severe myelosuppression and mucositis leading to increased risks for opportunistic pneumonias and aspiration pneumonitis are more often sequelae of conventional chemotherapy. Interstitial and alveolar lung disease patterns are the most frequent, and may manifest clinically as noncardiogenic pulmonary edema (NCPE), ARDS, pneumonitis, alveolar hemorrhage, and/or pulmonary fibrosis. PH, triggered by drug-induced thromboembolic phenomena or endothelial injury, is also well described. Any of these lung injury patterns as well as injury to the airways, pleura and mediastinum may induce changes in cardiac hemodynamics and adrenergic loads and, when severe, precipitate cardiac decompensation. Alternatively, pulmonary decompensation induced by chemotherapy-related myocarditis and heart failure is also reported following administration of some cancer agents, including the newer molecular targeted therapies.

Certain risk factors influence the occurrence and severity of lung injury as well as the latency periods between drug exposure and clinical symptoms. The significance of these factors varies with different agents and include advanced age, cumulative dose, concomitant or sequential radiotherapy, high-inspired supplemental oxygen supplementation, preexisting lung disease (in particular, fibrotic lung disease), and the use of multi-drug regimens.

The clinical manifestations of DILI are nonspecific. Dry cough, dyspnea, hypoxia, and low-grade fever, are common presenting symptoms which may progress insidiously over several weeks to 2 months after initiation of the first or subsequent cycles of therapy.[325] Symptom onset, however, varies widely. Acute and hyperacute hypersensitivity reactions have been reported following exposure to some drugs, such as paclitaxel or methotrexate. Delayed

reactions leading to pulmonary fibrosis may occur months to years after exposure to some agents, such as bleomycin, busulfan, cyclophosphamide, gemcitabine and BCNU as a late manifestation of DILI.[326–329] Bronchospasm and allergic reactions are common manifestations of infusion reactions which typically occur within minutes to hours of therapy. Late-onset manifestations, occurring 2 months to years after completion of the drug have been described following exposure busulfan, bleomycin, mitomycin C, cyclophosphamide, gemcitabine, and the nitrosoureas.[326–328,330] Wheezing with or without a concomitant rash may signal a hypersensitivity reaction. The lung examination is often clear, although bibasilar rales may be auscultated, particularly in the setting of pulmonary fibrosis.

Interstitial, alveolar or mixed infiltrates with bibasilar predominance are the most common radiographic findings. Focal nodular consolidations that mimic tumor involvement have also been described, particularly flowing bleomycin exposure. Pleural effusions are also seen, which are typically small to moderate in size and bilateral.

Both the clinical and radiographic manifestations of DILI are indistinguishable from other nondrug-related causes of lung damage. Moreover, there are no pathognomonic histopathologic findings or derangements in laboratory evaluations and respiratory function that are sufficient to establish the diagnosis. Competing diagnoses, including infection, aspiration pneumonitis, radiation injury, acute lung injury/ARDS, pulmonary edema, cancer relapse, pulmonary hemorrhage, and lymphangitic spread of tumor should be excluded. Thus, the diagnosis of DILI is largely based on the temporal association between drug exposure and the development of pulmonary injury once competing diagnoses have been excluded. The adverse cardiopulmonary reactions triggered by some of these agents may be severe and rapidly fatal. Therefore, the clinician must maintain a high index of suspicion and must be familiar with the well-described pulmonary toxicities triggered by classic chemotherapeutic agents as well as emerging toxicities associated with newer drugs.

Reductions in the diffusing capacity for carbon monoxide (DLCO) may represent the earliest and only derangement upon pulmonary function testing. With disease progression, a restrictive lung defect may be seen. Airflow obstruction, particularly following infusion reactions to taxanes and monoclonal antibody therapies has also been described. Recrudescence of clinical signs and symptoms following challenge testing establishes the diagnosis, however challenge testing is not recommended due to unpredictable and

TABLE 18-5 Lung injury patterns following cancer therapies: Conventional chemotherapy

PULMONARY SYNDROME	AGENT CLASS						
	ALKYLATING AGENTS	ANTI-METABOLITES	CYTOTOXIC ANTIBIOTICS	TOPOISO-MERASE INHIBITORS	PODOPHY-LLOTOXINS	TAXANES MICROTUBULE INHIBITORS	OTHER
Parenchymal Disease							
Interstitial Pneumonitis/ Pulmonary Fibrosis	Busulfan BCNU CCNU Cyclophosphamide Ifosphamide Temazolamide Oxaliplatin Melphalan	Methotrexate Azathioprine Cytarabine Fludarabine Azacitabine Gemcitabine	Bleomycin Mitomycin C	Topotecan Irinotecan Amrubicin Daunorubicin Liposomal Doxorubicin		Paclitaxel Docetaxel	ATRA Arsenic trioxide Procarbazine
Eosinophilic Pneumonia	Busulfan Cyclophosphamide Oxaliplatin	Methotrexate Cytarabine Fludarabine Gemcitabine Pentostatin	Bleomycin		Etoposide	Paclitaxel Docetaxel	
DAD/ARDS/ NCPE/DAH	Busulfan, Cyclophosphamide, Ifosphamide, Temazolamide, Oxaliplatin Melphalan	Methotrexate Azathioprine Cytarabine Fludarabine Azacitabine Gemcitabine Pentostatin Pemetrexed Zinostatin	Bleomycin Mitomycin C	Topotecan	Etoposide	Paclitaxel Docetaxel Vincristine Vinblastine Vindesine Vinorelbine Ixabepilone	ATRA Arsenic trioxide
Radiation Recall Pneumonitis		Gemcitabine	Bleomycin	Amrubicin Daunorubicin Liposomal Doxorubicin		Paclitaxel Docetaxel	
Granuloma formation	Oxaliplatin	Methotrexate					

Airway Disease							
Infusion Reaction/ bronchospasm	Cyclophosphamide Ifosphamide Carboplatin Cisplatin Oxaliplatin	Methotrexate Gemcitabine Pemetrexed	Bleomycin Mitomycin C	Amrubicin Daunorubicin Liposomal Doxorubicin	Etoposide Teniposide	Paclitaxel Docetaxel Vincristine Vinblastine Vindesine Vinorelbine	L-asparaginase
BOOP	Busulfan, Cyclophosphamide Ifosphamide Oxaliplatin	Methotrexate	Bleomycin	Topotecan			L-asparaginase
Vascular Disease							
Pulmonary hypertension		Zinostatin	Bleomycin Mitomycin C				
VTE/DVT							ATRA
Pleural Disease							
Pleural Effusion	Cyclophosphamide	Methotrexate Gemcitabine	Mitomycin			Docetaxel Paclitaxel	ATRA Arsenic trioxide Procarbazine
Pleural thickening	BCNU Bleomycin Cyclophosphamide						
Other							
Opportunistic Infections	Temozolamide	Methotrexate Fludarabine					
MetHemoglobinemia	Cyclophosphamide Ifosphamide						
Acute Chest pain Myocardial infarction			Bleomycin PEB: (Cisplatin/ Vincrstine/ Bleomycin) PVB: (Cisplatin/ vincristine/ bleomycin)				

TABLE 18-6 Lung injury patterns following cancer therapies: molecular targeted therapies and immune checkpoint inhibitors

PULMONARY SYNDROME	AGENT CLASS					
	MONOCLONAL ANTIBODIES	TYROSINE KINASE INHIBITORS	RAPAMYCIN INHIBITORS	PROTEOSOME INHIBITORS	IMMUNE MODULATORS CHECKPOINT INHIBITORS	OTHER
Parenchymal Disease						
	Cetuximab Panitumumab Alemtuzumab Rituximab Brentuximab	Gefitinib Erlotinib Imatinib Dasatinib Sorafenib Sunitunib Vandetanib Idelalisib Trametinib Crizotinib	Everolimus Temsirolimus	Bortezomib Carlfizomib	Thalidomide IL-2 Ipilimumab Nivolimab Pembrolizumab	
DAD/ARDS/NCPE/DAH	Cetuximab Panitumumab Alemtuzumab Rituximab Ofatumumab Ibritumomab Trastuzumab Pertuzumab Gemtuzumab	Gefitinib Erlotinib Imatinib Sorafenib Vandetanib Crizotinib Ruxolitinib	Everolimus Temsirolimus	Bortezomib	Thalidomide Lenolidomide CART inhibitiors Blinotumomab	
Radiation Recall Pneumonitis	Panitumumab	Erlotinib Vemurafenib		Bortezomib		
Granuloma formation	Ipilumumab		Everolimus		IFN-g Ipilimumab Nivolimab Pembrolizumab	
Hemoptysis	Bevacizumab Alemtuzumab Rituximab	Sorafenib Sunitunib Pazopanib			IL-2 TNF IFN-g	

Airway Disease						
Infusion Reaction/ bronchospasm	Cetuximab Panitumumab Bevacizumab Alemtuzumab Rituximab Obinutuzumab Ofatumumab Ibritumomab Trastuzumab Pertuzumab Gemtuzumab Ipilimumab Pembrolizumab				Ipilimumab Nivolimab Pembrolizumab	
BOOP	Rituximab			Bortezomib	Thalidomide IFN-g	
Vascular Disease						
Pulmonary hypertension		Dasatinib Bosutinib Ponatinib Pazopanib Crizotinib		Bortezomib Carlfizomib	IL-2 IFN-g	
VTE/DVT	Bevacizumab	Dasatinib Ponatinib Pazopanib Crizotinib			Thalidomide Lenolidomide	Palbociclib
Pleural Disease						
Pleural Effusion	Panitumumab	Imatinib Dasatinib Bosutinib			IL-2 IFN-g	
Pleural thickening						
Other						
Opportunistic Infections	Ofatumumab Ibritumomab	Idelalisib Trametinib Crizotinib Vemurafenib Ruxolitinib	Everolimus			

sometimes severe adverse reactions. The diagnosis of DILI thus relies on the temporal association between drug exposure and the development of lung injury, the presence of a recognized clinical pattern following exposure to a drug that is a known or suspected culprit, and the exclusion of competing diagnoses.[331–334]

Treatment of DILI requires discontinuation of the drug in most cases. Corticosteroid therapy may ameliorate symptoms in steroid-responsive lung injury patterns, such as hypersensitivity pneumonitis, eosinophilic pneumonia, and BOOP. Signs of severe acute, subacute or progressive pulmonary toxicity (dyspnea at rest, decrease in oxygen saturation below 90 or more than 4% below baseline) are indications for initiation of systemic corticosteroids in patients with steroid-responsive lung disease. Although there are no evidence-based guidelines for corticosteroid therapy in this setting, prednisone or its equivalent, dosed at 40–60 mg daily is generally used, unless the patient is mechanically ventilated. For those patients and patients with impending respiratory failure, intravenous methylprednisolone is preferred. Steroids are typically tapered over a 1–3 month time period, depending on the response to therapy. Any decision to reintroduce the offending agent must be based on the individual drug, the severity of the toxicity reaction, and the availability of alternative therapies. Interstitial edema, owing to injury to the epithelial and endothelial cells, may give way to alveolar edema, diffuse alveolar damage (DAD), and end-stage fibrotic lung as the disease progresses. In some cases, disease progression may continue despite corticosteroid therapy and drug withdrawal.

SPECIFIC CLINICOPATHOLOGIC SYNDROMES

INTERSTITIAL LUNG DISEASE (ILD) Interstitial lung disease is the most common pattern of DILD. Diverse histologic patterns of ILD exists, ranging from nonspecific interstitial pneumonitis (NSIP), hypersensitivity pneumonitis (HP), bronchiolitis obliterans with organizing pneumonia (BOOP), and granulomatous pneumonitis. HP is more appropriately referred to as an allergic or immunologic lung injury, as HP implies injury to the lung only as the result of inhaled organic dusts. Many of the patterns of ILD-related lung injury may progress to potentially life-threatening acute respiratory distress syndrome with its pathologic hallmark, diffuse alveolar damage. The various histopathologic patterns of ILD share many of the same symptoms of dry cough, dyspnea, fatigue, however the onset of symptoms, disease duration, and outcomes vary substantially from one form of ILD to the next. NSIP, the most frequent morphologic pattern of drug-induced IP, typically develops insidiously over hours to days following drug exposure. In chronic forms of ILD, symptoms may occur months to years following drug exposure. CT imaging is far superior to plain films in identifying ILD. Mixed alveolar-interstitial abnormalities on chest imaging studies are the most common radiographic findings, which classically localize to the peripheral and lower lung zones (Figure 18-12). A reduction in DL_{CO} and a restrictive defect on pulmonary function testing are supportive, but nonspecific findings.

The list of chemotherapeutic agents implicated in the development of drug-induced ILD is extensive

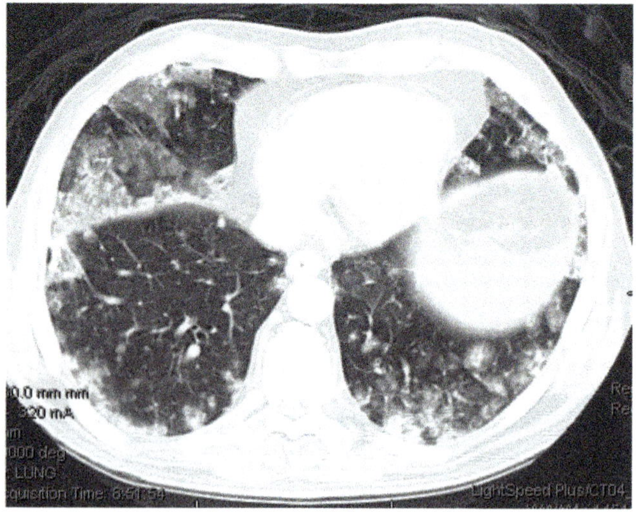

FIGURE 18-12 Gemcitabine-related lung toxicity. A 50-year-old man developed severe shortness of breath 11 days after completing his first cycle of gemcitabine for pancreatic carcinoma. Bronchoscopically obtained lung specimens were negative for malignancy and microbial pathogens. Lung biopsies suggested NSIP.

and includes most classes of the conventional chemotherapeutic agents, the molecular targeted therapies, biologic immunotherapy agents and the immune checkpoint inhibitor therapies.[335–348] The features of ILD may differ with each drug. Thus, a working knowledge of the characteristics of chemotherapy-related ILD is critical to improving outcomes. Several of these agents are discussed below.

Bleomycin is a key component in anticancer regimens that are frequently used in the treatment of many potentially curable cancers, including testicular germ-cell tumors and Hodgkin lymphoma (HL). Lung injury is the most frequent adverse effect of bleomycin toxicity, occurring with varying severity in 20%–46% of bleomycin-treated patients. The associated mortality rate of 1%–4% is felt to be unacceptably high, particularly in the setting of patients with curable cancers. Cytokine activation and free radical formation is thought to underlie the development of bleomycin-related lung toxicity. The bleomycin catalyzing enzyme, bleomycin hydrolase, is absent in lung and skin tissue, rendering these organs vulnerable to injury. Patterns of lung injury include acute allergic pneumonitis with peripheral eosinophilia resembling eosinophilic pneumonia, BOOP, acute chest pain syndrome, and PH associated with PVOD. Dose-dependent bleomycin interstitial pneumonitis (BIP) with progressive pulmonary fibrosis represent the most serious of bleomycin-related lung injury patterns.[349–351] The onset of BIP is typically signaled by dry cough and exertional dyspnea, which typically occur 4–10 weeks after bleomycin administration and may evolve over weeks to months. Bibasilar ground glass opacities are early findings on CT, which may give way to linear and subpleural nodular lesions as the disease progresses. Concomitant or sequential exposure to radiation or oxygen synergistically predisposes bleomycin-treated patients to severe lung injury. Bleomycin is a known radiosensitizing agent. This property potentiates the toxic effects of radiation on the lung, resulting in generalized pulmonary fibrotic reactions that may extend well outside of the radiation field.[352–356] The sequence of bleomycin-radiation combinations does not appear to influence the subsequent development of lung injury. The optimal interval between these two therapies that mitigate toxicity has not been established. Excess lung injury among patients treated with radiation therapy within a year of prior bleomycin exposure is well described in the literature.[353,356] Exposure to high inspired oxygen concentrations is also considered to be a risk factor for severe lung injury in bleomycin-treated patients.[357–361] Severe and sometimes fatal acute lung injury owing to bleomycin-oxygen synergism has been reported. Clinical symptoms of pneumonitis and respiratory failure precipitated by ARDS may occur as early as 18 hours after oxygen exposure in bleomycin-treated patients. Restriction of supplemental oxygen levels to <25% FIO_2 and postponing elective surgeries requiring general anesthesia and high inspired oxygen levels by > 3 months in bleomycin-exposed patients greatly decreased postoperative morbidity and mortality in one study.[362] However, the threshold dose and duration of supplemental oxygen as well as the interval between bleomycin and oxygen exposure that confer an increased risk of lung damage remains uncertain. In general, high oxygen exposures within the prior 6 months of bleomycin therapy are thought carry an increased risk of lung injury. Although the potentiation of lung toxicity by high inspired oxygen following bleomycin exposure has been inculpated in animal models, this association has been debated. Furthermore, the at risk interval following bleomycin exposure which confers increased susceptibility to pneumotoxicity has not been established. These unresolved issues pose particular problems for bleomycin-treated patients undergoing surgical procedures with general anesthesia and the intensivist caring for bleomycin-treated patients on mechanical ventilation. The risk of BIP with fibrosis exists for all dosage levels of bleomycin, but increases precipitously from 3%–5% with cumulative doses below 450 U to 17% when cumulative doses of the drug exceed 500 U.[363,364] Age greater than 70 years, bolus and intravenous routes of administration, multi-agent therapy, and uremia are other associated risk factors[356,365–368] Brentuximab vedotin, a CD30 targeted antibody-drug conjugate, has received recent FDA approval in the management of patients with refractory HL. Severe and sometimes fatale BIP has been observed when brentuximab is given in combination with bleomycin-based therapies.[369] Spontaneous reversal of clinical and laboratory abnormalities following bleomycin withdrawal is common with milder forms of BIP. Hemodynamic instability associated with PH may develop with disease progression, leading to ventilatory failure, cardiovascular collapse and death. The utility of steroid therapy in the management of advanced disease has not been proven.

ILD may also occur as a form of immune-mediated lung injury following immune checkpoint inhibitor therapy, including the cytotoxic T-lymphocyte antigen-4 (CTLA-4) inhibitor, and the programmed cell death-1 (PD-1) inhibitors (Figure 18-13). Rapidly fatal lung injury following immune checkpoint inhibition has been described. As with other forms of DILI, the clinical presentation may be nonspecific, and, thus urgent evaluation with pulmonary function tests, CT imaging of the chest, and bronchoscopy to exclude competing diagnoses is warranted.

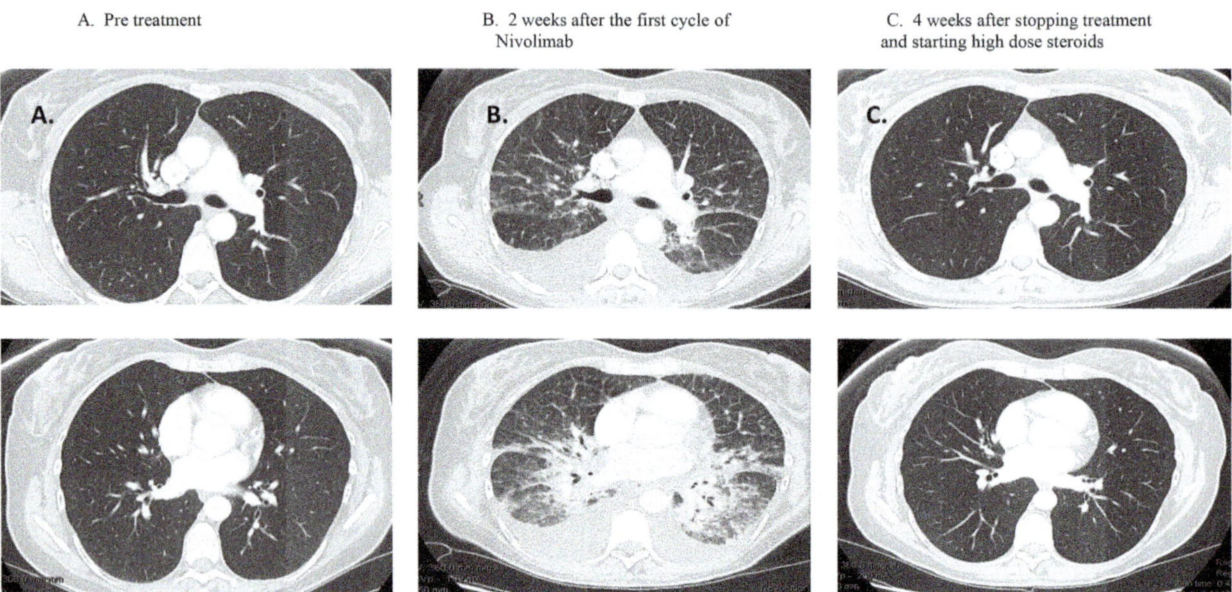

FIGURE 18-13 Nivolumab toxicity. A 45-year-old woman who developed severe dyspnea and cough 2 weeks after completing the first cycle of combination nivolumab therapy for metastatic melanoma. (A) Baseline chest radiograph is clear. (B) Two weeks after completing first cycle of therapy a CT of the chest demonstrated bilateral areas of consolidation and ground glass changes with bilateral small effusions. (C) Symptoms and radiographic changes resolved with discontinuation of nivolumab and ipilimumab and high dose steroid therapy.

■ Hypersensitivity-Like Reactions and Eosinophilic Lung Disease

Hypersensitivity-like reactions in the lung resembling hypersensitivity pneumonitis have been described following treatment with numerous chemotherapeutic agents. The drugs that have been most frequently implicated include methotrexate, bleomycin, etoposide, teniposide, and the taxane agents.[336,366,370–374] Patients typically present with fever, dyspnea, dry cough and BAL lymphocytosis following repeated exposure to the offending drug. The disease may appear as an acute, subacute, or chronic illness. Overall, the prognosis for patients with early stage disease is very favorable. Complete resolution of symptoms and radiographic findings is expected following steroid therapy and cessation of antigen exposure. Rarely, patients may develop chronic HP, which is usually progressive and irreversible. PH and cor pulmonale may develop as a result of end-stage, fibrotic lung disease.

Eosinophilic pneumonia following therapy with fludarabine, interleukin-2, methotrexate, bleomycin, procarbazine, and more recently, oxaloplatin is well documented.[375–378] Elevated eosinophils in peripheral blood and BAL fluid along with upper lobe-predominant homogeneous opacities are clues to the diagnosis (Figure 18-14). Drug withdrawal and initiation of high dose steroids typically yield favorable outcomes, although rapid progression to respiratory failure has been described.

■ Pleural Disease

Pleuroparenchymal reactions are most often described following treatment with methotrexate, docetaxel, gemcitabine, azathioprine, mitomycin, interleukin-2, ATRA, dasatanib, and interferon-γ. Pleural disease may manifest as isolated pleural effusions, but more often presents as a generalized pulmonary reaction that includes pulmonary infiltrates and effusions.[379] Cardiotoxicity with associated heart failure and pleural effusions is well described following anthrachycline- and nonanthracycline-based conventional chemotherapeutics and is an emerging concern following administration of the molecularly targeted therapies, particularly those that target the vascular-endothelial growth factor receptor (VEGF).[380,381] Pleural thickening may accompany pulmonary fibrosis as a late manifestation of cyclophosphamide, BCNU, or bleomycin toxicity.

■ Alveolar Lung Disease: Noncardiogenic Pulmonary Edema

Noncardiogenic pulmonary edema (NCPE) is an under-recognized and potentially fatal syndrome of anticancer therapy. Subacute symptoms of dry cough, tachypnea, fatigue, dyspnea and chest discomfort typically develop insidiously within hours or a few days of drug exposure. Patients may be markedly hypoxemic at presentation. The radiographic appearance of NCPE is similar to other causes of pulmonary edema,

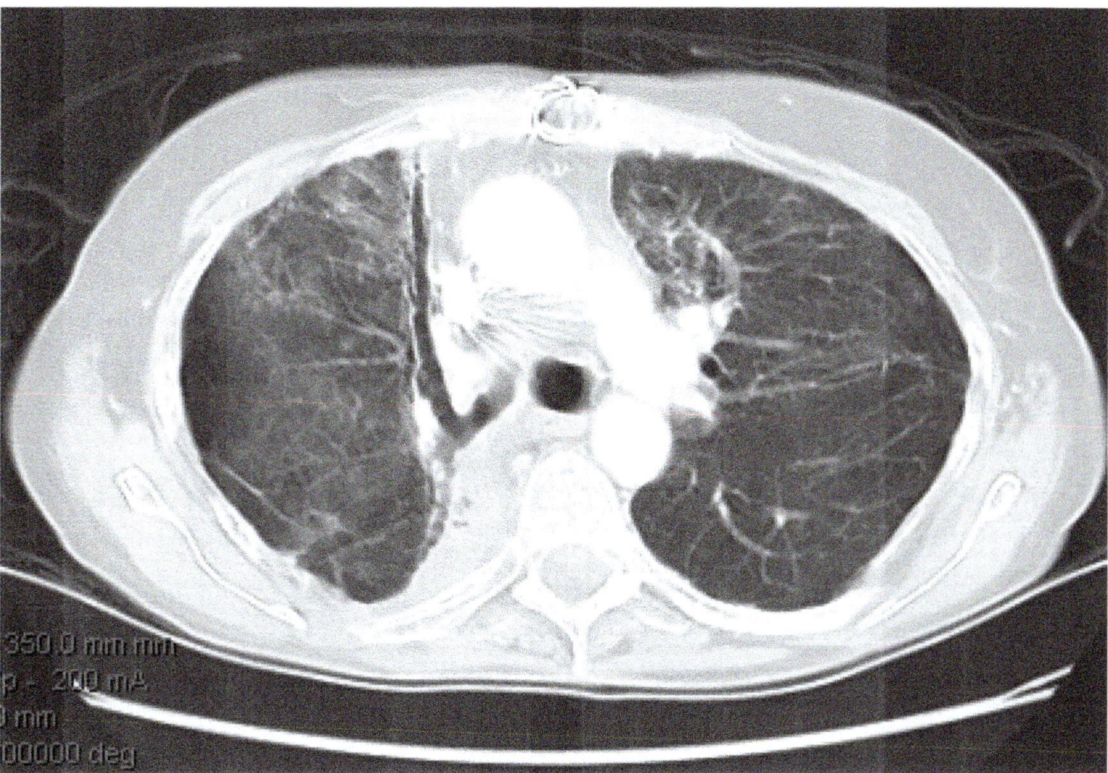

FIGURE 18-14   Methotrexate-related eosinophilic pneumonia. A 48-year-old woman presented 2 weeks after initiating methotrexate-based therapy for treatment of sarcoma with dry cough and severe shortness of breath. Work-up identified upper lobe predominant infiltrates with significant peripheral and BAL eosinophilia, consistent with methotrexate-related eosinophilic pneumonia. Symptoms improved with drug withdrawal and chronic steroid therapy. RUL volume loss and radiation scarring is noted, consistent with the patient's prior history of radiation therapy.

although the absence of cardiomegaly, pulmonary vascular redistribution and Kerley B lines on chest radiographs favors a noncardiogenic etiology. Drug-induced NCPE often occurs as an idiosyncratic reaction, independent of drug dosage or duration of therapy. Mild and self-limited reactions are common, although progression to ARDS with fatal outcomes occasionally occur. Cancer therapeutic agents that are recognized triggers of NCPE include the antimetabolites (Ara-C, gemcitabine, methotrexate), docetaxel, all-trans retinoic acid (ATRA) and the biologic response modifiers (interleukin-2, tumor necrosis factor) are frequently implicated in the development of drug-induced NCPE. NCPE is also recognized during therapy with some of the monoclonal antibodies, notably denileukin difitox and imatinib mesylate administration.[382,383] Injury to the pulmonary endothelial cells with associated pulmonary capillary leak is the postulated mechanism of drug-related NCPE. Underlying cardiac disease, when present, increases the risk of drug-induced NCPE and confounds the diagnosis. Treatment is supportive with supplemental oxygen, diuretics, positive end-expiratory pressure, and occasionally mechanical ventilation. Recovery is typically rapid following drug withdrawal. A role for steroids in the treatment of drug-related NCPE is uncertain. Symptom recurrence often develops following rechallenge with the offending drug. Pulmonary edema associated with cytokine release syndrome (CRS) is a potentially severe complication of T-cell activation produced by T-cell engaging immunotherapies, such as bi-specific T-cell engagers (BiTEs) and chimeric antigen receptor-modified T cells (CART).[384,385]

■ Pulmonary Vascular Disorders (PVD): Thromboembolic Disease, Pulmonary Hypertension, Pulmonary Veno-Occlusive Disease

The lungs receive virtually all of the cardiac output, which it distributes to the alveolar surface for gas exchange via an extensive vascular network. This expansive vascular surface area renders the lungs vulnerable to injury by blood-borne drugs. Blood flow through the lungs depends on a balance between intravascular volume and microvascular hydrostatic pressures. Drugs that impair left ventricular function, leading to increased left sided pressures or, alternatively, cause an increase in microvascular pressures or expansion of intravascular volume may result in excessive fluid leakage into the pulmonary interstitium. Other potential mechanisms of drug-induced vascular injury include vascular occlusion/spasm, increased permeability due to direct or indirect toxicity to the vascular endothelium, and immunologic mechanisms.

The major clinical manifestations of pulmonary vascular injury include PH, hemorrhage, and acute pulmonary edema. PH may occur as a consequence of direct vascular injury or, alternatively, as an indirect result of an embolic event. An example of pulmonary hypertension caused by direct vascular injury is PVOD), a process characterized by fibrous obliteration of pulmonary venules and small pulmonary veins (see below). PVOD is probably more common following chemotherapy than published reports indicate. The most incriminating data implicates bleomycin, BCNU in PVOD-related disease. An association with chest irradiation and other drugs, including mitomycin and bleomycin have also been suggested.[248,249,251–254,386–392] PVOD following bleomycin therapy is felt to be due to drug-induced endovascular damage and may result in severe pulmonary hypertension and cor pulmonale. This vascular lesion typically occurs in association with bleomycin-induced parenchymal lung disease, but may also occur as an isolated finding. The prognosis is poor. Most diagnoses are made at necropsy.[387,393] Emerging data suggests an association between the use of the cytotokine chemotherapeutic agents, IL-2 and interferon-γ, and the development of PAH.[394,395] These immunomodulatory agents may cause transient but substantial elevations in pulmonary artery pressures and right heart failure by stimulating the thromboxane cascade. Two tyrosine kinase inhibitors that target Bcr-Abl, dasatinib, and more recently, bosutinib, have been strongly implicated in the development of PAH. PAH has been reported in up to 10% of patients following dasatinib therapy. Pulmonary capillary wedge pressers (PCWP) are normal, thus establishing the diagnosis of precapillary pulmonary hypertension. Patients may present with severe PAH with associated cor pulmonale 8–48 months after initiation of one of these agents. Clinical and hemodynamic improvements following drug discontinuation are a unique feature of this form of PAH, however, pulmonary pressures may not fully normalize in up to 50% of patients following cessation of therapy. The efficacy of PAH-specific therapies has not been studied in any large randomized trials. Patients with dasatinib- or bosutinib-related PAH have been successfully treated with other Bcr-Abl inhibitors such nilotinib without recrudescence of PAH (Table 18-7).[396–399]

Vascular wall hypertrophy due to direct endothelial toxicity has been reported following Zinostatin therapy.[400] Indirect vascular injury caused by thrombosis is well documented following several chemotherapeutic agents, including tamoxifen, thalidomide, and its analog, lenalidomide.[401–403] Tamoxifen decreases protein C and antithrombin III levels.[404] The risk of thrombosis is enhanced 3-fold when this agent is given in combination with other chemotherapeutic drugs, such as cyclophosphamide, methotrexate and 5-flurouracil.[405,406] Thalidomide-based chemotherapy, given in combination with steroids, doxorubicin or BCNU confers a 14%–43% increase risk of thromboembolic phenomenon.[407–409] Increased rates of venous thromboembolism have also been associated with EGFR targeted therapies, such as panitumumab (see Figure 18-5), cetuximab, erlotinib, and vandetanib and the anti-lymphocyte kinase inhibitor, crizotinib.[410] Excess rates of arterial and venous thrombosis have been associated with anti-angiogenic therapies that target vascular endothelial growth factor, such as bevacizumab, pazopanib, axitinib, levantinib, and sunitinib.[411,412] Nilotinib and ponatinib are two BCR/ABL-targeted drugs primarily used in the treatment of CML and other Ph+ chromosome leukemias. Both agents have been associated with severe and progressive arterial occlusive disease (PAOD). One unique feature of vasculopathy associated with these agents is the persistence and progression of disease despite discontinuation of the drug. Peripheral vascular disease, cerebral ischemia, myocardial infarction and PH are prominent clinical features of this disease. Risk factors for PAOD are similar to those for the development of atherosclerotic disease. Thus, risk stratification strategies for cardiovascular disease is applicable for patients being considered for nilotinib- or ponatinib-based therapies. Standard cardiovascular treatment guidelines, including the use of statins and aspirin for patients who are at risk for cardiovascular disease are recommended, although there is no evidence of risk PAOD risk reduction in patients treated with one of these drugs.[413,414] Other agents, including the cyclin dependent kinase inhibitor palbociclib, are also associated with the development of pulmonary thromboembolism.[415]

■ Airway Disease: Bronchospasm/ Anaphylaxis

Chemotherapy-related bronchospasm has been described following the administration of taxanes (paclitaxel), platinum compounds (cisplatin, carboplatin, oxaliplatin), podophyllotoxins (teniposide, etoposide), asparaginase, procarbazine and, occasionally, doxorubicin and 6-mercaptopurine. Almost all epi-

TABLE 18-7   Adverse vascular events associated with molecular targeted therapies

AGENT	AGENT CLASS	MAJOR MOLECULAR TARGET(S)	VASCULAR ADVERSE EVENTS								
			NCPE	DVT/PE	PAOD	PTH	Systemic HTN	CP	MI	CHF	Other
Erlotinib*	TKI	**EGFR (HER-1)**		4%				12%	1%–2%		Increased Qtc-9%;
Vandetanib	TKI	**EGFR**, FLT-4, RET, KDR					33% (9%–10% grade 3–4)				CVA/ TIA-1%
Lapatanib	TKII	**HER2, EGFR**								1-2%	Increased Qtc-16%
Cetuximab	MoAb	**EGFR**									Increased Qtc
Panitumumab	MoAB	**EGFR**									Increased Qtc
Trastuzumab	MoAb	**EGFR, Her2/neu**						Monotherapy- 2%–7%; in combination with paclitaxel – 2%–13%; in combination with anthracyclines or cyclophosphamide 27%			
Sorafenib	TKI	**VEGF**, B-Raf, FLT-1-4, PDGFR, KIT, KDR, FGR					9%–41% (10% grade 3–4)	3%	1%	2%	
Sunitinib	TKI	**VEGF**, ABL-1, c-Kit, SRC, FLT-3,4, PDGFR, KIT, KDR, FGFR, c-smc		3%			27%–34% (10% grade 3–4)	13%	11%	4%–8%	
Pazopanib	TKI	**VEGF**, , ABL-1, c-Kit, FLT1,4, PDGFR-A,B, KDR, FGFR, c-fms		1-5%			40% (7% grade 3–4)	5%–10%	2%	11%	Increased Qtc-2%; Bradycardia 3%–19%

(continued)

TABLE 18-7 Adverse vascular events associated with molecular targeted therapies (*continued*)

AGENT	AGENT CLASS	MAJOR MOLECULAR TARGET(S)	VASCULAR ADVERSE EVENTS								
Axitinib	TKI	**VEGF,** c-Kit, FLT-1,4 PDGFR-A,B, KDR		1%–3%			40% (16% grade 3–4)	2%	1%		
Lenvatinib	TKII	**VEGF,** c-Kit, FLT-1,4 PDGFR-B, KDR, RET		3%			73%(44% grade 3–4)			2%–6%	Increased Qtc-9%;
Bevacizumab	MoAb	**VEGF**		3%–5%			4%–35%	xx	0.6—1.5%		CVA
Ramucirumab	MoAb	**VEGFR-2**					4%	7%–11%			
Imatinib	TKI	**ABL-1,** c-Kit, FLT-3, PDGFR-A,B					10%				
Dasatinib	TKI	**ABL-1,** PDGFR-A,B, KIT, FGFR2, SRC							4%		
Nilotinib	TKI	**ABL-1,** c-Kit, FLT-3, PDGFR-A,B			3%–4%	3%–4%	10%–11%	5%–9%	5%–9%		CVA/ TIA-1%–3%
Ponatinib	TKI	**ABL-1,** c-Kit, FLT-1,3,4, FDGR, PDGFR, KDR, SRC,TIE2		5%	8%	8%	53%–71%	2%	12%		
Bosutinib	TKI	**ABL-1,** FLT-1,2,3, FDGR, PDGFR-A,B, KDR, SRC									
Crizotinib	TKI	**ALK,** MET, Rosi	31%–49%	6%						2%	Increased Qtc-2%; Bradycardia 3%–19%

sodes have been associated with parenteral administration of these agents. Bronchospasm following paclitaxel and teniposide administration is thought to be due to a type 1-hypersensitivity reaction associated with mast cell degranulation.[416,417] Prophylaxis with histamine receptor antagonists and steroids prior to administration of taxane agents is now standard and has reduced the incidence of paclitaxel-induced bronchospasm from 30% to 2%.[416] In other cases, the mechanism of bronchospasm is unknown, but may result from a non-immune mediated release of histamine or cytokines. Bronchospasm typically occurs in conjunction with other symptoms, including flushing, alterations in heart rate and blood pressure, dyspnea, fever, pruritus, nausea, and occasionally rash. Severe, and occasionally life-threatening infusion reactions have been reported during intravenous infusion of monoclonal antibodies such as retuximab, transtuzumab, alemtuzumab, cetuximab, and gemtuzumab. Infusion-related anaphylactoid reactions have been described which warrant discontinuation of the drug. Finally, combination therapy with concurrent or sequential vinorelbine (or other vinca alkyloids) and mitomycin chemotherapy may rarely precipitate acute lung reactions characterized by cough, bronchospasm, flushing, dyspnea, abdominal pain, and hypotension. Airway symptoms typically improve with drug withdrawal and supportive therapy, such as supplemental oxygen, antihistamines, steroids, and nebulized β2-agonists. In selected cases, prophylaxis with steroids and antihistamines may permit successful rechallenge.

Broncholitis Obliterans with Organizing Pneumonia (BOOP) BOOP may complicate drug therapy as well as several cancer- and noncancer-related disorders, including infection, connective tissue diseases, and lung or stem cell transplantation. Among the chemotherapeutic agents associated with this type of lung injury, bleomycin, cyclophosphamide, doxorubicin, methotrexate, busulfan, mitomycin-C rituximab, oxaliplatin, and the interferons have been most frequently reported.[418–423] Patients may present 4–8 weeks following therapy with diffuse infiltrative opacities and often migratory pulmonary opacities on imaging studies. The response to steroid therapy is generally favorable; however, rapid steroid withdrawal may precipitate relapse.

OTHER FORMS OF DILD

An acute chest pain syndrome has been described during bleomycin infusion. This rare, self-limited disorder is characterized by substernal chest pressure that mimics myocardial infarction, although electrocardiographic and serologic evidence of myocardial injury are usually absent.[51] Symptom control is usually achieved with analgesics and may not recur with repeat administration of the drug. The etiology of bleomycin-related acute chest pain syndrome is unclear. Coronary artery vasospasm associated with bleomycin-related Reynaud's has been proposed, but remains unproven.[424] Acute myocardial infarction is a rare, but well described complication of two chemotherapy regimens PEB (cisplatin, etoposide, bleomycin) and PVB (cisplatin, vincristine, bleomycin).[425,426] Cisplatin-induced hypomagnesemia and direct endothelial damage is thought to play a major role in these events with the role of bleomycin being less clear.

■ Radiation-Induced Lung Injury

Clinically significant lung toxicity occurs in 5%–20% of patients following thoracic radiation. Lung injury has been reported following radiation treatment of primary as well as metastatic lesions in the thorax. Classic radiation pneumonitis (RP) represents an early manifestation of radiation-related lung toxicity, which typically develops insidiously over the initial 1 to 3 months and peaks at 3–4 months after radiotherapy. Radiation fibrosis (RF) appears later, usually at 6 months following thoracic irradiation and stabilizes over the ensuing year (Figure 18-15). These reactions are usually predictable, dose-dependent, and confined to the irradiated field. Fever, dyspnea, chest pain, and nonproductive cough, coupled with measurable changes in pulmonary function tests, including a reduction in lung volumes and transfer factor (DLCO), may be seen as early as 2–3 months after irradiation. These clinical manifestations vary with the volume of lung injured, the degree of preexisting lung injury and underlying pulmonary reserve. Hypoxic respiratory failure leading to fatal cardiopulmonary collapse has been reported in up to 8% of patients following thoracic radiation.[427,428] Radiographically, RP is signaled by the development diffuse haze and patchy areas of consolidation with or without air-bronchograms that coalesce over time to conform to the treatment portals. Later as RF develops, these changes give way to well-demarcated areas of volume loss, linear densities, bronchiectasis, retraction of the lung parenchyma, tenting and elevation of the hemidiaphragm, and ipsilateral pleural thickening. Ipsilateral pneumothorax and, occasionally, small pleural effusions also occur as late findings.

Other forms of radiation lung injury, including sporadic pneumonitis (SP) and radiation recall pneumonitis (RRP) are also recognized. SP occurs in approximately 5% of patients following radiation therapy and is thought to represent a type of hypersensitivity pneumonitis. Unlike classic radiation pneumonitis, SP is associated with diffuse involvement of both lung fields caused by a bilateral CD_4+

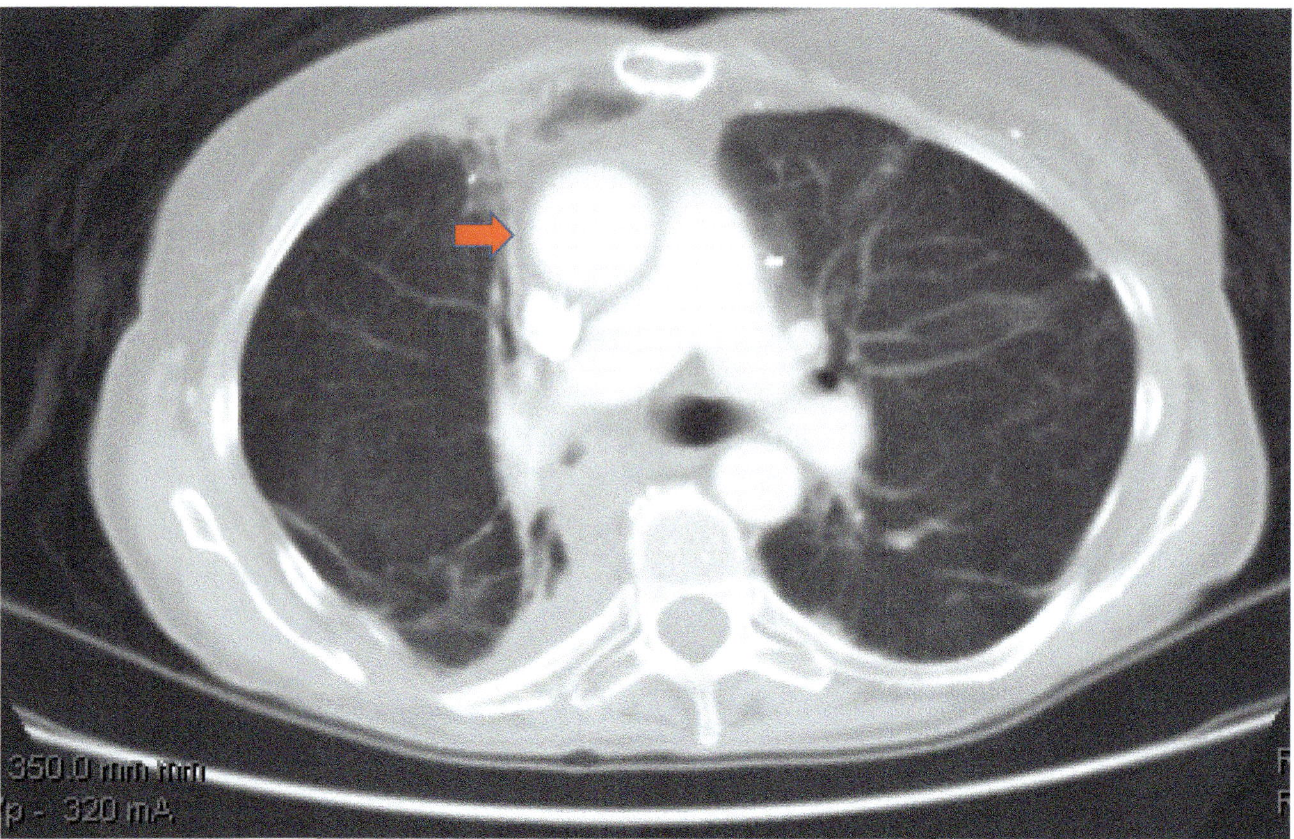

FIGURE 18-15 Radiation fibrosis. A 46-year-old man. CT scan performed 13 months following completion of chemoradiation therapy of sarcoma shows volume loss with bronchiectatic changes. The radiation fibrosis conforms to the straight-edged border that outlines the prior radiation port (arrow).

T-lymphocytic alveolitis. Symptoms of dyspnea and dry cough are disproportionate to the volume of lung irradiated and typically occur at 1–2 months following thoracic irradiation. Resolution of symptoms and radiographic changes is common, usually in 6–8 weeks, without any long-term sequelae.[429–431] Lung injury in RRP is characterized by the development of an acute inflammatory reaction within a previously irradiated area of pulmonary tissue shortly after application of certain chemotherapeutic agents. The drugs that are most often implicated in this reaction include the antracyclines, taxanes tamoxifen, gemcitabine, and erlotinib.[432–434] Withdrawal of the precipitating agent is recommended. The clinical utility of systemic corticosteroid therapy in this setting is unclear. Other rare, but serious complications of radiation-induced lung injury have been described, including PVOD, BOOP, and eosinophilic pneumonia (EP).[435,436] BOOP and EP have been reported following breast radiation. Both entities are characterized by migratory pulmonary infiltrates that may involve nonirradiated areas of the lung which typically develop 1–3 months after radiotherapy.

Modification of risk factors, such as total dose, dose per fraction of radiation, and the volume of lung irradiated, may mitigate the severity of radiation-induced lung injury. Preexisting lung disease, underlying pulmonary reserve, prior radiation therapy, as well as physical characteristics of the irradiation and beam arrangements may also influence the rate and severity of radiation-induced lung toxicity.[437] Total radiation doses that exceed 4000 cGy are almost always associated with radiographic evidence of lung injury.[438] In addition to the inherent propensity to produce lung toxicity, multimodality regimens that combine radiation with certain chemotherapeutic agents may potentiate an adverse radiation response in the lungs and shorten the latency period following radiation exposure.[439] These agents, known as radiation sensitizers, include mitomycin, cyclophosphamide, vincristine, adriamycin, bleomycin, gemcitabine, recombinant interferon-α, the taxanes, verafenib, and actinomycin D (Table 18-8).

It is generally agreed that a hyperfractionated course of radiation delivered to the smallest lung volume offers the lowest possibility of lung toxicity.

TABLE 18-8 Radiation sensitizing agents

RADIATION SENSITIZING AGENTS
Taxanes
Mitomycin
Cyclophosphamide
Vincristine
Adriamycin,
Bleomycin,
Gemcitabine
Interferon a
Taxanes
Verafenib
Actinomycin D

Other radiation strategies that are designed to limit radiation exposure to normal lung, such as conformal therapy and intensity-modulated radiation therapy (IMRT) are increasingly used. Systemic steroids are generally used in the management of symptomatic radiation pneumonitis, although no large body of data detailing the efficacy of corticosteroids in this setting is currently available and guidelines for steroid administration have not been firmly established. Prednisone dosed at 0.5–1 mg/kg of body weight is a reasonable starting dose in most patients, which may be tapered according to clinical response over the ensuing weeks. The late phase of pneumonitis may be refractory to even high dose steroids. No effective strategies for intervening in the late (fibrotic) phase of radiation lung injury have reported.

Cardiac impairment may also occur as a consequence of the effect of radiation on neighboring tissues, including the heart, pericardium, and large vessels. Pericarditis, coronary artery disease, cardiomyopathy, valvular heart disease, and conduction abnormalities may occur years after radiation therapy to the thorax. In a recent retrospective study, 29% of lung cancer patients with central tumors in which the heart was included in the radiation field developed cardiac complications, detected by myocardial perfusion imaging.[440] A prior history of congestive heart failure and/or conduction abnormalities were significantly associated with radiation-related cardiac abnormalities. The predominant cardiac complications included silent ischemia, arrhythmias, and pericardial effusions. Although this study was not sufficiently powered to determine if silent ischemia detected on myocardial perfusion imaging was predictive of subsequent cardiovascular ischemic events, other studies have clearly shown a significant increased risk of cardiac events, including myocardial infarction and congestive heart failure, years after thoracic radiation exposure.[441–443]

Congestive heart failure and/or a prior history of conduction abnormalities were significantly associated with future cardiac morbidity after radiation therapy. Multimodality therapy with thoracic radiation and anthracycline- or transtuzumab-based chemotherapy may also increase the risk of cardiotoxicity.[444–446] Cardiac volume sparing using conformal and IMRT radiation strategies, careful 3-dimensional treatment planning, and breath-holding techniques has been shown to reduce the volume of cardiac irradiation.[447,448] Physicians taking care of cancer patients treated with thoracic radiation must be aware of the potential direct and indirect adverse consequences of radiation therapy on the heart. Careful selection and close cardiac monitoring of patients with risk factors for cardiac injury following thoracic radiation is recommended.

LUNG INFECTIONS AND HEART-LUNG INTERACTIONS

Infections are common sequelae of aggressive immunosuppressive chemotherapy regimens. Among infections in this setting, pneumonias are the predominant presentation. The prevalence of pneumonias, including fatal pneumonias, has escalated as more aggressive cancer treatment protocols have been implemented. Adverse cardiac events, such as myocardial infarction, arrhythmias, and heart failure are major contributing factors to morbidity and mortality during hospitalization of the immunocompromised and the elderly patient for pneumonia. Among patients hospitalized for pneumonia, new or worsening heart failure has been reported in 10%–33%, arrhythmias in 6%–11%, and acute coronary syndrome in 5%–11%.[449] Conversely, among hospitalized patients admitted for atrial tachyarrythmias, pneumonia (7%) was second only to congestive heart failure (13%) as leading comorbid diagnoses.[450]

Pneumonia may trigger cardiac disease through direct and indirect pathophysiologic mechanisms. Acute inflammation associated with pneumonia may precipitate incident heart failure directly by acting as a myocardial depressant and by increasing left ventricular afterload and oxygen consumption. Pneumonia-related hypoxemia and tachycardia are associated with increased pulmonary arterial pressure, right ventricular afterload, and myocardial oxygen demand, which ultimately lead to shifts in the balance of myocardial metabolic supply and demand and compromised myocardial function.[449,451,452] Acute coronary syndrome in the setting of pneumonia may be triggered by hypoxia, increased sympathetic activity with associated alterations in circulatory volume and coronary vascular tone, and plaque rupture owing to increased inflammatory cytokines and destabilization of atherosclerotic plaques. These increased metabolic demands are particularly relevant among patients with preexisting heart failure and subclinical coronary artery disease, where myocardial infarction associated with demand ischemia may occur. Severe pneumonia, hyperlipidemia, hypoalbuminemia, older age, and renal disease, are recognized risk factors for cardiac disease among hospitalized patients with lung infection.[453,454] The recent recognition of cardiovascular disease as a significant component of morbidity and mortality in patients hospitalized for pneumonia has raised concerns regarding the need to broaden therapeutic strategies to include cardioprotective treatments, particularly in the elderly. Whether these treatment strategies would be effective in reducing the overall mortality of patients hospitalized for pneumonia has not been definitively studied.

Infections within the lung may disseminate to other organ systems, including the brain and heart. Cardiac involvement by lung infections is poorly characterized, in part owing to the fact that the diagnosis of many cardiac infections, including *Aspergillus* species and *Cytomegalovirus* are difficult to establish. Successful identification of underlying cardiac infections is confounded by the often indistinct interface between true cardiac pathogens and microorganisms that are usually considered to be contaminants, such as coagulase negative Staphylococci, a variety of fungi, and certain mycobacterial species. Moreover, many of these pathogens fail to elicit a significant inflammatory response, especially in the neutropenic patient. Thus, early signs and symptoms of cardiac infection may be muted. Simultaneous involvement of the lungs and other organ systems by infection and the development of co-morbid illnesses that mimic cardiac disease further confound the problem.

The most widely distributed cardiac infections among immunosuppressed patients are infections caused by viruses and toxoplasma, with bacterial and fungal pathogens occurring less frequently (Table 18-9). Specific cardiac structures appear to be differentially targeted, depending on the particular organism. For example, mycobacterial species, toxoplasma, and certain viral infections exhibit a tropism for the myocardium and pericardium. These organisms typically cause pericarditis with associated pericardial effusions. Bacterial and fungal pathogens may also involve the pericardium and tend to involve cardiac valvular structures rather than the heart muscles (Figure 18-16). An exception to this general rule is *Mycobacterium tuberculosis*, which has a propensity to affect the pericardium, leading to often hemorrhagic pericardial effusions and constrictive pericarditis.

Among the various immunosuppressed states associated with cardiac infections, HIV-related cardiac disease has been the most extensively studied. Rates of cardiac disease are more than 10-fold higher among patients with a clinical diagnosis of HIV-AIDS compared to the HIV-seropositive, non-AIDS patient.[455] HIV most commonly involves the pericardium, resulting pericarditis with associated pericardial effusion. HIV-related myocarditis has also been reported, occurring in approximately 1/3 of patients. Patients with low CD4 counts and/or end-stage disease are particularly susceptible to HIV-related pericardial and myocardial invasion by opportunistic infections, such as *Toxoplasma gondii*, *Cytomegalovirus (CMV)*, and *Herpes Simplex virus (HSV)*. These pathogens may initially manifest as a primary lung infection with subsequent extrapulmonary spread of disease. Bacteremic spread of disease has also been documented. Many of these lung pathogens also occur in the non-HIV setting as a sequela of hematopoietic stem cell transplantation (HSCT) or in association with various lymphoproliferative disorders, including lymphoma and chronic lymphocytic leukemia.

T. gondii, usually occurs as a late sequela of HSCT.[456–458] Patients typically present between the second and sixth month following stem cell transplantation with respiratory failure caused by bilateral interstitial pneumonitis. Risk factors include pretransplant toxoplasma seropositivity, allogeneic transplantation, and the presence of graft-versus-host disease (GVHD). Dissemination to other organ systems, including the brain and heart is common. Myocardial involvement occurs in nearly 70% of patients with disseminated toxoplasmosis, which may be signaled by the development of congestive heart failure or new onset bundle branch block. Central nervous system dissemination, manifested clinically as encephalitis with altered mental status and seizures, is a universal finding among AIDS patients with cardiac involvement. Focal areas of necrosis with collections of lymphocytes, plasma cells and histiocytes are seen on histologic examination of myocardial tissue. A paucity of inflammatory cells coupled with the presence of tissue eosinophils offers further clues to the diagnosis. The diagnosis is established by identification of tachyzoites or cysts in tissue smears. Serologic tests for toxoplasmosis have been unpredictable. Recently, polymerase chain reaction (PCR) amplification of specific T. gondii antigens or DNA sequences in blood, cerebrospinal fluid or bronchoalveolar lavage fluid has proven to be a useful tool in the early diagnosis of infections caused by this organism. Unfortunately, disseminated toxoplasma infection is most often diagnosed at autopsy. Pyrimethemine-sulfadiazine administration

TABLE 18-9   Lung-cardiac pathogens in the immunocompromised host

BACTERIA	COMMENTS
Staphylococcus aureus	Prominent cause of nosocomial endocarditis/pericarditis in transplant patients; significant pathogen in exit site and tunnel infections of central lines
Streptococcus pneumoniae	Prominent cause of nosocomial endocarditis, especially among transplant recipients Invasive pneumococcal infection, chronic steroid use, HIV augment risk
Enterococcus	Prominent cause of nosocomial endocarditis. Associated with right-sided catheter-related endocarditis. Outbreaks may be associated with poor hand washing. Vancomycin resistance a growing problem.
S. Viridans	Severe granulocytopenia and mucositis following transplantation augment risk. Other risk factrs include quinolone antibiotics, cimetidine, and antacid use. Penicillin resistance a growing problem
Listeria monocytogenes	Majority of adult cases (>70%) occur following transplantation amd among patients with HIV or leukemia. May affect both native and prosthetic valves. Mortality rate is 48%.
Gram negative rods	*Gram negative rods*
Nocardia	Endocarditis typically occurs as a complication of AIDS
Mycobacterial species	May cause tunnel infections of central lines. Increased risk among chronically immunosuppressed patients
Fungus	
Candida sp.	Associated with tunnel infections involving long lines/central venous catheters. Blood cultures are positive in 70% of patients.
Aspergillus sp.	May affect both native and prosthetic valves. Aspergillus induced coronary artery thrombosis leads to myocardial necrosis
Mucormycosis	AIDS patients and patients with prothetic valves are at greatest risk. Produces myocardial necrosis in a manner histologically similar to aspergillus endocarditis
Histoplasma capsulatum	Risk stratification is geographically determined. Severe/prolonged immunocompromised states confer highest risk
Virus	
Cytomegalovirus	Most common cause of viral myocarditis/pericarditis among transplanted patients. Other risk factors include hematologic malignancies and AIDS.
Ebstein-Barr virus	May cause life-threatening pneumonia with endocarditis among severely immunocompromised patients. EBV-induced dilated cardiomyopathymay occur early (within 1–3 months) following HSCT. Increased risk among seronegative recipients, active CMV infection, HIV seropositivity. Associated with post-transplant lymphoproliferative disorders
Adenovirus	May cause life-threatening pneumonia with endocarditis among severely immunocompromised patients.
HIV	May cause lymphocitic myocarditis, although role in cardiac infection is not fully defined.
Parasitic	
Toxoplasplasma gondii	May develop as late sequela of HSCT. Pretransplant seropositivity, presence of GVHD, allogeneic transplantation confer highest risk. May appear as widely disseminated and fatal disease

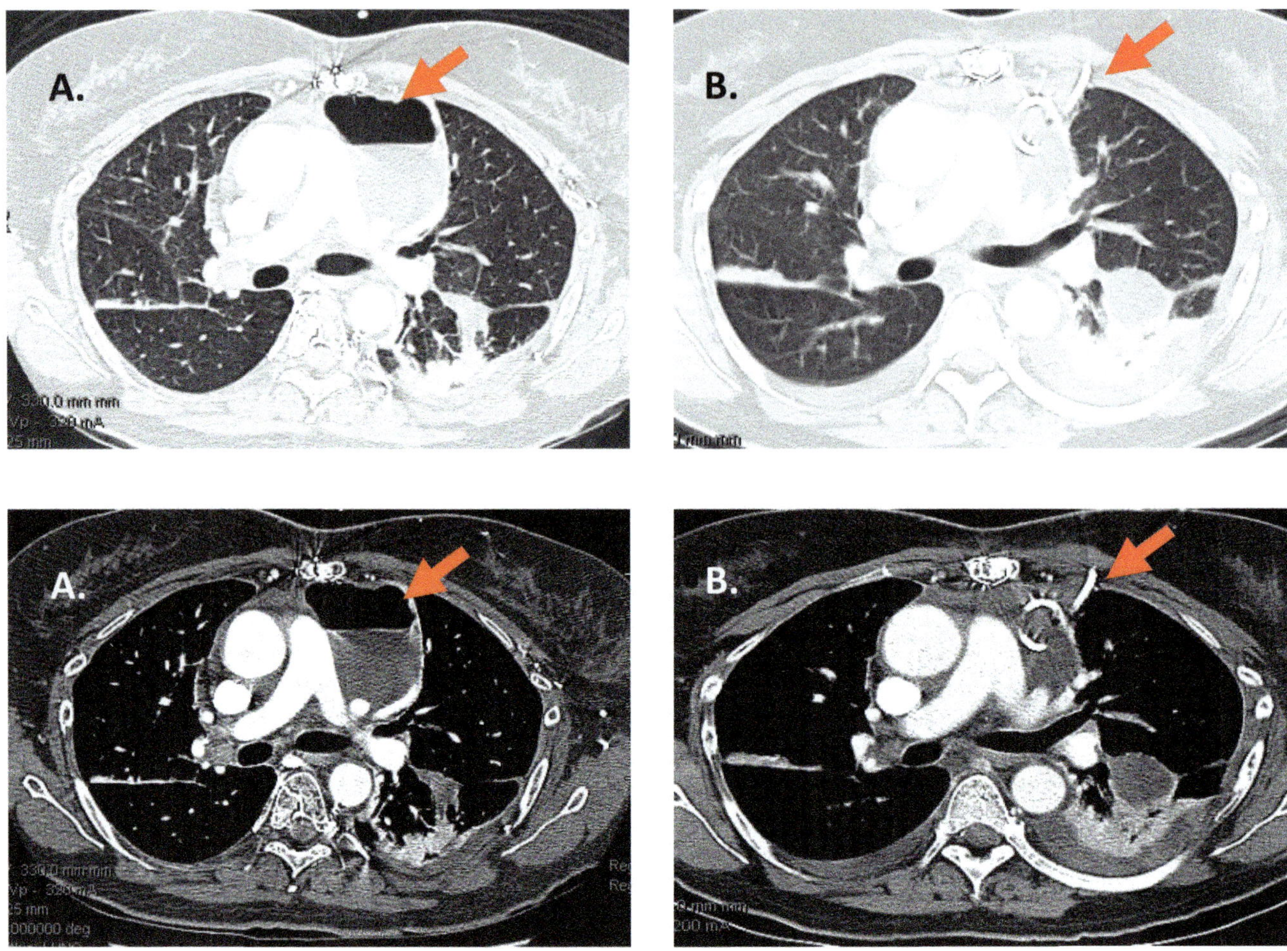

FIGURE 18-16 Pericardial abscess 10 months after surgical resection of a thymoma. The patient presented with a 3 day history of high spiking fevers and anterior substernal chest pain. CT imaging showed a large cavity with air-fluid level in the anterior mediastinum (A). Cultures of abscess grew *Aspergillus fumigates.* The abscess was drained percutaneously (B) and responded to aggressive antifungal therapy. A small left sided parapneumonic effusion with associated atelectasis is also seen.

remains the mainstay of therapy. Atovaquone or pryimethamine-clindamycin combinations are reasonable alternatives for patients who are intolerant of, or have failed first-line therapy.[459,460] The virulence of this pathogen in the setting of the immunocompromised host is underscored by mortality rates exceeding 90%.

Cytomegalovirus, a member of the herpes family of viruses, is an important cause of recalcitrant infections in immunocompromised patients.[461,462] Currently, CMV pneumonitis complicates 12%–20% of HSCT, with the highest period of post-transplant vulnerability occurring within the first 6–12 weeks of hematopoietic stem cell transplants (HSCT).[463,464] Although nosocomial acquisition of CMV disease through the use of infected blood or blood products occasionally occurs, reactivation of latent disease represents the predominant source of CMV infection.[465–467] CMV reactivation is tightly linked to impaired immunity. The

balance of evidence suggests that immune response to CMV is pivotal in limiting dissemination of the virus.[468] Although the virus may target a variety of organ systems, the apparent tropism of CMV for the lung may explain the higher rates of CMV pneumonitis in this group of patients versus other clinical manifestations of the disease. Clinical syndromes attributable to extrapulmonary CMV infection include gastrointestinal ulcerations, leukopenia, atypical lymphocytosis, hepatitis, arthritis, and carditis. Fatal CMV myocarditis and pericarditis with tamponade have been described as complications of hematologic malignancies.[469,470]

More often, cardiac involvement of disseminated CMV is seen among patients with AIDS. Susceptible patients typically present with fever, malaise, hypoxia, dyspnea, and dry cough. Radiographic changes are nonspecific and include diffuse interstitial infiltrates, ground-glass attenuation and nodule formation. Clinical signs and symptoms of CMV myocarditis range from asymptomatic myocardopathy to fulminant congestive heart failure. Intractable ventricular and supraventricular arrhythmias have also been reported.[469] CMV-related pericardial effusions are typically small and of no significant hemodynamic consequence. Symptomatic pericarditis and cardiac tamponade, however, have been documented rarely.[470] The diagnosis is suggested by isolation of CMV from cultures of peripheral blood buffy coat. Intranuclear inclusion bodies or cytomegalic cells within areas of inflammation and alveolar damage on sputum or BAL cytopathology or lung biopsy specimens are pathognomonic for CMV infection. These findings, coupled with unexplained cardiomyopathy or arrhythmias should heighten the suspicion for CMV-related cardiac disease in the high-risk patient. Unfortunately, the diagnosis is often made at necropsy. Pathologic examination of the heart typically demonstrates marked disruption and disintegration of muscle bands associated with cytomegalic inclusion bodies. Novel diagnostic strategies, including the use of nucleic acid probes and PCR amplification methods, in the diagnosis of CMV infection are currently being used for the early detection of viral disease.[471] Combined treatment with intravenous gancyclovir, together with immune globulin represents standard therapy for established disease. Alternatively, foscarnet, an inorganic pyrophosphate with equivalent clinical efficacy against CMV may represent a reasonable therapeutic option in patients who are intolerant of ganciclovir. The extent of lung injury parallels CMV viral load in the blood and also dictates the length of therapy. Three to six-week therapy is usually indicated for treatment of established disease.

Several other infections of viral etiology that may cause fulminant pneumonia and associated carditis in the immunocompromised host deserve mention. Adenovirus is a common cause of self-limited upper respiratory tract symptoms in children that may cause intractable pneumonia in the immunocompromised setting, particularly following HSCT. Adenoviral pneumonitis complicates 0.9%–6.5% of HSCT, often with devastating consequences.[472,473] Increased rates of adenoviral infections and disseminated disease are seen among recipients of T-cell-depleted bone marrow grafts and among patients who develop GVHD post transplantation. The clinical spectrum of disseminated adenoviral infections includes hepatitis, hemorrhagic cystitis, meningoencephalitis, tubulointerstitial nephritis, disseminated intravascular coagulation, hemorrhagic colitis, acute pericarditis, and acute myocarditis. Adenoviral myocarditis may lead to dilated

cardiomyopathy and refractory heart failure.[471] The diagnosis is suggested by the finding of viral inclusions, including "Cowdry A" or smudge cells on cytologic analysis of body fluids and tissues. PCR is currently being successfully employed in the rapid detection of adenoviral sequences. Various antiviral regimens have been tried, however, optimal therapy for this disease is not well defined. Epstein–Barr Virus (EBV), a ubiquitous human herpes virus, is the culpable infection that underlies the development of adolescent infectious mononucleosis. Typically an innocuous infection of negligible consequence in the normal host, EBV may cause life-threatening pneumonia among severely immunocompromised individuals. Other factors that enhance the risk of developing EBV-related pneumonia and associated disseminated disease include sero-negative recipient status and active CMV infection.[474–476] Impaired T-cell immune surveillance is characteristic of severe immune deficiency. EBV may induce uncontrolled proliferation of B-lymphocytes in the face of impaired immune surveillance, resulting in a heterogeneous group of post-transplant lymphoproliferative disorders (PTLD). The clinical manifestations of EBV-associated PTLD include asymptomatic seroconversion, monoclonal B-cell proliferation with nodal and extra-nodal tumors, and fulminant disseminated disease with sepsis. PTLD predominantly appears as a complication of solid organ transplants, but may be seen following hematopoietic transplants as well. Fulminant disease is most often seen among recipients of HLA-mismatched or T-cell depleted allografts, and among patients treated for GVHD.[477] Cardiac involvement occurs early, usually within the first 3 months following HSCT and is manifested as pericarditis or myocarditis with associated dilated cardiomyopathy. In addition, disseminated, EBV-associated non-Hodgkin's lymphoma following HSCT has been reported.[477,478] Patients may present with widespread, rapidly progressive, lymphomatous infiltration of the lungs, heart, gastrointestinal tract, central nervous system and kidneys. Fatal arrhythmias secondary to lymphomatous involvement of the cardiac conduction system have been reported.[478] Sudden cardiac death may occur in the absence prior signs of cardiac decompensation. Noninvasive imaging studies are useful in defining the extent of cardiac involvement, but cannot reliably distinguish tumor from other types on endocardial masses. Thus, the diagnosis relies on tissue biopsies, which should be performed early to enable specific therapy. Reductions in immunosuppressive therapy and the use of antiviral agents such as acyclovir or ganciclovir are routinely employed in the treatment of EBV-related PTLD following HSCT. This therapeutic approach, however, has not substantially changed the poor prognosis of patients with widely disseminated disease. Other viruses, including herpes simplex virus (HSV), respiratory syncitial virus (RSV) and influenza virus rarely cause myocardial disease.[479–482] Disease dissemination typically occurs in association with severe immunosuppression and as a result of viremia originating from the lungs or some other extracardiac site.

Invasive fungal infections are substantial threat to the successful treatment of patients with cancer, particularly the post-transplant setting and among patients with hematologic malignancies. Among the spectrum of fungal infections in this population of patients, pneumonias caused by Aspergillus species are the most common and the most life threatening. More than 300 different species of Aspergillus has been identified. The predominant species causing infection in humans include *A. Niger, A. fumigatus, A. nidulans,* and *A. clavatus. A. versicolor* is also recognized as an emerging cause of recalcitrant skin and lung lesions among patients with hematologic malignancies.[483–485] The predisposing role of neutropenia in the development of fungal pneumonias is well established. The degree of immune suppression, including the duration of neutropenia (> 7 days) and absolute neutrophil count (granulocyte counts of <1 x 10^9/l) act as tenacious substrates for the development of Aspergillus infection as well as other fungal disorders. Recipients of allogeneic stem cell transplants and T-cell depleted marrow allografts also show increased vulnerability to the development of fungal infections, presumably on the basis of associated delays in engraftment. Patients frequently present with vague symptoms of fever, dry cough, and dyspnea. Other signs and symptoms, such as focal wheezing, hemoptysis, pleuritic chest pain, and a pleural friction rub are highly suggestive. This constellation of findings, however, is seen in less than a third of patients. Radiographic findings of diffuse infiltrates and nodules are frequent, but nonspecific findings. Extrathoracic sites of Aspergillus infection include the sinuses, skin, frontal cortex, periorbital areas, as well as the heart. Blood-stream infection is also seen and heralds a poor prognosis. Wedge-shaped, pleural-based infiltrates consistent with the radiographic appearance of pulmonary infarction and CT evidence of an air-crescent or halo sign, when present, are helpful in discriminating Aspergillosis from other types of pneumonia. The propensity for Aspergillus to invade cardiac structures is recognized as one of the most virulent complications of disseminated disease. Cardiac involvement may occur as a consequence of hematogenous seeding or secondary to contiguous spread from pulmonary infections. Most cardiac structures are vulnerable to Aspergillus infection. The

histopathologic correlates of myocardial involvement include myocardial abscesses that may be either focal or diffuse. These lesions may extend from the myocardium into the endocardium, resulting in mural endocarditis. The predilection of Aspergillus to invade vessels may result in mycotic thrombosis and consequent ischemic necrosis of large portions of the heart.[486] Hemodynamic instability associated with Aspergillus myocarditis is poorly responsive to inotropic agents or antifungal therapy. The prognosis remains dismal despite aggressive therapy. Mucormycosis, an angioinvasive pathogen which belongs to the class of filamentous fungi, has been increasingly recognized as a cause of severe and often fatal infections, particularly among immunocompromised patients.

Although candidal species are considered commensal flora in humans, deeply invasive candidiasis decisively contributes to the morbidity of certain groups of patients, including recipients of HSCT and among patients with indwelling intravenous catheters. Increased colonization of candidal species in the oral cavity or gastrointestinal tract heightens the risk of systemic candidiasis.[487] Candida pneumonia is a rare disorder that commonly results from aspiration of upper airway contents or from hematogenous dissemination. Lung infections are typically caused by *Candida albicans,* although *C. glabrata, C. tropicalis* and *C. krusei* have been noted recently with increasing frequency.[488,489] Affected patients typically present with nonspecific symptoms of fever and dry cough. The chest radiograph may demonstrate micronodular lesions similar to that seen with pneumonias caused by Aspergillus. The presence of skin or sinus involvement or radiographic evidence of a halo sign helps to distinguish Aspergillus-associated pneumonia from that caused by Candida. Extrathoracic manifestations of Candida, including local invasion of the retina or mucosal surfaces of the gastrointestinal or genitourinary tracts, may suggest the diagnosis. The diagnosis of Candida pneumonia should be considered among patients with progressive infiltrates unresponsive to antibiotic therapy. Frequent upper airway contamination by Candida confounds the diagnosis, which usually requires histopathologic evidence of tissue invasion for confirmation. Hematogenous dissemination of Candida can spread to virtually organ. Candida, the most frequent cause of fungal carditis, tends to target cardiac valves. Embolization of valvular vegetations may occur, resulting in acute cerebrovascular events. Blood cultures are positive in more than 70% of patients. *C. albicans* is the most common species involved, however carditis owing to *C. tropicalis, C. parapsilopsis,* and *C. glabrata* have been sited with increased frequency. The therapeutic approach may involve surgery combined with systemic antifungal therapy. Treatment typically requires antifungal therapy with amphotericin B, lipid-complexed amphotericin B, or the triazole compounds combined with surgery.

Bacterial endocarditis in the cancer patient is a rare entity. The true prevalence of cancer-related bacterial endocarditis is unknown. Information regarding this disorder is primarily gleaned from case reports and small case series in the literature. Early and aggressive administration of antimicrobial therapy, resulting in either prevention or rapid control of bacteremia and endocardial seeding has putatively resulted in an overall decline in this disorder.

Catheter-related, right-sided nosocomial endocarditis has been described in 5% of recipients of HSCT.[490] Hemodialysis also portends a 2- to 3-fold increased risk of nosocomial endocarditis compared to the general population.[491] Increased rates of nosocomial endocarditis are seen with the use of intravenous catheters and following medico-surgical procedures. The predominant pathogens that are most frequently associated with nosocomial endocarditis are those that have the greatest propensity to adhere to damaged valves such as *Staphylococcus aureus*, *Streptococcus species* and enterococci, which comprise more than 80% of the pathogens responsible for this disease.

The triad of pneumococcal pneumonia, meningitis and endocarditis was first described by Heschl and subsequently by Osler more than a century ago. The usual portal of entry for pneumococcal endocarditis is the lungs, although occasionally the development of this disease may be attributed to extrapulmonary sites of infection. Risk factors for invasive pneumococcal disease include chronic glucocorticoid therapy, HIV and other chronic immunosuppressive illnesses, recent respiratory infection, and chronic pulmonary disease. The curtailment and clearance of pneumococcal infection involves humoral and cellular immune responses that are both local and systemic in distribution. For example, following the establishment of a pneumococcal infection, phagocytic effector cells are mobilized and activated, IgG and IgA antibodies directed against the pneumococcal capsule are generated and the complement pathways are activated. Thus, an array of immunologic defects that are commonly seen in the cancer patient, including impaired chemotaxis, qualitative and quantitative neutrophil defects, and impaired antibody generation may contribute to sustained bacteremia and/or invasive pneumococcal disease. In addition, the development of mucositis and its attendant enhanced propensity to aspirate following cancer chemotherapy, further augments the risk of developing serious invasive pneumococcal disease. Endocardial disease may develop after a transient

respite following pneumococcal pneumonia. Patients typically present with fever, sepsis, and cardiac failure secondary to valvular destruction several weeks following pneumonia. Once established, pneumococcal endocarditis typically follows an aggressive and relentless course. Hemodynamic instability associated with valvular vegetations may lead to acute valvular insufficiency. These frequently large vegetations show a predilection for the aortic valve.[492,493] Local valvular complications include abscess formation and perforation. The propensity to infect and rapidly destroy left-sided cardiac valves undoubtedly contributes to the poor outcome. In addition, extracardiac sequelae, such as systemic embolization are also seen at increased rates. Recent studies have confirmed the superior sensitivity of transesophageal (TEE) over transthoracic echocardiography in detecting valvular vegetations and abscess formation as well as in providing information regarding the competency of the valves and paravalvular structures. Optimum therapy for pneumococcal endocarditis involves a multidisciplinary approach, involving infectious disease specialists, cardiologists, and cardiac surgeons. Four to six weeks of antimicrobial therapy is advocated.[492,494] The choice of antimicrobial regimen is dictated by susceptibility testing and/or the prevalence of resistant pneumococcal strains in ones geographic area. A combined medical-surgical approach should be considered for patients with recalcitrant systemic infections caused by a surgically removable focus, intractable congestive heart failure secondary to valvular insufficiency and recurrent life-threatening embolization. Early valvular surgery may confer an improved survival.[492,495] Hemodialysis, intravenous catheters, medico-surgical procedures also confer an increased risk for endocarditis.[491] Catheter-related, right-sided nosocomial endocarditis has been described in 5% of recipients of HSCT.[490] Rates of endocarditis are 2- to 3-fold higher among patients undergoing hemodialysis compared to the general population. Pathogens that have the greatest propensity to adhere to damaged valves, such as *Staphylococcus aureus*, *Streptococcus species* and enterococci comprise more than 80% of the pathogens responsible for disease in these settings.

■ Disorders of Ventilatory Control

Lung failure versus pump failure ■ Disorders of ventilatory control may be due to "lung failure" or "pump failure". Both forms of injury may have devastating consequences on the heart. In lung failure, hypoxia caused by ventilation/perfusion abnormalities, shunts, or alterations of alveolar-capillary diffusion may lead to PH and cor pulmonale. A classic example of lung failure is ARDS. In other disorders, such as atelectasis, pulmonary embolism, and shunt associated with pulmonary edema, lung failure develops as a consequence of ventilatory/perfusion mismatch in the absence of ARDS.

Primary failure of alveolar ventilation leads to ventilatory pump failure, which is characterized by severe hypercapnia and acidosis with only mild hypoxemia. The major components of the ventilatory pump include the respiratory controllers of the drive to breathe located in the central nervous system (CNS), the chest wall (including the respiratory muscles), and the pathways that connect the central controllers with the respiratory muscles (spinal and peripheral nerves). Conditions that compromise specific components of the ventilatory pump such as impaired drive, inadequate neuromuscular competence, and increased respiratory system load and chest wall abnormalities are prevalent causes of pump failure in patients with cancer. The cardiac consequences of hypercapneic respiratory acidosis include increased sympathomimetic output, reduced cardiac contractility, tachycardia and increased preload. These perturbations may be clinically trivial under normal circumstances, but are poorly tolerated by the debilitated cancer patient and by patients with preexisting cardiac disease. Hypercapnia-induced increases in sympathomimetic output may potentiate cardiac arrhythmias. Beta blocker medications may impair compensation for the negative inotropic effects of hypercapnia and thus should be avoided, if possible. Hypercapnia-induced PH with associated right heart failure are also concerns. The vasodilatory effects of hypercapnia may result in significant hypotension, especially among patients with prior hypovolemia. Occasionally, conditions causing lung and pump failure coexist, resulting in severe cardiorespiratory impairments. This mixed picture is a common source of respiratory failure in the cancer patient. The major causes lung and pump failure in cancer are listed in Table 18-10. The diverse influence of lung failure on cardiovascular performance is discussed elsewhere in this chapter. The causes of ventilatory failure among cancer patients will be briefly discussed below.

Pump failure due to central nervous system disorders: Impaired drive ■ Pump failure owing to central depression of ventilatory drive may result from isolated insults to the central nervous system, such as medullary tumors or infarction, radiation to the base of the skull or following neurosurgical procedures for brainstem tumors, particularly those that are close to the floor of the fourth ventricle. Sedating or narcotic medications and occult hypothyroidism may have similar adverse effects. These insults may be sufficient to cause respiratory failure, but more often result in chronic respiratory insufficiency. Respiratory failure ensues with the introduction of an additional insult. Even small doses of narcotic or sedating medications in this setting may produce profound alveolar hypoventilation with associated hypercapneic respiratory failure.

Pump failure due to peripheral nervous system disorders: Inadequate neuromuscular competence ■ Conditions that cause neuromuscular dysfunction, such as primary neurologic diseases, spinal cord lesions, neuromuscular blocking drugs and muscle weakness may precipitate ventilatory failure by interrupting signal transmission from the CNS to the respiratory muscles. Severe ventilatory depression requiring artificial ventilatory support is expected following administration of neuromuscular blocking agents and has also been reported following chronic methadone use. Other drugs, such as sedatives, anxiolytics, hypnotics, and aminoglycosides typically produce severe respiratory depression only in the setting of preexisting neuromuscular diseases, such as myasthenia gravis and myasthenic paraneoplastic syndrome or after massive overdose. Chronic muscular weakness and fatigue are prominent complaints in the cancer population that may emerge from multifactorial etiologies. Malnutrition and cachexia are well-known complications of advanced cancer, which contributes decisively to depressed strength and endurance of the skeletal muscles, including the diaphragm.[496–498] In addition, hypoperfusion states (cardiogenic, septic, or hemorrhagic shock), excess lactate or hydrogen ion production, and severe anemia may potentiate cancer-related muscle fatigue and respiratory failure.

Profound generalized muscle weakness may occur as a sequela of prolonged steroid therapy or chemotherapy- and diuretic-induced electrolyte disturbances, such as hypophosphatemia, hypokalemia, and hypomagnesemia.[499,500] Beta-agonists, diuretics, and corticosteroids are common therapies in the cancer patient that may exacerbate hypophosphatemia and aggravate muscle weakness. The deleterious effects of chemotherapeutic agents and other drugs on the neuromuscular system are well described. Peripheral neuropathy incited by some biological therapy agents (bortezomib thalidomide), platinum-based agents, vinca alkaloids, taxanes, antimetabolites is well described in the literature. The deleterious effects of these drugs on lung function may be subtle in the absence of predisposing factors, such as preexisting neuromuscular abnormalities. Severe myopathy associated with myositis has been reported following immune checkpoint inhibitor therapies.[501] Finally, a number of paraneoplastic syndromes may cause diffuse neural dysfunction and respiratory failure in the cancer setting. Among these, Lambert-Eaton

TABLE 18-10   Major features of respiratory failure

	LUNG FAILURE – TYPE I	PUMP FAILURE – TYPE II
Name	Acute hypoxic respiratory failure	Ventilatory faliure
Underlying Cause	Ventilation/perfusion abnormalities, Shunts, Alterations of alveolar-capillary membrane	Alveolar hypoventilation Decreased area for gas exchange
Common associated diseases	ARDS, Pneumonia Pneumonitis Embolic phenomenon (thrombus, fat) ILD Pulmonary fibrosis Pulmonary hypertension Bronchiectasis	**Depressed CNS**—drugs, hypothyroidism, metabolic alkalosis, structural CNS lesions, idiopathic **Altered chest wall/neuromuscular system**-kyposcoliosis, Guillain–Barre, Amyotrophic lateral sclerosis, diaphragmatic fatigue, poliomyelitis, Myasthenia gravis, obesity hypoventilation syndrome, cervical cord injury, electrolyte disturbance (hypokalemia, hypophosphatemia, hypomagnesemia) **Lungs/airways**—severe ARDS, Severe asthma, emphysema
Major gas derangement	Hypoxemia, PaO2 <60 mmHg; PCO2 normal	Hypercapnea, PCO2 > 45; Hypoxemia

myasthenic syndrome (LEMS), which affects about 3% of patients with small-cell lung cancer, myasthenia gravis, which occurs in 10%–15% of patients with thymoma, and demyelinating peripheral neuropathy, seen in 50% of patients with the osteosclerotic form of plasmacytoma are most common. The respiratory insufficiency associated with these disorders is typically subacute and debilitating. Stressors such as infection or surgery in the setting of LEMS may precipitate acute, florid ventilatory failure.

COPD is a common co-morbidity of lung cancer. Diaphragmatic flattening and lung hyperinflation are characteristic disturbances in advanced COPD which contribute to compromised respiratory muscle performance and ventilatory failure. Ventilatory failure owing to diaphragmatic dysfunction may also occur following the use of anesthetic agents such as halothane, propofol, and nitrous oxide.[502,503] Surgeries to the head and neck cancer, anterior mediastinum, esophagus or lungs may cause persistent diaphragmatic dysfunction and ventilatory failure. Phrenic nerve invasion by lymphomas and cancers of the lung and head and neck may cause similar problems.

Pump failure due to increased work of breathing: Increased respiratory system load and chest wall abnormalities ▪ Ventilatory failure secondary to increased airway resistive workloads is a cardinal feature of advanced COPD. Other disorders associated with airway obstruction and increased airway resistance, including inflammation, edema, or physical obstruction of the airway by mucous, blood, or tumor may also precipitate ventilatory failure. Prior intubation, radiation to the head and neck, and intubation with a small (<7.5 mm internal diameter) endotracheal tube are common causes of proximal airway resistance in the cancer setting that may lead to ventilatory failure. Increased minute ventilation, owing to factors that contribute to excess carbon dioxide production (fever, respiratory distress, infection) or increased dead space ventilation (pulmonary embolism pre-existing lung disease, hypovolemia, PEEP) may also precipitate ventilatory failure. Finally, abnormalities involving the chest wall and thoracic spine caused by tumor, radiation or surgery may cause increased chest wall elastic loads, increased work of breathing and ventilatory failure.

HEART-LUNG INTERACTIONS IN THE CRITICALLY ILL PATIENT

▪ Cardiac Consequences of Ventilatory Failure

Many of the causes of lung and pump failure in the cancer setting may lead to cardiogenic and noncardiogenic shock with associated hemodynamic instability. More than 60% of cancer patients with ARDS, a common cause of lung failure, require positive pressure ventilation and pharmacologic circulatory support.[504] Mechanical ventilation, pharmacologic therapy for circulatory collapse, as well as the underlying lung pathology may all contribute to hemodynamic instability either through preload insufficiency or excessive afterload. The effects of positive pressure ventilation on the heart are triggered primarily by ventilator-induced changes in pleural pressure (Ppl) and trans-pulmonary pressure (TP). Conditions that decrease chest wall compliance, such as ascites, obesity, chest wall edema, anasarca, and large pleural effusions, may cause precipitous increases in Ppl. Changes in volume status, venous tone and resting intra-abdominal pressure influence intrapleural pressure and its effect on venous return. The effect of positive pressure ventilation on venous return is exaggerated when large tidal volumes or excessively high levels of PEEP are used. In addition, hypovolemic states and clinical settings of vasodilation that occur during sepsis, adrenal insufficiency, and shock may also amplify the reduction in venous return during positive pressure ventilation. Attenuations in RV preload results in decreased RV output, decreased pulmonary venous return to the left heart, reduced stroke volume and hypotension. Similarly, intra-abdominal hypertension mediated by a variety of cancer-related conditions, including sepsis, ascites, pancreatitis, and ileus can lead to reduced venous return and hypotension.

The influence of airway pressure and lung volume on cardiac function is particularly important to consider in the management of the critically ill patient requiring mechanical ventilation. Elevated airway pressures may have deleterious effects on stroke volume, particularly in the setting of hypovolemia or increase intra-abdominal pressures. Efforts to reduce Ppl by draining pleural or peritoneal fluids, and patient positioning may improve venous return. Ventilator strategies that limit tidal volumes and PEEP may also be of benefit in the management of these patients. Increased PVR secondary to mechanical ventilation or PEEP may overdistend the RV, resulting in ventricular interdependence and a stiff, poorly compliant LV. The net result is an increase in left atrial pressure, diminished LV preload and compliance, and reduced LV stroke volume and cardiac output. Pathologic states that are associated with ventricular interdependence include acute massive pulmonary embolism, pulmonary hypertension, tricuspid insufficiency, severe bronchospasm, atrial septal defect and pulmonary insufficiency. Large negative swings in intrathoracic pressure may also increase RV afterload by increasing PVR and impeding RV emptying. In addition, pericardial diseases such as tamponade and pericardial constriction may significantly restrain ventricular filling

and amplify the respiratory changes in ventricular volume. Adjustments in PEEP, mean airway pressures and lung protective ventilation strategies designed to mitigate lung overdistension by incorporating low tidal volumes and modes of ventilation may modulate some of these physiologic effects. Specific ventilator strategies are beyond the scope of this chapter. An overall synopsis of the cardiovascular effects of MV and the application of PEEP on intrathoracic pressures and cardiac output is given in Figure 18-17.

Importantly, during the state of ventricular interdependence, the clinically measured PAWP may not reliably reflect the state of LV preload. Hemodynamic measurements should be interpreted with caution in these situations in order to avoid the clinical error of interpreting a mechanically induced reduction of left ventricular diastolic compliance as left ventricular failure. Echocardiography may provide more accurate qualitative and quantitative assessments of LV volumes and function in these settings. The oversdistended RV may also compromise RV coronary blood flow, resulting in RV ischemia and deteriorating RV systolic function. Overly zealous fluid resuscitation in the setting of acute cor pulmonale may precipitate RV failure by inducing further distension of the RV and associated RV ischemia. Thus, the successful management of the patient's volume status requires maintenance of a fine balance between underfilling (inadequate preload) and volume overload. This therapeutic exercise is confounded by the fact that in the setting of altered biventricular compliance, intravascular pressure measurements for the assessment of volume status are often misleading. Measurements of central venous pressures (CVP) and PAPs during a positive pressure breath may offer rough estimates of volume status. During the respiratory cycle, early inspiratory increases in systolic blood pressures is seen due to movement of blood from the alveolar vessels into the left ventricle with a reduction in left ventricular afterload and rightward septal shift. This is followed by decreases in systolic pressures as the influence of PPV on venous return prevails.[505] PPV exerts a marked effect on arterial waveform variability (pulse pressure and systolic pressure) during states of volume depletion. This effect may be mitigated with fluid loading in volume responsive states. Dynamic changes in arterial waveform variables in mechanically ventilated patients may, in fact, prove to be more sensitive measure of fluid responsiveness than more conventional measurements, such as the CVP. These waveform measurements may help to guide decisions regarding fluid challenges in mechanically ventilated patients. Arterial waveform measurements in the setting of large variations in

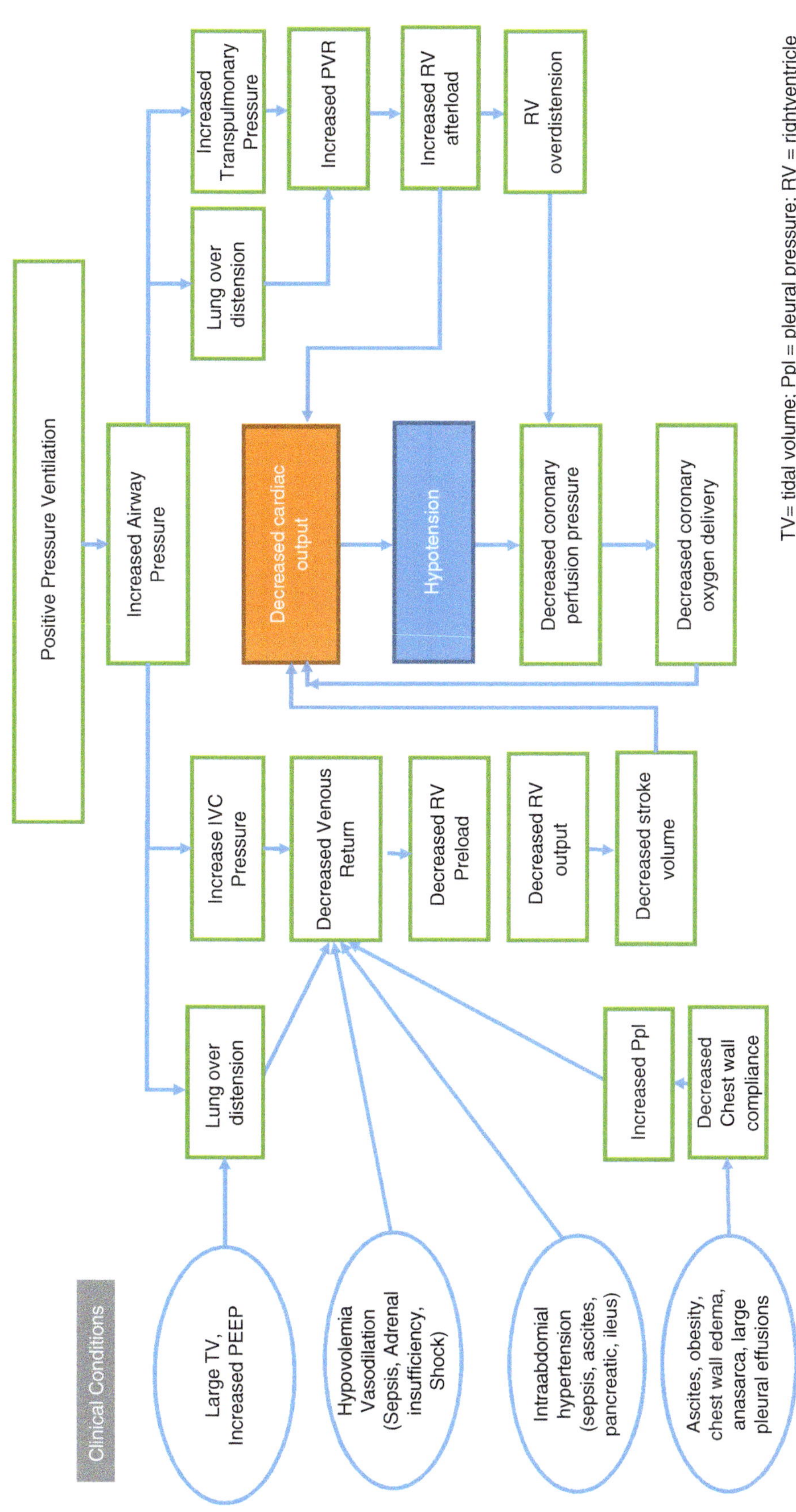

FIGURE 18-17 Effects of mechanical ventilation and the application of PEEP on the heart.

thoracic pressures, as seen in large pleural effusions or low tidal volumes during lung volume protective strategies for ARDS may lead to false positive and false negative tests, respectively, and should be interpreted with caution.[506,507] The need for fluid challenges in the critical ill setting should always take into account the effect of fluid administration on cardiac function and systemic perfusion.

Pharmacologic agents such as nitroprusside and nitroglycerine may also alter ventricular compliance by reducing RV preload and increasing LV compliance, resulting in decreased right ventricular end diastolic volume (RVEDP). The efficacy of vasopressor agents to augment blood pressure in low cardiac output states requires close monitoring of LVEDV (LV preload) by echocardiography, as many of these agents may simply increase LVEDP without a parallel increase in LVEDV and cardiac output.

CARDIAC CONSEQUENCES OF WEANING FROM THE VENTILATOR

Weaning patients from mechanical ventilation induces significant changes in intrathoracic pressures with profound consequences on cardiovascular function, particularly in patients with poor cardiac reserve. Excess airway secretions, ineffective cough, muscle weakness, and altered mental status are frequently sited causes of weaning failures. The cardiovascular consequences of weaning from mechanical ventilation are often overlooked. Studies have shown marked changes in transmural pulmonary artery occlusion pressure, PAP, hypoxic pulmonary vasoconstriction, cardiac output and LV afterload with attempted extubation, which may contribute to failure to wean among patients. These changes may lead to recurrent pulmonary edema, particularly in patients with poor left ventricular function. Echocardiography and biologic markers, such as BNP and NT-proBNP helpful in stratifying patients at risk for weaning failure and optimizing weaning strategies, particularly those patient with cardiac etiologies for failed extubation.[508–511] PH with associated acute cor pulmonale may also impede successful weaning from the ventilator. Pulmonary vasodilator therapies along with lung protective strategies may potentially reduce PAPs and facilitate weaning.

SUMMARY

The biological crosstalk between the heart and lungs represents a complex symbiosis under normal circumstances. This tightly wound inter-relationship quickly gives way to demanding diagnostic and therapeutic challenges in disease states in which derangements in and treatment strategies for one organ system may profoundly affect the performance of the other. Pulmonary hypertension with cor pulmonale are perhaps the most recognized cardiac consequences of pulmonary disease. The significance of other pulmonary disorders on the heart, including drug- and radiation-induced lung diseases, pneumonia, sleep-disordered breathing and COPD are increasingly recognized as contributors of cardiovascular morbidity and mortality. Mechanical ventilation profoundly underscores heart-lung interdependence. Alterations in cardiovascular function during mechanical ventilation occurs via intricate and often opposing mechanisms. The fine balance between heart-lung interactions is often challenged in the cancer setting due to sequelae of cancer or its treatment. Knowledge of these interactions is critical in the successful management of patients with cancer.

REFERENCES

1. Van Eeden S, Leipsic J, Paul Man SF, Sin D. The relationship between lung inflammation and cardiovascular disease. *Am J Respir Crit Care Med*. 2012;186:11–16.
2. Bradley TD, Floras JS. Sleep apnea and heart failure: Part II: central sleep apnea. *Circulation*. 2003;107:1822–1826.
3. Bradley TD, Floras JS. Sleep apnea and heart failure: Part I: obstructive sleep apnea. *Circulation*. 2003;107:1671–1678.
4. Wouters E, Reynaert NL, Dentener MA, Vernooy J. Systemic and local inflammation in asthma and chronic obstructive pulmonary disease: is there a connection? *Proc Am Thorac Soc*. 2009;6:638–647.
5. Ross R. Atherosclerosis is an inflammatory disease. *Am Heart J*. 1999;138:419–420.
6. Dourado V, Tanni SE, Vale SA, Faganello MM, Sanchez FF, Godoy I. Systemic manifestations in chronic obstructive pulmonary disease. *J Bras Pneumol*. 2006;32:161–171.
7. Fabbri LM, Rabe K. From COPD to chronic systemic inflammatory synrome? *Lancet*. 2007;370:797–799.
8. Yanbaeva DG, Dentener MA, Creutzberg EC, Wesseling G, Wouters E. Systemic effects of smoking. *Chest*. 2007;131:1557–1566.
9. Hansson GK, Libby P, Tabas I. Inflammation and plaque vulnerability. *J Intern Med*. 2015;278:483–493.
10. Alonso-Martínez JL, Llorente-Diez B, Echegaray-Agara M, Olaz-Preciado F, Urbieta-Echezarreta M, González-Arencibia C. C-reactive protein as a predictor of improvement and readmission in heart failure. *Eur J Heart Fail*. 2002;4:331–336.
11. Levine B, Kalman J, Mayer L, Fillit HM, Packer M. Elevated circulating levels of tumor necrosis factor in severe chronic heart failure. *N Engl J Med*. 1990;323:236–241.

12. Vila V, Martínez-Sales V, Almenar L, Lázaro IS, Villa P, Reganon E. Inflammation, endothelial dysfunction and angiogenesis markers in chronic heart failure patients. *Int J Cardiol.* 2008;130:276–277.

13. Sánchez-Lázaro IJ, Almenar L, Reganon E, et al. Inflammatory markers in stable heart failure and their relationship with functional class. *Int J Cardiol.* 2008;129:388–393.

14. Schneider C, Bothner U, Jick SS, Meier CR. Chronic obstructive pulmonary disease and the risk of cardiovascular diseases. *Eur J Epidemiol.* 2010;25:253–260.

15. Terzano C, Conti V, Di Stefano F, et al. Comorbidity, hospitalization, and mortality in COPD: results from a longitudinal study. *Lung.* 2010;188:321–329.

16. Panetta NL, Krachman S, Chatila W. Chronic obstructive pulmonary disease and its comorbidities. *Panminerva Med.* 2009;51:115–123.

17. Zvezdin B, Milutinov S, Koijicic M. A post-mortemanalysis of major causes of early death in patients hospitalizedwith chronic obstructive pulmonary disease. *Chest.* 2009;136:376–380.

18. Hansell A, Walk J, Soriano J. What do chronic obstructive pulmonary disease patients die from? A multiple cause coding analysis. *Eur Respir J.* 2003;22:809–814.

19. Sidney S, Sorel M, Quesenberry CP Jr, DeLuise C, Lanes S, Eisner MD. COPD and incident cardiovascular disease hospitalizations and mortality: Kaiser Permanente Medical Care Program. *Chest.* 2005;128:2068–2075.

20. Sin D, Man SF. Chronic obstructive pulmonary disease as a risk factor for cardiovascular morbidity and mortality. *Proc Am Thorac Soc.* 2005;2:8–11.

21. Hole DJ, Watt GC, Davey-Smith G, Hart CL, Gillis CR, Hawthorne V. Impaired lung function and mortality risk in men and women: findings from the Renfrew and Paisley prospective population study. *BMJ.* 1996;313:711–715.

22. Soriano JB, Rigo F, Guerrero D, et al. High prevalence of undiagnosed airflow limitation in patients with cardiovascular disease. *Chest.* 2010;137:333–340.

23. van Gestel Y, Goei D, Hoeks SE, et al. Predictive value of NT-proBNP in vascular surgery patients with COPD and normal left ventricular systolic function. *COPD.* 2010;7:70–75.

24. Donaldson GC, Hurst JR, Smith CJ, Hubbard RB, Wedzicha J. Increased risk of myocardial infarction and stroke following exacerbation of COPD. *Chest.* 2010;137:1091–1097.

25. Lappalainen U, Whitsett JA, Wert SE, Tichelaar JW, Bry K. Interleukin-1beta causes pulmonary inflammation, emphysema, and airway remodeling in the adult murine lung. *Am J Respir Cell Mol Biol.* 2005;32:311–318.

26. Kleinbongard P, Heusch G, Schulz R. TNFalpha in atherosclerosis, myocardial ischemia/reperfusion and heart failure. *Pharmacol Ther.* 2010;127:295–314.

27. Mukhopadhyay S, Hoidal JR, Mukherjee T. Role of TNFα in pulmonary pathophysiology. *Respir Res.* 2006;7:125.

28. Sun J, Sukhova1 GK, Wolters PJ, et al. Mast cells promote atherosclerosis by releasing proinflammatory cytokines. *Nat Med.* 2007;13:719–724.

29. Chung KF. Cytokines in chronic obstructive pulmonary disease. *Eur Respir J.* December 2001;34:50s–59s.

30. Robertson AK, Rudling M, Zhou X, Gorelik L, Flavell RA, Hansson G. Disruption of TGF-beta signaling in T cells accelerates atherosclerosis. *J Clin Invest.* 2003;112:1342–1350.

31. Bäck M, Hansson G. Leukotriene receptors in atherosclerosis. *Ann Med.* 2006;38:493–502.

32. Pardo A, Selman M. Proteinase-antiproteinase imbalance in the pathogenesis of emphysema: the role of metalloproteinases in lung damage. *Histol Histopathol.* 1999;14:227–233.

33. Bäck M, Weber C, Lutgens E. Regulation of atherosclerotic plaque inflammation. *J Intern Med.* 2015;278:462–482.

34. Bobika A. Transforming growth factor-betas and vascular disorders. *Arterioscler Thromb Vasc Biol.* 2006;26:1712–1720.

35. Navratilova Z, Kolek V, Petrek M. Matrix metalloproteinases and their inhibitors in chronic obstructive pulmonary disease. *Arch Immunol Ther Exp (Warsz).* 2015;2015:177–193

36. López-Sánchez M, Muñoz-Esquerre M, Huertas D, et al. Inflammatory markers and circulating extracellular matrix proteins in patients with chronic obstructive pulmonary disease and left ventricular diastolic dysfunction. *Clin Respir J.* 2017 Nov;11(6):859–866.

37. Beeh KM, Kornmann O, Buhl R, Culpitt SV, Giembycz MA, Barnes PJ. Neutrophil chemotactic activity of sputum from patients with COPD: role of interleukin 8 and leukotriene B4. *Chest.* 2003;123:1240–1247.

38. Bäck M. Review Leukotriene signaling in atherosclerosis and ischemia. *Cardiovasc Drugs Ther.* 2009;23:41–48.

39. Venugopal SK, Devaraj S, Jialal I. Effect of C-reactive protein on vascular cells: evidence for a proinflammatory, proatherogenic role. *Curr Opin Nephrol Hypertens.* 2005;14:33–37.

40. Jialal I, Devaraj S, Venugopal S. C-reactive protein: risk marker or mediator in atherothrombosis? *Hypertension.* 2004;44:6–11.

41. Mancini GB, Etminan M, Zhang B, Levesque LE, FitzGerald JM, Brophy J. Reduction of morbidity and mortality by statins, angiotensin-converting enzyme inhibitors, and angiotensin receptor blockers in patients with chronic obstructive pulmonary disease. *J Am Coll Cardiol.* 2006;47:2554–2560.

42. Mroz RM, Lisowski P, Tycinska A, et al. Anti-inflammatory effects of atorvastatin treatment in chronic obstructive pulmonary disease. A controlled pilot study. *J Physiol Pharmacol.* 2015;66:111–128.

43. Keddissi JJ, Younis WG, Chbeir EA, et al. The use of statins and lung function in current and former smokers. *Chest.* 2007;132:1764–1771.

44. Dobler CC, Wong KK, Marks G. Associations between statins and COPD: a systematic review. *BMC Pulm Med.* 2009;9:32–44.

45. Criner GJ1, Connett JE, Aaron SD, et al. Simvastatin for the prevention of exacerbations in moderate-to-severe COPD. *N Engl J Med*. 2014;370:2201–2210.

46. Mascitelli L, Pezzetta F. Inhibition of the renin-angiotensin system in patients with COPD and pulmonary hypertension. *Chest*. 2007;131:938; author reply 938–939.

47. Andreas S, Herrmann-Lingen C, Raupach T, et al. AngiotensinII blockers in obstructive pulmonary disease: a randomised controlled trial. *Eur Respir J*. 2006;27:972–979.

48. Dransfield MT, Rowe SM, Johnson JE, Bailey WC, Gerald L. Use of beta blockers and the risk of death in hospitalised patients with acute exacerbations of COPD. *Thorax*. 2008;63:301–305.

49. Chokroverty S. Adult sleep disorders. *Suppl Clin Neurophysiol*. 2004;57:534–544.

50. Sajkov D, McEvoy RD. Obstructive sleep apnea and pulmonary hypertension. *Prog Cardiovasc Dis*. 2009;51:363–370.

51. White D. New chemotherapy-induced pulmonary syndromes. *Pulm Perspect*. 1995;12:4–5.

52. Schiffman P, Trontell MC, Mazar MF, Edelman NH. Sleep deprivation decreases ventilatory response to CO2 but not load compensation. *Chest*. 1983;84:695–698.

53. Chen H, Tang YR. Sleep loss impairs inspiratory muscle endurance. *Am Rev Respir Dis*. 1989;140:907–909.

54. Cooper A, Gabor JY, PJ. H. Sleep in the critically ill patient. *Semin Respir Crit Care Med* 2001;22:153-164.

55. Rosenberg J, Wildschiødtz G, Pedersen MH, von Jessen F, H. K.. Late postoperative nocturnal episodic hypoxaemia and associated sleep pattern. *Br J Anaesth* 1994;72:145-150.

56. Gabor J, Cooper AB, Hanly PJ. Sleep disruption in the intensive care unit. *Curr Opin Crit Care*. 2001;7:21–27.

57. Knill R, Skinner MI, Novick T, Vandenberghe HM, Moote CA. The night of intense REM sleep after anesthesia and surgery increases urinary catecholamines. *Can J Anaesth*. 1990;37:S12.

58. Irwin M, Clark C, Kennedy B, Christian Gillin J, Ziegler M. Nocturnal catecholamines and immune function in insomniacs, depressed patients, and control subjects. *Brain Behav Immun*. 2003;15:365–372.

59. Vgontzas A, Zoumakis M, Papanicolaou DA, et al. Chronic insomnia is associated with a shift of interleukin-6 and tumor necrosis factor secretion from nighttime to daytime. *Metabolism*. 2002;51:887–892.

60. Knutson K, Van Cauter E, Rathouz PJ, et al. Association between sleep and blood pressure in midlife: the CARDIA sleep study. *Arch Intern Med*. 2009;169:1055–1061.

61. King C, Knutson KL, Rathouz PJ, Sidney S, Liu K, Lauderdale DS. Short sleep duration and incident coronary artery calcification. *JAMA*. 2008;300:2859–2866.

62. Sephton S, Sapolsky RM, Kraemer HC, Spiegel D. Diurnal cortisol rhythm as a predictor of breast cancer survival. *J Natl Cancer Inst*. 2000;92:994–1000.

63. Kripke D, Simons RN, Garfinkel L, Hammond EC. Short and long sleep and sleeping pills. *Is increased mortality associated? Arch Gen Psychiatry*. 1979;36:103–116.

64. Cleeland C. Cancer-related symptoms. *Semin Radiat Oncol*. 2000;10:175–190.

65. Stepanski EJ, Burgess HJ. Sleep and cancer. *Sleep Med Clin*. 2007:2:67–75.

66. Theobald D. Cancer pain, fatigue, distress, and insomnia in cancer patients. *Clin Cornerstone*. 2004;6:S15–S21.

67. Network N. Cancer-related fatigue. Clinical practice guidelines in oncology. *J Natl Compr Canc Netw*. 2003;1:308–331.

68. Davidson J, MacLean A, Brundage M, Schulze K. Sleep disturbance in cancer patients. *Soc Sci Med*. 2002;54:1309–1321.

69. Palesh OG, Roscoe JA, Mustian KM, et al. Prevalence, demographics, and psychological associations of sleep disruption in patients with cancer: university of Rochester Cancer Center-Community Clinical Oncology Program. *J Clin Oncol*. 2010;28:292–298.

70. Blask DE, Brainard GC, Dauchy RT, et al. Melatonin-depleted blood from premenopausal women exposed to light at night stimulates growth of human breast cancer xenografts in nude rats. *Cancer Res*. 2005;65:11174–11184.

71. Filipski E, Delaunay F, King VM, et al. Effects of chronic jet lag on tumor progression in mice. *Cancer Res*. 2004;64:7879–7885.

72. Hansen J, Stevens RG. Case-control study of shift-work and breast cancer risk in Danish nurses: impact of shift systems. *Eur J Cancer*. 2012;48:1722–1729.

73. Megdal SP, Kroenke CH, Laden F, Pukkala E, Schernhammer ES. Night work and breast cancer risk: a systematic review and meta-analysis. *Eur J Cancer*. 2005;41:2023–2032.

74. Straif K, Baan R, Grosse Y, et al. Carcinogenicity of shift-work, painting, and fire-fighting. *Lancet Oncol*. 2007;8:1065–1066.

75. Verkasalo PK, Lillberg K, Stevens RG, et al. Sleep duration and breast cancer: a prospective cohort study. *Cancer Res*. 2005;65:9595–9600.

76. Kakizaki M, Kuriyama S, Sone T, et al. Sleep duration and the risk of breast cancer: the Ohsaki Cohort Study. *Br J Cancer*. 2008;99:1502–1505.

77. Pinheiro SP, Schernhammer ES, Tworoger SS, Michels KB. A prospective study on habitual duration of sleep and incidence of breast cancer in a large cohort of women. *Cancer Res*. 2006;66:5521–5525.

78. Vogtmann E, Levitan EB, Hale L, et al. Association between sleep and breast cancer incidence among postmenopausal women in the Women's Health Initiative. *Sleep*. 2013;36:1437–1444.

79. Kushida C, Morgenthaler TI, Littner MR, et al. Practice parameters for the treatment of snoring and Obstructive Sleep Apnea with oral appliances: an update for 2005. *Sleep*. 2006;29:240–243.

80. Zamarron C, Valdes Cuadrado L, Alvarez-Sala R. Pathophysiologic mechanisms of cardiovascular disease in obstructive sleep apnea syndrome. *Pulm Med*. 2013;2013:521087.

81. Peker Y, Hedner J, Norum J, Kraiczi H, Carlson J. Increased incidence of cardiovascular disease in

middle-aged men with obstructive sleep apnea: a 7-year follow-up. *Am J Respir Crit Care Med*. 2002;166:159–165.

82. Schillaci G, Battista F, Fiorenzano G, et al. Obstructive sleep apnea and cardiovascular disease—A new target for treatment. *Curr Pharm Des*. 2015;21:3496–3504.

83. Kushida CA, Littner MR, Morgenthaler T, et al. Practice parameters for the indications for polysomnography and related procedures: an update for 2005. *Sleep*. 2005;28:499–521.

84. Lanfranchi PA, Somers VK, Braghiroli A, Corra U, Eleuteri E, Giannuzzi P. Central sleep apnea in left ventricular dysfunction: prevalence and implications for arrhythmic risk. *Circulation*. 2003;107:727–732.

85. Cowie MR, Woehrle H, Wegscheider K, et al. Rationale and design of the SERVE-HF study: treatment of sleep-disordered breathing with predominant central sleep apnoea with adaptive servo-ventilation in patients with chronic heart failure. *Eur J Heart Fail*. 2013;15:937–943.

86. Ponikowski P, Javaheri S, Michalkiewicz D, et al. Transvenous phrenic nerve stimulation for the treatment of central sleep apnoea in heart failure. *Eur Heart J*. 2012;33:889–894.

87. Bradley TD, Logan AG, Kimoff RJ, et al. Continuous positive airway pressure for central sleep apnea and heart failure. *N Engl J Med*. 2005;353:2025–2033.

88. Arzt M, Bradley TD. Treatment of sleep apnea in heart failure. *Am J Respir Crit Care Med*. 2006;173:1300–1308.

89. Sin DD, Logan AG, Fitzgerald FS, Liu PP, Bradley TD. Effects of continuous positive airway pressure on cardiovascular outcomes in heart failure patients with and without Cheyne-Stokes respiration. *Circulation*. 2000;102:61–66.

90. Anker SD, von Haehling S, Germany R. Sleep-disordered breathing and cardiovascular disease. *Indian Heart J*. 2016;68(suppl 1):S69–S76.

91. Pafili K, Steiropoulos P, Papanas N. The relationship between obstructive sleep apnoea and coronary heart disease. *Curr Opin Cardiol*. 2015;30:439–446.

92. Kohler M, Craig S, Pepperell JC, et al. CPAP improves endothelial function in patients with minimally symptomatic OSA: results from a subset study of the MOSAIC trial. *Chest*. 2013;144:896–902.

93. Koshino Y, Villarraga HR, Orban M, et al. Changes in left and right ventricular mechanics during the Mueller maneuver in healthy adults: a possible mechanism for abnormal cardiac function in patients with obstructive sleep apnea. *Circ Cardiovasc Imaging*. 2010;3:282–289.

94. Koshino Y, Satoh M, Katayose Y, et al. Sleep apnea and ventricular arrhythmias: clinical outcome, electrophysiologic characteristics, and follow-up after catheter ablation. *J Cardiol*. 2010;55:211–216.

95. Fletcher E. The relationship between systemic hypertension and obstructive sleep apnea: facts and theory. *Am J Med*. 1995;98:118–128.

96. Lavie P, Silverberg D, Oksenberg A, Hoffstein V. Obstructive sleep apnea and hypertension: from correlative to causative relationship. *J Clin Hypertens (Greenwich)*. 2001;3:296–301.

97. Somers V, Dyken ME, Clary MP, Abboud FM. Sympathetic neural mechanisms in obstructive sleep apnea. *J Clin Invest*. 1995;96:1897–1904.

98. Phillips BG, Somers VK. Hypertension and obstructive sleep apnea. *Curr Hypertens Rep* 2003;5:380-385.

99. Kato M, Roberts-Thomson P, Phillips BG, et al. Impairment of endothelium-dependent vasodilation of resistance vessels in patients with obstructive sleep apnea. *Circulation*. 2000;102:2607–2610.

100. Phillips B, Kato M, Narkiewicz K, Choe I, VK. S. Increases in leptin levels, sympathetic drive, and weight gain in obstructive sleep apnea. *Am J Physiol Heart Circ Physiol*. 2000;279:H234–H237.

101. Banno K, MH. K. Sleep apnea: clinical investigations in humans. *Sleep Med*. 2007;8:400–426.

102. Malone S, Liu PP, Holloway R, Rutherford R, Xie A, Bradley TD. Obstructive sleep apnoea in patients with dilated cardiomyopathy: effects of continuous positive airway pressure. *Lancet*. 1991;338:1480–1484.

103. Mooe T, Franklin KA, Wiklund U, Rabben T, Holmström K. Sleep-disordered breathing and myocardial ischemia in patients with coronary artery disease. *Chest*. 2000;117:1597–1602.

104. Andreas S, Schulz R, Werner GS, Kreuzer H. Prevalence of obstructive sleep apnoea in patients with coronary artery disease. *Coron Artery Dis*. 1996;7:541–545.

105. Gami A, Howard DE, Olson EJ, Somers VK. Day-night pattern of sudden death in obstructive sleep apnea. *N Engl J Med*. 2005;352:1206–1214.

106. Zwillich C, Devlin T, White D, Douglas N, Weil J, Martin R. Bradycardia during sleep apnea. Characteristics and mechanism. *J Clin Invest*. 1982;69:1286–1292.

107. Kanagala R, Murali NS, Friedman PA, et al. Obstructive sleep apnea and the recurrence of atrial fibrillation. *Circulation*. 2003;107:2589–2594.

108. Gottlieb DJ. Sleep apnea and the risk of atrial fibrillation recurrence: structural or functional effects? *J Am Heart Assoc*. 2014;3:e000654.

109. Almendros I, Montserrat JM, Ramirez J, et al. Intermittent hypoxia enhances cancer progression in a mouse model of sleep apnoea. *Eur Respir J*. 2012;39:215–217.

110. Hakim F, Wang Y, Zhang SX, et al. Fragmented sleep accelerates tumor growth and progression through recruitment of tumor-associated macrophages and TLR4 signaling. *Cancer Res*. 2014;74:1329–1337.

111. Nieto FJ, Peppard PE, Young T, Finn L, Hla KM, Farre R. Sleep-disordered breathing and cancer mortality: results from the Wisconsin Sleep Cohort Study. *Am J Respir Crit Care Med*. 2012;186:190–194.

112. Campos-Rodriguez F, Martinez-Garcia MA, Martinez M, et al. Association between obstructive sleep apnea and cancer incidence in a large multicenter Spanish cohort. *Am J Respir Crit Care Med*. 2013;187:99–105.

113. Rada R. Obstructive sleep apnea and head and neck neoplasms. *Otolaryngol Head Neck Surg*. 2005;132:794–799.

114. Faiz SA, Balachandran D, Hessel AC, et al. Sleep-related breathing disorders in patients with tumors in the head and neck region. *Oncologist*. 2014;19:1200–1206.

115. Baessler A, Nadeem R, Harvey M, et al. Treatment for sleep apnea by continuous positive airway pressure improves levels of inflammatory markers—A meta-analysis. *J Inflamm (Lond)*. 2013;10:13.

116. Patel SR, White DP, Malhotra A, Stanchina ML, Ayas NT. Continuous positive airway pressure therapy for treating sleepiness in a diverse population with obstructive sleep apnea: results of a meta-analysis. *Arch Intern Med*. 2003;163:565–571.

117. Kaneko Y, Floras JS, Usui K, et al. Cardiovascular effects of continuous positive airway pressure in patients with heart failure and obstructive sleep apnea. *N Engl J Med*. 2003;348:1233–1241.

118. Javaheri S. Effects of continuous positive airway pressure on sleep apnea and ventricular irritability in patients with heart failure. *Circulation*. 2000;101:392–397.

119. Kim Y, Koo YS, Lee HY, Lee SY. Can continuous positive airway pressure reduce the risk of stroke in obstructive sleep apnea patients? a systematic review and meta-analysis. *PLOS ONE*. 2016;11:e0146317.

120. Yaggi HK, Mittleman MA, Bravata DM, et al. Reducing cardiovascular risk through treatment of obstructive sleep apnea: 2 methodological approaches. *Am Heart J*. 2016;172:135–143.

121. Marin JM, Carrizo SJ, Vicente E, Agusti AG. Long-term cardiovascular outcomes in men with obstructive sleep apnoea-hypopnoea with or without treatment with continuous positive airway pressure: an observational study. *Lancet*. 2005;365:1046–1053.

122. Kasai T, Narui K, Dohi T, et al. Prognosis of patients with heart failure and obstructive sleep apnea treated with continuous positive airway pressure. *Chest*. 2008;133:690–696.

123. Monreal M, Fernandez-Llamanzares J, Pereandreau J. Occult cancer in patients with venous thromboembolism: which patients, which cancers? *Thromb Haemost*. 1997;78:1316.

124. Wanscher B, Frifelt J, Silverstein-Smith C. Thrombosis caused by polyurethane double-lumen subclavian superior vena cava catheter and hemodialysis. *Crit Care Med*. 1988;16:624.

125. Salzman E, Harris W. Prevention of venous thromboembolism in orthopaedic patients. *J Bone Joint Surg*. 1976;58:903–913.

126. Dalen J, Alpert J. Natural history of pulmonary embolism. *Prog Cardiovasc Dis*. 1975;17:257–270.

127. Goldhaber S. Pulmonary embolism. *N Engl J Med*. 1998;339:93–104.

128. Carson J, Kelley M, Duff A, et al. The clinical course of pulmonary embolism. *N Engl J Med*. 1992;326:1240–1245.

129. van Beek EJ, Kuijer PM, Buller HR, Brandjes DP, Bossuyt PM, ten Cate JW. The clinical course of patients with suspected pulmonary embolism. *Arch Intern Med*. 1997;157:2593–2598.

130. Kasper W, Konstantinides S, Geibel A. Prognostic significance of right ventricular afterload stress detected by echocardiography in patients with clinically suspected pulmonary embolism. *Heart*. 1997;77:346–349.

131. Moser K. Venous thromboembolism: state of the art. *Am Rev Respir Dis*. 1990;141:235.

132. Prudoni P, Lensing A, Buller H. Deep vein thrombosis and the incidence of subsequent symptomatic cancer. *N Engl J Med*. 1992;327:1128–1133.

133. Ribeiro A, Juhlin-Dannfelt A, Brodin LA, Holmgren A, Jorfeldt L. Pulmonary embolism: relation between the degree of right ventricle overload and the extent of perfusion defects. *Am Heart J*. 1998;135:868–874.

134. Investigators TP. Tissue plasminogen activator for the treatment of acute pulmonary embolism. *Chest*. 1990;97:528.

135. Stein P, Saltzman H, Weg J. Clinical characteristics of patients with acute pulmonary embolism. *Am J Cardiol*. 1991;68:1723–1724.

136. Ferrari E, AImbert, Chevalier T, Mihoubi A. The ECG in pulmonary embolism. Predictive value of negative T waves in precordial leads—80 case reports. *Chest*. 1997;111:537–543.

137. Chan TC, Vilke GM, Pollack M, Brady WJ. Electrocardiographic manifestations: pulmonary embolism. *J Emerg Med*. 2001;21:263–270.

138. Bounameaux H, De Moerloose P, Perrier A, Miron M. D-dimer testing in suspected venous thromboembolism: an update. *QJM*. 1997;90:437–442.

139. Goldhaber S, Simons G, Elliot C. Quantitative plasma D-Dimer levels among patients undergoing pulmonary angiography for suspected pulmonary embolism. *JAMA*. 1993;270:2819.

140. Ferretti G, Byanian D, Pison J, et al. Acute pulmonary embolism: rule of helical CT in 164 poatients with intermediate probability on ventilation-perfusion scintigraphy for the diagnosis of pulmonary embolism. *Radiology*. 1998;205:453–458.

141. Garg K, Kemp J, Wojcik D. Thromboembolic disease: comparison of combined CT pulmonary angiography and venography with bilateral leg sonography in 70 patients. *AJR Am J Roentgenol*. 2000;175:997.

142. Van Rossum A, Treurnet F, Rieft G, Smith S, Schepers-Bok R. Role of spiral volumetric computed tomography in the assessment of patients with clinical suspiciaon of pulmonary embolism and abnormal ventilation-perfusion scan. *Thorax*. 1996;51:23–28.

143. Hull R, Raskob G, Ginsberg J. A noninvasive strategy for the treatment of patients with suspected pulmonary embolism. *Arch Intern Med*. 1994;154:289.

144. Remy-Jardin M, Remy J, Deschildre F, et al. Diagnosis of pulmonary embolism with spiral CT. Comparison with pulmonary angiography and scintigraphy. *Radiology*. 1996;200:699–706.

145. Konstantinides SV. 2014 ESC Guidelines on the diagnosis and management of acute pulmonary embolism. *Eur Heart J*. 2014;35:31453–146.

146. Chong BH, Chong JH. Heparin-induced thrombocytopenia. *Expert Rev Cardiovasc Ther*. 2004;2:547–559.

147. Harenberg J, Jorg I, Fenyvesi T. Heparin-induced thrombocytopenia: pathophysiology and new treatment options. *Pathophysiol Haemost Thromb*. 2002;32:289–294.

148. Goor Y, Goor O, Eldor A. Heparin-induced thrombocytopenia with thrombotic sequelae: a review. *Autoimmun Rev*. 2002;1:183–189.

149. Prudoni P, Lensing A, Builler HR, et al. Comparison of subcutaneous low-molecular-weight heparin with

intraveneous standard heparin in proximal deep-vein thrombosis. *Lancet*. 1992;339:441–445.

150. Hull R, Raskob G, Pineo GF, et al. Subcutaneous low-molecular-weight heparin compared with continous intravenous heparin in the treatment of proximal-vein thrombosis. *N Engl J Med*. 1992;26:975–982.

151. Simmoneau G, Sors H, Charbonnier B. A comparison of low-molecular-weight heparin with unfractionated heparin for acute pulmonary embolism. *N Engl J Med*. 1997;337:663–669.

152. Investigators TC. Low-molecular-weight heparin in the treatment of patients with venous thromboembolism. *N Engl J Med*. 1997;337:657–662.

153. Siragusa S, Cosmi B, Piovella F, Hirsh J, Ginsberg JS. Low-molecular-weight heparins and unfractionated heparin in the treatment of patients with acute venous thromboembolism: results of a meta-analysis. *Am J Med*. 1996;100:269–277.

154. Gould MK, Dembitzer AD, Doyle RL, Hastie TJ, Garber AM. Low-molecular-weight heparins compared with unfractionated heparin for treatment of acute deep venous thrombosis. A meta-analysis of randomized, controlled trials. *Ann Intern Med*. 1999;130:800–809.

155. Dolovich LR, Ginsberg JS, Douketis JD, Holbrook AM, Cheah G. A meta-analysis comparing low-molecular-weight heparins with unfractionated heparin in the treatment of venous thromboembolism: examining some unanswered questions regarding location of treatment, product type, and dosing frequency. *Arch Intern Med*. 2000;160:181–188.

156. Breddin HK, Hach-Wunderle V, Nakov R, Kakkar VV. Effects of a low-molecular-weight heparin on thrombus regression and recurrent thromboembolism in patients with deep-vein thrombosis. *N Engl J Med*. 2001;344:626–631.

157. Warkentin TE, Levine MN, Hirsh J, et al. Heparin-induced thrombocytopenia in patients treated with low-molecular-weight heparin or unfractionated heparin. *N Engl J Med*. 1995;332:1330–1335.

158. Norrby K. Heparin and angiogenesis: a low-molecular-weight fraction inhibits and a high-molecular-weight fraction stimulates angiogenesis systemically. *Haemostasis*. 1993;23:141–149.

159. Douketis J, Kearon C, Bates S, Duku E, Ginsberg J. Risk of fatal pulmonary embolism in patients with treated venous thromboembolism. *JAMA*. 1998;279(6):458–462.

160. Schulman S, Staffan G, MD, Margareta G. The Duration of oral anticoagulant therapy after a second episode of venous thromboembolism. *N Engl J Med*. 1997;336:393–398.

161. Dalen J, Joseph A, Hirsh J. ThrombolytictTherapy for pulmonary embolism: is it effective? Is it safe? when is it indicated? *Arch Intern Med*. 1997;157:2550–2556.

162. Thomas M, Chauhan A, More R. Pulmonary embolism-an update on thrombolytic therapy. *QJM*. 2000;93:261–267.

163. Goldhaber S, Haire W, Feldstein M. Alteplase versus heparin in acute pulmonary embolism: randomized trial assessing right-ventricular function and pulmonary perfusion. *Lancet*. 1993;341:507–511.

164. Konstantinides S. Thrombolysis in submassive pulmonary embolism? Yes. *J Thromb Haemost*. 2003;1:1127–1129.

165. Konstantinides S. The case for thrombolysis in acute major pulmonary embolism: hemodynamic benefits and beyond. *Intensive Care Med*. 2002;28:1547–1551.

166. Investigators U. Urokinase pulmonary embolism trial. Phase I results: a cooperative study. *JAMA*. 1970;214:2163–2172.

167. Konstantinides S, Geibel A, Olschewski M. Association between thrombolytic treatment and the prognosis of hemodynamically stable patients with major pulmonary embolism. *Circulation*. 1997;96:882.

168. Konstantinides S, Geibel A, Olschewski M, et al. Association between thrombolytic treatment and the prognosis of hemodynamically stable patients with major pulmonary embolism: results of a multicenter registry. *Circulation*. 1997;96:882–888.

169. Goldhaber S, Heit J, Sharma G. Randomized controlled trial of recombinant tissue plasminogen activator versus urokinase in the treatment of acute pulmonary embolism. *Lancet*. 1988;2:293–298.

170. Tapson V, Davidson C, Bauman R. Rapid thrombolysis of massive pulmonary emboli without systemic fibrinogenolysis: intra-embolic infusion of thrombolytic therapy. *Am Rev Respir Dis*. 1992;146:A719.

171. Kanter D, Mikkola K, Patel S. Thrombolytic therapy for pulmonary embolism: frequency of intracanial hemorrhage and associated risk factors. *Chest*. 1997:1241.

172. Saveyev V. Massive pulmonary embolism: embolectomy or thrombolysis. *Int Angiol*. 1985;4:137–140.

173. Clarke D, Abrams L. Pulmonary embolectomy: a 25-year experience. *J Thorac Cardiovasc Surg*. 1986;92:442.

174. Meyer G, Sors H, Charbonnier B. The European Cooperative Study Group for Pulmonary Embolism. *J Am Coll Cardiol*. 1992;19:239–245.

175. Koning R, Cribier A, Gerber L. A new treatment for severe pulmonary embolism: percutaneous rheolytic thrombectomy. *Circulation*. 1997;96:2498–2500.

176. Greenfield L, Proctor M, Williams D. Long-term experience with transvenous catheter pulmonary embolectomy. *J Vasc Surg*. 1993;18:450–457.

177. Hoeper MM, Bogaard HJ, Condliffe R, et al. Definitions and diagnosis of pulmonary hypertension. *J Am Coll Cardiol*. 2013;62:D42–D50.

178. Galie N, Simonneau G. The fifth world symposium on pulmonary hypertension. *J Am Coll Cardiol*. 2013;62:D1–D3.

179. Ghofrani HA, D'Armini AM, Grimminger F, et al. Riociguat for the treatment of chronic thromboembolic pulmonary hypertension. *N Engl J Med*. 2013;369:319–329.

180. McGoon M, Gutterman D, Steen V, et al. American College of Chest Physicians.Screening, early detection, and diagnosis of pulmonary arterial hypertension: ACCP evidence-based clinical practice guidelines. *Chest* 2004;126(suppl):14S–34S.

181. MacNee W. Pathophysiology of cor pulmonale in chronic obstructive pulmonary disease. Part two. *Am J Respir Crit Care Med*. 1994;150:1158–1168.

182. MacNee W. Pathophysiology of cor pulmonale in chronic obstructive pulmonary disease. Part One. *Am J Respir Crit Care Med*. 1994;150:833–852.

183. Ahearn G, Tapson VF, Rebeiz A, Greenfield J Jr. Electrocardiography to define clinical status in primary pulmonary hypertension and pulmonary arterial hypertension secondary to collagen vascular disease. *Chest*. 2002;122:524–527.

184. D'Alonzo G, Barst R, Ayres S, et al. Survival in patients with primary pulmonary hypertension: results for a national prospective study. *Ann Inter Med*. 1991;115:343–349.

185. Ricciardi MJ, Knight BP, Martinez FJ, Rubenfire M. Inhaled nitric oxide in primary pulmonary hypertension: a safe and effective agent for predicting response to nifedipine. *J Am Coll Cardiol*. 1998;32:1068–1073.

186. Sitbon O, Brenot F, Denjean A, et al. Inhaled nitric oxide as a screening vasodilator agent in primary pulmonary hypertension. A dose-response study and comparison with prostacyclin. *Am J Respir Crit Care Med*. 1995;151:384–389.

187. Sitbon O, Humbert M, Jaïs X, et al. Long-term response to calcium channel blockers in idiopathic pulmonary arterial hypertension. *Circulation*. 2005;111:3105–3111.

188. Rich S, Dantzker D, Ayres S, et al. Primary pulmonary hypertension: a national prospective study. *Ann Inter Med*. 1987;107:216–223.

189. Sun X, Hansen J, Oudiz R, Wasserman K. Pulmonary function in primary pulmonary hypertension. *J Am Coll Cardiol*. 2003;41:1028–1035.

190. Raeside D, Chalmers G, Clelland J, et al. Pulmonary artery pressure variation in patients with connective tisuue disease: 24 hour ambulatory pulmonary artery pressure monitoring. *Thorax*. 1998;53:857–862.

191. D'Alonzo G, Dantzker D. Gas exchange alterations following pulmonary thromboembolism. *Clin Chest Med*. 1984;5:411.

192. Worsley D, Alvari A, Aronchick J. Chest radiographic findings in patients with acute pulmonary embolism: observations from the PIOPED study. *Radiology*. 1993;189:133–136.

193. Fedullo PF, Tapson VF. Clinical practice. The evaluation of suspected pulmonary embolism. *N Engl J Med*. 2003;349:1247–1256.

194. Mousseaux E, Meunier P, Azancott S, Dubayle P, Gaux JC. Cardiac metastatic melanoma investigated by magnetic resonance imaging. *Magn Reson Imaging*. 1998;16:91–95.

195. Baggen VJ, Leiner T, Post MC, et al. Cardiac magnetic resonance findings predicting mortality in patients with pulmonary arterial hypertension: a systematic review and meta-analysis. *Eur Radiol*. 2016;26:3771–3780.

196. Nagaya N, Nishikimi T, Uematsu M, et al. Plasma brain natriuretic peptide as a prognostic indicator in patients with primary pulmonary hypertension. *Circulation*. 2000;102:865–870.

197. Leuchte H, Holzapfel M, Baumgartner RA, et al. Clinical significance of brain natriuretic peptide in primary pulmonary hypertension. *J Am Coll Cardiol*. 2004;43:764–770.

198. Andreassen A, Wergeland R, Simonsen S, Geiran O, Guevara C, Ueland T. N-terminal pro-B-type natriuretic peptide as an indicator of disease severity in a heterogeneous group of patients with chronic precapillary pulmonary hypertension. *Am J Cardiol*. 2006;98:525–529.

199. Rubin L. Current concepts: primary pulmonary hypertension. *N Engl J Med*. 1997;336(2):111–117.

200. Farber H, Loscalzo J. Pulmonary arterial hypertension. *N Engl J Med*. 2004;16:1655–1665.

201. Montani D, Bergot E, Gunther S, et al. Pulmonary arterial hypertension in patients treated by dasatinib. *Circulation*. 2012;125:2128–2137.

202. Sztrymf B, Coulet F, Girerd B, et al. Clinical outcomes of pulmonary arterial hypertension in carriers of BMPR2 mutation. *Am J Respir Crit Care Med*. 2008;177:1377–1383.

203. Rosenzweig E, Barst RJ. Pulmonary arterial hypertension in children: a medical update. *Curr Opin Pediatr*. 2008;20:288–293.

204. Elliott C, Glissmeyer EW, Havlena GT, et al. Relationship of BMPR2 mutations to vasoreactivity in pulmonary arterial hypertension. *Circulation*. 2006;113:2509–2515.

205. Castro M, Krowka M, Schroeder D. Frequency and clinical implications of increased pulmonarty artery pressures in liver transplant patients. *Mayo Clin Proc*. 1996;71:543–551.

206. Rossi S, Gilbert-Barness E, Saari T. Pulmonary hypertension with coexisting portal hypertension. *Pediatr Pathol*. 1992;12:433049.

207. Janssen H, Haagsma E, vanUum S, et al. Extrahepatic portal vein thrombosis: aetiology and determinants of survival. *Gut*. 2001;49:720–724.

208. Machado RF, Farber HW. Pulmonary hypertension associated with chronic hemolytic anemia and other blood disorders. *Clin Chest Med*. 2013;34:739–752.

209. Robalino B, Moodie D. Association between primary pulmonary hypertensionand portal hypertension: analysis of its pathophysiology and clinicial, laboratory and hemodynamic manifestions. *J Am Coll Cardiol*. 1991;17:492.

210. Sitbon O, Lascoux-Combe C, Delfraissy JF, et al. Prevalence of HIV-related pulmonary arterial hypertension in the current antiretroviral therapy era. *Am J Respir Crit Care Med*. 2008;177:108–113.

211. Degano B, Yaici A, Le Pavec J, et al. Long-term effects of bosentan in patients with HIV-associated pulmonary arterial hypertension. *Eur Respir J*. 2009;33:92–98.

212. Ghofrani H, Barst RJ, Benza RL, et al. Future perspectives for the treatment of pulmonary arterial hypertension. *J Am Coll Cardiol*. 2009;51:S108–S117.

213. Ghamra ZW, Dweik RA. Primary pulmonary hypertension: an overview of epidemiology and pathogenesis. *Cleve Clin J Med*. 2003;70:S2–S8.

214. Giaid A. Nitric oxide and endothelin-1 in pulmonary hypertension. *Chest*. 1998;114:208S–212S.

215. Chen HI, Hu CT, Wu CY, Wang D. Nitric oxide in systemic and pulmonary hypertension. *J Biomed Sci*. 1997;4:244–248.

216. Perrella MA, Edell ES, Krowka MJ, Cortese DA, Burnett JC, Jr. Endothelium-derived relaxing factor in

pulmonary and renal circulations during hypoxia. *Am J Physiol*. 1992;263:R45–R50.

217. Smith AP, Demoncheaux EA, Higenbottam TW. Nitric oxide gas decreases endothelin-1 mRNA in cultured pulmonary artery endothelial cells. *Nitric Oxide*. 2002;6:153–159.

218. Dinh-Xuan AT. Endothelial modulation of pulmonary vascular tone. *Eur Respir J*. 1992;5:757–762.

219. Millatt LJ, Whitley GS, Li D, et al. Evidence for dysregulation of dimethylarginine dimethylaminohydrolase I in chronic hypoxia-induced pulmonary hypertension. *Circulation*. 2003;108:1493–1498.

220. Mehta S, Stewart DJ, Langleben D, Levy RD. Short-term pulmonary vasodilation with L-arginine in pulmonary hypertension. *Circulation*. 1995;92:1539–1545.

221. Nagaya N, Uematsu M, Oya H, et al. Short-term oral administration of L-arginine improves hemodynamics and exercise capacity in patients with precapillary pulmonary hypertension. *Am J Respir Crit Care Med*. 2001;163:887–891.

222. Giad A, Saleh D. Expession of endothelin-1 in the lungs of patients with pulmonary hypertension. *NEJM*. 1995;1993:1732–1739.

223. Tuder RM, Voelkel NF. Angiogenesis and pulmonary hypertension: a unique process in a unique disease. *Antioxid Redox Signal*. 2002;4:833–843.

224. Mehta JL, Bryant JL, Jr., Mehta P. Reduction of nitric oxide synthase activity in human neutrophils by oxidized low-density lipoproteins. Reversal of the effect of oxidized low-density lipoproteins by high-density lipoproteins and L-arginine. *Biochem Pharmacol*. 1995; 50:1181–1185.

225. Rubin L, Badesch D, Barst R, et al. Bosentan therapy for pulmonary arterial hypertension. *N Engl J Med*. 2002;346:896–903.

226. Fagan KA, McMurtry IF, Rodman DM. Role of endothelin-1 in lung disease. *Respir Res*. 2001;2:90–101. Epub 2001 Feb 2022.

227. Eddahibi S, Humbert M, Sediame S, et al. Imbalance between platelet vascular endothelial growth factor and platelet-derived growth factor in pulmonary hypertension. Effect of prostacyclin therapy. *Am J Respir Crit Care Med*. 2000;162:1493–1499.

228. Trembath RC, Harrison R. Insights into the genetic and molecular basis of primary pulmonary hypertension. *Pediatr Res*. 2003;53:883–888.

229. Simonneau G, Gatzoulis MA, Adatia I, et al. Updated clinical classification of pulmonary hypertension. *J Am Coll Cardiol*. 2013;62:D34–D41.

230. Meyrick B, Reid L. Hypoxia and incorporation of [3H]-thymidine by cells of the rat pulmonary arteries and alveolar wall. *Am J Pathol*. 1979;96:51–70.

231. Murray T, Chken L, Marshall B. Hypoxic contraction of cultured pulmonary vascular smooth muscles. *Am J Respir Cell Mol Biol*. 1990;3:457–465.

232. Cargill R, Kiely D, Clark R, Lipworth B. Hypoxaemia and release of endothelin-1. *Thorax*. 1995;50:1308–1310.

233. Brij S, Peacock A. Cellular responses to hypoxia in the pulmonary circulation. *Thorax*. 1998;53:1075–1079.

234. Peacock A, Dawes K, Shock A. Endothelin-1 and endothelin-3 induce chemotaxis and replication of pulmonary artery fibroblasts. *Am J Respir Cell Mol Biol*. 1992;7:492–499.

235. Christman B, McPherson C, Newman J. An imbalance between the exrection of thromboxane and prostacyclin metabolites in pulmonary hypertension. *NEJM*. 1992;327:214–221.

236. Egermayer P, Town G, Peacock A. Role of serotonin in the pathogenesis of acute and chronic pulmonary hypertension. *Thorax*. 1999;54(2):161–168.

237. Johnson R, Roodman G. Hematologic manifestations of malignancy. *Dis Mon*. 1989;35(11):721–768.

238. Breuer J, Georgaraki A, Seiverding L. Increased turnover of serotonin in children with pulmonary hypertension secondary to congenital heart disease. *Pediatr Cardiol*. 1996;17:214–219.

239. Abenhaim L. Appetite suppressant drugs and the risk of primary pulmonary hypertension. *NEJM*. 1996;335:609–616.

240. Voelkel N. Appetite suppressants and pulmonary hypertension. *Thorax*. 1997;52:563–567.

241. Wagenwoort C. *Primary Pulmonary Hypertension: Pathology*. London: Chapman and Hall; 1996.

242. Loyd JE, Atkinson JB, Pietra GG, Virmani R, Newman JH. Heterogeneity of pathologic lesions in familial primary pulmonary hypertension. *Am Rev Respir Dis*. 1988;138:952–957.

243. He H, Venema VJ, Gu X, Venema RC, Marrero MB, Caldwell RB. Vascular endothelial growth factor signals endothelial cell production of nitric oxide and prostacyclin through flk-1/KDR activation of c-Src. *J Biol Chem*. 1999;274:25130–25135.

244. Tuder RM, Chacon M, Alger L, et al. Expression of angiogenesis-related molecules in plexiform lesions in severe pulmonary hypertension: evidence for a process of disordered angiogenesis. *J Pathol*. 2001;195:367–374.

245. Simonneau G, Galiè N, Rubin LJ, et al. Clinical classification of pulmonary hypertension. *J Am Coll Cardiol*. 2004;43:5S–12S.

246. Simonneau G, Robbins IM, Beghetti M, et al. Updated clinical classification of pulmonary hypertension. *J Am Coll Cardiol*. 2009;54:S43–S54.

247. Frazier A, Franks TJ, Mohammed TL, Ozbudak IH, Galvin JR. From the Archives of the AFIP: pulmonary veno-occlusive disease and pulmonary capillary hemangiomatosis. *Radiographics*. 2007;27:867–882.

248. Hackman R, Madtes D, Petersen F, Clark J. Pulmonary venoocclusive disease following bone marrow transplantation. *Transplantation*. June 1989;47:989–992.

249. Trobaugh-Lotrario A, Greffe B, Deterding R, Deutsch G, Quinones R. Pulmonary veno-occlusive disease after autologous bone marrow transplant in a child with stage IV neuroblastoma: case report and literature review. *J Pediatr Hematol Oncol*. 2003;25:405–409.

250. Swift G, Gibbs A, Campbell I. Pulmonary veno-occlusive disease and Hodgkin's lymphoma. *Eur Respir J*. 1993;6:596–598.

251. Kramer M, Estenne M, Berkman N, et al. Radiation-induced pulmonary veno-occlusive disease. *Chest.* 1993;104(4):1282–1284.

252. Mukai M, Kondo M, Bohgaki T, Notoya A, Kohno M. Pulmonary veno-occlusive disease following allogeneic peripheral blood stem cell transplantation for chronic myeloid leukaemia. *Br J Haematol.* 2003;123:1.

253. Malhotra P, Varma S, Varma N, et al. Pulmonary veno-occlusive disease as a cause for reversible pulmonary hypertension in a patient with multiple myeloma undergoing peripheral blood stem cell transplantation. *Am J Hematol.* 2005;80:164–165.

254. Gagnadoux F, Capron F, Lebeau B. Pulmonary veno-occlusive disease after neoadjuvant mitomycin chemotherapy and surgery for lung carcinoma. *Lung Cancer.* 2002;36:213–215.

255. Willems E, Canivet JL, Ghaye B, et al. Pulmonary veno-occlusive disease in myeloproliferative disorder. *Eur Respir J.* 2009;33:213–216.

256. Mandel J, Mark EJ, Hales CA. Pulmonary veno-occlusive disease. *Am J Respir Crit Care Med.* 2000;162:1964–1973.

257. Wagenvoort CA, Wagenvoort N, Takahashi T. Pulmonary veno-occlusive disease: involvement of pulmonary arteries and review of the literature. *Hum Pathol.* 1985;16:1033–1041.

258. Weiner-Kronish J, Goldstein RS, Matthay R, Biondi J, Broadus V. Lack of association of pleural effusion with chronic pulmonary arterial and right artial hypertension. *Chest.* 1987;92:967–970.

259. Swensen SJ, Tashjian JH, Myers JL, et al. Pulmonary venoocclusive disease: CT findings in eight patients. *AJR Am J Roentgenol.* 1996;167:937–940.

260. Harris P, Heath D. *Pulmonary Veno-Occlusive Disease.* Philadelphia, PA: University of Pennsylvania Press; 1986.

261. Gugnani M, Pierson C, Vanderheide R, Girgis RE. Pulmonary edema complicating prostacyclin therapy in pulmonary hypertension associated with scleroderma: a case of pulmonary capillary hemangiomatosis. *Arthritis Rheum.* 2000;43:699–703.

262. Holcomb BW Jr, Loyd JE, Ely EW, Johnson J, Robbins IM. Pulmonary veno-occlusive disease: a case series and new observations. *Chest.* 2000;118:1671–1679.

263. Oudiz R. Pulmonary hypertension associated with left-sided heart disease. *Clin Chest Med.* 2007;28:233–241, x.

264. Paulus W, Tschöpe C, Sanderson JE, et al. How to diagnose diastolic heart failure: a consensus statement on the diagnosis of heart failure with normal left ventricular ejection fraction by the Heart Failure and Echocardiography Associations of the European Society of Cardiology. *Eur Heart J.* 2007;28:2539–2550.

265. Vachiery JL, Adir Y, Barbera JA, et al. Pulmonary hypertension due to left heart diseases. *J Am Coll Cardiol.* 2013;62:D100–D108.

266. Guazzi M, Arena R, Pinkstaff S, Guazzi MD. Six months of Sildenafil therapy improves heart rate recovery in patients with heart failure. *Int J Cardiol.* 2009;136:341–343.

267. Guazzi M, Tumminello G, Di Marco F, Fiorentini C, Guazzi MD. The effects of phosphodiesterase-5 inhibition with sildenafil on pulmonary hemodynamics and diffusion capacity, exercise ventilatory efficiency, and oxygen uptake kinetics in chronic heart failure. *J Am Coll Cardiol.* 2004;44:2339–2348.

268. Palmer SM, Robinson LJ, Wang A, Gossage JR, Bashore T, Tapson VF. Massive pulmonary edema and death after prostacyclin infusion in a patient with pulmonary veno-occlusive disease. *Chest.* 1998;113:237–240.

269. Humbert MM. Update in pulmonary arterial hypertension 2007. *Am J Respir Crit Care Med.* 2008;177:574–579.

270. Chaouat A, Bugnet AS, Kadaoui N, et al. Severe pulmonary hypertension and chronic obstructive pulmonary disease. *Am J Respir Crit Care Med.* 2005;172:189–194.

271. Banno K, Walld R, Kryger MH. Increasing obesity trends in patients with sleep-disordered breathing referred to a sleep disorders center. *J Clin Sleep Med.* 2005;1:364–366.

272. Arcasoy SM, Christie JD, Ferrari VA, et al. Echocardiographic assessment of pulmonary hypertension in patients with advanced lung disease. *Am J Respir Crit Care Med.* 2003;167:735–740.

273. Weitzenblum E, Chaouat A, Canuet M, Kessler R. Pulmonary hypertension in chronic obstructive pulmonary disease and interstitial lung diseases. *Semin Respir Crit Care Med.* 2009;30:458–470.

274. Sajkov D, Wang T, Saunders NA, Bune AJ, Mcevoy RD. Continuous positive airway pressure treatment improves pulmonary hemodynamics in patients with obstructive sleep apnea. *Am J Respir Crit Care Med.* 2002;165:152–158.

275. Seeger W, Adir Y, Barbera JA, et al. Pulmonary hypertension in chronic lung diseases. *J Am Coll Cardiol.* 2013;62:D109–D116.

276. Weitzenblum E, Sautegeau A, Ehrhart M, Mammosser M, Pelletier A. Long-term oxygen therapy can reverse the progression of pulmonary hypertension in patients with chronic obstructive pulmonary disease. *Am Rev Respir Dis.* 1985;131:493–498.

277. Group NOTT. Continuous or nocturnal oxygen therapy in hypoxemic chronic obstructive lung disease. *Ann Intern Med.* 1980;93:391–398.

278. Piazza G, Goldhaber SZ. Chronic thromboembolic pulmonary hypertension. *N Engl J Med.* 2011;364:351–360.

279. Pengo V, Lensing AW, Prins MH, et al. Incidence of chronic thromboembolic pulmonary hypertension after pulmonary embolism. *N Engl J Med.* 2004;350:2257–2264.

280. Lang IM. Chronic thromboembolic pulmonary hypertension—not so rare after all. *N Engl J Med.* 2004;350:2236–2238.

281. Piovella F, D'Armini AM, Barone M, Tapson VF. Chronic thromboembolic pulmonary hypertension. *Semin Thromb Hemost.* 2006;32:848–855.

282. Condliffe R, Kiely DG, Gibbs JS, et al. Prognostic and aetiological factors in chronic thromboembolic pulmonary hypertension. *Eur Respir J.* 2009;33:332–338.

283. Kim NH, Delcroix M, Jenkins DP, et al. Chronic thromboembolic pulmonary hypertension. *J Am Coll Cardiol.* 2013;62:D92–D99.

284. Keogh A, Mayer E, Benza RL, et al. Interventional and surgical modalities of treatment in pulmonary hypertension. *J Am Coll Cardiol.* 2009;54: S67–S77.

285. Jamieson S, Kapelanski DP, Sakakibara N, et al. Pulmonary endarterectomy: experience and lessons learned in 1,500 cases. *Ann Thorac Surg*. 2003;76:1457–1462.

286. O'Connell C, Montani D, Savale L, et al. Chronic thromboembolic pulmonary hypertension. *Presse Med*. 2015;44:e409–e416.

287. Dingli D, Utz JP, Krowka MJ, Oberg AL, Tefferi A. Unexplained pulmonary hypertension in chronic myeloproliferative disorders. *Chest*. 2001;120:801–808.

288. Garcia-Manero G, Schuster SJ, Patrick H, Martinez J. Pulmonary hypertension in patients with myelofibrosis secondary to myeloproliferative diseases. *Am J Hematol*. 1999;60:130–135.

289. Guilpain P, Montani D, Damaj G, et al. Pulmonary hypertension associated with myeloproliferative disorders: a retrospective study of ten cases. *Respiration*. 2008;76:295–302.

290. Popat U, Frost A, Liu E, et al. New onset of myelofibrosis in association with pulmonary arterial hypertension. *Ann Intern Med*. 2005;143:466–467.

291. Asosingh K, Farha S, Lichtin A, et al. Pulmonary vascular disease in mice xenografted with human BM progenitors from patients with pulmonary arterial hypertension. *Blood*. 2012;120:1218–1227.

292. Yan L, Chen X, Talati M, et al. Bone Marrow-derived cells contribute to pathogenesis of pulmonary arterial hypertension. *Am J Respir Crit Care Med*. 2016 Apr 15;193(8):898–909.

293. Faiz SA, Iliescu C, Lopez-Mattei J, Patel B, Bashoura L, Popat U. Resolution of myelofibrosis associated pulmonary artery hypertension following allogeneic hematopoietic stem cell transplantation. *Pulm Circ*. 2016;6:611–613.

294. Reich J. Concurrent sarcoidosis and lung cancer. *Chest*. 2009;136:943.

295. Cohen P, Kurzrock R. Sarcoidosis and malignancy. *Clin Dermatol*. 2007;25:326–333.

296. Li J, Safford RE, Aduen JF, Heckman MG, Crook JE, Burger CD. Pulmonary hypertension and thyroid disease. *Chest*. 2007;132:793–797.

297. Kashyap AS, Kashyap S. Thyroid disease and primary pulmonary hypertension. *JAMA*. 2001;285:2853–2854.

298. Anderson M, Kriett JM, Kapelanski DP, Tarazi R, Jamieson SW. Primary pulmonary artery sarcoma: a report of six cases. *Ann Thorac Surg*. 1995;59:1487–1490.

299. Mayer E, Kriegsmann J, Gaumann A, et al. Surgical treatment of pulmonary artery sarcoma. *J Thorac Cardiovasc Surg*. 2001;121:77–82.

300. Blackmon S, Rice DC, Correa AM, et al. Management of primary pulmonary artery sarcomas. *Ann Thorac Surg*. 2009;87:977–984.

301. Bakaeen F, Jaroszewski DE, Rice DC, et al. Outcomes after surgical resection of cardiac sarcoma in the multimodality treatment era. *J Thorac Cardiovasc Surg*. 2009;137:1454–1460.

302. Kruger A, Borowski M, Horst ER, deVivie P, Theissen P, Gross-Fengels W. Symptoms, diagnosis therapy of primary sarcomas of the pulmonary artery. *Thorac Cardiovasc Surg*. 1990;38:91–95.

303. Roberts K, Hamele-Bena D, Saqi A, Stein CA, Cole RP. Pulmonary tumor embolism: a review of the literature. *Am J Med*. 2003;115:228–232.

304. Veinot J, Ford S, Price R. Subacute cor pulmonale due to tumor embolization. *Chest*. 1992;102:323–327.

305. Goldhaber S, Dricker E, Buring J, et al. Clinical suspicion of autopsy-proven thrombotic and tumor pulmonary embolism in cancer patients. *Am Heart J*. 1987;114:1432.

306. Davis S, Mirick DK, Stevens RG. Night shift work, light and night, and risk of breast cancer. *J Natl Cancer Inst*. 2001;93:1557–1562.

307. Gutierrez-Macias A, Barandiaran KE, Ercoreca FJ, De Zarate MM. Acute cor pulmonale due to microscopic tumour embolism as the first manifestation of hepatocellular carcinoma. *Eur J Gastroenterol Hepatol*. 2002;14:775–777.

308. Singh S, Nath H, Pinkard N, Alexander C. Bronchioloalveolar carcinoma causing pulmonary hypertension a unique manifestation. *AJR Am J Roentgenol*. 1994;162(1):30–32.

309. Hibbert M, Braude S. Tumour microembolism presenting as "primary pulmonary hypertension". *Thorax*. 1997;52(11):1016–1017.

310. Lee J, Kim Y, Lee K, Chung M. Tuberculous fibrosing mediastinitis: radiologic findings (letter). *AJR Am J Roentgenol*. 1996;167:1598–1599.

311. Lagerstrom C, Mitchell H, Graham B, Hammon JJ. Chronic fibrosisng mediastinitis and superior vena caval obstruction from blastomycosis. *Ann Thorac Surg*. 1992;54:764–765.

312. Mole T, Glover J, Sheppard M. Sclerosing mediastinitis: a report on 18 cases. *Thorax*. 1995;50:280–283.

313. Dechambre S, Dorzee J, Fastrez J, Hanzen C, Van Houtte P, d'Odemont J. Bronchial stenosis and sclerosing mediastinitis: an uncommon complication of external thoracici radiotherapy. *Eur Respir J*. 1998;11:1188–1190.

314. Newman JH, Fanburg BL, Archer SL, et al. Pulmonary arterial hypertension: future directions: report of a National Heart, Lung and Blood Institute/Office of Rare Diseases workshop. *Circulation*. 2004;109:2947–2952.

315. Hoeper MM, McLaughlin VV, Dalaan AM, Satoh T, Galie N. Treatment of pulmonary hypertension. *Lancet Respir Med*. 2016;4:323–336.

316. Fuster V, Steele P, Edwards W, Gersh BJ, McGoon MD, Frye RL. Primary pulmonary hypertension: Natural history and importance of thrombosis. *Circulation*. 1984;70:580–587.

317. Galie N, Humbert M, Vachiery JL, et al. 2015 ESC/ERS Guidelines for the diagnosis and treatment of pulmonary hypertension: The Joint Task Force for the Diagnosis and Treatment of Pulmonary Hypertension of the European Society of Cardiology (ESC) and the European Respiratory Society (ERS): Endorsed by: Association for European Paediatric and Congenital Cardiology (AEPC), International Society for Heart and Lung Transplantation (ISHLT). *Eur Heart J*. 2016;37:67–119.

318. Reichenberger F, Pepke-Zaba J, McNeil K, Parameshwar J, Shapiro LM. Atrial septostomy in the treatment

of severe pulmonary arterial hypertension. *Thorax.* 2003;58:797–800.

319. McNeil K, Dunning J, Morrell NW. The pulmonary physician in critical care. 13: the pulmonary circulation and right ventricular failure in the ITU. *Thorax.* 2003;58:157–162.

320. Badesch D, Tapson V, McGoon M, et al. Continuous intravenous epoprostenol for pulmonary hypertension due to the scleroderma spectrum of disease: a randomized, controlled trial. *Ann Intern Med.* 2000;132(6):425–434.

321. Hoeper M, Galle N, Simonneau G, Rubin L. New treatments for pulmonary arterial hypertension. *Am J Respir Crit Care Med.* 2002;165:1209–1216.

322. Kaarteenaho R, Kinnula V. Diffuse alveolar damage: a common phenomenon in progressive interstitial lung disorders. *Pulm Med.* 2011;2011531302. doi: 10.1155/2011/531302.

323. Higenbottam T, Kuwano K, Nemery B, Fujita Y. Understanding the mechanism of drug-associated interstitial lung disease. *Br J Cancer.* 2004;91:S31–S37.

324. Delaunois L. Mechanisms in pulmonary toxicology. *Clin Chest Med.* 2004;25:1–14.

325. Vahid B, Marik PE. Infiltrative lung diseases: complications of novel antineoplastic agents in patients with hematological malignancies. *Can Respir J.* 2008;15:211–216.

326. Sostman H, Matthay R, Putnam C. Cytotoxic drug-induced lung disease. *Am J Med.* 1977;62:371–388.

327. White D, Rankin J, Stover D. Severe bleomycin-induced pneumonitis: clinical features and response to corticosteroids. *Chest.* 1984;86:723–728.

328. Cooper JA, White D, Matthay R. Drug-induced pulmonary disease. Part 1 Cytotoxic drugs. *Adv Intern Med.* 1986;42:231–268.

329. Rossi S, Erasmus JJ, McAdams HP, Sporn TA, Goodman PC. Pulmonary drug toxicity: radiologic and pathologic manifestations. *Radiographics.* 2000;20:1245–1259.

330. Uzel I, Ozguroglu M, Uzel B, et al. Delayed onset bleomycin-induced pneumonitis. *Urology.* 2005;66:195.

331. Camus P. Interstitial lung disease in patients with non-small-cell lung cancer: causes, mechanisms and management. *Br J Cancer.* 2004;91(suppl 2):S1–S2.

332. Camus P, Bonniaud P, Fanton A, Camus C, Baudaun N, Foucher P. Drug-induced and iatrogenic infiltrative lung disease. *Clin Chest Med.* 2004;25:479–519, vi.

333. Camus P, Fanton A, Bonniaud P, Camus C, Foucher P. Interstitial lung disease induced by drugs and radiation. *Respiration.* 2004;71:301–326.

334. Camus P, Kudoh S, Ebina M. Interstitial lung disease associated with drug therapy. *Br J Cancer.* 2004;91(suppl 2):S18–S23.

335. Steijfer S. Bleomycin-induced pneumonitis. *Chest.* 2001;120:617–624.

336. Zisman DA, McCune WJ, Tino G, Lynch JP, 3rd. Drug-induced pneumonitis: the role of methotrexate. *Sarcoidosis Vasc Diffuse Lung Dis.* 2001;18:243–252.

337. Inoue A, Saijo Y, Maemondo M, et al. Severe acute interstitial pneumonia and gefitinib. *Lancet.* 2003;361:137–139.

338. Kris MG, Natale RB, Herbst RS, et al. Efficacy of gefitinib, an inhibitor of the epidermal growth factor receptor tyrosine kinase, in symptomatic patients with non-small cell lung cancer: a randomized trial. *JAMA.* 2003;290:2149–2158.

339. Read W, Mortimer J, Picus J. Severe interstitial pneumonitis associated with docetaxel administration. *Cancer.* 2002;94:847–853.

340. Ostoros G, Pretz A, Fillinger J, Soltesz I, Dome B. Fatal pulmonary fibrosis induced by paclitaxel: a case report and review of the literature. *Int J Gynecol Cancer.* 2006;16:391–393.

341. Anderson P, Höglund M, Rödjer S. Pulmonary side effects of interferon-alpha therapy in patients with hematological malignancies. *Am J Hematol.* 2003;73:54–58.

342. Wagner S, Mehta AC, Laber DA. Rituximab-induced interstitial lung disease. *Am J Hematol.* 2007;82:916–919.

343. Takano T, Ohe Y, Kusumoto M, et al. Risk factors for interstitial lung disease and predictive factors for tumor response in patients with advanced non-small cell lung cancer treated with gefitinib. *Lung Cancer.* 2004;45:93–104.

344. Niho S, Kubota K, Goto K, et al. First-line single agent treatment with gefitinib in patients with advanced non-small-cell lung cancer: a phase II study. *J Clin Oncol.* 2006;24:64–69.

345. Liu V, White DA, Zakowski MF, et al. Pulmonary toxicity associated with erlotinib. *Chest.* 2007;132:1042–1044.

346. Atkins M, Kidalgo M, Stadler WM, et al. Randomized phase II study of multiple dose levels of CCI-779, a novel mamalian target of rapamycin kinase inhibitor, in patients with advanced refractory renal cell carcinoma. *J Clin Oncol.* 2004;2004:909–918.

347. Rothenburger M, Teerling E, Bruch C, et al. Calcineurin inhibitor-free immunosuppression using everolimus (Certican) in maintenance heart transplant recipients: 6 months' follow-up. *J Heart Lung Transplant.* 2007;26:250–257.

348. Yagüe X, Soy E, Merino B, Puig J, Fabregat M, Colomer R. Interstitial pneumonitis after oxaliplatin treatment in colorectal cancer. *Clin Transl Oncol.* 2005;7:515–517.

349. Jules-Elysee K, White DA. Bleomycin-induced pulmonary toxicity. *Clinics Chest Med.* 1990;11:1–20.

350. Lombard C, Churg A, Winokur S. Pulmonary veno-occlusive disease following therapy for malignant neoplasms. *Chest.* 1987;92:871–876.

351. Yousem S, Lifson JD, Colby TV. Chemotherapy-induced eosinophilic pneumonia. Relation to bleomycin. *Chest.* 1985;88:103–106.

352. Einhorn L, Krause M, Hornback N, Furnas B. Enhanced pulmonary toxicity with bleomycin and radiotherapy in oat cell lung cancer. *Cancer.* 1976;37:2414–2416.

353. Nygaard K, Smith-Erichsen N, Hatlevoll R, Refsum SB. Pulmonary complications after bleomycin, irradiation and surgery for esophageal cancer. *Cancer.* 1978;41:17–22.

354. Catane R, Schwade J, Turrisi A. Pulmonary toxicity after radiation and bleomycin: a review. *Int J Radiat Oncol Biol Phys.* 1979;5:1513–1528.

355. Kreisman H, Wolkove N. Pulmonary toxicity of antineoplastic therapy. *Semin Oncol.* 1992;19:508–520.

356. Samuels M, Johnson D, Holoye P. Large-dose bleomycin therapy and pulmonary toxicity: a possible role of prior radiotherapy. *JAMA*. 1976;235:1117–1120.

357. Luis M, Ayuso A, Martinez G, Souto M, Ortells J. Intraoperative respiratory failure in a patient after treatment with bleomycin: previous and current intraoperative exposure to 50% oxygen. *Eur J Anaesthesiol*. 1999;16:66–68.

358. Cersosimo R, Matthews SJ, Hong WK. Bleomycin pneumonitis potentiated by oxygen administration. *Drug Intell Clin Pharm*. 1985;19:921–923.

359. Goldiner P, Rooney S. In defense of restricting oxygen in bleomycin-treated surgical patients. *Anesthesiolgy*. 1984;61:225–227.

360. Goldiner PL, Schweizer O. The hazards of anesthesia and surgery in bleomycin-treated patients. *Semin Oncol*. 1979;6:121–124.

361. Ingrassia T, Ryu JH, Trastek VF, Rosenow EC. Oxygen-exacerbated bleomycin pulmonary toxicity. *Mayo Clin Proc*. 1991;66:548.

362. Mathes DD. Bleomycin and hyperoxia exposure in the operating room. *Anesth Analg*. 1995;8:624–629.

363. Blum R, Carter S, Agre K. A clinical review of bleomycin: a new antineoplastic agent. *Cancer*. 1973:904–913.

364. Cooper J, White D, Matthay R. State of the art: drug-induced pulmonary disease. *Am Rev Respir Dis*. 1986;133:321–340.

365. Sleijfer S. Bleomycin-induced pneumonitis. *Chest*. 2001;120:617–624.

366. Comis R. Bleomycin pulmonary toxicity: current status and future directions. *Semin Oncol*. 1992:64–70.

367. Parvinen L, Kilkku P, Makinen E. Factors affecting the pulmonary toxicity of bleomycin. *Acta Radiol*. 1983;22:417–421.

368. Simpson A, Paul J, Graham J, Kaye SB. Fatal bleomycin pulmonary toxicity in the west of Scotland 1991–95; a review of patients with germ cell tumors. *Br J Cancer*. 1998;78:1061–1066.

369. Younes A, Bartlett NL, Leonard JP, et al. Brentuximab vedotin (SGN-35) for relapsed CD30–positive lymphomas. *N Engl J Med*. 2010;363:1812–1821.

370. Parish JM, Muhm JR, Leslie KO. Upper lobe pulmonary fibrosis associated with high-dose chemotherapy containing BCNU for bone marrow transplantation. *Mayo Clin Proc*. 2003;78:630–634.

371. Willenbacher W, Mumm A, Bartsch HH. Late pulmonary toxicity of bleomycin. *J Clin Oncol*. 1998;16:3205.

372. Rubio C, Hill M, O'Brien M, Cunningham D. Idiopathic pneumonia syndrome after high-dose chemotherapy for relapsed Hodgkin's disease. *Br J Cancer*. 199775(7):1044–1048.

373. Wang G, Yang K, Perng R. Life-threatening hypersensitivity pneumonitis induced by docetaxel (taxotere). *Br J Cancer*. 2001;85:1247–1250.

374. Kouroussis C, Mavroudis D, Kakolyris S, et al. High incidence of pulmonary toxicity of weekly docetaxel and gemcitabine in patients with non-small cell lung cancer: results of a dose-finding study. *Lung Cancer*. 2004;44:363–368.

375. Trojan A, Meier R, Licht A, Taverna C. Eosinophilic pneumonia after administration of fludarabine for the treatment of non-Hodgkin's lymphoma. *Ann Hematol*. 2002;81:535–537.

376. Omar L, Najia S, Robert A, Elson P, Balk R. Methotrexate pulmonary toxicity. *Expert Opin Drug Saf*. 2005;4:723–730.

377. Mahmood T, Mudad R. Pulmonary toxicity secondary to procarbazine. *Am J Clin Oncol*. 2002;25:187–188.

378. Gagnadoux F, Roiron C, Carrie E, Monnier-Cholley L, Lebeau B. Eosinophilic lung disease under chemotherapy with oxaliplatin for colorectal cancer. *Am J Clin Oncol*. 2002;25:388–390.

379. Huggins JT, Sahn SA. Drug-induced pleural disease. *Clin Chest Med*. 2004;25:141–153.

380. Jensen SA, Hasbak P, Mortensen J, Sorensen JB. Fluorouracil induces myocardial ischemia with increases of plasma brain natriuretic peptide and lactic acid but without dysfunction of left ventricle. *J Clin Oncol*. 2010;28:5280–5286.

381. Grandin EW, Ky B, Cornell RF, Carver J, Lenihan DJ. Patterns of cardiac toxicity associated with irreversible proteasome inhibition in the treatment of multiple myeloma. *J Card Fail*. 2015;21:138–144.

382. Briasoulis E, Pavlidis N. Noncardiogenic pulmonary edema: an unusual and serious complication of anticancer therapy. *Oncologist*. 2001;6:153–161.

383. Roychowdhury D, Cassidy C, Peterson P, Arning M. A report on serious pulmonary toxicity associated with gemcitabine-based therapy. *Invest New Drugs*. 2002;20:311–315.

384. Barrett DM, Teachey DT, Grupp SA. Toxicity management for patients receiving novel T-cell engaging therapies. *Curr Opin Pediatr*. 2014;26:43–49.

385. Dai H, Wang Y, Lu X, Han W. Chimeric antigen receptors modified T-cells for cancer therapy. *J Natl Cancer Inst*. 2016;108:1–15.

386. Williams LM, Fussell S, Veith RW, Nelson S, Mason CM. Pulmonary veno-occlusive disease in an adult following bone marrow transplantation. Case report and review of the literature. *Chest*. 1996;109:1388–1391.

387. Rose A. Pulmonary veno-occlusive disease after chemotherapy with bleomycin. *Hum Pathol*. 1984;15:199.

388. Doll DC, Yarbro JW. Vascular toxicity associated with antineoplastic agents. *Semin Oncol*. 1992;19:580–596.

389. Lossos I, Breuer R, Or R, et al. Bacterial pneumonia in recipients of bone marrow transplantation: a five year prospective study. *Transplantation*. 1995;60:672–678.

390. Salzman D, Adkins DR, Craig F, Freytes C, LeMaistre CF. Malignancy-associated pulmonary veno-occlusive disease: report of a case following autologous bone marrow transplantation and review. *Bone Marrow Transplant*. 1996;18:755–760.

391. Veeraraghavan S, Koss MN, Sharma OP. Pulmonary veno-occlusive disease. *Curr Opin Pulm Med*. 1999;5:310–313.

392. Vansteenkiste J, Bomans P, Verbeken EK, Nackaerts KL, Demedts MG. Fatal pulmonary veno-occlusive disease possibly related to gemcitabine. *Lung Cancer*. 2001;31:83–85.

393. Knight B, Rose AG. Pulmonary veno-occlusive disease after chemotherapy. *Thorax*. 1985;40:874–875.

394. Fruehauf S, Steiger S, Topaly J, Ho AD. Pulmonary artery hypertension during interferon-alpha therapy for chronic myelogenous leukemia. *Ann Hematol.* 2001;80:308–310.

395. Car BD, Eng VM, Lipman JM, Anderson TD. The toxicology of interleukin-12: a review. *Toxicol Pathol.* 1999;27:58–63.

396. Mattei D, Feola M, Orzan F, Mordini N, Rapezzi D, Gallamini A. Reversible dasatinib-induced pulmonary arterial hypertension and right ventricle failure in a previously allografted CML patient. *Bone Marrow Transplant.* 2009;43:967–968.

397. Montani D, Dorfmuller P, Maitre S, et al. [Pulmonary veno-occlusive disease and pulmonary capillary hemangiomatosis]. *Presse Med.* 2010;39:134–143.

398. Guignabert C, Montani D. Key roles of Src family tyrosine kinases in the integrity of the pulmonary vascular bed. *Eur Respir J.* 2013;41:3–4.

399. Guignabert C, Dorfmuller P. Pathology and pathobiology of pulmonary hypertension. *Semin Respir Crit Care Med.* 2013;34:551–559.

400. Rosenow E. Drug-induced pulmonary disease. *Dis Mon.* 1994;40:253–310.

401. Sandler A. Bevacizumab in non small cell lung cancer. *Clin Cancer Res.* 2007;13:s4613–s4616.

402. Socinski M, Novello S, Sanchez J, et al. Efficacy and safety of sunitinib in previously treated, advanced non-small cell lung cancer (NSCLC): preliminary results of a multicenter phase II trial. *J Clin Oncol (Meeting Abstracts).* 2006;24:7001.

403. Procopio G, Verzoni E, Gevorgyan A, et al. Safety and activity of sorafenib in different histotypes of advanced renal cell carcinoma. *Oncology.* 2007;73:204–209.

404. Rogers JI, Murgo A, Fontana J, Raich P. *Chemotherapy for breast cancer decreased plasma protein C and protein S. J Clin Oncol.* 1988;6:276–281.

405. Pritchard KI, Paterson AH, Paul NA, Zee B, Fine S, Pater J. Increased thromboembolic complications with concurrent tamoxifen and chemotherapy in a randomized trial of adjuvant therapy for women with breast cancer. National Cancer Institute of Canada Clinical Trials Group Breast Cancer Site Group. *J Clin Oncol.* 1996;14:2731–2737.

406. Cuzick J, Forbes J, Edwards R, et al. First results from the International Breast Cancer Intervention Study (IBIS-I): a randomised prevention trialTamoxifen for prevention of breast cancer. *Lancet.* 2002;360:817–824.

407. Fine HA, Wen PY, Maher EA, et al. Phase II trial of thalidomide and carmustine for patients with recurrent high-grade gliomas. *J Clin Oncol.* 2003;21:2299–2304.

408. Zangari M, Siegel E, Barlogie B, et al. Thrombogenic activity of doxorubicin in myeloma patients receiving thalidomide: implications for therapy. *Blood.* 2002;100:1168–1171.

409. Zonder J. Thrombotic complications of myeloma therapy. *Hematology Am Soc Hematol Educ Program.* 2006:348–355.

410. Petrelli F, Cabiddu M, Borgonovo K, Barni S. Risk of venous and arterial thromboembolic events associated with anti-EGFR agents: a meta-analysis of randomized clinical trials. *Ann Oncol.* 2012;23:1672–1679.

411. Faruque LI, Lin M, Battistella M, et al. Systematic review of the risk of adverse outcomes associated with vascular endothelial growth factor inhibitors for the treatment of cancer. *PLOS ONE.* 2014;9:e101145.

412. Shah NP, Wallis N, Farber HW, et al. Clinical features of pulmonary arterial hypertension in patients receiving dasatinib. *Am J Hematol.* 2015;90:1060–1064.

413. Valent P, Hadzijusufovic E, Schernthaner GH, Wolf D, Rea D, le Coutre P. Vascular safety issues in CML patients treated with BCR/ABL1 kinase inhibitors. *Blood.* 2015;125:901–906.

414. Iliescu C, Grines CL, Herrmann J, et al. SCAI expert consensus statement: evaluation, management, and special considerations of cardio-oncology patients in the cardiac catheterization laboratory (Endorsed by the Cardiological Society of India, and Sociedad Latino Americana de Cardiologia Intervencionista). *Catheter Cardiovasc Interv.* 2016;87:895–899.

415. Finn RS, Crown JP, Lang I, et al. The cyclin-dependent kinase 4/6 inhibitor palbociclib in combination with letrozole versus letrozole alone as first-line treatment of oestrogen receptor-positive, HER2-negative, advanced breast cancer (PALOMA-1/TRIO-18): a randomised phase 2 study. *Lancet Oncol.* 2015;16:25–35.

416. Markman M. Management of toxicities associated with the administration of taxanes. *Expert Opin Drug Saf.* 2003;2:141–146.

417. Szebeni J, Alving CR, Savay S, et al. Complement activation-related pseudoallergy caused by liposomes, micellar carriers of intravenous drugs, and radiocontrast agentsformation of complement-activating particles in aqueous solutions of Taxol: possible role in hypersensitivity reactions. *Crit Rev Ther Drug Carrier Syst.* 2001;18:567–606.

418. Cooper J. Drug-induced lung disease. *Adv Intern Med.* 1997;42:231–268.

419. Kumar K, Russo MW, Borczuk AC, et al. *Significant pulmonary toxicity associated with interferon and ribavirin therapy for hepatitis C. Am J Gastroenterol.* 2002;97:2432–2440.

420. Cordier J. Cryptogenic organising pneumonia. *Eur Respir J.* November 2006;28:422–446.

421. Crespi C, Gualandi S, Piscaglia F, Bolondi L. Onset of bronchiolitis obliterans organizing pneumonia in a liver transplant recipient under peg-interferon and ribavirin treatment. *Intern Emerg Med.* 2008;3:77–80.

422. Biehn S, Kirk D, Rivera MP, Martinez AE, Khandani AH, Orlowski RZ. Bronchiolitis obliterans with organizing pneumonia after rituximab therapy for non-Hodgkin's lymphoma. *Hematol Oncol.* 2006;24:234–237.

423. Garrido M, O'Brien A, González S, Clavero JM, Orellana E. Cryptogenic organizing pneumonitis during oxaliplatin chemotherapy for colorectal cancer: case report. *Chest.* 2007;132:1997–1999.

424. Bokemeyer C, Berger CC, Kuczyk MA, Schmoll HJ. Evaluation of long-term toxicity after chemotherapy for testicular cancer. *J Clin Oncol.* 1996;14:2923–2932.

425. Lajer H, Daugaard G. Cisplatin and hypomagnesemia. *Cancer Treat Rev.* 1999;25:47–58.

426. van den Belt-Dusebout A, Nuver J, de Wit R, et al. Long-term risk of cardiovascular disease in 5-year survivors of testicular cancer. *J Clin Oncol*. 2006;24:467–475.

427. Rice D, Smythe WR, Liao Z, et al. Dose-dependent pulmonary toxicity after postoperative intensity-modulated radiotherapy for malignant pleural mesothelioma. *Int J Radiat Oncol Biol Phys*. 2007;69:350–357.

428. Graham MV, Purdy JA, Emami B, et al. Clinical dose-volume histogram analysis for pneumonitis after 3D treatment for non-small cell lung cancer (NSCLC). *Int J Radiat Oncol Biol Phys*. 1999;45:323–329.

429. Smith JC. Radiation pneumonitis. Case report of bilateral reaction after unilaternal irradiation. *Am Rev Respir Dis*. 1964;89:264–269.

430. Gibson PG, Bryant DH, Morgan GW, et al. Radiation-induced lung injury: a hypersensitivity pneumonitis? *Ann Intern Med*. 1988;109:288–291.

431. Abratt RP, Morgan GW. Lung toxicity following chest irradiation in patients with lung cancer. *Lung Cancer*. 2002;35:103–109.

432. Bostrom A, Sjölin-Forsberg G, Wilking N, Bergh JG. Radiation recall: another call with tamoxifen. *Acta Oncol*. 1999;38:955–959.

433. Schwarte S, Wagner K, Karstens JH, Bremer M. Radiation recall pneumonitis induced by gemcitabine. *Strahlenther Onkol*. 2007;183:215–217.

434. Schweitzer V, Juillard GJ, Bajada CL, Parker RG. Radiation recall dermatitis and pneumonitis in a patient treated with paclitaxel. *Cancer*. 1995;76:1069–1072.

435. Cottin V, Frognier R, Monnot H, A L, P D, JF C. Chronic eosinophilic pneumonia after radiation therapy for breast cancer. *Eur Respir J*. November 2004;23:9–13.

436. Cornelissen R, Senan S, Antonisse IE, et al. Bronchioliti3s obliterans organizing pneumonia (BOOP) after thoracic radiotherapy for breast carcinoma. *Radiat Oncol*. 2007;2:2.

437. Movsas B, Raffin TA, Epstein AH, Link CJ Jr. Pulmonary radiation injury. *Chest*. 1997;111:1061–1076.

438. Marks LB, Yu X, Vujaskovic Z, Small W Jr, Folz R, Anscher MS. Radiation-induced lung injury. *Semin Radiat Oncol*. 2003;13:333–345.

439. Phillips TL. Effects of chemotherapy and irradiation on normal tissues. *Front Radiat Ther Oncol*. 1992;26:45–54.

440. Gayed I, Gohar S, Liao Z, McAleer M, Bassett R, SW. Y. The clinical implications of myocardial perfusion abnormalities in patients with esophageal or lung cancer after chemoradiation therapy. *Int J Cardiovasc Imaging*. 2009;25:487–495.

441. Hancock S, Donaldson SS, Hoppe RT. Cardiac disease following treatment of Hodgkin's disease in children and adolescents. *J Clin Oncol*. 1993;11:1208–1215.

442. Pepine C, Sharaf B, Andrews TC, et al. Relation between clinical, angiographic and ischemic findings at baseline and ischemia-related adverse outcomes at 1 year in the Asymptomatic Cardiac Ischemia Pilot study. ACIP Study Group. *J Am Coll Cardiol*. 1997;29:1483–1489.

443. Darby S, McGale P, Taylor CW, Peto R. Long-term mortality from heart disease and lung cancer after radiotherapy for early breast cancer: prospective cohort study of about 300,000 women in US SEER cancer registries. *Lancet Oncol*. 2005;6:557–565.

444. Tsoutsou P, Koukourakis MI, Azria D, Belkacémi Y. Optimal timing for adjuvant radiation therapy in breast cancer: a comprehensive review and perspectives. *Crit Rev Oncol Hematol*. 2009;7:102–116.

445. Myrehaug S, Pintilie M, Tsang R, et al. Cardiac morbidity following modern treatment for Hodgkin lymphoma: supra-additive cardiotoxicity of doxorubicin and radiation therapy. *Leuk Lymphoma*. 2008;49:1486–1493.

446. Gallucci G, Capobianco AM, Coccaro M, Venetucci A, Suriano V, Fusco V. Myocardial perfusion defects after radiation therapy and anthracycline chemotherapy for left breast cancer: a possible marker of microvascular damage. Three cases and review of the literature. *Tumori*. 2008;94:129–133.

447. Lu H, Cash E, Chen MH, Chin L, Manning WJ, Harris J, Bornstein B. Reduction of cardiac volume in left-breast treatment fields by respiratory maneuvers: a CT study. *Int J Radiat Oncol Biol Phys*. 2000;47:895–904.

448. Korreman S, Pedersen AN, Nøttrup TJ, Specht L, Nyström H. Breathing adapted radiotherapy for breast cancer: comparison of free breathing gating with the breath-hold technique. *Radiother Oncol*. 2005;76:311–318.

449. Corrales-Medina VF, Madjid M, Musher D. Role of acute infection in triggering acute coronary syndromes. *Lancet Infect Dis*. 2010;10:83–92.

450. Wattigney WA, Mensah GA, Croft J. Increasing trends in hospitalization for atrial fibrillation in the United States, 1985 through 1999: implications for primary prevention. *Circulation*. 2003;108:711–716.

451. Chirinos JA, Segers P. Noninvasive evaluation of left ventricular afterload: part 1: pressure and flow measurements and basic principles of wave conduction and reflection. *Hypertension*. 2010;56:555–562.

452. Musher DM, Rueda AM, Kaka AS, Mapara S. The association between pneumococcal pneumonia and acute cardiac events. *Clin Infect Dis*. 2007;45:158–165.

453. Griffin AT, Wiemken TL, Arnold FW. Risk factors for cardiovascular events in hospitalized patients with community-acquired pneumonia. *Int J Infect Dis*. 2013;17:e1125–e1129.

454. Aliberti S, Ramirez JA. Cardiac diseases complicating community-acquired pneumonia. *Curr Opin Infect Dis*. 2014;27:295–301.

455. Harrity P, Subramanion R. *Human Immunodeficiency Virus Infection Cardiac Lesions*. Stanford, CT: Appleton & Lange; 1997.

456. de Medeiros BC, de Medeiros CR, Werner B, Loddo G, Pasquini R, Bleggi-Torres LF. Disseminated toxoplasmosis after bone marrow transplantation: report of 9 cases. *Transpl Infect Dis*. 2001;3:24–28.

457. Dawis MA, Bottone EJ, Vlachos A, Burroughs MH. Unsuspected Toxoplasma gondii empyema in a bone marrow transplant recipient. *Clin Infect Dis*. 2002;34:e37–e39.

458. Pomeroy C, Filice GA. Pulmonary toxoplasmosis: a review. *Clin Infect Dis*. 1992;14:863–870.

459. Katlama C, Mouthon B, Gourdon D, Lapierre D, Rousseau F. Atovaquone as long-term suppressive

therapy for toxoplasmic encephalitis in patients with AIDS and multiple drug intolerance. Atovaquone Expanded Access Group. *Aids*. 1996;10:1107–1112.

460. Torres RA, Weinberg W, Stansell J, et al. Atovaquone for salvage treatment and suppression of toxoplasmic encephalitis in patients with AIDS. Atovaquone/Toxoplasmic Encephalitis Study Group. *Clin Infect Dis*. 1997;24:422–429.

461. Winston D, Ho W, Champlin R. Cytomegalovirus infections after allogenic bone marrow transplantation. *Rev Infect Dis*. 1990;12:S776.

462. Jules-Elysee K, Stover D, Yahalom J, White DA, Gulati SC. Pulmonary complications in lymphoma patients treated with high-dose therapy and autologous bone marrow transplantation. *Am Rev Respir Dis*. 1992;146:485.

463. Nguyen Q, Champlin R, Giralt S, et al. Late cytomegalovirus pneumonia in adult allogeneic blood and marrow transplant recipients. *Clin Infect Dis*. 1999;28:618–623.

464. Goodrich JM, Bowden RA, Fisher L, Keller C, Schoch G, Meyers JD. Ganciclovir prophylaxis to prevent cytomegalovirus disease after allogeneic marrow transplant. *Ann Intern Med*. 1993;118:173–178.

465. Boeckh M, Leisenring W, Riddell SR, et al. Late cytomegalovirus disease and mortality in recipients of allogeneic hematopoietic stem cell transplants: importance of viral load and T-cell immunity. *Blood*. 2003;101:407–414. Epub 2002 Sep 2012.

466. Boeckh M, Nichols WG, Papanicolaou G, Rubin R, Wingard JR, Zaia J. Cytomegalovirus in hematopoietic stem cell transplant recipients: current status, known challenges, and future strategies. *Biol Blood Marrow Transplant*. 2003;9:543–558.

467. Wingard JR. Viral infections in leukemia and bone marrow transplant patients. *Leuk Lymphoma*. 1993;11:115–125.

468. Reddehase MJ. The immunogenicity of human and murine cytomegaloviruses. *Curr Opin Immunol*. 2000;12:390–396.

469. Adachi N, Kiwaki K, Tsuchiya H, Migita M, Yoshimoto T, Matsuda I. Fatal cytomegalovirus myocarditis in a seronegative ALL patient. *Acta Paediatr Jpn*. 1995;37:211–216.

470. Razzouk BI, Patrick CC, Marina N. Cytomegalovirus causing pericarditis with tamponade in an adolescent with cancer. *Med Pediatr Oncol*. 1996;26:70.

471. Bowles NE, Ni J, Kearney DL, et al. Detection of viruses in myocardial tissues by polymerase chain reaction. evidence of adenovirus as a common cause of myocarditis in children and adults. *J Am Coll Cardiol*. 2003;42:466–472.

472. Flomenberg P, Babbitt J, Drobyski WR, et al. Increasing incidence of adenovirus disease in bone marrow transplant recipients. *J Infect Dis*. 1994;169:775–781.

473. Bruno B, Gooley T, Hackman RC, Davis C, Corey L, Boeckh M. Adenovirus infection in hematopoietic stem cell transplantation: effect of ganciclovir and impact on survival. *Biol Blood Marrow Transplant*. 2003;9:341–352.

474. Herzig KA, Juffs HG, Norris D, et al. A single-centre experience of post-renal transplant lymphoproliferative disorder. *Transpl Int*. 2003;16:529–536.

475. Basgoz N, Preiksaitis JK. Post-transplant lymphoproliferative disorder. *Infect Dis Clin North Am*. 1995;9:901–923.

476. Dharnidharka VR, Sullivan EK, Stablein DM, Tejani AH, Harmon WE. Risk factors for posttransplant lymphoproliferative disorder (PTLD) in pediatric kidney transplantation: a report of the North American Pediatric Renal Transplant Cooperative Study (NAPRTCS). *Transplantation*. 2001;71:1065–1068.

477. Claviez A, Tiemann M, Wagner HJ, Dreger P, Suttorp M. Epstein-Barr virus-associated post-transplant lymphoproliferative disease after bone marrow transplantation mimicking graft-versus-host disease. *Pediatr Transplant*. 2000;4:151–155.

478. Ottaviani G, Matturri L, Rossi L, Jones D. Sudden death due to lymphomatous infiltration of the cardiac conduction system. *Cardiovasc Pathol*. 2003;12:77–81.

479. Takehana H, Inomata T, Kuwao S, et al. Recurrent fulminant viral myocarditis with a short clinical course. *Circ J*. 2003;67:646–648.

480. Maisch B, Ristic AD, Portig I, Pankuweit S. Human viral cardiomyopathy. *Front Biosci*. 2003;8:s39–s67.

481. Checchia PA, Appel HJ, Kahn S, et al. Myocardial injury in children with respiratory syncytial virus infection. *Pediatr Crit Care Med*. 2000;1:146–150.

482. Alsolaiman MM, Alsolaiman F, Bassas S, Amin DK. Viral encephalitis associated with reversible asystole due to sinoatrial arrest. *South Med J*. 2001;94:540–541.

483. Anaissie EJ, Stratton SL, Dignani MC, et al. Pathogenic molds (including Aspergillus species) in hospital water distribution systems: a 3-year prospective study and clinical implications for patients with hematologic malignancies. *Blood*. 2003;101:2542–2546. Epub 2002 December 2545.

484. McWhinney P, Kibbler C, Hamon M, et al. Progress in the diagnosis and management of aspergillosis in bone marrow transplantation: 13 years' experience. *Clin Infect Dis*. 1993;17:397–404.

485. Reijula K, Tuomi T. Mycotoxins of aspergilli: exposure and health effects. *Front Biosci*. 2003;8:s232–s235.

486. Hori M, Knight L, Carvalho P, Stevens D. Aspergillar myocarditis and acute coronary artery occlusion in an Immunocompromised patient. *West J Med*. 1991;155:525–527.

487. Guiot HF, Fibbe WE, van 't Wout JW. Risk factors for fungal infection in patients with malignant hematologic disorders: implications for empirical therapy and prophylaxis. *Clin Infect Dis*. 1994;18:525–532.

488. Goodman JL, Winston DJ, Greenfield RA, et al. A controlled trial of fluconazole to prevent fungal infections in patients undergoing bone marrow transplantation. *N Engl J Med*. 1992;326:845–851.

489. Saubolle MA. Fungal pneumonias. *Semin Respir Infect*. 2000;15:162–177.

490. Martino P, Girmenia C, Venditti M, et al. Spontaneous pneumothorax complicating pulmonary mycetoma in patients with acute leukemia. *Rev Infect Dis*. 1990;12:611–617.

491. Abbott KC. Excess cardiovascular mortality in chronic dialysis patients. *Am J Kidney Dis*. 2002;40:1349–1350.

492. Aronin SI, Mukherjee SK, West JC, Cooney EL. Review of pneumococcal endocarditis in adults in the penicillin era. *Clin Infect Dis*. 1998;26:165–171.

493. Powderly WG, Stanley SL Jr, Medoff G. Pneumococcal endocarditis: report of a series and review of the literature. *Rev Infect Dis*. 1986;8:786–791.

494. Lefort A, Mainardi JL, Selton-Suty C, Casassus P, Guillevin L, Lortholary O. Streptococcus pneumoniae endocarditis in adults. A multicenter study in France in the era of penicillin resistance (1991–1998). The Pneumococcal Endocarditis Study Group. *Medicine (Baltimore)*. 2000;79:327–337.

495. Alexiou C, Langley SM, Stafford H, Haw MP, Livesey SA, Monro JL. Surgical treatment of infective mitral valve endocarditis: predictors of early and late outcome. *J Heart Valve Dis*. 2000;9:327–334.

496. Arora NS, Rochester DF. Effect of body weight and muscularity on human diaphragm muscle mass, thickness, and area. *J Appl Physiol*. 1982;52:64–70.

497. Ottery FD. Definition of standardized nutritional assessment and interventional pathways in oncology. *Nutrition*. 1996;12:S15–S19.

498. Nitenberg G, Raynard B. Nutritional support of the cancer patient: issues and dilemmas. *Crit Rev Oncol Hematol*. 2000;34:137–168.

499. Polla B, D'Antona G, Bottinelli R, Reggiani C. Respiratory muscle fibres: specialisation and plasticity. *Thorax*. 2004;59:808–817.

500. van Balkom RH, van der Heijden HF, van Herwaarden CL, Dekhuijzen PN. Corticosteroid-induced myopathy of the respiratory muscles. *Neth J Med*. 1994;45: 114–122.

501. Ito A, Kondo S, Tada K, Kitano S. Clinical development of immune checkpoint inhibitors. *Biomed Res Int*. 2015;2015:605478.

502. Fauroux B, Cordingley J, Hart N, et al. Depression of diaphragm contractility by nitrous oxide in humans. *Anesth Analg*. 2002;94:340–345, table of contents.

503. Shaw IC, Mills GH, Turnbull D. The effect of propofol on airway pressures generated by magnetic stimulation of the phrenic nerves. *Intensive Care Med*. 2002;28:891–897.

504. Mekontso DA, Boissier F, Charron C, et al. Acute cor pulmonale during protective ventilation for acute respiratory distress syndrome: prevalence, predictors, and clinical impact. *Intensive Care Med*. 2016 May;42(5):862–870.

505. Guervilly C, Forel JM, Hraiech S, et al. Right ventricular function during high-frequency oscillatory ventilation in adults with acute respiratory distress syndrome. *Crit Care Med*. 2012;40:1539–1545.

506. Marik PE, Cavallazzi R, Vasu T, Hirani A. Dynamic changes in arterial waveform derived variables and fluid responsiveness in mechanically ventilated patients: a systematic review of the literature. *Crit Care Med*. 2009;37:2642–2647.

507. Mesquida J, Kim HK, Pinsky MR. Effect of tidal volume, intrathoracic pressure, and cardiac contractility on variations in pulse pressure, stroke volume, and intrathoracic blood volume. *Intensive Care Med*. 2011;37:1672–1679.

508. Chien JY, Lin MS, Huang YC, Chien YF, Yu CJ, Yang PC. Changes in B-type natriuretic peptide improve weaning outcome predicted by spontaneous breathing trial. *Crit Care Med*. 2008;36:1421–1426.

509. Grasso S, Leone A, De Michele M, et al. Use of N-terminal pro-brain natriuretic peptide to detect acute cardiac dysfunction during weaning failure in difficult-to-wean patients with chronic obstructive pulmonary disease. *Crit Care Med*. 2007;35:96–105.

510. Zapata L, Vera P, Roglan A, Gich I, Ordonez-Llanos J, Betbese AJ. B-type natriuretic peptides for prediction and diagnosis of weaning failure from cardiac origin. *Intensive Care Med*. 2011;37:477–485.

511. Moschietto S, Doyen D, Grech L, Dellamonica J, Hyvernat H, Bernardin G. Transthoracic Echocardiography with Doppler Tissue Imaging predicts weaning failure from mechanical ventilation: evolution of the left ventricle relaxation rate during a spontaneous breathing trial is the key factor in weaning outcome. *Crit Care*. 2012;16:R81.

19 Cardiac Emergencies Among Cancer Patients

Carmen P. Escalante ■ *Sai-Ching Jim Yeung*

Managing cardiac problems among cancer patients in emergency settings is complex and challenging. Several factors that contribute to the development of malignancy—tobacco use, physical inactivity, and a high-fat diet—are also risk factors for atherosclerotic heart disease. Moreover, cancer and cancer treatments may lead directly or indirectly to myocardial dysfunction, ischemia, or dysrhythmia. A review of the causes of death among cancer patients found that 4% died of cardiac problems; of these, 90% died of atherosclerosis-related ischemic heart disease.[1] In addition to acute and chronic medical problems common among the general population, cancer patients can have cardiac problems specifically related to malignancy or cancer therapy.[2] Because cancer incidence increases with age, cancer patients may have important preexisting comorbid conditions such as hypertension, hypercholesterolemia, valvular problems, and coronary artery disease.[3] They may also have occult cardiac diseases that remain undiagnosed until they cause symptoms, usually presenting as unstable angina, myocardial dysfunction, or cardiac dysrhythmia.

GENERAL APPROACH TO CARDIAC EMERGENCIES AMONG CANCER PATIENTS

When a cancer patient presents to an emergency center or other acute care facility with an emergent cardiac problem, consideration of the status of the malignancy is essential to providing appropriate care. A suitable treatment plan should take into account the extent of the malignancy, the response to the current cancer treatment, and the overall prognosis, as well as the patient's and the family's wishes (Figure 19-1). Cancer survivors with cured or stable disease should be treated as aggressively as any other patient. For such patients, acute cardiac management, including invasive interventional treatments, should not be withheld because of a history of malignancy. However, for patients with advanced cancer and a short expected lifespan, palliative and supportive therapies are often appropriate, with the focus on enhancing patient comfort and quality of life.

Cancer patients with cardiac symptoms should be evaluated promptly with a review of the chief complaints, measurement of vital signs, and a focused physical examination. The history should include the duration, acuity, and severity of symptoms, previous cardiac problems, and a review of cardiac risk factors. Patients should have the benefits of continuous cardiac monitoring, and in most cases 12-lead electrocardiography (ECG) should be performed.

Cancer patients in an unstable condition who are appropriate candidates for cardiopulmonary resuscitation (CPR) may be treated according to standard guidelines that are readily accessible on the Internet. For patients who are not candidates for CPR, discussion of resuscitation status with the patient or his or her proxy or family members will be necessary. Resuscitation status should be discussed and confirmed, if possible, with the primary oncologist or the physician most familiar with the patient's overall health status and prognosis. Often there have been previous discussions of resuscitation status even when documentation of those discussions is not clearly discernable from the medical record.

SUDDEN CARDIOPULMONARY ARREST AMONG CANCER PATIENTS

■ Causes

Sudden cardiopulmonary arrest among cancer patients may be related to the malignancy, antineoplastic therapy, or comorbid nonmalignant diseases (e.g., coronary artery disease). A review of 28 cases of sudden death among Japanese cancer patients showed that half died of acute myocardial infarction (MI) and one third died of cancer-related complications (including cardiac involvement by cancer).[4] In some cases, identification of specific probable causes leading to the cardiopulmonary arrest may enable the physician to tailor the resuscitative efforts to fit the specific need of the patient, thereby resulting in successful resuscitation.

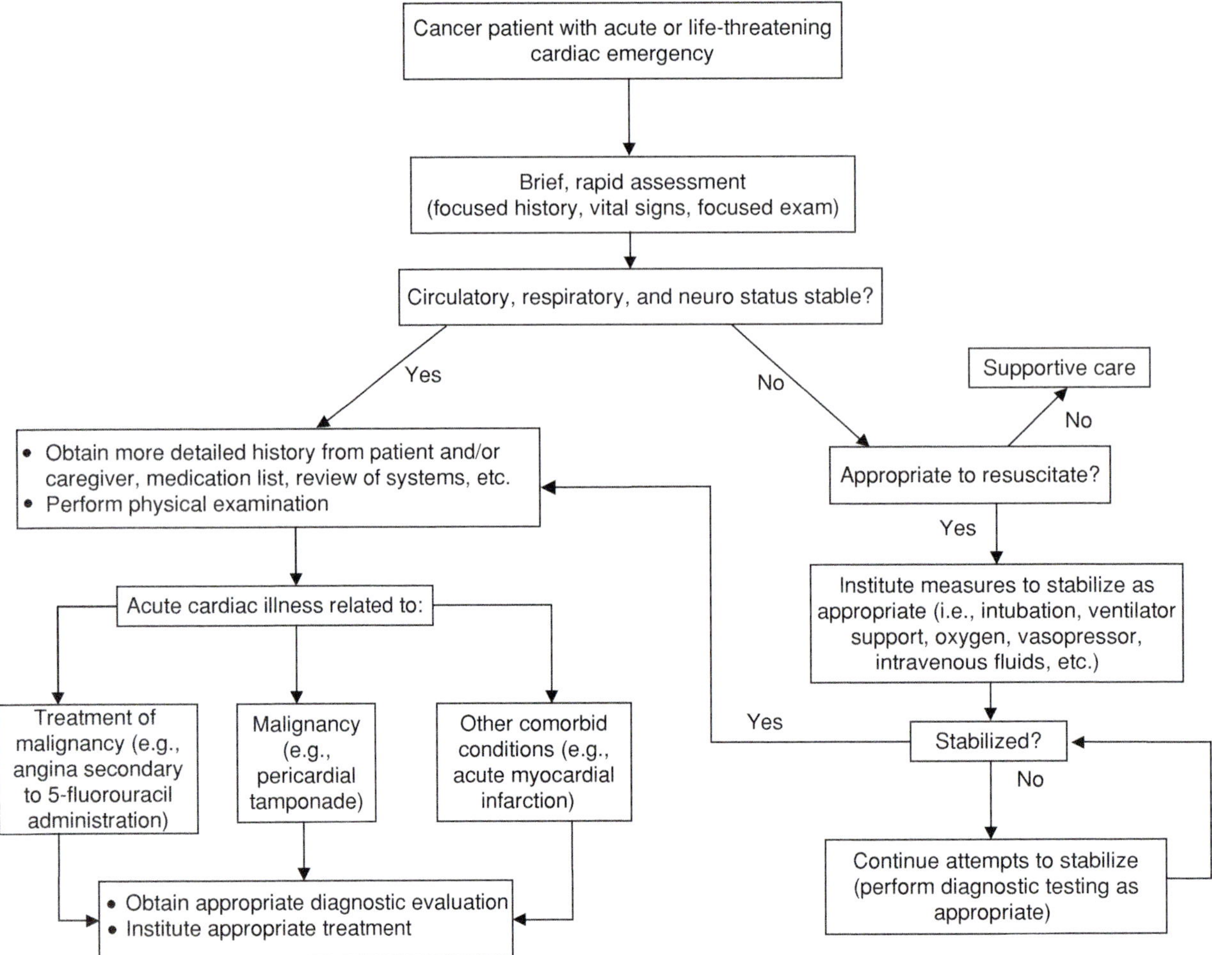

FIGURE 19-1   Approach to cardiac emergencies among cancer patients.

Tumor-related causes ■ Malignant pericardial effusion with tamponade may be the first manifestation of metastatic disease. Among patients with cardiac tamponade, knowledge or suspicion of the precipitating cause must guide the physician's resuscitative effort and focus those efforts on alleviating the mechanical impediment to cardiac filling and emptying. In cases of cardiac tamponade, resuscitative efforts will not succeed until pericardiocentesis is performed to relieve the pressure on the cardiac chambers. Pulseless electrical activity (PEA) may be an important clue to tamponade for patients with cardiac arrest and may be important in identifying the etiology; prompt recognition and intervention may be life-saving. Patients who are successfully resuscitated from cardiac arrest due to cardiac tamponade may have a relatively good short-term prognosis. However, these patients tend to experience recurrent effusion, and the long-term prognosis depends more on the extent of the metastatic disease.

Carcinoid crisis (or acute carcinoid syndrome) is an uncommon but preventable and treatable cause of cardiopulmonary arrest among cancer patients.[5] Patients with carcinoid crisis may experience refractory hypotension, dysrhythmias, and bronchospasm due to massive release of serotonin and other vasoactive peptides from the tumor.[6,7] Carcinoid crisis can be aborted or treated effectively with octreotide (Sandostatin), a somatostatin analogue. The usual dose is 150 to 500 μg given intravenously.[8] Carcinoid crisis may be precipitated by anesthesia, biopsy, surgery, chemotherapy, or adrenergic drugs (e.g., dopamine and epinephrine).

Tumors also can induce dysrhythmias by secretion of hormone mediators (e.g., pheochromocytomas can secrete catecholamines, and carcinoid tumors can secrete serotonin) or by direct mechanical irritation or compression of the heart or pericardium.[9] Dysrhythmias associated with myocardial or metastatic tumors,[10] coronary obstruction by tumor,[11] acute heart failure due to blood flow obstruction by atrial or ventricular metastasis,[12] and massive tumor embolization[13,14] have all been reported as causes of sudden cardiopulmonary arrest.

Cardiac amyloidosis can also lead to intractable congestive heart failure (CHF), dysrhythmias, conduction disturbances, and sudden death.[15–17] Other tumor-related causes of cardiopulmonary arrest include tumor- or malignancy-induced hemorrhage, malignancy-induced loss of lung function with or without secondary pulmonary hypertension, lymphangitic spread of the tumor, airway obstruction, and loss of brain stem function.[18,19]

Treatment-related causes ■ Among the treatment-related causes of cardiopulmonary arrest among patients with cancer, both chemotherapy and radiotherapy can be contributing factors.

Antineoplastic chemotherapeutic agents cannot differentiate malignant forms of cells and may cause complications that can lead to cardiopulmonary arrest.[9] Angina, MI, CHF, hypotension, dysrhythmia, and sudden death have all been reported as complications of treatment with various cytotoxic chemotherapy drugs.[20] Anthracyclines (doxorubicin, daunorubicin, epirubicin, and idarubicin), mitoxantrone, and mitomycin are known to injure cardiomyocytes, leading to cardiomyopathy. Although the long-term cardiotoxicity of anthracyclines depends on the cumulative dose,[21] these drugs may also cause acute adverse effects, and electrocardiographic and rhythm changes (mostly benign) have been noted in as many as 30% of patients treated with doxorubicin.[22,23] Sudden cardiopulmonary arrest has been reported but is exceedingly rare, despite some early reports of rates of cardiac arrest approaching 1% for patients who had received doxorubicin.[24–26] High-dose cyclophosphamide may cause acute ventricular dysrhythmia, cardiomyopathy, pericardial effusion, and cardiac arrest.[27] Fluorouracil has been associated with acute coronary vasospasm leading to angina and MI.[28,29] Vasospasm or worsening angina in a patient receiving fluorouracil can be treated with calcium channel blockers and transdermal nitroglycerin.[30] Hypotension, dysrhythmia, and sudden death have also been reported with cytokines (interleukin-2)[31] and interferons,[32] as well as with monoclonal antibodies.[33] Severe electrolyte abnormalities (hyperkalemia, hypokalemia, hypomagnesemia,[34] hypocalcemia) resulting from the toxic effects of chemotherapy (nephrotoxicity,[34] gastrointestinal toxicity such as nausea, vomiting, and diarrhea,[34] tumor lysis syndrome,[35] etc.) may also lead to cardiac arrest. Fatal ventricular arrhythmia has also been reported in rare cases of graft-versus-host disease of the heart.[36]

Irradiation of the chest can have adverse effects on the pericardium and the heart.[9,37,38] Pericarditis may occur shortly after or months to years after exposure of the chest to radiation; the symptoms may be confused with those of angina, especially when such patients are seen for the first time in an emergency center. Radiotherapy may eventually lead to pericardial effusion, tamponade, or pericardial fibrosis. Exposure of the heart to radiation may result in electrocardiographic changes, including T-wave abnormalities and atrial or, less frequently, ventricular dysrhythmias. Cardiac exposure to radiation therapy is also associated with accelerated atherosclerosis, coronary artery endarteritis, medial fibrosis, intimal proliferation, MI, and sudden death.[37,39] Patients with restrictive cardiomyopathy,[37] dysrhythmia,[40] and valvular diseases[40,41] resulting from radiation therapy may present to the emergency room months or years after irradiation of the chest.

■ Resuscitation

When cardiopulmonary arrest results from an acute potentially reversible insult (e.g., pulmonary embolus, cardiac tamponade, choking, aspiration, medication effects or toxicities, or cardiac dysrhythmia) as opposed to end-stage diseases, resuscitation is more likely to be successful.[42] The rate of successful resuscitation for cancer patients in cardiopulmonary arrest is generally lower than that for the general population, as is the likelihood that resuscitated cancer patients will be discharged from the hospital. However, such statistics are based on the population selected for resuscitation at any given institution and vary considerably.[5,43,44] A French study found that 14% of cancer patients who experienced return of spontaneous circulation after cardiac arrest survived for 6 months or longer.[45] A review of 41 patients who underwent CPR in our Emergency Center after out-of-hospital cardiac arrest found that 18 (43%) were admitted to the intensive care unit (ICU) alive but only two (4.9%) were discharged alive to their home.[46] The overall probability of surviving inpatient resuscitation is approximately one in three, and the probability of being discharged alive is one in eight.[47] Therefore, a patient who does not have end-stage cancer but who is in cardiopulmonary arrest should be resuscitated as vigorously as any noncancer patient. However, when cardiopulmonary arrest occurs as the expected final event of end-stage cancer, resuscitation will not succeed.[48]

Assessment of prognosis may be difficult or impossible when a cancer patient presents to a health care facility in cardiopulmonary arrest or impending arrest, because the physician providing the emergency care may have never seen the patient before. In such cases, the decision to initiate or continue resuscitative efforts should be based on the patient's apparent physical condition and, if known, the events leading to or preceding the cardiopulmonary arrest. Continuing resuscitation should be based on markers of outcome, including the duration of the arrest, the initial and ongoing cardiac rhythm, the presence of rigor mortis or algor mortis, the cancer-related prognosis, the prospects of cancer therapy (i.e., the options available for treating the cancer), performance status, nutritional status, comorbid conditions, patient age, potential quality of life, and expressed directives of the patient or family.[49] The fact that an ambulance is summoned to transport a dying cancer patient to an emergency center may indicate that the acute event is unexpected, that the family is not aware of or has not come to terms with the patient's terminal condition, or that the patient or family is seeking relief from suffering during the last moments of life.

Once a decision has been made to resuscitate a cancer patient who is in cardiopulmonary arrest, most physicians and health care providers follow the algorithms outlined in the advanced cardiac life support (ACLS) protocols,[50,51] with emphasis on the maintenance of airway, breathing, and circulation. However, these protocols may require modification if the patient's malignant disease severely hampers the resuscitative effort: bulky tumor in the orolaryngeal area may make intubation impossible and dictate the need for early tracheostomy; severe thrombocytopenia greatly predisposes the patient to traumatic and hemorrhagic complications of chest compressions; and extensive bone metastasis in the chest may lead to multiple fractures or flail chest during chest compressions. Fear of such complications should not be considered contraindications to resuscitation, but such preexisting conditions may dictate modifications in the standard resuscitation protocols that may be implemented with the intent of improving outcome for any individual patient. Some special circumstances of resuscitation may occur among cancer patients: anaphylaxis, electrolyte imbalance, cardiac tamponade, pulmonary embolism, and opioid overdose. These special circumstances may be handled as recommended in the American Heart Association (AHA) guidelines.[52,53] Post–cardiac arrest care[54] should be initiated if there is return of spontaneous circulation and should be continued in the ICU.

ACUTE CORONARY SYNDROME

Coronary artery disease (CAD) remains the leading cause of death in the United States, causing more deaths each year than cancer. Because cardiac and neoplastic diseases have a number of risk factors in common (e.g., old age, tobacco use, physical inactivity, high-fat diet, diabetes mellitus, and obesity), CAD and cancer often coexist. Patients with cancer frequently present with new onset of symptoms consistent with CAD or exacerbation of previously diagnosed CAD. Developing the differential diagnosis for patients with cancer who present with symptoms consistent with CAD is problematic, because symptoms are confusing. Instituting treatment for an acute cardiac problem must not be delayed, but the likelihood of a non-cardiac etiology is much higher among this population, and the risks associated with modern therapy for emergency cardiovascular care and intervention are also higher.

In the context of cardiac emergencies, the term *acute coronary syndrome* (ACS) refers to a range of acute ischemic cardiac conditions ranging from unstable angina to acute MI.[55,56] Unstable angina includes new-onset angina, angina at rest, exacerbation of angina, and postinfarction angina. Non–ST-segment elevation myocardial infarction (NSTEMI) and ST-segment elevation myocardial infarction (STEMI) are on the severe side in the spectrum of ACS.

CAUSES AND RISK FACTORS

ACS results from an imbalance between oxygen demand and supply. It may accelerate rapidly when myocardial perfusion is decreased because of thrombus formation due to atherosclerotic plaque disruption, thus resulting in narrowing of the coronary artery lumen. Acute MI results from restriction of coronary blood flow to a degree that leads to ischemic death of the myocardium. Among cancer patients, most cases of acute MI are probably secondary to atherosclerotic coronary disease and thus may respond to thrombolytic therapy. Emboli to a coronary artery can occur more frequently among cancer patients, and this form of MI should be included in the differential diagnosis of a patient presenting to the emergency room with ACS.[57,58]

Chemotherapeutic agents such as anthracyclines (doxorubicin, daunorubicin, epirubicin, and idarubicin), mitoxantrone, cyclophosphamide, fluorouracil, capecitabine, bevacizumab, trastuzumab, sunitinib, lapatinib, and sorafenib may induce cardiomyopathy.[2,59] The risk of MI is increased by antiangiogenic agents such as bevacizumab[60,61] and sunitinib.[62] Additionally, fluorouracil is known to cause myocardial ischemia secondary to coronary vasospasm.[63–67] Patients with preexisting atherosclerotic CAD appear to be more susceptible to this phenomenon. Ongoing administration of these chemotherapeutic agents should be suspended when the cancer patient presents with symptoms suggestive of ACS.

Cancer patients with anemia, fever, and infection may be more susceptible to ACS than the general population. It is unclear whether this susceptibility is purely a greater burden with respect to a fixed oxygen supply or whether other relationships are also involved. Patients undergoing radiotherapy with the radiation field overlying the heart are at higher risk of early advanced CAD or accelerated stenosis in epicardial arteries.[68] These arteries are thickened and have a smaller lumen. Microvascular injury due to irradiation causes fibrosis and ischemic cardiomyopathy.[68–72]

Other rare factors and events associated with an increased risk of acute MI among cancer patients include extreme hyperleukocytosis in leukemias,[73] hyperadrenergic stimulation due to pheochromocytoma in the presence of preexisting CAD,[74] and left atrial myxomas.[75,76] Cardiac metastases can also lead to chest pain and changes on the standard ECG that mimic those seen with acute MI.[77] Patients with metastatic cancer involving the heart may have ECG abnormalities that resemble those seen with myocardial ischemia.[78] Inverted symmetrical T waves suggesting ongoing myocardial ischemia may be seen in patients with intracranial hemorrhage.

In the absence of guidelines specific for cancer patients, risk stratification using the predictors of short-term risk of death or nonfatal MI among patients with non–ST-segment elevation (NSTE) ACS should guide the clinical management.[55]

■ Treatment

Management approaches to ACS that do not take the patient's cancer care into account may expose the patient to unnecessary invasive procedures or actions that can delay the treatment of cancer. Cancer patients presenting to an emergency center with symptoms compatible with ACS should be evaluated and treated according to the American College of Cardiology (ACC) and AHA practice guidelines (Figure 19-2).[55,56] Immediate (<10 min) assessment should include determining vital signs and oxygen saturation, establishing intravenous access, obtaining a brief targeted history, and performing a physical examination. Blood should be drawn for laboratory studies, including electrolytes, coagulation profile, and measurement of cardiac enzyme activity—e.g., a cardiac-specific troponin (troponin I) level and/or the cardiac fraction of creatine phosphokinase—with or

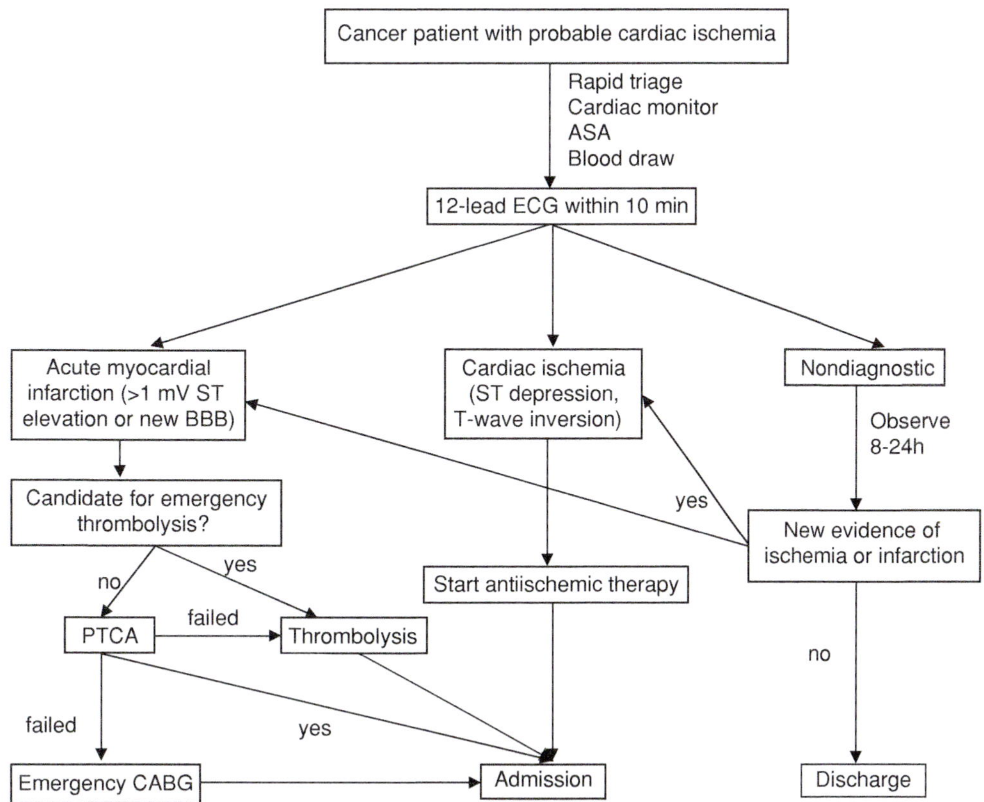

FIGURE 19-2   Emergency care of patients with acute coronary syndromes. ASA, acetylsalicylic acid; BBB, bundle branch block; CABG, coronary artery bypass grafting; ECG, electrocardiogram; PTCA, percutaneous transluminal coronary angioplasty.

without measurement of C-reactive protein levels. The patients should undergo continuous cardiac monitoring for rhythm disturbances and evidence of continued or increasing ischemia. During the assessment, potential noncardiac causes of symptoms should be carefully reviewed for the exclusion of conditions that can mimic ACS: aortic dissection, pulmonary embolism, pneumothorax, and pericarditis. If findings indicate a noncardiac cause, the appropriate evaluation should be pursued. The likelihood that the signs and symptoms indicate acute cardiac ischemia can be assessed on the basis of published ACC/AHA guidelines.[79]

The following therapies should be initiated promptly in the absence of contraindications: supplemental oxygen, sublingual nitroglycerin, morphine or another appropriate opiate for pain not eliminated by nitroglycerin, and aspirin. Nitroglycerin cannot be used if the patient has taken phosphodiesterase-5 inhibitors (sildenafil, vardenafil, and tadalafil). Ticlopidine may be an alternative if aspirin cannot be used because of true allergy. Aspirin therapy has been shown to significantly improve the 7-day survival cancer patients with ACS and thrombocytopenia ($<100,000/\mu L$) without severe bleeding complications.[80] However, the risks and benefits of antiplatelet therapies for cancer patients with ACS and severe thrombocytopenia (for instance, $<25,000/\mu L$) has not been studied. Oral β-adrenergic blockers are recommended in the absence of contraindications (overt heart failure, high risk of cardiogenic shock, bradycardia, atrioventricular [AV] block, and asthma), and intravenous loading may be indicated for refractory angina, hypertension, and tachycardia. Non-aspirin non-steroidal anti-inflammatory drugs (NSAIDs) are contraindicated for patients with ACS.

Patients with definitive or possible ACS but normal initial findings on 12-lead ECG or cardiac biomarker studies should be observed with cardiac monitoring. Serial ECG and cardiac biomarker studies should be repeated 8 to 12 hours after the onset of symptoms. If the results of these tests are normal, the patient should be scheduled for an exercise or pharmacologic stress test either before or shortly after discharge.

Patients with intermediate short-term risk of death or MI[55] should be admitted to the hospital for treatment. An early invasive strategy is preferred for patients with initially stabilized unstable angina/NSTEMI, refractory angina, or hemodynamic or electrical instability, but the decision must be individualized on the basis of the potential impact of invasive cardiac procedures on ongoing oncologic care and whether the patient would consent to or is likely to survive revascularization procedures/operations. Anticoagulation is indicated for ACS patients with intermediate or high short-term risk of death or MI. Fondaparinux and bivalirudin may be preferable to low molecular weight heparin and unfractionated heparin for cancer patients with ACS who are at high risk of bleeding. Antiplatelet therapy is also indicated for these patients. For patients with non–ST elevation ACS, aspirin (acetylsalicylic acid, ASA) should be administered shortly after initial assessment. Clopidogrel is the substitute for patients allergic to ASA, and its loading dose is 600 mg. Clopidogrel offers ischemic benefits but will increase the risk of bleeding complications for patients who require a coronary artery bypass procedure. The monoclonal antibody abciximab (c7E3 Fab) is a noncompetitive inhibitor of fibrinogen, whereas eptifibatide (a cyclic heptapeptide) and tirofiban (a nonpeptide), which are small-molecule inhibitors of the glycoprotein 2b/3a receptor, have short half-lives, giving them a rapid "on-off" effect.

Triple antiplatelet therapy with ASA, clopidogrel, and glycoprotein 2b/3a receptor inhibitors may benefit ACS patients who are at increased risk of bleeding and do not require coronary artery bypass surgery.[55] How to safely manage antiplatelet therapy for cancer patients with ACS and various degrees of thrombocytopenia requires further investigation.

Patients with clear ECG evidence of acute MI (ST-segment elevation >1 mV or new left bundle branch block) should be evaluated for immediate reperfusion therapy. When such therapy is deemed appropriate, it should be initiated immediately. Ideally, thrombolytic therapy should be administered within 30 minutes after the patient arrives in the emergency center of a hospital without percutaneous coronary intervention (PCI) capability, and percutaneous transluminal coronary angioplasty should be performed within 90 minutes after the patient arrives at the emergency center.[56] These patients should be rapidly transported out of the emergency center for early invasive or conservative management depending on their risk profiles. The risk of death due to acute MI depends greatly on the duration of symptoms. The greatest benefit of thrombolytic therapy is observed when therapy is initiated within 3 hours of the onset of symptoms, although substantial benefit is still observed if therapy is initiated within 12 hours.

For cancer patients, the risk of bleeding should be taken into account, and the status of the malignancy (presence of underlying coagulopathy, platelet count, site of tumor and location of metastases, and history of previous bleeding) should also be considered. Thrombolytic agents are contraindicated for patients with primary or metastatic brain lesions (Table 19-1). Among other subsets of cancer patients, the risk of complications associated with thrombolytic therapy is probably also increased, although definitive prospective studies of the risks for these patients have not been undertaken. For patients with acute MI, percutaneous

TABLE 19-1 Special circumstances in cardiopulmonary resuscitation

Pulmonary Embolism (PE)	Thrombolysis may be considered when arrest is suspected to be caused by PE. With confirmed PE leading to cardiac arrest, thrombolysis or surgical/mechanical embolectomy is a reasonable option. Thrombolysis can be beneficial even when chest compressions have been provided.	
Opioid Overdose	Empiric naloxone treatment is recommended for all unresponsive opioid-associated life-threatening emergencies. Resuscitative measures (high-quality chest compressions plus ventilation) should take priority over naloxone. Naloxone may be continued in postarrest care to antagonize long-acting opioids.	
Anaphylaxis	Epinephrine (0.2 to 0.5 mg intramuscularly [IM] every 5 to 15 minutes if no improvement) by IM or intravenous (IV) injection should be given early to all patients with severe systemic allergic reaction, especially hypotension, airway swelling, or difficulty breathing. Early in resuscitation, plans should be made for advanced airway management, including tracheotomy, etc. Vasogenic shock may require large-volume IV fluid resuscitation and pressors. Adjuvant medications include H_1 and H_2 antagonists, inhaled β-adrenergic agonists, and IV corticosteroids.	
Life-Threatening Electrolyte Disturbances	Empirical IV push of calcium chloride or gluconate may be considered when hyperkalemia or hypermagnesemia is suspected as the cause of cardiac arrest. For cardiotoxicity-related cardiac arrest, 1 to 2 g $MgSO_4$ IV push is recommended. For hypokalemia, IV bolus administration of potassium is not recommended.	
Cardiac Tamponade	Emergency pericardiocentesis without imaging guidance during cardiac arrest may be helpful.	

Source: Selected from the Appendix of Callaway CW, 2015[54] on the basis of relevance to cancer patients.

transluminal coronary angioplasty may be used as primary therapy, in combination with thrombolytic therapy, or as rescue therapy after failure of thrombolysis treatment. When thrombolytic therapy is contraindicated (Table 19-2), primary percutaneous transluminal coronary angioplasty may still be an option. Other pharmacotherapy should include ASA unless it is absolutely contraindicated, beta-adrenergic blockers, nitrates, and an antithrombin regimen (Table 19-3). For cancer patients with severe thrombocytopenia, the risks and benefits of antiplatelet and anticoagulation therapies should be further investigated.

DYSRHYTHMIA

As intimated above, serious dysrhythmia can deteriorate to hemodynamically unstable forms and can precipitate cardiopulmonary arrest and death. Dysrhythmia is a common problem for cancer patients and demands urgent or emergent evaluation.[9] Dysrhythmia may be related to malignancy or treatment of the malignancy, or it may be the result of other unrelated medical problems.

Symptoms of dysrhythmia also can be subtle and intermittent. When such symptoms exist, they are generally in the form of palpitations or the hemodynamic effects of the cardiac rhythm disturbance. Clinically significant signs and symptoms of these hemodynamic effects include isolated or recurrent loss of consciousness (syncope), lightheadedness, dizziness, chest pain, dyspnea, and transient or persistent acute neurological deficits. Nonhemodynamic effects include palpitations and peripheral vascular or central nervous system embolism, as well as palpitations that may be quite troublesome to the patient.

Sustained dysrhythmia can be diagnosed electrocardiographically with relative ease. However, dysrhythmia is often transient, and transient or intermittent dysrhythmia may present a diagnostic challenge. An electrocardiographic rhythm strip or a brief period of continuous monitoring does not exclude the possibility of a latent and potentially serious rhythm disturbance. When symptoms (palpitations, syncope, etc.) suggest dysrhythmia, Holter monitoring for longer periods of time in the emergency room setting is indicated to try to capture the arrhythmic events and diagnose the

TABLE 19-2   Contraindications to thrombolytic therapy

Absolute contraindications
Any previous intracranial hemorrhage
Active bleeding or bleeding diathesis (not including menses)
Structural cerebral vascular lesion or abnormality
Aortic dissection
Intracranial malignant tumors (primary or metastatic)
Ischemic cerebrovascular accident within 3 months (except acute event within 4.5 hours)
Significant closed-head or facial trauma within 3 months
Intracranial or intraspinal surgery within 2 months
Severe uncontrolled hypertension (unresponsive to emergency therapy)
For streptokinase, previous treatment within the previous 6 months
Known allergy to thrombolytic drugs
Relative contraindications
Active peptic ulcer disease
Anticoagulation
Major surgery within 3 weeks
Ischemic cerebrovascular accident >3 months before presentation, dementia, or other known intracranial pathology
Pregnancy
Traumatic or prolonged cardiopulmonary resuscitation (>10 min)
History of chronic, severe, poorly controlled hypertension
Severe uncontrolled hypertension at presentation (>180/110 mmHg)
Internal bleeding within 2–4 weeks
Vascular puncture at noncompressible sites

Source: Table based on O'Gara et al, 2013.[126]

TABLE 19-3   Medications for the acute management of myocardial infarction

DRUG	INITIAL DOSE
Platelet aggregation inhibitors	
Aspirin	160 to 325 mg orally in the emergency room Tablets should be chewed if enteric-coated
Clopidogrel	Loading dose 600 mg orally
Prasugrel	60 mg as early as possible
Ticagrelor	180 mg as early as possible
Eptifibatide	(double bolus) IV bolus of 180 µg/kg followed by an infusion of 2 µg/kg/min; a second 180 µg/kg bolus is administered 10 min after the first bolus
Ticlopidine	250 mg po
Tirofiban	(high-bolus dose) 25-mcg/kg IV bolus, then 0.15 µg/kg/min
Abciximab	0.25 mg/kg IV bolus administered 10-60 minutes before PCI, followed by 0.125 µg/kg/min IV (maximum 10 µg/min)

DRUG	INITIAL DOSE
β-adrenergic receptor antagonists	
Esmolol	A 1-minute loading dose of 500 μg/kg IV followed by infusion of 50 to 150 μg/kg/min; titrate to achieve 30% reductions in heart rate and derived rate-pressure products
Metoprolol tartrate	5 mg IV every 5 minutes up to 15 mg IV total as tolerated; titrate to heart rate and BP
Propranolol	5 to 8 mg IV at <1 mg/min
Thrombolytics	
Tenecteplase	Single IV weight-based bolus
Recombinant human tissue plasminogen activator (Alteplase)	15 mg IV bolus; 0.75 mg/kg over 30 min (maximum 50 mg), then 0.5 mg/kg over 60 min IV up to a total of 100 mg
Reteplase	10 units IV bolus followed by a second 10-unit IV bolus given 30 min apart
Streptokinase	1.5 million units over 30 to 60 min IV
Anti-thrombotic therapy	
Fondaparinux	Not recommended as a sole anticoagulant for primary PCI; 1 mg/kg subcutaneously every 12 h;
Enoxaparin	0.3 mg/kg IV if the last subcutaneous dose was >8 h before PCI
Unfractionated heparin	With GP IIb/IIIa receptor antagonist: IV bolus 50 to 70 units/kg With no GP IIb/IIIa receptor antagonist: IV bolus 70 to 100 units/kg
Nitrates	
Ongoing chest pain	0.4 mg sublingually every 5 min up to 3 doses as BP allows
IV nitroglycerin for acute myocardial infarction, congestive heart failure, persistent ischemic chest pain, or hypertension	IV infusion at 10 μg/min; titrate to desired BP effect
Angiotensin-converting enzyme inhibitors	
Captopril	6.25–12.5 mg po tid to start; titrate to 25–50 mg tid as tolerated
Enalapril	1 mg enalapril IV over 2 hours; then 5 to 20 mg/day
Lisinopril	2.5–5 mg/d to start; titrate to 10 mg/d or higher as tolerated
Ramipril	2.5 mg bid to start; titrate to 5 mg po bid as tolerated
Morphine	4–8 mg IV initially, with lower doses in elderly; 2–8 mg IV every 5–15 min if needed

Sources: Table based on O'Gara et al, 2013[126]; Ryan et al, 1999[127]

bid, two times per day; BP, blood pressure; GP, glycoprotein; IV, intravenous; PCI, percutaneous coronary intervention; po, by mouth; tid, three times per day problem. Analysis of cardiac rhythm may be more complicated for cancer patients than for those without malignancy because cancer patients often exhibit exaggerated respiratory variations of the electrical axis and because changes in both mean QRS and P-wave voltage and axis can be confused with heart rhythm disturbances. Such changes may be due to pleural or pericardial effusions, pulmonary surgery (pneumonectomy or lobectomy), or radiation-induced lung damage.

■ Causes

Primary dysrhythmia, arising from cardiac and pericardial involvement, may be focal or diffuse. Myocardial ischemia; increased intracardiac pressure and wall stress; congestive, hypertrophic, and infiltrative cardiomyopathy; and fibrosis related to aging are common causes of primary dysrhythmia for all patients. Among cancer patients, dysrhythmia can also be caused by primary or metastatic malignant intracardiac tumors,[81,82] amyloid infiltration,[83] myocarditis,[84] pericarditis,[85] pericardial constriction,[86] and cardiomyopathy related to antitumor agents, especially anthracyclines.[22]

Secondary dysrhythmia can be caused by general toxic reactions to drugs[87]; increased sympathetic states, such as those related to severe anxiety, hyperthyroidism, and mediator release (pheochromocytoma and carcinoid tumors)[9]; derangements of electrolyte metabolism[9]; and radiation-induced damage to the heart.[86] Some cancer drugs are especially arrhythmogenic (Table 19-4); in addition, many cancer patients are treated with antifungal agents,[88–91] antiprotozoans,[92] antibiotics,[93,94] and opioids (e.g., methadone), which have also been reported to be associated with rhythm disturbances.

■ Treatment

Therapy for dysrhythmia should be based on both urgency and etiology. In the case of hemodynamically stable secondary dysrhythmias, immediate measures should consist of restoration of normal body chemistry through correction of metabolic derangements (particularly homeostasis of potassium, calcium, and magnesium) and removal of culprit drugs or substances. Specific treatment aimed at reversing the causative factor should be initiated. When treatment aimed at controlling the cardiac rhythm is believed to be necessary, standard guidelines for management of dysrhythmia should be followed. Commonly used antiarrhythmic drugs are listed in Table 19-5.

Paroxysmal supraventricular tachycardia may be reverted to sinus rhythm in some cases by carotid sinus massage or other vagal maneuvers. Adenosine administered as one or two rapidly infused boluses under electrocardiographic monitoring is frequently effective in restoring sinus rhythm. The drug may also be used to help determine the mechanism of the dysrhythmia when the nature of the disturbance is unclear from electrocardiographic rhythm or monitoring strips. Careful analysis of standard ECGs usually obviates the use of adenosine as a diagnostic tool.

Primary dysrhythmia ■ Dysrhythmias that originate from structural cardiac abnormalities are much more difficult to control than dysrhythmias of metabolic etiology, especially for cancer patients. Such primary dysrhythmias are likely to persist over long periods and to progress to high-grade and life-threatening dysrhythmias. In the emergency setting, therapeutic goals are geared towards stabilizing the hemodynamic and respiratory status, discovering correctable pathologies, and controlling the symptoms. Emergent consultation with cardiologists and emergent diagnostic or interventional procedures may be necessary.

Patients in an unstable condition should be treated with aggressive pharmacological or electrical interventions, and such interventions should generally follow established algorithms or guidelines set by the AHA.[95] These interventions include administration of a vasopressor such as vasopressin or epinephrine to support blood pressure (if necessary); administration of antiarrhythmic drugs, such as amiodarone, lidocaine, and procainamide hydrochloride; electrical cardioversion or defibrillation; airway management; ventilation with oxygen; administration of intravenous fluid; and chest compression (if necessary). Emergency treatment of torsades de pointes differs from the standard treatment for other types of ventricular tachycardia and entails expedient administration of intravenous magnesium, electrical cardioversion, electrical overdrive pacing, or pharmacological overdrive pacing with isoproterenol, as well as the administration of phenytoin or lidocaine.[96]

Secondary dysrhythmia ■ Stable secondary dysrhythmia is unlikely to deteriorate into a life-threatening or catastrophic problem. Frequently, secondary dysrhythmia presents as either ventricular ectopy, in bigeminy, trigeminy or other coupled patterns, or as supraventricular ectopy, most often as intermittent or sustained supraventricular tachycardia. Isolated premature ventricular complexes do not necessarily require treatment. Beta-adrenergic blockers may help correct these arrhythmias. When control with a beta-blocker is not satisfactory and additional intervention is needed, antiarrhythmic agents such as propafenone and acebutolol are sometimes preferred over amiodarone, which has an extremely long pharmacokinetic half-life. Nevertheless, amiodarone

TABLE 19-4 Chemotherapeutic drugs associated with dysrhythmias and other cardiac problems

	A FIB/ A FLUT/ SVT	AVB	BRADYCARDIA	V FIB/ VT	↑QTC/ TORSADE	HTN	ACS/ MI	PE	CHF	MYOCARDITIS	PERICARDITIS/ EFFUSION
Alkylating agents											
Busulfan	x	x									x
Cisplatin	x	x	x						x		
Cyclophosphamide	x		x	x			x		x	x	x
Mitomycin									x		
Antimetabolites											
Capecitabine				x			x				
Fluorouracil	x			x			x				
Gemcitabine	x						x		x		
Methotrexate							x	x			x
Fludarabine									x		x
Cytarabine									x		
Anthracyclines											
Daunorubicin		x							x	x	x
Doxorubicin	x		x	x	x				x		
Mitoxantrone	x						x		x		
Idarubicin	x						x		x		
Epirubicin		x	x	x					x		
Antimicrotubule agents											
Docetaxel	x		x				x		x		
Paclitaxel	x	x	x	x			x	x	x		
Vinorelbine							x				
Vincristine							x				
Vinblastine							x				

(continued)

TABLE 19-4 Chemotherapeutic drugs associated with dysrhythmias and other cardiac problems (*continued*)

	A FIB/ A FLUT/ SVT	AVB	BRADYCARDIA	V FIB/ VT	↑QTC/ TORSADE	HTN	ACS/ MI	PE	CHF	MYOCARDITIS	PERICARDITIS/ EFFUSION
HER2 blockers											
Lapatinib				x			x		x		
Trastuzumab	x								x		
Pertuzumab									x		
Antiangiogenic agents											
Bevacizumab						x	x	x	x		
Sunitinib	x				x	x	x	x	x		
Sorafenib				x	x	x	x		x		
Pazopanib			x		x	x					
Thalidomide	x	x	x	x			x	x	x		x
Lenalidomide	x						x	x	x		
Pomalidomide	x						x	x	x		
Other TKIs											
Imatinib	x				x	x	x		x		
Erlotinib					x						
Nilotinib					x	x					
Dasatinib					x		x		x		x
Crizotinib			x		x			x			
Ceritinib			x		x						x
Lenvatinib				x		x	x		x		
Pazopanib			x	x		x	x		x		
Ponatinib	x	x	x			x	x	x	x		
Vemurafenib	x				x						
Vandetanib					x	x			x		
Proteasome inhibitors											
Bortezomib	x	x	x	x	x		x		x		x
Carfilzomib	x						x		x		x

	A FIB/ A FLUT/ SVT	AVB	BRADYCARDIA	V FIB/ VT	↑QTC/ TORSADE	HTN	ACS/ MI	PE	CHF	MYOCARDITIS	PERICARDITIS/ EFFUSION
Miscellaneous											
Arsenic Trioxide				x	x						
Alemtuzumab		x							x		
Rituximab	x			x							
Interferon-gamma	x	x		x			x		x		x
Interleukin-2	x		x	x			x			x	x
Irinotecan			x					x			
Tretinoin			x			x	x		x	x	x
Panobinostat					x		x				
Ipilimumab										x	x

QTc, prolongation of QT corrected; A Fib, atrial fibrillation; A Flut, atrial flutter; AVB, atrial ventricular block; BBB, bundle branch block; CHF, congestive heart failure; HER2, human epidermal growth factor receptor 2; HTN, hypertension; MI, myocardial infarction; PVC, premature ventricular contraction; PE, pulmonary embolism; SVT, supraventricular tachycardia; TKI, tyrosine kinase inhibitor; V Fib, ventricular fibrillation; VT, ventricular tachycardia

TABLE 19-5 Commonly used intravenous antiarrhythmic drugs

NAME	CLASS	DOSE	INDICATION
Adenosine	Nucleoside	6 mg IV over <3 sec followed by normal saline 20-ml bolus; second dose and third dose of 12 mg 2 min apart prn	Narrow complex PSVT; PSVT due to atrioventricular node or sinus node reentry
Amiodarone	Class III antiarrhythmic	Cardiac arrest: 300 mg IVP; 150 mg IVP q 3 to 5 min up to 2.2 g/day Stable wide complex tachycardia: 150 mg IV over 10 min; repeat q 10 min prn; maintenance infusion 0.5 mg/min; up to 2.2 g/day	Supraventricular or ventricular tachydysrhythmias; control of rapid atrial tachydysrhythmia in patients with low left ventricular ejection fraction when digoxin is ineffective
Atropine	Anticholinergic	0.5 to 1 mg IVP q 3 to 5 min prn up to 0.04 mg/kg	Symptomatic sinus bradycardia; Mobitz type I atrioventricular block; asystole
Digoxin	Digitalis glycoside	Loading dose: 10 to 15 μg/kg lean body weight in divided doses	To slow ventricular response in atrial fibrillation or atrial flutter; PSVT
Diltiazem	Calcium channel blocker	0.25 mg/kg IV over 2 min; second dose 0.35 mg/kg IV over 2 min, 15 min later prn; maintenance: 5 to 15 mg/h by titration	To slow ventricular response in atrial fibrillation or atrial flutter; PSVT; to terminate atrioventricular nodal reentrant tachycardia
Esmolol	β-blocker	0.5 mg/kg over 1 min; then infuse at 0.05 mg/kg/min; titrate up to maximum of 0.3 mg/kg/min	PSVT, atrial fibrillation or atrial flutter; reduce incidence of ventricular fibrillation in myocardial infarction or unstable angina
Ibutilide	Class III antiarrhythmic	1 mg IV over 10 min; repeat in 10 min prn	Supraventricular tachycardia including atrial fibrillation or flutter; effective for conversion of atrial fibrillation or flutter of relatively brief duration
Isoproterenol	β-agonist	Infuse 2 to 10 μg/min titrate	Symptomatic bradycardia; torsades de pointes refractory to magnesium; β-blocker overdose

NAME	CLASS	DOSE	INDICATION
Lidocaine	Local anesthetic	1 to 1.5 mg/kg IVP; repeat 0.5 to 0.75 mg/kg IVP q 5 to 10 min up to total of 3 mg/kg prn; maintenance: 30 to 50 µg/kg/min IV	Ventricular tachycardia or ventricular fibrillation; wide-complex tachycardia; significant ventricular ectopy; torsades de pointes
Metoprolol	β-blocker	5 mg slow IVP q 5 min up to a total of 15 mg	PSVT, atrial fibrillation or atrial flutter; reduce incidence of ventricular fibrillation in myocardial infarction or unstable angina
Procainamide hydrochloride	Class IA antiarrhythmic	20 to 50 mg/min up to a total dose of 17 mg/kg	Recurrent ventricular fibrillation or ventricular tachycardia
Propranolol	β-blocker	0.1 mg/kg slow IVP in 3 divided doses 2 to 3 min apart	PSVT, atrial fibrillation, or atrial flutter; reduce incidence of ventricular fibrillation in myocardial infarction or unstable angina
Quinidine gluconate	Class IA antiarrhythmic	Intermittent bolus doses of 80 mg every 5 to 10 min or 10 mg/min IV infusion up to 400 mg	Supraventricular and ventricular dysrhythmias
Verapamil	Calcium channel blocker	2.5 to 5 mg IV over 2 min; repeat q 15 to 30 min prn up to a total of 20 mg	PSVT, atrial fibrillation, or atrial flutter

IV, intravenous; IVP, intravenous push; prn, as needed; PSVT, paroxysmal supraventricular tachycardia; q, every

should be considered when short-acting agents have failed or when patients exhibit a low left-ventricular ejection fraction. However, amiodarone should be administered with caution to patients with hepatic insufficiency and patients with underlying thyroid disease.[97] Amiodarone may occasionally cause hypotension, bradycardia, and QT prolongation that may precipitate episodes of torsades de pointes.[97] Except for beta-adrenergic blockers, many antiarrhythmic drugs—especially those in classes IA, IC, and III—are also potentially proarrhythmic.[98] Cardiac monitoring should be performed during the initiation of antiarrhythmic therapy because of cancer patients' increased susceptibility to proarrhythmic adverse effects resulting from preexisting metabolic derangements and the concomitant use of or exposure to other proarrhythmic agents.

Supraventricular tachycardia is the most common dysrhythmia among cancer patients. Sustained supraventricular dysrhythmia among cancer patients is often difficult to correct with drug therapy.[99] Although pharmacological agents are used to regulate or terminate the abnormal heart rhythm, elective, synchronized cardioversion under short-acting general anesthesia should be considered early and planned appropriately when pharmacologic agents are not successful.[100] The initial energy level recommended by the AHA for cardioversion is 100 Joules, but this level may not be high enough to convert atrial fibrillation. Higher energy levels (>200 J) for cardioversion may be appropriate for cancer patients who have concomitant effusions or fluid retention, and for those who are substantially overweight.[101] Lower initial shock energy levels (i.e., 50 to 100 J) may be used to convert atrial flutter. If sinus rhythm can be restored within 48 hours of the onset of supraventricular tachycardia, anticoagulation therapy may be unnecessary. In the absence of clear evidence as to the time of onset of dysrhythmia, anticoagulation therapy should be administered before cardioversion. Transesophageal echocardiography may exclude the presence of intracardiac thrombi before elective synchronized cardioversion.[102]

ACUTE HEART FAILURE

Acute failure of cardiac pump function may be precipitated by a variety of factors, including severe hypertension, cardiac ischemia, MI, dysrhythmia, flow obstruction by tumor, pulmonary embolism, pericardial tamponade, and valvular failure. Heart failure among cancer patients may or may not be related to cancer therapy. Many cancer patients are elderly, with preexisting valvular problems or ischemic cardiomyopathy. Cardiotoxic chemotherapy can decrease cardiac contractility (Table 19-4). Radiation therapy can cause heart attack and heart failure. Immunotherapy with antibodies that target immune checkpoints has been reported to cause autoimmune myocarditis.[103,104]

The cardinal symptoms of decompensated CHF are fatigue, dyspnea, orthopnea, and peripheral edema. Among cancer patients, these same symptoms may also be caused by a variety of other factors, such as pulmonary diseases, airway obstruction, hypoalbuminemia, and portal hypertension. In the general population, approximately 30% of patients with CHF also have CAD,[105] and morbidity and mortality rates are higher for these patients than for those without CAD.

In the diagnosis of acute CHF, physical examination, ECG, chest radiography, and measurement of cardiac enzyme activity and brain natriuretic peptide (B-type natriuretic peptide, BNP) levels are helpful. On physical examination, signs suggestive of CHF may include severe changes in blood pressure, jugular venous distention, bibasilar rales on lung auscultation, diastolic (S3) or presystolic (S4) heart sounds on cardiac auscultation, cardiac murmurs, hepatojugular reflux, and dependent peripheral edema. The ECG provides information about evidence of active myocardial ischemia or old MIs. Chest radiography is helpful for detecting pulmonary causes of symptoms and may provide radiologic evidence of cardiogenic pulmonary edema. Measurement of cardiac enzyme activity may reveal myocardial damage, and BNP levels are diagnostic of CHF.[106–108] BNP measurements are highly sensitive but only moderate specific in the detection of CHF.[109] Echocardiography is extremely valuable in confirming the diagnosis of CHF and often aids in determining the etiology.

Patients with CHF and symptoms consistent with severe hypertension, hypotension, cardiac ischemia, hypoxia, or dysrhythmias should be promptly moved to a critical care area in the emergency center. Monitoring of cardiac rhythm, blood pressure, and pulse oximetry should be initiated. The management of acute CHF in the emergency setting is a clinical challenge. Supplemental oxygen and intravenous access should be initiated. Therapy should be aimed at improving hemodynamic function and may include diuretics, inotropic agents, vasodilators, and natriuretic peptides. The administration of nitrates (e.g., nitroglycerin) and a loop diuretic may induce the resolution of acute symptoms and hemodynamic dysfunction. Nesiritide is not recommended for routine use for patients with acute decompensated heart failure.[110] New pharmacotherapy for chronic heart failure includes ivabradine (an I_f channel blocker) and sacubitril/valsartan (angiotensin-receptor neprilysin inhibitors), but their roles in the acute management of heart failure among cancer patients are not clear. For patients with acute CHF and pulmonary edema who are at increased risk of or who have contraindications to endotracheal intubation, noninvasive ventilation modalities such as continuous positive airway pressure and bilevel positive airway pressure may help avoid endotracheal intubation.[111]

PERICARDIAL TAMPONADE

Pericardial tamponade occurs when pericardial fluid accumulates to the point that it compromises hemodynamics.[75,112] Among cancer patients, two mechanisms can lead to the accumulation of excess fluid in the pericardial space: obstruction of lymphatic drainage, and excessive fluid secretion from tumor nodules on pericardial surfaces. Mesothelioma is the most common malignancy that arises from the pericardium.[113] Carcinoma of the lung and malignant thymoma may involve the pericardium by direct extension. More frequently, malignancies invade the pericardium by retrograde lymphangitic spread or hematogenous dissemination (e.g., carcinomas of the lung and breast).[113] Malignant melanoma is the neoplasm most likely to metastasize to the heart. Lymphomas (both Hodgkin and non-Hodgkin), leukemias, and gastrointestinal neoplasms may also cause pericardial effusion.[114]

Nonneoplastic causes of pericardial tamponade include pericardial abscess,[115] candidal pericarditis,[116] and complications of central venous catheterization.[117,118]

SYMPTOMS AND SIGNS

Although malignant pericardial effusion is occasionally the first clinical manifestation of malignancy, it is usually a late finding among patients with known metastatic disease. More than two thirds of patients with malignant pericardial effusion exhibit no symptoms.[113,114] Among symptomatic patients, the most common complaints are shortness of breath, pleuritic chest pain, orthopnea, and general weakness. Findings from physical examination may range from a complete absence of abnormalities to tachycardia, hypotension, jugular venous distention, hepatomegaly, and peripheral edema. The classic findings of cardiac tamponade are determined not only by the quantity of pericardial fluid but also by the rapidity of fluid accumulation.[119] Pulsus paradoxus, an exaggeration of the usually normal decrease in systolic blood pressure with inspiration, is a classic finding of cardiac tamponade but is nonspecific because it is also seen among patients with lung cancer, clinically significant chronic lung disease, or cor pulmonale of other etiologies.[120]

■ Diagnosis

Because the symptoms and physical findings of pericardial tamponade are frequently nonspecific, a definitive diagnosis usually requires additional testing. Electrical alternans in ECGs, when present, is a very helpful finding; the variation in electrical amplitude results when the heart swings closer to and farther away from the chest wall during a swinging cycle that spans two cycles of cardiac activity.[121] Two-dimensional echocardiography is the most useful test for diagnosing pericardial effusion and evaluating the hemodynamic significance of a pericardial effusion, i.e., the presence or absence of cardiac tamponade. Collapse or compression of the right atrium, diastolic collapse of the right ventricle, and cardiac "rocking" (a side-to-side or front-to-back movement of the heart) are often observed in association with cardiac tamponade. Alterations in the respiratory variation of Doppler flow patterns across the mitral and tricuspid valves are helpful in evaluating the hemodynamic effects of pericardial effusions. Computed tomography or magnetic resonance imaging studies frequently detect pericardial effusions as an incidental finding. These studies provide information about the location (loculated or not) and size of pericardial effusion but cannot provide adequate assessment of the functional significance of the pericardial effusion with respect to hemodynamics, because these are factors related to intrapericardial pressure rather than to the extent of the effusion.

■ Treatment

Initial treatment of a patient with malignant pericardial effusion depends on the patient's hemodynamic stability. In the resuscitation of cardiac arrest, emergency pericardiocentesis without ultrasound guidance may be helpful for patients with pericardial tamponade if an ultrasound machine is not readily available (Table 19-1).[52] For patients with hemodynamic compromise, echocardiography-guided pericardiocentesis, with placement of a drainage catheter into the pericardial space, may be performed emergently in the emergency center or electively in either an ICU or a cardiac laboratory. Complications are infrequent but may include massive pericardial bleeding (when a coronary artery is damaged) and pneumothorax (especially among patients with emphysema). Pericardial fluid can be drained from the catheter, and the catheter can remain in place until less than 50 ml of fluid drains over 24 hours. In many instances (about 70% of cases),[122] fluid will not reaccumulate once the catheter has been removed; if fluid accumulation recurs, either repeated pericardiocentesis or surgical intervention to create a pleuropericardial window may be necessary. The recurrence rate of pericardiotomy is approximately 5%.[122] The results of cytologic testing of pericardial fluid are positive for metastatic disease in only 70% to 80% of patients with malignant pericardial effusion, and negative findings from cytology do not rule out malignancy as the cause.

The pleuropericardial window procedure is usually performed in an operating room, but it can be performed in a hospital room or an ICU with administration of local anesthesia. A laparoscopic transdiaphragmatic approach for creating a pericardioperitoneal shunt has also been described.[123]

■ Syncope

Syncope is defined as isolated or recurrent transient loss of consciousness and is due to generalized cerebral ischemia. Among cancer patients, both oncologic and nononcologic etiologies may lead to syncope. Because of the focus of this text, the discussion in this chapter will be limited to cardiac causes of syncope (Table 19-6).

TABLE 19-6 Differential diagnosis of syncope due to cardiac disorders

Electrical disorders
    Atrial dysrhythmias
    Conduction defects (sinoatrial or atrioventricular)
    Valvular abnormalities (aortic stenosis, prosthetic valve dysfunction)
    Ventricular dysrhythmias
Other obstructions
    Atrial myxoma
    Chest mass
    Congenital heart disease
    Hypertrophic cardiomyopathies
    Impaired venous return
        Abdominal or thoracic masses
        Cough syncope
    Low-output cardiac failure
        Cardiomegalies (cardiomyopathy secondary to doxorubicin use)
        Myocardial infarction
        Congenital diseases
    Pericardial tamponade
    Pulmonary hypertension

Source: Adapted from Drislane FW. Transient events. *In:* M. A. Samuels, S. Feske (eds), *Office Practice of Neurology*, p 112. New York: Churchill Livingstone, Inc, 1996[128]

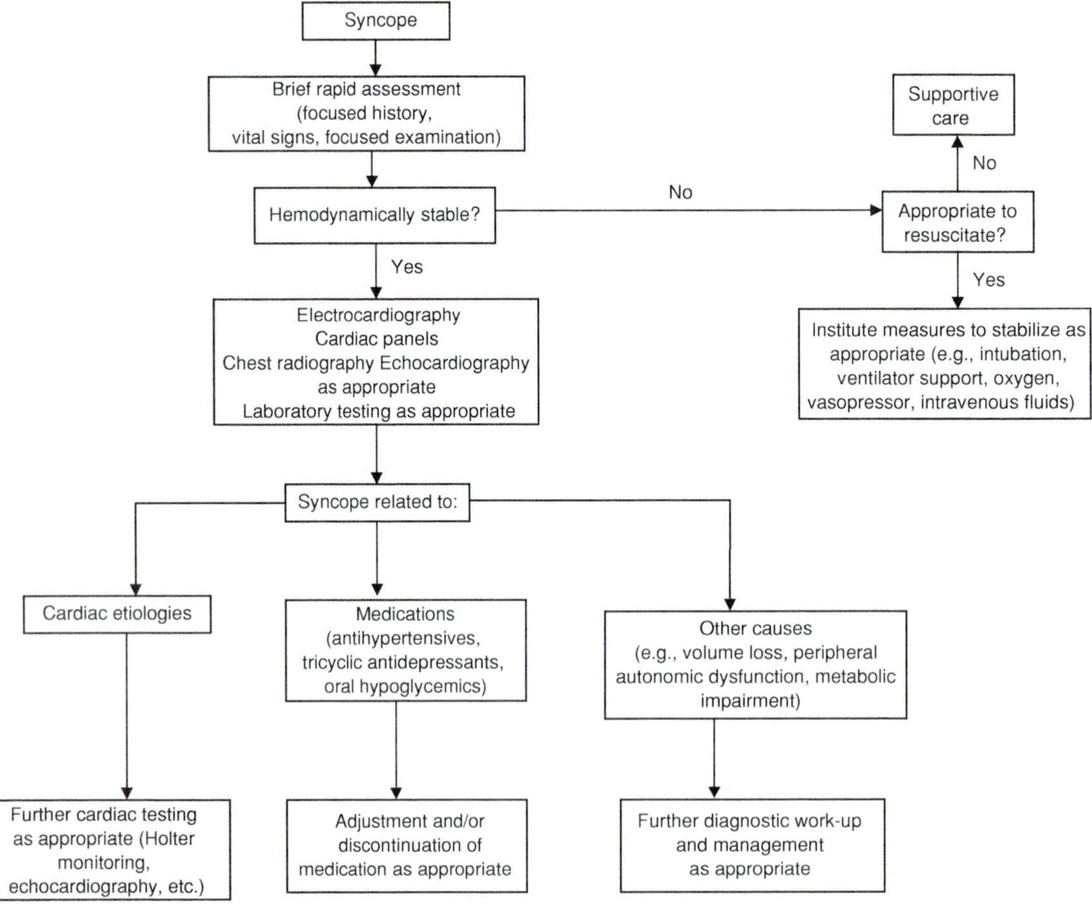

Figure 19-3 Approach to syncope among cancer patients, with a focus on cardiac etiologies.

When a patient presents with syncope, a cardiac cause should be investigated. Some cardiac causes of syncope are truly emergent, and in these cases the patient should be rapidly assessed and stabilized while the ongoing evaluation proceeds (Figure 19-3). Examples may include acute MI, pericardial tamponade, and ventricular dysrhythmias. The extent of the malignancy and the overall prognosis should be considered during both the evaluation and the interventional phases. Patients with advanced malignancy and predicted shortened life span may be best treated with appropriate supportive measures. For others, management should be similar to management for patients experiencing syncope without a diagnosis of malignancy. For patients with syncope believed to be from a cardiac etiology, further testing may include prolonged (Holter) cardiac monitoring, electrophysiologic studies, echocardiography, non-pharmacologic or pharmacologic stress testing, and coronary angiography.

The medical history and the results of physical examination, laboratory tests, and ECG can often establish the cause of the syncopal event.[124] ECG may be helpful in identifying rate and rhythm disturbances (heart block and atrial and ventricular dysrhythmias), long QT syndrome, or ongoing cardiac ischemia. If the cause remains unknown after this initial evaluation, further evaluation should be based on the findings of these initial studies.[125] For some patients, the cause of the syncopal event may remain unknown even with an appropriate and sometimes extensive diagnostic work-up. Those patients should be followed up closely with attention to any additional symptoms that arise.

Medications for patients with syncope should be reviewed carefully. Many cardiac medications may cause changes in sympathetic and vagal tones to the heart, leading to orthostatic hypotension. Patients taking multiple cardiac medications may experience drug interactions resulting in syncope. Frequently, cancer patients experience substantial weight loss because of their malignancy or the effects of their treatment. For patients with substantial weight loss, readjusting the dosage of medications, especially antihypertensives and oral hypoglycemics, may be necessary.

Orthostatic hypotension as a cause of syncope is not unusual among cancer patients. Although tilt-table studies are often used to detect orthostatic hypotension, measuring blood pressure with the patient sitting and standing is often sufficient to establish the diagnosis and is much less costly. Many of these patients remain symptomatic, but simple guidance that includes sitting on the side of the bed for a few moments and modestly increasing sodium intake may make a considerable difference.

SUMMARY

The emergency cardiac care of cancer patients differs from that of the general population in a number of ways. First, the likelihood that a typical cardiac symptom may be a manifestation of cancer must always be considered. Second, the risks of standard cardiac interventions may be considerably greater for cancer patients. Although clear indications of a cardiac etiology should not impede prompt intervention, reflection on the risk-benefit relationship is especially prudent for these patients. Last, cancer patients may have a greatly reduced life expectancy, and zealous intervention to reduce risks that may be totally appropriate for patients without cancer may be burdensome and fruitless for cancer patients. Inappropriate intervention may even delay crucial anticancer treatment for these patients. Whatever the cardiac situation, treating a cancer patient demands insight into the various attributable mechanisms and novel treatment strategies in the setting of the patient's life expectancy.

REFERENCES

1. Inagaki J, Rodriguez V, Bodey GP. Proceedings: causes of death in cancer patients. *Cancer*. 1974;33(2):568–573.
2. Yeh ET, Chang HM. Oncocardiology-past, present, and future: a review. *JAMA Cardiol*. 2016;1(9):1066–1072.
3. Mistiaen WP. Cancer in heart disease patients: what are the limitations in the treatment strategy? *Future Cardiol*. 2013;9(4):535–547.
4. Chinen K, Kurosumi M, Ohkura Y, Sakamoto A, Fujioka Y. Sudden unexpected death in patients with malignancy: a clinicopathologic study of 28 autopsy cases. *Pathol Res Pract*. 2006;202(12):869–875.
5. Mehta AC, Rafanan AL, Bulkley R, Walsh M, DeBoer GE. Coronary spasm and cardiac arrest from carcinoid crisis during laser bronchoscopy. *Chest*. 1999;115(2):598–600.
6. Kahil ME, Brown H, Fred HL. The carcinoid crisis. *Arch Intern Med*. 1964;114:26–28.
7. Westberg G, Ahlman H, Nilsson O, Illerskog A, Wängberg B. Secretory patterns of tryptophan metabolites in midgut carcinoid tumor cells. *Neurochem Res*. 1997;22(8):977–983.
8. Kvols LK. Therapy of the malignant carcinoid syndrome. *Endocrinol Metab Clin North Am*. 1989;18(2):557–568.
9. Keefe DL. Cardiovascular emergencies in the cancer patient. *Semin Oncol*. 2000;27(3):244–255.
10. Ottaviani G, Rossi L, Ramos SG, Matturri L. Pathology of the heart and conduction system in a case of sudden death due to a cardiac fibroma in a 6-month-old child. *Cardiovasc Pathol*. 1999;8(2):109–112.
11. Bussani R, Silvestri F. Images in cardiovascular medicine. Sudden death in a woman with fibroelastoma of the aortic valve chronically occluding the right coronary ostium. *Circulation*. 1999;100(21):2204.

12. Murakami T, Komiya A, Mikata K, Kaneko S, Ikeda I. Cardiac metastasis of renal pelvic cancer. *Int J Urol*. 2007;14(3):240–241.

13. Idir M, Oysel N, Guibaud JP, Labouyrie E, Roudaut R. Fragmentation of a right atrial myxoma presenting as a pulmonary embolism. *J Am Soc Echocardiogr*. 2000;13(1):61–63.

14. Chan GS, Ng WK, Ng IO, Dickens P. Sudden death from massive pulmonary tumor embolism due to hepatocellular carcinoma. *Forensic Sci Int*. 2000;108(3):215–221.

15. King D, Sheard JD, Silas JH. Cardiac amyloidosis in the presence of Bence-Jones proteinuria and normal serum immunoglobulins. *Br J Clin Pract*. 1993;47(6):336–337.

16. Skadberg BT, Bruserud O, Karwinski W, Ohm OJ. Sudden death caused by heart block in a patient with multiple myeloma and cardiac amyloidosis. *Acta Med Scand*. 1988;223(4):379–383.

17. Wahlin A, Olofsson BO, Eriksson A, Backman C. Myeloma-associated cardiac amyloidosis. A case report. *Acta Med Scand*. 1984;215(2):189–192.

18. Sanchez-Hermosillo E, Sikirica M, Carter D, Valigorsky JM. Sudden death due to undetected mediastinal germ cell tumor. *Am J Forensic Med Pathol*. 1998;19(1):69–71.

19. Opeskin K, Ruszkiewicz A, Anderson RM. Sudden death due to undiagnosed medullary-pontine astrocytoma. *Am J Forensic Med Pathol*. 1995;16(2):168–171.

20. Yeh ET, Tong AT, Lenihan DJ, et al. Cardiovascular complications of cancer therapy: diagnosis, pathogenesis, and management. *Circulation*. 2004;109(25):3122–3131.

21. Steinherz L, Steinherz P. Delayed cardiac toxicity from anthracycline therapy. *Pediatrician*. 1991;18(1):49–52.

22. Bristow MR, Billingham ME, Mason JW, Daniels JR. Clinical spectrum of anthracycline antibiotic cardiotoxicity. *Cancer Treat Rep*. 1978;62(6):873–879.

23. Dindogru A, Barcos M, Henderson ES, Wallace HJ Jr. Electrocardiographic changes following adriamycin treatment. *Med Pediatr Oncol*. 1978;5(1):65–71.

24. Wortman JE, Lucas VS Jr, Schuster E, Thiele D, Logue GL. Sudden death during doxorubicin administration. *Cancer*. 1979;44(5):1588–1591.

25. O'Bryan RM, Luce JK, Talley RW, Gottlieb JA, Baker LH, Bonadonna G. Phase II evaluation of adriamycin in human neoplasia. *Cancer*. 1973;32(1):1–8.

26. Couch RD, Loh KK, Sugino J. Sudden cardiac death following adriamycin therapy. *Cancer*. 1981;48(1):38–39.

27. Mills BA, Roberts RW. Cyclophosphamide-induced cardiomyopathy: a report of two cases and review of the English literature. *Cancer*. 1979;43(6):2223–2226.

28. Ensley JF, Patel B, Kloner R, Kish JA, Wynne J, al-Sarraf M. The clinical syndrome of 5-fluorouracil cardiotoxicity. *Invest New Drugs*. 1989;7(1):101–109.

29. Gradishar W, Vokes E, Schilsky R, Weichselbaum R, Panje W. Vascular events in patients receiving high-dose infusional 5-fluorouracil-based chemotherapy: the University of Chicago experience. *Med Pediatr Oncol*. 1991;19(1):8–15.

30. Oleksowicz L, Bruckner HW. Prophylaxis of 5-fluorouracil-induced coronary vasospasm with calcium channel blockers. *Am J Med*. 1988;85(5):750–751.

31. Sievers EL, Lange BJ, Sondel PM, et al. Feasibility, toxicity, and biologic response of interleukin-2 after consolidation chemotherapy for acute myelogenous leukemia: a report from the Children's Cancer Group. *J Clin Oncol*. 1998;16(3):914–919.

32. Sonnenblick M, Rosin A. Cardiotoxicity of interferon. A review of 44 cases. *Chest*. 1991;99(3):557–561.

33. Keefe DL. Trastuzumab-associated cardiotoxicity. *Cancer*. 2002;95(7):1592–1600.

34. Bashir H, Crom D, Metzger M, Mulcahey J, Jones D, Hudson MM. Cisplatin-induced hypomagnesemia and cardiac dysrhythmia. *Pediatr Blood Cancer*. 2007;49(6):867–869.

35. Van Der Klooster JM, Van Der Wiel HE, Van Saase JL, Grootendorst AF. Asystole during combination chemotherapy for non-Hodgkin's lymphoma: the acute tumor lysis syndrome. *Neth J Med*. 2000;56(4):147–152.

36. Roberts SS, Leeborg N, Loriaux M, et al. Acute graft-versus-host disease of the heart. *Pediatr Blood Cancer*. 2006;47(5):624–628.

37. Vallebona A. Cardiac damage following therapeutic chest irradiation. Importance, evaluation and treatment. *Minerva Cardioangiol*. 2000;48(3):79–87.

38. Benoff LJ, Schweitzer P. Radiation therapy-induced cardiac injury. *Am Heart J*. 1995;129(6):1193–1196.

39. Gyenes G. Radiation-induced ischemic heart disease in breast cancer—a review. *Acta Oncol*. 1998;37(3):241–246.

40. Knight CJ, Sutton GC. Complete heart block and severe tricuspid regurgitation after radiotherapy. Case report and review of the literature. *Chest*. 1995;108(6):1748–1751.

41. Raviprasad GS, Salem BI, Gowda S, Leidenfrost R. Radiation-induced mitral and tricuspid regurgitation with severe ostial coronary artery disease: a case report with successful surgical treatment. *Cathet Cardiovasc Diagn*. 1995;35(2):146–148.

42. Sculier JP, Markiewicz E. Cardiopulmonary resuscitation in medical cancer patients: the experience of a medical intensive-care unit of a cancer centre. *Support Care Cancer*. 1993;1(3):135–138.

43. Rozenbaum EA, Shenkman L. Predicting outcome of inhospital cardiopulmonary resuscitation. *Crit Care Med*. 1988;16(6):583–586.

44. Hendrick JM, Pijls NH, van der Werf T, Crul JF. Cardiopulmonary resuscitation on the general ward: no category of patients should be excluded in advance. *Resuscitation*. 1990;20(2):163–171.

45. Champigneulle B, Merceron S, Lemiale V, et al. What is the outcome of cancer patients admitted to the ICU after cardiac arrest? Results from a multicenter study. *Resuscitation*. 2015;92:38–44.

46. Hwang JP, Patlan J, de Achaval S, Escalante CP. Survival in cancer patients after out-of-hospital cardiac arrest. *Support Care Cancer*. 2009;18(1):51–55.

47. Ebell MH, Becker LA, Barry HC, Hagen M. Survival after in-hospital cardiopulmonary resuscitation. A meta-analysis. *J Gen Intern Med*. 1998;13(12):805–816.

48. Ewer MS, Kish SK, Martin CG, Price KJ, Feeley TW. Characteristics of cardiac arrest in cancer patients as a predictor of survival after cardiopulmonary resuscitation. *Cancer*. 2001;92(7):1905–1912.

49. Morris JC, Holland JF. Oncologic emergencies. In: Holland JF, Frei E, Bast RC, Kufe DW, Pollock RE, Weichelbaum RR, eds. *Cancer Medicine*. 5th ed. Hamilton, Ontario, Canada: BC Decker, Inc; 2000:2433–2453.

50. Donnino MW, Navarro K, Berg K, Brooks SC, Crider J, et al. *Advanced Cardiovascular Life Support (ACLS) Provider Manual*. 16th ed. Dallas, TX: American Heart Association, Inc; 2016.

51. ACLS Training Center. Algorithms for advanced cardiac life support 2018. https://www.acls.net/aclsalg. htm. Accessed April 1, 2018.

52. Lavonas EJ, Drennan IR, Gabrielli A, et al. Part 10: special circumstances of resuscitation: 2015 American Heart Association guidelines update for cardiopulmonary resuscitation and emergency cardiovascular care. *Circulation*. 2015;132(18 suppl 2):S501–S518.

53. Vanden Hoek TL, Morrison LJ, Shuster M, et al. Part 12: cardiac arrest in special situations: 2010 American Heart Association guidelines for cardiopulmonary resuscitation and emergency cardiovascular care. *Circulation*. 2010;122(18 suppl 3):S829–S861.

54. Callaway CW, Donnino MW, Fink EL, et al. Part 8: post-cardiac arrest care: 2015 American Heart Association guidelines update for cardiopulmonary resuscitation and emergency cardiovascular care. *Circulation*. 2015;132(18 suppl 2):S465–S482.

55. Amsterdam EA, Wenger NK, Brindis RG, et al. ACC/ AHA task force members; society for cardiovascular angiography and interventions and the society of thoracic surgeons. 2014 AHA/ACC guideline for the management of patients with non-ST-elevation acute coronary syndromes: executive summary: a report of the American College of Cardiology/American Heart Association Task Force on Practice Guidelines. *Circulation*. 2014;130(25):2354–2394.

56. O'Gara PT, Kushner FG, Ascheim DD, et al. 2013 ACCF/ AHA guideline for the management of ST-elevation myocardial infarction: executive summary: a report of the American College of Cardiology Foundation/ American Heart Association Task Force on Practice Guidelines. *Circulation*. 2013;127(4):529–555.

57. Ackermann DM, Hyma BA, Edwards WD. Malignant neoplastic emboli to the coronary arteries: report of two cases and review of the literature. *Hum Pathol*. 1987;18(9):955–959.

58. Pineda AM, Mihos CG, Nascimento FO, Santana O, Lamelas J, Beohar N. Coronary embolization from a left atrial myxoma containing malignant lymphoma cells. *Tex Heart Inst J*. 2015;42(6):565–568.

59. Escalante CP, Chang YC, Liao K, et al. Epidemiology section of the mucositis study group of the multinational association of supportive care in cancer, 2013. Meta-analysis of cardiovascular toxicity risks in cancer patients on selected targeted agents. *Support Care Cancer*. 2016;24(9):4057–4074.

60. Patel JN, Jiang C, Hertz DL, et al. Bevacizumab and the risk of arterial and venous thromboembolism in patients with metastatic, castration-resistant prostate cancer treated on Cancer and Leukemia Group B (CALGB) 90401 (Alliance). *Cancer*. 2015;121(7):1025–1031.

61. Scappaticci FA, Skillings JR, Holden SN, et al. Arterial thromboembolic events in patients with metastatic carcinoma treated with chemotherapy and bevacizumab. *J Natl Cancer Inst*. 2007;99(16):1232–1239.

62. Jang S, Zheng C, Tsai HT, et al. Cardiovascular toxicity after antiangiogenic therapy in persons older than 65 years with advanced renal cell carcinoma. *Cancer*. 2016;122(1):124–130.

63. de Forni M, Malet-Martino MC, Jaillas P, et al. Cardiotoxicity of high-dose continuous infusion fluorouracil: a prospective clinical study. *J Clin Oncol*. 1992;10(11):1795–1801.

64. Freeman NJ, Costanza ME. 5-Fluorouracil-associated cardiotoxicity. *Cancer*. 1998;61(1):36–45.

65. Keefe DL, Roistacher N, Pierri MK. Clinical cardiotoxicity of 5-fluorouracil. *J Clin Pharmacol*. 1993;33(11):1060–1070.

66. Ensley J, Kish J, Tapazoglou E, et al. 5-Fluorouracil infusions associated with an ischemic cardiotoxicity syndrome [abstract 554]. *Proc Am Soc Clin Oncol*. 1986;5:142.

67. Wacker A, Lersch C, Scherpinski U, Reindl L, Seyfarth M. High incidence of angina pectoris in patients treated with 5-fluorouracil. A planned surveillance study with 102 patients. *Oncology*. 2003;65(2):108–112.

68. McEniery PT, Dorosti K, Schiavone WA, Pedrick TJ, Sheldon WC. Clinical and angiographic features of coronary artery disease after chest irradiation. *Am J Cardiol*. 1987;60(13):1020–1024.

69. Tracy GP, Brown DE, Johnson LW, Gottlieb AJ. Radiation-induced coronary artery disease. *JAMA*. 1974;228(13):1660–1662.

70. Simon EB, Ling J, Mendizabal RC, Midwall J. Radiation-induced coronary artery disease. *Am Heart J*. 1984;108(4 pt 1):1032–1034.

71. Silverberg GD, Britt RH, Goffinet DR. Radiation induced carotid artery disease. *Cancer*. 1978;41(1):130–137.

72. Stewart JR, Fajardo LF. Radiation-induced heart disease: an update. *Prog Cardiovasc Dis*. 1984;27(3):173–194.

73. Cohen Y, Amir G, Da'as N, Gillis S, Rund D, Polliack A. Acute myocardial infarction as the presenting symptom of acute myeloblastic leukemia with extreme hyperleukocytosis. *Am J Hematol*. 2002;71(1):47–49.

74. Biccard BM, Gopalan PD. Phaeochromocytoma and acute myocardial infarction. *Anaesth Intensive Care*. 2002;30(1):74–76.

75. Lazaros G, Latsios G, Tsalamandris S, et al. Cardiac myxoma and concomitant myocardial infarction. *Embolism, atherosclerosis or combination? Int J Cardiol.* 2016;205:124–126.

76. Sachithanandan A, Badmanaban B, McEneaney D, MacGowan SW. Left atrial myxoma presenting with acute myocardial infarction. *Eur J Cardiothorac Surg.* 2002;21(3):543.

77. Daher IN, Luh JY, Duarte AG. Squamous cell lung cancer simulating an acute myocardial infarction. *Chest.* 2003;123(1):304–306.

78. Ewer MS, Ali MK. Critical cardiologic considerations in the cancer patient. *Crit Care Clin.* 1988;4(1):41–60.

79. Neumar RW, Shuster M, Callaway CW, et al. Part 1: executive summary: 2015 American Heart Association Guidelines Update for Cardiopulmonary Resuscitation and Emergency Cardiovascular Care. *Circulation.* 2015;132(18 suppl 2):S315–S367.

80. Sarkiss MG, Yusuf SW, Warneke CL, et al. Impact of aspirin therapy in cancer patients with thrombocytopenia and acute coronary syndromes. *Cancer.* 2007;109(3):621–627.

81. Lopez FF, Mangi A, Mylonakis E, Chen JL, Schiffman FJ. Atrial fibrillation and tumor emboli as manifestations of metastatic leiomyosarcoma to the heart and lung. *Heart Lung.* 2000;29(1):47–49.

82. Vaduganathan M, Patel NK, Lubitz SA, Neilan TG, Dudzinski DM. A "malignant" arrhythmia: cardiac metastasis and ventricular tachycardia. *Tex Heart Inst J.* 2016;43(6):558–559.

83. Mathew V, Olson LJ, Gertz MA, Hayes DL. Symptomatic conduction system disease in cardiac amyloidosis. *Am J Cardiol.* 1997;80(11):1491–1492.

84. Pentz WH. Advanced heart block as a manifestation of a paraneoplastic syndrome from malignant thymoma. *Chest.* 1999;116(4):1135–1136.

85. Donnelly MS, Weinberg DS, Skarin AT, Levine HD. Sick sinus syndrome with seroconstrictive pericarditis in malignant lymphoma involving the heart: a case report. *Med Pediatr Oncol.* 1981;9(3):273–277.

86. Slama MS, Le Guludec D, Sebag C, et al. Complete atrioventricular block following mediastinal irradiation: a report of six cases. *Pacing Clin Electrophysiol.* 1991;14(7):1112–1118.

87. Pai VB, Nahata MC. Cardiotoxicity of chemotherapeutic agents: incidence, treatment and prevention. *Drug Saf.* 2000;22(4):263–302.

88. Wassmann S, Nickenig G, Böhm M. Long QT syndrome and torsade de pointes in a patient receiving fluconazole. *Ann Intern Med.* 1999;131(10):797.

89. Tholakanahalli VN, Potti A, Hanley JF, Merliss AD. Fluconazole-induced torsade de pointes. *Ann Pharmacother.* 2001;35(4):432–434.

90. Coley KC, Crain JL. Miconazole-induced fatal dysrhythmia. *Pharmacotherapy.* 1997;17(2):379–382.

91. Tsai WC, Tsai LM, Chen JH. Combined use of astemizole and ketoconazole resulting in torsade de pointes. *J Formos Med Assoc.* 1997;96(2):144–146.

92. Otsuka M, Kanamori H, Sasaki S, et al. Torsades de pointes complicating pentamidine therapy of Pneumocystis carinii pneumonia in acute myelogenous leukemia. *Intern Med.* 1997;36(10):705–708.

93. Anderson ME, Mazur A, Yang T, Roden DM. Potassium current antagonist properties and proarrhythmic consequences of quinolone antibiotics. *J Pharmacol Exp Ther.* 2001;296(3):806–810.

94. Shaffer D, Singer S, Korvick J, Honig P. Concomitant risk factors in reports of torsades de pointes associated with macrolide use: review of the United States Food and Drug Administration Adverse Event Reporting System. *Clin Infect Dis.* 2002;35(2):197–200.

95. Link MS, Berkow LC, Kudenchuk PJ, et al. Part 7: adult advanced cardiovascular life support: 2015 American Heart Association Guidelines Update for Cardiopulmonary Resuscitation and Emergency Cardiovascular Care. *Circulation.* 2015;132(18 suppl 2):S444–S464.

96. Thomas SH, Behr ER. Pharmacological treatment of acquired QT prolongation and torsades de pointes. *Br J Clin Pharmacol.* 2016;81(3):420–427.

97. Epstein AE, Olshansky B, Naccarelli GV, Kennedy JI Jr, Murphy EJ, Goldschlager N. Practical management guide for clinicians who treat patients with amiodarone. *Am J Med.* 2016;129(5):468–475.

98. Frumin H, Kerin NZ, Rubenfire M. Classification of antiarrhythmic drugs. *J Clin Pharmacol.* 1989;29(5):387–394.

99. Gibbs HR, Swafford J, Nguyen HD, Ewer MS, Ali MK. Postoperative atrial fibrillation in cancer surgery: preoperative risks and clinical outcome. *J Surg Oncol.* 1992;50(4):224–227.

100. Page RL, Joglar JA, Caldwell MA, et al. 2015 ACC/AHA/HRS guideline for the management of adult patients with supraventricular tachycardia: a report of the American College of Cardiology/American Heart Association Task Force on Clinical Practice Guidelines and the Heart Rhythm Society. *J Am Coll Cardiol.* 2016;67(13):e27–e115.

101. Gallagher MM, Guo XH, Poloniecki JD, Guan Yap Y, Ward D, Camm AJ. Initial energy setting, outcome and efficiency in direct current cardioversion of atrial fibrillation and flutter. *J Am Coll Cardiol.* 2001;38(5):1498–1504.

102. Benetos G, Bonou M, Toutouzas K, Diamantopoulos P, Viniou N, Barbetseas J. Advances in anticoagulation management of patients undergoing cardioversion of nonvalvular atrial fibrillation. *Hamostaseologie.* 2017;37(4):277–285.

103. Johnson DB, Balko JM, Compton ML, et al. Fulminant myocarditis with combination immune checkpoint blockade. *N Engl J Med.* 2016;375(18):1749–1755.

104. Laubli H, Balmelli C, Bossard M, Pfister O, Glatz K, Zippelius A. Acute heart failure due to autoimmune myocarditis under pembrolizumab treatment for metastatic melanoma. *J Immunother Cancer.* 2015;3:11.

105. Lettman NA, Sites FD, Shofer FS, Hollander JE. Congestive heart failure patients with chest pain:

incidence and predictors of acute coronary syndrome. *Acad Emerg Med*. 2002;9(9):903–909.

106. Latini R, Masson S, de Angelis N, Arnand I. Role of brain natriuretic peptide in the diagnosis and management of heart failure: current concepts. *J Card Fail*. 2002;8(5):288–299.

107. Maisel A. B-type natriuretic peptide measurements in diagnosing congestive heart failure in the dyspneic emergency department patient. *Rev Cardiovasc Med*. 2002;3(suppl 4):S10–S17.

108. Wieczorek SJ, Wu AH, Christenson R, et al. A rapid B-type natriuretic peptide assay accurately diagnoses left ventricular dysfunction and heart failure: a multicenter evaluation. *Am Heart J*. 2002;144(5):834–839.

109. Lader E. BNP levels had high sensitivity but moderate specificity for detecting congestive heart failure in the emergency department. *ACP J Club*. 2003;138(1):23.

110. O'Connor CM, Starling RC, Hernandez AF, et al. Effect of nesiritide in patients with acute decompensated heart failure. *N Engl J Med*. 2011;365(1):32–43.

111. Panacek EA, Kirk JD. Role of noninvasive ventilation in the management of acutely decompensated heart failure. *Rev Cardiovasc Med*. 2002;3(suppl 4):S35–S40.

112. Ewer MS, Durand JB, Swafford J, Yusuf SW. Emergency cardiac problems. In: Yeung SC, Escalante CP, eds. *Oncologic Emergencies*. Hamilton, Ontario, Canada: BC Decker, Inc; 2002:304–314.

113. Warren WH. Malignancies involving the pericardium. *Semin Thorac Cardiovasc Surg*. 2000;12(2):119–129.

114. McKenna RJ Jr, Ali MK, Ewer MS, Frazier OH. Pleural and pericardial effusions in cancer patients. *Curr Probl Cancer*. 1985;9(6):1–44.

115. Muto M, Ohtsu A, Boku N, Takoro J, Yoshida S. Streptococcus milleri infection and pericardial abscess associated with esophageal carcinoma: report of two cases. *Hepatogastroenterology*. 1999;46(27):1782–1784.

116. Rabinovici R, Szewczyk D, Ovadia P, Greenspan JR, Sivalingam JJ. Candida pericarditis: clinical profile and treatment. *Ann Thorac Surg*. 1997;63(4):1200–1204.

117. Yavaşcaoğlu B, Yilmazlar A, Korfali G, Senkaya I. Pericardial tamponade as a delayed lethal complication of central venous catheterization. *Eur J Anaesthesiol*. 2001;18(7):487–489.

118. Murray BH, Cohle SD, Davison P. Pericardial tamponade and death from Hickman catheter perforation. *Am Surg*. 1996;62(12):994–997.

119. Kralstein J, Frishman W. Malignant pericardial diseases: diagnosis and treatment. *Am Heart J*. 1987;113(3):785–790.

120. Hoit BD, Shaw D. The paradoxical pulse in tamponade: mechanisms and echocardiographic correlates. *Echocardiography*. 1994;11(5):477–487.

121. Calkins J, Amsterdam E. Images in cardiology: electrical alternans and its resolution in an adult with a large pericardial effusion. *Clin Cardiol*. 2004;27(12):701.

122. Labbé C, Tremblay L, Lacasse Y. Pericardiocentesis versus pericardiotomy for malignant pericardial effusion: a retrospective comparison. *Curr Oncol*. 2015;22(6):412–416.

123. Pataki N, Szelig L, Horvath OP, Biki B, Molnar TF. Pericardial drainage using the transdiaphragmatic route: refinement of the laparoscopic technique. *Surg Endosc*. 2002;16(7):1105.

124. Linzer M, Yang EH, Estes NA 3rd, Wang P, Vorperian VR, Kapoor WN. Diagnosing syncope. Part 1: value of history, physical examination and electrocardiography. Clinical Efficacy Assessment Project of the American College of Physicians. *Ann Intern Med*. 1997;126(12):989–996.

125. Linzer M, Yang EH, Estes NA 3rd, Wang P, Vorperian VR, Kapoor WN. Diagnosing syncope. Part 2: unexplained syncope. Clinical Efficacy Assessment Project of the American College of Physicians. *Ann Intern Med*. 1997;127(1):76–86.

126. O'Gara PT, Kushner FG, Ascheim DD, et al. 2013 ACCF/AHA guideline for the management of ST-elevation myocardial infarction: a report of the American College of Cardiology Foundation/American Heart Association Task Force on Practice Guidelines. *Circulation*. 2013 Jan 29;127(4):e362–425.

127. Ryan TJ, Antman EM, Brooks NH, et al. 1999 Update: ACC/AHA guidelines for the management of patients with acute myocardial infarction: executive summary and recommendations. *Circulation*. 1999;100(9):1016–1030.

128. Drislane FW. Transient events. In: Samuels MA, Feske S, eds. *Office Practice of Neurology*. New York, NY: Churchill Livingstone, Inc; 1996:112.

20 Cardiac Considerations for Treating Cancer in Infants and Children

Neha Bansal ▪ Rofida Nofal ▪ Sanjeev Aggarwal ▪ Vivian I. Franco ▪ Emma R. Lipshultz ▪ Stephen E. Sallan ▪ Steven E. Lipshultz

INTRODUCTION

Between 2007 and 2011, the incidence of childhood cancer increased by 0.6% per year, making it the second most common cause of death among children 1 to 14 years old.[1] However, mortality rates for childhood cancer have declined by 67% over the past four decades, from 6.3 per 100,000 population in 1970 to 2.1 in 2011.[1] The 5-year survival rate for all forms of pediatric cancers also increased from 58% to 83% between 2004 and 2010.[1] As of 2005, nearly one-fourth of the almost 330,000 survivors of childhood cancer have survived longer than 30 years since diagnosis.[2]

The reduction in mortality rates is largely attributable to improved treatments and high rates of participation in clinical trials. Unfortunately, the same treatments that cure cancer also increase the risk of adverse effects on other organ systems, especially the cardiovascular system.[3] The application and dosing of cancer therapies were originally limited by acute cardiac complications (Table 20-1). Newer treatment protocols that limit chemotherapy dosing and use more accurate radiation targeting have reduced the incidence of acute cardiac complications to less than 1%.[4] However, it is now clear that the cardiotoxicity of treatment is not limited to acute complications and that the long-term survivors are at risk of cardiovascular complications for the rest of their lives (Table 20-1).[5–10]

Cardiovascular-related disease is the leading cause of morbidity and mortality among survivors after cancer itself.[10–14] Survivors are significantly more likely than their siblings to report congestive heart failure, myocardial infarction, pericardial disease, or valvular abnormalities ($p<0.001$).[15] Among 1853 adult survivors of childhood cancer, cardiomyopathy was present in 7.4%, coronary artery disease in 3.8%, valvular regurgitation or stenosis in 28.0%, and conduction or rhythm abnormalities in 4.4%.[16] Treatment-related cardiotoxicity has even been identified as a leading indication for heart transplant among young adults.[17] Anthracycline-containing regimens and radiation treatment especially have been associated with an increased risk of these cardiovascular complications.[11,12,14,15,17,18]

A large proportion of survivors exposed to known cardiotoxic treatments have subclinical cardiotoxicity[6–9,19] that ranges from pericardial or valvular damage associated with cardiac exposure to radiation to decreased left ventricular (LV) systolic and diastolic functions associated with anthracyclines.[6–9] This cardiotoxicity appears to be progressive and leads to clinical cardiovascular disease.[8] Several factors are associated with subclinical cardiotoxicity, including higher cumulative doses of anthracyclines and cardiac radiation; a higher dose rate of anthracycline administration; use of concomitant cardiotoxic therapies, such as vinca alkaloids; younger age at treatment; increasing time since treatment; female sex; elevated concentrations of serum cardiac troponin T (cTnT) or N-terminal probrain natriuretic peptide (NT-proBNP) during anthracycline therapy; and congestive heart failure (HF) during anthracycline therapy.[18,20,21]

Neither the frequency nor the rate of progression from subclinical changes to symptomatic cardiac disease nor the risk factors for such progression are completely known. In addition to cancer therapy-induced cardiac and vascular damage, some survivors may also be at increased risk of several traditional atherosclerotic disease risk factors, such as obesity, physical inactivity, and metabolic abnormalities.[10,22,23] This combined effect of myocardial damage and increased disease risk among survivors remains poorly defined, and additional studies are necessary for informing clinical practice.

The adverse effects of cancer treatment may be especially problematic among children.[24] Cancer therapies, aimed at stopping the rapid division of neoplastic cells, also potentially interfere with normal tissue growth, as clearly evidenced by long-term cancer survivors who never attain normal height.[25] Children's developmental immaturity does not allow them to compensate for therapy-related insults. Thus, HF rates are higher among children than among adults treated with the same anthracycline dose, adjusted for body size.[26] However, survivors of childhood cancers live longer than do adults with cancer, and long-term adverse effects of cancer treatments among these children will be determined only with lifelong follow-up studies. Currently, most survivors live for at least

TABLE 20-1   Characteristics of various types of anthracycline-associated cardiotoxicity

CHARACTERISTIC	ACUTE CARDIOTOXICITY	EARLY ONSET, CHRONIC PROGRESSIVE CARDIOTOXICITY	LATE ONSET, CHRONIC PROGRESSIVE CARDIOTOXICITY
Onset	Within the first week of anthracycline treatment	<1 year after completion of anthracycline therapy	>1 year after completion of anthracycline therapy
Risk factor dependence	Unknown	Yes	Yes
Clinical features in adults	Transient depression of myocardial contractility; myocardial necrosis (cTnT elevation); arrhythmia	Dilated cardiomyopathy; arrhythmia	Dilated cardiomyopathy; arrhythmia
Clinical features in children	Transient depression of myocardial contractility; myocardial necrosis (cTnT elevation); arrhythmia	Restrictive cardiomyopathy, dilated cardiomyopathy, or both; arrhythmia	Restrictive cardiomyopathy, dilated cardiomyopathy, or both; arrhythmia
Course	Usually reversible on discontinuation of anthracycline	Can be progressive	Can be progressive

Sources: From: Lipshultz SE, Alvarez JA, Scully RE. Anthracycline-associated cardiotoxicity in survivors of childhood cancer. *Heart* 2008;94:525–33. Adapted with permission from Adams MJ, Lipshultz SE. Pathophysiology of anthracycline- and radiation-associated cardiomyopathies: implications for screening and prevention. *Pediatr Blood Cancer.* 2005;44(7): 600–606. Copyright Wiley-Liss, Inc.

a decade after successful treatment of their original cancer.[27] Thus, small subclinical changes can become more severe over a lifetime and can cause marked cardiovascular morbidity that adult patients do not experience.

Understanding the acute and chronic cardiovascular complications of long-term cancer survivors is important for oncologists, cardiologists, and other health care providers caring for such patients, not only after cancer treatment but also when treatment options are selected at diagnosis. In this chapter, we review the treatment-related cardiovascular complications associated with treating childhood cancers and propose methods for preventing, screening, and treating these patients. We conclude with a discussion of lifetime cardiovascular risk among survivors and of necessary research.

CARDIOTOXIC THERAPIES

Certain treatments of childhood cancer are cardiotoxic, especially anthracyclines, radiation therapy with cardiac exposure, and tyrosine kinase inhibitors.[28] The most common presentation of HF for both adults and children is often dilated cardiomyopathy, in which the LV is dilated and its function is reduced. However, among survivors, the cardiotoxic manifestations of both anthracycline treatment and cardiac exposure to radiation are often similar to a restrictive-like cardiomyopathy. The pathophysiology probably differs and is most simply described as a myocardial disease in which the LV fails to properly fill during diastole because of impaired LV relaxation and stretching. Often resulting from myocardial stiffness, impaired stretching means that the LV cannot accommodate an appropriate volume of blood at a normal filling pressure. For these survivors, LV dysfunction is often the result of both reduced LV systolic performance and diastolic dysfunction with altered LV filling. This reduced LV function is caused by various abnormalities, including a reduction in the number of cardiomyocytes and damage to the remaining cardiomyocytes and stem cells that can normally produce additional cardiomyocytes.

■ Anthracyclines

For several decades, anthracyclines have effectively treated a variety of hematologic and solid tumors in

TABLE 20-2 Risk Factors for anthracycline-related cardiotoxicity

RISK FACTOR	NOTES	REFERENCES
Cumulative anthracycline dose	Cumulative doses >500 mg/m² associated with statistically significantly elevated long-term risk	Lipshultz et al.[8]; Krischer et al.[6]; Lipshultz et al.[9]; Lipshultz et al.[10]
Length of interval after therapy	Incidence of clinically relevant cardiotoxicity increases progressively after therapy	Lipshultz et al.[8]; Lipshultz et al.[9]; Lipshultz et al.[10]
Rate of anthracycline administration	Prolonged administration to minimize circulating dose volume may decrease toxicity; results are mixed	Lipshultz et al.[102]
Individual anthracycline dose	Higher individual anthracycline doses are associated with increased risk of late cardiotoxicity, even when cumulative doses are limited	Lipshultz et al.[9]; Lipshultz et al.[10]
Type of anthracycline	Liposomal encapsulated preparations may reduce cardiotoxicity; results for anthracycline analogues and cardiotoxicity differences are conflicting	Wouters et al.[100]; Barry et al.[20]; VanDalen et al.[100]
Radiation therapy	Cumulative radiation dose >30 Gy; before or concomitant anthracycline treatment	Giantris et al.[31]; Adams et al.[21]
Concomitant therapy	Trastuzumab, cyclophosphamide, bleomycin, vincristine, amsacrine, and mitoxantrone may increase susceptibility/toxicity; others agents have also been implicated	Giantris et al.[31]; Barry et al.[20]
Pre-existing cardiac risk factors	Hypertension; ischemic, myocardial, or valvular heart disease; previous cardiotoxic treatment	Barry et al.[20]
Comorbid conditions	Diabetes, obesity, renal dysfunction, pulmonary disease, sepsis, infection, endocrinopathies, electrolyte and metabolic abnormalities, and pregnancy	Barry et al.[20]
Age	Both young and advanced age at treatment are associated with elevated risk	Lipshultz et al.[8]; Lipshultz et al.[9]
Sex	Females are at greater risk than males	Lipshultz et al.[9]
Additional factors	Trisomy 21; African American ancestry	Krischer et al.[6]

Source: From: Lipshultz SE, Alvarez JA, Scully RE. Anthracycline-associated cardiotoxicity in survivors of childhood cancer. *Heart.* 2008;94:525–533.

children. Anthracyclines such as doxorubicin, daunorubicin, epirubicin, and idarubicin have been instrumental in improving the survival rates for children and are part of first-line therapy for many childhood cancer treatment protocols. In fact, more than half of childhood cancer survivors have been treated with anthracyclines.[29] Clinically important cardiotoxicity is a serious limitation of this medication and had led to the use of lower doses for children.[20,30] This potential

for long-term cardiotoxicity is well established, and its awareness among providers is crucial both during and after the treatment of children with cancer.[17]

Anthracycline cardiotoxicity can be categorized at the time of presentation as either acute or chronic; chronic cases are further categorized as early or late onset (Table 20-2).[31] Acute toxicity presents within hours or days of treatment, often as conduction abnormalities and arrhythmias, including ST-segment and

T-wave changes, tachycardia, and premature ventricular contractions.[31–34] At high doses of anthracyclines, acute LV dysfunction can occur and sometimes causes HF. Histologically, cardiac tissue exhibits fewer myofibrils than normal, cellular dropout, and mitochondrial distortion.[35] However, because the endomyocardial biopsies required for this analysis increases the risks of complications among children, they are seldom used to evaluate children for evidence of anthracycline toxicity.

Some histologic abnormalities may be transient, disappearing after cancer therapy, whereas others may be persistent and may progress for years after treatment. In fact, severe cardiotoxicity detected during or shortly after treatment, even with an intervening asymptomatic period, is strongly associated with eventual HF. A follow-up study of survivors treated with anthracyclines and with acute HF found that all recovered temporarily, although nearly half later experienced recurrent HF.[6] Reducing the dose of anthracyclines substantially reduced the incidence of acute cardiac complications, to less than 1%. However, chronic LV dysfunction remains an important clinical concern.[4]

Although the estimated incidence of chronic HF among survivors treated with anthracyclines ranges from 1% to 16%, the true rate may be even higher with longer follow-up.[8,36] In addition to these cases of symptomatic LV dysfunction, chronic anthracycline cardiotoxicity also often manifests itself as subclinical abnormalities in LV structure and function. These subclinical changes may in some cases progress to HF and cardiac death. Such effects may also leave survivors more vulnerable to eventual cardiovascular insults that are not related to anthracycline, such as ischemic heart disease.

Among 115 survivors of acute lymphoblastic leukemia (ALL) or osteogenic sarcoma treated with the anthracycline doxorubicin 6 years previously, LV wall thickness was decreased relative to body-surface area.[6–8] Such changes are often inversely proportional to the LV wall stress placed on LV cardiomyocytes; this stress impairs their systolic performance, limits LV contractility, and can ultimately reduce cardiac output. This LV wall stress is referred to as *LV afterload* and is directly proportional to LV dimension and blood pressure and inversely proportional to LV wall thickness. In this study, the reduced LV wall thickness z-score was related to increased LV afterload among more than half of survivors, although LV dimension and LV pressure remained normal.

The intrinsic ability of the heart to contract, regardless of external LV wall stress, such as LV afterload, depends on load-independent LV contractility, which is measured as the LV stress-velocity index. This index is termed *load-independent LV contractility*. The above-mentioned study of ALL patients found that LV load-independent contractility was below normal for nearly one-fifth of patients, a finding indicating that cardiomyocyte dysfunction was common. As a measure of the strength of systolic contraction, LV fractional shortening depends on both LV wall stress and LV contractility. LV fractional shortening was reduced among one-fourth of the survivors studied. Additionally, reductions in LV fractional shortening were related to decreased health of the cardiomyocytes and to LV contractility among half of survivors and to elevated LV wall stress and LV afterload among the others. These findings clearly indicate that, 6 years after anthracycline treatment, many survivors have markedly abnormal LV systolic function that is related to both increased LV afterload and decreased LV contractility.

A follow-up study of these survivors 8 years after treatment found that younger age at diagnosis and increased follow-up time were associated with decreased LV wall thickness (Figure 20-1).[7] Higher individual anthracycline dosages were associated with increased LV dimension, which indicates LV dilation. Decreased LV wall thickness and increased LV dimensions contributed to increased LV afterload, which was elevated in relation to these risk factors among these survivors. This increased LV afterload indicates that the LV walls are under increased stress during contraction, and the heart must overcome such stress to ensure normal LV systolic performance and

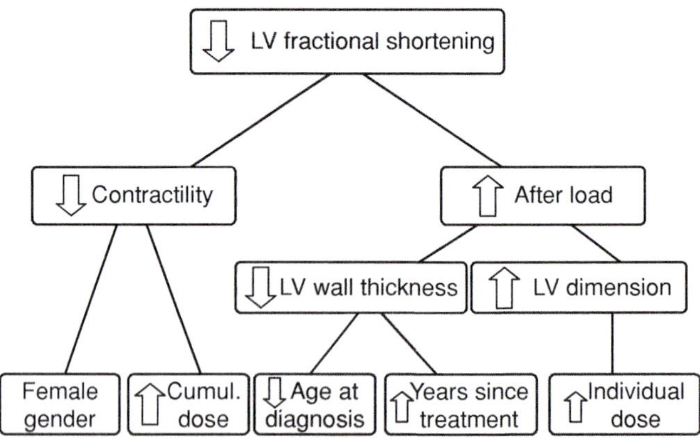

FIGURE 20-1 Factors associated with cardiac abnormalities and progression to left ventricular dysfunction in childhood cancer survivors treated with anthracyclines. LV, left ventricular. (Reproduced by permission. Wouters KA, Kremer LC, Miller TL, Herman EH, Lipshultz SE. Protecting against anthracycline-induced myocardial damage: a review of the most promising strategies. *Br J Haematol.* 2005;131:561–578.)

cardiac output. Female sex and increased cumulative anthracycline dose were also associated with reduced LV contractility, a finding indicating unhealthy heart muscle (Figure 20-1). Reduced LV contractility could ultimately reduce LV systolic performance and cardiac output.

Another follow-up study of these patients 12 years after treatment found that the anthracycline-related abnormalities of LV structure and function had progressed as LV mass and LV contractility progressively declined (Figure 20-2).[8] Left ventricular mass continued to decline with subsequent elevations in LV afterload, a finding indicating continually increasing LV wall stress that would require increasing compensation by LV cardiomyocytes to maintain LV systolic performance. Left ventricular contractility also continued to decline, a finding indicating that the health of cardiac muscle cells in the LV worsened over time. Especially troubling

were declines in LV systolic function, measured as reduced LV fractional shortening and blood pressure values, which may portend future premature cardiovascular morbidity. This study also found that even survivors who received low cumulative doses of anthracyclines were still at risk of chronic cardiotoxicity years after therapy. There is no safe dose of anthracyclines.

A mean 17.3-year follow-up of these 115 survivors found that the LV dimension-to-body-surface area had decreased and that the LV thickness-to-body-surface area subsequently increased, resulting in a normal LV thickness-to-dimension ratio, a finding indicating ventricular remodeling (Figure 20-3). This shrinking ratio of myocardial cavity to body-surface area (which we have called *Grinch Syndrome*, indicating a heart too small for body size) is chronic cardiomyopathy, which may result in HF, heart transplant, or premature death among long-term survivors.[37]

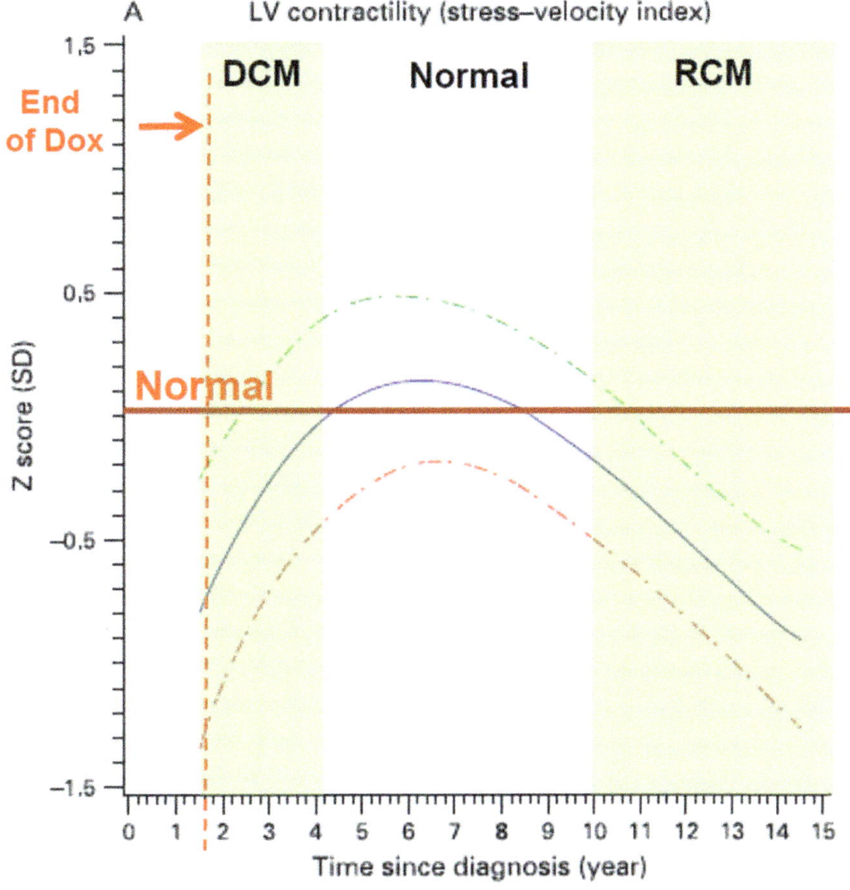

FIGURE 20-2 Changes in left ventricular structure and function over time, reported as Z-scores, from a study of 115 survivors of childhood acute lymphoblastic leukemia. Solid line, overall group mean; dashed lines, upper and lower bounds of the 95% confidence interval for left ventricular contractility (LV stress-velocity index). Dox, doxorubicin; DCM, dilated cardiomyopathy; RCM, restrictive cardiomyopathy (Modified from Lipshultz SE, Lipsitz SR, Sallan SE, et al. Chronic progressive cardiac dysfunction years after doxorubicin therapy for childhood acute lymphoblastic leukemia. *J Clin Oncol.* 2005;23:2629–263.)

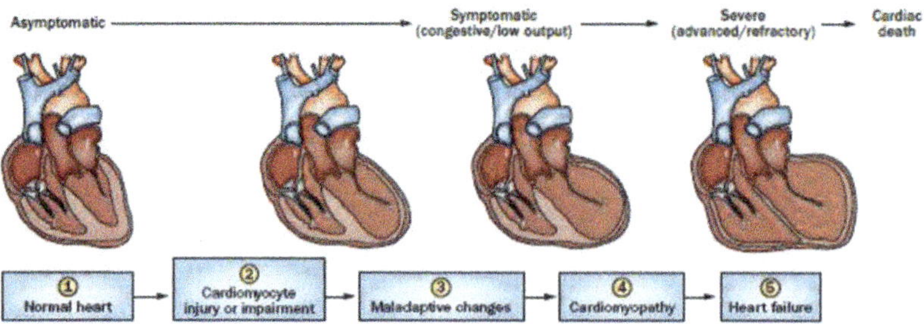

FIGURE 20-3 Stages in the development of pediatric ventricular dysfunction. (Permission from Nature Publishing Group, Lipshultz SE, et al. *Nat Rev Clin Oncol.* 2013;10:697–710.)

The restrictive-like nature of anthracycline cardiotoxicity may be important because it suggests that theories and treatments based on studies of dilated cardiomyopathy may not improve our understanding of anthracycline cardiotoxicity over a lifetime.[38] Abnormal LV structure and function, as well as a restrictive-like cardiomyopathy pattern, have also been found in other long-term follow-up studies of anthracycline-treated survivors.[39–41]

In addition to echocardiographic findings, histological evidence also indicates the impact of chronic anthracycline cardiotoxicity. Endomyocardial biopsies from survivors with chronic anthracycline cardiotoxicity exhibit both individual cardiac myocyte hypertrophy and cytoplasmic and nuclear enlargement.[5,6] These biopsies have also shown various degrees of interstitial fibrosis, which may partially explain the restrictive-like cardiomyopathy seen among survivors, although individual cardiomyocyte hypertrophy with inadequate LV wall thickness suggests that an inadequate LV mass initiates the restrictive physiology. These findings are consistent with those of echocardiography.

Treatment-related damage probably results in both cardiac cell death and permanent injury to many remaining cardiac cells. The remaining myocytes become hypertrophied by trying to compensate for those lost, but when this compensation is no longer adequate to maintain an LV mass appropriate for the somatic size of the child, LV wall thickness is reduced relative to body-surface area. This reduction may be worsened by increased apoptosis and by reduced numbers and function of cardiac stem cells. Reduced LV wall thickness increases LV wall stress and may eventually impair LV systolic performance and cardiac output. This chain of LV abnormalities, in which the remaining cardiomyocytes cannot maintain an appropriate LV wall thickness, may be exacerbated by situations such as growth hormone supplementation, pregnancy, exercise, anemia, viral infections, and additional chemotherapy, all of which increase

cardiac demands. Survivors treated with anthracyclines should be monitored carefully before or during such subsequent potential sequential stresses.

The cellular mechanisms underlying these echocardiographic, histologic, and symptomatic changes suggest that the creation of oxygen free radicals may damage the cells.[42–44] Anthracyclines readily enter cells through passive diffusion and reach intracellular concentrations several hundred times higher than those in extracellular compartments. Intracellularly, anthracyclines can undergo a series of redox reactions that result in a self-perpetuating cycle in which reactive oxygen radicals are produced. Intracellular anthracyclines may also form complexes with intracellular iron, and these complexes can produce free radicals. Reactive oxygen species and free radicals are then capable of causing DNA damage and lipid peroxidation.

Anthracyclines also have a high affinity for the mitochondrial membrane and the inner mitochondrial membrane lipid, cardiolipin.[45] This affinity can lead to anthracycline accumulation within the mitochondria, an accumulation that may impair mitochondrial membrane stability or mitochondrial DNA damage through intercalation. Such changes may subsequently impair the cell's ability to produce energy, as well as its ability to handle added oxidative stress.[43,46–48]

Several other mechanisms of anthracycline-related cardiotoxicity have been proposed, including the induction of apoptosis, the production of vasoactive amines, the formation of toxic metabolites, the upregulation of nitric oxide synthetase, and the inhibition of transcription and translation.[49–51] The findings of a recent study have shed some light on the relative sensitivity of younger tissue cells to chemotherapy medications.[52] The mitochondria of the heart and brain tissues of young mice and humans are primed for apoptosis, predisposing them to undergo cell death in response to genotoxic damage. This apoptotic machinery is almost absent from adult mitochondria, rendering them *apoptosis refractory*. Thus, young pediatric cancer patients are subject to severe adverse effects of radiation and chemotherapy from which older adults are relatively spared.[52]

Over the past several years, topoisomerase-IIβ (Top2β) alterations have been considered as a possible mechanism of doxorubicin-mediated cardiotoxicity.[53,54] As the only Top2 gene in the heart tissue, this Top2β has also been well established as the molecular target of the anticancer activity of anthracyclines.[55] The Top2β-doxorubicin-DNA ternary cleavage complex induces DNA double-strand breaks, causing cell death.[56] In mice, cardiomyocyte-specific deletion of Top2β protects cardiomyocytes from doxorubicin-induced DNA double-strand breaks and transcriptome changes, which result in defective mitochondria and the generation of reactive oxygen species.[53] Furthermore, peripheral blood leukocyte Top2β expression has been found to be higher among anthracycline-sensitive patients (with LV ejection fraction [LVEF] ≥ 10% lower than baseline and LVEF < 50%, even though these patients received a cumulative doxorubicin dose ≤ 250 mg/m^2) than among anthracycline-resistant patients (who received a cumulative doxorubicin dose ≥ 450 mg/m^2 with an LVEF ≥ 50%), a finding suggesting the potential use of Top2β as a surrogate marker of susceptibility to anthracycline-induced cardiotoxicity.[57] Furthermore, again in mice, deleting Top2β from cardiomyocytes prevented anthracycline-induced cardiotoxicity.[53] These insights into molecular changes may lead to new strategies for preventing anthracycline-induced cardiotoxicity by targeting Top2β.[58]

Because cardiac abnormalities do not develop in all children exposed to anthracyclines, and because the clinical severity of such abnormalities varies greatly, determining the factors that may increase their likelihood is greatly important. As stated above, higher cumulative doses of anthracyclines, higher anthracycline dose rates, the concomitant use of cardiotoxic therapies (such as mediastinal irradiation), younger age at treatment, increasing time since treatment, female sex, elevations in serum cTnT or NT-proBNP concentrations during anthracycline therapy, and HF during anthracycline therapy are risk factors for anthracycline cardiotoxicity.[18,39]

The strong association between the cumulative anthracycline dose and cardiotoxicity appears to become more important with time from treatment, as shown in a study of nearly 5000 survivors treated with anthracyclines who described their cardiac health at up to 30 years after treatment (Table 20-2, Figure 20-3).[15] Genetic factors can detect patients who are at higher risk of anthracycline cardiotoxicity and so may be useful in preventing cardiotoxicity.[59] This hypothesis is supported by the greater cardiac susceptibility of patients with trisomy 21 and of black patients.[4,59,60]

Despite these population-based risk factors, determining the individual risk for a specific patient is still limited. Thus, at present, all children who are treated with anthracycline should be followed closely for cardiotoxicity during and after treatment, including long-term follow-up into adulthood. The risk factors presented above are currently used to guide the frequency of follow-up examinations and may also help increase our understanding of the underlying pathophysiologic mechanisms.

RADIOTHERAPY

Irradiating the heart during cancer treatments can lead to a spectrum of cardiovascular abnormalities during follow-up. Radiation exposure can damage the pericardium, myocardium, conduction system, valves, and coronary arteries.[61] Microcirculatory damage in the heart is believed to be a common and initiating step for several forms of radiation-induced cardiac pathology because it reduces blood flow to areas of the myocardium and pericardium and leads to ischemia and subsequent fibrosis of affected tissues.[62]

Radiation-induced endothelial injury is probably responsible for coronary artery damage.[62] The mechanisms underlying damage to avascular cardiac valves are less clear; however, chronic inflammation probably contributes.[57,61] Radiation-induced pathology can have diverse clinical manifestations, including coronary artery disease, pericarditis, cardiomyopathy, valvular disease, and conduction abnormalities. Cardiac irradiation can also potentiate the cardiotoxicity of anthracycline therapy.[61]

Four studies that compared cardiac-related mortality rates among survivors to those among the general population[63] found a 22–68-fold increase in risk of cardiac death. The reported frequency of symptomatic cardiovascular disease varied widely, probably because of differences in study design, quality, and populations, but some of these studies found cardiac or cardiovascular disease in more than 20% of survivors. At 11 years after treatment, 10% of survivors treated with cardiac irradiation had coronary artery disease, and another 6% had clinically important valvular abnormalities. Of those with coronary artery disease, all had at least one traditional coronary artery disease risk factor, such as diabetes, hypertension, or high cholesterol, but higher radiation dose was also a risk factor. After 30 years, nearly 12% of those survivors in the highest-dose radiation group (a cumulative radiation dose greater than 3500 cGy) reported having HF, and 6% reported having had

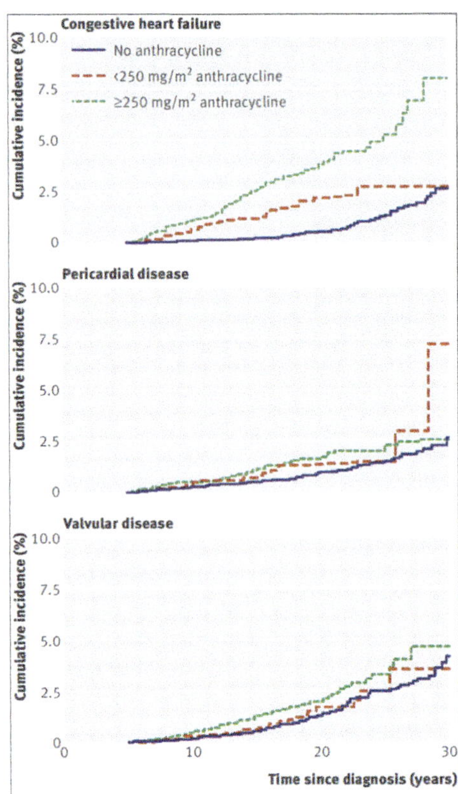

FIGURE 20-4 Cumulative incidence of cardiac disorders among childhood cancer survivors, by average cardiac radiation dose. (A) Congestive heart failure. (B) Pericardial disease. (C) Valvular disease. (From: Mulrooney DA, Yeazel MW, Kawashima T, et al. Cardiac outcomes in a cohort of adult survivors of childhood and adolescent cancer: retrospective analysis of the Childhood Cancer Survivor Study cohort. *BMJ.* 2009;339:b46067.)

a myocardial infarction (Figure 20-4). Even those patients who had been treated as children with the lowest cumulative doses of cardiac irradiation (< 500 cGy) often reported cardiac-related disease with subsequent follow-up (Figure 20-4).

A more detailed clinical evaluation of 48 asymptomatic survivors of Hodgkin disease 14 years after treatment with cardiac irradiation found that, in addition to the increased risk of symptomatic cardiac disease or death, subclinical abnormalities in cardiac structure and function were even more common.[9] Although all survivors described their health as good or better, 47 of the 48 had at least one cardiac abnormality, and 21 had marked intracardiac valvular defects. These survivors also exhibited substantial reductions in LV mass, LV wall thickness, LV end-diastolic dimensions, and LV end-systolic wall stress, findings suggesting that these patients have a restrictive cardiomyopathy. Of the 48 survivors, 20 had evidence of LV diastolic dysfunction consistent with a restrictive cardiomyopathy.

Only 4 had been treated with anthracyclines, a finding indicating that their cardiomyopathy is probably the result of cardiac irradiation.[9] A follow-up study of 21 of these 48 patients recently concluded that maximum oxygen consumption appears to be associated with future poor quality of life ($P = 0.02$).[64] A more recent study of 2617 survivors of Hodgkin lymphoma found a median interval of 19 years between cancer diagnosis and coronary heart disease.[65] This study also found a linear relationship between radiation dose and the incidence of coronary heart disease.

Patients with cardiac complications due to irradiation often require surgery. A retrospective cohort study of 173 patients with a documented history of cancer requiring chest irradiation found that short-term and long-term mortality rates were higher than those among 305 matched patients without radiation exposure who underwent similar surgical procedures.[66] During a mean (± SD) follow-up of 7.6 (± 3) years, 58% of 173 patients in the radiation-associated heart disease group died, whereas 28% of the 305 patients in the comparison group died ($P < 0.001$). This study also found that the incidence of proximal coronary artery disease and valvular heart disease was higher among patients exposed to radiation than among the comparison group.

TYROSINE KINASE INHIBITORS

Tyrosine kinase inhibitors (TKIs) are a rapidly growing chemotherapeutic drug class with high anticancer activity; they are used to treat a variety of cancers. The ubiquitous nature of the tyrosine kinases and their implication in nearly all types of cancer development make them a target for therapeutic intervention.[67,68] TKIs are not completely selective for cancer cells and can produce cardiac adverse effects, including arrhythmia, myocardial injury, and HF.[69,70] Although these drugs are still primarily used to treat adults, they are attracting greater interest in treating children, among whom their cardiac effects are unknown.

Alterations in tyrosine kinase pathways in cardiac cells may vary across TKIs, as may the progression from TKI inhibition to cardiomyocyte dysfunction and cardiac disease. Most of what is known about the potential cardiotoxic effects of TKIs comes from studies of the two most commonly used TKIs, trastuzumab and imatinib.[70–72] Trastuzumab inhibits the HER2 receptor, which is overexpressed in 20%–30% of human breast cancers and is associated with more-aggressive disease.[73] Although effective, trastuzumab is associated with an increased incidence of HF, both when used as monotherapy and when used with other known cardiotoxic treatments, such as anthracyclines and alkylating agents.[74] Although trastuzumab use is likely to remain more limited to treating breast cancer, which occurs predominantly in women, TKIs are now increasingly being used to treat a variety of childhood cancers.[75,76] Short- and long-term monitoring of the cardiac status of children exposed to TKIs will be an important part of evaluating these treatments.

Imatinib is highly effective in treating several types of cancer, most notably chronic myelogenous leukemia. Imatinib has been associated with cardiac injury, but only rarely.[72] Cardiac troponin T concentrations may indicate cardiac damage after imatinib treatment, and the severity of the cardiac injury can be influenced by arterial blood pressure.[77] Despite a lack of evidence-based guidelines, patients with cardiac disease or those who are at risk of LV dysfunction should be carefully monitored during treatment with imatinib because many patients who have imatinib-related HF also appear to have had other risk factors before treatment, such as HF or coronary artery disease.[78]

A retrospective study of 219 sarcoma patients treated with imatinib found that cardiac complications were rare.[79] Less-severe cardiotoxic effects, such as edema or effusions, occurred in 8.2% of these patients. A recent prospective study of 59 patients with chronic myeloid leukemia treated with imatinib for 3.4 years found no evidence of myocardial deterioration.[80] Although similar reports show that imatinib is less cardiotoxic than other chemotherapies, such as the anthracyclines, the long-term consequences of this therapy are still largely unknown, especially when it is administered with other cardiotoxic agents.

CARDIAC MONITORING

The cardiac status of survivors can be monitored with several techniques before, during, and after cancer treatment, but little evidence guides the use of these techniques.[81] The clinical utility of monitoring depends on whether it occurs before, during, or after treatment and on which strategies are being used. For patients who will be treated with known cardiotoxic therapies, such as anthracyclines or cardiac irradiation, baseline and follow-up echocardiography focused on relevant cardiac data for the therapy used can help identify cardiotoxicity, although its value may be limited during therapy and it is resource-intense.

As in other cardiac disorders, readily available serum biomarkers, such as cTnT, are being increasingly used to detect acute cardiotoxicity during treatment. Additionally, biomarkers such as NT-proBNP, a

measure of cardiomyopathy related to increased production of this peptide in relation to LV pressure or volume overload, and highly sensitive C-reactive protein, a generalized measure of inflammation that may be associated with cardiac disease, may be useful in the ongoing cardiac evaluation of these patients and in detecting long-term cardiotoxicity. However, despite the utility of echocardiography and biomarker assays for cardiac monitoring, regular histories and physical examinations remain essential.

ECHOCARDIOGRAPHY

Echocardiography is the most common method of monitoring the cardiac status of children with cancer.[82] Nearly all treatment protocols that include anthracyclines require a pretreatment echocardiogram for collecting baseline measurements of cardiac structure and function.[82] However, the utility of echocardiography in monitoring patients with preexisting echocardiographic abnormalities has recently been questioned.[83] Furthermore, echocardiographic measures of LV systolic performance, including those obtained with newer techniques of myocardial two-dimensional (2D) strain echocardiography, are not related to biomarker concentrations of myocardial injury during anthracycline therapy.[84,85] These measurements may be affected by cytokine-mediated myocardial depression and abnormal LV loading conditions.[84,86] These confounding factors have rendered echocardiographic measurements acquired during chemotherapy less predictive of late cardiotoxicity among long-term survivors; they are not nearly as useful in this regard as are cTnT and NT-proBNP concentrations.

Echocardiographic measurements may help to determine which patients are more vulnerable than others to cardiotoxic therapies and to provide comparisons for newer measurements, but measurements obtained during therapy have not yet been validated for this purpose. The goal is to detect as early as possible any subtle cardiotoxic changes that increase the risk of cardiovascular disease progression. Newer techniques, such as Doppler echocardiography, cardiac strain, and strain rate, have recently been used in conjunction with cardiac biomarkers to accomplish this task.[19,86–89]

Subclinical echocardiographic changes in LV structure and function depend on several factors that are not cardiac-related, including LV afterload and preload, but that can vary greatly among children undergoing chemotherapy.[81] A more recent study found no relationship between myocardial 2D strain echocardiography findings and cTnT or NT-pro-BNP concentrations.[86]

To some degree, this finding may reflect the ability of echocardiography to detect cellular changes only after they have caused macroscopic changes in either LV structure or function.[90,91] Despite this limited ability, many childhood cancer treatment protocols still require echocardiography at various points during treatment.[84] Unfortunately, such testing may actually be harmful if abnormal results change cancer treatment and therefore may lead to reduced oncologic effectiveness among patients who do not have clinical cardiovascular disease. The overall success of childhood cancer therapy should be defined by the life-long balance of oncologic effectiveness with toxicities and late effects, with quality of life taken into account.[81]

After cancer treatment, echocardiography is the main method used to detect cardiotoxicity among survivors. Recommendations for surveillance often conflict, given the limitations of echocardiography.[92] Current guidelines from the Children's Oncology Group recommend life-long echocardiographic screening every 3 to 5 years for survivors treated with anthracyclines or cardiac irradiation.[93,94] These guidelines take into account various risk factors, including age at treatment, other therapies received, and cumulative dose, to determine the frequency of follow-up. In contrast, Scottish Intercollegiate Guidelines recommend screening every 2 to 3 years for patients at higher risk of anthracycline-induced cardiotoxicity but do not recommend a screening duration.[95] The American Heart Association recommends close monitoring of cardiac function, but its guidelines do not specify the modality or frequency of screening.[96] Although recommended echocardiographic testing may detect subclinical cardiac abnormalities in many survivors, the meaning of such abnormalities for individual survivors is still unclear, as is how to slow or stop these changes from progressing to clinically apparent disease. In fact, recently, the efficacy and cost-effectiveness of these screening guidelines have been questioned.[97,98] The implementation of these strategies must also be considered because many survivors do not adhere to current screening guidelines, although physician involvement increases adherence.[99]

SERUM CARDIAC TROPONIN CONCENTRATIONS

The inability of echocardiography to reliably detect cardiac damage among childhood cancer patients led to investigations of serum concentrations of cTnT as a more sensitive marker of acute anthracycline-related cardiac damage (Table 20-1).[90,91,100,101] Serum cardiac troponin levels are now widely used in diagnosing and managing ischemic heart disease in adults. They also provide valuable clinical information about many other types of cardiac damage in children.[102–106]

The protein cTnT is a cardiac-specific isoform present in both the contractile unit of the cardiac myocyte and the cytoplasm. Normally, serum concentrations of cTnT are undetectable by standard assays beyond the newborn period. Elevated (> or = 0.5 ng/ml) concentrations indicate cardiac myocyte damage, although newer, more sensitive tests may able to detect lower concentrations; however, the implications of any underlying cardiomyocyte damage are less clear.[105]

Serum cTnT concentrations were significantly elevated during therapy in 6 of 10 children with ALL treated with anthracyclines. This result contrasts with that of 5 children who had been treated with anthracyclines but at the time of the study were being treated with other chemotherapeutic agents; none of these children had elevated serum cTnT concentrations. The serum cTnT elevations in the group still being treated with anthracyclines were strongly correlated with LV end-diastolic dimension and LV wall thickness measurements taken 9 months after treatment.[90]

These findings are consistent with those obtained from animal models, in which cTnT concentrations were elevated in response to doxorubicin.[91,100] Additionally, these studies found that cTnT concentrations were related to both the dose of doxorubicin and the severity of the findings from cardiac histopathologic examination. Additional histologic examinations showed that cardiac cells with the most pathologic changes were also those with the smallest amounts of remaining intracellular cTnT. These findings are consistent with the hypothesis that anthracyclines damage cardiomyocytes and release intracellular cTnT into the circulation.

The findings presented above support the use of serum cTnT concentrations to measure cardiac damage in several studies of patients with childhood cancer treated with anthracyclines.[84,107–109] One study found that lower cTnT concentrations during treatment were associated with improved cardiac structure and function as measured by echocardiography 4 years later.[101] These findings are evidence of the value of serum cTnT measurements in monitoring survivors who are being treated with anthracyclines, and these measurements are now being increasingly used worldwide.[110–113] Among 134 children being treated with moderate-dose anthracyclines for high-risk ALL, elevated serum cTnT concentrations during the first 90 days of anthracycline treatment were significantly associated with reduced LV end-diastolic posterior wall thickness and LV mass and with increased LV remodeling 4 years later.[101]

SERUM NT-PROBNP CONCENTRATIONS

Echocardiography is the most accepted method of monitoring survivors for cardiac abnormalities after treatment, but used alone it may yield incomplete results, and it is resource-intensive.[81,82] The desire to use echocardiography more judiciously, to confirm ambiguous echocardiographic results, and to detect abnormalities not apparent on echocardiography has led to studies of the family of biomarkers related to BNP. These biomarkers may also assist in monitoring childhood cancer patients during therapy because, unlike serum cTnT elevations that indicate myocardial damage, elevated concentrations of BNP and related markers indicate increased myocardial stress that may precede myocardial damage.

The protein BNP is produced by the ventricles in response to increased cardiac stress and is an attractive option for monitoring survivors because of this physiologic relationship with cardiac function and because of the low cost and wide availability of assays. In addition to BNP, the N-terminal peptide of BNP, NT-proBNP, is secreted simultaneously but has a longer half-life and is often used for the same purpose. Several studies of pediatric HF have found that BNP is an important diagnostic and prognostic tool.[114,115]

Among 200 children with ALL treated with doxorubicin, serum NT-proBNP concentrations measured after treatment were associated with elevated concentrations of serum cTnT and abnormal LV fractional shortening.[101,116] In this study, a higher proportion of patients had elevated NT-proBNP concentrations than had elevated cTnT concentrations, a finding suggesting that NT-proBNP may be more sensitive than cTnT alone in determining which survivors are at higher risk of future anthracycline-related cardiomyopathy. Of the 134 children described above who were treated with moderate-dose anthracyclines for high-risk ALL, elevated serum concentrations of NT-proBNP, indicating cardiomyopathy during the first 90 days of treatment, were correlated with abnormal LV thickness-to-dimension ratios 4 years later (Figure 20-5). Furthermore, during and after treatment the percentage of patients with elevated NT-proBNP concentrations was higher than that of patients with elevated cTnT concentrations.[101]

Even among childhood leukemia survivors treated with low-dose anthracycline, higher concentrations of NT-pro-BNP may detect cardiotoxicity earlier than does echocardiography.[117] The relationships between these hormones and cardiac abnormalities among survivors treated with anthracyclines have been found consistently, although they were not consistent in the outcomes examined or the hormone assays used. A recent meta-analysis found that serum concentrations of BNP were significantly higher after treatment with anthracyclines among patients with cardiotoxicity than among those without cardiotoxicity.[118] NT-pro-BNP concentrations are now used worldwide to surveil cancer survivors for cardiotoxicity.[85,86,111,118–122]

■ Serum Concentrations of hs-CRP and NT-proBNP

Systemic inflammation is not only associated with increased rates of cardiovascular disease among adults but may also be a unique mechanism underlying other cardiac-related diseases, including pediatric cardiomyopathy and anthracycline-related cardiotoxicity.[115] Concentrations of high-sensitivity C-reactive protein (hs-CRP) are an easily measured marker of systemic inflammation and are commonly used in a variety of clinical settings.[115] Among 19 children with HF, who were separated into three groups on the basis of symptom severity, hs-CRP concentrations were associated with decreased LV function and also discriminated between symptom severity groups.[115] Furthermore, concentrations of hs-CRP were significantly higher among 201 survivors than among sibling control subjects.[10] Another study found that the percentage of patients in the doxorubicin-only group who had elevated hs-CRP concentrations was higher 6 months after the initiation of treatment than at baseline and was also significantly higher than that among the dexrazoxane-treated group by the end of treatment.[101] Serum hs-CRP concentrations may be valuable for detecting survivors who are at higher risk of subsequent cardiac disease but who would otherwise be missed.

TRADITIONAL RISK FACTORS FOR CARDIOVASCULAR DISEASE

Survivors, like the general population, may exhibit one or more of the traditional risk factors for atherosclerosis and cardiovascular disease and, thus, for cardiovascular complications and ischemic heart damage. In addition, some survivors may be at higher risk of these traditional atherosclerotic risk factors, a finding adding to the risk of cardiovascular disease beyond that directly related to cancer therapies, such as irradiation. The prevalence of these traditional atherosclerotic risk factors among survivors and the additional cardiovascular risk are associated with a history of childhood cancer and specific treatments, especially cranial irradiation because of its association with endocrine abnormalities.

The most commonly studied traditional and modifiable atherosclerotic risk factors are obesity, tobacco

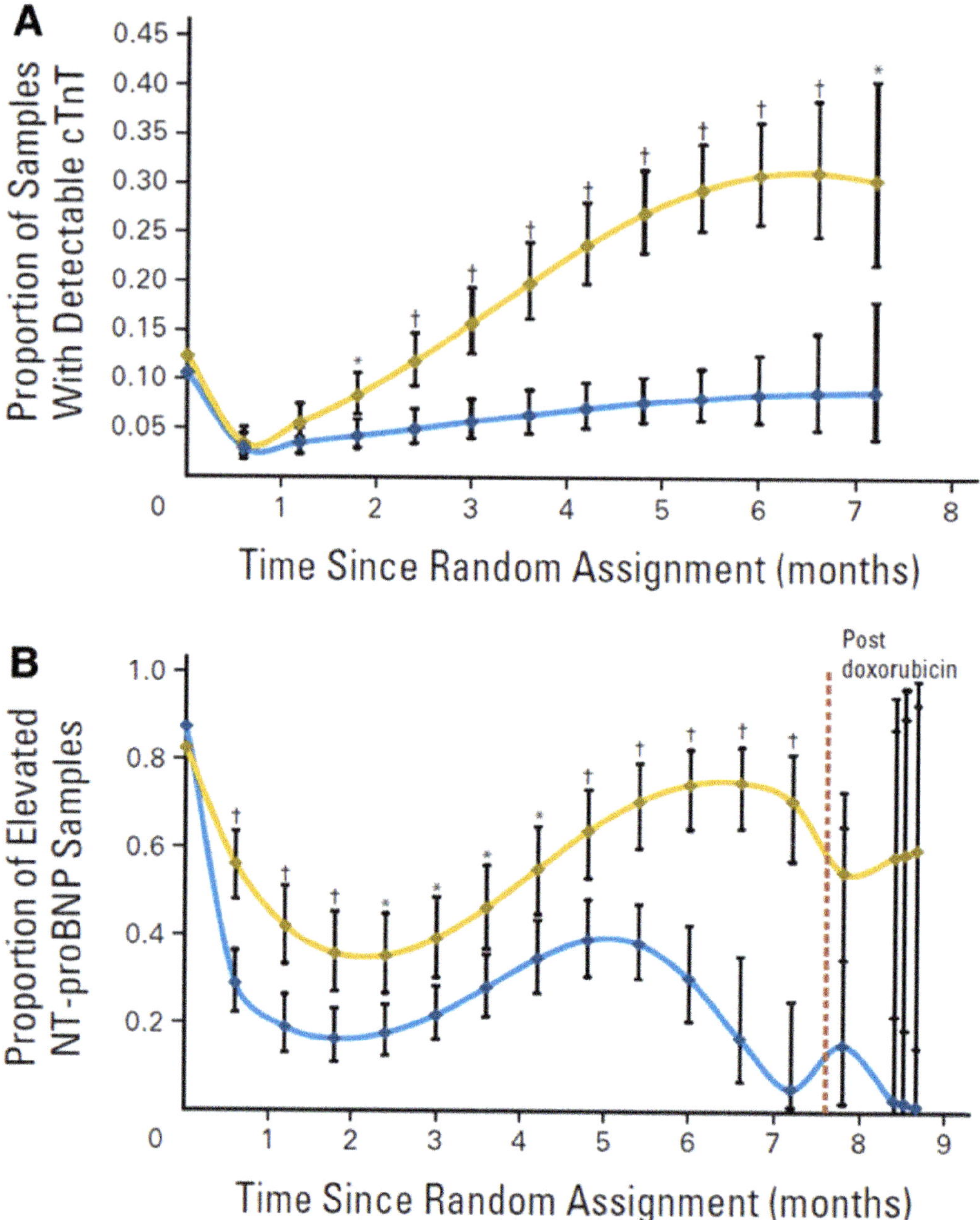

FIGURE 20-5 Model-based estimated probability of having (A) an increased cardiac troponin T concentration or (B) an elevated N-terminal pro-brain natriuretic peptide (NT-proBNP) concentration in patients treated with doxorubicin, with or without dexrazoxane. Blue line, doxorubicin-dexrazoxane group; gold line, doxorubicin group. Vertical bars show 95% confidence intervals. Increased cardiac troponin T (cTnT) concentration is defined as a value higher than 0.01 ng/ mL. *, $P \leq 0.05$ vs. dexrazoxane group; †, $P \leq 0.001$vs. dexrazoxane group. Results of an overall test for dexrazoxane effect during treatment were statistically significant ($P < 0.001$). Increased NT-proBNP concentration is defined as a value of 150 pg/mL or higher for children less than 1 year old and of 100 pg/mL or higher for children aged 1 year or older. *, $P \leq 0.05$ vs. dexrazoxane group; †, $P \leq 0.001$ vs. dexrazoxane group. Results of an overall test for dexrazoxane effect were statistically significant ($P < 0.001$) during treatment but were not statistically significant after treatment ($P = 0.24$). (Permission from American Society of Clinical Oncology. Lipshultz SE, et al. Lipshultz SE, Miller TL, Scully RE, et al. Changes in cardiac biomarkers during doxorubicin treatment of pediatric patients with high-risk acute lymphoblastic leukemia: associations with long-term echocardiographic outcomes. *J Clin Oncol.* 2012 Apr 1;30(10):1042–1049. doi: 10.1200/JCO.2010.30.3404. Epub 2012 Feb 27.)

use, diabetes mellitus, dyslipidemia, and physical inactivity. An improved understanding of the lifetime cardiovascular risk associated with these factors in cancer survivors may help guide current treatment decisions and determine the potential additional cardiovascular risk associated with specific cancer therapies, such as prophylactic cranial irradiation.[123] For survivors, who may already be at increased risk of atherosclerotic disease or who are less able to compensate for atherosclerotic disease, knowing how these risk factors affect overall long-term cardiovascular risk may inform preventive or therapeutic interventions.

■ Obesity

Over the past 30 years, childhood obesity (body mass index [BMI] ≥ 30, the adult definition of obesity) has become an increasingly serious public health concern in the United States. In 2012, almost 17% of 2- to 19-year-olds were obese, as were almost 14% of adolescents aged 12 to 19 years.[124] Childhood overweight and obesity are especially troubling because they are associated with poor health outcomes, such as coronary artery disease, hypertension, and diabetes and because they are strongly associated with obesity in adulthood, which is associated with an increased risk of atherosclerotic disease and death. According to the American Heart Association Childhood Obesity Research Summit, "Obesity contributes to a significant burden in terms of chronic diseases, rising healthcare costs, and, most importantly, disability and premature death. It appears that this burden will increase in the future."[125]

Studies of obesity among survivors have found similarly troubling increases, a finding suggesting that survivors may be at higher risk of obesity because of their cancer. The largest report to date of nearly 8000 survivors who were more than 20 years old and alive at the time of the baseline questionnaire assessment found that nearly 13% were obese, with a BMI higher than 30, and that another 28% were overweight, with a BMI between 25 and 30.[126] This study also found that survivors, despite a high prevalence of obesity, were not more likely to be obese than the general population, although certain groups were at higher risk, such as survivors of ALL. However, other studies have found no increased risk for being underweight or overweight or obese among survivors than among the rest of the population[127]; these studies included ALL survivors.[128] Among 893 childhood cancer survivors in the Netherlands, only girls had a significantly higher incidence of obesity.[129] Children with high BMI, those younger at the time of cancer diagnosis, and those treated with cranial irradiation were at highest risk of a high BMI after treatment.[129]

Survivors treated with cranial irradiation are decidedly at increased risk of obesity. Many studies show treatment-related damage to the hypothalamic-pituitary axis, with subsequent growth hormone deficiency and eventual obesity. However, some studies report a higher risk of being overweight[130] or underweight,[131] whereas others have found that the weight distribution among these survivors is similar to that of the general population.[132] However, it is clear that obesity is prevalent among survivors of all types of childhood cancer and may predispose this group to future health problems, especially atherosclerotic disease, which may be especially problematic because these patients are less able to compensate for ischemic cardiac insults.

TOBACCO USE

Cigarette smoking is an important preventable risk factor for cardiovascular disease and death, as well as all-cause mortality. High-risk behaviors, such as abusing cigarettes, alcohol, energy drinks, or illicit drugs, may increase the risk of late cardiotoxicity.[18] A systematic review of the health behaviors of survivors found that most studies have reported lower rates of smoking among survivors relative to the general population, although these rates are still high enough to warrant concern and interventions.[133] As many as 17% of all survivors and of the general population in the United States are active smokers.[134] However, a more recent study reported that almost 35% of adult survivors smoke cigarettes, despite the additional risks associated with their history of cancer and its treatment.[135] Moreover, in the United States, the smoking prevalence among adult survivors was significantly higher than among the control group of adults with no history of cancer, especially among women, and the prevalence varied markedly by geographic region.[135]

INSULIN RESISTANCE AND DYSLIPIDEMIA

The increasing prevalence of obesity and the decreasing amount of physical activity have increased the prevalence of insulin resistance and overt diabetes. In 2012, the prevalence of diabetes in United States was 14.3%.[136] Diabetes, an important risk factor for cardiovascular disease, triples the risk of ischemic heart disease in 45- to 64-year-olds. A recent report involving more than 8000 survivors found that they were nearly twice as likely to report having diabetes as their sibling controls.[137] Exposure to total body irradiation, abdominal irradiation, or cranial irradiation was associated with increased reporting of diabetes, even after the analyses were adjusted for BMI and level of physical activity. This result suggests that traditional prevention methods may be only partially effective and that new approaches may be necessary for minimizing the cardiovascular and health complications associated with insulin resistance and diabetes among survivors.

Diabetes mellitus eventually developed in 157 (7%) of 2265 Hodgkin lymphoma survivors.[138] The cumulative incidence after 30 years was 8.3%.[138] A cross-sectional study found that 319 childhood cancer survivors at least 5 years after diagnosis had more adiposity, lower lean body mass, and higher levels of total cholesterol, low-density lipoprotein cholesterol, and triglyceride concentration than did 208 sibling control subjects. Survivors were also less insulin-sensitive than control subjects.[139]

The American Heart Association and other committees charged with reducing cardiovascular risk among high-risk children have concluded that treating diabetes mellitus or insulin resistance is likely to be as effective among childhood cancer survivors as among the general population, unless the underlying causes of impaired glucose metabolism are different, such as abnormalities in the hypothalamus-pituitary axis.[140]

Another study comparing childhood cancer survivors to their siblings found that the incidence of insulin resistance was significantly higher among those treated with platinum-based chemotherapy plus cranial radiotherapy and among those treated with steroids but no platinum-based chemotherapy.[141] A recent review concluded that hypothalamic irradiation determines growth hormone deficiency and hypogonadism.[142] Moreover, irradiation can disrupt the appetite-regulating center, leading to hyperphagia and, thus, to obesity. These conditions create insulin resistance, which contributes to the development of metabolic syndrome and diabetes mellitus.

Another effect of irradiation or chemotherapy is that it may directly damage pancreatic beta cells, thereby disrupting insulin secretion.[142] Complicating matters further for many survivors is the fact that treatment-related cardiotoxicity may leave survivors more vulnerable to cardiovascular disease.[8] Survivors may also have other, less-common metabolic risk factors, such as vitamin D deficiency, that increase their total cardiovascular risk.[143]

Aggressive and early intervention is warranted to reduce the risk in this population as much as possible. A 16-year follow-up of 340 long-term survivors of childhood cancer found that 20% had hypercholesterolemia, 6% had hypertriglyceridemia, and 8% were obese. Total body irradiation and growth hormone deficiency increased the risk of both hypercholesterolemia and hypertriglyceridemia. The risk of hypercholesterolemia was also higher among survivors who underwent autologous hematopoietic stem cell transplant or platinum-based chemotherapy.[144]

A study of 50 survivors with abnormal cholesterol concentrations at an average of 13 years after cancer diagnosis found that mean high-density lipoprotein (HDL) cholesterol concentrations, which are associated with decreased cardiovascular risk, were lower than those among age- and sex-matched control subjects.[22] The results of this study also suggested that dyslipidemia is associated with endocrine dysfunction and possibly with growth hormone deficiency.

Another study involving 23 patients who had undergone bone marrow transplant as children found that, at a median follow-up of 20 years, 17 patients had abnormally low concentrations of HDL cholesterol and abnormally high concentrations of low-density lipoprotein (LDL) cholesterol.[145] Another study involving more than 200 survivors found that the mean concentration of LDL cholesterol was higher than that among 70 healthy siblings.[10] However, these cholesterol abnormalities were found in studies involving adults and show that increased concentrations of LDL cholesterol and decreased concentrations of HDL cholesterol are strongly associated with atherosclerosis and future cardiovascular complications.

Both lifestyle modifications and medications can improve LDL cholesterol and HDL cholesterol concentrations.[146] Although these lifestyle modifications and medications have yet to be tested among survivors, they have greatly reduced the risk of cardiovascular disease and death for the general population.[147] It is hoped that these interventions will also improve outcomes for survivors, who are already at higher risk of elevated LDL cholesterol and reduced HDL cholesterol concentrations.[140]

PHYSICAL INACTIVITY

Physical inactivity is associated with a higher risk of cardiovascular disease, as are other traditional atherosclerotic disease risk factors, such as insulin resistance, dyslipidemia, and obesity. Several medical associations, including the American Academy of Pediatrics, recommend physical activity, and several organizations, including the U.S. Department of Health and Human Services, have issued exercise guidelines.[148] Among 1000 children whose physical activity was measured with an accelerometer, levels of physical activity decreased markedly between 9 and 15 years of age. By the age of 15 years, nearly 70% of children exercised less than the current guideline recommendation of 1 hour per day.[149]

Although physical activity is uncommon among the general population, it appears to be even less common among survivors. A survey of nearly 10,000 survivors and 3,000 of their siblings showed that survivors were more likely than their siblings to be physically inactive, had not engaged in leisure-time physical activity in the past month, and were less likely than their siblings to meet recommended physical activity guidelines.[150] This survey and others have found that some survivors may be unable to comply with these guidelines because of physical limitations due to cancer-related surgery or treatment-related cardiac damage.[151] It is hoped that appropriate and safe increases in the physical activity of survivors will decrease their cardiovascular risk.[151–153]

TREATING ANTHRACYCLINE-ASSOCIATED CARDIOTOXICITY

Long-term survivors of childhood cancers are a growing sector of the population, and most of them have been exposed to anthracyclines. Current screening tests have detected a large and increasing number of asymptomatic and symptomatic cardiac complications, which create a great need for validated therapies that can prevent and treat the cardiotoxicity associated with cancer therapy.[93] Given that these cardiac complications are often progressive, medical interventions are potentially of great benefit to survivors. Such interventions are often used, and the opportunities for and value of expanding their use are large.[36]

Drugs that are often used, and for which relevant clinical data exist, are angiotensin-converting enzyme (ACE) inhibitors, beta blockers, and growth hormone therapy. These therapies, however, appear to be of unknown or limited benefit in reducing the morbidity and mortality rates associated with anthracycline-related cardiotoxicity in children. Knowing the natural progression of anthracycline-related structural changes, in which dilated cardiomyopathy becomes restrictive cardiomyopathy, is essential for tailoring therapy because many medications used to treat heart failure caused by dilated cardiomyopathy are inappropriate for treating those caused by restrictive cardiomyopathy.[154]

Currently, there is no standard therapy for anthracycline-related cardiotoxicity. The goal of therapy is to prevent or slow LV remodeling rather than to treat the cause of cardiomyopathy.[155] Testing new therapies in this population is important because anthracycline-related cardiotoxicity differs markedly from other forms of pediatric and adult heart disease, and this difference probably limits the appropriateness of generalizing results across populations. This situation emphasizes the need for new and specific strategies for treating anthracycline-related cardiotoxicity and suggests that methods of preventing these complications would be of great clinical utility.

◼ Treatment with ACE Inhibitors

As discussed above, the use of serial echocardiography to monitor survivors exposed to anthracyclines has shown that elevated LV afterload may precede clinically apparent LV dysfunction and is largely the result of decreased LV mass and LV wall thickness. The increased stress placed on the remaining cardiac myocytes has been hypothesized to further exacerbate decreased LV wall thickness and to contribute to the progression to HF.[38,156] Thus, interventions that reduce LV afterload, such as ACE inhibitors, were expected to break the cycle of events leading to anthracycline-related cardiotoxicity.[157] This hypothesis was supported by the effectiveness of ACE inhibitors in treating other forms of pediatric ventricular dysfunction and their incorporation into guidelines for treating pediatric HF.[158] However, the fact that ACE inhibitors do not provide a sustained benefit in treating survivors with anthracycline-related cardiotoxicity raises concerns that the risks of these drugs may outweigh their benefit in this population.[38]

The preventiOn of left Ventricular dysfunction with Enalapril and caRvedilol in patients submitted to intensive ChemOtherapy for the treatment of Malignant hEmopathies (OVERCOME) trial randomly assigned 90 adult patients with normal baseline cardiac function to receive either enalapril and carvedilol before and after high-dose chemotherapy or no cardiovascular drugs. At 6-months' follow-up, LVEF was significantly more preserved in the treatment group than in the control group.[159]

A retrospective review of serial echocardiogram images obtained from long-term survivors being treated with the ACE inhibitor enalapril provided the first evidence that ACE inhibitors may not be as effective as hypothesized.[160] This study examined all 18 survivors who had been treated with enalapril after treatment with doxorubicin at Boston Children's Hospital from 1984 to 1989; 6 of these survivors were in HF at the beginning of therapy. As expected, during the first few years of enalapril therapy the mean LV afterload was significantly reduced and was strongly related to reductions in diastolic blood pressure. Mean LV fractional shortening also improved, although LV wall thickness did not. After patients had taken the drug for 6 to 10 years, these improvements were no longer evident. Mean LV wall thickness steadily declined. All

6 patients who were in HF when enalapril therapy was initiated had died or undergone heart transplant, and 7 of the 12 originally asymptomatic patients had progressed to HF. The results of this study indicate that, although ACE inhibitors may exert some short-term benefit, they do not prevent the progression of disease and do not alter the pathologic process of decreasing LV wall thickness relative to body-surface area.

These findings were confirmed by the results of a randomized trial involving 135 survivors treated with enalapril.[161] Despite initial reductions in LV afterload in the enalapril group, neither LV fractional shortening nor LV contractility improved. Additionally, adverse events were more common among the enalapril group than among a control group and included dizziness or hypotension in 22% and fatigue in 10%. This trial, however, had several limitations, including a median follow-up of only 2.8 years, the use of a surrogate outcome not validated in this population, and maximal cardiac index on exercise testing. Thus, the trial does not provide definitive evidence of benefit for this population.

That these studies did not find a clear clinical benefit for ACE inhibitors suggests that the proven and suspected risks associated with their use should be evaluated more completely.[38] In addition to well-described risks, such as cough and symptoms of hypotension, other issues may be associated with the use of these drugs to treat survivors, especially because this group is expected to have a lifetime of accumulated exposure. The issues include but are not limited to cost, drug interactions, risk of second neoplasms, chronic neurohormonal suppression, and psychosocial concerns.[38] The findings also suggest that the results of studies of other forms of pediatric ventricular dysfunction may not be generalizable to survivors with anthracycline-related cardiotoxicity. This suggestion highlights the unique restrictive-like pattern often seen in anthracycline-related cardiotoxicity.

TREATMENT WITH BETA BLOCKERS

The use of beta blockers to treat survivors with LV dysfunction is largely supported by pathophysiological theories, generalizations from studies involving either adults or children with other forms of cardiac disease, and descriptive reports of their use in survivors.[20] The blockade of sympathetic stimulation to the heart and reduced cardiac demand are hypothesized to slow the progression of anthracycline-related cardiotoxicity. Specifically, carvedilol is attractive because it simultaneously reduces cardiac demand, as a nonselective beta blocker, and LV afterload, as an alpha-1 blocker through systemic vasodilation.

Carvedilol effectively treats other forms of pediatric HF. Among 24 children with dilated cardiomyopathy and LV dysfunction, carvedilol was well tolerated and was associated with substantial improvements in LV ejection fraction and mean LV sphericity index.[162] These findings are consistent with those of other studies and suggest that carvedilol improves LV performance.[163,164] A randomized trial involving 25 adults treated with doxorubicin with or without carvedilol pretreatment found that, after 6 months, mean ejection fraction was preserved in the carvedilol group but was significantly decreased in the doxorubicin-only group.[165] A randomized trial involving 50 children with newly diagnosed ALL treated with doxorubicin with or without carvedilol pretreatment found that pretreatment reduced LV systolic function and increased plasma troponin I and lactate dehydrogenase concentrations. Pretreatment with carvedilol significantly increased systolic function and inhibited doxorubicin-induced increases in plasma troponin I and lactate dehydrogenase concentrations. However, the follow-up period was short.[166]

TREATMENT WITH GROWTH HORMONE

For many survivors, growth hormone deficiency can be the result of treatment-related exposures, such as cranial irradiation.[9] The cranial irradiation associated with cardiac risk among cancer patients may also be related to growth hormone deficiency.[10] For these survivors, growth hormone replacement therapy may help address the anthropomorphic issues related to this deficiency. Growth hormone supplementation is also likely to have cardiac consequences that are especially relevant to survivors with treatment-related cardiotoxicity.[167] However, the added cardiac demands associated with growth hormone use may overwhelm the remaining cardiac myocytes.[168] Growth hormone may induce LV growth and reduce LV afterload.[169] Such changes could possibly be beneficial by slowing or preventing the progression of anthracycline cardiotoxicity.[167] This hypothesis is supported by the results of small pilot studies involving adults with cardiomyopathy and HF, although these findings have not been confirmed by larger randomized controlled trials.[167]

A retrospective review involving 34 survivors treated with growth hormone therapy and 86 similar untreated patients found that growth hormone therapy was associated with significant increases in both LV mass and LV wall thickness, although these gains were lost when therapy was discontinued.[167] Neither increased LV mass nor LV wall thickness was associated with decreased LV afterload, however, because of a simultaneous expansion in LV end-diastolic dimensions.[167] Additionally, load-independent LV function, as measured by LV contractility, did not improve.[167] These results preclude the use of growth hormone therapy for the sole purpose of treating older children for anthracycline cardiotoxicity.

When the risk of premature cardiovascular disease is reduced, the trade-offs between treating growth hormone–deficient survivors with growth hormone replacement therapy and the risk of cancer recurrence or a second malignancy are unknown. The timing of growth hormone administration may be important when optimal windows for effective cardiac therapy are assessed. Other points that must be addressed are the duration of therapy and the effectiveness of growth hormone as prophylaxis for anthracycline-related cardiotoxicity.

Survivors may need growth hormone therapy for reasons other than as potential therapy for anthracycline-related cardiotoxicity. In such a case, baseline and serial echocardiographic images should be acquired so that any cardiac complications can be detected. The effects of administering growth hormone therapy before anthracycline-related cardiotoxicity occurs are unknown.

TREATMENT WITH MECHANICAL SUPPORT

If medical management fails, mechanical support can be used. Such support includes pacemakers, ventricular assist devices, implantable defibrillators, and extracorporeal membranous oxygenation. However, as many as 40% of patients experience complications associated with these interventions, such as coagulopathy, infection, and neurological complications.[101] Cardiac transplant is indicated when there are no other options.[170]

PREVENTING ANTHRACYCLINE CARDIOTOXICITY

Anthracyclines have contributed greatly to improvements in childhood cancer survival. Additionally, the ability to use even higher doses of anthracyclines without the fear of cardiac complications could provide a new strategy for further improving survival rates.[171] Given that current medical interventions do little to stop or slow the progression of treatment-related cardiotoxicity, efforts to prevent this toxicity remain of great clinical interest.[171] Although some preventive methods have not been as successful

as hoped, the cardioprotectant dexrazoxane and several other strategies continue to hold great promise in helping prevent anthracycline-related cardiotoxicity.[171,172] Other prevention methods are being investigated in animal models and in trials involving adults. Nevertheless, such strategies will require specific testing in childhood cancer patients before they can be used to treat these patients (Figure 20-6).[171]

TREATMENT WITH LIPOSOMAL FORMULATIONS OF ANTHRACYCLINES

One of the strategies proposed to decrease anthracycline-related cardiotoxicity is liposomal encapsulation, which alters the tissue distribution and pharmacokinetics of the liposome agents. Liposomal formulations of anthracyclines include liposomal daunorubicin, liposomal doxorubicin (D-99), and pegylated liposomal doxorubicin. Liposomal formulations allow the anthracycline molecule to penetrate selectively through the impaired vasculature; this penetration increases the concentration of the drug in the tumor and reduces exposure of the sensitive tissues of the heart muscle to the drug. The slow release of the drug coupled with the alteration of tissue distribution may reduce peak plasma doxorubicin concentrations in heart muscle.[173] The risk of anthracycline-induced cardiotoxicity is considerably lower with liposomal doxorubicin formulations than with conventional doxorubicin. However, because few studies have compared liposomal daunorubicin with conventional anthracyclines, their relative effect is unknown.[173–175]

A multicenter therapy-optimization trial (Acute Myeloblastic Leukemia–Berlin-Frankfürt-Münster [AML-BFM] 2004) randomly assigned 521 children with AML to induction therapy with either liposomal daunorubicin or idarubicin. Event-free 5-year overall survival rates and the cumulative incidence of relapse were similar in both groups, but treatment-related mortality rates were lower with daunorubicin (2 of 257 patients) than with idarubicin (10 of 264 patients; $P = 0.04$). Grade 3/4 cardiotoxicity occurred rarely after induction (daunorubicin, 4 patients; idarubicin, 5 patients). Only 1 patient treated with daunorubicin and 3 patients treated with idarubicin experienced subclinical or mild cardiomyopathy during follow-up. The study concluded that overall antileukemic activity was similar with both drugs and that treatment-related mortality rates were lower with liposomal daunorubicin than with idarubicin.[174] An open-label, single-arm phase II trial of elderly patients with diffuse large

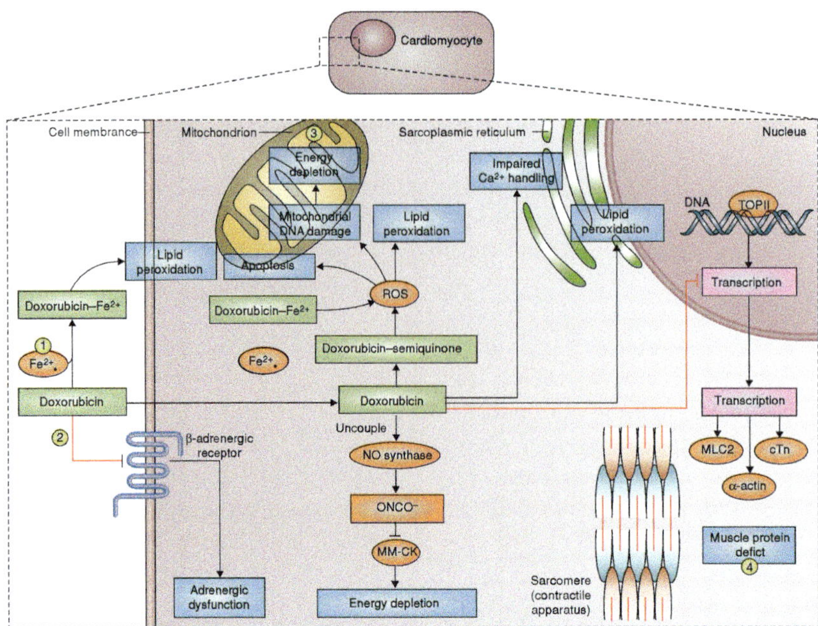

FIGURE 20-6 Potential opportunities for cardioprotection. cTn, cardiac troponin; MLC-2, myosin light chain 2; MM-CK, myofibrillar isoform of the CK enzyme; NO, nitric oxide; ROS, reactive oxygen species; TOPII, topoisomerase II;. (Adapted from Lipshultz SE, Cochran TR, Franco VI, Miller TL. Treatment-related cardiotoxicity in survivors of childhood cancer. *Nat Rev Clin Oncol*. 2013 Dec;10(12):697–710. Used with permission from The Nature Publishing Group.)

B-cell lymphoma substituted a conventional anthracycline with pegylated liposomal doxorubicin and reached similar conclusions.[175]

TREATMENT WITH ANTHRACYCLINE DERIVATIVES

Epirubicin, idarubicin, and mitoxantrone are structural analogues of anthracyclines that are believed to be less cardiotoxic than the original anthracyclines. A meta-analysis of studies treating adults with anthracyclines concluded that the risk of clinical cardiotoxicity with doxorubicin and epirubicin treatment was twice that of mitoxantrone treatment.[176] Among 115 adults treated with idarubicin (IDA)-based therapy (> 150 mg/m²) for AML or myelodysplasia, the incidence of cardiac damage was 5% at a median follow-up of 225 days after the last IDA dose (range, 15 to 1110 days). However, among patients treated with IDA-based therapy, the LV ejection fraction decreased by at least 10% in 18% of patients and by at least 7% in 15% of patients.[177]

A separate study of patients with advanced-stage breast cancer found that none of 37 IDA-treated patients and 3 of 19 doxorubicin-treated patients experienced clinical cardiotoxicity.[178] However, studies using these drugs to treat children are still lacking.[179]

TREATMENT WITH CONTINUOUS ANTHRACYCLINE INFUSION

Although the cellular mechanisms of anthracycline cardiotoxicity are not completely understood, changing from a bolus to a continuous infusion of anthracyclines was believed to provide some cardiac benefit by lowering peak serum concentrations, thereby reducing the exposure of cardiac cells to the drug without losing its effectiveness.[180] Observational studies involving children found that higher dosages were associated with cardiotoxicity, independent of the effect of total dose.[7] In addition, continuous infusion limited the acute cardiotoxicity among adults treated with anthracyclines, and some observational studies involving children reached similar findings.[180,181] This evidence led many researchers to begin using continuous infusion protocols for children, despite a lack of evidence for long-term cardioprotective efficacy.[182]

A randomized controlled trial of doxorubicin administered as a continuous infusion over 48 hours versus as a bolus infusion for children with high-risk ALL found no cardiac-related benefit of continuous infusion.[180] At a median of 1.5 years after diagnosis, both groups had similar LV mass, LV wall thickness, LV end-diastolic dimension, and LV fractional shortening values. In addition, some these patients treated at the Dana-Farber Cancer Institute had undergone a more detailed echocardiographic evaluation that also found no difference between groups in LV contractility as measured by the LV stress-velocity index. Similar findings were also reached by a retrospective review of 111 patients treated either with continuous anthracycline infusion over 6 hours or with bolus infusion in a treatment protocol that was dependent on the number of years during which the patient had received treatment.[182] Again, 5 years after treatment, both groups of children exhibited similar LV wall thickness, LV fractional shortening, LV end-diastolic dimension, and LV contractility, as measured by the LV stress-velocity index. An additional retrospective review of 44 children with cancer treated with anthracycline given either as a continuous infusion over 24 hours or as a bolus infusion also found no statistically significant differences between groups in echocardiographic characteristics 7 years after diagnosis.[183] A multicenter randomized trial treated 102 children with high-risk ALL with either continuous infusion or bolus infusion of doxorubicin. At a median follow-up of 8 years, the groups did not differ in cardiac function, mass, or wall thickness. At 10 years, event-free survival rates did not differ between the groups.[184]

Continuous infusion is not without risks.[180] Not only is it associated with longer hospital stays, the need for central catheter placement, and additional costs, it may also be associated with an increased incidence of complications, such as mucositis, psychological effects, and thromboembolic events.[180] Given these risks, and given the fact that several studies have found no cardiac-related benefit, continuous infusion should not be used to limit cardiotoxicity among childhood cancer patients.[171,180]

TREATMENT WITH DEXRAZOXANE

Dexrazoxane is a diketopiperazine hydrolyzed to form an open ring. It acts as a chelating agent, reducing the number of metal ions that can complex with anthracyclines.[185] As a consequence, dexrazoxane is believed to act as a free radical scavenger. In addition, it can change the configuration of topoisomerase 2β, thereby preventing anthracyclines from binding to the enzyme.[186]

Patients treated with dexrazoxane exhibited significantly ($P = 0.001$) lower mitochondrial DNA copy numbers per cell than did those who were not treated with dexrazoxane.[187,188] An elevated number of mitochondrial DNA copies indicates cardiac mitochondrial dysfunction.[189] Dexrazoxane reduces acute cardiotoxic effects for adults treated with anthracyclines and is

currently recommended by the American Society of Clinical Oncology to prevent cardiotoxicity in specific adult-cancer treatment protocols.[171]

However, the possibility that dexrazoxane could decrease clinical response and increase the incidence of secondary malignancy was a concern. Given the differences between adults and children in the mechanisms leading to cardiotoxicity and the possibility that dexrazoxane could interfere with the oncologic efficacy of anthracyclines, studies of a potential cardioprotective effect for children were necessary before dexrazoxane could be considered a part of routine clinical practice for treating children with cancer.[172,190] Balancing the cardioprotective effect of dexrazoxane with any potential negative impact of the agent on the effectiveness of anthracyclines will be the main determinant of its use in treating children.

Early studies showed that children, adolescents, and young adults treated with dexrazoxane plus doxorubicin exhibited less subclinical cardiotoxicity,[191] better myocardial responses, better LV performance,[192–196] and fewer cardiac events[196] than did patients who were not treated with dexrazoxane. A randomized trial using dexrazoxane to treat children with ALL found that elevated cTnT concentrations occurred among significantly fewer (21% of 82 children) patients treated with both doxorubicin and dexrazoxane than among patients (50% of 76 children) treated with doxorubicin alone. Differences between the groups began to emerge between 61 and 120 days after the start of therapy and persisted throughout the rest of the treatment period (Figures 20-7 and 20-8).[84] As treatment progressed, the differences between groups became even greater. Between days 181 and 240, nearly half of those treated with doxorubicin alone exhibited an elevated cTnT concentration, as opposed to fewer than 10% of those treated with both doxorubicin and dexrazoxane. This protective effect was also present when only extremely high cTnT values (> 0.025 ng/mL) were considered elevated.

In 2011, the Committee for Medicinal Products for Human Use of the European Medicines Agency evaluated the use of dexrazoxane to prevent anthracycline-induced cardiotoxicity among children.[197] The Committee concluded that the safety and efficacy of dexrazoxane had not been established for children and that there was a risk of second malignant neoplasm (SMNs). As a result, the European Medicines Agency recommended that dexrazoxane be contraindicated for patients younger than 18 years.

Since this recommendation, evidence supporting the administration of dexrazoxane to children has been accumulating. A meta-analysis found that HF occurred in 11 (1.4%) of 769 adults and children

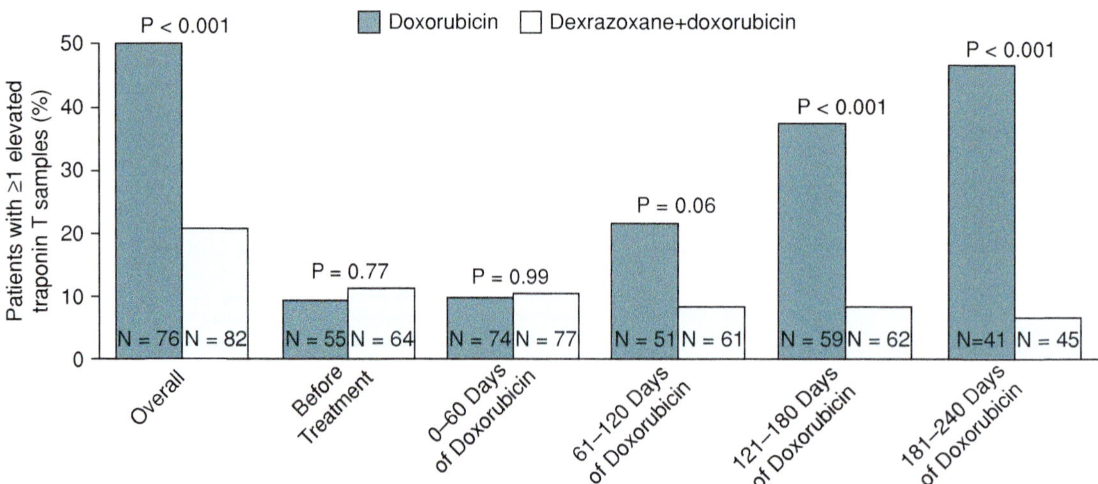

FIGURE 20-7 Percentage of patients with at least one elevated cardiac troponin T concentration overall, before treatment with doxorubicin, and during treatment. (From: Lipshultz SE, Rifai N, Dalton VM, Levy DE, et al. The effect of dexrazoxane on myocardial injury in doxorubicin-treated children with acute lymphoblastic leukemia. *N Engl J Med.* 2004 Jul 8;351(2):145–153.)

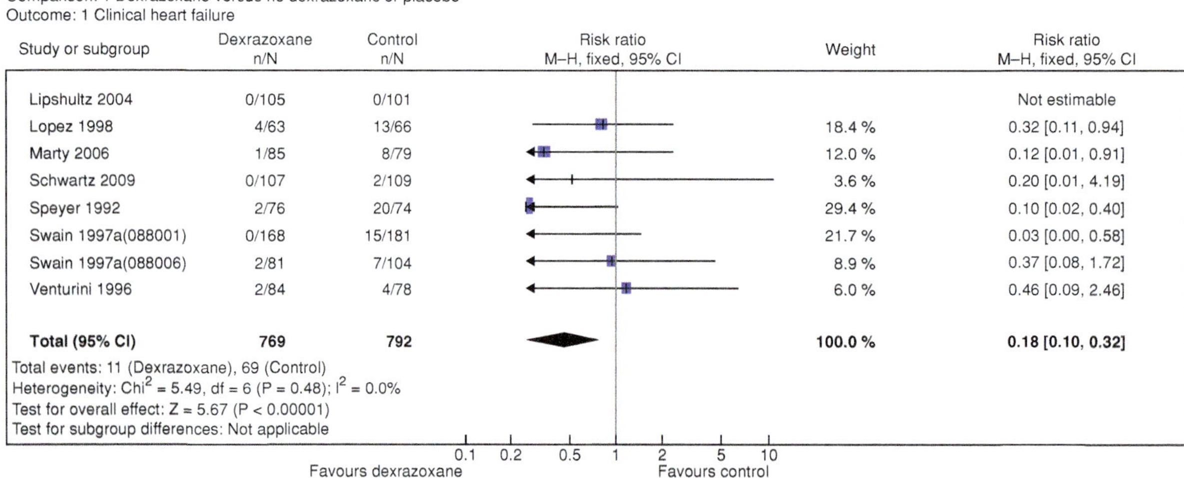

FIGURE 20-8 Relative risk of clinical heart failure in 8 randomized trials involving children, 158 of whom were treated with anthracycline, with or without dexrazoxane, or placebo. CI, confidence interval; M-H, Mantel Haenszel method. (van Dalen EC, Caron HN, Dickinson HO, Kremer LC. Cardioprotective interventions for cancer patients receiving anthracyclines. *Cochrane Database Syst Rev* 2011 (6):CD003917.)

receiving dexrazoxane plus anthracycline and in 69 (8.7%) of 792 patients treated with anthracycline alone, a finding indicating that dexrazoxane clearly exerts a cardioprotective benefit ($P < 0.001$).[198] The findings of another meta-analysis involving a pooled sample of 2015 adults and children undergoing chemotherapy were similar in terms of the cardioprotective benefit of dexrazoxane.[199] A recent systematic review and meta-analysis of 26 publications from 17 randomized and nonrandomized studies involving children and adolescents treated with anthracyclines indicated that

dexrazoxane reduced clinical cardiotoxicity rates (relative risk (RR), 0.29; $P = .001$) and clinical and subclinical cardiotoxic effects (RR = 0.43; $P < .001$).[200]

Another group reviewed 10 studies of children and adolescents treated with anthracyclines and found that response rates and survival times were similar in groups treated with or without dexrazoxane. Mean survival rates ranged from 71% to 87% among patients treated with dexrazoxane and from 73% to 86% among patients treated without dexrazoxane.[201] A multicenter randomized trial involving 205 children with high-risk

ALL treated with doxorubicin found that dexrazoxane provided long-term cardioprotection without compromising oncological efficacy.[194]

Concerns regarding whether dexrazoxane increases the risk of SMNs arose primarily from findings by Tebbi and colleagues, who treated 478 children for Hodgkin lymphoma and found 10 SMNs, 8 in the dexrazoxane group, after 58 months of follow-up.[202] However, their long-term follow-up study involving 225 low-risk patients found that the 8-year event-free survival rate was not associated with dexrazoxane administration.[203] Another study found that, at 6-year follow-up, event-free survival rates were identical for patients with ALL who were or were not treated with dexrazoxane, and the risk of recurrence or SMNs was not increased (Figure 20-9).[204] A recent study using male mice concluded that dexrazoxane plays a protective role in decreasing the incidence of doxorubicin-induced aneuploidy because of its radical-scavenging activity; thus, dexrazoxane averts SMNs and abnormal reproductive outcomes.[205]

The Children's Oncology Group combined data from three randomized clinical trials[202,203,206] involving a total of 1008 children with leukemia or lymphoma, 507 of whom had been treated with dexrazoxane. At a median follow-up of 12.6 years, the study found that dexrazoxane was not associated with overall mortality rates or with differential causes of death.[207] A retrospective analysis of 15,532 cancer patients from 43 Pediatric Health Information System

children's hospitals found that the SMN rate was 0.21% for the dexrazoxane group and 0.55% for the non-dexrazoxane group. Dexrazoxane was not associated with the risk of SMNs.[208]

A recent report from the Children's Oncology Group showed that, among 537 pediatric pateints treated with anthracyclines for T-cell acute lymphoblastic leukemia or advanced-stage lymphoblastic non-Hodgkin lymphoma, and randomly assigned to pretreatement with dexrazoxane bolus, dexrazoxane exhibited cardioprotective effects without compromising antitumor efficacy or increasing the incidence of tocxicities. Although 8 of 11 secondary malignancies occurred in the dexrazoxane group, the difference from the control group was not statistically significant.[209] Another report from the Children's Oncology Group showed that dexrazoxane not only exerted a cardioprotective effect among patients with nonmetastatic osteosarcoma but also allowed safe increases in the cummulative doses of doxorubicin.[210]

Despite evidence supporting the cardioprotective effects of dexrazoxane, in the United States only 2% of children with AML were treated with this agent between 1999 and 2009.[211] In August 2014, the FDA designated dexrazoxane as an orphan drug for "prevention of cardiomyopathy for children and adolescents 0 through 16 years of age treated with anthracyclines."[212] Currently, both the Dana-Farber Cancer Institute Acute Lymphoblastic Leukemia Consortium and the Children's Oncology Group include dexrazoxane in their research protocols that involve anthracyclines.[201]

Dexrazoxane appears to be more cardioprotective for female patients, a finding supported by the results of studies using animal models.[194,213] These findings highlight the fact that sex is a risk factor for both anthracycline-related cardiotoxicity and reduced cardioprotection from dexrazoxane. Much remains unknown about the mechanisms underlying such differences.[194] Although the most efficient method of administration and the optimal dose remain to be determined, dexrazoxane clearly benefits children treated with anthracyclines.[204,214]

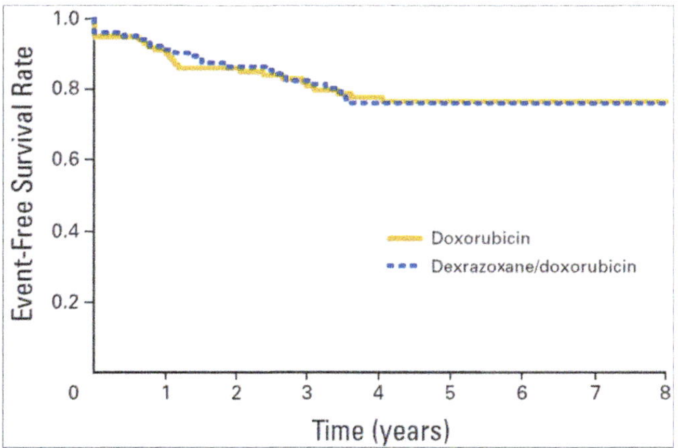

FIGURE 20-9 Event-free survival among 205 children with acute lymphoblastic leukemia treated with doxorubicin with or without dexrazoxane. (Barry EV, Vrooman LM, Dahlberg SE, Neuberg DS, Asselin BL, Athale UH, Clavell LA, et al. Absence of secondary malignant neoplasms in children with high-risk acute lymphoblastic leukemia treated with dexrazoxane. *J Clin Oncol: Official Journal of the American Society of Clinical Oncology.* 2008 Mar 1;26(7):1106–1111.)

TREATMENT WITH AMIFOSTINE

Amifostine is a broad-spectrum cytoprotective agent that scavenges oxygen free radicals. Animal studies have found that cardiac function improves when amifostine is administered with doxorubicin.[215] However, among 28 children with osteosarcoma treated with amifostine and doxorubicin, cardiac function did not differ markedly from that of children treated with placebo. Still, 2 of 28 patients in the placebo group and none of the 28 children in the treatment group experienced subclinical HF.[216] Recommendations regarding amifostine treatment require larger studies for standardization.[155]

TREATMENT WITH METABOLIC SUPPLEMENTS

The low cost and ease of administration of metabolic dietary supplements make them attractive for helping protect children against cardiotoxicity during cancer treatment. Of particular interest in protecting against anthracycline cardiotoxicity are coenzyme Q and L-carnitine.[171] Both molecules are found naturally in the mitochondria and are important to their proper function. That these agents might protect against the mitochondrial dysfunction and pathologic changes caused by anthracycline exposure is supported by their successful use in treating other medical conditions in both children and adults.[171]

L-carnitine helps transport energy-rich, long-chain fatty acids through the mitochondria and thus is essential to cellular energy production. Among 38 children treated with anthracyclines, those with abnormal results on stress echocardiography exhibited significantly lower concentrations of serum L-carnitine.[217] The authors suggested that these decreased concentrations probably reflect physiological differences that may predispose certain children to the cardiotoxic effects of anthracyclines.[217] Among rats treated concomitantly with doxorubicin and L-carnitine, the 120-day cardiac mortality rate was reduced from 53% to 8%.[218] L-carnitine was found to prevent acute anthracycline-associated echocardiographic changes and increases in serum levels of creatine kinase isoenzyme MB (CK-MB).[219,220]

Coenzyme Q is present in large quantities in the inner mitochondrial membrane, where it is important for energy production. The results of small studies involving human subjects suggest that coenzyme Q supplementation is cardioprotective.[171] Among 20 children treated with anthracyclines for either ALL or non-Hodgkin lymphoma, the decline in LV fractional shortening was slower among those receiving coenzyme Q than among those not receiving it.[221] In addition, several studies involving adults have found that coenzyme Q decreases LV dysfunction without affecting oncologic efficacy, although it exerted no beneficial effect in randomized trials involving adults with HF.[20,171] The evidence does not support considering either L-carnitine or coenzyme Q as the standard of care.[176]

CONCLUSIONS

Many children and adolescents with cancer are treated with cardiotoxic agents. Although these agents have greatly improved survival rates, they do lead to cardiovascular complications. Acute, clinically important cardiotoxicity caused by frontline treatment protocols for childhood cancer is now rare, but chronic cardiovascular problems related to treatment have become an important cause of morbidity and mortality for long-term cancer survivors. Treatment-induced cardiomyopathy can occur during treatment or as long as months or years thereafter. Given that chemotherapy-induced cardiac damage is often irreversible, treatment strategies aimed at preventing or reducing this damage are important. Such strategies include using cardioprotective agents, such as dexrazoxane; limiting or changing chemotherapy dosing schedules; screening patients for additional cardiovascular risk factors; and performing serial monitoring to detect the signs and symptoms of cardiac damage during therapy and follow-up.

Future research should focus on refining chemotherapy protocols so as to minimize cardiovascular and other adverse effects while maintaining acceptable rates of response to treatment. In addition to the development of validated biomarkers for the risk of late cardiotoxic-related events and new drugs with fewer cardiotoxic effects, the use of cardioprotective strategies is vital if we are to continue improving both the short-term and the long-term health of children with cancer.

REFERENCES

1. Siegel RL, Miller KD, Jemal A. Cancer statistics, 2015. *CA Cancer J Clin*. 2015;65(1):5–29.
2. Mariotto AB, Rowland JH, Yabroff KR, et al. Long-term survivors of childhood cancers in the United States. *Cancer Epidemiol Biomarkers Prev*. 2009;18(4):1033–1040.
3. Scully RE, Lipshultz SE. Anthracycline cardiotoxicity in long-term survivors of childhood cancer. *Cardiovasc Toxicol*. 2007;7(2):122–128.
4. Krischer JP, Epstein S, Cuthbertson DD, Goorin AM, Epstein ML, Lipshultz SE. Clinical cardiotoxicity following anthracycline treatment for childhood cancer: the Pediatric Oncology Group experience. *J Clin Oncol*. 1997;15(4):1544–1552.
5. Goorin AM, Chauvenet AR, Perez-Atayde AR, Cruz J, McKone R, Lipshultz SE. Initial congestive heart failure, six to ten years after doxorubicin chemotherapy for childhood cancer. *J Pediatr*. 1990;116(1):144–147.
6. Lipshultz SE, Colan SD, Gelber RD, Perez-Atayde AR, Sallan SE, Sanders SP. Late cardiac effects of doxorubicin therapy for acute lymphoblastic leukemia in childhood. *N Engl J Med*. 1991;324(12):808–815.

7. Lipshultz SE, Lipsitz SR, Mone SM, et al. Female sex and drug dose as risk factors for late cardiotoxic effects of doxorubicin therapy for childhood cancer. *N Engl J Med*. 1995;332(26):1738–1743.

8. Lipshultz SE, Lipsitz SR, Sallan SE, et al. Chronic progressive cardiac dysfunction years after doxorubicin therapy for childhood acute lymphoblastic leukemia. *J Clin Oncol*. 2005;23(12):2629–2636.

9. Adams MJ, Lipsitz SR, Colan SD, et al. Cardiovascular status in long-term survivors of Hodgkin's disease treated with chest radiotherapy. *J Clin Oncol*. 2004;22(15):3139–3148.

10. Lipshultz SE, Landy DC, Lopez-Mitnik G, et al. Cardiovascular status of childhood cancer survivors exposed and unexposed to cardiotoxic therapy. *J Clin Oncol*. 2012;30(10):1050–1057.

11. Oeffinger KC, Mertens AC, Sklar CA, et al. Childhood Cancer Survivor Study. Chronic health conditions in adult survivors of childhood cancer. *N Engl J Med*. 2006;355(15):1572–1582.

12. Mertens AC, Liu Q, Neglia JP, et al. Cause-specific late mortality among 5-year survivors of childhood cancer: the Childhood Cancer Survivor Study. *J Natl Cancer Inst*. 2008;100(19):1368–1379.

13. Garwicz S, Anderson H, Olsen JH, et al. Association of the Nordic Cancer Registries; Nordic Society for Pediatric Hematology Oncology. Late and very late mortality in 5-year survivors of childhood cancer: changing pattern over four decades—experience from the Nordic countries. *Int J Cancer*. 2012;131(7):1659–1666.

14. Tukenova M, Guibout C, Oberlin O, et al. Role of cancer treatment in long-term overall and cardiovascular mortality after childhood cancer. *J Clin Oncol*. 2010;28(8):1308–1315.

15. Mulrooney DA, Yeazel MW, Kawashima T, et al. Cardiac outcomes in a cohort of adult survivors of childhood and adolescent cancer: retrospective analysis of the Childhood Cancer Survivor Study cohort. *BMJ*. 2009;339:b4606.

16. Mulrooney DA, Armstrong GT, Huang S, et al. Cardiac outcomes in adult survivors of childhood cancer exposed to cardiotoxic therapy: a cross-sectional study. *Ann Intern Med*. 2016;164(2):93–101.

17. Levitt G, Anazodo A, Burch M, Bunch K. Cardiac or cardiopulmonary transplantation in childhood cancer survivors: an increasing need? *Eur J Cancer*. 2009;45(17):3027–34.

18. Lipshultz SE, Adams MJ. Cardiotoxicity after childhood cancer: beginning with the end in mind. *J Clin Oncol*. 2010;28(8):1276–1281.

19. Leger K, Slone T, Lemler M, et al. Subclinical cardiotoxicity in childhood cancer survivors exposed to very low dose anthracycline therapy. *Pediatr Blood Cancer*. 2015;62(1):123–127.

20. Barry E, Alvarez JA, Scully RE, Miller TL, Lipshultz SE. Anthracycline-induced cardiotoxicity: course, pathophysiology, prevention and management. *Expert Opin Pharmacother*. 2007;8(8):1039–1058.

21. Adams MJ, Lipshultz SE. Pathophysiology of anthracycline- and radiation-associated cardiomyopathies: implications for screening and prevention. *Pediatr Blood Ccancer*. 2005;44(7):600–606.

22. Talvensaari KK, Lanning M, Tapanainen P, Knip M. Long-term survivors of childhood cancer have an increased risk of manifesting the metabolic syndrome. *J Clin Endocrinol Metab*. 1996;81(8):3051–3055.

23. Landy DC, Miller TL, Lopez-Mitnik G, et al. Aggregating traditional cardiovascular disease risk factors to assess the cardiometabolic health of childhood cancer survivors: an analysis from the Cardiac Risk Factors in Childhood Cancer Survivors Study. *Am Heart J*. 2012;163(2):295–301.e2.

24. Alvarez JA, Scully RE, Miller TL. Long-term effects of treatments for childhood cancers. *Curr Opin Pediatr*. 2007;19(1):23–31.

25. Didcock E, Davies HA, Didi M, Ogilvy Stuart AL, Wales JK, Shalet SM. Pubertal growth in young adult survivors of childhood leukemia. *J Clin Oncol*. 1995;13(10):2503–2507.

26. Von Hoff DD, Rozencweig M, Layard M, Slavik M, Muggia FM. Daunomycin-induced cardiotoxicity in children and adults. A review of 110 cases. *Am J Med*. 1977;62(2):200–208.

27. Silverman LB, Stevenson KE, O'Brien JE, et al. Long-term results of dana-farber cancer institute ALL consortium protocols for children with newly diagnosed acute lymphoblastic leukemia (1985-2000). *Leukemia*. 2010;24(2):320–334.

28. Simbre VC, Duffy SA, Dadlani GH, Miller TL, Lipshultz SE. Cardiotoxicity of cancer chemotherapy: implications for children. *Paediatr Drugs*. 2005;7(3):187–202.

29. Lipshultz SE, Alvarez JA, Scully RE. Anthracycline associated cardiotoxicity in survivors of childhood cancer. *Heart*. 2008;94(4):525–533.

30. Nysom K, Holm K, Lipsitz SR, et al. Relationship between cumulative anthracycline dose and late cardiotoxicity in childhood acute lymphoblastic leukemia. *J Clin Oncol*. 1998;16(2):545–550.

31. Giantris A, Abdurrahman L, Hinkle A, Asselin B, Lipshultz SE. Anthracycline-induced cardiotoxicity in children and young adults. *Crit Rev Oncol Hematol*. 1998;27(1):53–68.

32. Yeh ET, Tong AT, Lenihan DJ, et al. Cardiovascular complications of cancer therapy: diagnosis, pathogenesis, and management. *Circulation*. 2004;109(25):3122–3131.

33. Steinberg JS, Cohen AJ, Wasserman AG, Cohen P, Ross AM. Acute arrhythmogenicity of doxorubicin administration. *Cancer*. 1987;60(6):1213–1218.

34. Horacek JM, Jakl M, Horackova J, Pudil R, Jebavy L, Maly J. Assessment of anthracycline-induced cardiotoxicity with electrocardiography. *Exp Oncol*. 2009;31(2):115–117.

35. Billingham ME, Mason JW, Bristow MR, Daniels JR. Anthracycline cardiomyopathy monitored by morphologic changes. *Cancer Treat Rep*. 1978;62(6):865–872.

36. Kremer LC, van Dalen EC, Offringa M, Voûte PA. Frequency and risk factors of anthracycline-induced

clinical heart failure in children: a systematic review. *Ann Oncol*. 2002;13(4):503–512.

37. Lipshultz SE, Scully RE, Stevenson KE, et al. Hearts too small for body size after doxorubicin for childhood ALL: grinch syndrome [abstract]. *J Clin Oncol*. 2014;32(suppl 15):10021.

38. Lipshultz SE, Colan SD. Cardiovascular trials in long-term survivors of childhood cancer. *J Clin Oncol*. 2004;22(5):769–773.

39. Armenian SH, Gelehrter SK, Vase T, et al. Screening for cardiac dysfunction in anthracycline-exposed childhood cancer survivors. *Clin Cancer Res*. 2014;20(24): 6314–6323.

40. Sorensen K, Levitt GA, Bull C, Dorup I, Sullivan ID. Late anthracycline cardiotoxicity after childhood cancer: a prospective longitudinal study. *Cancer*. 2003;97(8):1991–1998.

41. Ganame J, Claus P, Uyttebroeck A, et al. Myocardial dysfunction late after low-dose anthracycline treatment in asymptomatic pediatric patients. *J Am Soc Echocardiogr*. 2007;20(12):1351–1358.

42. Horenstein MS, Vander Heide RS, L'Ecuyer TJ. Molecular basis of anthracycline-induced cardiotoxicity and its prevention. *Mol Genet Metab*. 2000;71(1-2):436–444.

43. Lebrecht D, Setzer B, Ketelsen UP, Haberstroh J, Walker UA. Time-dependent and tissue-specific accumulation of mtDNA and respiratory chain defects in chronic doxorubicin cardiomyopathy. *Circulation*. 2003;108(19):2423–2429.

44. Minotti G, Menna P, Salvatorelli E, Cairo G, Gianni L. Anthracyclines: molecular advances and pharmacologic developments in antitumor activity and cardiotoxicity. *Pharmacol Rev*. 2004;56(2):185–229.

45. Nicolay K, van der Neut R, Fok JJ, de Kruijff B. Effects of adriamycin on lipid polymorphism in cardiolipin-containing model and mitochondrial membranes. *Biochim Biophys Acta*. 1985;819(1):55–65.

46. Ashley N, Poulton J. Mitochondrial DNA is a direct target of anti-cancer anthracycline drugs. *Biochem Biophys Res Commun*. 2009;378(3):450–455.

47. Wallace KB. Doxorubicin-induced cardiac mitochondrionopathy. *Pharmacol Toxicol*. 2003;93(3):105–115.

48. Thompson KL, Rosenzweig BA, Zhang J, et al. Early alterations in heart gene expression profiles associated with doxorubicin cardiotoxicity in rats. *Cancer Chemother Pharmacol*. 2010;66(2):303–314.

49. Chen B, Peng X, Pentassuglia L, Lim CC, Sawyer DB. Molecular and cellular mechanisms of anthracycline cardiotoxicity. *Cardiovasc Toxicol*. 2007;7(2):114–121.

50. Ito H, Miller SC, Billingham ME, et al. Doxorubicin selectively inhibits muscle gene expression in cardiac muscle cells in vivo and in vitro. *Proc Natl Acad Sci USA*. 1990;87(11):4275–4279.

51. Peng X, Chen B, Lim CC, Sawyer DB. The cardiotoxicology of anthracycline chemotherapeutics: translating molecular mechanism into preventative medicine. *Mol Interv*. 2005;5(3):163–171.

52. Sarosiek KA, Fraser C, Muthalagu N, et al. Developmental regulation of mitochondrial apoptosis by c-Myc governs age- and tissue-specific sensitivity to cancer therapeutics. *Cancer Cell*. 2017;31(1):142–156.

53. Zhang S, Liu X, Bawa-Khalfe T, et al. Identification of the molecular basis of doxorubicin-induced cardiotoxicity. *Nat Med*. 2012;18(11):1639–1642.

54. Khiati S, Dalla Rosa I, Sourbier C, et al. Mitochondrial topoisomerase I (top1mt) is a novel limiting factor of doxorubicin cardiotoxicity. *Clin Cancer Res*. 2014;20(18):4873–4881.

55. Tewey KM, Rowe TC, Yang L, Halligan BD, Liu LF. Adriamycin-induced DNA damage mediated by mammalian DNA topoisomerase II. *Science*. 1984;226(4673):466–468.

56. Lyu YL, Kerrigan JE, Lin CP, et al. Topoisomerase IIbeta mediated DNA double-strand breaks: implications in doxorubicin cardiotoxicity and prevention by dexrazoxane. *Cancer Res*. 2007;67(18):8839–8846.

57. Ong DS, Aertker RA, Clark AN, et al. Radiation-associated valvular heart disease. *J Heart Valve Dis*. 2013;22(6):883–892.

58. Vejpongsa P, Yeh ET. Topoisomerase 2β: a promising molecular target for primary prevention of anthracycline-induced cardiotoxicity. *Clin Pharmacol Ther*. 2014;95(1):45–52.

59. Aminkeng F, Ross CJ, Rassekh SR, et al. CPNDS Clinical Practice Recommendations Group. Recommendations for genetic testing to reduce the incidence of anthracycline-induced cardiotoxicity. *Br J Clin Pharmacol*. 2016;82(3):683–695.

60. Krischer JP, Cuthbertson DD, Epstein S, Goorin AM, Epstein ML, Lipshultz SE. Risk factors for early anthracycline clinical cardiotoxicity in children: the Pediatric Oncology Group experience. *Prog Pediatr Cardiol*. 1998;8(2):83–90.

61. Adams MJ, Lipshultz SE, Schwartz C, Fajardo LF, Coen V, Constine LS. Radiation-associated cardiovascular disease: manifestations and management. *Semin Radiat Oncol*. 2003;13(3):346–356.

62. Adams MJ, Hardenbergh PH, Constine LS, Lipshultz SE. Radiation-associated cardiovascular disease. *Crit Rev Oncol Hematol*. 2003;45(1):55–75.

63. van der Pal HJ, van Dalen EC, Kremer LC, Bakker PJ, van Leeuwen FE. Risk of morbidity and mortality from cardiovascular disease following radiotherapy for childhood cancer: a systematic review. *Cancer Treat Rev*. 2005;31(3):173–185.

64. Adams MJ, Ng AK, Mauch P, Lipsitz SR, Winters P, Lipshultz SE. Peak oxygen consumption in Hodgkin's lymphoma survivors treated with mediastinal radiotherapy as a predictor of quality of life 5 years later. *Prog Pediatr Cardiol*. 2015;39(2, Part A):93–98.

65. van Nimwegen FA, Schaapveld M, Cutter DJ, et al. Radiation dose-response relationship for risk of coronary heart disease in survivors of Hodgkin lymphoma. *J Clin Oncol*. 2016;34(3):235–243.

66. Wu W, Masri A, Popovic ZB, et al. Long-term survival of patients with radiation heart disease undergoing cardiac surgery: a cohort study. *Circulation*. 2013;127(14):1476–1485.

67. Krause DS, Van Etten RA. Tyrosine kinases as targets for cancer therapy. *N Engl J Med*. 2005;353(2):172–187.

68. Drake JM, Lee JK, Witte ON. Clinical targeting of mutated and wild-type protein tyrosine kinases in cancer. *Mol Cellular Biol*. 2014;34(10):1722–1732.

69. Guglin M, Cutro R, Mishkin JD. Trastuzumab-induced cardiomyopathy. *J Card Fail*. 2008;14(5):437–444.

70. Baron KB, Brown JR, Heiss BL, et al. Trastuzumab-induced cardiomyopathy: incidence and associated risk factors in an inner-city population. *J Card Fail*. 2014;20(8):555–559.

71. Tan-Chiu E, Yothers G, Romond E, et al. Assessment of cardiac dysfunction in a randomized trial comparing doxorubicin and cyclophosphamide followed by paclitaxel, with or without trastuzumab as adjuvant therapy in node-positive, human epidermal growth factor receptor 2-overexpressing breast cancer: NSABP B-31. *J Clin Oncol*. 2005;23(31):7811–7819.

72. Kerkelä R, Grazette L, Yacobi R, et al. Cardiotoxicity of the cancer therapeutic agent imatinib mesylate. *Nat Med*. 2006;12(8):908–916.

73. Toikkanen S, Helin H, Isola J, Joensuu H. Prognostic significance of HER-2 oncoprotein expression in breast cancer: a 30-year follow-up. *J Clin Oncol*. 1992;10(7):1044–1048.

74. Sivagnanam K, Rahman ZU, Paul T. Cardiomyopathy associated with targeted therapy for breast cancer. *Am J Med Sci*. 2016;351(2):194–199.

75. Lee-Sherick AB, Zhang W, Menachof KK, et al. Efficacy of a Mer and Flt3 tyrosine kinase small molecule inhibitor, UNC1666, in acute myeloid leukemia. *Oncotarget*. 2015;6(9):6722–6736.

76. Furman WL, Navid F, Daw NC, et al. Tyrosine kinase inhibitor enhances the bioavailability of oral irinotecan in pediatric patients with refractory solid tumors. *J Clin Oncol*. 2009;27(27):4599–4604.

77. Herman EH, Knapton A, Rosen E, et al. A multifaceted evaluation of imatinib-induced cardiotoxicity in the rat. *Toxicol Pathol*. 2011;39(7):1091–1106.

78. Atallah E, Durand JB, Kantarjian H, Cortes J. Congestive heart failure is a rare event in patients receiving imatinib therapy. *Blood*. 2007;110(4):1233–1237.

79. Trent JC, Patel SS, Zhang J, et al. Rare incidence of congestive heart failure in gastrointestinal stromal tumor and other sarcoma patients receiving imatinib mesylate. *Cancer*. 2010;116(1):184–192.

80. Estabragh ZR, Knight K, Watmough SJ, et al. A prospective evaluation of cardiac function in patients with chronic myeloid leukaemia treated with imatinib. *Leuk Res*. 2011;35(1):49–51.

81. Lipshultz SE, Sanders SP, Goorin AM, Krischer JP, Sallan SE, Colan SD. Monitoring for anthracycline cardiotoxicity. *Pediatrics*. 1994;93(3):433–437.

82. van Dalen EC, van den Brug M, Caron HN, Kremer LC. Anthracycline-induced cardiotoxicity: comparison of recommendations for monitoring cardiac function during therapy in paediatric oncology trials. *Eur J Cancer*. 2006;42(18):3199–3205.

83. Mina A, Rafei H, Khalil M, Hassoun Y, Nasser Z, Tfayli A. Role of baseline echocardiography prior to initiation of anthracycline-based chemotherapy in breast cancer patients. *BMC Cancer*. 2015;15:10.

84. Lipshultz SE, Rifai N, Dalton VM, et al. The effect of dexrazoxane on myocardial injury in doxorubicin-treated children with acute lymphoblastic leukemia. *N Engl J Med*. 2004;351(2):145–153.

85. Malik A, Jeyaraj PA, Calton R, et al. Are biomarkers predictive of anthracycline-induced cardiac dysfunction? *Asian Pac J Cancer Prev*. 2016;17(4):2301–2305.

86. Mavinkurve-Groothuis AM, Marcus KA, Pourier M, et al. Myocardial 2D strain echocardiography and cardiac biomarkers in children during and shortly after anthracycline therapy for acute lymphoblastic leukaemia (ALL): a prospective study. *Eur Heart J Cardiovasc Imaging*. 2013;14(6):562–569.

87. Pudil R, Horacek JM, Strasova A, Jebavy L, Vojacek J. Monitoring of the very early changes of left ventricular diastolic function in patients with acute leukemia treated with anthracyclines. *Exp Oncol*. 2008;30(2):160–162.

88. Burdick J, Berridge B, Coatney R. Strain echocardiography combined with pharmacological stress test for early detection of anthracycline induced cardiomyopathy. *J Pharmacol Toxicol Methods*. 2015;73:15–20.

89. Moon TJ, Miyamoto SD, Younoszai AK, Landeck BF. Left ventricular strain and strain rates are decreased in children with normal fractional shortening after exposure to anthracycline chemotherapy. *Cardiol Young*. 2014;24(5):854–865.

90. Lipshultz SE, Rifai N, Sallan SE, et al. Predictive value of cardiac troponin T in pediatric patients at risk for myocardial injury. *Circulation*. 1997;96(8):2641–2648.

91. Herman EH, Lipshultz SE, Rifai N, et al. Use of cardiac troponin T levels as an indicator of doxorubicin-induced cardiotoxicity. *Cancer Res*. 1998;58(2):195–197.

92. Kremer LC, Mulder RL, Oeffinger KC, et al. International Late Effects of Childhood Cancer Guideline Harmonization Group. A worldwide collaboration to harmonize guidelines for the long-term follow-up of childhood and young adult cancer survivors: a report from the International Late Effects of Childhood Cancer Guideline Harmonization Group. *Pediatr Blood Cancer*. 2013;60(4):543–549.

93. Shankar SM, Marina N, Hudson MM, et al; Cardiovascular Disease Task Force of the Children's Oncology Group. Monitoring for cardiovascular disease in survivors of childhood cancer: report from the Cardiovascular Disease Task Force of the Children's Oncology Group. *Pediatrics*. 2008;121(2):e387–e396.

94. Landier W, Bhatia S, Eshelman DA, et al. Development of risk-based guidelines for pediatric cancer survivors: the Children's Oncology Group long-term follow-up guidelines from the Children's Oncology Group late effects committee and nursing discipline. *J Clin Oncol*. 2004;22(24):4979–4990.

95. Wallace WH, Thompson L, Anderson RA. Guideline Development Group. Long term follow-up of survivors

of childhood cancer: summary of updated SIGN guidance. *BMJ.* 2013;346:f1190.

96. Hunt SA, Abraham WT, Chin MH, et al. American College of Cardiology; American Heart Association Task Force on Practice Guidelines; American College of Chest Physicians; International Society for Heart and Lung Transplantation; Heart Rhythm Society. ACC/AHA 2005 Guideline Update for the Diagnosis and Management of Chronic Heart Failure in the Adult: a report of the American College of Cardiology/American Heart Association Task Force on Practice Guidelines (Writing Committee to Update the 2001 Guidelines for the Evaluation and Management of Heart Failure): developed in collaboration with the American College of Chest Physicians and the International Society for Heart and Lung Transplantation: endorsed by the Heart Rhythm Society. *Circulation.* 2005;112(12):e154–e235.

97. Wong FL, Bhatia S, Landier W, et al. Cost-effectiveness of the Children's Oncology Group long-term follow-up screening guidelines for childhood cancer survivors at risk for treatment-related heart failure. *Ann Intern Med.* 2014;160(10):672–683.

98. Ramjaun A, AlDuhaiby E, Ahmed S, et al. Echocardiographic detection of cardiac dysfunction in childhood cancer survivors: how long is screening required? *Pediatr Blood Cancer.* 2015;62(12):2197–2203.

99. Cox CL, Hudson MM, Mertens A, et al. Medical screening participation in the childhood cancer survivor study. *Arch Intern Med.* 2009;169(5):454–462.

100. Herman EH, Zhang J, Lipshultz SE, et al. Correlation between serum levels of cardiac troponin-T and the severity of the chronic cardiomyopathy induced by doxorubicin. *J Clin Oncol.* 1999;17(7):2237–2243.

101. Lipshultz SE, Miller TL, Scully RE, et al. Changes in cardiac biomarkers during doxorubicin treatment of pediatric patients with high-risk acute lymphoblastic leukemia: associations with long-term echocardiographic outcomes. *J Clin Oncol.* 2012;30(10):1042–1049.

102. Moran AM, Lipshultz SE, Rifai N, et al. Non-invasive assessment of rejection in pediatric transplant patients: serologic and echocardiographic prediction of biopsy-proven myocardial rejection. *J Heart Lung Transplant.* 2000;19(8):756–764.

103. Chiang VW, Burns JP, Rifai N, Lipshultz SE, Adams MJ, Weiner DL. Cardiac toxicity of intravenous terbutaline for the treatment of severe asthma in children: a prospective assessment. *J Pediatr.* 2000;137(1):73–77.

104. Lipshultz SE, Somers MJ, Lipsitz SR, Colan SD, Jabs K, Rifai N. Serum cardiac troponin and subclinical cardiac status in pediatric chronic renal failure. *Pediatrics.* 2003;112(1 pt 1):79–86.

105. Lipshultz SE, Wong JC, Lipsitz SR, et al. Frequency of clinically unsuspected myocardial injury at a children's hospital. *Am Heart J.* 2006;151(4):916–922.

106. Lipshultz SE, Simbre VC 2nd, Hart S. Frequency of elevations in markers of cardiomyocyte damage in otherwise healthy newborns. *Am J Cardiol.* 2008;102(6):761–766.

107. Herman EH, Zhang J, Rifai N, et al. The use of serum levels of cardiac troponin T to compare the protective activity of dexrazoxane against doxorubicin- and mitoxantrone-induced cardiotoxicity. *Cancer Chemotherapy Pharmacol.* 2001;48(4):297–304.

108. Cardinale D, Sandri MT, Colombo A, et al. Prognostic value of troponin I in cardiac risk stratification of cancer patients undergoing high-dose chemotherapy. *Circulation.* 2004;109(22):2749–2754.

109. Cheung YF, Yu W, Cheuk DK, et al. Plasma high sensitivity troponin T levels in adult survivors of childhood leukaemias: determinants and associations with cardiac function. *PLOS ONE.* 2013;8(10):e77063.

110. Bryant J, Picot J, Baxter L, Levitt G, Sullivan I, Clegg A. Use of cardiac markers to assess the toxic effects of anthracyclines given to children with cancer: a systematic review. *Eur J Cancer.* 2007;43(13):1959–1966.

111. Mavinkurve-Groothuis AM, Kapusta L, Nir A, Groot-Loonen J. The role of biomarkers in the early detection of anthracycline-induced cardiotoxicity in children: a review of the literature. *Pediatr Hematol Oncol.* 2008;25(7):655–664.

112. Stevens PL, Lenihan DJ. Cardiotoxicity due to chemotherapy: the role of biomarkers. *Curr Cardiol Rep.* 2015;17(7):603.

113. Ylänen K, Poutanen T, Savukoski T, Eerola A, Vettenranta K. Cardiac biomarkers indicate a need for sensitive cardiac imaging among long-term childhood cancer survivors exposed to anthracyclines. *Acta Paediatr.* 2015;104(3):313–319.

114. Rusconi PG, Ludwig DA, Ratnasamy C, et al. Serial measurements of serum NT-proBNP as markers of left ventricular systolic function and remodeling in children with heart failure. *Am Heart J.* 2010;160(4):776–783.

115. Ratnasamy C, Kinnamon DD, Lipshultz SE, Rusconi P. Associations between neurohormonal and inflammatory activation and heart failure in children. *Am Heart J.* 2008;155(3):527–533.

116. Berridge BR, Pettit S, Walker DB, et al. A translational approach to detecting drug-induced cardiac injury with cardiac troponins: consensus and recommendations from the Cardiac Troponins Biomarker Working Group of the Health and Environmental Sciences Institute. *Am Heart J.* 2009;158(1):21–29.

117. Mladosievicova B, Urbanova D, Radvanska E, Slavkovsky P, Simkova I. Role of NT-proBNP in detection of myocardial damage in childhood leukemia survivors treated with and without anthracyclines. *J Exp Clin Cancer Res.* 2012;31:86.

118. Wang YD, Chen SX, Ren LQ. Serum B-type natriuretic peptide levels as a marker for anthracycline-induced cardiotoxicity. *Oncol Lett.* 2016;11(5):3483–3492.

119. Sherief LM, Kamal AG, Khalek EA, Kamal NM, Soliman AA, Esh AM. Biomarkers and early detection of late onset anthracycline-induced cardiotoxicity in children. *Hematology.* 2012;17(3):151–156.

120. Lenihan DJ, Stevens PL, Massey M, et al. The utility of point-of-care biomarkers to detect cardiotoxicity during anthracycline chemotherapy: a feasibility study. *J Card Fail.* 2016;22(6):433–438.

121. Zidan A, Sherief LM, El-Sheikh A, et al. NT-proBNP as early marker of subclinical late cardiotoxicity after doxorubicin therapy and mediastinal irradiation in childhood cancer survivors. *Dis Markers*. 2015;2015:513219.

122. Mavinkurve-Groothuis AM, Groot-Loonen J, Bellersen L, et al. Abnormal NT-pro-BNP levels in asymptomatic long-term survivors of childhood cancer treated with anthracyclines. *Pediatr Blood Cancer*. 2009;52(5):631–636.

123. LeClerc JM, Billett AL, Gelber RD, et al. Treatment of childhood acute lymphoblastic leukemia: results of Dana-Farber ALL Consortium Protocol 87-01. *J Clin Oncol*. 2002;20(1):237–246.

124. Ogden CL, Carroll MD, Kit BK, Flegal KM. Prevalence of childhood and adult obesity in the United States, 2011-2012. *JAMA*. 2014;311(8):806–814.

125. Daniels SR, Jacobson MS, McCrindle BW, Eckel RH, Sanner BM. American Heart Association childhood obesity research summit: executive summary. *Circulation*. 2009;119(15):2114–2123.

126. Meacham LR, Gurney JG, Mertens AC, et al. Body mass index in long-term adult survivors of childhood cancer: a report of the childhood cancer survivor study. *Cancer*. 2005;103(8):1730–1739.

127. Warner EL, Fluchel M, Wright J, et al. A population-based study of childhood cancer survivors' body mass index. *J Cancer Epidemiol*. 2014;2014:531958.

128. Lindemulder SJ, Stork LC, Bostrom B, et al. Survivors of standard risk acute lymphoblastic leukemia do not have increased risk for overweight and obesity compared to non-cancer peers: a report from the Children's Oncology Group. *Pediatr Blood Cancer*. 2015;62(6):1035–1041.

129. van Santen HM, Geskus RB, Raemaekers S, et al. Changes in body mass index in long-term childhood cancer survivors. *Cancer*. 2015;121(23):4197–4204.

130. Lustig RH, Post SR, Srivannaboon K, et al. Risk factors for the development of obesity in children surviving brain tumors. *J Clin Endocrinol Metab*. 2003;88(2):611–616.

131. Schulte F, Bartels U, Bouffet E, Janzen L, Hamilton J, Barrera M. Body weight, social competence, and cognitive functioning in survivors of childhood brain tumors. *Pediatr Blood Cancer*. 2010;55(3):532–539.

132. Razzouk BI, Rose SR, Hongeng S, et al. Obesity in survivors of childhood acute lymphoblastic leukemia and lymphoma. *J Clin Oncol*. 2007;25(10):1183–1189.

133. Clarke SA, Eiser C. Health behaviours in childhood cancer survivors: a systematic review. *Eur J Cancer*. 2007;43(9):1373–1384.

134. Emmons K, Li FP, Whitton J, et al. Predictors of smoking initiation and cessation among childhood cancer survivors: a report from the childhood cancer survivor study. *J Clin Oncol*. 2002;20(6):1608–1616.

135. Asfar T, Dietz NA, Arheart KL, et al. Smoking behavior among adult childhood cancer survivors: what are we missing? *J Cancer Surviv*. 2016;10(1):131–141.

136. Menke A, Casagrande S, Geiss L, Cowie CC. Prevalence of and trends in diabetes among adults in the United States, 1988-2012. *JAMA*. 2015;314(10):1021–1029.

137. Meacham LR, Sklar CA, Li S, et al. Diabetes mellitus in long-term survivors of childhood cancer. Increased risk associated with radiation therapy: a report for the childhood cancer survivor study. *Arch Intern Med*. 2009;169(15):1381–1388.

138. van Nimwegen FA, Schaapveld M, Janus CP, et al. Risk of diabetes mellitus in long-term survivors of Hodgkin lymphoma. *J Clin Oncol*. 2014;32(29):3257–3263.

139. Steinberger J, Sinaiko AR, Kelly AS, et al. Cardiovascular risk and insulin resistance in childhood cancer survivors. *J Pediatr*. 2012;160(3):494–499.

140. Kavey RE, Allada V, Daniels SR, et al. American Heart Association Expert Panel on Population and Prevention Science; American Heart Association Council on Cardiovascular Disease in the Young; American Heart Association Council on Epidemiology and Prevention; American Heart Association Council on Nutrition, Physical Activity, and Metabolism; American Heart Association Council on High Blood Pressure Research; American Heart Association Council on Cardiovascular Nursing; American Heart Association Council on the Kidney in Heart Disease; Interdisciplinary Working Froup on Quality of Care and Outcomes Research. Cardiovascular risk reduction in high-risk pediatric patients: a scientific statement from the American Heart Association Expert Panel on Population and Prevention Science; the Councils on Cardiovascular Disease in the Young, Epidemiology and Prevention, Nutrition, Physical Activity and Metabolism, High Blood Pressure Research, Cardiovascular Nursing, and the Kidney in Heart Disease; and the Interdisciplinary Working Group on Quality of Care and Outcomes Research: endorsed by the American Academy of Pediatrics. *Circulation*. 2006;114(24):2710–2738.

141. Baker KS, Chow EJ, Goodman PJ, et al. Impact of treatment exposures on cardiovascular risk and insulin resistance in childhood cancer survivors. *Cancer Epidemiol Biomarkers Prev*. 2013;22(11):1954–1963.

142. Bizzarri C, Bottaro G, Pinto RM, Cappa M. Metabolic syndrome and diabetes mellitus in childhood cancer survivors. *Pediatr Endocrinol Rev*. 2014;11(4):365–373.

143. Revuelta Iniesta R, Rush R, Paciarotti I. Systematic review and meta-analysis: prevalence and possible causes of vitamin D deficiency and insufficiency in pediatric cancer patients. *Clin Nutr*. 2016;35(1):95–108.

144. Felicetti F, D'Ascenzo F, Moretti C, et al. Prevalence of cardiovascular risk factors in long-term survivors of childhood cancer: 16 years follow up from a prospective registry. *Eur J Prev Cardiol*. 2015;22(6):762–770.

145. Gurney JG, Ness KK, Sibley SD, et al. Metabolic syndrome and growth hormone deficiency in adult survivors of childhood acute lymphoblastic leukemia. *Cancer*. 2006;107(6):1303–1312.

146. Expert Panel on Detection, Evaluation, and Treatment of High Blood Cholesterol in Adults. Executive Summary of The Third Report of The National Cholesterol Education Program (NCEP) Expert Panel on Detection, Evaluation, And Treatment of High Blood Cholesterol In Adults (Adult Treatment Panel III). *JAMA*. 2001;285(19):2486–2497.

147. Grundy SM, Cleeman JI, Merz CN, et al. Implications of recent clinical trials for the National Cholesterol Education Program Adult Treatment Panel III Guidelines. *J Am Coll Cardiol*. 2004;44(3):720–732.

148. Council on Sports Medicine and Fitness; Council on School Health. Active healthy living: prevention of childhood obesity through increased physical activity. *Pediatrics*. 2006;117(5):1834–1842.

149. Nader PR, Bradley RH, Houts RM, McRitchie SL, O'Brien M. Moderate-to-vigorous physical activity from ages 9 to 15 years. *JAMA*. 2008;300(3):295–305.

150. Ness KK, Leisenring WM, Huang S, et al. Predictors of inactive lifestyle among adult survivors of childhood cancer: a report from the childhood cancer survivor study. *Cancer*. 2009;115(9):1984–1994.

151. Berdan CA, Tangney CC, Scala C, Stolley M. Childhood cancer survivors and adherence to the American Cancer Society guidelines on nutrition and physical activity. *J Cancer Surviv*. 2014;8(4):671–679.

152. Li HC, Chung OK, Ho KY, Chiu SY, Lopez V. Effectiveness of an integrated adventure-based training and health education program in promoting regular physical activity among childhood cancer survivors. *Psychooncology*. 2013;22(11):2601–2610.

153. Cox CL, Montgomery M, Oeffinger KC, et al. Promoting physical activity in childhood cancer survivors: results from the childhood cancer survivor study. *Cancer*. 2009;115(3):642–654.

154. Lipshultz SE, Diamond MB, Franco VI, et al. Managing chemotherapy-related cardiotoxicity in survivors of childhood cancers. *Paediatr Drugs*. 2014;16(5):373–389.

155. Akam-Venkata J, Franco VI, Lipshultz SE. Late cardiotoxicity: issues for childhood cancer survivors. *Curr Treat Options Cardiovasc Med*. 2016;18(7):47.

156. Grenier MA, Fioravanti J, Truesdell SC, Mendelsohn AM, Vermilion RP, Lipshultz SE. Angiotensin-converting enzyme inhibitor therapy for ventricular dysfunction in infants, children and adolescents: a review. *Prog Pediatr Cardiol*. 2000;12(1):91–111.

157. Silber JH. Role of afterload reduction in the prevention of late anthracycline cardiomyopathy. *Pediatr Blood Cancer*. 2005;44(7):607–613.

158. Rosenthal D, Chrisant MR, Edens E, et al. International society for heart and lung transplantation: practice guidelines for management of heart failure in children. *J Heart Lung Transplant*. 2004;23(12):1313–1333.

159. Bosch X, Rovira M, Sitges M, et al. Enalapril and carvedilol for preventing chemotherapy-induced left ventricular systolic dysfunction in patients with malignant hemopathies: the OVERCOME trial (preventiOn of left Ventricular dysfunction with Enalapril and caRvedilol in patients submitted to intensive ChemOtherapy for the treatment of Malignant hEmopathies). *J Am Coll Cardiol*. 2013;61(23):2355–2362.

160. Lipshultz SE, Lipsitz SR, Sallan SE, et al. Long-term enalapril therapy for left ventricular dysfunction in doxorubicin-treated survivors of childhood cancer. *J Clin Oncol*. 2002;20(23):4517–4522.

161. Silber JH, Cnaan A, Clark BJ, et al. Enalapril to prevent cardiac function decline in long-term survivors of pediatric cancer exposed to anthracyclines. *J Clin Oncol*. 2004;22(5):820–828.

162. Rusconi P, Gómez-Marin O, Rossique-González M, et al. Carvedilol in children with cardiomyopathy: 3-year experience at a single institution. *J Heart Lung Transplant*. 2004;23(7):832–838.

163. Bruns LA, Chrisant MK, Lamour JM, et al. Carvedilol as therapy in pediatric heart failure: an initial multicenter experience. *J Pediatr*. 2001;138(4):505–511.

164. Williams RV, Tani LY, Shaddy RE. Intermediate effects of treatment with metoprolol or carvedilol in children with left ventricular systolic dysfunction. *J Heart Lung Transplant*. 2002;21(8):906–909.

165. Kalay N, Basar E, Ozdogru I, et al. Protective effects of carvedilol against anthracycline-induced cardiomyopathy. *J Am Coll Cardiol*. 2006;48(11):2258–2262.

166. El-Shitany NA, Tolba OA, El-Shanshory MR, El-Hawary EE. Protective effect of carvedilol on adriamycin-induced left ventricular dysfunction in children with acute lymphoblastic leukemia. *J Card Fail*. 2012;18(8):607–613.

167. Landy DC, Miller TL, Lipsitz SR, et al. Cranial irradiation as an additional risk factor for anthracycline cardiotoxicity in childhood cancer survivors: an analysis from the cardiac risk factors in childhood cancer survivors study. *Pediatr Cardiol*. 2013;34(4):826–834.

168. Lipshultz SE, Vlach SA, Lipsitz SR, Sallan SE, Schwartz ML, Colan SD. Cardiac changes associated with growth hormone therapy among children treated with anthracyclines. *Pediatrics*. 2005 Jun;115(6):1613–1622.

169. Shaddy RE, Olsen SL, Bristow MR, et al. Efficacy and safety of metoprolol in the treatment of doxorubicin-induced cardiomyopathy in pediatric patients. *Am Heart J*. 1995;129(1):197–199.

170. Ward KM, Binns H, Chin C, Webber SA, Canter CE, Pahl E. Pediatric heart transplantation for anthracycline cardiomyopathy: cancer recurrence is rare. *J Heart Lung Transplant*. 2004;23(9):1040–1045.

171. Wouters KA, Kremer LC, Miller TL, Herman EH, Lipshultz SE. Protecting against anthracycline-induced myocardial damage: a review of the most promising strategies. *Br J Haematol*. 2005;131(5):561–578.

172. Lipshultz SE. Dexrazoxane for protection against cardiotoxic effects of anthracyclines in children. *J Clin Oncol*. 1996;14(2):328–331.

173. Yildirim Y, Gultekin E, Avci ME, Inal MM, Yunus S, Tinar S. Cardiac safety profile of pegylated liposomal doxorubicin reaching or exceeding lifetime cumulative doses of 550 mg/m2 in patients with recurrent ovarian and peritoneal cancer. *Int J Gynecol Cancer*. 2008;18(2):223–227.

174. Creutzig U, Zimmermann M, Bourquin JP, et al. Randomized trial comparing liposomal daunorubicin with idarubicin as induction for pediatric acute myeloid leukemia: results from Study AML-BFM 2004. *Blood*. 2013;122(1):37–43.

175. Oki Y, Ewer MS, Lenihan DJ, et al. Pegylated liposomal doxorubicin replacing conventional doxorubicin

in standard R-CHOP chemotherapy for elderly patients with diffuse large B-cell lymphoma: an open label, single arm, phase II trial. *Clin Lymphoma Myeloma Leuk*. 2015;15(3):152–158.

176. Smith LA, Cornelius VR, Plummer CJ, et al. Cardiotoxicity of anthracycline agents for the treatment of cancer: systematic review and meta-analysis of randomised controlled trials. *BMC Cancer*. 2010;10:337.

177. Anderlini P, Benjamin RS, Wong FC, et al. Idarubicin cardiotoxicity: a retrospective study in acute myeloid leukemia and myelodysplasia. *J Clin Oncol*. 1995;13(11):2827–2834.

178. Martoni A, Piana E, Guaraldi M, et al. Comparative phase II study of idarubicin versus doxorubicin in advanced breast cancer. *Oncology*. 1990;47(5):427–432.

179. Pellicori P, Calicchia A, Lococo F, Cimino G, Torromeo C. Subclinical anthracycline cardiotoxicity in patients with acute promyelocytic leukemia in long-term remission after the AIDA protocol. *Congest Heart Fail*. 2012;18(4):217–221.

180. Lipshultz SE, Giantris AL, Lipsitz SR, et al. Doxorubicin administration by continuous infusion is not cardioprotective: the Dana-Farber 91-01 acute lymphoblastic leukemia protocol. *J Clin Oncol*. 2002;20(6):1677–1682.

181. Berrak SG, Ewer MS, Jaffe N, et al. Doxorubicin cardiotoxicity in children: reduced incidence of cardiac dysfunction associated with continuous-infusion schedules. *Oncol Rep*. 2001;8(3):611–614.

182. Levitt GA, Dorup I, Sorensen K, Sullivan I. Does anthracycline administration by infusion in children affect late cardiotoxicity? *Br J Haematol*. 2004;124(4):463–468.

183. Gupta M, Steinherz PG, Cheung NK, Steinherz L. Late cardiotoxicity after bolus versus infusion anthracycline therapy for childhood cancers. *Med Pediatr Oncol*. 2003;40(6):343–347.

184. Lipshultz SE, Miller TL, Lipsitz SR, et al. Dana-Farber Cancer Institute Acute Lymphoblastic Leukemia Consortium. Continuous versus bolus infusion of doxorubicin in children with ALL: long-term cardiac outcomes. *Pediatrics*. 2012;130(6):1003–1011.

185. Zuppinger C, Timolati F, Suter TM. Pathophysiology and diagnosis of cancer drug induced cardiomyopathy. *Cardiovasc Toxicol*. 2016;7(2):61–66.

186. Vejpongsa P, Yeh ET. Prevention of anthracycline-induced cardiotoxicity: challenges and opportunities. *J Am Coll Cardiol*. 2014;64(9):938–945.

187. Lipshultz SE, Anderson LM, Miller TL, et al. Dana-Farber Cancer Institute Acute Lymphoblastic Leukemia Consortium. Impaired mitochondrial function is abrogated by dexrazoxane in doxorubicin-treated childhood acute lymphoblastic leukemia survivors. *Cancer*. 2016;122(6):946–953.

188. Lipshultz SE, Miller TL, Gerschenson M, et al. Effect of dexrazoxane on impaired mitochondrial structure and function in doxorubicin-treated childhood ALL survivors [abstract]. *J Clin Oncol*. 2012;30(suppl):9530.

189. Hasinoff BB, Herman EH. Dexrazoxane: how it works in cardiac and tumor cells. Is it a prodrug or is it a drug? *Cardiovasc Toxicol*. 2016;7(2):140–144.

190. Sallan SE, Lipshultz SE. Wise up: do not do it without protection! *Pediatr Blood Cancer*. 2005;45(7):872–873.

191. Wexler LH, Andrich MP, Venzon D, et al. Randomized trial of the cardioprotective agent ICRF-187 in pediatric sarcoma patients treated with doxorubicin. *J Clin Oncol*. 1996;14(2):362–72.

192. Paiva MG, Petrilli AS, Moisés VA, Macedo CR, Tanaka C, Campos O. Cardioprotective effect of dexrazoxane during treatment with doxorubicin: a study using low dose dobutamine stress echocardiography. *Pediatr Blood Cancer*. 2005;45(7):902–908.

193. de Matos Neto RP, Petrilli AS, Silva CM, et al. Left ventricular systolic function assessed by echocardiography in children and adolescents with osteosarcoma treated with doxorubicin alone or in combination with dexrazoxane. *Arq Bras Cardiol*. 2006;87(6):763–771.

194. Lipshultz SE, Scully RE, Lipsitz SR, et al. Assessment of dexrazoxane as a cardioprotectant in doxorubicin-treated children with high-risk acute lymphoblastic leukaemia: long-term follow-up of a prospective, randomised, multicentre trial. *Lancet Oncol*. 2010;11(10):950–961.

195. Choi HS, Park ES, Kang HJ, et al. Dexrazoxane for preventing anthracycline cardiotoxicity in children with solid tumors. *J Korean Med Sci*. 2010;25(9):1336–1342.

196. Kang M, Kim KI, Song YC, Shin WG, Oh JM. Cardioprotective effect of early dexrazoxane use in anthracycline treated pediatric patients. *J Chemother*. 2012;24(5):292–296.

197. European Medicines Agency. Assessment report Dexrazoxane-containing medicinal products. http://www.ema.europa.eu/docs/en_GB/document_library/Referrals_document/Dexrazoxane_31/WC500120340.pdf. Accessed October 2, 2017.

198. van Dalen EC, Caron HN, Dickinson HO, Kremer LC. Cardioprotective interventions for cancer patients receiving anthracyclines. *Cochrane Database Syst Rev*. 2008;(2):CD003917.

199. Kalam K, Marwick TH. Role of cardioprotective therapy for prevention of cardiotoxicity with chemotherapy: a systematic review and meta-analysis. *Eur J Cancer*. 2013;49(13):2900–2909.

200. Shaikh F, Dupuis LL, Alexander S, Gupta A, Mertens L, Nathan PC. Cardioprotection and second malignant neoplasms associated with dexrazoxane in children receiving anthracycline chemotherapy: a systematic review and meta-analysis. *J Natl Cancer Inst*. 2015;108(4). doi:10.1093/jnci/djv357

201. Lipshultz SE, Franco VI, Sallan SE, et al. Dexrazoxane for reducing anthracycline-related cardiotoxicity in children with cancer: an update of the evidence. *Prog Pediatr Cardiol*. 2014;36(1-2):39–49.

202. Tebbi CK, London WB, Friedman D, et al. Dexrazoxane-associated risk for acute myeloid leukemia/myelodysplastic syndrome and other secondary malignancies in pediatric Hodgkin's disease. *J Clin Oncol*. 2007;25(5):493–500.

203. Tebbi CK, Mendenhall NP, London WB, et al. Response-dependent and reduced treatment in lower risk Hodgkin lymphoma in children and adolescents,

results of P9426: a report from the Children's Oncology Group. *Pediatr Blood Cancer*. 2012;59(7):1259–1265.

204. Barry EV, Vrooman LM, Dahlberg SE, et al. Absence of secondary malignant neoplasms in children with high-risk acute lymphoblastic leukemia treated with dexrazoxane. *J Clin Oncol*. 2008;26(7):1106–1111.

205. Attia SM, Ahmad SF, Bakheet SA. Impact of dexrazoxane on doxorubicin-induced aneuploidy in somatic and germinal cells of male mice. *Cancer Chemother Pharmacol*. 2016;77(1):27–33.

206. Schwartz CL, Constine LS, Villaluna D, et al. A risk-adapted, response-based approach using ABVE-PC for children and adolescents with intermediate- and high-risk Hodgkin lymphoma: the results of P9425. *Blood*. 2009;114(10):2051–2059.

207. Chow EJ, Asselin BL, Schwartz CL, et al. Late mortality after dexrazoxane treatment: a report from the Children's Oncology Group. *J Clin Oncol*. 2015;33(24):2639–2645.

208. Seif AE, Walker DM, Li Y, et al. Dexrazoxane exposure and risk of secondary acute myeloid leukemia in pediatric oncology patients. *Pediatr Blood Cancer*. 2015;62(4):704–709.

209. Asselin BL, Devidas M, Chen L, et al. Cardioprotection and safety of dexrazoxane in patients treated for newly diagnosed T-cell acute lymphoblastic leukemia or advanced-stage lymphoblastic non-Hodgkin lymphoma: a report of the Children's Oncology Group Randomized Trial Pediatric Oncology Group 9404. *J Clinical Oncol*. 2016;34(8):854–862.

210. Schwartz CL, Wexler LH, Krailo MD, et al. Intensified chemotherapy with dexrazoxane cardioprotection in newly diagnosed nonmetastatic osteosarcoma: a report from the Children's Oncology Group. *Pediatr Blood Cancer*. 2016;63(1):54–61.

211. Walker DM, Fisher BT, Seif AE, et al. Dexrazoxane use in pediatric patients with acute lymphoblastic or myeloid leukemia from 1999 and 2009: analysis of a national cohort of patients in the Pediatric Health Information Systems database. *Pediatr Blood Cancer*. 2013;60(4):616–620.

212. US Food and Drug Administration. Search orphan drug designations and approvals. https://www.accessdata.fda.gov/scripts/opdlisting/oopd/. Accessed October 3, 2017.

213. Herman E, Knapton A, Zhang J, Hiraragi H, Lipshultz S. Gender is a factor that can impact the severity of doxorubicin (DXR) toxicity in spontaneously hypertensive rats (SHR). *FASEB J*. 2008;22(1 suppl):719.6.

214. Hutchins KK, Siddeek H, Franco VI, Lipshultz SE. Prevention of cardiotoxicity among survivors of childhood cancer. *Br J Clin Pharmacol*. 2017;83(3):455–465.

215. Nazeyrollas P, Frances C, Prevost A, et al. Efficiency of amifostine as a protection against doxorubicin toxicity in rats during a 12-day treatment. *Anticancer Res*. 2003;23(1A):405–409.

216. Gallegos-Castorena S, Martinez-Avalos A, Mohar-Betancourt A, Guerrero-Avendaño G, Zapata-Tarrés M, Medina-Sansón A. Toxicity prevention with amifostine in pediatric osteosarcoma patients treated with cisplatin and doxorubicin. *Pediatr Hematol Oncol*. 2007;24(6):403–408.

217. Hauser M, Gibson BS, Wilson N. Diagnosis of anthracycline-induced late cardiomyopathy by exercise-spiroergometry and stress-echocardiography. *Eur J Pediatr*. 2001;160(10):607–610.

218. Ginsberg JP, Womer RB. Preventing organ-specific chemotherapy toxicity. *Eur J Cancer*. 2005;41(17):2690–2700.

219. De Leonardis V, Neri B, Bacalli S, Cinelli P. Reduction of cardiac toxicity of anthracyclines by L-carnitine: preliminary overview of clinical data. *Int J Clin Pharmacol Res*. 1985;5(2):137–142.

220. De Leonardis V, De Scalzi M, Neri B, Bartalucci S, Cinelli P. Echocardiographic assessment of anthracycline cardiotoxicity during different therapeutic regimens. *Int J Clin Pharmacol Res*. 1987;7(4):307–311.

221. Iarussi D, Auricchio U, Agretto A, et al. Protective effect of coenzyme Q10 on anthracyclines cardiotoxicity: control study in children with acute lymphoblastic leukemia and non-Hodgkin lymphoma. *Mol Aspects Med*. 1994;15(suppl):s207–s212.

21 Infectious Endocarditis in Cancer Patients

Eduardo Yepez Guevara ■ *Jose Banchs* ■ *David J. Tweardy* ■ *Javier Adachi*

Infectious endocarditis (IE) is defined as an infection of the endocardial surface of the heart from which the heart valves are most commonly affected. In the last two decades, its prevalence has changed from presenting more frequently in a young population with rheumatic heart disease to the elderly with multiple associated comorbidities and exposed to multiple hospitalizations and invasive procedures like placement of cardiac devices and/or prosthetic heart valves. *Staphylococcus aureus* is currently the most common microorganism involved due to health care exposure, invasive procedures, intravascular catheters and intracardiac devices (Figure 21-1).[1–3]

Patients with active malignancy share the same risk factors as the general population but also are immunosuppressed and receive chemotherapy. A recent Spanish study reported IE to be more frequent in patients with solid tumors (80.6%) than hematological malignancies (19.4%) and most common neoplasms were coming from colon, prostate, lymphoma and urothelial tumors.[4] This episodes were more often nosocomial and related to vascular access.[4]

In-hospital mortality is 14%–22%, and the three risk factors reported as associated with 30-day mortality were *S. aureus* infection, new onset heart failure and non-surgical therapy.[2]

MICROORGANISMS INVOLVED IN IE

The most common organisms involved in acute IE are the same in patients with active malignancy than in the general population. Therefore, it is very important to obtain a detailed epidemiological and exposure history.[1,2]

Staphylococci are still the most common microorganisms involved. *Staphylococcus aureus* is most common in nosocomial IE and associated with catheter related infections. *Staphylococcus lugdunensis,* unlike other coagulase negative staphylococci causes a rare but destructive form of IE that involves native valves with multiple and bulky vegetations. Fortunately, this organism is still very susceptible to penicillin.[1,2]

Viridans Group Strep organisms are commonly present during bacteremia in line related infections, mucositis and granulocytopenia. *Streptococcus gallolyticus* (bovis) has been associated with occult colorectal cancer. Endocarditis has been diagnosed in 18%–62% of cases in the presence of bacteremia and usually occurs in elderly males and involves multiple valves.[1,5]

Enterococcus faecalis is involved in >90% of cases of IE due to enterococci. It presents in elderly population (>65yo) more common from gastrointestinal and genitourinary sources and hospital acquired. It has been also associated with colorectal cancer as *Streptococcus bovis.*[1,2,6]

The non-HACEK gram-negative organisms are rare causes of IE occurring in 1.8%–2.5% of the cases. In cancer patients can be attributed to line related infections and bacterial translocation due to mucositis and colitis during chemotherapy. The organisms involved are enterobacteriaceae, mainly *E. coli, Pseudomonas and Klebsiella pneumonia.* Non-typhi salmonella has been also implicated in case reports of immunocompromised patients with acute IE.[1,7,8]

Fungal organisms are involved in less than 2% of the cases and more common are Candida and Aspergillus (Figure 21-2). Other less frequent include endemic mycosis like cryptococcus, histoplasma, coccidioides, and blastomyces. *Histoplasma capsulatum* has been reported in prosthetic heart valve infections.[9,10] The risk factors associated include the prolonged use of broad spectrum antibiotics, prolonged neutropenia, parenteral nutrition, diabetes mellitus, previous valve surgery, prosthetic heart valve and central vascular access.[10] Fungal IE is associated with high risk of embolic events and *Candida spp.* organisms are the most frequently involved.[9,11]

Non-albicans candida (*Candida parapsilosis, Candida tropicalis, Candida glabrata*) IE is increasing in prevalence due to increased use of azoles.[9,10]

Aspergillus is considered one of the etiologies of culture negative IE.[1,3] *Aspergillus fumigatus* occurs in two thirds of the cases of Aspergillus endocarditis mostly in patients with prosthetic heart valves, immunocompromised and with hematological malignancies.[10] Other mold infections reported were due to *Lomentospora prolificans* (*Scedosporium prolificans*) and *Fusarium solani.*[12–14]

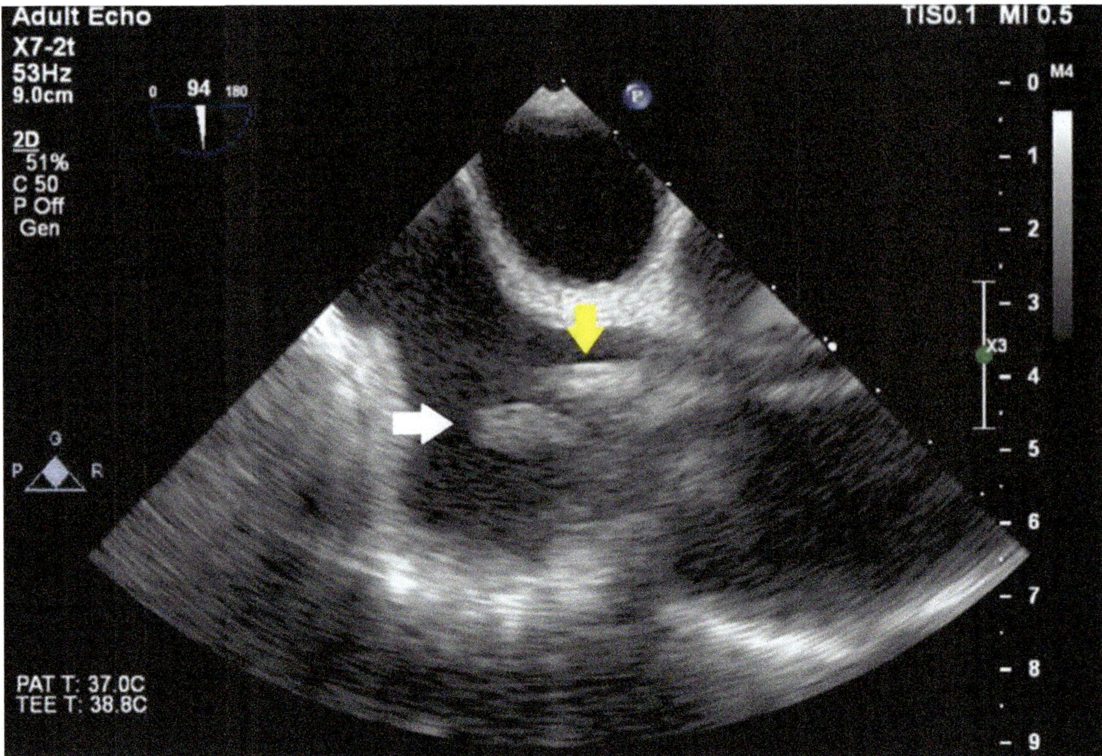

FIGURE 21-1 TEE bi-caval view, in a 55-year-old patient with pancreatic cancer and persistent blood cultures, of a large (1.1 cm) echo density typical of a vegetation (white arrow) in a pacemaker catheter (yellow arrow). It has dynamic mobility during the cardiac cycle concerning for risk of embolization.

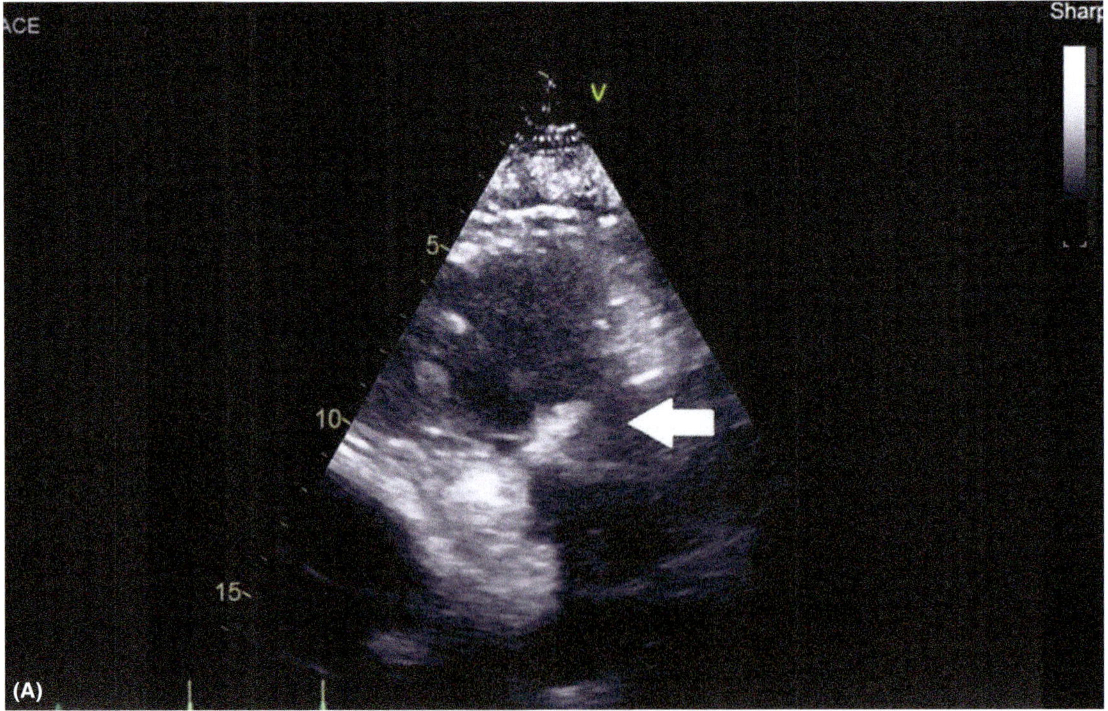

FIGURE 21-2 (A) Right parasternal view on trans-thoracic echocardiogram of a 41-year-old man with fever and shortness of breath. The white arrow points to a large echo density in the tricuspid valve. *(continued)*

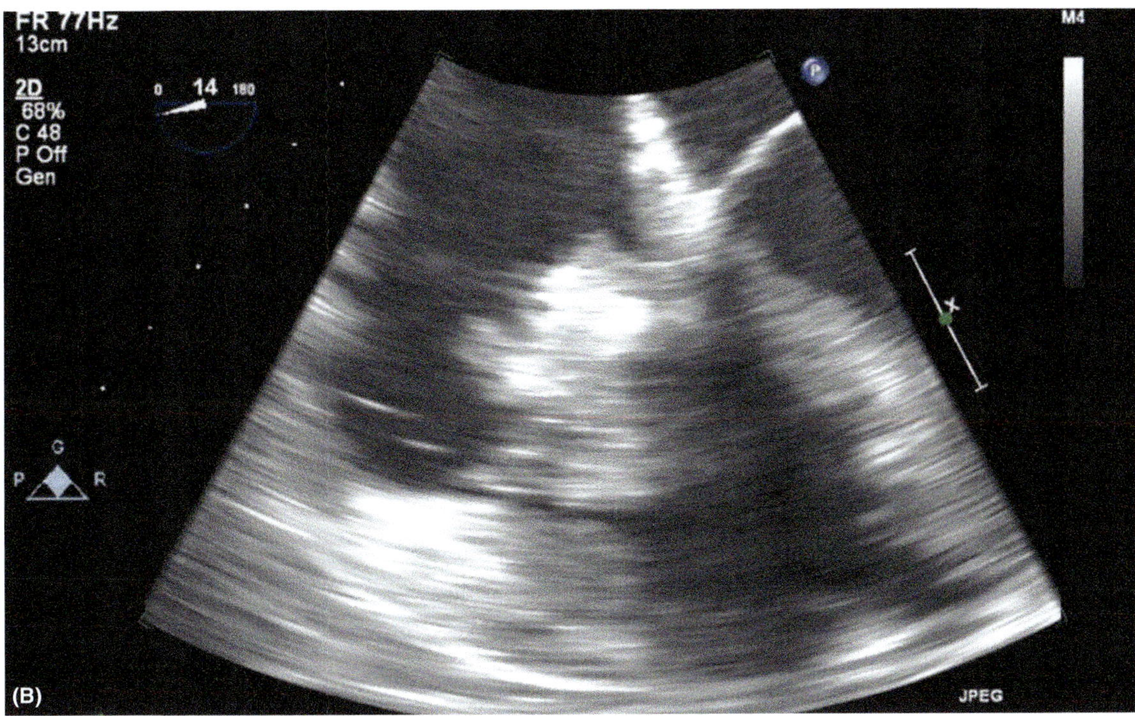

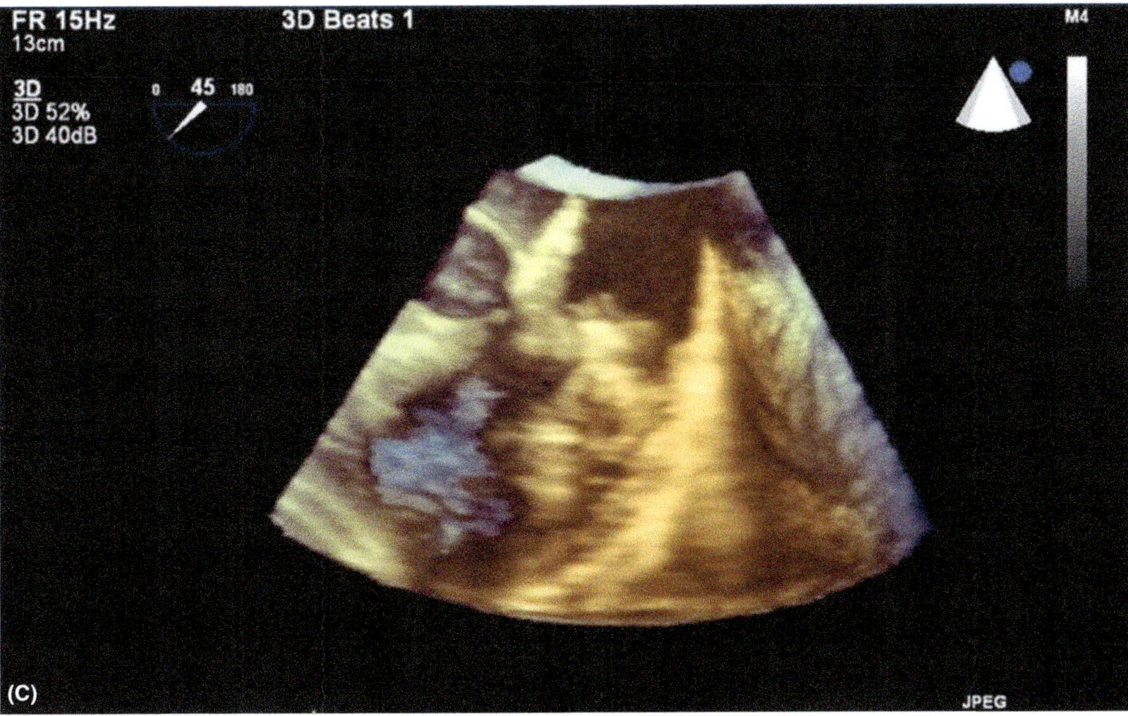

FIGURE 21-2 *(continued)* (B) 2D-TEE performed within 24 hrs shows a large >3 cm mass attached to the tricuspid valve, with components noted in all 3 leaflets, (C) 3D-TEE shows involvement of the papillary muscles. The vegetation was characteristic of fungal endocarditis.

Mycobacterial endocarditis is still very rare but is mostly associated with the nontuberculous rapid growth organisms like *M. abscessus, M. chelonae, M. fortuitum* and *M. mucogenicum.*[15] Rare cases of slow growing mycobacteria causing endocarditis have been reported including *M. tuberculosis.* Cases of *M. chimaera* prosthetic valve endocarditis and myocarditis have been reported in Europe in patients after open heart surgery.[16]

DIAGNOSIS OF IE

■ Clinical

Up to 90% of patients present with fever and 25% with clinical embolic phenomena (lung, brain, and spleen) at the time of diagnosis. Elderly and immunocompromised patients can be afebrile and have an atypical presentation.[1,3]

Diagnosis is still based in the modified Duke criteria with a sensitivity of 80% in native valve IE and much lower for prosthetic valve endocarditis.

Compared to the U.S. guidelines, the European include two major diagnostic criteria involving positive imaging for IE (PET C/T and cardiac CT) (Table 21-1).[1,3]

■ Echocardiography

It is still the initial imaging of choice, starting with a transthoracic echocardiography (TTE).

The sensitivity for diagnosis of vegetations in native valves is 70% for TTE and 96% for transesophageal echocardiography (TEE) and for prosthetic valves is 50% for TTE and 92% for TEE. Specificity is around 90% for both TTE and TEE (Figure 21-3).[1,3]

Three echocardiographic findings are major criteria in the diagnosis of IE: Vegetation, abscess or pseudoaneurysm and a new dehiscence of a prosthetic valve.[3]

Patients who require an initial TEE are the ones with high clinical suspicion, suboptimal quality of TTE (COPD, morbid obesity, previous thoracic or cardiovascular surgery), prosthetic heart valves,

TABLE 21-1 Definition of infectious endocarditis by modified Duke criteria

MODIFIED DUKE CRITERIA[1,3]	DEFINITIONS OF THE TERMS USED IN THE MODIFIED DUKE CRITERIA[1,3]
Definitive IE	**Major Criteria**

Pathological criteria:
 	
• Microorganisms demonstrated by culture or on histological examination of a vegetation, a vegetation that has embolized, or an intracardiac abscess specimen; or
• Pathological lesions; vegetation or intracardiac abscess confirmed by histological examination showing active endocarditis
 	
Clinical criteria
 	
• 2 major criteria; or
• 1 major criterion and 3 minor criteria; or
• 5 minor criteria
	1. **Blood cultures positive for IE:**
	  a. **Typical microorganisms consistent with IE from 2 separate blood cultures:**
	    • *Viridans streptococci, Streptococcus gallolyticus (Streptococcus bovis),* HACEK group, *Staphylococcus aureus;* or
	    • Community acquired enterococci, in the absence of a primary focus; or
	  b. **Microorganisms consistent with IE from persistently positive blood cultures:**
	    • At least 2 positive blood cultures of blood samples drawn >12h apart; or
	    • All of 3 or a majority of ≥4 separate blood cultures (with 1st and last samples drawn ≥1 hr apart); or
	  c. **Single positive blood culture for *Coxiella burnetii* or phase I IgG antibody titer ≥1:800**
	
	2. **Imaging positive for IE:**
	  a. Echocardiogram positive for IE: vegetation, abscess, pseudoaneurysm, intracardiac fistula, valvular perforation or aneurysm, new partial dehiscence of prosthetic valve.

MODIFIED DUKE CRITERIA[1,3]	DEFINITIONS OF THE TERMS USED IN THE MODIFIED DUKE CRITERIA[1,3]
	b. Abnormal activity around the site of prosthetic valve implantation detected by 18F-FDG PET/CT (only if prosthesis was implanted for >3 months) or radiolabeled leukocytes SPECT/CT **c.** Definitive paravalvular lesions by cardiac CT
Possible IE	**Minor Criteria**
• 1 major criterion and 1 minor criterion; or • 3 minor criteria	**a.** Predisposing heart condition or injection drug use **b.** Fever: Temperature >38C **c.** Vascular phenomena, including those detected by imaging; Major arterial emboli, septic pulmonary infarcts, infectious (mycotic) aneurysms, intracranial hemorrhage, conjunctival hemorrhages, and Janeway lesions.
Rejected IE	
• Firm alternate diagnosis; or • Resolution of symptoms suggesting IE with antibiotic therapy for ≤4 days; or • No pathological evidence of IE at surgery or autopsy, with antibiotic therapy for ≤4 days; or • Does not meet criteria for possible IE, as above	**d.** Immunologic phenomena: glomerulonephritis, Osler's nodes, Roth's spots and rheumatoid factor. **e.** Microbiological evidence: Positive blood culture that does not meet above criteria or serological evidence of active infection with organism consistent with IE.

Source: Adapted from Baddour et al.[1]; Habib et al.[3]

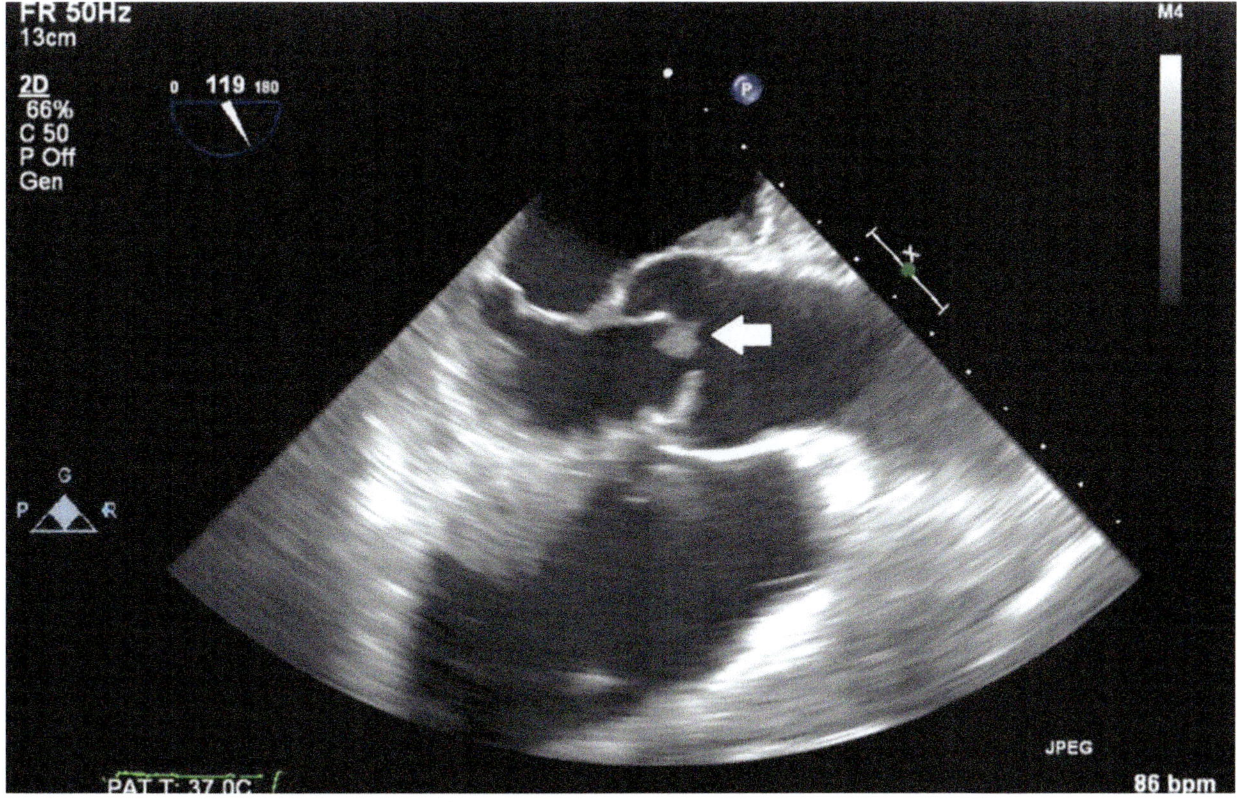

FIGURE 21-3 TEE of a 61-year-old man showing a small (7 mm) vegetation on the tip of the aortic valve non-coronary leaflets. TTE from 24 hrs prior did not reveal any abnormalities.

congenital heart disease, prior endocarditis or intracardiac devices.[1,3]

A TEE should follow a positive TTE for detection of complications in patients with high risk echocardiographic features like large or mobile vegetations, valvular insufficiency, and suggestion of perivalvular extension or secondary ventricular dysfunction (Figure 21-2A, B, C).[1]

Repeat TTE or TEE is recommended at the end of treatment in 5–7 days of a prior negative imaging if there is still high clinical suspicion or if a new complication ensues (new murmur, embolic event, heart failure, abscess, atrioventricular block).[1-3]

Intraoperative echocardiography after cardiopulmonary bypass is also recommended in all cases of IE undergoing surgery to document adequacy of the valve replacement, persistence of leaks and closure of fistulous tracts.[1,3]

Patients with *S. aureus* bacteremia at low risk of IE will not benefit from TEE if this four clinical criteria are present: Nosocomial or central line associated bacteremia, no intracardiac or prosthetic devices, no clinical signs of endocarditis and short duration of bacteremia <48–72 hrs.[17]

In patients with enterococcal bacteremia, a NOVA (number of positive blood cultures, unknown origin of bacteremia, prior heart valve disease and auscultation of a heart murmur) score <4 points suggests a very low risk for IE and a TEE can be obviated.[18]

Other diagnostic imaging modalities had been evaluated in many studies and reported in the European guidelines.[3]

Ekg-Gated Multi-Slice Computed Tomography (Ct) / Cardiac Ct

It is recommended for evaluation of prosthetic heart valve infections. It has a similar or more diagnostic accuracy than TEE to detect perivalvular abscess, pseudoaneurysms, and fistulae including information on anatomy and extension. It also helps in the preoperative non-invasive diagnosis of coronary artery disease before heart valve replacement.[1-3]

EKG-Gated Cardiac Magnetic Resonance Imaging

Anecdotal data and case reports are available in the literature, but no studies of diagnostic accuracy. The presence of artifacts with prosthetic materials is the main disadvantage of EKG-gated cardiac MRI.[2]

18F-Fluorodeoxyglucose Positron Emission Tomography (PET)/CT

Studies have found 18F-fluorodeoxyglucose PET/CT useful in the detection of peripheral emboli and metastatic infectious events. It is also helpful in patients with prosthetic valve infections or infections related to intracardiac devices.[2,3] A false positive result can be seen in patients who have undergone recent cardiac surgery (<1–3 months) due to the postoperative inflammatory response, soft atherosclerotic plaques, vasculitis, primary cardiac tumors, cardiac metastasis, and foreign body reactions.[2,3]

Radiolabeled White Blood Cell Single-Photon Emission Ct (Spect)

The use of radiolabeled leukocytes (^{111}In or ^{99m}Tc) is more specific for the detection of IE than FDG PET/CT, and it adds value in the diagnosis of prosthetic valve or cardiac device-related IE.[3]

Blood Cultures

It is recommended that at least three sets of blood cultures be obtained from a peripheral vein in 30-minute intervals. Negative blood cultures are more commonly present after prior use of antimicrobials; therefore, it is necessary to get blood cultures right before starting antimicrobial therapy.

Repeat blood cultures should be taken 48–72 hrs after starting therapy to evaluate the effectiveness of treatment and continued until bloodstream infection is cleared.[1,3]

Serology

Serology is useful in culture-negative IE, as outlined in Table 21-2.

Histopathology

The pathological examination of resected valvular tissue or fragment of emboli and the presence of a positive valvular tissue/emboli fragment culture remain the gold standard.[3] Immunohistochemical staining with the use of monoclonal or polyclonal antibodies may help in the identification of the species involved. Specific stains have been developed for *Bartonella* spp., *Coxiella burnetii,* and *T. whipplei.*[19]

TABLE 21-2   Investigation of rare causes of blood culture-negative infective endocarditis

PATHOGEN	DIAGNOSTIC PROCEDURES
Brucella **spp.**	Blood cultures, serology culture, immunohistology and PCR of surgical material.
Coxiella burnetii	Serology (IgG Phase I> 1:800), tissue culture, immunohistology and PCR of surgical material.
Bartonella **spp.**	Blood cultures, serology, culture, immunohistology and PCR of surgical material.
Tropheryma whipplei	Histology and PCR of surgical material.
Mycoplasma **spp.**	Serology, culture, immunohistology and PCR of surgical material
Legionella **spp.**	Blood cultures, serology, culture, immunohistology and PCR of surgical material.
Fungi	Blood cultures, serology, histology, GMS stains, PCR of surgical material

Source: From Habib et al., 2015.[3]

■ Molecular Methods

These are proposed in the context of culture-negative IE when there is a high clinical and epidemiological suspicion.[19] The use of mass spectrometry (MALDI-TOF) can be considered in centers with this capability and has the potential advantage of speeding up identification of the microorganisms involved.[3]

PCR assays, where the 16SrRNA region of bacteria, mycobacteria and fungi are amplified by the use of next generation sequencing, are being used in the identification of the organisms causing IE in culture negative patients. Better sensitivity is obtained from the use of cardiac valvular tissue. Its use on whole blood samples has also been reported in some cases but with very low sensitivity and rarely contributing to diagnosis. The current use of PCR assays is limited by detection of non-viable organism DNA or contamination during the collection process; therefore, any results require clinical correlation (Table 21-2).[1,3,19,20]

TREATMENT

Treatment of acute IE should be started as soon as possible with empirical antimicrobials according to epidemiological and history data obtained from patient.

In general, patients with native valve or late prosthetic valve IE (>1 year of surgery) will be infected by staphylococci, streptococci, and enterococci. In patients with early prosthetic valve IE and healthcare-associated IE, we need to treat for MRSA, enterococci, non-HACEK gram-negative pathogens and fungal organisms.[3]

The duration of therapy will depend on etiology, whether native or prosthetic heart valve, and if any complications are present. The first day of therapy is considered the first day of negative blood cultures in cases with prior positive cultures[2,3] or the first day after valve surgery if resected valve tissue is culture positive or in the presence of perivalvular abscess.[1]

STREPTOCOCCI[1,3]

Viridans group streptococci (VGS), *Streptococcus gallolyticus*, *Abiotrophia defective*, and *Granulicatella* species:

- If these organisms are highly susceptible to penicillin (MIC <0.125 µg/mL): Monotherapy with penicillin G, ceftriaxone, or vancomycin (if unable to tolerate penicillin) for 4 weeks is recommended in native valve IE. The desired vancomycin trough level should be between 10 and 15 µg/mL.

Intravenous gentamycin can be added to penicillin G or ceftriaxone to reduce the total duration of therapy to 2 weeks, except in patients with intra-cardiac or extracardiac abscess, creatinine clearance <20 mL/min or nutritionally deficient streptococci.

In prosthetic valve IE, the duration of therapy extends to 6 weeks and gentamycin is added to either penicillin G or ceftriaxone for the first 2 weeks of therapy.

- If these organisms are intermediate or highly resistant to penicillin (MIC ≥0.125 µg/mL)

In native valve IE, the duration of therapy is 4 weeks with penicillin G or ceftriaxone accompanied by IV gentamycin in the first 2 weeks or vancomycin for 4 weeks.

In prosthetic valve IE, the duration of therapy is 6 weeks of penicillin G or ceftriaxone accompanied with gentamycin for the whole duration of therapy. Another option is vancomycin for 6 weeks.

STAPHYLOCOCCI[1,3]

- Native valve with oxacillin-susceptible strains

MSSA cause a significant proportion of IE and more than 90% of isolates produce β-lactamase enzyme causing an inoculum effect in high bacterial load infections.[17]

Nafcillin, oxacillin, or cefazolin are recommended for 6 weeks in left sided and complicated right-sided IE.[1]

Two weeks of therapy alone in isolated tricuspid valve IE can be given if all this conditions apply: MSSA, good response to treatment, no metastatic sites of infection or empyema, no cardiac or extracardiac complications, no left sided or prosthetic valve infection, <20 mm valve vegetation, no severe immunosuppression (CD4 <200).[1,3]

An alternative therapy recommended in the European guidelines is 1 week of intravenous trimethroprim-sulfamethoxazole and clindamycin followed by 5 weeks of oral trimethroprim-sulfamethoxazole.[3]

- Native valve with oxacillin-resistant strains

Vancomycin or daptomycin are recommended for 6 weeks of therapy.

Daptomycin at doses of 6 mg/kg/day has been approved for right sided IE and has proven more effective than vancomycin for MSSA bacteremia and MRSA with vancomycin MIC >1 µg/mL.[1,3,21] Higher doses at 8–10 mg/kg/day have been recommended for left-sided IE and complicated infections.

- Prosthetic valve with oxacillin-susceptible strains

In general, the total duration of therapy is 6 weeks with the addition of rifampin after 3–5 days of effective antibiotic therapy and once bacteremia has been cleared.[1,3]

Nafcillin, oxacillin, first-generation cephalosporin, or vancomycin with rifampin for a minimum of 6 weeks is recommended with gentamycin for the first 2 weeks of therapy.

- Prosthetic valve with oxacillin-resistant strains

Vancomycin with rifampin for 6 weeks with gentamycin for the first 2 weeks.

If resistance to gentamycin is detected, another aminoglycoside or, in susceptible isolates, a fluoroquinolone can be used.

ENTEROCOCCI IE[1,3]

E. faecalis still accounts for 97% of cases of IE and is less frequently multidrug resistant.

In native valve IE with less than 3 months of symptoms and creatinine clearance >50 mL/min: 4 weeks of therapy is recommended with ampicillin or penicillin G with gentamycin.

In prosthetic valve IE or more than 3 months of symptoms: 6 weeks of therapy with ampicillin or penicillin G with gentamycin if creatinine clearance is >50 mL/min. If creatinine clearance <50 mL/min: Double beta-lactam therapy with ampicillin and ceftriaxone is recommended in E. faecalis IE.

The combination of ampicillin and ceftriaxone act synergistically by saturating different penicillin binding proteins and producing marked impairment in cell wall synthesis. It is also less nephrotoxic and now if the preferred combination regimen in IE due to enterococcus.

If enterococcus is resistant to penicillin or patient does not tolerate beta lactams, vancomycin with gentamycin for 6 weeks is indicated.

Linezolid or daptomycin for at least 6 weeks is an option in vancomycin resistant enterococci.

Daptomycin at doses of 10–12 mg/kg/day in combination with ampicillin or ceftaroline can be considered in patients with persistent bacteremia, enterococcal strains with high MICs to daptomycin (3 µg/mL) or recurrent aortic valve IE due to E. faecalis.[1,22]

HACEK MICROORGANISMS

Unless susceptibility to these drugs is detected, these organisms are considered ampicillin and penicillin resistant. Ceftriaxone is recommended for 4–6 weeks in native valve or prosthetic valve IE, respectively. Ciprofloxacin, levofloxacin or moxifloxacin is an option if patients are unable to tolerate cephalosporins.

NON-HACEK GRAM-NEGATIVE ORGANISMS

Early surgery with combination of beta-lactam with either an aminoglycoside or fluoroquinolone for at least 6 weeks is recommended.[3]

FUNGAL IE

Effective treatment requires a combination of antifungals for more than 6 weeks with early surgery. The initial regimen has to include amphotericin B with or without flucytosine in combination with an echinocandin or an azole.[1,23] Some experts recommend long-term or lifelong suppressive therapy with azoles after completion of therapy.[1,23]

CULTURE-NEGATIVE IE

As discussed before, the previous administration of antimicrobial agents is a major cause of culture negative IE. Other confirmed factors are fastidious bacteria (Coxiella, Bartonella, Legionella, Mycoplasma, etc.), fungi, or non-cultivatable agents.[1]

It is found that up to 20% of proven infectious endocarditis cases can have negative blood cultures,[24] therefore the importance of evaluation of epidemiological factors, prior history and previous infections is worth stressing.[1]

In acute native valve IE the empirical treatment needs to cover for *S. aureus*, B-hemolytic streptococci and aerobic gram-negative bacilli. Vancomycin and cefepime can be used in this cases. In a subacute presentation, additional coverage for VGS, HACEK, and enterococci is needed therefore the use of vancomycin with ampicillin-sulbactam is recommended.[1]

In patients with early (<1 year) prosthetic valve IE, a regimen that includes vancomycin, cefepime, gentamycin, and rifampin is recommended for coverage of staphylococci, enterococci, and aerobic gram-negative bacilli. If PVE is of late presentation the regimen can be simplified to Vancomycin and ceftriaxone.[1]

Antimicrobial therapy can be tailored if microorganisms are finally identified by serology, mass spectrometry, next-generation sequencing of 16srRNA.

MARANTIC ENDOCARDITIS

Marantic endocarditis is considered within the group of nonbacterial thrombotic endocarditis and does not cause destructive changes to the affected valve.[3] In an old large autopsy series, it was found that adenocarcinoma was the most frequent histologic type of related neoplasm, and common sites were from lung, pancreas, and gastric cancer although adenocarcinoma of unknown primary has also been reported.[25] Other review of cases continue to associate it more with solid tumors, being a part of a paraneoplastic phenomena, and more often involving the left side of the heart (aortic more often than mitral valve) in previously undamaged heart valves.[26] Marantic endocarditis has the same initial diagnostic workup to rule out IE, but its diagnosis also depends on a significant clinical suspicion, the presence of a vegetation not responding to antibiotic treatment and multiple systemic emboli.[3]

Its treatment consists of therapy directed to the underlying malignancy and systemic anticoagulation if not contraindicated.[3]

INDICATIONS FOR SURGERY

Valve surgery is indicated in patients with complicated left-sided IE despite adequate antimicrobial therapy and presence of three main indications: heart failure, uncontrolled infection or prevention of embolism. In the case of right-sided IE, right heart failure due to severe tricuspid regurgitation, poor or lack of response to medical therapy, tricuspid valve vegetations >20 mm and recurrent pulmonary embolism are indications for surgery. Initial medical management is recommended then valve repair rather than replacement.[1] The timing of surgery depends on the severity of this complications going from emergent (within 24 hrs), urgent (7 days) to elective (within 2 weeks) or early (within the hospitalization and before completion of full course of antibiotics) as per U.S. guidelines (Table 21-3).[1,3]

COMPLICATIONS OF ACUTE IE[1,3]

- **Periannular extension of infection:** This complication is more common in aortic than mitral and tricuspid IE.

- **Metastatic foci of infection:** Initial management and control of metastatic foci of infection must be done before valve surgery.

- **Embolic/Hemorrhagic stroke**: If surgical valve repair is indicated, delayed surgery (>1 month) is recommended in hemorrhagic stroke and severe neurological damage. Microbleeds (MRI T2 hypointensities <10 mm) are excluded from this timing consideration.

TABLE 21-3 Indications for surgery in infective endocarditis despite adequate antimicrobial therapy

INDICATION FOR SURGERY	AHA CLASS/LEVEL RECOMMENDATION	ESC CLASS/LEVEL RECOMMENDATION	NVE	PVE	TIME OF SURGERY
Left- sided IE					
Heart Failure with signs or symptoms	I (B)	I (B)	+	+	Early (AHA) Urgent (ESC)
Cardiogenic shock	N/A	I (B)	+	+	Emergency (ESC)
Refractory pulmonary edema	N/A	I (B)	+	+	Emergency (ESC)
Locally uncontrolled infection (abscess, false aneurysm, fistula, enlarging vegetation)	N/A	I (B)	+	+	Urgent (ESC)
Persistent infectiona	I (B)	IIa (B)	+	+	Early (AHA) Urgent (ESC)
IE caused by fungi or highly resistant organisms	I (B)	I (C)	+	+	Early (AHA) Urgent/elective (ESC)
Heart block, annular, aortic root abscess, or destructive penetrating lesions	I (B)	N/A	+	+	Early (AHA) Urgent (ESC)
Recurrent emboli with persistent, large (>10 mm) or enlarging vegetations	IIa (B)	I (B)	+	+	Early (AHA) Urgent (ESC)
Severe valvular regurgitation or stenosis and mobile vegetation >10 mm with low operative risk	IIa (B)	IIa (B)	+	+	Early (AHA) Urgent (ESC)
Mobile vegetation >10 mm involving anterior mitral valve leaflet and other indications for surgery	IIa (C)	N/A	+	+	Early (AHA)
Mobile vegetation >10 mm	IIb (C)	N/A		+	Early (AHA)
Very large vegetation >30 mm	N/A	IIa (B)	+	+	Urgent (ESC)
Large Vegetation >15 mm	N/A	IIb (C)	+	+	Urgent (ESC)

INDICATION FOR SURGERY	AHA CLASS/LEVEL RECOMMENDATION	ESC CLASS/LEVEL RECOMMENDATION	NVE	PVE	TIME OF SURGERY
PVE caused by staphylococci or non-HACEK gram-negative bacteria	N/A	IIa (C)		+	Urgent/elective (ESC)
Relapsing PVE	IIA (C)	N/A		+	Early (AHA)
Right-sided IE					
Microorganisms difficult to eradicate or bacteremia >7 days. S. aureus, P. aeruginosa, fungi	IIa (C)	IIa (C)			
Persistent tricuspid valve vegetations >20 mm after recurrent pulmonary emboli with or without concomitant right heart failure	IIa (C)	IIa (C)			
Right heart failure due to severe tricuspid regurgitation with poor response to diuretic therapy	IIa (C)	IIa (C)			

NVE: Native valve endocarditis
PVE: Prosthetic valve endocarditis
[a]Persistent bacteremia or fever lasting >5–7 days after starting appropriate antimicrobial therapy. Provided that other sites of infection and fever have been excluded.
Sources: Adapted from Baddour LM et al., 2015[1]; Habib G et al., 2015[3]; Bin Abdulhak AA, Tleyjeh IM, 2017.[27]

- **Mycotic aneurisms**: These can be located intracranially or extracranially with management based on careful risk assessment in each instance. These can be located intracranially or extracranially with management based on careful risk assessment in each instance. There is no consensus between continuing conservative management with antimicrobial therapy alone or proceeding with endovascular therapies (such as embolization, stenting, or coiling) in unruptured intracranial aneurysms; given their friable thin walls and proclivity to rupture. Ruptured infectious aneurysms are treated by open surgical procedures including bypass using Saphenous vein, aneurysmal clipping or even endovascular.[28,29]

- **Heart conduction abnormalities**: This complication is uncommon, occurring in 1%–15% of cases, and it represents the occurrence of perivalvular abnormalities. Patients in cardiac monitoring present from first degree AV block to complete bundle branch block. A new onset tachyarrhythmia may be caused by an ischemic event from an embolization of a vegetation into a coronary artery. New onset atrial fibrillation is more common in the elderly.

■ Risk factors for relapse of IE[3]

The major risk factors for relapse of IE are as follows:

- Inadequate antimicrobial treatment: Agent, dose, and duration.

- Resistant or fastidious microorganisms; *Brucella* spp, *Legionella* spp. *Chlamydia* spp, *Mycoplasma* spp, *Mycobacterium* spp, *Bartonella* spp, *Coxiella Burnetii*, fungi.

- Polymicrobial infection in an intravenous drug abuser.

- Empirical antimicrobial therapy for blood culture negative IE.

- Periannular extension.

- Prosthetic valve IE.

- Resistance to conventional antibiotic regimens.

- Positive valve culture.

- Persistence of fever at the seventh postoperative day.

- Chronic dialysis.

REFERENCES

1. Baddour LM, Wilson WR, Bayer AS, et al. Infective endocarditis in adults: diagnosis, antimicrobial therapy, and management of complications: a scientific statement for healthcare professionals from the American Heart Association. *Circulation*. 2015;132(15):1435–1486.

2. Gomes A, Glaudemans A, Touw DJ, et al. Diagnostic value of imaging in infective endocarditis: a systematic review. *Lancet Infect Dis*. 2017;17(1):e1–e14.

3. Habib G, Lancellotti P, Antunes MJ, et al. 2015 ESC guidelines for the management of infective endocarditis: the task force for the management of infective endocarditis of the European Society of Cardiology (ESC). Endorsed by: European Association for Cardio-Thoracic Surgery (EACTS), the European Association of Nuclear Medicine (EANM). *Eur Heart J*. 2015;36(44):3075–3128.

4. Fernandez-Cruz A, Munoz P, Sandoval C, et al. Infective endocarditis in patients with cancer: a consequence of invasive procedures or a harbinger of neoplasm?: a prospective, multicenter cohort. *Medicine (Baltimore)*. 2017;96(38):e7913.

5. Jans C, Boleij A. The road to infection: host-microbe interactions defining the pathogenicity of streptococcus bovis/streptococcus equinus complex members. *Front Microbiol*. 2018;9:603.

6. Corredoira J, Garcia-Pais MJ, Coira A, et al. Differences between endocarditis caused by Streptococcus bovis and Enterococcus spp. and their association with colorectal cancer. *Eur J Clin Microbiol Infect Dis*. 2015;34(8):1657–1665.

7. Noureddine M, de la Torre J, Ivanova R, et al. [Left-sided endocarditis due to gram-negative bacilli: epidemiology and clinical characteristics]. *Enferm Infecc Microbiol Clin*. 2011;29(4):276–281.

8. Ortiz D, Siegal EM, Kramer C, Khandheria BK, Brauer E. Nontyphoidal cardiac salmonellosis: two case reports and a review of the literature. *Tex Heart Inst J*. 2014;41(4):401–406.

9. Reyes HA, Carbajal WH, Valdez LM, Lozada C. Successful medical treatment of infective endocarditis caused by Candida parapsilosis in an immunocompromised patient. *BMJ Case Rep*. 2015; doi: 10.1136/bcr-2015-212128.

10. Tattevin P, Revest M, Lefort A, Michelet C, Lortholary O. Fungal endocarditis: current challenges. *Int J Antimicrob Agents*. 2014;44(4):290–294.

11. Riddell Jt, Kauffman CA, Smith JA, et al. Histoplasma capsulatum endocarditis: multicenter case series with review of current diagnostic techniques and treatment. *Medicine (Baltimore)*. 2014;93(5):186–193.

12. Kassar O, Charfi M, Trabelsi H, Hammami R, Elloumi M. Fusarium solani endocarditis in an acute leukemia patient. *Med Mal Infect*. 2016;46(1):57–59.

13. Kelly M, Stevens R, Konecny P. Lomentospora prolificans endocarditis—case report and literature review. *BMC Infect Dis*. 2016;16:36.

14. Kuroki K, Murakami T. Aspergillus endocarditis in a native valve without prior cardiac surgery. *Gen Thorac Cardiovasc Surg*. 2012;60(11):771–773.

15. Yuan SM. Mycobacterial endocarditis: a comprehensive review. *Rev Bras Cir Cardiovasc*. 2015;30(1):93–103.

16. Kohler P, Kuster SP, Bloemberg G, et al. Healthcare-associated prosthetic heart valve, aortic vascular graft, and disseminated Mycobacterium chimaera infections subsequent to open heart surgery. *Eur Heart J*. 2015;36(40):2745–2753.

17. Heriot GS, Cronin K, Tong SYC, Cheng AC, Liew D. Criteria for identifying patients with staphylococcus aureus bacteremia who are at low risk of endocarditis: a systematic review. *Open Forum Infect Dis*. 2017;4(4):ofx261.

18. Bouza E, Kestler M, Beca T, et al. The NOVA score: a proposal to reduce the need for transesophageal echocardiography in patients with enterococcal bacteremia. *Clin Infect Dis*. 2015;60(4):528–535.

19. Subedi S, Jennings Z, Chen SC. Laboratory approach to the diagnosis of culture-negative infective endocarditis. *Heart Lung Circ*. 2017;26(8):763–771.

20. Oberbach A, Schlichting N, Feder S, et al. New insights into valve-related intramural and intracellular bacterial diversity in infective endocarditis. *PLOS ONE*. 2017;12(4):e0175569.

21. Nannini EC, Singh KV, Arias CA, Murray BE. In Vivo effects of cefazolin, daptomycin, and nafcillin in experimental endocarditis with a methicillin-susceptible staphylococcus aureus strain showing an inoculum effect against cefazolin. *Antimicrob Agents Chemother*. 2013;57(9):4276–4281.

22. Beganovic M, Luther MK, Rice LB, Arias CA, Rybak MJ, LaPlante KL. A review of combination antimicrobial therapy for enterococcus faecalis bloodstream infections and infective endocarditis. *Clin Infect Dis*. 2018 67(2):303–309.

23. Pasha AK, Lee JZ, Low SW, Desai H, Lee KS, Al Mohajer M. Fungal Endocarditis: update on diagnosis and management. *Am J Med*. 2016;129(10):1037–1043.

24. Werner M, Andersson R, Olaison L, Hogevik H. A clinical study of culture-negative endocarditis. *Medicine (Baltimore)*. 2003;82(4):263–273.

25. El-Shami K, Griffiths E, Streiff M. Nonbacterial thrombotic endocarditis in cancer patients: pathogenesis, diagnosis, and treatment. *Oncologist*. 2007;12(5):518–523.

26. Mazokopakis EE, Syros PK, Starakis IK. Nonbacterial thrombotic endocarditis (marantic endocarditis) in cancer patients. *Cardiovasc Hematol Disord Drug Targets*. 2010;10(2):84–86.

27. Bin Abdulhak AA, Tleyjeh IM. Indications of surgery in infective endocarditis. *Curr Infect Dis Rep*. 2017;19(3):10.

28. Piccirilli M, Prizio E, Canizzato D, et al. The only case of mycotic anerysm of the ICA: clinical-radiological remarks and review of literature. *J Clin Neurosci*. 2017;38:62–66.

29. Ragulojan R, Grupke S, Fraser JF. Systematic review of endocascular, surgical and conservative options for infectious intracranially aneurysms and cardiac considerations. *J Stroke Cerebrovasc Dis*. 2019;28(3):838–844.

22 Magnetic Resonance Imaging and Therapeutic Radiation in Cancer Patients with Implanted Pacemaker or Defibrillator Devices

Kaveh Karimzad

INTRODUCTION

It is estimated that 50%–75% of patients with Cardiac Implantable Electronic Devices (CIEDs) will require magnetic resonance imaging (MRI) sometime during their lifetime after implantation of the device.[1] MRI has emerged as the preferred imaging modality and the primary tool for the assessment and evaluation of both malignant and benign tumors. Previously the presence of an implanted pacemaker or defibrillator was considered a contraindication for performance of MRI, but this practice has changed recently with availability of MRI conditional devices; two large prospective trials have demonstrated safety of MRI in patients with magnetic resonance non-conditional devices.[2,3]

EFFECTS OF MAGNETIC RESONANCE IMAGING ON CARDIAC IMPLANTABLE ELECTRONIC DEVICES

A recently published Heart Rhythm Society Expert Consensus Statement on MRI and radiation exposure in patients with CIEDs has provides an important summary of the effects of static and magnetic fields as well as RF energy generated by MRI on hardware and software components of CIEDs.[4] The potential effects of MRI on these devices is now sufficiently well-defined so that the implications for cancer patients can be appreciated.

Electromagnetic Interference (EMI) from radiofrequency energy pulses or changing magnetic field gradients may cause over-sensing errors which results in inappropriate function, particularly failure to pace the CIED devices appropriately. In the electromagnetic field generated by MRI imagers, CIED device leads may act as an antennas resulting in artefactual potentials sufficiently large to trigger sensing. Pacemakers or defibrillators thereby oversense the noise caused by

EMI, and the inappropriate inhibition of pacing due to oversensing can result in profound bradycardia or asystole in a pacing-dependent patient. EMI can be inappropriately detected as ventricular tachycardia or ventricular fibrillation in a patient with defibrillator which in turn results in the administration of an inappropriate ICD shock.

High energy EMI can lead to electrical or power-on reset. Reset is a safety back up mode of pacing in case of catastrophic failure of the device. The pacing and tachy-therapy parameters during reset mode is unique to each manufacturer; pacing mode during reset is a backup demand mode which might be inhibited due to oversensing of EMI. Electrical reset is very concerning in a pacemaker dependent patient during MRI because of change in the mode of pacing from asynchronous (no sensing) to demand pacing during the reset. During demand mode, pacing can be inhibited due to oversensing caused by EMI which then results in potentially lethal asystole in the pacemaker dependent patient. Also tachyarrhythmia therapy would be activated in reset mode which could result in inappropriate shock due to oversensing. For these reasons reset must be recognized promptly and addressed emergently during MRI to prevent life-threatening consequences.

The electrical current in the conductive wires of CIEDs caused by gradient magnetic field can results in myocardial capture and possible atrial or ventricular arrhythmia. A prospective multi-center study designed to determine the risks of performing non-thoracic 1.5T MRI scanning for patients with implanted pacemakers and ICDs exists under the name "MagnaSafe."[5] MagnaSafe investigators seek to determine the rates of temporary and permanent device parameter changes, including changes in lead threshold, lead impedance and battery voltage. Registry results reported six cases of atrial fibrillation and atrial flutter out of 1500 MRIs in patients with non-conditional pacemaker and defibrillators.[3] Instances of ventricular tachycardia in patients undergoing MRI have not been reported in the literature.

Changes in sensing and capture threshold have been reported in a recently published study by Nazarian et al., which showed decrease in P wave amplitude, increase in atrial capture threshold, increase in right ventricular capture threshold and increase in left ventricular capture threshold on 3%–4% of patients during long term follow up.[6] These changes in lead parameters were not clinically significant and did not require device revision or reprogramming. These changes in lead parameters are believed to be the result of lead component heating of and subsequent thermal tissue damage.[7] CIED leads do not contain any significant amount of ferromagnetic material. As a result movement of CIED leads are extremely unlikely in the magnetic field of MRI.[4]

In regard to cardiac devices and potential risks associated with MRI, there are two important definitions: MR conditional systems pose no known hazard under specified conditions of use. These conditions includes MRI field conditions, specific lead and generator combinations and MRI mode programming. It is important to mention that no CIED has an MRI safe designation. An MRI safe object such as a plastic has no hazard in any MRI environment. MR non-conditional system include all CIED systems other than those that meet MR conditional labeling, including patients with a mix of conditional generator and non-conditional leads.

Over the last several years engineers have made certain changes in lead and generator technology to reduce the risks associated with MRI which has resulted in MR conditional labeling of these devices by Food and Drug Administration (FDA). The majority of patients with CIEDs, however, still have MR non-conditional systems.

MANAGEMENT OF CANCER PATIENTS WITH MAGNETIC RESONANCE CONDITIONAL CARDIAC IMPLANTABLE ELECTRONIC DEVICES DURING MAGNETIC RESONANCE IMAGING

Prior to performing MRI in cancer patients with CIEDs, risks and benefits should be evaluated. There should be a close communication between ordering physician (often an oncologist), radiologist and cardiologist with the knowledge of CIED programming and management. It should be determined if the CIED system is MR conditional or not and there should be full knowledge about implanted leads including abandoned lead, fractured leads, recalled leads and

epicardial leads. Device programming, battery status and lead parameters should be evaluated prior to MRI. Also the patient's underlying rhythm and pacemaker dependency should be understood to determine the most appropriate mode of pacing during the procedure.

As an example of an algorithm of how patients can be managed, their initial visit is at a cardiac device clinic for interrogation of the device. During that visit MR conditionality can be evaluated, device and lead performance and pacemaker dependency status to determined, and the risk of performing MRI in that particular patient estimated. Subsequently these parameters are communicated to the radiologist who then determines if an MRI is the best and most appropriate test, and that there are no alternative imaging modalities. This algorithm, while developed in response to the needs of cancer patients, may provide a prudent path for the non-cancer patient as well.

MR conditional generators have an MRI-mode which can be turned on and off before and after the scan. The features of this mode are pre-scan device check, asynchronous or non-sensing mode, increased pacing output during scan, disabling of tachycardia detection, shock therapy and restoration of pre-scan programming and values after the scan.[4] Most MR conditional systems are approved for 1.5 Tesla MRI scanners in normal operating mode but some newer systems are FDA-approved for 3T scanning. Most are approved for full body scanning including thorax and cardiac MRI.

Abandoned leads, lead extenders, lead remnants, fractured leads and epicardial leads make a system MR non-conditional even if the patient has an implanted MRI conditional system. In fact in our institution these are few contraindications for patients with CIEDs who are referred for MRI. Langman et al. demonstrated in an in vitro study abandoned pacemaker leads showed greater lead tip heating compared to leads attached to a generator.[8] Patients with abandoned nonfunctional leads and epicardial leads were excluded from two recently published large prospective studies on safety of performing MRI in patients with MR non-conditional systems.[3,5,6] A recently published study from University of Michigan reported no major complication in a small number of patients who underwent MRI with abandoned leads.[9] Higgins et al., in a small clinical study performed MRI in 19 patients with abandoned pacemaker and defibrillator leads and reported no adverse event.[10] No specific cancer-related reports are available, but these studies are deemed highly relevant to the cancer population that share clinical imaging needs.

Recently published Heart Rhythm Society (HRS) consensus statement on management of patients undergoing MRI has clearly recommended that an institutional workflow algorithm be applied, and that it should be used for patients with MR conditional as well as those with non-conditional devices.[4] Even though there has been several clinical and in vitro studies showing safety of MR conditional devices when appropriate conditions of use are followed, there are many combinations of CIEDs and scanning parameters that must be taken into account. Careful attention in needed even in MR conditional systems, as it is impossible to predict every situation that might be encountered during MRI. This may have even greater relevance for the cancer patient who may have a number of risk factors for complications, and for this reason existence of an institutional protocol or algorithm is essential. Close collaboration between the MR imaging specialist and a cardiologist with in depth knowledge in CIEDs management and programming should form an integral part of the institutional workflow. The appropriateness, benefits and necessity of MRI should be evaluated by MR imaging specialist in comparison to alternative imaging modalities.

Continuous monitoring of patients cardiac rhythm and transcutaneous pulse oximetry are required during MRI scan. ECG monitoring might not be reliable and difficult to interpret in some cases due to electrical artifact caused by certain MR sequences. In these situation pulse oximetry is very important because in most cases it is not affected by different MR sequences and can show us any change in pulse rate. Due to possibility of unexpected scenarios like ventricular pacing inhibition in an intermittently pacing-dependent patient or ventricular tachycardia in a patient with defibrillator when tachycardia detection and shock therapy is deactivated, it is recommended that personnel with advanced cardiac life support (ACLS) skills be present for the duration of device reprogramming during MRI even in patients with MR conditional CIED systems.

HRS document recommends that personnel with skill to program CIED should be available and can be reached for scan in patients with MRI conditional systems but it is generally not necessary for such person to be present for the duration of MRI scan itself. In our institution a person who is skilled in programming and managing CIEDs is always present during MRI scan even for patients with MR conditional systems.

The main determinant factors in programming MR conditional CIEDs during MRI are pacemaker dependency status and underlying heart rate. In these devices turning MRI mode "on" automatically deactivate advanced or adaptive pacing features and defibrillator tachycardia detection and shock

therapies. CIED should be programmed asynchronous (non-sensing mode) in pacemaker dependent patient to overcome the issue of oversensing EMI and possibility of pacing inhibition and asystole. Program pacing rate may be set slightly faster than rate of pacing during reset in pacemaker dependent patients with ventricular pacing so as to detect power on reset during MRI; pacemaker dependency is defined as showing no underlying rhythm when checking the device at VVI with lower rate of 35 bpm. In patients with sinus node dysfunction with sinus bradycardia and predominantly atrial pacing and normal AV nodal conduction, the device may be programmed in an asynchronous atrial pacing mode (AOO) to prevent potential hemodynamically significant bradycardia during the MRI. In patients who are not pacemaker dependent with minimal pacing, it is reasonable to program the device to a non-pacing mode (ODO or OVO).

MANAGEMENT OF PATIENTS WITH MAGNETIC RESONANCE NON-CONDITIONAL CARDIAC IMPLANTABLE ELECTRONIC DEVISES DURING MAGNETIC RESONANCE IMAGING

Over last several years many small cohorts of patients with non-conditional CIEDs undergoing MRI have been reported.[11–16] Overall MR scanning was safe with some minor issues but with no life threatening complications reported. Two recently published large prospective studies have addressed the safety of performing MRI in patients with non-conditional CIED systems. In MagnaSafe multicenter registry MRI was performed in 1000 patients with pacemaker and 500 patients with defibrillator.[3] All CIED systems were non-conditional, the study only enrolled patients undergoing non-thoracic MRI. Patients with abandoned leads, nonfunctional leads, and devices in Elective Replacement Indicator (ERI) were excluded. Pacemaker dependent patients with pacemaker (28%) were included but pacemaker dependent patients with defibrillator were excluded in this study. No deaths, lead failures, or loss of capture or ventricular tachycardia occurred during MRI. One ICD generator had to be replaced immediately because it could not be interrogated after MRI. There were six cases of self-terminating atrial fibrillation and atrial flutter during or immediately after the MRI procedure. Partial reset was reported in six cases (five patients) affecting the patient, or the lead or the device identification information. There was no reported case of full electrical reset with programming changes during MRI.

In another large prospective study from Johns Hopkins University by Nazarian et al., 1509 patients with nonconditional pacemaker and defibrillators undergoing MRI were studied.[6] As was the case in the MagnaSafe trial, patients with abandoned leads, epicardial leads, as well as pacemaker dependent patients with defibrillators without asynchronous pacing capacity were excluded. No long term clinically significant adverse event was reported. Electrical reset to back up mode of pacing occurred in nine patients. In one patient with pacemaker could not be reprogrammed after reset and it had to be replaced. This patient's pacemaker generator had less than one month battery life remaining prior to MRI. Changes in device parameters was reported immediately after MRI in long term follow up. Only one patient out of eight with power-on reset had transient inhibition of pacing with asymptomatic pause. The most common notable change immediately after MRI was decrease in P wave amplitude in 1% of patients. Increase in atrial capture threshold, right ventricular capture threshold and left ventricular lead capture threshold was reported in 3%–4% of patients during long term follow up. These changes were not clinically significant and did not require device revision or reprogramming. The main determinants of changes in device parameters were lead length, number of scans and anatomical region of scanning. There are some small studies that suggested thoracic MRI has higher risk than non-thoracic MRI due to proximity of magnetic field to the device, but in Johns Hopkins study there was no association between region of imaging and changes in device parameters during long term follow up.[17] Longer right ventricular leads had larger reduction in right ventricular sensing during long term follow up. While these studies were not undertaken on cancer patients, patients with malignant disease now undergo MRI with increasing frequency, and when imaging is undertaken with observation, prudence, and caution, it has a low incidence of complications. Cancer patients should not have crucial imaging denied because of the presence of implantable devices.

To optimize these procedures, especially in cancer patients, and minimize associated risks, there should be an institutional policy in place with close collaboration and communication of MR imaging specialist and cardiologist with in depth knowledge of CIED programming and management, as well as with the referring oncologist who may in the best position to balance risks and benefits. The radiologist should determine if MRI is the preferred imaging study with no acceptable alternative imaging modality. The radiologist, cardiologist and referring physician should have a clear understanding of risks and benefits of MRI in a patient with nonconditional CIED system, and the patient should be fully informed and comprehend the need for imaging information as well as the risks. Documentation of the informed consent interaction should constitute an integral part of the medical record.

The recently-released HRS consensus statement on safety of MRI in patients with CIEDs has clearly mentioned that patients with non-conditional CIED systems can undergo MRI if this imaging modality is the best test for the condition and there is an institutional protocol and a designated responsible MR specialist and physician with knowledge and skills to program and manage patients with CIED. Patients with fractured, epicardial and abandoned leads are excluded as there is no adequate data to support the safety of MRI in patients with these leads. As discussed previously, continuous ECG and pulse oximetry monitoring should be done during MRI with careful attention to pulse oximetry for any changes in heart rate other than programmed pacing rate as ECG might not be interpretable in most cases due to electrical artifact caused by different MR sequences.

In non-conditional CIED systems advanced or adaptive features like magnet mode, rate response, noise discrimination and ventricular sense response should be manually deactivated. In patients with defibrillators, tachycardia detection and shock therapy should be deactivated. Asynchronous mode of pacing (DOO, AOO or VOO) should be programmed for pacemaker dependent patient. The rate of pacing should be programmed in a way that it does not compete with underlying rhythm and avoid competitive pacing. Programming the rate slightly faster than the reset mode enables the diagnoses of a power-on reset during MRI in a pacemaker dependent patient. One possible dangerous situation is programming the device to the asynchronous mode with ventricular pacing in a patient with cardiomyopathy and high burden of ventricular ectopy. In such patients there is a possibility of vulnerable-period ventricular activation and induction of ventricular arrhythmia. Patients who are not pacemaker dependent and have a reliable intrinsic rhythm of more than 40 bpm with no symptoms of hemodynamic instability can be programmed to a non-pacing mode (OVO, ODO) or an inhibited mode (VVI).

A cardiac device specialist with the skills to program the CIED should be present during MRI in these patients. A cardiologist with ability to insert temporary transvenous pacer catheter and in depth knowledge of CIED programming should be present in the control room during MRI for patients with nonconditional CIED systems who are pacemaker dependent. For patients who are not pacemaker dependent, the cardiologist with above mentioned skills should be immediately available in premises of MR suite. Ideally, fluoroscopy should be available in the event it is needed for insertion of a temporary pacing device and line.

At the MD Anderson Cancer center, we have monitored and managed close to 700 cancer patients with CIEDs (pacemaker, defibrillator and CRT devices) undergoing MRI over the last 8–9 years. Our volume is steadily increasing and currently we manage 3 patients weekly on average. Most of our patients have MR non-conditional devices. We exclude patients with abandoned, epicardial and fractured leads. Also patients with subcutaneous defibrillator have been traditionally excluded, but evolving designations of new devices may alter this relative contra-indication. Patients with generator at elective replacement indicator (ERI) may be considered for generator changes prior to undergoing MRI. In our series of patients there has not been a case of death, ventricular tachycardia, lead malfunction, loss of pacing, inhibition of pacing due to power on reset, inappropriate defibrillator shock or need for temporary pacer insertion; a single case of complete malfunction of a non-conditional defibrillator in a pacemaker non-dependent patient who had to undergo subsequent defibrillator generator change. In instances where pacemakers do not have the programmable feature to disable magnet response, MRI with asynchronous pacing at an appropriate magnet response rate was programmed. In our series, one MRI had to be aborted because reported symptoms of chest discomfort in a patient with biventricular defibrillator. Episode of chest pain was transient and lasted only few seconds, patient described it as stabbing. Device interrogation showed unchanged sensing and capture function of all leads, cardiac enzymes were negative and echocardiogram did not reveal any evidence of pericardial effusion. Brain followed by pelvis MRI for prostate cancer constitute the majority of MRIs in patients with CIEDs. In regard to patients with implantable loop recorder, there is no need for monitoring during MRI, as the loop recorder can be interrogated and rhythm analyzed prior to MRI to assess and download any previously recorded event as artifacts may be recorded during MRI that can result in the deletion of previously recorded relevant events.

RADIATION THERAPY IN PATIENTS WITH IMPLANTED PACEMAKER OR DEFIBRILLATOR DEVICES

■ Introduction

With an aging population and increased use of pacemaker and defibrillators, the number of patients with these devices who present for radiation therapy for treatment or their cancer is increasing; high-volume radiation therapy centers, therefore, treat an increasingly large proportion of patients with implanted cardiac devices that may be impacted by radiation therapy. Modern devices have metal-oxide semiconductors, which allows for the building of smaller devices, but these may show increased susceptibility to direct damage by radiation. Damage usually occurs in the silicon and silicon oxide insulators of cardiac devices.[18]

Most common external beam radiation in clinical practice is photon-based radiation, but other types, including electrons, protons and rarely neutrons may be encountered. It is important to distinguish between Gy which is defined as the absorption of one joule of radiation energy per kilogram of matter, and MV (beam energy) which basically shows the penetrating power of radiation. Neutrons are produced at higher beam energies during photon therapy (>10 MV) and at all clinically used energies with proton therapy. Additionally, the method of delivery during proton therapy can determines the amount of secondary neutrons with higher levels with passive scattering as oppose to pencil beam scanning.

EFFECTS OF RADIATION ON CARDIAC IMPLANTABLE ELECTRONIC DEVICES WITH PHOTON THERAPY

American Association of Physics in Medicine (AAPM) published the initial guidelines regarding management of CIEDs in patients undergoing radiation therapy in 1994.[19] In that report the recommendation was based on cumulative dose delivered to the device which was set at threshold dose of 2 Gy. Patients whose devices would receive more than 2 Gy were categorized as high risk. Most of the recommendations and treatment protocols in radiation oncology literature is based on this 2 Gy threshold. With contemporary devices it appears that there is minimal association between device failure and cumulative dose delivered to the device.[20,21] Recent studies has shown that permanent damage is very rare and most reported malfunctions are recoverable resets to device memory, constituting a soft reset.

Electromagnetic interference during radiation therapy has the theoretical potential to cause inhibition of pacing due to oversensing or inappropriate ICD shock, but it does not appear to have any clinical effect. There has not been a reported case of inappropriate ICD shock or inhibition of pacing in patients undergoing radiation therapy in literature. There are different practices in high-volume centers regarding deactivation of shock therapy during magnetic radiation, but without any evidence of clinically significant oversensing due to EMI during radiation, deactivation of ICD tachy-therapy may not be necessary. There have been reports of changes in pacing thresholds due to radiation.[22]

It appears that strongest predictor of device malfunction during photon therapy radiation is beam energy. Zaremba et al. demonstrated a 5-fold increase in device malfunction during photon therapy with beam energy > 15 MV.[16] In this review the cumulative tumor dose was not associated with device malfunction. Scatter radiation can also cause reset due to neutron exposure. Scatter neutrons increase with increased photon beam energy. Conventional patient shielding options usually do not protect against neutron scatter exposure.

In a retrospective study performed at MD Anderson by Grant et al., 215 patients underwent 249 courses of radiation therapy with 6–18 MV photon, electron or Gamma Knife. The authors reported 15 cases of neutron related reset, including memory reset in 5, parameter reset requiring reprogramming in 8 and unrecoverable reset requiring CIED replacement in 2 patients. Interestingly this is the only in vivo study in the literature which reported oversensing. Three patients including one with inappropriate VT detection and one who experienced a device charge by a defibrillator that could be aborted prior to delivery, were reported.[21] Device reset in this study only occurred with neutron producing treatment (>10 MV). Device malfunction did not correlate with cumulative dose to the device.

EFFECTS OF RADIATION ON CARDIAC IMPLANTABLE ELECTRONIC DEVICES WITH PROTON THERAPY

Secondary neutrons are produced in all energies of proton therapy, and especially so with passively scattered proton therapy. The largest in vivo study addressing the issue of implantable cardiac device malfunction with proton therapy was performed at MD Anderson.[23] Gomez et al., reviewed 42 patients undergoing proton therapy. Five device reset were noted in 4 patients. All patients who had device reset were receiving passive scattering therapy to thorax and none were pacemaker dependent. Normal function were restored in all reset patients without clinical effect. The incidence of reset was 10% for all patients and 25% for patients receiving thoracic radiation.

MANAGEMENT OF PATIENTS WITH CARDIAC IMPLANTABLE ELECTRONIC DEVICES DURING RADIATION THERAPY

Traditionally cumulative radiation dose and direct exposure have been considered as the primary determinant factor of device malfunction. However, the two recent large observational studies noted above have shown that production of secondary neutrons due to high beam energy of photon therapy (>10 MV) or proton therapy is the strongest indicator of CIED malfunction in contemporary devise.[15,16] Most device malfunctions are in form of memory reset (soft reset) or parameter changes requiring reprogramming. It worth mentioning that different device vendors has diverging opinions and recommendations regarding management of CIEDs during radiation. These recommendations are not necessarily consistent with the new body of evidence in the literature. The Heart Rhythm Society has recently released a very useful document addressing the issue of CIEDs management during radiation therapy.[4]

Over the last several years high volume radiation therapy centers have presented management algorithms for patients with CIEDs undergoing radiation therapy. The algorithm used at The MD Anderson Cancer Center was established more than a decade ago and was modelled to some extend after the algorithm used at the University of Michigan.[24] The most comprehensive guideline for management of patients with CIEDs undergoing radiation was published in 2012 from the Netherlands.[25] Their guidelines were based on the assumption that the chance of device failure increases with increasing dose of radiation (cumulative absorbed dose). This assumption is based on older and smaller studies, but as noted above, two new large observational studies published in 2015 clearly demonstrated that device malfunctions are due to neutron producing radiation like high energy beam photon therapy and proton therapy.[15,16] In the Netherlands' guideline cumulative dose and pacing dependency have been combined to categorize patients into low, medium and high risk groups. A practical feature of the MD Anderson algorithm is pulse check method to minimize the frequency of visits to the device clinic during radiation therapy. If it is clinically possible, the lower rate limit is programed to be slightly faster than the reset mode and we ask the radiation therapy team to check the heart rate after each radiation fraction. Lower rate of pacing is unique to each device company and it is usually in the 65–70 bpm window. The device is programmed to a lower rate of 75 to enable the detection of a reset by checking the pulse rate, and avoiding the need for interrogations. If the detected heart rate is lower than the programed lower rate, the device can be checked promptly for damage or for documented reset. This method is very useful in a pacemaker-dependent patient, but it is not helpful if the patient's intrinsic heart rate is faster than programed lower rate limit. The technique is limited in those instances where programming the lower rate at 75 bpm results in significant increase in right ventricular pacing in a patient with depressed left ventricular systolic function. In such patients more frequent device checks may be essential.

A complete CIED evaluation should be performed prior to initiation of radiation treatment to assess if the patient is pacemaker dependent and to check battery status, sensing and capture function. Close communication between radiation oncology and device management teams is crucial. The device management team should be aware of the radiation plan, and if the patient is expected to receive neutron producing radiation like high energy beam photon therapy (>10 MV) or proton therapy. These patients should have more frequent device checks during radiation especially if they are pacemaker dependent. In general non-neutron producing radiation is preferred over neutron producing treatment in patients with CIEDs to minimize the risk of device reset especially in pacemaker

dependent patients. Other important information like absorbed radiation dose to the device and proximity of radiation field to the device should be provided to the device management team.

In MD Anderson algorithm (Figure 22-1), the initial question that needs to be addressed is the necessity of device repositioning. The only situation when device repositioning is necessary is when the CIED in its current location interferes with the required radiation dose to be administered to the tumor or lymph node. Other factors that might favor device relocation are pacemaker dependency and treatment with neutron producing radiation therapy with device in direct radiation field. The decision to reposition a CIED should be made after discussing details with the patient and radiation oncology team (Figure 22-2). Overall prognosis, underlying cardiac function and ability to tolerate the procedure should be considered. Lead extraction should be preferably avoided in view of the risk for potentially life threatening complications. Lead extenders and subcutaneous tunneling techniques are preferred over lead extraction.

At MD Anderson we manage 10–15 patients undergoing radiation therapy on a monthly basis. Device relocation is rarely needed. We almost exclusively use lead extenders to move the device to contralateral pectoral site for device repositioning. Most

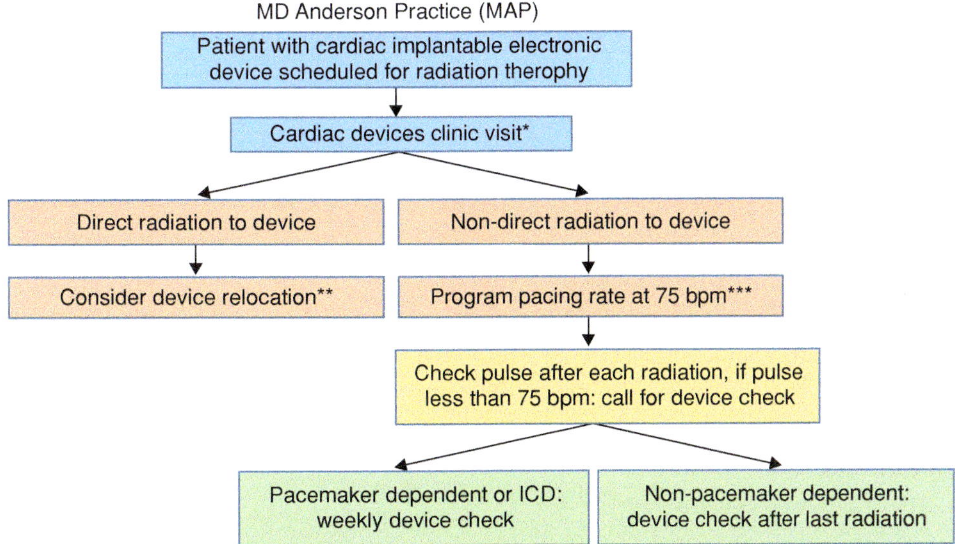

FIGURE 22-1 The MD Anderson algorithm for evaluation and management of patients with implanted electronic devices who are to receive therapeutic radiation. *Notes:* *Enrollment in remote monitoring if available; **Factors favoring relocation: pacemaker dependency, device interfering with effective radiation dose to tumor and neutron producing radiation; ***If pacing at 75 bpm not possible: (1) Pacemaker dependent, ICD and neutron producing radiation: weekly; (2) Nonpacemaker-dependent, every 2 weeks.

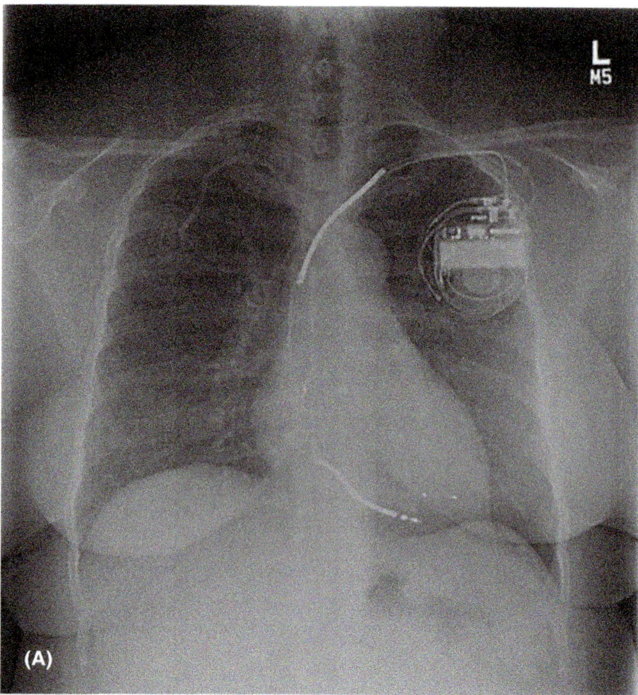

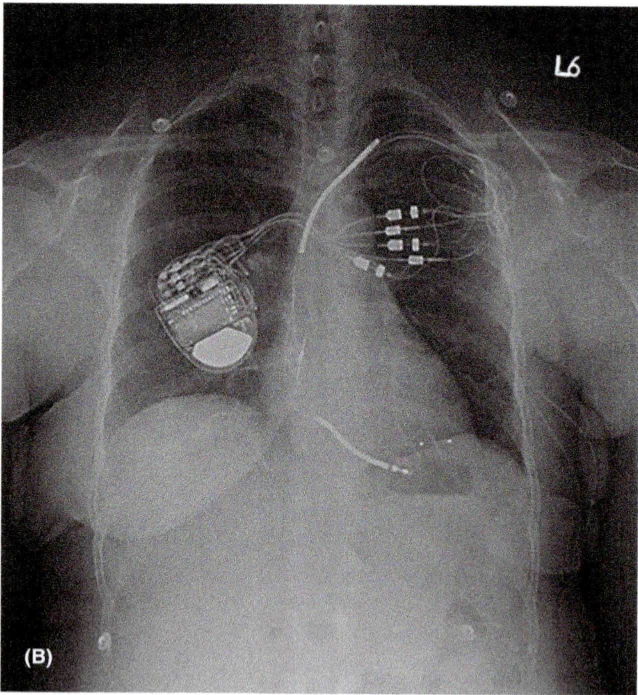

FIGURE 22-2 (A and B) Image of a patient with a bi-ventricular pacemaker initially on the left side (A) that was moved to the right side using lead extenders (B) to allow left-sided radiation for breast cancer.

of our device relocation cases were for patients with breast cancer followed by lung cancer. In patients with breast cancer we coordinate with breast surgeon to perform relocation under general anesthesia at the time of mastectomy. Figure 22-2 depicts chest X-ray images of a patient who responded to biventricular pacing with improvement in left ventricular systolic function from 25% to 45%. She subsequently was diagnosed left-sided breast cancer. The device at its initial location would have precluded the recommended radiation treatment to the tumor bed and lymph nodes. Her device was moved to the right pectoral site at the time of mastectomy using subcutaneous tunneling technique and five lead extenders.

If we determine that the device is not in the direct radiation field, we use the pulse check method (We program the pacing rate at 75 beats per minute which is a slightly faster than the reset mode for all device manufacturers). Subsequently, radiation treatment is continued and we ask the radiation therapy team to the check the heart rate after each radiation fraction. If the heart rate is less than 75 beats per minute, we immediately check the device for reset. But if the heart rate is more than 75 beats per minute after each radiation fraction, we proceed to the next treatment. Device interrogation would be performed at the completion of radiation treatment. When the pulse check method is not possible, more frequent device checks should be performed, as follows: Weekly check for pacemaker-dependent patients, ICD patients and those receiving neutron producing radiation; device check every two weeks for non-pacemaker-dependent patients. Figure 22-2 summarizes this approach.

REFERENCES

1. Kalin R, Stanton MS. Current clinical issues for MR scanning of pacemaker and defibrillator patients. *Pacing Clin Electrophysiol.* 2005;28:326–328.
2. Nazarian S, Hansford R, Roguin A, et al. A prospective evaluation of a protocol for magnetic resonance imaging of patients with implanted cardiac devices. *Ann Intern Med.* 2011;155(7):415–424.
3. Russo RJ, Costa HS, Silva PD, et al. Assessing the risks associated with MRI in patients with a pacemaker or defibrillator. *N Engl J Med.* 2017;376:755–764.
4. Indik JH, Gimbel JR, Abe H, et al. 2017 HRS expert consensus statement on magnetic resonance imaging and radiation exposure in patients with cardiovascular implantable electronic devices. *Heart Rhythm.* 2017;14(7):e97–e153.
5. Determining the Safety of MRI for Patients with Pacemakers and Implantable Cardioverter-Defibrillators. https://magnasafe.org/images/MagnaSafe_Registry_Summary_Page_7-2012.pdf. Accessed April 10, 2019.
6. Nazarian S, Hansford R, Rashsepar AA, et al. Safety of magnetic resonance imaging in patients with cardiac devices. *N Eng J Med.* 2017;377:2555–2564.

7. Luechinger R, Zeijlemaker VA, Pederson EM, et al. In vivo heating of pacemaker leads during magnetic resonance imaging. *Eur Heart J.* 2005;26:376–383.

8. Langman DA, Goldberg IB, Finn JP, et al. Pacemkaer lead tip heating in abandoned and pacemaker attached leads at 1.5 Tesla MRI. *J Magn Reson Imaging.* 2011;33:426–431.

9. Horwood L, Attili A, Luba F, et al. Magnetic resonance imaging in patients with cardiac implanted electronic devices: focus on contraindications to magnetic resonance imaging protocol. *Europace.* May 1, 2017;19:812–817.

10. Higgins JV, Gard JJ, Sheldon SH, et al. Safety and outcomes of magnetic resonance imaging in patients with abandoned pacemaker and defibrillator leads. *Pacing Clin Electrophysiol.* 2014;37:1284–1290.

11. Burk PT, Ghanbari H, Alexander PB, et al. A protocol for patients with cardiovascular implantable devices undergoing magnetic resonance imaging (MRI): should defibrillation threshold testing be performed post MRI. *J interve Card Electropysiol.* 2010;28(1):59–66.

12. Junttila MJ, Fishman JE, Lopera GA, et al. Safety of serial MRI in patients with implantable cardiac defibrillators. *Heart.* 2011;97(22):1852–1856.

13. Martin ET, Coman JA, Shellock FG, et al. Magnetic resonance imaging and cardiac safety at 1.5-Tesla. *J AM Coll Cardiol.* 2004;43(7):1315–1324.

14. Mollerus M, Albin G, Lipinski M et al. Cardiac biomarkers in patients with permanent pacemakers and defibrillators undergoing an MRI scan. *Pacing Clin Electrophysiol.* 2008;31(10):1241–1245.

15. Naehle CP, Strach K, Thomas D, et al. Magnetic resonance imaging at 1.5-T in patients with implantable cardioverter -defibrillator. *J AM Coll Cardiol.* 2009;54(6):549–555.

16. Sommer T, Naehle CP Yang A, et al. Strategy for safe performance of extra-thoracic magnetic resonance imaging at 1.5 Tesla in the presence of cardiac pacemaker in non-pacemaker dependent patients: a prospective study with 115 examinations. *Circulation.* 2006;114(12):1285–1292.

17. Gimbel JR, Kanal E. Can patients with implantable pacemakers safely undergo magnetic resonance imaging? *J Am Coll Cardiol.* 2004;43:1325–1327.

18. Baumann R, Hossain T, Murata S, Kitagawa I. Boron compounds as a dominant source of alpha particles in semiconductor devices. Paper presented at: *Reliability Physics Symposium, 33rd Annual Proceeding IEEE international,* April 4-6, 1995; Las Vegas, NV. http://irps.org/wp-content/uploads/past-conference/1990s/1995-ToC.pdf

19. Marbach JR, Sontag MR, Van Dyk J, et al. Management of radiation oncology patients with implanted cardiac pacemakers: report of AAPM task group No. 34. American association of physics in Medicine. *Med Phys.* 1994;21:85–90.

20. Brambatti M, Mathew R, Strang B, et al. Management of patients with implantable cardioverter-defibrillators and pacemakers who require radiation therapy. *Heart Rhythm.* 2015;12:2148–2154.

21. Grant JD, Jensen GL, Tang C, et al. Radiotherapy-induced malfunction in contemporary cardiovascular implantable electronic devices: clinical incidence and predictors. *JAMA Oncol.* 2015;1:624–632.

22. Zaremba T, Jakobsen AR, Sogaard M, et al. Risk of device malfunction in cancer patients with implantable cardiac devices undergoing radiotherapy: a population-based cohort study. *Pacing Clin Electrophysiol.* 2015;3:342–356.

23. Gomez DR, Poenisch F, Pinnix CC, et al. Malfunctions of implantable cardiac devices in patients receiving proton beam therapy: incidence and predictors. *Int J Radiat Oncol Biol Phys.* 2013;87:570–575.

24. Makkar A, Prisciandaro J, Agrawal S, et al. Effect of radiation therapy on permanent pacemaker and implantable cardioverter-defibrillator function. *Heart Rhythm.* 2012;9:1964–1968.

25. Hurkmans CW, Knegjens JL, Oei BS, et al. Dutch Society of Radiotherapy and Oncology (NVRO). Management of radiation oncology patients with a pacemaker or ICD: a new comprehensive practical guideline in the Netherlands. *Radiat Oncol.* 2012;7:198.

26. The University of Texas MD Anderson Cancer Center; https://www.mdanderson.org/for-physicians/clinical-tools-resources/clinical-practice-algorithms/clinical-management-algorithms.html

23 Cardiovascular Interventions for Cancer Patients

Ezequiel Muñoz ▪ *Brian Greet* ▪ *Konstantinos Marmagkiolis* ▪ *Cezar Iliescu*

INTRODUCTION

The evolution of cancer therapeutics has led to significant increases in the survival rates of those affected: cancer death rates decreased by 1.8% per year from 2002 through 2011 for men and by 1.4% per year for women. Current estimates posit that the number of people living beyond a cancer diagnosis in 2014 was 14.5 million, and that estimate is expected to increase to 19 million by the year 2024.[1] With such advances, it is also estimated that one of every 570 young adults between the ages of 20 and 30 years in the United States will be a survivor of a childhood cancer.[2] Although the armamentarium of treatment options has increased over recent years via therapeutics such as radiotherapy, chemotherapy, surgery, and immunotherapy, there has also been an increase in potential adverse reactions, because many of these agents exert untoward effects on the cardiovascular system. Such effects include accelerated epicardial disease, heart failure, stroke, and dysrhythmia.[3-5] These treatment effects, coupled with the direct complications of many cancers on the cardiovascular system, have led to the burgeoning field of cardio-oncology.

Unique issues arise when cancer patients require interventional cardiovascular procedures. Such issues include timing procedures in relation to the oncologic treatment course; addressing the wide range of comorbid diseases, including thrombocytopenia (TP) and paraneoplastic disease; difficulties with vascular access; coagulopathies; and the absence of outcome-driven data regarding interventions for these patients. Often, a combined medical and interventional approach is required for achieving the best balance of these patients' risk–benefit profile.[3]

The intent of the following chapter is to highlight the challenges posed, the tools available, and the methods used to optimize interventional cardiovascular care for cancer patients.

▪ Malignancy and Coronary Disease

Cancer patients are known to be at increased risk of coronary heart disease. Three main causes, including the hypercoagulable state of malignancies and the vascular effects of chemotherapy and radiation, have been linked.

Hypercoagulable state and coronary artery disease in cancer patients ▪ The hypercoagulable state among cancer patients depends on several clinical factors, such as the site of the primary cancer and the stage of the disease.[6] Published studies documenting the risk of thrombosis by cancer type show that pancreatic and brain malignancies have the highest risk of association with thrombotic events (Figure 23-1).[7]

Emerging data have enhanced our understanding of cancer-associated thrombosis (Figure 23-2). The mechanisms are likely to be multiple and may be directly related to the induction of thrombin generation by tumor cells and to the stimulation of prothrombic activity by normal host tissues as a secondary response to the cancer.[8] Malignancy is known to cause an up-regulation of tumor-derived cytokines, including interleukin (IL)-8 and platelet-activating factor (PAF), which trigger a torrent of downstream events. Recently, neutrophil extracellular traps (NETs), a part of the innate immune system, have been implicated in experiments as a potential cause of this procoagulable state.[9] The link between cancer, thrombosis, and NETs was first established by Demers and colleagues in 2012 and has been directly implicated in the impairment of cardiac and renal vascular function in mouse models.[9] During the process of NET formation, negatively charged chromatin and associated histones are deposited within the vasculature. These NETs then provide a scaffold and a stimulus for thrombus formation.[10] Administration of heparin and deoxyribonuclease (DNase) has been shown to promote the restoration of normal function in peripheral vessels and to dismantle NETs in tumor-bearing mice.[10]

Cancer cells may activate platelets in vitro by contact, by releasing platelet stimulators such as adenosine diphosphate (ADP) and thromboxane A2, and by generating thrombin through the activity of tumor-associated procoagulants.[8]

Cytokines such as tumor necrosis factor (TNF) and IL-1, whose production is often elevated in cancer patients, contribute to endothelial cell damage

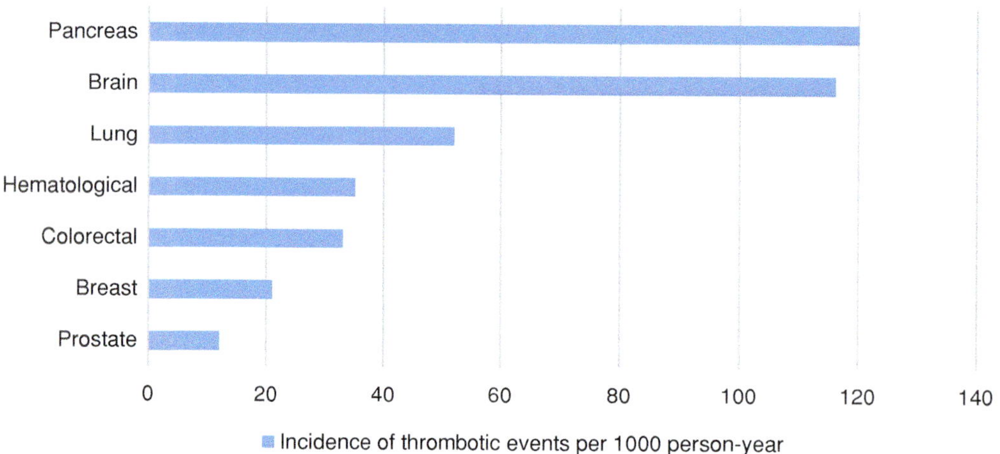

FIGURE 23-1   Incidence of thrombotic events per 1000 person-years according to cancer type.

and to the expression of E selectin, PAFs, and tissue factor.[8]

Solid tumors growing outside the blood vasculature may also increase the permeability of the microvasculature, allowing fibrinogen and other plasma-clotting proteins to leak into the extravascular space, where procoagulants associated with tumor cells or with benign stromal cells can initiate clotting and subsequent fibrin deposition.[8]

Vascular effects of chemotherapy ■ Of paramount importance to the interventional cardiologist is a knowledge of those agents that cause vascular toxicity. Vasospasm has been reported among patients being treated with pyrimidine analogues, including fluorouracil (5-FU) and capecitabine. Fluorouracil has

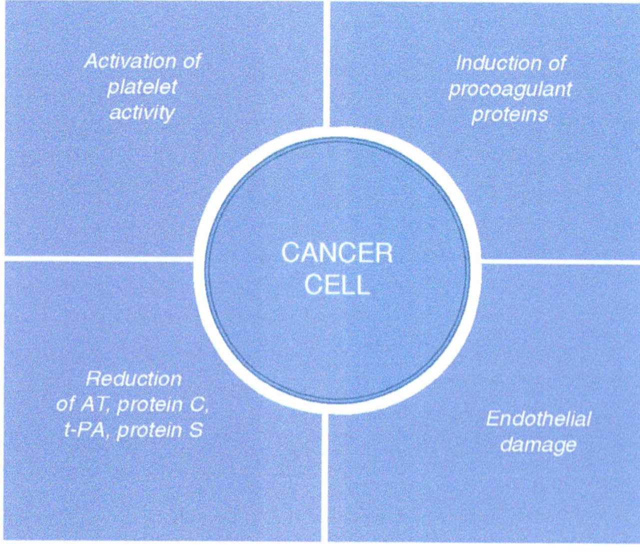

FIGURE 23-2   Procoagulant effects of cancer cells. AT, antithrombin; tPA, tissue plasminogen activator.

been shown to trigger abnormal vasoreactivity at the initiation of therapy,[11] possibly because of endothelial damage and alterations in molecular signaling pathways that control vascular smooth muscle tone.[12,13] Some studies have found that preexisting coronary disease is a risk factor for vascular toxicity; however, this condition has also been reported among patients without preexisting disease. Rarely, myocardial infarction, cardiogenic shock, and cardiac arrest have been reported to occur with an incidence of up to 2%.[13]

Recently, a large meta-analysis bound that bevacizumab, a vascular endothelial growth factor (VEGF) inhibitor, is associated with an increased incidence of ischemic heart disease. The overall incidence was 1%, which reflected a relative risk of 2.49 compared to control subjects.[14] Additional meta-analyses have also reported an association between bevacizumab and an elevated risk of arterial thrombotic events, including unstable coronary syndrome and myocardial infarction.[15,16] The postulated mechanism behind ischemic heart disease is believed to be endothelial cell–mediated VEGF depletion with induction of endothelial dysfunction and the downstream effects of vasoconstriction, inflammation, platelet activation, and vascular remodeling.

Studies evaluating sunitinib have shown that as many as 70% of patients treated with this agent experience a reduction in coronary flow reserve that appears to be related to duration of therapy.[17] In experimental animal models, sunitinib administration has led to microvascular impairment and rarefication of microvascular pericytes and capillaries.[18,19] Additionally, an abnormal vasofunctional balance may play a role in the reduction of coronary flow via endothelial nitric oxide synthase uncoupling along with an increase in the production of mitochondrial superoxide and endothelin 1.[18,20]

Sorafenib administration has been associated with coronary vasospasm in multiple vessels.[21,22] It has also been implicated in the progression of coronary artery disease, and animal models have shown that sorafenib induces myocyte necrosis.[23,24]

The tyrosine kinase inhibitors nilotinib and ponatinib have been associated with the progression of atherosclerosis and an increase in the incidence of ischemic events.[25,26] They have also been shown to involve multiple vascular territories in patients with no known coronary disease.[27–29]

A number of case reports have shown that the taxanes, including paclitaxel and docetaxel, are a rare cause of acute coronary syndrome.[30–32] Vasospasm has been implicated as the key mechanism, with underlying coronary artery disease as a likely predisposing factor.

Cisplatin has been associated with acute coronary thrombosis, at times in multiple coronary territories. It has been associated with a 1.5- to 7-fold higher long-term risk of coronary artery disease and myocardial infarction.[33–35] Often co-administered with cisplatin, both bleomycin and vinblastine can cause aggravation of endothelial dysfunction and can induce endothelial apoptosis.[36,37]

Finally, both aromatase inhibitors and androgen-deprivation therapy with gonadotropin-releasing hormone agonists have been found to increase overall cardiovascular risk.[38–41]

Vascular effects of chemotherapy agents are summarized in Table 23-1.

■ Cardiovascular Effects of Radiation Therapy

Cardiovascular effects of radiation therapy can be either nonvascular or vascular.

Nonvascular effects of radiation therapy ■ Radiation therapy, a mainstay of treatment for breast, lung, and esophageal cancers and lymphoma, was an under-recognized cause of serious cardiac disease until the mid-1990s, when its association with coronary artery disease (CAD) was fully characterized.[43] Although cardiac involvement is common at radiation doses higher than 30 Gy, the impact of lower doses of radiation is less clear.[44] Cardiac manifestations of radiation-induced injury range from occult subclinical histopathological changes to irreversible injury resulting in substantial morbidity and mortality. Overall cardiac mortality rates are higher among patients undergoing radiation therapy for Hodgkin disease or breast cancer.[45]

Both early- and late-onset pericardial disease due to radiation therapy are relatively common. The average incidence of acute pericarditis in association with thoracic irradiation has been drastically reduced to approximately less than 5% of cases at present and is most common during the first few weeks after initiation of treatment.[43] More commonly, late-onset pericarditis is usually encountered within 10 years after radiation therapy and affects as many as 20% of patients.

TABLE 23-1 Vascular effects of chemotherapy agents

CHEMOTHERAPY AGENT	VASCULAR EFFECT	INCIDENCE OF ISCHEMIA (%)[42]
5-fluorouracil	• Vasospasm • Myocardial infarction	• 1.3–4.1
Bevacizumab	• Unstable angina • Myocardial infarction • Arterial thrombosis	• 0.6–1.5
Capecitabine	• Vasospasm	• 3.0–9.0
Cisplatin	• Acute coronary thrombosis	
Docetaxel	• Vasospasm	• 1.7–5.0
GnRH agonists	• Increased cardiovascular risk	
Nilotinib	• Ischemic events • Progression of atherosclerosis	• < 2.0
Paclitaxel	• Vasospasm	• < 1.5
Ponatinib	• Ischemic events • Progression of atherosclerosis	• 13.0–53.0
Sorafenib	• Vasospasm	• 2.7–3.0
Sunitinib	• Microvascular impairment	

GnRH, gonadotropin-releasing hormone

Radiation is also known to cause fibrosis of the pericardium. Pericardial fibrosis is a process in which collagen deposition occurs within the parietal pericardium with replacement of the peripheral adipose layer. The once relatively thin adipose layer (0.5 mm) can be replaced and its thickness can increase to as much as 8 mm. These changes can result in a stiff pericardial sac that can cause a constrictive physiology. The incidence of constriction ranges from 4% to 20% and is highly dependent on radiation dosage.[43]

Myocardial fibrosis is an uncommon finding, often associated with radiation doses higher than 30 Gy. The process involves the diffuse, often patchy proliferation of bands of collagen separating and replacing normal myocytes as a result of damage to the endothelium of the myocardial blood capillaries. Findings can often be subclinical for years and are commonly detected incidentally as evidence of systolic or diastolic dysfunction on echocardiography.[44] If found, common areas of regional wall motion abnormalities include the inferior wall, although diffuse hypokinesis is often present.[43] The incidence of overt failure increases with the co-administration of anthracyclines and high-dose radiation therapy.[44]

Valvular heart disease can develop in patients undergoing radiation therapy and most often in those who received more than 30 Gy at early age, predominantly during childhood, adolescence, and early adulthood.[46] Pathologic findings include diffuse or focal leaflet fibrosis and thickening, along with calcification. The area most commonly involved is the mitral-aortic curtain.[47] Subclinical manifestation of valvular disease is often associated with an average latency of 11.5 years after radiation treatment. Symptomatic valvular disease generally appears later, with an average latency period of 16.5 years.[47]

VASCULAR EFFECTS OF RADIATION THERAPY

Radiation therapy has been associated with a twofold increase in the risk of death due to CAD among patients with Hodgkin disease or breast cancer.[48,49] The risk of fatal myocardial infarction (MI) is generally highest 5 to 10 years after initial radiation therapy. This risk is higher for patients receiving higher radiation doses, those receiving radiation at younger ages (childhood, adolescence, and early adulthood), or those with preexisting comorbid coronary disease.[44] Although its pathophysiologic mechanism is similar to that of native coronary disease and involves the accumulation of lipid-containing macrophages and the intimal proliferation of myofibroblasts, the plaques associated with radiation-associated coronary disease are more fibrous than those associated with native coronary disease. Endothelial cells are highly susceptible to the effects of ionizing radiation, and experimental models have shown that both cholesterol plaques and thromboses can form within days after radiation exposure.[50,51] In addition, luminal obstruction and loss of capillaries are frequently found in patients who have been treated with radiation therapy.[43]

As many as 20% of patients treated with radiation therapy for Hodgkin lymphoma will experience severe stenosis of the ostium (Figure 23-3) of the left main or the right coronary system 2 or more decades later, and some of these diagnoses are missed with conventional

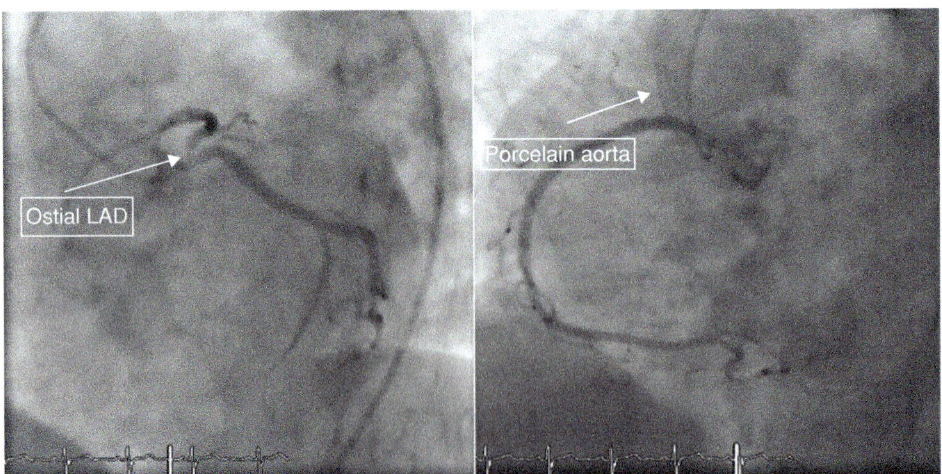

FIGURE 23-3 A 64-year-old woman who underwent excision of a spinal tumor at the age of 14 and was subsequently treated with radiation therapy to this area was evaluated for invasive mammary carcinoma 50 years later before the initiation of cancer therapy. An elective coronary angiogram (left) shows the ostial left anterior descending (LAD) artery. Fluoroscopy (right) shows the porcelain aorta.

stress testing.[51,52] Coronary disease has been found as early as 5 years after treatment in breast cancer survivors treated with radiation therapy for left-sided cancers.[53] Also unique to radiation-induced coronary disease is its predilection for the left main coronary artery and the proximal segment of the right coronary artery.[46]

Head and neck tumors that require treatment with radiation therapy have been found be associated with an increased risk of ischemic stroke and carotid arterial disease (Figure 23-4).[54–57] Case series have supported the use of carotid artery stenting to treat patients with this type of radiation-induced disease.[58–60] Supraclavicular and mediastinal irradiation has been associated with both carotid artery disease and subclavian stenosis, as supported by a retrospective study involving Hodgkin lymphoma patients. The prevalence of carotid artery disease, subclavian artery disease, or both was 7.4% at 17 years after radiation therapy.[61]

Although reported less frequently, peripheral artery disease (PAD) is a concern for those undergoing radiation therapy for a variety of extracardiac malignancies.[62–64] The mechanism of radiation-induced vascular injury is believed to be similar to that of coronary vascular injury. Very few data are available regarding the use of percutaneous intervention in such cases.

SCREENING CANCER PATIENTS FOR CARDIOVASCULAR DISEASE

Compared to the general population, oncology patients are a unique population with different prevalence and incidence rates of cardiovascular disease. It is therefore difficult to generalize earlier screening studies involving these patients. Thus, various medical societies have formulated recommendations for the proper screening of oncology patients, as highlighted in Table 23-2. Nonetheless, the best time to initiate surveillance is unclear, and no consensus yet exists.

Ideally, patients should undergo a baseline cardiovascular assessment before the initiation of oncologic therapy. However, such an assessment is often not feasible for a multitude of reasons.

The Children's Oncology Group recommends that all children who were treated with either radiation therapy or anthracycline undergo an annual history and physical examination. Noninvasive surveillance with either electrocardiography (ECG) or multi-gated acquisition (MUGA) imaging are recommended once the survivor enters long-term follow-up (usually 2 years after completion of therapy) and is repeated at a frequency ranging from 1 to 5 years as determined by the patient's age at first treatment and the dose of anthracycline administered. In addition, patients treated either with 40 Gy of radiation therapy or with 30 Gy of radiation therapy plus anthracyclines concomitantly should undergo a stress test 5 to 10 years after completing radiation therapy.[65]

The International Late Effects of Childhood Cancer Guideline from the Harmonization Group differs from these recommendations in that it does not base screening intervals on the patient's age at initiation of therapy. Surveillance is recommended for those treated with a cumulative dose of more than 250 mg/m^2 of anthracyclines and is considered reasonable for those treated with more than 100 mg/m^2 but less than 250 mg/m^2 of anthracycline. Surveillance is also recommended for

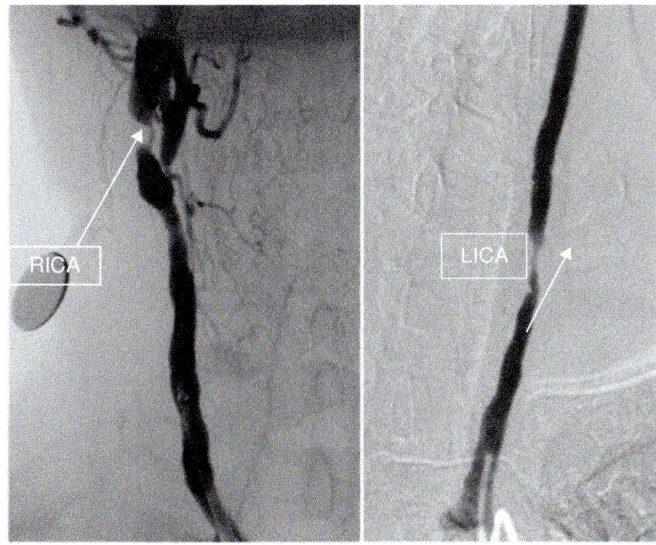

FIGURE 23-4 Bilateral (right internal carotid artery [RICA] and left internal carotid artery [LICA]) radiation-induced carotid stenosis in a patient with thyroid cancer, as demonstrated by angiograms.

TABLE 23-2 Recommendations for cardiovascular screening of cancer patients. LVEF, left ventricular ejection fraction

SOCIETY	CONDITIONS			SCREENING FREQUENCY FOR NONINVASIVE IMAGING	RECOMMENDED TEST(S)
The Children's Oncology Group[65]	Initiation of combined radiotherapy and anthracycline therapy beginning when the patient is less than 5 years old			Every year	Annual history and physical examination Initiate 2 years after completion of therapy: Electrocardiography **and** Echocardiography (preferred for those who have been treated with radiation) **or** Multi-gated acquisition (MUGA) imaging
	Anthracycline without irradiation			Every year	
	Age at first dose	Total dose (mg/m^2)			
	< 1 year	≥ 200			
	1–4 years	≥ 300			
	> 5 years				
	Age at first dose	Total dose (mg/m^2)		Every 2 years	
	< 1 year	< 200			
	1–4 years	≥ 100 to < 300			
	> 5 years	≥ 200 to < 300			
	Age at first dose	Dose (mg/m^2)		Every 5 years	
	1–4 years	< 100			
	> 5 years	< 200			
International Guideline Harmonization Group for Late Effects of Childhood Cancer[66]	Children and adolescents treated with anthracyclines or radiotherapy			Initiate 2 years after completion of cardiotoxic therapy and continue every 5 years thereafter	History and physical examination Echocardiography (first choice) Cardiac magnetic resonance imaging (alternative) Radionuclide angiography (second alternative)
	Survivors treated with a combination of chest irradiation and anthracyclines				
	Female survivors of childhood cancer who have asymptomatic cardiomyopathy			During pregnancy and delivery	

SOCIETY	CONDITIONS	SCREENING FREQUENCY FOR NONINVASIVE IMAGING	RECOMMENDED TEST(S)
The American Society of Echocardiography and the European Association of Cardiovascular Imaging[67]	During and after therapy, screen patients with the following: • A high risk for development of drug-induced cardiomyopathy (decrease in LVEF of 10 percentage points or more, to a value < 53%) • Risk factors for cardiovascular disease • Known left ventricular dysfunction • > 65 years of age • Treatment with high doses of anthracyclines (> 350 mg/m^2) or combination chemotherapy with anthracyclines and other drugs		History and physical examination Electrocardiography Echocardiography
Society for Cardiovascular Angiography and Interventions (SCAI) Expert Consensus Statement[3]	**Prechemotherapy cardioprotection:** • Patients with coronary artery disease may benefit from prophylactic treatment with beta blockers, angiotensin antagonists, statins, or dexrazoxane[69] • For patients with a history of hypertension, blood pressure should be managed with angiotensin-converting enzyme 1 (ACE1) and beta blockers (especially carvedilol or nebivolol) • Patients with intermediate to high cardiovascular risk (based on cardiovascular risk scores) who are undergoing cardiotoxic therapy should be referred to a cardiologist or a cardio-oncologist before treatment initiation • For patients with established coronary artery disease (CAD), adding or continuing beta blockers may be beneficial[70] • For detecting high-risk patients, screening via echocardiographic studies and cardiac biomarkers is encouraged **Chemoprotection before irradiation** • The use of aspirin and statins should be encouraged for oncologic patients with coronary artery disease, if these drugs can be tolerated*. • Patients with head and neck malignancies or lymphoma who are being treated with supraclavicular irradiation because of their increased risk of cerebrovascular events should undergo carotid artery screening • Stress testing is advised for long-term surveillance of radiation-induced heart disease, but coronary angiography may be preferable		

*Some oncology patients may be taking hepatotoxic agents and may exhibit an increased risk of bleeding or impairment of liver function.

those treated with 35 Gy or more of radiation therapy and is considered reasonable for those treated with more than 15 Gy but less than 35 Gy. In addition, patients who were treated with the combination of 15 Gy or more of radiation and 100 mg/m^2 or more of anthracycline therapy should also undergo surveillance. This surveillance process should start 2 years after completion of therapy and should be repeated every 5 years; more frequent surveillance is reasonable for high-risk survivors. The preferred modality of surveillance, in addition to history and physical examination, is echocardiography, followed by cardiac magnetic resonance imaging (MRI) and, finally, by radionuclide angiography.[66]

The American Society of Echocardiography (ASE) and the European Association of Cardiovascular Imaging (EACI) have also published a consensus document with recommendations for imaging studies for adult patients during and after cancer therapy. Their guidelines include baseline screening (history, physical examination, ECG, and echocardiography) for those at high risk, defined as those with established or risk factors for cardiovascular disease, those with left ventricular (LV) dysfunction, and those who are older than 65 years. Those who are treated with more than 240 mg/m² of anthracycline should undergo left ventricular function assessment before each subsequent cycle of therapy. All patients treated with anthracyclines should undergo imaging once at the end of therapy and again 6 months after its completion. Patients treated with trastuzumab should undergo echocardiography every 3 months during therapy. If a patient's LV function falls below 53%, if global longitudinal strain decreases beyond the lower limits of normal, or if a test for troponins is positive during or near the time of administration of therapy, consultation with a cardiologist is recommended, primarily so that both the oncologist and the cardiologist can reevaluate the risk/benefit ratio of continuing chemotherapy. Patients whose echocardiography results have not changed at 6 months after treatment should undergo annual evaluations, with initiation of repetition of imaging as clinically necessary. The guideline statement also recommends cardiac MRI for those whose echocardiography results are suboptimal.[67]

In a separate document, the ASE and the EACI released an expert consensus on multimodality imaging for those who have undergone radiotherapy. Recommendations include a yearly targeted clinical history and physical examination, along with screening with echocardiography for high-risk asymptomatic patients 5 years after exposure and for all other patients 10 years after exposure. High-risk patients are defined as those who underwent therapy at a young age (childhood, adolescence, and early adulthood), those with cardiovascular risk factors or preexisting cardiovascular disease, those exposed to high doses of radiation (> 30 Gy), those treated concomitantly with chemotherapy, and those who underwent anterior or left chest irradiation without shielding. After that initial screening, all patients should undergo noninvasive imaging studies every 5 years. Additionally, the group recommends noninvasive stress testing 5 to 10 years after therapy for high-risk patients. For patients who may have pericardial constriction, cardiac MRI is suggested for additional diagnostic purposes.[68]

In its consensus statement on cardiac catheterization for cardio-oncology patients, the Society for Cardiovascular Angiography and Interventions (SCAI) also released recommendations about screening of patients undergoing chemotherapy or radiotherapy. For those undergoing chemotherapy with the potential for vasotoxicity, a yearly history and physical examination is recommended. The recommendations for patients without symptoms are coronary computed tomography angiography (CCTA) and carotid ultrasonography every 5 years and ankle brachial index testing annually if they have been treated with therapies that pose a persistent vascular risk. Patients with symptoms of coronary disease should undergo coronary angiography, and those who have indications of symptomatic cerebrovascular disease should undergo carotid ultrasonography with or without carotid magnetic resonance angiography and cerebral MRI. Patients with symptomatic PAD disease should undergo CCTA with distal run-off.[3]

If patients are undergoing mediastinal or thoracic irradiation, SCAI recommends screening thoracic echocardiography for those with at least one risk factor for radiation-induced heart disease; those with no such risk factors should undergo this screening test every 10 years. Risk factors for radiation-induced heart disease are age less than 15 years or more than 60 years at initiation of radiotherapy, anterior or left chest wall irradiation, tumor in or next to the heart, lack of shielding, high-dose radiotherapy fraction of more than 2 Gy per day or a cumulative dose of more than 30 Gy, concomitant chemotherapy, any cardiovascular risk factor, and preexisting CAD. In addition, patients should undergo a screening exercise echocardiography stress test or CCTA every 5 years, with earlier evaluation at 2 years for patients older than 60 years and those with one or more cardiovascular risk factors or known CAD. Patients who have undergone radiation therapy and may have pericardial effusion or restriction, valvular heart disease, or cardiomyopathy should undergo transthoracic echocardiography with hemodynamic catheterization as necessary. Patients with arrhythmia should undergo ECG and either Holter monitor testing or event monitoring. Finally, patients who may have CAD should undergo coronary angiography. Those who are being considered for cardiothoracic surgery should undergo gated chest CT for detecting mediastinal fibrosis, porcelain aorta, or patency of the internal mammary arteries.[3]

CHEMOTHERAPY CARDIOPROTECTION

Continuous doxorubicin infusion (48–72 hr), liposomal doxorubicin administration, and dexrazoxane administration have been shown to help limit the cardiotoxicity of anthracyclines. The antitumor properties of anthracyclines have been shown to be caused by an area-under-the-curve (AUC) effect as opposed to a peak plasma level. Compared with continuous administration, bolus delivery of anthracyclines has been shown to result in a higher anthracycline concentration within the heart but with a similar AUC effect. As such, it has been shown that the efficacy of continuous infusion of anthracyclines is similar to that of bolus dosing but is associated with a lower incidence of cardiotoxicity. Liposomal doxorubicin works by restricting administration to the inside of vessel walls of organs with tight capillary junctions, thus reducing overall toxicity. Dexrazoxane works by changing the configuration of topoisomerase 2β and preventing anthracyclines from binding to the topoisomerase 2β complex.[71-73]

The efficacy of prophylaxis with angiotensin-converting enzyme (ACE) inhibitors, angiotensin receptor blockers, and beta blockers in the primary prevention of anthracycline toxicity has been evaluated in randomized controlled trials. Most of these trials have shown promising results, blunting overall reductions in left ventricular ejection fraction (LVEF) over time. These studies, however, are generally limited by their lack of long-term follow-up.[70,74,75]

Studies using beta blockers and ACE inhibitors for secondary prevention of anthracycline toxicity in high-risk patients have yielded promising results, showing a decrease in the decline of LVEF. Results were better when therapy was initiated earlier.[76,77]

CARDIOPROTECTION BEFORE IRRADIATION

For patients with elevated cardiovascular risk or with known cardiac disease, therapy should be initiated according to current American Heart Association/American College of Cardiology (AHA/ACC) guidelines.[3]

■ Preoperative Evaluation of Oncology Patients with Coronary Disease

Providing operative care for patients with an oncologic diagnosis is a common requirement for cardiologists. Proper risk stratification and perioperative management are important facets of care in avoiding perioperative and postoperative cardiac complications.

The 2014 ACC/AHA guidelines for the perioperative management of patients undergoing noncardiac surgery recommend an algorithmic approach. For those undergoing nonemergent surgery who do not have acute coronary syndrome but do have a serious valvular abnormality, active arrhythmia, or decompensated heart failure, the risk of perioperative cardiac events should be quantified to determine whether any risk exceeds 1%. The ACC/AHA emphasizes 3 potential means of quantifying this risk.[78]

The Revised Cardiac Risk Index (RCRI) is a validated and accepted tool for assessing the perioperative risk of major cardiac complications (myocardial infarction, pulmonary edema, ventricular fibrillation or primary cardiac arrest, and complete heart block).[79] Components of the score are shown in Figure 23-5.

The American College of Surgeons National Surgical Quality Improvement Program (ACS-NSQIP) has developed 2 newer tools. The patients included in each of these cohorts were treated at more than 525 participating hospitals in the United States, and the data were gathered from more than 1 million surgical procedures. The first of these tools is the Myocardial Infarction and Cardiac Arrest (MICA) risk prediction rule, created in 2011.[80] Unlike the RCRI, the MICA tool considers the specific surgical procedure being undertaken. Outcomes are also defined slightly differently than in the RCRI: e.g., cardiac arrest is defined as *chaotic cardiac rhythm* requiring the initiation of basic or advanced life support, and MI is defined as at least one of the following: documented ECG findings of MI, ST elevation of at least 1 mm in more than 1 contiguous lead, new left bundle-branch block, new Q wave in at least 2 contiguous leads, or a serum troponin level more than 3 times normal if ischemia is suspected. The use of a validation cohort in this trial suggests that the predictive value of the MICA score is better than that of the traditional RCRI scoring system.[81]

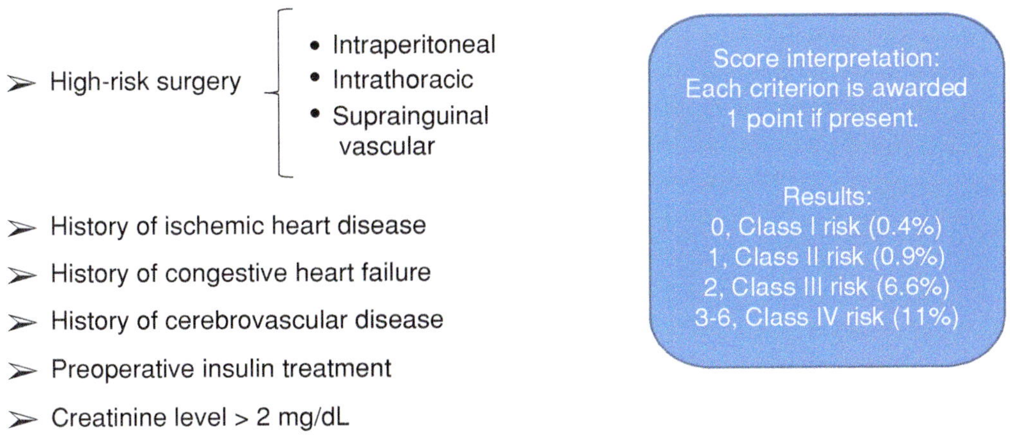

FIGURE 23-5 The Revised Cardiac Risk Index (RCRI) score.

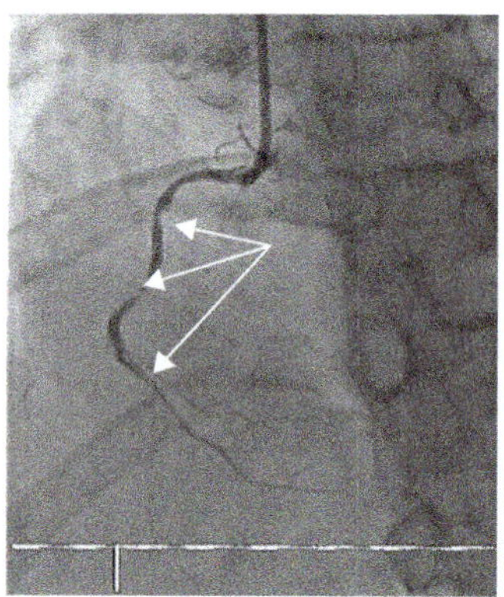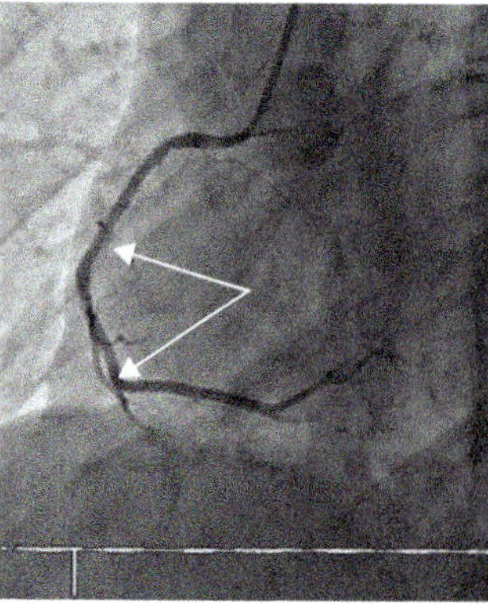

FIGURE 23-6 Coronary angiogram of a 64-year-old woman with a history of chronic lymphocytic leukemia and idiopathic thrombocytopenia purpura who had undergone treatment with FCR (fludarabine, cyclophosphamide, rituximab) that was currently in remission and who presented with cardiac arrest. The image shows diffuse disease throughout the right coronary artery (RCA), and the patient underwent successful RCA stenting.

The ACS-NSQIP surgical risk calculator is another validated approach for quantifying risk preoperatively.[82] The calculator includes 21 patient-specific variables (e.g., age, sex, body mass index) and provides risk stratification for events such as major adverse cardiovascular events (MACE), death, and 8 additional outcomes.[83]

Once risk stratification has been performed and baseline functional status has been assessed, if further cardiac evaluation is warranted, a staged approach is suggested by the most recent SCAI guidelines. These guidelines recommend initial assessment of coronary anatomy (invasive coronary angiography or CCTA) and physiology (stress test, cardiac positron emission tomography [PET], and fractional flow reserve [FFR] testing), followed by an interdisciplinary plan that best balances the patient's risks and benefits for preoperative intervention and the patient's upcoming surgery.[3]

Determining the optimal timing for elective surgery is more difficult when patients have recently undergone percutaneous coronary intervention (PCI), particularly the placement of a drug-eluting stent (DES). The risk of postoperative MI and death is substantially elevated for patients treated with a stent who subsequently stop taking dual antiplatelet therapy at the time of the procedure. For patients treated with a bare metal stent (BMS), it may be safe to stop administration of one of the antiplatelet agents 4 to 6 weeks after stent implantation, but dual antiplatelet therapy (DAPT) must be continued for at least 3 to 6 months (preferably 1 year) for those treated with a DES, even if surgery is performed. Additional risk stratification for determining when antiplatelet therapy should be

stopped is possible with optical coherence tomography (OCT) (see below).

CANCER PATIENTS WITH STABLE ANGINA

Patients with stable angina and an oncologic diagnosis should be treated with goal-directed medical therapy for initial treatment, because no survival advantage has yet been demonstrated for PCI.[84] If patients' anginal symptoms progress despite optimal goal-directed therapy, the severity of cardiac disease, the stage of the malignancy, and the condition of the patient should dictate whether PCI or coronary artery bypass grafting (CABG) is a reasonable option for palliation of chest pain. PCI is generally preferable to CABG for patients with aggressive malignancy or widespread disease, whereas CABG can be considered for patients with a potential cure or a good overall prognosis (see discussion of PCI and CABG below).

■ Cancer Patients with Acute Coronary Syndrome

Cancer patients with acute coronary syndrome are a heterogeneous group with a wide spectrum of clinical variables. Tailoring treatment and balancing risk will not only ensure that patients who will benefit most receive appropriate treatment but will also avoid potentially hazardous treatment for those with a good prognosis.

Acute coronary syndrome constitutes multiple clinical presentations that are compatible with acute myocardial ischemia, including unstable angina (UA), non–ST-elevation myocardial infarction (NSTEMI), and ST-elevation myocardial infarction (STEMI). In the spectrum of acute coronary syndrome, the ACS, the ACC, and the AHA have defined UA/NSTEMI by ECG ST-segment depression or by prominent T-wave inversion or the presence of biomarkers of necrosis (e.g., troponin) in the absence of ST-segment elevation and in the appropriate clinical setting (chest discomfort or anginal equivalent).[85]

Acute coronary syndrome, and more specifically STEMI, carries a higher mortality rate for patients with an oncologic diagnosis than for those without such a diagnosis (Figure 23-6). In particular, the mortality rate is 3-fold higher for patients with a malignancy diagnosed within 6 months of STEMI who undergo PCI than for those with a malignancy diagnosed more than 6 months ago. This higher mortality rate could be explained by the presence of anemia, a very common condition among cancer patients.[86] Anemia is known to predict cardiovascular death and heart failure among patients with STEMI because of the increased myocardial oxygen demand associated with the increased stroke volume and tachycardia that are necessary for maintaining adequate systemic delivery of oxygen.[87]

Cancer is a known predictor of stent thrombosis because of the development of a hypercoagulable state.[88] This condition is a treatment challenge because antithrombotic therapy and vascular access increase the risk of bleeding, which may worsen the anemia exhibited by many of these patients, thus increasing the risk of heart failure. Nonetheless, antithrombotic treatment is essential for avoiding the ischemic complications associated with hypercoagulability.[86]

A multicenter study by Velders and colleagues studied the outcomes of 208 patients with cancer who experienced STEMI that was treated with PCI. The authors recommended placing a bare-metal stent (BMS) or an everolimus-eluting stent (because of a faster endothelization rate) to decrease the risk of stent thrombosis.[86]

The National Heart, Lung, and Blood Institute (NHLBI) acute coronary syndrome registry yielded similar findings: cancer was one of the strongest independent predictors of in-hospital death and 1-year mortality.[89]

One of the largest single-center studies to date involved 456 cancer patients presenting with either STEMI or NSTEMI. Only 3.3% of these patients underwent PCI. The most common presenting symptoms were dyspnea (44%), chest pain (30.3%), and hypotension (23%). Medical management varied greatly: 46% were treated with aspirin, 48% with beta blockers, and 21% with statins. The administration of either aspirin or beta blockers was an independent predictor of improved survival rates. Those who underwent PCI exhibited a trend toward increased survival rates. Overall, however, the 1-year survival rate was only 26%. Selection bias was probably a confounding variable in this analysis given the likelihood that patients whose condition is clinically more stable and who have a better prognosis will receive more-aggressive care.[90]

Conservative versus early invasive strategy ■ Conservative treatment involves intense medical management followed by noninvasive tests for determining which patients may require coronary angiography. Intense medical management includes bed rest, oxygen, opiate analgesics for pain relief, and antiischemic and antiplatelet or antithrombotic drugs. In the general population, the use of aspirin, beta blockers, statins, and coronary revascularization improves the outcome of patients with acute MI. Similar results have been observed among patients with cancer.[42]

Patients with either UA or NSTEMI with 3 or more high-risk features (Box 23-1) for adverse outcomes

may derive the greatest benefit from an early invasive approach[91] that has been adapted for cancer patients at the University of Texas MD Anderson Cancer Center (UTMDACC): the modified Thrombosis in Myocardial Infarction (TIMI) score.

If patients present with acute myocardial infarction, placement of an intra-aortic balloon pump (IABP) should be performed for cardiogenic shock; for hemodynamic support during catheterization, angioplasty, or both; before high-risk surgical procedures; for mechanical complications of MI; or for refractory UA after MI.[42]

A proposed schema for interventional management of acute coronary syndrome management in cancer patients is shown in Figure 23-7.

Cancer patients who present to an emergency center with symptoms compatible with a diagnosis of acute coronary syndrome should be fully treated according to the ACC/AHA Practice Guidelines. The diagnosis of cancer should not be an important contraindication to treatment.[42]

ENDOVASCULAR TREATMENT OF CANCER PATIENTS WITH THROMBOCYTOPENIA

Thrombocytopenia is a common problem among cancer patients; as many as 10% to 25% of cancer patients with solid tumors have platelet counts lower than 100,000/mL.[92] Baseline TP increases the risk of bleeding and of other adverse cardiac events.[93] Among oncology patients, TP has been associated with an increased propensity for thrombus formation, and

---

BOX 23-1 High-risk features that should lead to consideration of an early invasive approach for cancer patients with acute coronary syndrome

High-risk features

- Age > 70 years

- Elevated troponin levels

- ST segment changes

- Thrombosis In Myocardial Infarction score ≥ 3

- Known coronary artery disease

- Sustained ventricular tachycardia

- Depressed left ventricular function (ejection fraction < 40)

- Previous percutaneous coronary intervention

- Previous coronary artery bypass grafting

- History of previous chest irradiation

- Known prothrombotic chemotherapy

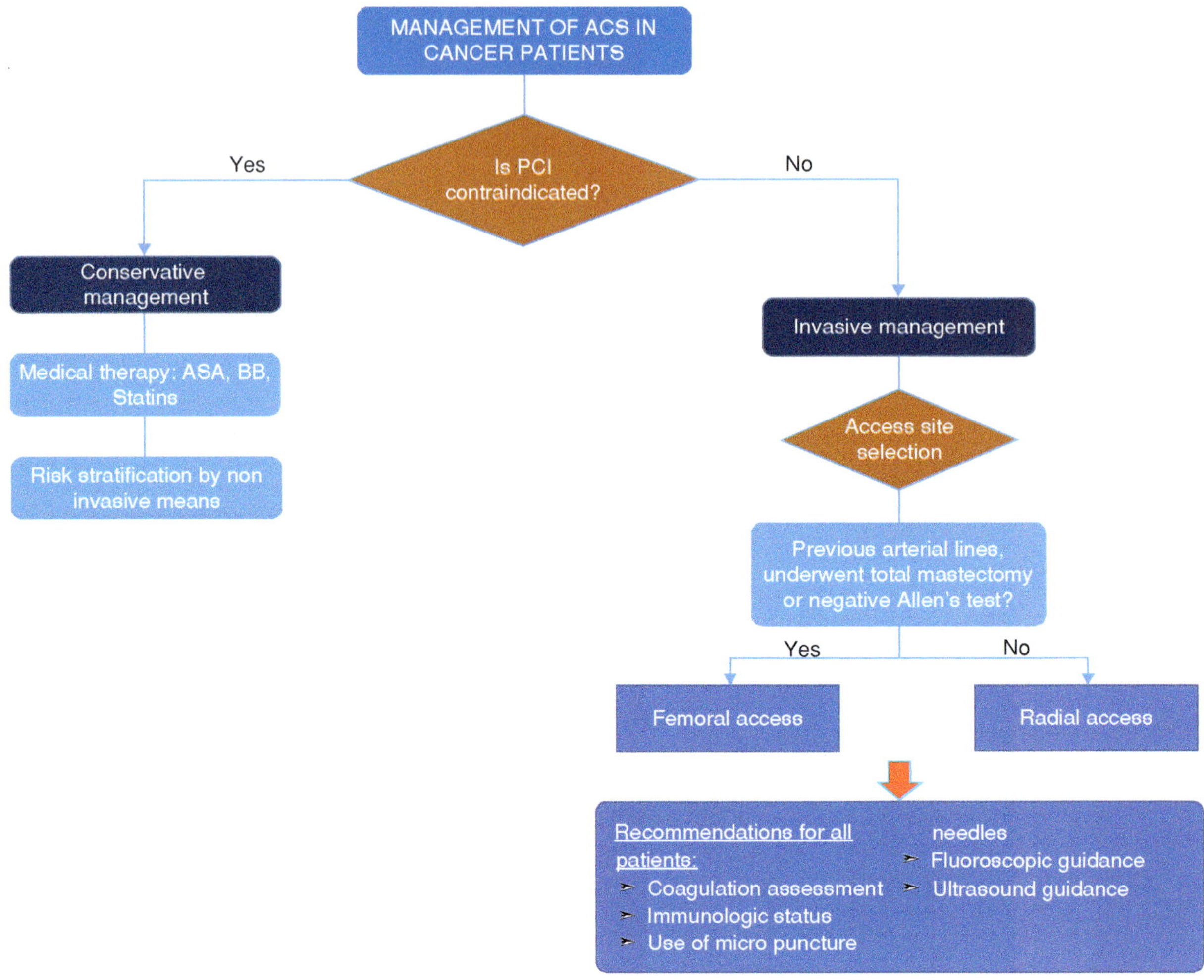

FIGURE 23-7 Management of acute coronary syndrome in cancer patients: percutaneous coronary intervention. ACS, acute coronary syndrome; ASA, acetylsalicylic acid; BB, beta blocker; PCI, percutaneous coronary intervention.

platelet function rather than count may be the determining factor.[94]

The cause of thrombosis among cancer patients with TP is multifactorial.[95] One potential pathway involves the induction of megakaryocytopoiesis. Odell and coworkers[96] studied the stimulation of megakaryocytopoiesis by acute TP and found large platelets in the circulation within 12 hours after the induction of TP; nearly half of all platelets were large by 18 hours after the induction of TP.[96] Mean platelet volumes are substantially elevated among patients with acute MI and stroke despite a decrease in the overall platelet count.[97,98] Other mechanisms of thrombosis in the setting of TP include the involvement of microparticles derived from platelets upon activation of the coagulation cascade. Elevated platelet microparticle levels have been found in patients with idiopathic thrombocytopenic purpura (ITP) and acute coronary syndrome in the context of a low platelet count.[99]

The recommended revascularization approach for patients with TP is shown in Figure 23-8. Prophylactic platelet transfusion is not indicated if the platelet count is higher than 10,000/mL; however, transfusions at higher levels may be necessary for patients with fever, hyperleukocytosis, a rapid decrease in platelet count, or coagulation abnormalities.[95] For patients with solid tumors who are undergoing treatment for bladder, gynecologic, or colorectal tumors or melanoma; for those with necrotic tumors, a higher platelet threshold of 20,000/mL may be necessary. Responsiveness should be assessed shortly after transfusion by follow-up platelet counts, and histocompatible platelets must be available for alloimmunized patients.

If patients do not respond to 2 ABO-compatible transfusions of platelet concentrates stored for less than 72 hours, the suspicion for alloimmune-refractory TP should be high. In such a case, platelets should be selected from donors who are HLA-A and HLA-B matched.

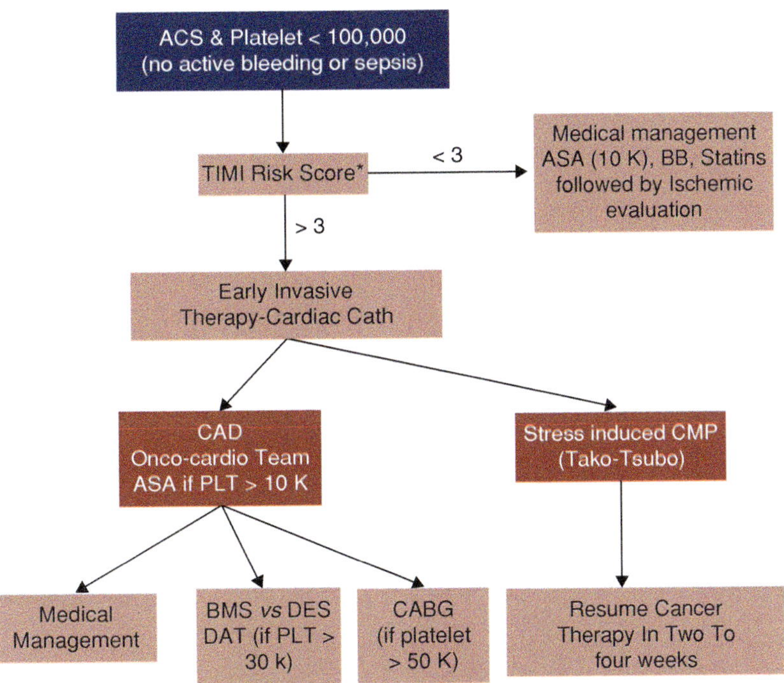

FIGURE 23-8 Recommended revascularization approach for patients with thrombocytopenia at the University of Texas MD Anderson Cancer Center. ACS, acute coronary syndrome; ASA, acetylsalicylic acid; BB, beta blocker; BMS, bare-metal stent; CABG, coronary artery bypass grafting; CAD, coronary artery disease; CMP, cardiomyopathy; DAPT, dual antiplatelet therapy; DES, drug-eluting stent; PLT, platelets; TIMI, Thrombolysis in Myocardial Infarction score.

Current available clinical experience and conference consensus documents do not specify a minimal platelet level that poses an absolute contraindication to coronary angiography.[100] Additionally, most interventional procedures may be performed if patients have a platelet count of 40,000 to 50,000/mL in the absence of comorbid coagulation abnormalities.[3]

Aspirin therapy has been shown to be of benefit even for patients with TP.[85] A case series of cancer patients with TP who were undergoing PCI found that bleeding is minimal with the use of meticulous access technique, micropuncture, and careful hemostasis.[95,101] According to SCAI guidelines and the revascularization approach taken at the UTMDACC, all acute coronary syndrome patients with platelet counts higher than 10,000/mL are treated with aspirin; treatment with PCI is an option for those with platelet counts higher than 30,000/mL, PCI is a potential option; and CABG is an additional option for those with platelet counts higher than 50,000/mL. Patients are given an initial dose of 30 to 50 U/kg of heparin when platelet counts are lower than 50,000/mL, and additional heparin is administered if the activated clotting time (ACT) is lower than 250 seconds. Patients with platelet counts higher than 50,000/mL are given a standard dose of either 50 to 70 U/kg of heparin or bivalirudin. Clopidogrel is the $P2Y_{12}$

inhibitor of choice for these patients as long as platelet counts are higher than 30,000/mL. If platelet counts are lower than 50,000/mL, the duration of DAPT may be restricted to 2 weeks after balloon angioplasty alone, 4 weeks after BMS placement, and 6 months after placement of a second- or third-generation DES if optimal stent expansion is confirmed by intravascular ultrasonography (IVUS) or OCT. Therapeutic platelet transfusions are recommended for patients with TP in whom bleeding develops during or after cardiac catheterization.[3]

Although few data are available for cancer patients, thromboelastography (TEG) testing should be considered for patients with CAD and platelet counts lower than 30,000/mL. The results of such testing may assist in clinical decision making with regard to platelet transfusion and the use of DAPT. Such data have been extrapolated from other patient populations, namely cardiovascular and liver transplant patients.[85,102]

VASCULAR ACCESS CONSIDERATIONS

One of the most common causes of morbidity and mortality associated with cardiac catheterization is related to vascular access. Vascular access and its potential for bleeding complications is a subject of great importance, especially in the care of patients with cancer.[103] All patients should be fully assessed, with an evaluation of coagulation and immunologic status before a procedure is performed so that potential complications can be avoided. Ultrasound guidance, micropuncture needles, and fluoroscopic guidance help to minimize procedure-related complications.[104,105]

Table 23-3 compares the 2 main access sites for cardiac catheterization.[3,106–111]

■ Fractional Flow Reserve, Intravascular Ultrasonography, and Optical Coherence Tomography for Cancer Patients

Because coronary angiography provides only a 2-dimensional image, it is an imperfect tool for accurately evaluating left main coronary artery (LMCA) stenosis. For cancer patients, treatment delays of 2 to 4 weeks may substantially affect patient survival. FFR and IVUS have considerably improved diagnostic accuracy for CAD and are frequently used to gauge the severity of LMCA disease in the general population. The measurement of functional importance of a given lesion is essential because the absence of inducible myocardial ischemia is associated with excellent outcomes after medical treatment.[112]

Fractional flow reserve–guided percutaneous coronary intervention ■ In the general population, a FFR of 0.80 or lower is more than 90% accurate in indicating hemodynamically significant stenosis. In the Fractional Flow Reserve versus Angiography for Multivessel Evaluation 2 (FAME 2) study, De Bruyne and colleagues[113] examined the clinical outcomes of patients with CAD treated with optimal medical therapy alone and those treated with both PCI and optimal medical therapy. Patients with hemodynamically significant stenosis were included in the study and were randomly assigned to one of the 2 groups. Results showed that patients treated with both PCI and optimal medical therapy had a better prognosis, lower rates of urgent revascularization, and a lower risk of death and MI than did patients treated with optimal medical therapy alone. In contrast with the Clinical Outcomes Utilizing Revascularization and Aggressive Drug Evaluation (COURAGE) trial, the FAME 2 study demonstrated that FFR-guided PCI is important in the treatment of ischemic coronary disease and can help guide coronary revascularization.[114] A meta-analysis[115] of 19 studies that used FFR levels to guide treatment of ischemic coronary disease provided further validation by suggesting that it is safe to defer treatment of patients with normal FFR and those being treated for abnormal FFR levels.

Intravascular ultrasonography ■ Because of its advantages in spatial resolution and imaging of the vascular wall, IVUS is superior to angiography in determining the severity of lesions and allows better characterization of luminal processes than does conventional angiography (Figure 23-9).[116] Additionally, it allows

TABLE 23-3 Considerations for vascular access

	FEMORAL ACCESS SITE	RADIAL ACCESS SITE
Recommendations/ Advantages	Patients who have abnormal results on an Allen test, who have had multiple previous arterial lines, and who have undergone total mastectomy	Lower risk of bleeding and increased patient satisfaction Preferred access site if the patient is a candidate for both radial and femoral access
Complications/Disadvantages	Associated with a higher risk of bleeding Puncture outside the middle of the common femoral artery may lead to retroperitoneal hemorrhage, pseudoaneurysm, arteriovenous fistula, thrombosis, or extensive bleeding	Technical difficulty and increased risk of radiation exposure
Special considerations	Vascular closure devices do not seem to result in less bleeding than manual compression but do increase the risk of local infections and delayed epithelization Femoral angiography recommended for identifying potential access complications after transfemoral access	

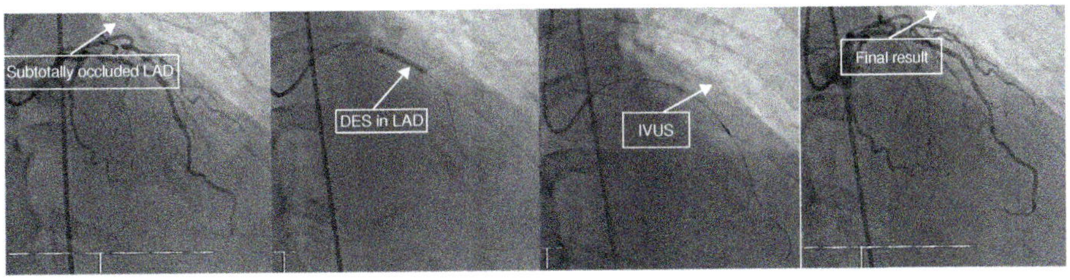

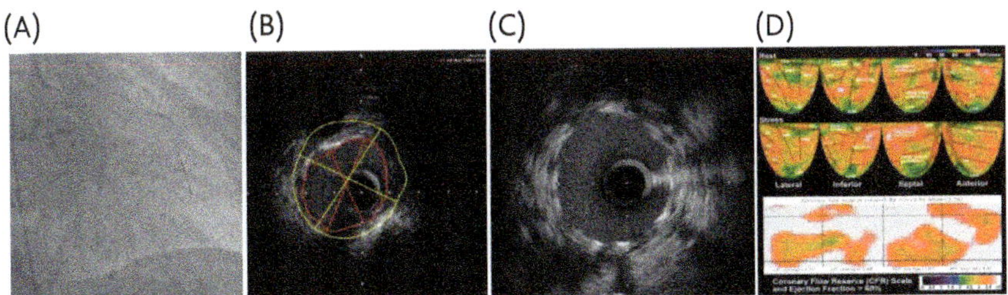

FIGURE 23-9   Intravenous ultrasound (IVUS)-guided placement of a stent in a patient with hematological malignancy and chronic thrombocytopenia for non–ST-elevation myocardial infarction. DES, drug-eluting stent; LAD, left anterior descending (artery).

FIGURE 23-10   A 45-year-old man with metastatic malignant melanoma underwent video-assisted thoracoscopic lobectomy of the right lower lobe. Flash pulmonary edema and non–ST-elevation myocardial infarction with left main disease; diagnosis was facilitated by angiogram (A). Intravascular ultrasound images confirmed severe ostial left main disease (B). Six months after successful placement of a drug-eluting stent (C), a follow-up cardiac positron emission tomography scan (D) showed normal flow in the left anterior descending artery and the circumflex territory with a mild nontransmural scar at the apex and normal ejection fraction (60%).

earlier detection of procedure-related complications and suboptimal stent expansion.[117,118]

Multiple studies have demonstrated that IVUS-guided stent placement may decrease restenosis rates and reduce the incidence of adverse clinical outcomes after implantation of a BMS.[119,120] Jang and coworkers[117] published the results of a meta-analysis of studies investigating the use of IVUS in placing a DES and concluded that, compared with angiography-guided PCI, IVUS-guided DES implantation decreases the incidence of serious cardiac events, stent thrombosis, and target lesion revascularization. IVUS has also been shown to be helpful in detecting stent underexpansion, malpositioning, incomplete lesion coverage, and residual plaque.[117]

IVUS-derived minimal lumen area (MLA) is an anatomical metric used to evaluate the severity of CAD. Nascimento and colleagues[121] performed a meta-analysis to determine whether this anatomical metric could serve as a surrogate for the functional evaluation provided by FFR. They found that, compared to FFR, a cross-sectional measurement of MLA by IVUS may be slightly more suitable in helping to defer revascularization but is not useful for recommending revascularization. This meta-analysis was limited, however, by substantial heterogeneity among the included trials.

■ The Experience at the University of Texas MD Anderson Cancer Center with Fractional Flow Reserve and Intravascular Ultrasonography for Left Main Disease

Researchers at UTMDACC have analyzed the data obtained from a series of cancer patients who underwent coronary angiography because of acute coronary syndrome or abnormal results on cardiovascular stress tests. Among patients with clinically significant angiographic disease of the LMCA (> 50% stenosis), as determined by quantitative coronary angiography (QCA), either FFR or IVUS was performed. Revascularization was performed if the FFR value was higher than 0.75 or if IVUS detected an absolute cross-sectional area larger than 7 mm^2 for symptomatic disease or larger than 6 mm^2 for asymptomatic disease. When these IVUS and FFR cut-off values were used, interventions were deferred for 50% of patients, and cancer therapy was resumed without interruption. All patients in the deferred intervention group were able to complete cancer treatment without clinically significant cardiac events at a follow-up of up to 6 months.

For cancer patients with concomitant left main (LM) disease (Figure 23-10), assessment of severity solely on the basis of coronary angiography results is suboptimal. Further evaluation with IVUS and FFR can detect a subgroup of patients for whom intervention can be safely deferred. This approach facilitates cancer treatment and reduces the duration of hospital stay and the overall costs of medical care.

Optical coherence tomography ■ OCT is a novel imaging technique that uses an optical analogue of ultrasound (infrared light emission) to provide cross-sectional images of tissue at a resolution of 10 to 20 μm or more. It can be used to evaluate the coronary arteries for diagnostic purposes (Figure 23-11).[122] Because it yields high-resolution images, it enables the differentiation of the various layers of the coronary arterial vessel wall and accurate classification of tissue characteristics. Such characteristics include the identification of fibrous areas that are homogeneous and signal-rich, fibro-calcified areas that are signal-poor with well-defined borders, and lipid-rich areas that are signal-poor with diffuse borders.[123]

Compared to IVUS and coronary angiography, OCT has the advantages of better plaque characterization and lower interobserver variability in luminal dimensions and intimal thickness.[122] Likewise, OCT can identify lipid-rich plaque and thin-cap fibroatheroma, which account for more than 80% of clinically relevant plaque ruptures.

Given its high accuracy and reproducibility, OCT has been the modality of choice for stent analysis in the assessment of strut apposition to the luminal wall.[124] Reports of discrepancies between OCT and IVUS in stent assessment indicate that OCT shows a smaller luminal area but a larger in-stent tissue coverage area than IVUS.[125]

OCT is very useful for cancer patients when discontinuation of antiplatelet therapy is necessary in the perioperative or periprocedural period. OCT findings can support management decisions by detecting a subgroup of patients with adequate strut apposition and endothelialization. Such findings support a decrease in the risk of acute in-stent thrombosis and help guide temporary discontinuation of antiplatelet therapy.[126]

■ Procedural and Postprocedural Considerations for Cancer Patients Undergoing Percutaneous Coronary Intervention

Performing PCI for patients with an oncologic diagnosis requires balancing lesion characteristics, cancer stage, and therapy, with the understanding that cancer is a prothrombotic and proinflammatory state associated with an elevated risk of stent thrombosis and, potentially, of in-stent restenosis. BMS or the newer-generation DES are the preferred agents for revascularization. Bifurcating lesions and overlapping stents, given their elevated risk of stent thrombosis (ST), should be avoided if possible. Noncompliant high-pressure (> 16 atm) balloons should be used in conjunction with IVUS or OCT to ensure apposition, adequate stent expansion, and avoidance of edge dissection. The experience with OCT at UTMDACC has demonstrated that incomplete stent coverage or apposition, underexpansion of the stent, and in-stent restenosis are common problems among cancer patients and may lead to an increased number of adverse events.[3] Dual antiplatelet agents have recently been shown to be beneficial when administered for more than 1 year; however, this finding has not been validated in cancer patients.[127]

For all patients undergoing PCI, an ACT of more than 250 sec should be maintained throughout the

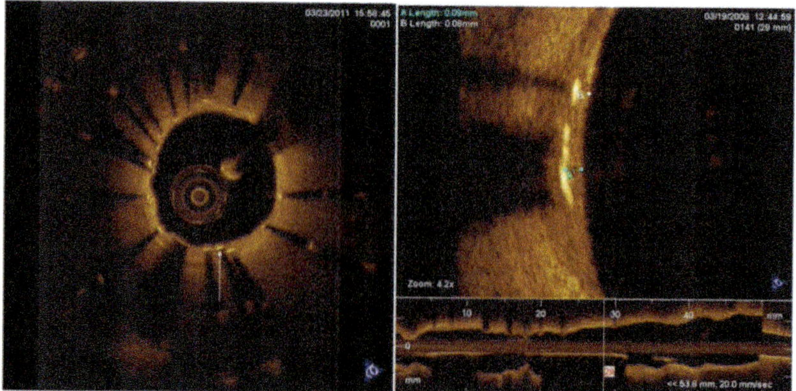

FIGURE 23-11 Optical coherence tomography images of everolimus-coated drug-eluting stents showing neointimal coverage at 1 month after placement. Dual antiplatelet therapy was discontinued so that cancer therapy could be administered.

procedure.[124] For patients with severe TP (platelet count < 50,000/mL), lower doses of unfractionated heparin (30–50 U/kg) may achieve a therapeutic ACT.[128]

For patients who require urgent surgery, balloon angioplasty without stenting or BMS placement is preferred as the best method for limiting the interruption of DAPT.

Endothelialization among patients undergoing chemotherapy may be delayed and impaired; therefore, patients being treated with such agents may benefit from an extension of DAPT.[129] Therapeutic agents such as thalidomide and cisplatinum are known to be prothrombotic and therefore may increase the risk of clots if DAPT administration is stopped. If patients require urgent surgical procedures, the administration of at least one antiplatelet agent should be continued if possible.

Comorbid gastrointestinal and digestive tract tumors can also cause substantial problems for patients being treated with DAPT. Coronary disease has been found to be an independent predictor of advanced colon cancer.[130,131] Bleeding is a known risk for patients with gastrointestinal malignancy and those for whom cessation of antiplatelet therapy has been necessary, because these patients have exhibited an elevated incidence of cardiac complications after PCI.[132] Balloon angioplasty with delayed stenting after recovery from cancer surgery may be a viable alternative, but its use has not yet been well validated.[129]

CORONARY ARTERY BYPASS GRAFTING

CABG is a viable approach for revascularization. An added advantage of CABG for cancer patients is that no prolonged antiplatelet therapy is necessary; thus, CABG reduces the risk of bleeding risk for these patients, who have a predisposition for bleeding.[129] CABG has been performed along with tumor resection as either a simultaneous or a 2-stage procedure. This technique reduces hospitalization stays and costs and avoids repeat thoracotomy, complications, and delays in further treatment for malignancy.[134-135]

Hemodynamic assessment of lesion severity by FFR or cardiac PET could limit the number of bypass grafts necessary and thus decrease the on-pump time or allow an off-pump procedure (left internal mammary artery [LIMA] to left anterior descending [LAD] artery), thereby decreasing the recovery time and the rate of procedural complications and allowing earlier resumption of cancer therapy.

Cancer patients with radiation-induced fibrosis of the chest wall and vasculature may experience impaired wound healing postoperatively.[136]

■ Pericardiocentesis

Pericardiocentesis is often recommended for cancer patients for both palliative and diagnostic purposes.

TP is a frequent comorbid condition among patients undergoing pericardiocentesis. With careful technique and the use of procedures such as micropuncture, the risks of pericardiocentesis can be substantially reduced. A study performed at UTMDACC involved 212 cancer patients who underwent pericardiocentesis. The results showed a low overall complication rate with no significant differences in outcomes between patients with or without TP.[137]

An algorithm for pericardiocentesis in the setting of TP has been developed at UTMDACC. The initial decision is predicated on the urgency of the procedure. If time permits, TEG can be useful in guiding the management of blood products. Either echocardiography or chest CT can assist in the determination of the best approach for accessing the pericardial fluid. If the effusion is more than 8 cm away from the subxiphoid space, or if clinically substantial hepatomegaly is present, a transapical or lateral approach is preferred (Figure 23-12).

Once pericardiocentesis has been performed, El Haddad and coworkers[137] recommend catheter drainage for 3 to 5 days.

Surgical approaches, such as pericardial window, pericardioperitoneal shunt, and pericardiectomy, are associated with the highest success rates for drainage, ranging from 87% to 100%, with low complication and mortality rates.[138,139] The overall success rate for percutaneous pericardiocentesis alone, with or without catheter drainage, is 60%, but the complication rate (8%) is higher than that for a surgical approach (1%–2%).[139]

BALLOON PERICARDIOTOMY

Malignant effusions are known to be an independent risk factor for later reaccumulation of an effusion, which is reported to occur in 36% to 62% of cases.[140,141] Balloon pericardiotomy allows the creation of a pericardial window by balloon inflation. This procedure has the advantage of being fast, simple, and effective in preventing recurrence.[142] A subxiphoid approach is standard. A dilating balloon containing 30% of radiographic contrast is advanced over the guide wire into the pericardial border and is manually inflated to create a window.[143] After the procedure, echocardiography and chest radiography are recommended for assessing the possible reaccumulation of pericardial fluid or iatrogenic left pleural effusion. This technique is being adopted by some centers as the initial approach to malignant pericardial effusions.[3,142]

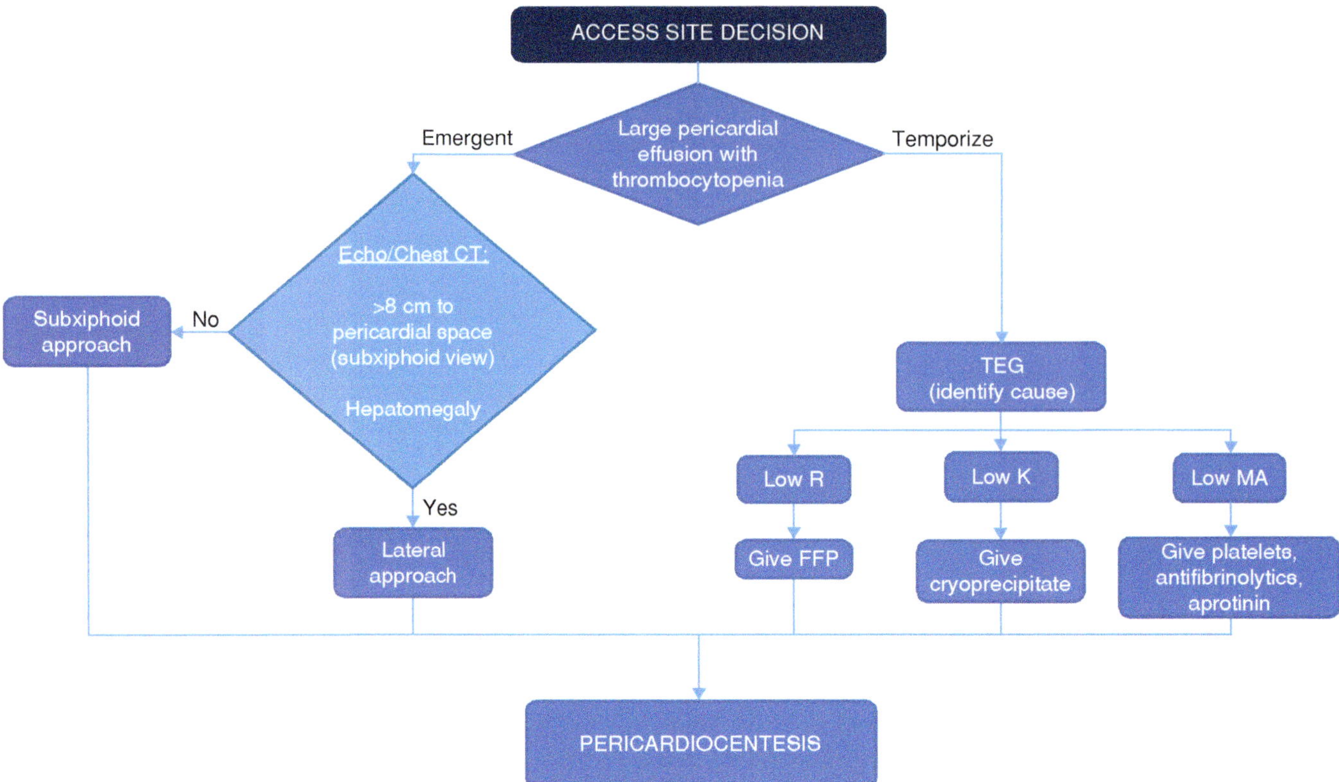

FIGURE 23-12 Access site decision algorithm for pericardiocentesis in patients with thrombocytopenia. CT, computed tomography; echo, echocardiography; FFP, fresh frozen plasma; K, clot formation time; MA, maximal amplitude; R, reaction time; TEG, thromboelastography.

ENDOMYOCARDIAL BIOPSY

The AHA/ACC guidelines name 14 clinical scenarios for which diagnostic endomyocardial biopsy (EMB) is indicated. Many of these scenarios affect cancer patients (Box 23-2, Clinical Scenarios for Which the AHA/ACC Guidelines Recommend Endomyocardial Biopsy).[144]

Multiple studies have shown a complication rate of less than 2%. Such complications are cardiac tamponade, pneumothorax, atrial fibrillation, and ventricular arrhythmia.[145,146] Although the mortality rate associated with EMB is largely related to the risk of perforation, this risk is very low.[146]

The risks of EMB depend on the clinical condition of the patient, the experience of the operator, and the availability of expertise in cardiac pathology.[147] Five to ten 2-mm samples must be taken from one region of the right ventricular septum. In general, at least 4 or 5 samples are submitted for light microscopic examination, and more may be submitted for transmission electron microscopy in the context of suspected anthracycline cardiotoxicity.[148,149]

Transmission electron microscopy may also be helpful in assessing suspected infiltrative disorders such as amyloidosis, glycogen storage diseases, lysosomal storage diseases, and, occasionally, viral myocarditis.[147] One or more samples may be frozen for molecular studies, immunofluorescence analysis, or immunohistochemical testing.[147]

The use of fluoroscopy in combination with guidance by transthoracic echocardiography, transesophageal echocardiography, or intracardiac echocardiography may result in samples of better quality, the use of lower amounts of radiation, and earlier detection of complications.[147]

BALLON AORTIC VALVULOPLASTY AND TRANSCATHETER AORTIC VALVE IMPLANTATION

Aortic stenosis in cancer patients portends a worsened survival rate in those left unrepaired, as demonstrated by Yusuf and coworkers[150] Valvular disease, specifically aortic stenosis, is therefore of great concern for oncology patients, especially those who are older. The incidence of aortic stenosis increases dramatically with patients' age: its incidence ranges from 2% to 7% for those older than 65 years to more than 15% for those older than 90.[151,152]

BOX 23-2   Clinical Scenarios for Which the AHA/ACC Guidelines Recommend Endomyocardial Biopsy

- New-onset heart failure of less than 2 weeks' duration associated with a normal-sized or a dilated left ventricle and hemodynamic compromise
- New-onset heart failure of 2 weeks' to 3 months' duration associated with a dilated left ventricle and new ventricular arrhythmias, second- or third-degree heart block, or failure to respond to usual care within 1 to 2 weeks
- Heart failure of more than 3 months' duration associated with a dilated left ventricle and new ventricular arrhythmias, second- or third-degree heart block, or failure to respond to usual care within 1 to 2 weeks
- Heart failure associated with a dilated cardiomyopathy of any duration associated with suspected allergic reaction, eosinophilia, or both
- Heart failure associated with suspected anthracycline cardiomyopathy
- Heart failure associated with unexplained restrictive cardiomyopathy
- Suspected cardiac tumors
- Unexplained cardiomyopathy in children
- New-onset heart failure of 2 weeks' to 3 months' duration associated with a dilated left ventricle, without new ventricular arrhythmias or second- or third-degree heart block, that responds to usual care within 1 to 2 weeks
- Heart failure of more than 3 months' duration associated with a dilated left ventricle, without new ventricular arrhythmias or second- or third-degree heart block, that responds to usual care within 1 to 2 weeks
- Heart failure associated with unexplained hypertrophic cardiomyopathy
- Suspected arrhythmogenic right ventricular dysplasia or cardiomyopathy
- Unexplained ventricular arrhythmias
- Unexplained atrial fibrillation

Various therapeutic options exist for aortic stenosis, such as balloon aortic valvuloplasty, surgical aortic valve replacement (SAVR), and transcatheter aortic valve replacement (TAVR). SAVR is considered the current treatment of choice for patients with severe symptomatic aortic stenosis (AS), regardless of age. The surgical risk for elderly patients with multiple comorbid conditions, however, can be very high. Cancer patients with severe AS are commonly excluded from surgical procedures, perhaps because of the prohibitive anatomy (mediastinal fibrosis, severe lung disease, porcelain aorta, scar tissue from previous surgical procedures).[153]

Balloon aortic valvuloplasty (BAV) is considered a palliative option for patients with increased perioperative risk, those who require an urgent noncardiac surgery (such as oncology patients), and those who will undergo open heart surgery and are in a hemodynamically unstable condition.[154] However, the effects of BAV are transient, usually lasting from 3 to 6 months.

TAVR may be a viable option for cancer patients with acceptable prognoses and severely symptomatic AS.[3] However, because data regarding the use of TAVR for cancer patients are currently unavailable, cancer patients are excluded from most TAVR programs.[155]

CONCLUSIONS

Cancer patients can experience additional comorbid conditions caused by previous therapy. These conditions should be considered when treatment is provided.

For patients undergoing concomitant cardiovascular disease and cancer treatment, the decisional therapeutic process is more complex and should include all of the teams involved in their care (oncology, internal medicine, emergency medicine, critical care, surgery, radiology).

For patients free of cancer or those battling the disease, multiple available interventional tools could provide the additional information and treatment that are necessary for to increasing cardiovascular and overall survival.

REFERENCES

1. Kohler BA, Sherman RL, Howlader N, et al. Annual report to the nation on the status of cancer, 1975-2011, featuring incidence of breast cancer subtypes by race/ethnicity, poverty, and state. *J Natl Cancer Inst.* 2015;107(6):djv048.

2. Aziz NM, Oeffinger KC, Brooks S, Turoff AJ. Comprehensive long-term follow-up programs for pediatric cancer survivors. *Cancer.* 2006;107(4):841–848.

3. Iliescu CA, Grines CL, Herrmann J, et al. SCAI Expert consensus statement: evaluation, management, and special considerations of cardio-oncology patients in the cardiac catheterization laboratory (endorsed by the Cardiological Society of india, and Sociedad Latinoamericana de Cardiología Intervencionista). *Catheter Cardiovasc Interv.* 2016;87(5):E202–223.

4. Putt M, Hahn VS, Januzzi JL, et al. Longitudinal changes in multiple biomarkers are associated with cardiotoxicity in breast cancer patients treated with doxorubicin, taxanes, and trastuzumab. *Clin Chem.* 2015;61(9):1164–1172.

5. Raschi E, Vasina V, Ursino MG, Boriani G, Martoni A, De Ponti F. Anticancer drugs and cardiotoxicity: Insights and perspectives in the era of targeted therapy. *Pharmacol Ther.* 2010;125(2):196–218.

6. Falanga A, Marchetti M, Russo L. The mechanisms of cancer-associated thrombosis. *Thromb Res.* 2015;135(suppl 1):S8–S11.

7. Wilhelm M. Risk of venous thromboembolism in patients with cancer treated with cisplatin: a systematic review and meta-analysis [German]. *Strahlenther Onkol.* 2013;189(8):704–705.

8. Blann AD, Dunmore S. Arterial and venous thrombosis in cancer patients. *Cardiol Res Pract.* 2011;2011:394740.

9. Demers M, Krause DS, Schatzberg D, et al. Cancers predispose neutrophils to release extracellular DNA traps that contribute to cancer-associated thrombosis. *Proc Natl Acad Sci USA.* 2012;109(32):13076–13081.

10. Fuchs TA, Brill A, Duerschmied D, et al. Extracellular DNA traps promote thrombosis. *Proc Natl Acad Sci USA.* 2010;107(36):15880–15885.

11. Südhoff T, Enderle MD, Pahlke M, et al. 5-Fluorouracil induces arterial vasocontractions. *Ann Oncol.* 2004;15(4):661–664.

12. Stewart T, Pavlakis N, Ward M. Cardiotoxicity with 5-fluorouracil and capecitabine: more than just vasospastic angina. *Intern Med J.* 2010;40(4):303–307.

13. Polk A, Vistisen K, Vaage-Nilsen M, Nielsen DL. A systematic review of the pathophysiology of 5-fluorouracil-induced cardiotoxicity. *BMC Pharmacol Toxicol.* 2014;15:47.

14. Chen XL, Lei YH, Liu CF, et al. Angiogenesis inhibitor bevacizumab increases the risk of ischemic heart disease associated with chemotherapy: a meta-analysis. *PLOS ONE.* 2013;8(6):e66721.

15. Schutz FA, Je Y, Azzi GR, Nguyen PL, Choueiri TK. Bevacizumab increases the risk of arterial ischemia: a large study in cancer patients with a focus on different subgroup outcomes. *Ann Oncol.* 2011;22(6):1404–1412.

16. Ranpura V, Hapani S, Chuang J, Wu S. Risk of cardiac ischemia and arterial thromboembolic events with the angiogenesis inhibitor bevacizumab in cancer patients: a meta-analysis of randomized controlled trials. *Acta Oncol.* 2010;49(3):287–297.

17. Sen F, Yildiz I, Basaran M, et al. Impaired coronary flow reserve in metastatic cancer patients treated with sunitinib. *J BUON.* 2013;18(3):775–781.

18. Kappers MH, van Esch JH, Sluiter W, Sleijfer S, Danser AH, van den Meiracker AH. Hypertension induced by the tyrosine kinase inhibitor sunitinib is associated with increased circulating endothelin-1 levels. *Hypertension.* 2010;56(4):675–681.

19. Chintalgattu V, Rees ML, Culver JC, et al. Coronary microvascular pericytes are the cellular target of sunitinib malate-induced cardiotoxicity. *Sci Transl Med.* 2013;5(187):187ra69.

20. Winnik S, Lohmann C, Siciliani G, et al. Systemic VEGF inhibition accelerates experimental atherosclerosis and disrupts endothelial homeostasis—implications for cardiovascular safety. *Int J Cardiol.* 2013;168(3):2453–2461.

21. Porto I, Leo A, Miele L, Pompili M, Landolfi R, Crea F. A case of variant angina in a patient under chronic treatment with sorafenib. *Nat Rev Clin Oncol.* 2010;7(8):476–480.

22. Naib T, Steingart RM, Chen CL. Sorafenib-associated multivessel coronary artery vasospasm. *Herz.* 2011;36(4):348–351.

23. Pantaleo MA, Mandrioli A, Saponara M, et al. Development of coronary artery stenosis in a patient with metastatic renal cell carcinoma treated with sorafenib. *BMC Cancer.* 2012;12:231.

24. Duran JM, Makarewich CA, Trappanese D, et al. Sorafenib cardiotoxicity increases mortality after myocardial infarction. *Circ Res.* 2014;114(11):1700–1712.

25. Aichberger KJ, Herndlhofer S, Schernthaner GH, et al. Progressive peripheral arterial occlusive disease and other vascular events during nilotinib therapy in CML. *Am J Hematol.* 2011;86(7):533–539.

26. Quintás-Cardama A, Kantarjian H, Cortes J. Nilotinib-associated vascular events. *Clin Lymphoma Myeloma Leuk.* 2012;12(5):337–340.

27. Tefferi A. Nilotinib treatment-associated accelerated atherosclerosis: when is the risk justified? *Leukemia.* 2013;27(9):1939–1940.

28. Coon EA, Zalewski NL, Hoffman EM, Tefferi A, Flemming KD. Nilotinib treatment-associated cerebrovascular disease and stroke. *Am J Hematol.* 2013;88(6):534–535.

29. Tefferi A, Letendre L. Nilotinib treatment-associated peripheral artery disease and sudden death: yet another reason to stick to imatinib as

front-line therapy for chronic myelogenous leukemia. *Am J Hematol*. 2011;86(7):610–611.

30. Schrader C, Keussen C, Bewig B, von Freier A, Lins M. Symptoms and signs of an acute myocardial ischemia caused by chemotherapy with Paclitaxel (Taxol) in a patient with metastatic ovarian carcinoma. *Eur J Med Res*. 2005;10(11):498–501.

31. Esber C, Breathett K, Sachak T, Moore S, Lilly SM. Acute myocardial infarction in patient with triple negative breast cancer after paclitaxel infusion: a case report. *Cardiol Res*. 2014;5(3,4):108–111.

32. Rawal G, Yadav S, Kumar R. Paclitaxel induced acute ST elevation myocardial infarction: a rare case report. *J Clin Diagnos Res*. JDCR.. 2016;10(10):xd01–xd02.

33. Berliner S, Rahima M, Sidi Y, et al. Acute coronary events following cisplatin-based chemotherapy. *Cancer Invest*. 1990;8(6):583–586.

34. Jafri M, Protheroe A. Cisplatin-associated thrombosis. *Anticancer Drugs*. 2008;19(9):927–929.

35. Karabay KO, Yildiz O, Aytekin V. Multiple coronary thrombi with cisplatin. *J Invasive Cardiol*. 2014;26(2): E18–E20.

36. Gallagher H, Carroll WM, Dowd M, Rochev Y. The effects of vinblastine on endothelial cells. *Endothelium*. 2008;15(1):9–15.

37. Stefenelli T, Kuzmits R, Ulrich W, Glogar D. Acute vascular toxicity after combination chemotherapy with cisplatin, vinblastine, and bleomycin for testicular cancer. *Eur Heart J*. 1988;9(5):552–556.

38. Amir E, Seruga B, Niraula S, Carlsson L, Ocaña A. Toxicity of adjuvant endocrine therapy in postmenopausal breast cancer patients: a systematic review and meta-analysis. *J Natl Cancer Inst*. 2011;103(17): 1299–1309.

39. Nanda A, Chen MH, Braccioforte MH, Moran BJ, D'Amico AV. Hormonal therapy use for prostate cancer and mortality in men with coronary artery disease-induced congestive heart failure or myocardial infarction. *JAMA*. 2009;302(8):866–873.

40. Nguyen PL, Chen MH, Goldhaber SZ, et al. Coronary revascularization and mortality in men with congestive heart failure or prior myocardial infarction who receive androgen deprivation. *Cancer*. 2011;117(2):406–413.

41. Parekh A, Chen MH, Graham P, et al. Role of androgen deprivation therapy in early salvage radiation among patients with prostate-specific antigen level of 0.5 or less. *Clin Genitourin Cancer*. 2015;13(1):e1–e6.

42. Iliescu C, Iliescu G, Marmagkiolis K. Myocardial ischemia and acute coronary syndrome in cancer patients. In: Plana JC, Lopez Fernandez T, Gomez de Diego JJ, Garcia Fernancez MA, Pinto FJ, eds. *Cardio-Oncology–Theory Book + Case Study Book*. Madrid: CTO Editorial, S.L.; 2015.

43. Heidenreich PA, Kapoor JR. Radiation induced heart disease: systemic disorders in heart disease. *Heart*. 2009;95(3):252–258.

44. Darby SC, Cutter DJ, Boerma M, et al. Radiation-related heart disease: current knowledge and future prospects. *Int J Radiat Oncol Biol Phys*. 2010;76(3):656–665.

45. Carver JR, Shapiro CL, Ng A, et al. ASCO Cancer Survivorship Expert Panel. American Society of Clinical Oncology clinical evidence review on the ongoing care of adult cancer survivors: cardiac and pulmonary late effects. *J Clin Oncol*. 2007;25(25):3991–4008.

46. Glanzmann C, Kaufmann P, Jenni R, Hess OM, Huguenin P. Cardiac risk after mediastinal irradiation for Hodgkin's disease. *Radiother Oncol*. 1998; 46(1):51–62.

47. Gujral DM, Lloyd G, Bhattacharyya S. Radiation-induced valvular heart disease. *Heart*. 2016;102(4):269–276.

48. Hancock SL, Tucker MA, Hoppe RT. Factors affecting late mortality from heart disease after treatment of Hodgkin's disease. *JAMA*. 1993;270(16):1949–1955.

49. Henry-Amar M, Hayat M, Meerwaldt JH, et al. Causes of death after therapy for early stage Hodgkin's disease entered on EORTC protocols. EORTC Lymphoma Cooperative Group. *Int J Radiat Oncol Biol Phys*. 1990; 19(5):1155–1157.

50. Stewart FA, Heeneman S, Te Poele J, et al. Ionizing radiation accelerates the development of atherosclerotic lesions in ApoE-/- mice and predisposes to an inflammatory plaque phenotype prone to hemorrhage. *Am J Pathol*. 2006;168(2):649–658.

51. Lee MS, Finch W, Mahmud E. Cardiovascular complications of radiotherapy. *Am J Cardiol*. 2013;112(10): 1688–1696.

52. Orzan F, Brusca A, Conte MR, Presbitero P, Figliomeni MC. Severe coronary artery disease after radiation therapy of the chest and mediastinum: clinical presentation and treatment. *Br Heart J*. 1993;69(6):496–500.

53. Taylor CW, Nisbet A, McGale P, Darby SC. Cardiac exposures in breast cancer radiotherapy: 1950s-1990s. *Int J Radiat Oncol Biol Phys*. 2007;69(5):1484–1495.

54. Bahl A, Ghoshal S, Sharma SC. Increased risk of ischemic stroke in young nasopharyngeal carcinoma patients. in regard to Lee et al. (Int J Radiat Oncol Biol Phys 2011;81:e833–e838). *Int J Radiat Oncol Biol Phys*. 2012;82(4):1321.

55. Lam WW, Leung SF, So NM, et al. Incidence of carotid stenosis in nasopharyngeal carcinoma patients after radiotherapy. *Cancer*. 2001;92(9):2357–2363.

56. Dorresteijn LD, Kappelle AC, Boogerd W, et al. Increased risk of ischemic stroke after radiotherapy on the neck in patients younger than 60 years. *J Clin Oncol*. 2002;20(1):282–288.

57. Cheng SW, Ting AC, Lam LK, Wei WI. Carotid stenosis after radiotherapy for nasopharyngeal carcinoma. *Arch Otolaryngol Head Neck Surg*. 2000;126(4):517–521.

58. Al-Mubarak N, Roubin GS, Iyer SS, Gomez CR, Liu MW, Vitek JJ. Carotid stenting for severe radiation-induced extracranial carotid artery occlusive disease. *J Endovasc Ther*. 2000;7(1):36–40.

59. Ting AC, Cheng SW, Yeung KM, et al. Carotid stenting for radiation-induced extracranial carotid artery occlusive disease: efficacy and midterm outcomes. *J Endovasc Ther*. 2004;11(1):53–59.

60. Houdart E, Mounayer C, Chapot R, Saint-Maurice JP, Merland JJ. Carotid stenting for radiation-induced stenoses: a report of 7 cases. *Stroke*. 2001; 32(1):118–121.

61. Bowers DC, McNeil DE, Liu Y, et al. Stroke as a late treatment effect of Hodgkin's disease: a report from

the Childhood Cancer Survivor Study. *J Clin Oncol.* 2005;23(27):6508–6515.

62. Milutinovic J, Darcy M, Thompson KA. Radiation-induced renovascular hypertension successfully treated with transluminal angioplasty: case report. *Cardiovasc Intervent Radiol.* 1990;13(1):29–31.

63. Saka B, Bilge AK, Umman B, et al. Bilateral renal artery stenosis after abdominal radiotherapy for Hodgkin's disease. *Int J Clin Pract.* 2003;57(3):247–248.

64. Jurado JA, Bashir R, Burket MW. Radiation-induced peripheral artery disease. *Catheter Cardiovasc Interv.* 2008;72(4):563–568.

65. Friedman DL, Hudson MM, Landier W. Keeping your heart healthy after treatment for childhood cancer. Health link: children's Oncology Group. Heart health 2013. http://survivorshipguidelines.org/pdf/healthlinks/English/heart_health_Eng.pdf. Accessed October 9, 2017.

66. Armenian SH, Hudson MM, Mulder RL, et al. International Late Effects of Childhood Cancer Guideline Harmonization Group. Recommendations for cardiomyopathy surveillance for survivors of childhood cancer: a report from the International Late Effects of Childhood Cancer Guideline Harmonization Group. *Lancet Oncol.* 2015;16(3):e123–e136.

67. Plana JC, Galderisi M, Barac A, et al. Expert consensus for multimodality imaging evaluation of adult patients during and after cancer therapy: a report from the American Society of Echocardiography and the European Association of Cardiovascular Imaging. *Eur Heart J Cardiovasc Imaging.* 2014;15(10):1063–1093.

68. Lancellotti P, Nkomo VT, Badano LP, et al. European Society of Cardiology Working Groups on Nuclear Cardiology and Cardiac Computed Tomography and Cardiovascular Magnetic Resonance; American Society of Nuclear Cardiology; Society for Cardiovascular Magnetic Resonance; Society of Cardiovascular Computed Tomography. Expert consensus for multi-modality imaging evaluation of cardiovascular complications of radiotherapy in adults: a report from the European Association of Cardiovascular Imaging and the American Society of Echocardiography. *Eur Heart J Cardiovasc Imaging.* 2013;14(8):721–740.

69. Vejpongsa P, Yeh ET. Prevention of anthracycline-induced cardiotoxicity: challenges and opportunities. *J Am Coll Cardiol.* 2014;64(9):938–945.

70. Kaya MG, Ozkan M, Gunebakmaz O, et al. Protective effects of nebivolol against anthracycline-induced cardiomyopathy: a randomized control study. *Int J Cardiol.* 2013;167(5):2306–2310.

71. Gabizon AA. Stealth liposomes and tumor targeting: one step further in the quest for the magic bullet. *Clin Cancer Res.* 2001;7(2):223–225.

72. Pacciarini MA, Barbieri B, Colombo T, Broggini M, Garattini S, Donelli MG. Distribution and antitumor activity of adriamycin given in a high-dose and a repeated low-dose schedule to mice. *Cancer Treat Rep.* 1978;62(5):791–800.

73. Valdivieso M, Burgess MA, Ewer MS, et al. Increased therapeutic index of weekly doxorubicin in the therapy of non-small cell lung cancer: a prospective, randomized study. *J Clin Oncol.* 1984;2(3):207–214.

74. Georgakopoulos P, Roussou P, Matsakas E, et al. Cardioprotective effect of metoprolol and enalapril in doxorubicin-treated lymphoma patients: a prospective, parallel-group, randomized, controlled study with 36-month follow-up. *Am J Hematol.* 2010;85(11): 894–896.

75. Kalay N, Basar E, Ozdogru I, et al. Protective effects of carvedilol against anthracycline-induced cardiomyopathy. *J Am Coll Cardiol.* 2006;48(11):2258–2262.

76. Lipshultz SE, Lipsitz SR, Sallan SE, et al. Long-term enalapril therapy for left ventricular dysfunction in doxorubicin-treated survivors of childhood cancer. *J Clin Oncol.* 2002;20(23):4517–4522.

77. Cardinale D, Colombo A, Lamantia G, et al. Anthracycline-induced cardiomyopathy: clinical relevance and response to pharmacologic therapy. *J Am Coll Cardiol.* 2010;55(3):213–220.

78. Fleisher LA, Fleischmann KE, Auerbach AD, et al. 2014 ACC/AHA guideline on perioperative cardiovascular evaluation and management of patients undergoing noncardiac surgery: executive summary: a report of the American College of Cardiology/American Heart Association task force on practice guidelines. Developed in collaboration with the American College of Surgeons, American Society of Anesthesiologists, American Society of Echocardiography, American Society of Nuclear Cardiology, Heart Rhythm Society, Society for Cardiovascular Angiography and Interventions, Society of Cardiovascular Anesthesiologists, and Society of Vascular Medicine. Endorsed by the Society of Hospital Medicine. *J Nucl Cardiol.* 2015;22(1):162–215.

79. Lee TH, Marcantonio ER, Mangione CM, et al. Derivation and prospective validation of a simple index for prediction of cardiac risk of major noncardiac surgery. *Circulation.* 1999;100(10):1043–1049.

80. Surgical Risk Calculator. http://www.surgicalriskcalculator.com/miorcardiacarrest/. Accessed July 7, 2019.

81. Gupta PK, Gupta H, Sundaram A, et al. Development and validation of a risk calculator for prediction of cardiac risk after surgery. *Circulation.* 2011;124(4): 381–387.

82. American College of Surgeons National Surgical Quality Improvement Program. Surgical risk calculator. http://riskcalculator.facs.org/. Accessed July 7, 2019.

83. Cohen ME, Ko CY, Bilimoria KY, et al. Optimizing ACS NSQIP modeling for evaluation of surgical quality and risk: patient risk adjustment, procedure mix adjustment, shrinkage adjustment, and surgical focus. *J Am Coll Surg.* 2013;217(2):336–346.e1.

84. Hueb W, Lopes N, Gersh BJ, et al. Ten-year follow-up survival of the Medicine, Angioplasty, or Surgery Study (MASS II): a randomized controlled clinical trial of 3 therapeutic strategies for multivessel coronary artery disease. *Circulation.* 2010;122(10):949–957.

85. Anderson JL, Adams CD, Antman EM, et al. 2012 ACCF/AHA focused update incorporated into the ACCF/AHA 2007 guidelines for the management of patients with unstable angina/non-ST-elevation myocardial infarction: a report of the American College of Cardiology Foundation/American Heart Association task force on practice guidelines. *J Am Coll Cardiol.* 2013;61(23):e179–e347.

86. Velders MA, Boden H, Hofma SH, et al. Outcome after ST elevation myocardial infarction in patients with cancer treated with primary percutaneous coronary intervention. *Am J Cardiol.* 2013;112(12):1867–1872.

87. Sabatine MS, Morrow DA, Giugliano RP, et al. Association of hemoglobin levels with clinical outcomes in acute coronary syndromes. *Circulation.* 2005; 111(16):2042–2049.

88. van Werkum JW, Heestermans AA, Zomer AC, et al. Predictors of coronary stent thrombosis: the Dutch stent thrombosis registry. *J Am Coll Cardiol.* 2009;53(16):1399–1409.

89. Abbott JD, Ahmed HN, Vlachos HA, Selzer F, Williams DO. Comparison of outcome in patients with ST-elevation versus non-ST-elevation acute myocardial infarction treated with percutaneous coronary intervention (from the National Heart, Lung, and Blood Institute Dynamic Registry). *Am J Cardiol.* 2007;100(2): 190–195.

90. Yusuf SW, Daraban N, Abbasi N, Lei X, Durand JB, Daher IN. Treatment and outcomes of acute coronary syndrome in the cancer population. *Clin Cardiol.* 2012;35(7):443–450.

91. Milosevic A, Vasiljevic-Pokrajcic Z, Milasinovic D, et al. Immediate versus delayed invasive intervention for Non-STEMI patients: the RIDDLE-NSTEMI study. *JACC Cardiovasc Interv.* 2016;9(6):541–549.

92. Elting LS, Rubenstein EB, Martin CG, et al. Incidence, cost, and outcomes of bleeding and chemotherapy dose modification among solid tumor patients with chemotherapy-induced thrombocytopenia. *J Clin Oncol.* 2001;19(4):1137–1146.

93. Hakim DA, Dangas GD, Caixeta A, et al. Impact of baseline thrombocytopenia on the early and late outcomes after ST-elevation myocardial infarction treated primary angioplasty: analysis from the Harmonizing Outcomes with Revascularization and Stents in Acute Myocardial Infarction (HORIZONS-AMI) trial. *Am Heart J.* 2011;161(2):391–396.

94. Luzzatto G, Schafer AI. The prethrombotic state in cancer. *Semin Oncol.* 1990;17(2):147–159.

95. Yusuf SW, Iliescu C, Bathina JD, Daher IN, Durand JB. Antiplatelet therapy and percutaneous coronary intervention in patients with acute coronary syndrome and thrombocytopenia. *Tex Heart Inst J.* 2010;37(3):336–340.

96. Odell TT, Murphy JR, Jackson CW. Stimulation of megakaryocytopoiesis by acute thrombocytopenia in rats. *Blood.* 1976;48(5):765–775.

97. O'Malley T, Langhorne P, Elton RA, Stewart C. Platelet size in stroke patients. *Stroke.* 1995;26(6):995–999.

98. Cameron HA, Phillips R, Ibbotson RM, Carson PH. Platelet size in myocardial infarction. *Br Med J (Clin Res Ed).* 1983;287(6390):449–451.

99. VanWijk MJ, VanBavel E, Sturk A, Nieuwland R. Microparticles in cardiovascular diseases. *Cardiovasc Res.* 2003;59(2):277–287.

100. Schiffer CA, Anderson KC, Bennett CL, et al. American Society of Clinical Oncology. Platelet transfusion for patients with cancer: clinical practice guidelines of the American Society of Clinical Oncology. *J Clin Oncol.* 2001;19(5):1519–1538.

101. Iliescu C, Durand JB, Kroll M. Cardiovascular interventions in thrombocytopenic cancer patients. *Tex Heart Inst J.* 2011;38(3):259–260.

102. Kwak YL, Kim JC, Choi YS, Yoo KJ, Song Y, Shim JK. Clopidogrel responsiveness regardless of the discontinuation date predicts increased blood loss and transfusion requirement after off-pump coronary artery bypass graft surgery. *J Am Coll Cardiol.* 2010;56(24):1994–2002.

103. Ellis SG, Bhatt D, Kapadia S, Lee D, Yen M, Whitlow PL. Correlates and outcomes of retroperitoneal hemorrhage complicating percutaneous coronary intervention. *Catheter Cardiovasc Interv.* 2006;67(4):541–545.

104. Bangalore S, Bhatt DL. Femoral arterial access and closure. *Circulation.* 2011;124(5):e147–e156.

105. Ben-Dor I, Maluenda G, Mahmoudi M, et al. A novel, minimally invasive access technique versus standard 18-gauge needle set for femoral access. *Catheter Cardiovasc Interv.* 2012;79(7):1180–1185.

106. Fefer P, Matetzky S, Gannot S, et al. Predictors and outcomes associated with radial versus femoral access for intervention in patients with acute coronary syndrome in a real-world setting: results from the Acute Coronary Syndrome Israeli Survey (ACSIS) 2010. *J Invasive Cardiol.* 2014;26(8):398–402.

107. Sciahbasi A, Fischetti D, Picciolo A, et al. Transradial access compared with femoral puncture closure devices in percutaneous coronary procedures. *Int J Cardiol.* 2009;137(3):199–205.

108. Belli AM, Cumberland DC, Knox AM, Procter AE, Welsh CL. The complication rate of percutaneous peripheral balloon angioplasty. *Clin Radiol.* 1990;41(6):380–383.

109. Kim D, Orron DE, Skillman JJ, et al. Role of superficial femoral artery puncture in the development of pseudoaneurysm and arteriovenous fistula complicating percutaneous transfemoral cardiac catheterization. *Cathet Cardiovasc Diagn.* 1992;25(2):91–97.

110. Sherev DA, Shaw RE, Brent BN. Angiographic predictors of femoral access site complications: implication for planned percutaneous coronary intervention. *Catheter Cardiovasc Interv.* 2005;65(2):196–202.

111. Krishnasamy VP, Hagar MJ, Scher DJ, Sanogo ML, Gabriel GE, Sarin SN. Vascular closure devices: technical tips, complications, and management. *Tech Vasc Interv Radiol.* 2015;18(2):100–112.

112. Hachamovitch R, Berman DS, Shaw LJ, et al. Incremental prognostic value of myocardial perfusion single photon

emission computed tomography for the prediction of cardiac death: differential stratification for risk of cardiac death and myocardial infarction. *Circulation*. 1998;97(6):535–543.

113. De Bruyne B, Pijls NH, Kalesan B, et al. FAME 2 Trial Investigators. Fractional flow reserve-guided PCI versus medical therapy in stable coronary disease. *N Engl J Med*. 2012;367(11):991–1001.

114. Fihn SD, Blankenship JC, Alexander KP, et al. 2014 ACC/AHA/AATS/PCNA/SCAI/STS focused update of the guideline for the diagnosis and management of patients with stable ischemic heart disease: a report of the American College of Cardiology/American Heart Association Task Force on Practice Guidelines, and the American Association for Thoracic Surgery, Preventive Cardiovascular Nurses Association, Society for Cardiovascular Angiography and Interventions, and Society of Thoracic Surgeons. *J Am Coll Cardiol*. 2014;64(18):1929–1949.

115. Nascimento BR, Belfort AF, Macedo FA, et al. Meta-analysis of deferral versus performance of coronary intervention based on coronary pressure-derived fractional flow reserve. *Am J Cardiol*. 2015;115(3):385–391.

116. Mintz GS, Pichard AD, Kovach JA, et al. Impact of preintervention intravascular ultrasound imaging on transcatheter treatment strategies in coronary artery disease. *Am J Cardiol*. 1994;73(7):423–430.

117. Jang JS, Song YJ, Kang W, et al. Intravascular ultrasound-guided implantation of drug-eluting stents to improve outcome: a meta-analysis. *JACC Cardiovasc Interv*. 2014;7(3):233–243.

118. Abizaid AS, Mintz GS, Abizaid A, et al. One-year follow-up after intravascular ultrasound assessment of moderate left main coronary artery disease in patients with ambiguous angiograms. *J Am Coll Cardiol*. 1999;34(3):707–715.

119. Fitzgerald PJ, Oshima A, Hayase M, et al. Final results of the Can Routine Ultrasound Influence Stent Expansion (CRUISE) study. *Circulation*. 2000;102(5):523–530.

120. Oemrawsingh PV, Mintz GS, Schalij MJ, Zwinderman AH, Jukema JW, van der Wall EE. TULIP Study. Intravascular ultrasound guidance improves angiographic and clinical outcome of stent implantation for long coronary artery stenoses: final results of a randomized comparison with angiographic guidance (TULIP Study). *Circulation*. 2003;107(1):62–67.

121. Nascimento BR, de Sousa MR, Koo BK, et al. Diagnostic accuracy of intravascular ultrasound-derived minimal lumen area compared with fractional flow reserve—meta-analysis: pooled accuracy of IVUS luminal area versus FFR. *Catheter Cardiovasc Interv*. 2014;84(3):377–385.

122. Khandhar SJ, Yamamoto H, Teuteberg JJ, et al. Optical coherence tomography for characterization of cardiac allograft vasculopathy after heart transplantation (OCTCAV study). *J Heart Lung Transplant*. 2013;32(6):596–602.

123. Guddeti RR, Matsuo Y, Matsuzawa Y, et al. Clinical implications of intracoronary imaging in cardiac allograft vasculopathy. *Circ Cardiov Imaging*. 2015;8(1):1–8. doi:10.1161/CIRCIMAGING.114.002636.

124. Staico R, Costa MA, Chamié D, et al. Very long-term follow-up of strut apposition and tissue coverage with Biolimus A9 stents analyzed by optical coherence tomography. *Int J Cardiovasc Imaging*. 2013;29(5):977–988.

125. Capodanno D, Prati F, Pawlowsky T, et al. Comparison of optical coherence tomography and intravascular ultrasound for the assessment of in-stent tissue coverage after stent implantation. *EuroIntervention*. 2009;5(5):538–543.

126. Iliescu C, LeBeau JT, Silva G, et al. Optical coherence tomography–guided antiplatelet therapy in patients with coronary artery disease and cancer: the PROTECT-OCT registry. *J Am Coll Cardiol*. 2013;61(suppl S):E1128.

127. Mauri L, Kereiakes DJ, Yeh RW, et al. DAPT study investigators. Twelve or 30 months of dual antiplatelet therapy after drug-eluting stents. *N Engl J Med*. 2014;371(23):2155–2166.

128. Rao SV, Tremmel JA, Gilchrist IC, et al. Society for cardiovascular angiography and intervention's transradial working group. Best practices for transradial angiography and intervention: a consensus statement from the society for cardiovascular angiography and intervention's transradial working group. *Catheter Cardiovasc Interv*. 2014;83(2):228–236.

129. Krone RJ. Managing coronary artery disease in the cancer patient. *Prog Cardiovasc Dis*. 2010;53(2):149–156.

130. Neugut AI, Lebwohl B. Is the prevalence of colorectal neoplasm higher in patients with coronary artery disease? *Nat Clin Pract Oncol*. 2008;5(5):248–249.

131. Chan AO, Jim MH, Lam KF, et al. Prevalence of colorectal neoplasm among patients with newly diagnosed coronary artery disease. *JAMA*. 2007;298(12):1412–1419.

132. Shivaraju A, Patel V, Fonarow GC, Xie H, Shroff AR, Vidovich MI. Temporal trends in gastrointestinal bleeding associated with percutaneous coronary intervention: analysis of the 1998-2006 Nationwide Inpatient Sample (NIS) database. *Am Heart J*. 2011;162(6):1062–1068.e5.

133. Tsuji Y, Morimoto N, Tanaka H, et al. Surgery for gastric cancer combined with cardiac and aortic surgery. *Arch Surg*. 2005;140(11):1109–1114.

134. Ozsöyler I, Yilik L, Bozok S, et al. Off-pump coronary artery bypass surgery in patients with coronary artery disease and malign neoplasia: results of ten patients and review of the literature. *Heart Vessels*. 2006;21(6):365–367.

135. Schoenmakers MC, van Boven WJ, van den Bosch J, van Swieten HA. Comparison of on-pump or off-pump coronary artery revascularization with lung resection. *Ann Thorac Surg*. 2007;84(2):504–509.

136. Brown ML, Schaff HV, Sundt TM. Conduit choice for coronary artery bypass grafting after mediastinal radiation. *J Thorac Cardiovasc Surg*. 2008;136(5):1167–1171.

137. El Haddad D, Iliescu C, Yusuf SW, et al. Outcomes of cancer patients undergoing percutaneous pericardiocentesis for pericardial effusion. *J Am Coll Cardiol*. 2015;66(10):1119–1128.

138. Toth I, Szucs G, Molnar TF. Mediastinoscope-controlled parasternal fenestration of the pericardium: definitive surgical palliation of malignant pericardial effusion. *J Cardiothorac Surg*. 2012;7:56.

139. Jama GM, Scarci M, Bowden J, Marciniak SJ. Palliative treatment for symptomatic malignant pericardial effusion. *Interact Cardiovasc Thorac Surg.* 2014;19(6):1019–1026.

140. Tsang TS, Seward JB, Barnes ME, et al. Outcomes of primary and secondary treatment of pericardial effusion in patients with malignancy. *Mayo Clin Proc.* 2000;75(3):248–253.

141. Laham RJ, Cohen DJ, Kuntz RE, Baim DS, Lorell BH, Simons M. Pericardial effusion in patients with cancer: outcome with contemporary management strategies. *Heart.* 1996;75(1):67–71.

142. Ruiz-García J, Jiménez-Valero S, Moreno R, et al. Percutaneous balloon pericardiotomy as the initial and definitive treatment for malignant pericardial effusion. *Rev Esp Cardiologia (English Ed).* 2013;66(5):357–363.

143. Virk SA, Chandrakumar D, Villanueva C, Wolfenden H, Liou K, Cao C. Systematic review of percutaneous interventions for malignant pericardial effusion. *Heart.* 2015;101(20):1619–1626.

144. Elliott P, Arbustini E. The role of endomyocardial biopsy in the management of cardiovascular disease: a commentary on joint AHA/ACC/ESC guidelines. *Heart.* 2009;95(9):759–760.

145. Fowles RE, Mason JW. Endomyocardial biopsy. *Ann Inter Med.* 1982;97(6):885–894.

146. Deckers JW, Hare JM, Baughman KL. Complications of transvenous right ventricular endomyocardial biopsy in adult patients with cardiomyopathy: a seven-year survey of 546 consecutive diagnostic procedures in a tertiary referral center. *J Am Coll Cardiol.* 1992;19(1):43–47.

147. Cooper LT, Baughman KL, Feldman AM, et al. American Heart Association; American College of Cardiology; European Society of Cardiology; Heart Failure Society of America; Heart Failure Association of the European Society of Cardiology. The role of endomyocardial biopsy in the management of cardiovascular disease: a scientific statement from the American Heart Association, the American College of Cardiology, and the European Society of Cardiology. Endorsed by the Heart Failure Society of America and the Heart Failure Association of the European Society of Cardiology. *J Am Coll Cardiol.* 2007;50(19):1914–1931.

148. Billingham ME, Mason JW, Bristow MR, Daniels JR. Anthracycline cardiomyopathy monitored by morphologic changes. *Cancer Treat Rep.* 1978;62(6):865–872.

149. Torti FM, Bristow MR, Howes AE, et al. Reduced cardiotoxicity of doxorubicin delivered on a weekly schedule. Assessment by endomyocardial biopsy. *Ann Intern Med.* 1983;99(6):745–749.

150. Yusuf SW, Sarfaraz A, Durand JB, Swafford J, Daher IN. Management and outcomes of severe aortic stenosis in cancer patients. *Am Heart J.* 2011;161(6):1125–1132.

151. Iung B, Baron G, Butchart EG, et al. A prospective survey of patients with valvular heart disease in Europe: the Euro Heart Survey on valvular heart disease. *Eur Heart J.* 2003;24(13):1231–1243.

152. Pedersen WR, Klaassen PJ, Pedersen CW, et al. Comparison of outcomes in high-risk patients >70 years of age with aortic valvuloplasty and percutaneous coronary intervention versus aortic valvuloplasty alone. *Am J Cardiol.* 2008;101(9):1309–1314.

153. Bach DS, Cimino N, Deeb GM. Unoperated patients with severe aortic stenosis. *J Am Coll Cardiol.* 2007;50(20):2018–2019.

154. Kogoj P, Devjak R, Bunc M. Balloon aortic valvuloplasty (BAV) as a bridge to aortic valve replacement in cancer patients who require urgent non-cardiac surgery. *Radiol Oncol.* 2014;48(1):62–66.

155. Bavaria JE, Szeto WY, Roche LA, et al. The progression of a transcatheter aortic valve program: a decision analysis of more than 680 patient referrals. *Ann Thorac Surg.* 2011;92(6):2072–2076.

24 Psychosocial Considerations in Treating the Cancer Patient with Heart Disease

Anecita P. Fadol

INTRODUCTION

It is not uncommon for a patient to receive a dual diagnosis of cancer and heart disease. A cancer diagnosis by itself is associated with a variety of psychosocial challenges; however, having both diagnoses can result in multiplicative psychosocial issues, including fear, anxiety, depression, anger, denial, and intense uncertainty.

Patients with cancer often face fear of death or disability, fear of being an economic burden to the family, and fear and uncertainty about the future. It is not surprising that many patients with a cancer diagnosis exhibit signs of acute stress reactions. After the cancer diagnosis, treatment may involve multiple bodily assaults resulting from chemotherapy, radiation therapy, and surgery with all its attendant possibility of physical deformity. In addition to disrupting patients' social and work life, these treatments may even limit their ability to care for themselves or to live independently. Furthermore, cancer treatments may result in adverse cardiac problems, such as acute myocardial infarction (AMI), atrial fibrillation, or congestive heart failure (CHF), and these problems can lead to discontinuation of cancer treatment. These complex emotional reactions may affect quality of life, compliance with therapy, hospital length of stay, healthcare costs, morbidity rates, and even mortality rates.

In 2008, the Institute of Medicine (IOM) report entitled Cancer Care for the Whole Patient[1] recommend that all cancer care include the provision of appropriate integrated psychosocial services. However, despite substantial evidence that patients with cancer can have serious psychosocial problems for which evidence-based treatment is available, many patients still do not receive adequate psychosocial care.[2] The principal goal of psychosocial care is to recognize and address the effects of cancer and its treatment on the mental status and emotional well-being of patients, their family members, and their professional caregivers.

This chapter addresses the treatment of the most common psychosocial issues as an essential component of good-quality care for patients with cancer and heart disease. It also provides a general framework for assessment and suggests practical intervention strategies. This information will help clinicians to 1) recognize the importance of addressing psychosocial issues in successfully implementing a treatment plan, 2) routinely screen for psychosocial risk factors, 3) improve patients' quality of life (QoL) by managing comorbid psychological disorders, and 4) communicate with behavioral specialists who can help to address the social issues that may affect patients' plan of care.

■ Coping with a Cancer Diagnosis

Receiving a diagnosis of cancer is a life-changing event that brings with it a host of psychological reactions. Emotional reactions of anger and sadness related to having one's life dramatically interrupted and to the need to face the challenge of making meaningful adjustments are common. The costly treatment can consume the family's resources and pose an important challenge. The individual response may vary from patient to patient and may be influenced by the patient's personality factors, character traits, social support system, and other sociodemographic factors. With this stressful event, the patient may experience anxiety, depression, and a host of other symptoms.

Anxiety in a cardiac patient with cancer ■ Anxiety is defined as a negative affective state resulting from an individual's perception of threat and is characterized by perceived inability to predict, control, or gain the preferred results in given situations.[3] Although anxiety is considered an adaptive response to the threat of living with a chronic illness, it is not benign if it persists or is extreme.[4] Convincing evidence shows that anxiety is associated with high rates of medically unexplained symptoms and increased utilization of healthcare resources.[5–7] Moreover, anxiety disorders are strongly and independently associated with chronic medical illness,[8] low levels of physical health–related QoL, and physical disability.[9,10] The disability and the related poor physical and economic outcomes associated with anxiety disorders may be as great as those caused by depression. Kessler and colleagues[11] reported that the association between various anxiety disorders and depression is equal to or greater than the association between a chronic physical condition and depression.

Among patients with cancer, anxiety is a common response to threats of uncertainty, suffering, and mortality, and it fluctuates at crucial points in the disease trajectory. In a minority of patients, anxiety can persist at an excessive and uncomfortable level.[12] Clinical consequences are multifold, including less-effective medical decision-making, exacerbation of medical symptoms, and disruption in cancer care.[13-15] Among patients with cardiovascular disease (CVD), anxiety disorders are also common and are as disabling as depressive disorders.[16,17] Anxiety can hinder psychosocial adaptation and physical recovery after an acute event.[4]

For a patient with cancer and cardiovascular disease, anxiety can be caused by several factors (Table 24-1). The prevalence of anxiety among patients who have experienced an acute cardiac event is approximately 70% to 80%, and this anxiety persists chronically in approximately 20% to 25% of patients with CVD.[16] In patients with cancer, the cancer diagnosis itself is a source of anxiety, causing psychological distress, fear, dread, and sadness. Prevalence rates of anxiety and depressive disorders among cancer patients are generally in the range of 10% to 30%, and in many cases the rates of various anxiety disorders are equivalent to or greater than those of depression.[18-20] However, the rates of anxiety disorders vary depending on the type and stage of cancer, treatment regimens, time since diagnosis, sex, and methods used to diagnose psychiatric illness. No data are available

TABLE 24-1   Causes of anxiety among patients with cancer and heart disease

CAUSES OF ANXIETY AMONG PATIENTS WITH CANCER AND HEART DISEASE
Situational
Diagnosis of cancer
Diagnosis of cardiomyopathy or heart failure as a complication of cancer therapy
Awaiting results of tests
Preparation for frightening diagnostic procedures
Disease-Related
Severe symptoms related to treatment
Uncontrolled pain
Treatment-Related
Anxiety-producing drugs (antiemetics)
Frightening or painful procedures (MRI, CT scanning, surgery)
Anticipation of the adverse effects of chemotherapy

MRI, magnetic resonance imaging; CT, computed tomography

about the prevalence of anxiety disorders in patients with dual diagnoses of cancer and heart disease. In the validation study of a symptom assessment instrument, the MD Anderson Symptom Inventory–Heart Failure (MDASI-HF), 58 of the 156 patients with cancer and heart failure who participated in the study reported moderate (n = 33; 21%) or severe (n = 25; 16%) anxiety.[21]

Mechanisms of anxiety ■ Several proposed mechanisms may result in anxiety among cardiac patients with cancer. The endocrine and metabolic changes associated with cancer or its treatment, cancer prognosis, individual coping style, and social support systems may trigger anxiety in the patient.[22] Some medications commonly used in the treatment of cancer, such as glucocorticoids, are associated with a variety of symptoms, including anxiety.[23] A study of patients with mixed types of cancer found that anxiety disorders were associated with female sex and poor social support systems.[18] A history of major depression and feelings of helplessness or hopelessness can trigger anxiety among women with breast cancer.[24]

As a result of chronic stress and other negative emotions associated with the cancer diagnosis, anxiety may lead to activation of the hypothalamic–pituitary–adrenal (HPA) axis and the sympathetic nervous system.[25] Increases in the activity of the sympathetic nervous system and the release of plasma catecholamines may damage the vascular endothelium and lead to the release of fatty acids at levels higher than that necessary to meet metabolic requirements. Excess HPA activation may increase the severity of inflammation.[26] Anxiety is also hypothesized to increase cardiovascular reactivity to stress, thereby leading to greater strain on the heart as a result of increases in resting heart rate, blood pressure, baroreflex dysfunction, and variability in ventricular repolarization.[27-29] The combined effects of the sympathetic nervous system, HPA axis hyperactivity, and the altered sympathovagal control of the heart increase the risk of incident CVD and reduce the threshold for cardiac ischemia, arrhythmias, and sudden cardiac death.[30] Some evidence suggests that acute anxiety episodes in extreme emotional states may actually trigger AMI.[31]

Depression in heart disease and cancer ■ Depression is the most common emotional distress experienced by patients with chronic diseases such as heart disease and cancer.[5,32-36] Even among healthy persons, depression may be a risk factor for the development of heart disease and stroke.[32,34,37,38] A World Health Organization survey of 245,404 adults from 60 countries found that patients with comorbid depression reported worse overall health than those with diabetes, asthma, or CVD alone.[39] Major depression and elevated depressive symptoms are associated with a poorer prognosis for patients with coronary heart disease (CHD) and with higher rates of serious cardiac events and all-cause mortality after MI, unstable angina, and coronary artery bypass surgery.[30,34,40–42]

The National Cancer Institute defines depression as a mental condition marked by ongoing feelings of sadness, despair, loss of energy, sleep disorders, and difficulty dealing with the normal activities of daily life.[43] Patients with preexisting heart disease who receive a diagnosis of cancer may experience severe depression, although there is a paucity of research data to support this notion. Most studies of depression involve either cardiovascular patients or cancer patients, not patients with a dual diagnosis of both diseases. In the validation study of the MDASI-HF, 41 of the 156 patients with cancer and heart failure reported moderate (16%, n = 25) or severe (10%, n = 16) depression.[21]

Depression in a cancer patient is frequently not recognized because it is often seen as a natural reaction to the diagnosis; therefore, it is largely under detected and untreated. Patients often do not present with the complaint of depression and in many cases may deny it. Instead, patients may present with somatic symptoms, including gastrointestinal distress, pain, fatigue, or social withdrawal from family and friends.

Depression can affect treatment compliance and efficacy and may also affect the patient's cancer prognosis and the progression of cardiac disease.

Prevalence of depression ■ The prevalence of depression is markedly and consistently higher among patients with heart disease, stroke, and cancer than among the general population.[5,32,–36,44,45] Results of the National Health Interview Survey, which involved 30,801 adults, showed that the prevalence of depression ranged from 7.9% to 17% among patients with chronic medical conditions.[46] The study also found that the coexistence of major depression and chronic conditions is associated with higher rates of ambulatory care visits, emergency department visits, days spent in bed because of illness, and functional disability. Major depression and elevated depressive symptoms are associated with a poorer prognosis for patients with coronary heart disease.[41,42] Depression is related to poor QoL, poor recovery after a somatic event, and higher mortality rates.[47,48]

Depression is three times more common among patients after an AMI than among the general community.[49] Prevalence estimates among patients hospitalized for unstable angina, bypass surgeries, and angioplasty are similar to those among patients with AMI, but higher levels of depression are reported among patients with congestive heart failure.[34,50] The rate of subsequent cardiovascular events was 31% higher among patients with baseline depressive symptoms than among those without depressive symptoms.[51] Sixty to seventy percent of hospitalized patients who have and are subsequently found to have depression remain depressed even 1 to 4 months after hospital discharge.[32] Depression is associated with at least twice the risk of cardiac events over the first 1 to 2 years after an MI.[34,50]

Among patients with cancer, the prevalence of depressive disorders has been estimated to be as much as four times higher than among the general population, and it varies widely depending on several factors, including age, sex, time, and stage of cancer diagnosis, as well as the availability of social support and a social network.[35,52,53] The prevalence of depression appears to be higher among patients with cancers that carry poorer prognoses, such as pancreatic, oropharyngeal, and breast cancer.[35] In a retrospective study of breast cancer patients, 20% to 27% of patients were found to have depression, and 13.1% of these exhibited signs of major depression in the palliative stage of their disease.[54,55] Among patients with head and neck cancer, 26% were found to have depression; of those, more than 50% had psychiatric disorders in the advanced and palliative stages of their disease.[56,57] The prevalence of depression has been shown to be higher among women with cardiac disease, and evidence suggests that young women may be at a particularly high risk of depression after AMI.[38,58,59]

The risk of depression is also highest among patients with a history of previous psychological disorders, alcoholism, increased physical impairment, unmanaged pain, treatment regimens containing certain medications, concurrent illnesses that produce depressive symptoms, or a lack of social support. The patient's social support and the types of coping strategies involved can modulate the intensity and the expression of depression among cancer patients.[53] Although the prevalence of depression is higher among patients with cancer and heart disease, it is frequently undiagnosed. The clinicians should routinely screen these patients for depression, because untreated depression results in higher healthcare costs, decreased compliance, and decreased QoL.

Clinical symptoms of depression ■ The clinical symptoms of depression among patients with cancer and heart disease vary among individual patients and are different from those encountered among healthy persons. Among healthy persons, depression is usually manifested by somatic symptoms such as insomnia, appetite changes resulting in anorexia and weight loss, fatigue, poor concentration, and a loss of interest in previously enjoyable activities. These symptoms, however, are of little value in diagnosing depression among patients with cancer and heart disease because these symptoms can be a manifestation of the disease itself or of the sequelae of the cancer therapy. Certain psychological features, such as sadness, anhedonia, hopelessness, helplessness, low self-esteem, guilt feelings, and suicidal ideation, are more common relevant symptoms. A study of patients with metastatic breast cancer found that disturbed sleep was an indicator of worsening depression.[60] A text revision of the Diagnostic and Statistical Manual of Mental Disorders IV (DSM-IV), known as the DSM-IV-TR, published in 2000, recommends that the symptoms of a major depressive episode should include at least five of the nine possible symptoms of depression (Table 24-2).

Medications and depression ■ Numerous medications for heart disease, such as antihypertensive agents, analgesics, and anti-inflammatory agents, can produce depressive side effects (Table 24-3). In addition, antineoplastic agents (i.e., interferon alpha, interleukin 2), hormones (i.e., corticosteroids), sedatives, and tranquilizers that are often used in cancer treatment can also cause depression. Corticosteroids that are frequently included in the chemotherapy protocols can cause mood disturbances, including emotional lability

TABLE 24-2 Symptoms of major depression

1. Ongoing feelings of sadness or despair most of the day for two weeks
2. Loss of interest in most activities (anhedonia)
3. Weight loss or decrease in appetite
4. Insomnia or hypersomnia
5. Psychomotor agitation or retardation
6. Fatigue or loss of energy
7. Feelings of worthlessness or excessive or inappropriate guilt
8. Decreased ability to concentrate
9. Recurrent thoughts of death or suicidal ideation

and depression. Patients with uncontrolled pain are particularly prone to depressive symptoms; however, appropriate pain management should be instituted before a diagnosis of depression is made.

Biological and behavioral mechanisms of depression ■ Several factors have been proposed to explain the occurrence of depression among patients with cancer and heart disease. Certain chemotherapeutic regimens can cause metabolic and endocrine alterations resulting in depression. Other factors leading to depression are the use of immune-response modifiers, chronic

TABLE 24-3 Medications that may cause depression as an adverse effect

DRUG CLASSIFICATION	EXAMPLES
Antineoplastic agents	Interferon-alpha Interleukin-2 Procarbazine (Matulane) Vinblastine (Velban)
Analgesics/Anti-inflammatory agents	Opiates (morphine) Baclofen Indomethacin (Indocin)
Anticonvulsants	Phenobarbital Phenytoin (Dilantin)
Antihypertensive agents	Clonidine (Catapres) Methyldopa (Aldomet) Propanolol (Inderal)
Antiparkinsonism agents	Levodopa (Sinemet)
Hormones	Adrenocorticotropic hormone Corticosteroids
Sedatives	Barbiturates Diazepam Ethanol

pain, and the consequences of invasive and extensive surgeries.

Certain biological and behavioral mechanisms have been proposed as explanations for the link between depression and CHD. When compared to persons without depression, depressed patients with CHD frequently exhibit higher levels of biomarkers that have been found to predict cardiac events or to promote atherosclerosis. Several studies involving patients with coronary artery disease (CAD) and depression have reported reduced heart rate variability, a finding suggesting increased sympathetic activity.[61] Additionally, increased levels of C-reactive protein, interleukin-6, intercellular adhesion molecule, and fibrinogen suggest an increased inflammatory response.[62,63] There is also reported evidence of increases in HPA axis dysfunction and in plasma factor 4 and β-thromboglobulin levels; these increases suggest increased platelet activation and impaired vascular function.[64–66] The behavioral characteristics manifested by depressed patients, which include poor adherence to diet, exercise, and medication, tobacco use, social isolation, and chronic life stress,[67,68] may also contribute to the progression of CAD.

Screening for depression among patients with heart disease and cancer ■ Most cardiology practices do not routinely assess depression, except for research purposes. Current evidence indicates that only approximately half of cardiovascular physicians report that they treat their patients for depression, and not all patients who are recognized to be depressed are treated.[69] Some physicians are reluctant to treat depression among patients with CHD because they believe that depression after an acute cardiac event is a "normal" reaction to a stressful life event and that it will resolve after the patient has been discharged from the hospital and has returned to his or her normal activities. However, in many cases, depression may occur before and continue after an acute cardiac event.[70] The American Heart Association Science Advisory for Depression and Coronary Heart Disease recommends that cardiologists consider depression in the management of CHD, regardless of whether they treat the depression themselves or refer the patient to a healthcare provider who is qualified to treat it.[71]

Several instruments have been published for use in screening patients with CVD or cancer for anxiety and depression (Table 24-4). In oncology, the three most commonly used screening instruments for detecting depression are the Hospital Anxiety and Depression Scale; the Hamilton Rating Scale for Depression, with a sensitivity of 81.3% and a specificity of 87.5%; and the Brief Edinburgh Depression Scale, with a sensitivity of 72% and a specificity of 83%.[72–76]

The two self-report measures recommended for epidemiologic studies of CHD patients are the Beck Depression Inventory (BDI) and the Inventory of Depressive Symptomatology, Self-Report.[77–79] The BDI has been found to be an adequate screening tool for DSM-IV Major Depressive Disorder among patients with MI.[80]

A self-administered Patient Health Questionnaire (PHQ) (Figure 24-1) is available for assessing the severity of depression even in a busy clinical practice. The PHQ-9 is a brief depression-screening instrument with good psychometric properties for patients with CHD; it can provide a provisional diagnosis and severity score that can be used for selecting and monitoring treatment.[81–84] A PHQ-9 score of 10 or higher indicates a high probability of depression, and patients with these scores should be referred to a psychologist or a psychiatrist for a more comprehensive clinical evaluation to determine whether other mental disorders

TABLE 24-4 Most commonly used screening instruments for anxiety or depression

INSTRUMENT	DOMAINS OR FACTORS
Beck Depression Inventory[77,78]	Behavioral, cognitive, and somatic components of depression
Brief Edinburgh Depression Scale (BEDS)[76]	Two factors relating to blame, guilt, subjective sadness, and thoughts of self-harm
Center for Epidemiological Studies-Depression Scale (CES-D)[116]	Frequency of depressive symptoms. Four factors: negative affect and mood, positive mood and well-being, somatic, interpersonal
Hospital Anxiety and Depression Scale (HADS)[117]	Self-screen to rate severity of depression and anxiety
Profile of Mood States (POMS)[118]	Six subscales: tension-anxiety, depression-dejection, anger-hostility, vigor-activity, fatigue-inertia, and confusion-bewilderment
Patient Health Questionnaire 9 (PHQ 9)[86]	Symptoms of depression
Patient Health Questionnaire 2 (PHQ 2)[119]	Symptoms of depression

PATIENT HEALTH QUESTIONNAIRE (PHQ-9)

NAME: ____ DATE: ________________________

Over the *last 2 weeks,* how often have you been
bothered by any of the following problems?
(use "✓" to indicate your answer)

	Not at all	Several days	More than half the days	Nearly every day
1. Little interest or pleasure in doing things	0	1	2	3
2. Feeling down, depressed, or hopeless	0	1	2	3
3. Trouble falling or staying asleep, or sleeping too much	0	1	2	3
4. Feeling tired or having little energy	0	1	2	3
5. Poor appetite or overeating	0	1	2	3
6. Feeling bad about yourself—or that you are a failure or have let yourself or your family down	0	1	2	3
7. Trouble concentrating on things, such as reading the newspaper or watching television	0	1	2	3
8. Moving or speaking so slowly that other people could have noticed. Or the opposite—being so fidgety or restless that you have been moving around a lot more than usual	0	1	2	3
9. Thoughts that you would be better off dead, or of hurting yourself in some way	0	1	2	3

add columns :   +   +

(Healthcare professional: For interpretation of TOTAL, **TOTAL:** ________
please refer to accompanying scoring card.)

10. If you checked off *any* problems, how *difficult* have these problems made it for you to do your work, take care of things at home, or get along with other people?	Not difficult at all ________ Somewhat difficult ________ Very difficult ________ Extremely difficult ________

PHQ-9 is adapted from PRIME MD TODAY, developed by Drs Robert L. Spitzer, Janet B.W. Williams, Kurt Kroenke, and colleagues, with an educational grant from Pfizer Inc. For research information, contact Dr Spitzer at rls8@columbia. edu. Use of the PHQ-9 may only be made in accordance with the Terms of Use available at *http://www.pfizer.com.* Copyright ©1999 Pfizer Inc. All rights reserved. PRIME MD TODAY is a trademark of Pfizer Inc.

ZT274388

FIGURE 24-1   The patient health questionnaire (PHQ-9).

(i.e., anxiety) are present and to develop a suitable treatment plan.[71] A two-item screening tool, the PHQ-2, is recommended for identifying currently depressed patients within a CVD population.[84,85] The PHQ-2 questionnaire uses the first two items of the PHQ-9. Specifically, it asks patients how often they have experienced the following problems over the past two weeks: 1) having little interest or pleasure in doing things, and 2) feeling down, depressed, or hopeless. If the patient answers yes to either or both questions, all nine questions of the PHQ-9 should be asked.[86]

Barriers to effective assessment ■ Anxiety and mood disorders among patients with cancer and heart disease are often untreated or inadequately treated because of time or training constraints or because providers do not ask about psychological distress or consider it important. There are several barriers to effective assessment and intervention for anxiety and depression. First, many providers believe that anxiety and depression are natural reactions to the diagnosis of cancer rather than a comorbid and serious condition. Second, patients contribute to undertreatment of these disorders by trivializing their symptoms of fear, anxiety, or helplessness/hopelessness, or because they believe that these symptoms are an expected part of their diagnosis and treatment. Third, many patients are reluctant to share their emotional symptoms with busy healthcare professionals for fear that reporting these symptoms may divert the focus of treatment away from their cancer diagnosis. Fourth, providers often feel uncomfortable about probing into a patient's psychological distress because they are not prepared to deal with the patient's emotional response. Fifth, many providers believe that emotional issues should be managed by a clinical psychologist or psychiatrist. Sixth, patients are concerned about having a psychiatric diagnosis in their electronic medical record.

Management of depression ■

Psychosocial Interventions The management of depression and anxiety among cardiac patients with cancer is complicated, as is the management of other comorbid conditions. The evidenced-based management strategies include psychoeducational or psychosocial interventions and pharmacologic therapy.[87] Psychoeducational and psychosocial interventions include cognitive behavioral therapy, patient education and information, counseling and psychotherapy, behavioral therapy, and supportive interventions.[88]

Cognitive behavioral therapy (CBT) is defined as any specific psychological or psychosocial intervention that is relatively brief, goal-oriented, based on the learning principles of behavioral change, and directed at effecting change in a specific clinical outcome.[89] CBT is an effective treatment for depression and anxiety among patients with heart disease and those with a wide range of cancers.[89,90] It is usually prescribed for patients who cannot tolerate antidepressants or who prefer nonpharmacologic therapy. These patients should be referred to a psychiatrist or a qualified psychotherapist.

Some evidence suggests that other interventions, such as relaxation therapies, may be effective for patients with mild to moderate heart failure and cancer.[91–94] Exercise and exercise-based rehabilitation are effective for patients with ischemic heart disease and depression or anxiety.[91,92]

In general, published studies recommend and support the use of a combination of psychotherapy and pharmacological treatment.[52,87] Many patients with moderate to severe depression respond better to a combination of psychotherapy and antidepressant therapy than to either treatment alone.[71] The Enhancing Recovery in Coronary Heart Disease Patients (ENRICHD) study, a randomized controlled trial, recommended at least 12 to 16 sessions of CBT over 12 weeks for the remission of moderate to severe depression.[95,96] Pharmacologic psychotherapy, which includes antidepressant drugs and physical activity such as aerobic exercise, was found to be effective for moderate, severe, or recurrent depression.[97]

Pharmacologic Interventions Clinical practice guidelines published by the National Comprehensive Cancer Network, the National Health and Medical Research Council of Australia, and the American Psychiatric Association support the benefits of medication intervention in the management of depression.[93,98,99] The drugs most commonly used to treat depression among patients with cancer and heart disease, as shown by published studies, are tricyclic antidepressants (TCAs) and selective serotonin reuptake inhibitors (SSRIs).[100] Some cancer patients are treated with serotonin–norepinephrine reuptake inhibitors (SNRIs) or nonadrenergic and specific serotonergic antidepressants (NaSSAs).

The incidence of adverse effects is lower for SSRIs than for TCAs; thus, TCAs are preferable for patients with cancer and heart disease. Studies in patients after myocardial infarction that measured depression at less than five weeks showed less benefit for antidepressants, most likely because these drugs do not reach a therapeutic level for four to eight weeks. Some epidemiological studies have shown discord between the use of antidepressant drugs and associated cardiac risk, but randomized clinical trials have demonstrated that two SSRIs, sertraline and citalopram, are safe for patients with CHD.[101] A post hoc analysis of the ENRICHD study found that the incidence of death or recurrent MI was 42% lower for patients treated with an SSRI than for depressed patients not treated with an antidepressant.[100] The Sertraline Antidepressant Heart Attack Randomized Trial (SADHART) found that treatment with sertraline reduced platelet activation more than did other antiplatelet therapies, including clopidogrel.[102]

Impact of depression on patient management ▪ Regardless of etiology, depression has the same effect on patient management. The behavioral manifestations of depression, such as loss of interest and apathy, are associated with poorer adherence to medication regimens and with poorer compliance with medical treatment regimens.[103–105] Depression also reduces patients' motivation to participate in cardiac rehabilitation programs aimed at modifying cardiac risk factors that can result in higher healthcare utilization and costs and in reduced QoL.[41,50,106]

Although currently no direct evidence suggests that screening for depression improves outcomes among cardiovascular populations, depression has been linked with increased rates of morbidity and mortality, poorer risk factor modification, lower rates of cardiac rehabilitation, and reduced QoL. Therefore, it is important to routinely assess cardiac patients for depression and to initiate appropriate intervention for those most in need of treatment and support services.

Given the evidence of the increased rates of morbidity and mortality associated with depression and anxiety among cardiac patients with cancer, these psychosocial issues must be tackled so that these outcomes can be avoided, as well as simply to relieve the suffering that accompanies depression. Because of the complicated interactions among comorbid conditions, it is necessary to develop integrated disease-management systems for depression among patients with cancer and cardiac disease and to test the cost-effectiveness of these systems. The current system of providing care to these patients is linear: that is, the patient's physical disease is treated first, and then the patient is referred for mental health care, or vice versa.[107] This model of care is neither efficient nor cost-effective. An integrated disease-management system could include screening and monitoring for depressive symptoms, educational strategies about the diagnosis, and a stepped or tiered model for direct referral to a psychiatrist or psychologist as appropriate. Because of the chronic, recurring nature of symptoms of depression and the frequent occurrence of depression in association with CVD, it is especially important to identify safe and effective treatments for patients with depression and CVD.

cardiotoxic effects of cancer therapy. Patients with heart failure experience a substantial number of symptoms as a direct or indirect result of the disease, its treatment, and its associated comorbid conditions that are often complex, multifactorial, and challenging to manage. The cardinal symptoms of dyspnea and fatigue may mask the symptoms associated with distress related to anxiety and depression. Considerable evidence confirms the high prevalence of anxiety and depression among patients with cancer and heart failure (HF).[109–111] On the other hand, distress may amplify symptoms without associated physiologic aberrations. The patient's personality traits and psychosocial issues, such as mood, anxiety, and psychotic illnesses, may also alter the perception of somatic symptoms associated with chronic illnesses such as HF.

Screening for depression is usually not routine for patients with HF. Although they are aware of the prevalence and impact of depressive disorder among cardiac patients, cardiologists usually do not use the terms *anxiety* or *depression* to label psychological issues so as not delve into psychological terminology.[69] In fact, patients themselves are often reluctant to use these terms to describe their symptoms. Instead, healthcare providers are encouraged to preferentially use the term *distress* when they suspect that unpleasant feelings or emotions are associated with somatic symptoms or may interfere with a patient's ability to cope with HF symptoms and their treatment.[69,112] A literature review has shown that somatic symptoms are strongly associated with depression and anxiety, as are certain physiologic measures.[5] It has been demonstrated that patients with HF who experience depressive symptoms often underestimate their functional limitations and their self-reports of diminished functional activity and ability.[112] One study found no statistically significant direct link between depressive symptoms and New York Heart Association (NYHA) functional class, but the results of other studies suggest that patients with symptoms of depression are more likely to be assigned to a higher NYHA class[112]: patients with depressive symptoms were more likely to be assigned to NYHA class III or IV, whereas those with no depressive symptoms were more likely to be assigned to Class II.[101]

PSYCHOSOCIAL CONSIDERATIONS FOR PATIENTS WITH CANCER AND HEART FAILURE

Many chemotherapeutic agents that are used to treat cancer have cardiotoxic adverse effects[108] that can lead to heart failure as a complication. Heart failure is a common comorbid condition among patients with cancer because of ischemic heart disease or the

▪ Disease-Management Programs for Patients with Cancer and Heart Failure

Multidisciplinary disease-management programs have evolved to become models of care that address complex issues associated with chronic disease conditions such as HF and cancer. Both conditions are generally considered progressive diseases that in certain cases can occur not as isolated processes but rather as multiple confounding factors that form barriers to successful management. Patients have complex needs: they often experience substantial physical limitations and require complicated symptom management that impedes compliance with prescribed therapy and subsequently affects their QoL. Optimal management requires a holistic approach adapted to each patient's physiologic, psychosocial, behavioral, and financial factors, all of which may influence clinical outcomes.

The effectiveness of a program for managing HF as a comorbid condition for cancer patients has not been evaluated. However, numerous studies have reported the benefits of HF disease-management programs in reducing the frequency of hospital admissions and improving QoL.[113–118] These considerations provided the rationale for the development of the Heart Success Program, a collaborative multifaceted approach to disease management for patients with cancer and heart failure at the MD Anderson Cancer Center.

Heart success program ■ Although most disease-management programs are referred to as heart *failure* programs, the MD Anderson Cancer Center chose the term *Heart Success Program* to describe its collaborative approach to the management of cancer patients with HF. The word *success* was intentionally chosen to place a positive spin on the negative stigma

associated with HF. The program was designed to provide comprehensive care across the continuum; it includes a process-improvement framework that facilitates benchmarking and outcomes measurement and provides a venue for conducting research. Currently, because there is a paucity of research data to support evidenced-based practice for cancer patients with HF, the program uses the current American College of Cardiology/American Heart Association (ACC/AHA) guidelines for the evaluation and management of these unique patients.[114] However, cancer patients were excluded from the clinical trials that provided evidence for the formulation of this guideline.

The Heart Success Program model (Figure 24-2) was established to provide a structure for the management of cancer patients with HF. The principles underpinning this model were based on fostering teamwork, collaboration, and communication across the continuum of care among the multiple disciplines involved in providing care to cancer patients with HF. Patients and their families are the core of this program's multidisciplinary team approach. Through comprehensive education, patients are empowered to take better control of their situation, and this control improves compliance with pharmacologic therapy and treatment strategies designed specifically for each patient.

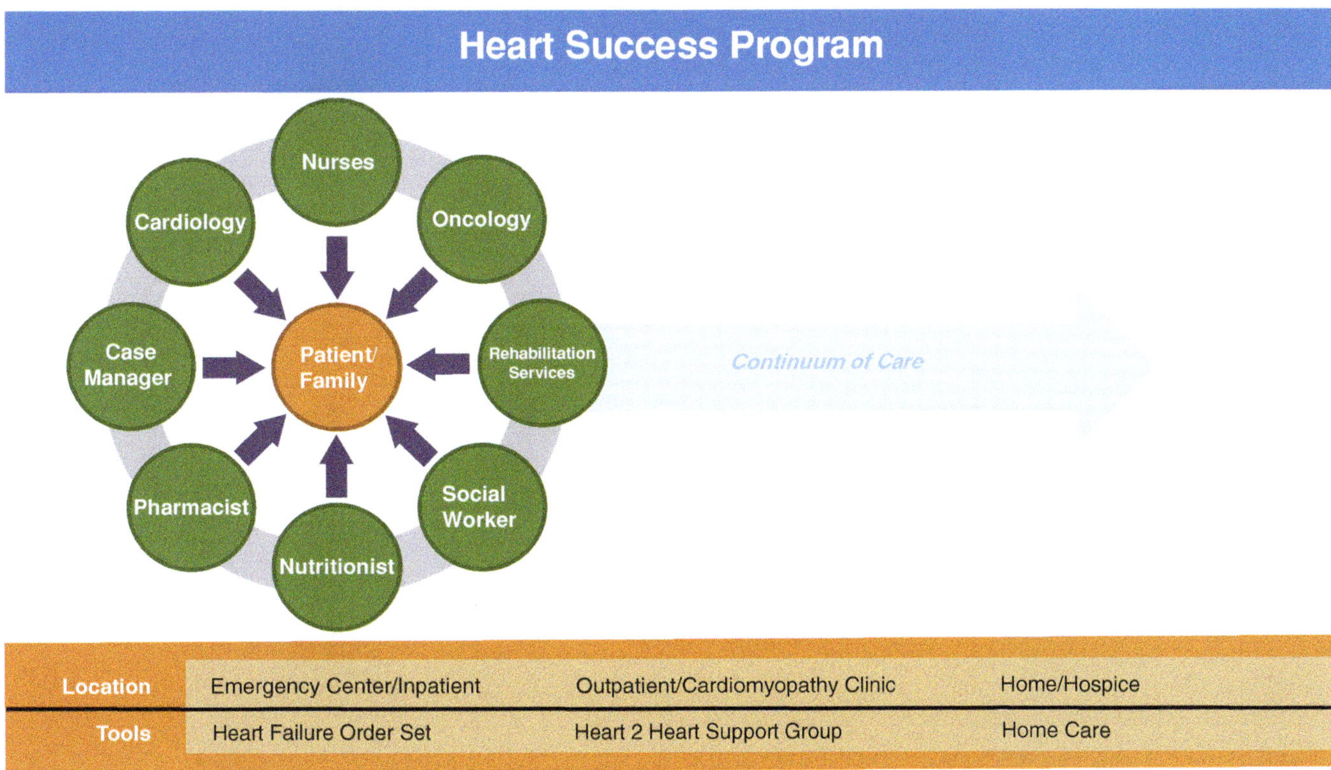

FIGURE 24-2 The heart success program model.

Draft

PLEASE USE A
BLACK INK PEN

Date: ☐☐ / ☐☐ / ☐☐
(month) (day) (year)

Subject's Initials: _____________

Study Subject #: ☐☐☐☐

Study Name: _________________________
____

Protocol #: _________________________

PI: _________________________________

Revision: 08/29/08

M. D. Anderson Symptom Inventory - Heart Failure (MDASI - HF)

Part I. How severe are your symptoms?

People with cancer frequently have symptoms that are caused by their disease or by their treatment. Patients with heart failure may have similar symptoms. We ask you to rate how severe the following symptoms have been *in the last 24 hours*. Please fill in the circle below from 0 (symptom has not been present) to 10 (the symptom was as bad as you can imagine it could be) for each item.

	NOT PRESENT 0	1	2	3	4	5	6	7	8	9	AS BAD AS YOU CAN IMAGINE 10
1. Your pain at its WORST?	○	○	○	○	○	○	○	○	○	○	○
2. Your fatigue (tiredness) at its WORST?	○	○	○	○	○	○	○	○	○	○	○
3. Your nausea at its WORST?	○	○	○	○	○	○	○	○	○	○	○
4. Your disturbed sleep at its WORST?	○	○	○	○	○	○	○	○	○	○	○
5. Your feeling of being distressed (upset) at its WORST?	○	○	○	○	○	○	○	○	○	○	○
6. Your shortness of breath at its WORST?	○	○	○	○	○	○	○	○	○	○	○
7. Your problem with remembering things at its WORST?	○	○	○	○	○	○	○	○	○	○	○
8. Your problem with lack of appetite at its WORST?	○	○	○	○	○	○	○	○	○	○	○
9. Your feeling drowsy (sleepy) at its WORST?	○	○	○	○	○	○	○	○	○	○	○
10. Your having a dry mouth at its WORST?	○	○	○	○	○	○	○	○	○	○	○
11. Your feeling sad at its WORST?	○	○	○	○	○	○	○	○	○	○	○
12. Your vomiting at its WORST?	○	○	○	○	○	○	○	○	○	○	○
13. Your numbness or tingling at its WORST?	○	○	○	○	○	○	○	○	○	○	○

Page 1 of 2

Copyright 2000 The University of Texas M. D. Anderson Cancer Center
All rights reserved.

FIGURE 24-3 The MD Anderson symptom inventory–heart failure instrument. *(continued)*

4946

Date : ☐☐ / ☐☐ / ☐☐
(month) (day) (year)

Participant Initials ☐☐

PLEASE USE
BLACK INK PEN

Study Participant # ☐☐☐

MDASI-HF: Bridging the Symptom Management Gap in Patients with Cancer and Concurrent Heart Failure to Improve Outcomes.
Protocol: 2007-0722
PI: Anecita Fadol
Revision: 01/12/2009

Time Point:
☐ Baseline ☐ 1st Month ☐ 2nd Month ☐ 3rd Month

Heart Failure (HF)

	NOT PRESENT 0	1	2	3	4	5	6	7	8	9	AS BAD AS YOU CAN IMAGINE 10
14. Your problem with **abdominal bloating** at its WORST?	○	○	○	○	○	○	○	○	○	○	○
15. Your problem with **ankle swelling** at its WORST?	○	○	○	○	○	○	○	○	○	○	○
16. Your difficulty **sleeping without adding more pillows under your head** at its WORST?	○	○	○	○	○	○	○	○	○	○	○
17. Your problem with **lack of energy** at its WORST?	○	○	○	○	○	○	○	○	○	○	○
18. Your problem with **racing heartbeat (palpitation)** at its WORST?	○	○	○	○	○	○	○	○	○	○	○
19. Your problem with **nighttime cough** at its WORST?	○	○	○	○	○	○	○	○	○	○	○
20. Your problem with **waking up at night with difficulty breathing** at its WORST?	○	○	○	○	○	○	○	○	○	○	○
21. Your problem with **sudden weight gain** at its WORST?	○	○	○	○	○	○	○	○	○	○	○

Part II. How have your symptoms interfered with your life?

Symptoms frequently interfere with how we feel and function. How much have your symptoms interfered with the following items in the last 24 hours:

	Did not Interfere 0	1	2	3	4	5	6	7	8	9	Interfered Completely 10
22. **General activity?**	○	○	○	○	○	○	○	○	○	○	○
23. **Mood?**	○	○	○	○	○	○	○	○	○	○	○
24. **Work (including work around the house)?**	○	○	○	○	○	○	○	○	○	○	○
25. **Relations with other people?**	○	○	○	○	○	○	○	○	○	○	○
26. **Walking?**	○	○	○	○	○	○	○	○	○	○	○
27. **Enjoyment of life?**	○	○	○	○	○	○	○	○	○	○	○

Page 2 of 2

Copyright 2000 The University of Texas M. D. Anderson Cancer Center
All rights reserved.

FIGURE 24-3 *(continued)* The MD Anderson symptom inventory–heart failure instrument.

Strategies for improving symptom management ■ To recognize symptoms, patients must be able to detect a change in symptom status. Early identification of symptoms and initiation of timely intervention are crucial components of a cost-effective disease-management approach for patients with chronic conditions. In fact, improvement of symptoms rather than long-term survival is a preferred therapeutic outcome for many patients with HF.[115] Unfortunately, clinical practice does not widely use symptom-based instruments to manage HF. Symptom recognition can be improved by reviewing the typical symptoms of HF with patients and their families during clinic visits.

Several educational strategies are used to reinforce patient teaching, including a video presentation about symptoms of HF; a patient-education booklet developed specifically for this patient population, called "Heart Success: A Resource Guide for Individuals Living with Cancer and Heart Failure"; a health diary including weight monitoring; and telephone follow-up. Weight monitoring is emphasized for patients with HF so that early signs of volume overload can be detected. Patients are encouraged to weigh themselves daily and to take note of a weight gain of more than two pounds per day for two consecutive days or more than five pounds in a week. Should such a weight gain occur, patients are instructed to contact their healthcare provider for guidance about the titration of diuretics. This titration is more complicated among cancer patients because nausea, vomiting, or diarrhea may occur with chemotherapy and must be taken into account before the dosage of diuretics is adjusted. Clearly, monitoring symptoms is an integral component of care for cancer patients with HF. To assist patients with such monitoring, Fadol and colleagues developed and validated the MDASI-HF (Figure 24-3), which is specifically designed for this unique patient population.[21]

The MDASI-HF is a 27-item symptom-assessment instrument for cancer patients with concurrent HF. The MDASI-HF exhibits documented reliability (Cronbach's alpha, .94 on 21 mean severity items; .89 on 13 core cancer symptoms; .83 on heart failure symptoms, and .92 on interference items. Criterion validity indicates a strong correlation of scores with measurements of both European Cooperative Oncology Group (ECOG) performance status ($r = .628$ for 21 mean severity items; .622 for 13 core items; .548 for HF items; and .645 for interference items) and NYHA functional classification ($r = .645$ for 21 mean severity items; .622 for 13 core items; .590 for 8 heart failure items; and .588 for 6 interference items). All correlations were statistically significant ($P < .0001$). The MDASI-HF can be used to identify symptom occurrence and to enhance the provider's understanding of the prevalence and severity of symptoms from the patient's perspective.

CONCLUSIONS

The psychosocial challenges that confront patients with cancer and heart disease are enormous and complicated. Awareness of the psychosocial risk profile that may increase the risk of cardiac events and the resulting pathophysiological dysfunction should enhance the clinician's opportunity for early intervention and should inform clinical judgment about which patients are at risk. The exact causes of the spectrum of symptoms that characterize these psychological issues are difficult to ascertain, given the overlap of the symptoms of cancer and HF and the adverse effects of therapy. Routine screening of these patients for psychosocial problems may enhance the opportunity for early referral and intervention.

Effective management requires a concerted effort and interdisciplinary collaboration among all healthcare providers involved in the management of these patients.

REFERENCES

1. Rozanski A, Blumenthal JA, Kaplan J. Impact of psychological factors on the pathogenesis of cardiovascular disease and implications for therapy. *Circulation*. 1999;99(16):2192–217.
2. Fann JR, Ell K, Sharpe M. Integrating psychosocial care into cancer services. *J Clin Oncol*. 2012;30(11):1178–1186.
3. Barlow DH. *Anxiety and It's Disorders: The Nature and Treatment of Anxiety and Panic*. New York, NY: The Guilford Press; 1988.
4. Kubzansky LD, Kawachi I. Going to the heart of the matter: do negative emotions cause coronary heart disease? *J Psychosom Res*. 2000;48(4–5):323–337.
5. Katon W, Lin EH, Kroenke K. The association of depression and anxiety with medical symptom burden in patients with chronic medical illness. *Gen Hosp Psychiatry*. 2007;29(2):147–155.
6. Marciniak MD, et al. The cost of treating anxiety: the medical and demographic correlates that impact total medical costs. *Depress Anxiety*. 2005;21(4):178–184.
7. McLaughlin TP, et al. Overlap of anxiety and depression in a managed care population: prevalence and association with resource utilization. *J Clin Psychiatry*. 2006;67(8):1187–1193.
8. Sareen J, et al. Disability and poor quality of life associated with comorbid anxiety disorders and physical conditions. *Arch Intern Med*. 2006;166(19):2109–2116.
9. Kroenke K, et al. Anxiety disorders in primary care: prevalence, impairment, comorbidity, and detection. *Ann Intern Med*. 2007;146(5):317–325.
10. Sareen J, et al. The relationship between anxiety disorders and physical disorders in the U.S. National Comorbidity Survey. *Depress Anxiety*. 2005;21(4):193–202.

11. Kessler RC. Epidemiology of women and depression. *J Affect Disord*. 2003;74(1):5–13.

12. Mitchell AJ, et al. Prevalence of depression, anxiety, and adjustment disorder in oncological, haematological, and palliative-care settings: a meta-analysis of 94 interview-based studies. *Lancet Oncol*. 2011;12(2):160–174.

13. Latini DM, et al. The relationship between anxiety and time to treatment for patients with prostate cancer on surveillance. *J Urol*. 2007;178(3 pt 1):826–831; discussion 831–832.

14. Andrykowski MA. The role of anxiety in the development of anticipatory nausea in cancer chemotherapy: a review and synthesis. *Psychosom Med*. 1990;52(4):458–475.

15. Greer JA, et al. Behavioral and psychological predictors of chemotherapy adherence in patients with advanced non-small cell lung cancer. *J Psychosom Res*. 2008;65(6):549–552.

16. Moser DK. Psychosocial factors and their association with clinical outcomes in patients with heart failure: why clinicians do not seem to care. *Eur J Cardiovasc Nurs*. 2002;1(3):183–188.

17. Stein MB, et al. Functional impact and health utility of anxiety disorders in primary care outpatients. *Med Care*. 2005;43(12):1164–1170.

18. Stark D, et al. Anxiety disorders in cancer patients: their nature, associations, and relation to quality of life. *J Clin Oncol*. 2002;20(14):3137–3148.

19. Kangas M, Henry JL, Bryant RA. The course of psychological disorders in the 1st year after cancer diagnosis. *J Consult Clin Psychol*. 2005;73(4):763–768.

20. Roth A, et al. Assessing anxiety in men with prostate cancer: further data on the reliability and validity of the Memorial Anxiety Scale for Prostate Cancer (MAX-PC). *Psychosomatics*. 2006;47(4):340–347.

21. Fadol A, et al. Psychometric testing of the MDASI-HF: a symptom assessment instrument for patients with cancer and concurrent heart failure. *J Card Fail*. 2008;14(6):497–507.

22. Smith EM, Gomm SA, Dickens CM. Assessing the independent contribution to quality of life from anxiety and depression in patients with advanced cancer. *Palliat Med*. 2003;17(6):509–513.

23. Raison CL, Miller AH. Depression in cancer: new developments regarding diagnosis and treatment. *Biol Psychiatry* 2003;54(3):283–294.

24. Okamura M, et al. Psychiatric disorders following first breast cancer recurrence: prevalence, associated factors and relationship to quality of life. *Jpn J Clin Oncol*. 2005;35(6):302–309.

25. Kubzansky LD, Davidson KW, Rozanski A. The clinical impact of negative psychological states: expanding the spectrum of risk for coronary artery disease. *Psychosom Med*. 2005;67(suppl 1):S10–S14.

26. Pitsavos C, et al. Anxiety in relation to inflammation and coagulation markers, among healthy adults: the ATTICA study. *Atherosclerosis*. 2006;185(2):320–326.

27. Carpeggiani C, et al. Personality traits and heart rate variability predict long-term cardiac mortality after myocardial infarction. *Eur Heart J*. 2005;26(16):1612–1617.

28. Fleet, R, et al. Myocardial perfusion study of panic attacks in patients with coronary artery disease. *Am J Cardiol*. 2005;96(8):1064–1068.

29. Rozanski A, et al. The epidemiology, pathophysiology, and management of psychosocial risk factors in cardiac practice: the emerging field of behavioral cardiology. *J Am Coll Cardiol*. 2005;45(5):637–651.

30. Carney RM, Freedland KE, Veith RC. Depression, the autonomic nervous system, and coronary heart disease. *Psychosom Med*. 2005;67(suppl 1):S29–S33.

31. Wittstein IS, et al. Neurohumoral features of myocardial stunning due to sudden emotional stress. *N Engl J Med*. 2005;352(6):539–548.

32. Bush DE, et al. Post-myocardial infarction depression. *Evid Rep Technol Assess (Summ)*. 2005;(123):1–8.

33. Sorensenf C, et al. Postmyocardial infarction mortality in relation to depression: a systematic critical review. *Psychother Psychosom*. 2005;74(2):69–80.

34. Frasure-Smith N, Lesperance F. Recent evidence linking coronary heart disease and depression. *Can J Psychiatry*. 2006;51(12):730–737.

35. Evans DL, et al. Mood disorders in the medically ill: scientific review and recommendations. *Biol Psychiatry*. 2005;58(3):175–189.

36. Bruce M. A systematic and conceptual review of post-traumatic stress in childhood cancer survivors and their parents. *Clin Psychol Rev*. 2006;26(3):233–256.

37. Fleet R, Lavoie K, Beitman BD. Is panic disorder associated with coronary artery disease? A critical review of the literature. *J Psychosom Res*. 2000;48(4–5):347–356.

38. Arthur HM. Depression, isolation, social support, and cardiovascular disease in older adults. *J Cardiovasc Nurs*. 2006;21(5 suppl 1):S2–S7; quiz S8–S9.

39. Moussavi S, et al. Depression, chronic diseases, and decrements in health: results from the World Health Surveys. *Lancet*. 2007;370(9590):851–858.

40. Frasure-Smith N, Lesperance F. Reflections on depression as a cardiac risk factor. *Psychosom Med*. 2005;67(suppl 1):S19–S25.

41. Parashar S, et al. Time course of depression and outcome of myocardial infarction. *Arch Intern Med*. 2006;166(18):2035–2043.

42. Carney RM, et al. Depression and five year survival following acute myocardial infarction: a prospective study. *J Affect Disord*. 2008;109(1–2):133–138.

43. National Cancer Institute. [cited 2009 July 11, 2009]. https://www.cancer.gov/about-cancer/coping/feelings/depression-hp-pdq/Accessed February 13, 2019.

44. Turner-Stokes L, Hassan N. Depression after stroke: a review of the evidence base to inform the development of an integrated care pathway. Part 1: diagnosis, frequency and impact. *Clin Rehabil*. 2002;16(3):231–247.

45. Hackett ML, et al. Frequency of depression after stroke: a systematic review of observational studies. *Stroke*. 2005;36(6):1330–1340.

46. Egede LE. Major depression in individuals with chronic medical disorders: prevalence, correlates and association with health resource utilization, lost productivity and functional disability. *Gen Hosp Psychiatry*. 2007;29(5):409–416.

47. de Jonge P, et al. Depressive symptoms in elderly patients predict poor adjustment after somatic events. *Am J Geriatr Psychiatry*. 2004;12(1):57–64.

48. Schulz R, Drayer RA, Rollman BL. Depression as a risk factor for non-suicide mortality in the elderly. *Biol Psychiatry*. 2002;52(3):205–225.

49. Thombs BD, et al. Prevalence of depression in survivors of acute myocardial infarction. *J Gen Intern Med*. 2006;21(1):30–38.

50. Rutledge T, et al. Depression in heart failure a meta-analytic review of prevalence, intervention effects, and associations with clinical outcomes. *J Am Coll Cardiol*. 2006;48(8):1527–1537.

51. Whooley MA. Depression and cardiovascular disease: healing the broken-hearted. *JAMA*. 2006;295(24):2874–2881.

52. Rodin G, et al. The treatment of depression in cancer patients: a systematic review. *Support Care Cancer*. 2007;15(2):123–136.

53. Pasquini M, Biondi M. Depression in cancer patients: a critical review. *Clin Pract Epidemol Ment Health*. 2007;3:2.

54. Lee KC, et al. Tamoxifen treatment and new-onset depression in breast cancer patients. *Psychosomatics*. 2007;48(3):205–210.

55. Wilson KG, et al. Depression and anxiety disorders in palliative cancer care. *J Pain Symptom Manage*. 2007;33(2):118–129.

56. McCaffrey JC, et al. Alcoholism, depression, and abnormal cognition in head and neck cancer: a pilot study. *Otolaryngol Head Neck Surg*. 2007;136(1):92–97.

57. Miovic M, Block S. Psychiatric disorders in advanced cancer. *Cancer*. 2007;110(8):1665–1676.

58. Pilote L, et al. A comprehensive view of sex-specific issues related to cardiovascular disease. *Cmaj*. 2007;176(6):S1–S44.

59. Mallik S, et al. Depressive symptoms after acute myocardial infarction: evidence for highest rates in younger women. *Arch Intern Med*. 2006;166(8):876–883.

60. Palesh OG, et al. A longitudinal study of depression, pain, and stress as predictors of sleep disturbance among women with metastatic breast cancer. *Biol Psychol*. 2007;75(1):37–44.

61. Carney RM, et al. Depression, heart rate variability, and acute myocardial infarction. *Circulation*. 2001;104(17):2024–2028.

62. Lesperance F, et al. The association between major depression and levels of soluble intercellular adhesion molecule 1, interleukin-6, and C-reactive protein in patients with recent acute coronary syndromes. *Am J Psychiatry*. 2004;161(2):271–277.

63. Empana JP, et al. Contributions of depressive mood and circulating inflammatory markers to coronary heart disease in healthy European men: the Prospective Epidemiological Study of Myocardial Infarction (PRIME). *Circulation*. 2005;111(18):2299–2305.

64. Taylor CB, et al. Psychophysiological and cortisol responses to psychological stress in depressed and non-depressed older men and women with elevated cardiovascular disease risk. *Psychosom Med*. 2006;68(4):538–546.

65. Serebruany VL, et al. Enhanced platelet/endothelial activation in depressed patients with acute coronary syndromes: evidence from recent clinical trials. *Blood Coagul Fibrinolysis*. 2003;14(6):563–567.

66. Sherwood A, et al. Impaired endothelial function in coronary heart disease patients with depressive symptomatology. *J Am Coll Cardiol*. 2005;46(4):656–659.

67. Thomas AJ, Kalaria RN, O'Brien JT. Depression and vascular disease: what is the relationship? *J Affect Disord*. 2004;79(1–3):81–95.

68. Everson-Rose SA, Lewis TT. Psychosocial factors and cardiovascular diseases. *Annu Rev Public Health*. 2005;26:469–500.

69. Feinstein RE, et al. A national survey of cardiovascular physicians' beliefs and clinical care practices when diagnosing and treating depression in patients with cardiovascular disease. *Cardiol Rev*. 2006;14(4):164–169.

70. Glassman AH, et al. Onset of major depression associated with acute coronary syndromes: relationship of onset, major depressive disorder history, and episode severity to sertraline benefit. *Arch Gen Psychiatry*. 2006;63(3):283–288.

71. Lichtman JH, et al. Depression and coronary heart disease: recommendations for screening, referral, and treatment: a science advisory from the American Heart Association Prevention Committee of the Council on Cardiovascular Nursing, Council on Clinical Cardiology, Council on Epidemiology and Prevention, and Interdisciplinary Council on Quality of Care and Outcomes Research: endorsed by the American Psychiatric Association. *Circulation*. 2008;118(17):1768–1775.

72. Walker J, et al. Performance of the Hospital Anxiety and Depression Scale as a screening tool for major depressive disorder in cancer patients. *J Psychosom Res*. 2007;63(1):83–91.

73. Teunissen SC, et al. Are anxiety and depressed mood related to physical symptom burden? A study in hospitalized advanced cancer patients. *Palliat Med*. 2007;21(4):341–346.

74. Pasquini M, et al. Detection and treatment of depressive and anxiety disorders among cancer patients: feasibility and preliminary findings from a liaison service in an oncology division. *Depress Anxiety*. 2006;23(7):441–448.

75. Guo Y, et al. The diagnosis of major depression in patients with cancer: a comparative approach. *Psychosomatics*. 2006;47(5):376–384.

76. Lloyd-Williams M, Shiels C, Dowrick C. The development of the Brief Edinburgh Depression Scale (BEDS) to screen for depression in patients with advanced cancer. *J Affect Disord*. 2007;99(1–3):259–264.

77. Diwan S, et al. Effectiveness of cervical epidural injections in the management of chronic neck and upper extremity pain. *Pain Physician*. 2012;15(4):E405–E434.

78. Beck AT, et al. An inventory for measuring depression. *Arch Gen Psychiatry*. 1961;4:561–571.

79. Rush AJ, et al. The Inventory of Depressive Symptomatology (IDS): psychometric properties. *Psychol Med*. 1996;26(3):477–486.

80. Strik JJ, et al. Sensitivity and specificity of observer and self-report questionnaires in major and minor depression

following myocardial infarction. *Psychosomatics*. 2001; 42(5):423–428.

81. Gilbody S, et al. Screening for depression in medical settings with the Patient Health Questionnaire (PHQ): a diagnostic meta-analysis. *J Gen Intern Med*. 2007;22(11):1596–1602.

82. Stafford L, Berk M, Jackson HJ. Validity of the Hospital Anxiety and Depression Scale and Patient Health Questionnaire-9 to screen for depression in patients with coronary artery disease. *Gen Hosp Psychiatry*. 2007;29(5):417–424.

83. McManus D, Pipkin SS, Whooley MA. Screening for depression in patients with coronary heart disease (data from the Heart and Soul Study). *Am J Cardiol*. 2005;96(8):1076–1081.

84. Davidson KW, et al. Assessment and treatment of depression in patients with cardiovascular disease: national heart, lung, and blood institute working group report. *Ann Behav Med*. 2006;32(2):121–126.

85. Whooley MA, et al. Case-finding instruments for depression. Two questions are as good as many. *J Gen Intern Med*. 1997;12(7):439–445.

86. Kroenke K, Spitzer RL, Williams JB. The PHQ-9: validity of a brief depression severity measure. *J Gen Intern Med*. 2001;16(9):606–613.

87. Williams S, Dale J. The effectiveness of treatment for depression/depressive symptoms in adults with cancer: a systematic review. *Br J Cancer*. 2006;94(3):372–390.

88. Fulcher CD, et al. Putting evidence into practice: interventions for depression. *Clin J Oncol Nurs*. 2008;12(1):131–140.

89. Osborn RL, Demoncada AC, Feuerstein M. Psychosocial interventions for depression, anxiety, and quality of life in cancer survivors: meta-analyses. *Int J Psychiatry Med*. 2006;36(1):13–34.

90. Wulsin LR. Is depression a major risk factor for coronary disease? A systematic review of the epidemiologic evidence. *Harv Rev Psychiatry*. 2004;12(2):79–93.

91. van Dixhoorn J, White A. Relaxation therapy for rehabilitation and prevention in ischaemic heart disease: a systematic review and meta-analysis. *Eur J Cardiovasc Prev Rehabil*. 2005;12(3):193–202.

92. Rees K, et al. Exercise based rehabilitation for heart failure. *Cochrane Database Syst Rev*. 2004(3):CD003331.

93. National Health and Medical Research Council, Australia. Psychosocial Clinical Practice Guidelines: Support and Counselling for Women with Breast Cancer. 2000. http://www.nhmrc.gov.au/guidelines/publications/cp61

94. National Health and Medical Research Council, Australia. Psychosocial Clinical Practice Guidelines for the Psychosocial care of Adults with Cancer. 2003. http://www.nhmrc.gov.au/guidelines/publications/cp90

95. Berkman LF, et al. Effects of treating depression and low perceived social support on clinical events after myocardial infarction: the Enhancing Recovery in Coronary Heart Disease Patients (ENRICHD) randomized trial. *JAMA*. 2003;289(23):3106–3116.

96. Thase ME, et al. Cognitive therapy versus medication in augmentation and switch strategies as second-step treatments: a STAR*D report. *Am J Psychiatry*. 2007;164(5):739–752.

97. Lesperance F, et al. Effects of citalopram and interpersonal psychotherapy on depression in patients with coronary artery disease: the Canadian Cardiac Randomized Evaluation of Antidepressant and Psychotherapy Efficacy (CREATE) trial. *JAMA*. 2007;297(4):367–379.

98. National Comprehensive Cancer Network. NCCN Guidelines for Supportive Care. Version 3.2012. http://www.nccn.org/professionals/physician_gls/pdf/distress.pdf

99. American Psychiatric Association. http://psychiatry-online.org/guidelines

100. Taylor CB, et al. Effects of antidepressant medication on morbidity and mortality in depressed patients after myocardial infarction. *Arch Gen Psychiatry*. 2005;62(7):792–798.

101. Sherwood A, et al. Relationship of depression to death or hospitalization in patients with heart failure. *Arch Intern Med*. 2007;167(4):367–373.

102. Serebruany VL, et al. Relationship between release of platelet/endothelial biomarkers and plasma levels of sertraline and N-desmethylsertraline in acute coronary syndrome patients receiving SSRI treatment for depression. *Am J Psychiatry*. 2005;162(6):1165–1170.

103. Gehi A, et al. Depression and medication adherence in outpatients with coronary heart disease: findings from the Heart and Soul Study. *Arch Intern Med*. 2005;165(21):2508–2513.

104. Rieckmann N, et al. Persistent depressive symptoms lower aspirin adherence after acute coronary syndromes. *Am Heart J*. 2006;152(5):922–927.

105. DiMatteo MR, Lepper HS, Croghan TW. Depression is a risk factor for noncompliance with medical treatment: meta-analysis of the effects of anxiety and depression on patient adherence. *Arch Intern Med*. 2000;160(14):2101–2107.

106. Ziegelstein RC, et al. Patients with depression are less likely to follow recommendations to reduce cardiac risk during recovery from a myocardial infarction. *Arch Intern Med*. 2000;160(12):1818–1823.

107. Kathol RG, Clarke D. Rethinking the place of the psyche in health: toward the integration of health care systems. *Aust N Z J Psychiatry*. 2005;39(9):816–825.

108. Yeh ET, Bickford CL. Cardiovascular complications of cancer therapy: incidence, pathogenesis, diagnosis, and management. *J Am Coll Cardiol*. 2009;53(24):2231–2247.

109. Scherer M, et al. Psychological distress in primary care patients with heart failure: a longitudinal study. *Br J Gen Pract*. 2007;57(543):801–807.

110. Haworth JE, et al. Prevalence and predictors of anxiety and depression in a sample of chronic heart failure patients with left ventricular systolic dysfunction. *Eur J Heart Fail*. 2005;7(5):803–808.

111. Konstam V, Moser DK, De Jong MJ. Depression and anxiety in heart failure. *J Card Fail*. 2005;11(6):455–463.

112. Skotzko CE. Symptom perception in CHF: (why mind matters). *Heart Fail Rev*. 2009;14(1):29–34.

113. McAlister FA, et al. Multidisciplinary strategies for the management of heart failure patients at high risk for admission: a systematic review of randomized trials. *J Am Coll Cardiol*. 2004;44(4):810–819.

114. Hunt SA, et al. 2009 Focused update incorporated into the ACC/AHA 2005 Guidelines for the Diagnosis and Management of Heart Failure in Adults A Report of the American College of Cardiology Foundation/American Heart Association Task Force on Practice Guidelines Developed in Collaboration With the International Society for Heart and Lung Transplantation. *J Am Coll Cardiol*. 2009;53(15):e1–e90.

115. Stanek EJ, et al. Preferences for treatment outcomes in patients with heart failure: symptoms versus survival. *J Card Fail*. 2000;6(3):225–232.

116. Radloff LS. The CES-D scale for research in the general popluation. *Applied Psychological Measurement*. 1977;1(3):385–401.

117. Hamilton M. A rating scale for depression. *J Neurol Neurosurg Psychiatry*. 1960;23:56–62.

118. McNair DM, Lorr M, Doppleman LF. *POMS Manual for the Profiles of Mood States*. San Diego: Educational and Testing Service; 1971.

119. Kroenke K, Spitzer RL, Williams JB. The Patient Health Questionnaire-2: validity of a two-item depression screener. *Med Care*. 2003;41(11):1284–1292.

25 Preoperative Assessment of the Cancer Patient for Noncardiovascular Surgery

Marc A. Rozner ▪ Shital Vachhani ▪ Teresa Moon ▪ January Y. Tsai*

INTRODUCTION/BACKGROUND

In 1846, four years after Crawford Long publicly demonstrated the use of ether anesthetic, the field of surgical anesthesia became accepted by the medical profession and the general public. This new specialty was viewed as an innovative step in the treatment of surgical patients, and with the development of this specialty came studies of complications and untoward events associated with the use of anesthetic agents. Since then, efforts to improve anesthetic (and therefore surgical) safety have included the following: 1) advances in anesthetic pharmacology, 2) better understanding of the pharmacokinetics and pharmacodynamics of anesthetic agents, 3) development and use of "smart" monitoring devices, 4) improved training of personnel, 5) reliable automated drug delivery systems, and 6) preoperative evaluation and management by an anesthesiologist of patients scheduled to undergo a surgical procedure.

From the perspective of an anesthesiologist, it is not surprising that preoperative anesthesia evaluation and risk assessment have become an integral part of the anesthetic management of a patient about to undergo a surgical procedure. Few physicians, other than anesthesiologists, have spent time in the operating room monitoring patients' vital signs and physiologic function while controlled trauma (i.e., surgery) is taking place. Furthermore, many consultant physicians and medical care providers believe, albeit without confirmatory data, that multiple preoperative consultations and interventions will reduce or eliminate perioperative complications. Yet rarely does a preoperative consultation identify new disease that affects perioperative outcome.[1]

Additionally, anesthesiologists and surgeons are less likely than cardiologists to believe that a cardiologist's advice will have a positive impact on perioperative management, but surgeons have reported a greater obligation to follow a cardiologist's recommendations, even when the surgeon disagrees with those recommendations.[2] Despite the results of published studies, many practitioners continue in their previously learned ways, believing that some "study" does not apply to their patients. As an example, some consultants continue to recommend placement of pulmonary artery catheters, which may actually harm patients.[3-5] Sometimes, a nonanesthesiologist consultant will recommend one anesthetic choice over another, but there remains a paucity of controlled studies to validate any such statement.

At many hospitals, especially tertiary care centers, the anesthesia preoperative clinic is often the last stop for any patient on the journey to any procedure that will require an anesthetic. Frequently, these visits take place more than 24 hours before surgery. For many tertiary care centers, the anesthesia preoperative clinic serves to bring the entire patient's medical history together. This behavior results from the usual tertiary care practice; that is, patients receive nontertiary care from their primary (and sometimes far-away) practitioners. Many of these patients have no institutional physician other than their surgeon, and, at places such as a cancer center, the patients bring records related to their cancer but not to their other medical problems. Because cancer patients frequently have other diseases in addition to their cancer, the preoperative anesthesiologist is charged with reviewing the medical history, performing a limited physical examination, determining whether comorbid diseases have been addressed satisfactorily, and arranging appropriate tests and consultations when indicated. As a result, the request for cardiology consultation often arises from this preoperative center visit.

For many years, anesthesiologists have been asked to assist in the assignment of risk for an operative procedure. This practice appears to have been "codified" in 1941 with the development of the New York Society of Anesthesiologists physical status scale, first published by Saklad.[6] Although the physical status score of the American Society of Anesthesiologists

*The editors note with sadness the passing of Dr. Marc Rozner before the revision of this chapter was completed. They acknowledge and appreciate the contributions of Drs. Vachhani, Moon, and Tsai in completing the update of this important contribution to *Cancer and the Heart*.

TABLE 25-1   The American Society of Anesthesiologists physical status classification system

P1	A normal healthy patient
P2	A patient with mild systemic disease without functional impairment
P3	A patient with severe systemic disease; functional impairment is present
P4	A patient with severe systemic disease that is a constant threat to life
P5	A moribund patient who is not expected to survive without the operation
P6	A declared brain-dead patient whose organs are being removed for donation

Source: From American Society of Anesthesiologists.[7]

(ASA PS) (Table 25-1) has been modified a few times and is sometimes used by nonanesthesiologists,[7–9] the ASA PS scale is fundamentally static and global in nature. It takes into account a large number of factors, many of which are subtle, and most of which are "known" only to anesthesiologists. The ASA PS offers little guidance for identifying or modifying individual risk factors for the perioperative period. Nevertheless, it serves the specialty well, and its predictive value for operative mortality in a contemporary dataset endures.[10,11]

The goal of the anesthesia-provided preoperative visit is to ascertain the patient's comorbid conditions, to attempt to modify the identified risk factors to optimize the patient's medical condition within a reasonable timeframe, and sometimes to discuss modifying the patient's treatment plan with the patient's other providers. For the cancer patient, all of these activities often take place within 2 to 3 days of the patient's initial presentation to the cancer center, and the patient undergoes surgery shortly thereafter. Many of the patients who present to MD Anderson Cancer Center for a second opinion also enter the operating room within a few days of their initial visit.

Most anesthesiologists believe that previous treatments for malignancy—whether surgical, chemotherapeutic, or radiotherapeutic—can affect a patient's comorbid diseases and surgical risk. Cardiologists have begun to formally address this field as well, as exemplified in a monograph by Albini and associates regarding the cardiotoxicity of cancer therapy in the setting of cardiovascular disease.[12,13] Additionally, certain tumors can cause physiologic disturbances by virtue of their secretory potentials or paraneoplastic syndromes, or because of simple mass effect (e.g., increased intracranial pressure from a space-occupying mass). Adverse effects due to secretory products include "tumor fever" from cytokine release,[14] hypotension and bronchospasm from metastatic carcinoid tumors,[15] and hypermetabolic syndromes from thyroid cancers[16] or pheochromocytoma.[17] Adverse effects of paraneoplastic syndromes include Eaton-Lambert syndrome,[18] cancer-associated retinopathy,[19] hypercalcemia of malignancy syndrome,[20] and complex regional pain syndromes.[21]

GOALS OF PREOPERATIVE EVALUATION

The evaluation and preoperative preparation of the cancer patient must always balance the urgency of operative intervention with the need to treat an intercurrent medical problem that will clearly affect the patient's perioperative course.[22] After all, patients with pancreatic cancer who have a mean life expectancy of 12 months and concurrent unstable coronary artery disease may not benefit from a Whipple procedure (pancreatectomy) if they experience a perioperative myocardial infarction and die shortly after the surgical procedure. Thus, issues in the preoperative anesthesia assessment of a cancer patient are similar to those in any preoperative clinic but frequently include extensive discussions with other physicians who will care for the patient.

The goals of preoperative anesthesia assessment are as follows:

1. Obtain pertinent information about patients' medical and social history and relevant records and tests, perform a physical examination according to anesthesia needs, determine whether further testing or consultation is required, assign risk (ASA PS Classification), and take steps to modify risks when possible;

2. Discuss clinically significant abnormal findings that are likely to increase patients' perioperative risk with the surgeon and, if need be, an oncologist, cardiologist, internist, or neurologist relative to risks and benefits of investigation, treatment, and the resulting delay(s). Occasionally, surgery is planned for pregnant patients, necessitating the inclusion of an obstetrician;

3. Educate patients (and their family members) about the various forms of anesthetics that could be used during the procedure, the benefits and risks of these choices, and the reasons for choosing one over the others. For example, recent Enhanced Recovery After Surgery

initiatives involve regional techniques and some nonopioid medications as part of a multimodal approach to pain management. This modality, including risks and benefits, is described in detail to the patient during the preoperative visit, because Enhanced Recovery programs have been associated with statistically significant decreases in length of hospital stay and in the incidence of hospital-acquired infections[23];

4. Prepare patients (and their family members) for entrance into the operating environment by explaining the equipment used, the personnel expected to be present, and the reasons that surgery can take longer than scheduled. For patients with clinically significant comorbid conditions, discussions of possible adverse events, intensive care unit (ICU) admission, and palliative measures that may be needed also take place;

5. Review consent to administer an anesthetic from patients or guardians;

6. Ensure that the minimal guidelines for laboratory screening (Table 25-2) and testing (Table 25-3) have been met;

7. Determine whether a pregnancy test will be required for women of childbearing age who have not been surgically sterilized. Although denial of pregnancy to the twentieth week of gestation occurs in 1 of 475 deliveries,[24] most preoperative anesthesiologists accept and document an immediate denial to the question "Is there any chance that you could be pregnant?" without laboratory testing. For patients who cannot provide this assurance, a test for urine levels of beta human chorionic gonadotropin (beta-hCG) is ordered. Although routine testing has been advocated by some clinicians,[25] it can lead to inappropriate surgical delays.[26] There is also a small risk (1 per 1,000 to 10,000 tests) of false-positive results,[27,28] a risk that may be increased in the setting of some malignancies[29] and can delay a surgical procedure. Management of a positive result from a pregnancy test includes the possible delay of the surgical procedure because of the need for repeat testing to ensure a rising titer;

8. Document the visit in a form acceptable to any institutional needs and to any governmental or commercial payer;

9. Provide guidance for the day-of-surgery use of ambulatory drugs. Because there is ample evidence that both angiotensin-converting enzyme (ACE)-inhibiting drugs and angiotensin receptor antagonists can provoke profound hypotension during the induction of anesthesia,[30-32] patients are often advised not to take these drugs on the day of surgery. For example, the multicenter prospective VISION study by Roshanov and colleagues evaluated 14,687 patients and found that withholding this class of drugs before major noncardiac surgery was associated with decreased mortality rates and fewer postoperative vascular events.[33] Nevertheless, the current American College of Cardiology/American Heart Association (ACC/AHA) guideline states, with Class IIa evidence, that the continuation of ACE inhibitors or angiotensin-receptor blockers is reasonable. Many centers ask patients to

---

TABLE 25-2 Minimal preoperative screening guidelines at MD Anderson Cancer Center

TEST	APPLICATION
CBC	Any surgical procedure with a risk of major bleeding or if previous CBC values are older than 1 year
BUN/Cr	Any operation involving the kidneys, ureters, bladder, or urethra. Values are acceptable for 3 months in the absence of changes in clinical condition or treatment regimens
ECG	Any patient at least 55 years old, within 1 year of surgery, or as indicated by medical history
T&S	Any surgical procedure with a risk of major bleeding (e.g., any body cavity entrance, all open intracranial neurosurgery, excision of a clinically significant sarcoma mass)

CBC, Complete blood count (hematological) to include white blood cell count, hemoglobin level, and platelet counts

BUN/Cr, Determination of the blood urea nitrogen level and the creatinine concentration

ECG, Standard 12-lead electrocardiogram

T&S, A type and screen test to include blood type and Rh determination as well as an indirect Coombs test.

TABLE 25-3 Preoperative diagnostic testing guidelines at MD Anderson Cancer Center

TEST	APPLICATION
Electrolytes, BUN/Cr	Hypertension Use of diuretics Use of digitalis Bowel obstruction History of renal dysfunction Diabetes Values up to six months old are acceptable in the absence of changes in clinical condition or chemotherapeutic treatment regimens
Glucose	Reasonable evidence that the glucose concentration is < 300 mg/dl at the time of surgery for patients with diabetes or patients undergoing steroid therapy
Coagulation Studies	Prothrombin (PT) and activated partial thromboplastin time (aPTT) studies are indicated for patients taking anticoagulant medications or for patients with a history of coagulation problems
Platelet Aggregation Study	Use of Clopidogrel (Plavix) within 5 days of surgery
ECG	History of coronary artery disease or congestive heart failure (unless there is a documented ECG result within the previous 6 months and no new symptoms) Clinically significant risk factors for perioperative ischemia, such as hypertension and diabetes mellitus Abnormal physical examination findings suggesting cardiac abnormalities
Chest X-ray	Signs or symptoms of active pulmonary disease

refrain from taking oral and injectable hypoglycemic agents, especially insulin glargine (Lantus) and insulin detemir (Levemir), so that undesired hypoglycemia can be avoided during surgery. For patients scheduled to undergo a procedure requiring nothing by mouth (NPO) status on the day before surgery (e.g., embolization to reduce bleeding), the doses of these injectable insulins and other long-acting oral hypoglycemic agents may be reduced or withheld for two nights. There are many new antithrombotic drugs with evolving recommendations for length of avoidance before elective surgery. Many clinicians refer to the perioperative guidelines of Douketis and co-workers.[34] In general, the risk of bleeding is weighed against the risk of detrimental thrombotic events after cessation of therapy, and discontinuation of therapy for elective surgery should be as brief as possible.[35]

CHEMOTHERAPY AND RADIATION THERAPY

Many patients with cancer have undergone chemotherapy, radiation therapy (RT), or both during their cancer treatment, yet few available studies provide guidance about preoperative evaluation, anesthetic choice, or anesthetic management for these patients. Nevertheless, there are clear relationships between particular types of chemotherapy or RT and certain physiologic derangements.

Chemotherapy

Although chemotherapy is discussed extensively in other chapters, certain issues recur that can cause surgical delays or exacerbate comorbid conditions. Many chemotherapeutic agents are associated with the development of cardiomyopathy or other clinically significant cardiovascular events, and these effects may remain subclinical until the patient is put under stress.[12] For the cancer patient with any history of heart failure or other unexplained dyspnea on exertion, a complete cardiology evaluation seems prudent. The condition of these patients seems to improve when they are taking regimens such as beta blockers, ACE inhibitors, and diuretics.[36–38] Some patients may also benefit from the initiation of cardiac pacing or cardiac resynchronization therapy (CRT).[39] Whether delaying elective surgery to institute these therapies will improve perioperative outcome has not been studied, but for patients with significant cardiomyopathy the benefits of beta blockade can be identified within 14 days of initiation of this therapy.[40]

Other agents with specific perioperative issues include the following:

Anthracyclines: Anthracyclines are commonly used in the neoadjuvant treatment of breast cancer and can cause considerable dose-dependent myocyte injury that may not become evident for months to years after the first exposure.[41] Early adverse effects include dysrhythmia, repolarization changes, pericarditis, and myocarditis. Late cardiotoxicity involves cardiomyopathy and heart failure. These agents should be considered for patients with unexpected or unexplained perioperative electrocardiogram (ECG) changes or poor functional status.

Bleomycin: The use of this agent is complicated primarily by pulmonary toxic effects, which include interstitial pneumonitis and pulmonary fibrosis.[41] In his review intended for an anesthesiology audience, Mathes states that the incidence of pulmonary toxic effects increases with creatinine clearance lower than 35 ml/min, concurrent cyclophosphamide use, or a history of chest irradiation.[42] The US Food and Drug Administration (FDA) black box warning states that the incidence of pulmonary fibrosis increases among elderly patients or those taking a total dose of more than 400 units. Although perioperative oxygen restriction has been suggested to reduce postoperative pulmonary morbidity, Donat and Levy found that intravenous fluid management, including transfusion, appears to be the most important factor affecting postoperative pulmonary morbidity and overall clinical outcome, regardless of oxygen administration.[43]

Platins: Cisplatin (and to a lesser extent, carboplatin and oxaliplatin) can induce nephrotoxicity manifested by elevations in blood urea nitrogen (BUN), creatinine, and serum uric acid levels. Magnesium wasting and hypomagnesemia can be found in a substantial number of patients treated with cisplatin.[44] Preoperative evaluation and preparation include demonstration of appropriate electrolyte balance, probably including a magnesium level, to ascertain the degree of renal insult. Prolonged Q-T intervals and rapid atrial fibrillation have been described after cisplatin infusion,[45] and renal impairment in the presence of antifungal therapy (a common treatment in cancer hospitals) can produce prolonged Q-T intervals and cardiac arrhythmias.[46] Because several case reports now describe the development of acute thrombosis in the setting of cisplatin administration, increased attention to perioperative deep vein thrombosis (DVT) may be warranted.[47–51]

5-Fluorouracil (FU)/capecitabine: Administration of 5-FU and its oral prodrug, capecitabine, have reportedly resulted in hemodynamically significant bradycardia.[52] A handful of anesthesia procedures at MD Anderson Cancer Center have been aborted because of sudden and profound intraoperative bradycardia without a clear inciting event. Some of those patients received temporary transvenous pacemakers to allow completion of surgery. Certainly, a specific combination of anesthetic agents alone could potentially cause this response. Because we are currently unable to predict which patients are at higher risk of bradycardia, perioperative recognition of this clinical possibility and the need for rapid establishment of an adequate pulse are necessary.

Thalidomide: Thalidomide appears to cause clinically significant sinus bradycardia in a small number of patients,[52–54] and this condition may necessitate pacemaker implantation, especially in the perioperative period. Other adverse events most frequently associated with thalidomide administration include somnolence, fatigue, peripheral neuropathy, and thromboembolism.[55]

■ Radiation Therapy

Radiation therapy is an integral part of cancer management, and it is often combined with chemotherapy and surgery. Many cancer patients undergo staged preoperative chemotherapy and radiotherapy 4 to 6 weeks before definitive surgery. Two specific issues related to RT deserve attention in any preoperative evaluation.

First, the myocardium or coronary arteries can suffer damage from radiation delivered to the chest. The potential adverse effects of mediastinal irradiation are numerous and include coronary artery disease, pericarditis, cardiomyopathy, valvular disease, and conduction abnormalities (see also Chapter 7).[56,57] A significantly higher risk of death due to ischemic heart disease has been reported for patients treated with RT to the chest for Hodgkin's disease and breast cancer,[58] although some investigators continue to argue with these findings, because it appears that the nature of the malignancy (e.g., breast cancer versus lymphoma), the treatment protocol, and the total radiation dose to the heart play an important role in these adverse events.[59,60] Damage to the endothelial cells in the coronary arteries has been proposed as one mechanism for heart disease after chest irradiation. Factors affecting the extent of coronary artery perfusion defects in radiation-induced coronary artery disease include the percentage of the left ventricle irradiated, concurrent hormonal treatment, and a history of hypercholesterolemia.[61] The risk of radiotherapy increases when it is combined with doxorubicin and the other anthracycline agents, because they appear to exert a synergistic toxic effect on the myocardium.[58,62]

The assessment of heart disease for patients who have undergone RT begins with an evaluation of their functional status (see next section). This assessment can include stress myocardial perfusion tests, echocardiography to evaluate pericardial or valvular disease, and echocardiography or multiple-gated acquisition (MUGA) scans to evaluate left ventricular ejection fraction (LVEF) when indicated. But no study has documented the usefulness of any of these tests in directing any specific interventions that should be instituted solely because of the surgical procedure.[1]

The second issue relates to patients who have undergone irradiation of the head and neck area, which can produce both trismus and limited neck extension. Although some patients will continue to demonstrate a normal airway on physical examination, it is often difficult to perform intubation on these patients in the operating room. Therefore, alternatives to direct laryngoscopy must be readily available for these patients. At our institution, many of these patients undergo elective fiberoptic intubation, indirect intubation, or videolaryngoscopy. Cardiologists should consider this issue of unanticipated difficult airway if they are planning conscious sedation for a procedure such as transesophageal echocardiography (TEE), because these patients have an increased incidence of obstructive sleep apnea,[63] which may predispose them to an increased incidence of complications.[64]

IMMUNOTHERAPY

Immunomodulators or immune checkpoint inhibitors are generally better tolerated than their cytotoxic conventional chemotherapeutic counterparts. Common adverse effects involve the gastrointestinal tract, skin, endocrine system, liver, and lungs. The few available reports of cardiac toxicity describe autoimmune myocarditis.[65] Rates of myocarditis in Phase I trials range from 1 of 207 patients to 1 of 475 patients who subsequently died of myocarditis.[66,67] Others report autoimmune myocarditis leading to left ventricular dysfunction and congestive heart failure (CHF),[65] Takotsubo syndrome,[68] or pericarditis.[69] Current package inserts for these immunomodulators do not include specific recommendations for monitoring or managing potential cardiac toxicities.

CARDIAC EVALUATION OF THE CANCER PATIENT WITH HEART DISEASE

The purpose of surgical risk assessment is to provide physicians and patients with information that will assist them in weighing the relative risks and benefits of proposed treatment plans. The previously mentioned ASA PS score has not, however, been validated for cancer patients, and it does not take into account their comorbid conditions, the physiologic issues surrounding exposure to chemotherapy and radiotherapy, or the complexity of the surgical procedure that will result. For example, multiple previous abdominal surgeries[70] or cancer therapy[71] can lead to the formation of adhesions, which will increase the operative time of abdominal surgery, exacerbate bowel swelling, and increase intraoperative fluid requirements. All of these conditions may lead to larger numbers of postoperative problems. Some of these issues are now addressed in the American College of Surgeons National Surgical Quality Improvement Program (ACS NSQIP)[72] universal surgical risk estimation tool, which is based on data from 393 hospitals and more than 1.4 million patients (www.riskcalculator.facs.org). This risk calculator includes variables such as ASA PS score, presence of disseminated cancer, and functional status. It reports "your risk, average risk, and chance of outcome" information that allows clinicians and patients to easily estimate perioperative risk and facilitate decision making.[73] The Eastern Cooperative Oncology Group (ECOG) has also introduced a six-point score for cancer population outcomes based on performance status. In a review of more than 2500 patients after cancer surgery, Young and associates suggest that the ASA PS score could, in fact, be used as a proxy for ECOG scores in the surgical setting.[74] Nevertheless, these predictive tools refer to the general cancer population instead of to patients with specific cancers. Also not well studied are the effects of noncancer comorbid conditions (e.g., coronary artery disease, cardiomyopathy, brittle diabetes, etc.) on the outcomes of cancer therapy, whether surgical or medical. This issue is discussed by Adachi and colleagues, whose case-control study found that overweight patients with gastric cancer exhibit a higher incidence of hypertension and diabetes, longer operative times, and a higher incidence of cancer recurrence and death.[75]

As improved anesthetic agents and techniques have reduced the complication rates associated with anesthesia, predicting and preventing perioperative morbidity and mortality due to cardiac disease has become the Holy Grail for many cardiologists, anesthesiologists, and internists. One of the earliest reports to assign levels of risk associated with cardiac disease in surgical patients was published by Goldman and co-workers in 1977, and it is likely that every cardiologist, anesthesiologist, internist, and surgeon who is interested in the classification of perioperative risk has read this paper many times.[76]

The current working document for preoperative evaluation of the cardiac patient for noncardiac surgery was published by the ACC/AHA in 1996[77] and now in its fourth revision, published in 2014.[78] Provided the patient does not require an emergent procedure and is not currently experiencing an acute coronary event, the 2014 ACC/AHA guideline recommends a stepwise approach that combines the assessment of patient comorbid conditions and surgical risk with the NSQIP calculator and then categorizes patients as either low risk (< 1% risk of major adverse cardiac events [MACE], such as that associated with cataract surgery) or elevated risk (> 1% risk of MACE). This binary choice eliminates the Intermediate category, which is usually conservatively treated as a high-risk group anyway. The new guideline also clarifies surgical timing: emergent, in which life or limb is threatened and surgery should occur within 6 hours; time-sensitive (most cancer patients), in which a delay of more than 1 to 6 weeks will negatively affect outcome; and elective, in which surgery can be delayed for as long as a year without repercussions.

Although these guidelines are well-accepted, much of medical practice is based on "usual and customary behavior," and the use of guidelines to change this physician practice remains difficult.[79,80] At the Anesthesiology Assessment Center, we continue to see patients who have undergone some sort of cardiac evaluation (stress testing, echocardiography, coronary angiography, percutaneous coronary intervention, or cardiac revascularization surgery), even though they did not meet the guideline criteria for such testing, and they are unlikely to benefit from the intervention. These scenarios are complicated by financial and medical issues that are beyond the scope of this document. It is important to keep in mind, however, that every medical test and intervention has a potential

downside, a point of particular significance to the patient with an unfavorable stress test result who has a complication during follow-up or during clean cardiac catheterization, or the patient for whom a delay in cancer surgery resulted in the spread of their disease. The ACC/AHA Guideline Update for exercise testing states that the rate of myocardial infarction or death as a result of exercise stress testing is 1 per 2500 tests.[81] In their review of exercise testing, Surawicz and Knilans cite a variety of studies suggesting that for every 20,000 exercise tests there are at least one death and 16 nonfatal complications requiring hospitalization.[82] Recently, the concept of the "lifetime attributable risk of cancer" due to the radiation delivered during these tests has surfaced, because these risks remain clinically significant.[83]

Finally, patients who do not exhibit ischemia during a stress test are often considered low risk. However, some of these patients have clinically significant cardiac disease factors and experience clinically significant cardiac morbidity or mortality rates[84,85]; therefore, additional medical management may be indicated. Although previous guidelines encouraged the initiation of therapy with a beta blocker, the current ACC/AHA guideline specifically recommends that beta blocker therapy not be initiated on the day of surgery.[78]

Preoperative Echocardiographic Evaluation

According to ACC guidelines, the routine use of echocardiography to determine ejection fraction should be avoided, because little additional information can be gained from these studies.[78] Nevertheless, many perioperative consultants continue to order echocardiograms or MUGA scans in the setting of exposure to cardiotoxic chemotherapy, especially drugs of the anthracycline class. These studies can delay a patient's surgical procedure, and such testing of patients with adequate functional status, normal findings from a cardiac examination, and no history of cardiomyopathy should be discouraged.

Serum Biomarkers

For patients who may have a cardiomyopathy, serologic screening for elevated levels of B-type natriuretic peptide (BNP) may be more efficient than referring the patient for echocardiography or radionuclide testing.[86,87] BNP testing appears to be a low-cost, rapid assessment with considerable prognostic value,[88–91] although little guidance is available about preoperative treatment of elevated serum concentrations of BNP, and poor renal function reduces the usefulness of BNP testing.[92] No studies have examined the sensitivity and specificity of this test for patients who have received chemotherapy. However, Zustovich and associates found elevated BNP levels in patients with non–small-cell lung cancer after chemotherapy and suggest that elevated BNP levels could indicate subclinical cardiac damage.[93] BNP also seems to be a useful predictor of postoperative complications such as postthoracotomy atrial fibrillation.[94] High serum levels of C-reactive protein (CRP) has been shown to predict survival in renal cell cancer patients and may be a useful adjunct in predicting perioperative complications,[95] although other risk factors, including coronary artery calcium score, probably offer no additional benefit.[96]

■ Stratification for Preoperative Cardiac Stress Testing

The ACC/AHA Guidelines provide expert opinion about the referral of patients for stress testing.[78] These criteria take into account patient risk factors (Table 25-4), patient functional status, and operative risk factors in an effort to predict which patients should undergo preoperative noninvasive cardiac stress testing. However, the weight attributed to each risk factor is unknown, as is the specific algorithm used to create the derived value. The introduction of the Surgeon Adjustment Score allows modification of the risk calculator result on the basis

of the surgeon's subjective assessment.[73] Although the gestalt of a seasoned surgeon with a history of excellent clinical outcomes may be unparalleled, the resulting prediction is no longer evidence-based or reproducible.

Several reports suggest that the use of the ACC guidelines reduces laboratory testing and the costs associated with preoperative evaluation without increasing the complication rate.[97] On the other hand, another report suggests that the criteria used in these guidelines for selecting patients for noninvasive cardiac stress testing are too broad and lead to increased testing without benefit.[98] Furthermore, one of the most common reasons for ordering stress testing is abnormal findings from an electrocardiogram; these findings do not appear to be related to the risk of a postoperative cardiac complication.[99] The most complicated issues relating to these guidelines and cancer patients include previous exposure to cardiotoxic chemotherapy, because these patients may be markedly deconditioned and have cardiomyopathy unrelated to coronary artery disease. In addition, patients who have undergone chest wall (mediastinal or breast) irradiation may exhibit accelerated development of coronary artery disease. As a result, patients who have undergone cardiotoxic chemotherapy or chest wall irradiation are more likely to undergo noninvasive stress testing, but, again, stress testing appears to be indicated only when patients' functional status has been impaired (i.e., inability to perform 4 metabolic

TABLE 25-4 Patient risk assignments at MD Anderson Cancer Center

ACTIVE CARDIAC CONDITIONS	CLINICAL RISK FACTORS
Decompensated CHF	History of ischemic heart disease
Unstable coronary syndromes	Stable CAD
-recent MI (< 30 days)	-after CABG
-unstable angina	-after PCI
-large "area of risk" by noninvasive study	Stable angina
Clinically significant arrhythmia	Previous MI
-high-grade AV block	History of CHF or compensated CHF
-ventricular arrhythmias with concomitant heart disease	History of cerebrovascular disease
-uncontrolled ventricular rate in supraventricular arrhythmia	Diabetes
	Renal insufficiency
	History of cardiotoxic chemotherapy
Severe valvular disease	History of chest wall irradiation

Source: Criteria have been adapted from the American College of Cardiology/American Heart Association (ACC/AHA) guideline update for perioperative cardiovascular evaluation for noncardiac surgery, 2017[68] for use at the Anesthesiology Assessment Center at The University of Texas MD Anderson Cancer Center.

AV, atrioventricular; CABG, coronary artery bypass grafting; CAD, coronary artery disease; CHF, congestive heart failure; MI, myocardial infarction; PCI, percutaneous coronary artery intervention (either simple angioplasty or stent placement).

equivalents [METs] of exercise) or when they are scheduled for major surgery.

Cardiopulmonary exercise testing (CPET) can be a useful tool for evaluating functional capacity before elevated-risk surgery for patients who are unable to participate in traditional tests or when it is difficult to ascertain their functional capacity from their history. Peak oxygen uptake and oxygen update at the anaerobic threshold may predict perioperative adverse events, but the lack of conclusive scientific data precludes the routine adoption of CPET at this time.[78,100]

Preoperative Cardiac Stress Testing

Although preoperative cardiac stress testing is not the domain of anesthesiologists, the preoperative consultant (who often *is* an anesthesiologist) must determine whether a stress test is indicated, and the consultant anesthesiologist should be able to reasonably interpret stress test data. Preoperative stress testing often delays the patient's surgical procedure, and it may not actually provide the intended information. For example, Pryma and colleagues retrospectively reviewed patient results during a 3-month period.[101] During this interval, 162 patients (7.7% of the surgical population) underwent some sort of stress testing. Over the first 7 postoperative days, 4 of these patients experienced cardiac events, but only 1 of them demonstrated an abnormal preoperative stress test result.

Furthermore, it is not entirely clear that invasive management of occlusive coronary artery disease actually improves perioperative outcome.[102,103] The following are important points that should be remembered and possibly communicated to the operative staff.

1. Heart rate is the principal determinant of myocardial oxygen demand.

2. Unlike most other tissues in the body, the heart extracts nearly all of the oxygen from the blood that passes through the myocardium (i.e., there is little or no oxygen reserve, unlike the ability of other vascular beds to increase oxygen extraction).

3. The only way to meet an increased oxygen demand by the myocardium is to increase oxygen delivery, which depends upon cardiac output (stroke volume and heart rate), hemoglobin concentration, oxygen saturation, and arterial partial pressure of oxygen Pao_2 (Pao_2 becomes increasingly important as the hemoglobin concentration declines)

In tests that increase the heart rate in order to provoke myocardial ischemia (exercise, dobutamine), a maximal heart rate for age (MHRA) and a target heart rate should be calculated. A retrospective study suggests that negative results from dobutamine stress echocardiography have a 100% negative predictive value for perioperative cardiac events, provided that no resting wall motion abnormality is present, regardless of the achieved heart rate.[104]

The reporting of stress testing has not been standardized, and shortcuts in reporting are frequently taken. The scribbled note "Normal stress test, cleared for surgery" on a prescription pad from any consultant is inadequate. At a minimum, every stress test report should include the following:

Indication for testing
Type of test and evaluation
Duration of exercise, if exercise was used
Heart rate achieved and percentage of MHRA (if heart rate tests)
Reason for stopping the test
Patient's symptoms during the test
Interpretation of test
Ejection fraction, wall motion, and end-systolic and end-diastolic volumes (nuclear study or echocardiography)
Follow-up recommendations guided by the test results

As with any test, stress testing can yield false-negative or false-positive results. Factors commonly associated with false-positive results from a treadmill stress test include severe anemia, left ventricular hypertrophy, hypertension, hypokalemia, and antiarrhythmic drug use (e.g., digoxin, quinidine, and procainamide).[82,105] Factors associated with normal stress test results despite the presence of coronary artery disease (CAD) include recent (< 24 hour) caffeine consumption,[106] inadequate heart rate response, or balanced ischemia.[85] Because of interpretive complexities, anesthesiologists and surgeons should be part of the discussion when multiple options (some nonsurgical) are available for a patient. Any patient whose exercise duration is less than 4 minutes upon reaching 80% MHRA should be evaluated for cardiomyopathy (rather than simple deconditioning) by nuclear scan or echocardiography before an elective procedure, especially for high-risk surgical procedures.

Contraindications to exercise testing generally include poor exercise conditioning (debilitation), lower-extremity peripheral vascular disease, severe hypertension, and clinically significant valvular stenosis. In general, if a stress test is indicated to rule out

CAD, one can identify a suitable testing modality on the basis of patient characteristics.

It is important to remember that stress testing will usually indicate which patients have hemodynamically significant (> 70%) stenosis in an epicardial vessel. Small-vessel disease (such as that present in patients with diabetes), left ventricular hypertrophy, elevated left ventricular end-diastolic pressure, or an epicardial vessel stenosis of less than 70% can produce abnormal stress test results without positive findings from angiography. Thus, the patient with abnormal stress test results but a coronary angiogram that shows no lesions amenable to intervention should be considered at higher risk than the patient with normal stress test results, especially when multiple risk factors for CAD are present (e.g., male sex, advanced age, family history of CAD, history of hypertension, sedentary lifestyle, and diabetes).

Finally, the patient with stable disease and one or more epicardial vessel lesions in the occlusive range of 50% to 70% often experience supply versus demand inequality, especially at high heart rates, which can be present postoperatively. Additionally, many of these patients also have underlying systolic dysfunction, diastolic dysfunction, or both, which can be exacerbated by postoperative hypotension, anemia, hypercarbia, hypoxemia, or hypertension, leading to myocardial infarction (MI).[107]

PREOPERATIVE REVASCULARIZATION

Although determining the presence of epicardial disease by using some form of cardiac stress testing seems to be relatively straightforward, the treatment of patients with a variety of lesions is not. There is considerable disagreement among practitioners regarding the use of medical management, percutaneous coronary intervention (PCI), and coronary artery bypass grafting (CABG) to treat these patients.[108] Many studies, however, shed considerable light on this issue. A multicenter study by McFalls and associates involved 462 Veterans Administration patients with clinically significant angiographic epicardial lesions (but without unstable coronary disease, left main lesions, significant cardiomyopathy, or aortic stenosis) who were scheduled for abdominal or infrainguinal vascular surgery. The patients were randomly assigned to PCI, CABG, or medical management before surgery.[109] The researchers found no difference in the postoperative 30-day rate of MI (12% intervention group vs. 14% medical management group, $P = 0.37$) and no difference in mortality rates at 32 months after surgery

(22% intervention group vs. 23% medical management group, $P = 0.92$). They did find, however, that the vascular surgical event was significantly delayed for the intervention group compared to the medical management group. They also reported 10 deaths in the intervention group and 1 death in the medical management group after random assignment but before vascular surgery, and that 21 patients who were originally assigned to medical management underwent a coronary artery intervention procedure during the study's follow-up period.

The recent placement of a coronary artery stent has been shown to substantially increase the risk of perioperative MI and death,[110,111] especially for patients who have undergone an inadequate course of dual antiplatelet therapy (DAPT).[112] A retrospective review of 899 cases showed that the risk of ischemic e vents after noncardiac surgery within 30 days of placement of a bare metal stent (BMS) was highest within 30 days of placement and lowest 90 days after placement.[113] Similarly, for 520 patients with drug eluting stents (DES) (Taxus, Boston Scientific; Cypher, Johnson and Johnson, Cordis; Endeavor, Medtronic; Xience, Abbott), the risk of ischemic events gradually declined over time, with a rate of 6.4% during the first 90 days after placement and a rate of 3.3% 365 days after placement.[114] The 2016 ACC/AHA guideline for the duration of DAPT among patients with CAD emphasizes the importance of weighing the risk of stent thrombosis against the risk of delaying surgery. Acknowledging that the newer-generation DES are associated with a lower risk of stent thrombosis, the duration of DAPT has also been modified to "optimally at least 6 months." The Patterns of Non-adherence to Antiplatelet Regimens in Stented Patients (PARIS) registry shows that optimal continuation of DAPT (6 months) is not associated with an increased incidence of MACE.[115] The duration of DAPT for patients with a BMS has not changed (30 days).[116]

THE CANCER PATIENT WITH A CARDIAC IMPLANTED ELECTRICAL DEVICE (CIED)

As noted above, improvements in surgical techniques, anesthetic care, and the management of comorbid diseases have increased the number of cancer patients who are considered good candidates for surgical procedures. This willingness also extends to patients with CIEDs. At the MD Anderson Cancer Center's Anesthesiology Assessment Center, approximately 340 patients with traditional pacemakers and 130 patients with implanted defibrillators are seen per year, composing almost 2% of all preoperative patients in the center.[117]

For this patient population, indications for implantation of a CIED include traditional reasons such as bradycardia and diseases of the atrioventricular node. Some patients receive a cardiac device because of a complication associated with their cancer or cancer therapy: e.g., thalidomide-related bradycardia, sino-atrial block from epirubicin, or heart failure from anthracycline exposure. Expanding implant indications for traditional pacemakers, defibrillators, anti–atrial fibrillation devices, and CRT devices will probably increase the number of cancer patients who have an implanted device.[118–121] Because the arrhythmia burden of anthracycline-induced dilated cardiomyopathy is similar to that of dilated cardiomyopathy in the absence of chemotherapy, Mazur and associates suggest that the clinical management of these patients may also be similar.[122] Perioperative patients with CIEDs require special consideration due to their combination of physical status and exposure to physiologic trespass and device dysfunction from sources of electromagnetic interference. In general, Kramer and associates found that the presence of a CIED is an independent predictor of frailty and poorer functional status.[123] Although few other studies have evaluated perioperative outcomes for patients with CIEDs, of 65 operative patients with pacemakers, Pili-Fluori and colleagues report postoperative MI in 7 patients, LV failure in 2 patients, and clinically significant arrhythmia in 2 patients, with 2 deaths (3%).[124] In addition, Trankina and co-workers performed a retrospective chart review and found that 32 of 169 patients (19%) exhibited changes in pacemaker status after surgery, which they attributed to electrosurgical cautery exposure.[125] These changes in device behavior may result in patient exposure to untreated malignant arrhythmias. Whether these findings are unique to cancer patients or are applicable to all presurgical patients remains unknown. Also, no systematic evaluation of any relationship between chemotherapy and pacemaker behavior has been published, but there is one report of a pacing threshold increase in the setting of chemotherapy.[126]

The 2011 Heart Rhythm Society/American Society of Anesthesiologists Expert Consensus Statement provides guidance for the perioperative management of patients with CIEDs.[127] The timing of preoperative and postoperative checks is described, as are situations requiring intraoperative reprogramming. All CIEDs should be comprehensively evaluated both before and after surgery, especially when an electrosurgical unit is used. At the MD Anderson Cancer Center, patients present to the Cardiac Device Clinic where the CIED Team evaluates the device and formulates a perioperative plan with the anesthesia and surgical teams. Several groups advocate simplified algorithms to minimize unnecessary device interrogation and reprogramming.[128,129] Avoidance of overly onerous requirements for busy clinicians tasked with the care of these patients should be weighed against the possibility that failure to obtain basic information about a patient's device may result in harm. Rozner and colleagues reported that 33% of 172 patients had not had an appropriate, timely visit to their cardiologist prior to their first presentation for surgery.[130] They also found that a comprehensive evaluation of each pacemaker revealed a pacemaker problem in 16% (27 patients) of first-visit patients. In one-third of these problems (9 patients), a pacemaker replacement for battery depletion was needed prior to the patient's elective procedure, and 4 of these 9 patients had a note from a cardiologist indicating that the patient was "cleared for anesthesia and surgery." Likewise, there was a "cleared for surgery" note from an internal medicine specialist in 3 of the 9 patients.

Establishing baseline normal CIED function is important not only to maintain a consistent level of care for patients who may not otherwise seek routine, recommended follow-up, but it also provides operating room staff with the necessary information to anticipate and appropriately manage the effects of commonly used AV nodal blocking drugs, electrosurgery, and other sources of electromagnetic interference that can result in urgent or emergent bradycardia or asystole in patients with pacemakers or inappropriate shock in patients with defibrillators.[131] In an ongoing protocol, we have noticed that many perioperative patients have misidentified CIEDs (i.e., defibrillators identified as pacemakers), in some instances resulting in puzzling device behavior. While most institutions and hospitals cannot feasibly maintain an active Cardiac Device Clinic, ours also serves to provide education and clinical support for our staff who want to provide quality, safe patient care but whose academic expertise may not lie in the evolving field of implanted cardiac devices. Finally, the postoperative assessment is important to ensure normal postoperative device function, to identify events that may have gone unnoticed intraoperatively, such as large volume blood transfusion resulting in elevated pacing threshold or inappropriate shock resulting in battery depletion, and to reprogram devices that may have needed preoperative programming changes. As CIED technology improves, the indications for immediate postoperative checks with apparent appropriate device function may change.

NEOPLASMS WITH SPECIAL PREOPERATIVE NEEDS

As mentioned above, certain cancers, especially endocrine neoplasms, can create or exacerbate underlying cardiovascular disease. It seems fitting, then, in this chapter, to briefly review these issues.

Pheochromocytomas arise from neural crest tissues, and they often become symptomatic owing to their secretory products. Although mainly arising in the adrenal glands, pheochromocytomas can be found anywhere along the sympathetic chain. There have been occasional reports of these tumors in the heart, primarily in the right atrium.[132,133] These neoplasms can arise spontaneously[134] or as a part of a syndrome or familial basis.[135] Because many of these tumors secrete catecholamines, patients can exhibit cardiac arrhythmia, ventricular hypertrophy, or outright cardiomyopathy.[136] Preoperative assessment thus includes a detailed cardiovascular history and physical, and echocardiography may demonstrate left ventricular hypertrophy[137] or the appearance of hypertrophic obstruction.[138] It appears that ventricular hypertrophy resolves with removal of the tumor.

Preoperative management consists of blood pressure and heart rate control. Traditionally, peripheral alpha blockade has been advocated to control blood pressure, although there remains controversy about the choice of drug. A retrospective review by Kocak and colleagues reported 49 patients treated with phenoxybenzamine, prazosin, or doxazocin with no difference in outcome, although this review had little power to detect differences.[139] Most anesthesiologists expect that a beta blocker will be added to the patient's drug regimen to control heart rate after adequate alpha blockade has been established, and many prefer to use shorter-acting cardioselective agents. The duration of preoperative treatment is unclear; Russell and associates have suggested that 5 to 7 days of treatment is adequate.[140] Intraoperative issues are primarily attributed to volume contraction from prolonged hypertension, hemodynamic swings, and heart rate issues until the neoplasm outflow vessels are ligated. Hypotension after the withdrawal of catecholamines is treated with vasopressors and volume expansion.

Recent advances in surgical technique and pharmacologic agents, however, have been postulated to minimize hemodynamic insults and perioperative mortality rates. Lentschener and co-workers reviewed studies published during the past 15 years and reported a perioperative mortality rate of close to zero when surgery is performed by experienced teams.[141] Fewer ICU admissions are reported with minimally invasive resection and decreased operative times.

Some studies have shown no significance difference in stroke volume variation between patients who receive prophylactic intravenous hydration and those who do not, a finding suggesting that hypotension after adrenal resection is due to decreased vascular tone and not to intravascular volume status. Additionally, intraoperative use of calcium channel blockers with a short half-life allows rapid titration of therapy. In some cases, careful intraoperative monitoring and management of blood pressure has not resulted in differences in intraoperative hemodynamics and mortality rates even when preoperative alpha- and beta-blocking drugs were not administered.

Metastatic carcinoid tumors are another secretory tumor with cardiovascular effects. In general, carcinoid tumors of the portal circulation do not appear to cause symptoms until the metabolic capacity of the liver is overwhelmed. Of course, carcinoid tumors can also arise in the lungs, the ovaries, or the rectum. Carcinoid heart disease, consisting primarily of right-sided valvular disease, occurs in many patients with the carcinoid syndrome.[142] Although tricuspid insufficiency is the most common finding, both pulmonic and tricuspid stenosis have been observed. Left-sided valvular lesions are rare.[143] Because carcinoid-associated valvular disease and right heart failure are important predictors of postoperative morbidity and mortality, it seems prudent to obtain, at a minimum, echocardiographic evaluation of the patient with carcinoid syndrome.[15] Histamine-releasing pharmacologic agents should generally be avoided during the perioperative period.[144] Some anesthesiologists believe that intraoperative monitoring with TEE is more useful than such monitoring with a pulmonary artery catheter, but no evidence exists upon which to base any recommendations. Drugs that can be used to treat perioperative bronchospasm and hypotension include somatostatin, cyproheptadine, ketanserin, and methysergide,[145,146] although ketanserin is not available in the United States. Of these agents, octreotide may be associated with the lowest perioperative complication rate.[15]

The patient with an intracardiac mass is often challenging to the operating room team. These tumors are most often diagnosed by transthoracic echocardiography or TEE during an evaluation for heart failure symptoms.[147] Masses in the heart can be thrombus, vegetation, or metastatic lesions from breast, lung, melanoma, or lymphoma, or they can be primary cardiac tumors.[148] For malignant tumors involving the heart, there are no studies evaluating the role of adjuvant therapy. Surgical management nearly always includes cardiopulmonary bypass and cardiac arrest, and intraoperative management frequently includes the use of TEE.[149] Autotransplantation is sometimes indicated.

SUMMARY

The preoperative evaluation of a patient with cancer must take into account the severity of the cancer disease, chemotherapeutic exposure, radiation exposure, and comorbid nonmalignant diseases. In addition, many cancer operations are part of a staged intervention for these patients; that is, the surgical procedure must be performed in a timely manner to complement the delivery of chemotherapy or radiation therapy. In the cancer patient, the discovery of untreated comorbid disease must lead to a discussion between the patient's oncologist, the surgeon, and the specialist who will be treating the comorbid condition. In such a setting, it is not appropriate to proceed to the operating room without such a discussion, nor is it appropriate to delay any procedure without speaking to the patient's other caregivers. As Ewer points out, the goal of every physician should be to achieve the best outcome with the lowest risk.[22] Although anesthesiologists prefer to anesthetize patients only after any coexisting medical conditions have been successfully mitigated, some cancer operations, while not true emergencies, cannot wait for interventions that could delay the procedure and allow the cancer to spread.

REFERENCES

1. Katz RI, Cimino L, Vitkun SA. Preoperative medical consultations: impact on perioperative management and surgical outcome. *Can J Anaesth*. 2005;52(7):697–702.
2. Katz RI, Barnhart JM, Ho G, Hersch D, Dayan SS, Keehn L. A survey on the intended purposes and perceived utility of preoperative cardiology consultations. *Anesth Analg*. 1998;87(4):830–836.
3. Sandham JD, Hull RD, Brant RF, et al. A randomized, controlled trial of the use of pulmonary-artery catheters in high-risk surgical patients. *N Engl J Med*. 2003;348(1):5–14.
4. Barone JE, Tucker JB, Rassias D, Corvo PR. Routine perioperative pulmonary artery catheterization has no effect on rate of complications in vascular surgery: a meta-analysis. *Am Surg*. 2001;67(7):674–679.
5. Bonazzi M, Gentile F, Biasi GM, et al. Impact of perioperative haemodynamic monitoring on cardiac morbidity after major vascular surgery in low risk patients. A randomised pilot trial. *Eur J Vasc Endovasc Surg*. 2002;23(5):445–451.
6. Saklad M. Grading of patients for surgical procedures. *Anesthesiology*. 1941;2:281–284.
7. American Society of Anesthesiologists. ASA physical status classification system. https://www.asahq.org/resources/clinical-information/asa-physical-status-classification-system Accessed February 24, 2018.
8. Culver DH, Horan TC, Gaynes RP, et al. Surgical wound infection rates by wound class, operative procedure, and patient risk index. National Nosocomial Infections Surveillance System. *Am J Med*. 1991;91(3B):152S–157S.
9. Goldmann DA, Weinstein RA, Wenzel RP, et al. Strategies to prevent and control the emergence and spread of antimicrobial-resistant microorganisms in hospitals. A challenge to hospital leadership. *JAMA*. 1996;275(3):234–240.
10. Vacanti CJ, VanHouten RJ, Hill RC. A statistical analysis of the relationship of physical status to postoperative mortality in 68,388 cases. *Anesth Analg*. 1970;49(4):564–566.
11. Hopkins TJ, Raghunathan K, Barbeito A, et al. Associations between ASA Physical Status and postoperative mortality at 48 h: a contemporary dataset analysis compared to a historical cohort. *Perioperative Medicine*. 2016;5(29). https://doi.org/10.1186/s13741-016-0054-z.
12. Yeh ET, Bickford CL. Cardiovascular complications of cancer therapy: incidence, pathogenesis, diagnosis, and management. *J Am Coll Cardiol*. 2009;53(24):2231–2247.
13. Albini A, Pennesi G, Donatelli F, Cammarota R, De Flora S, Noonan DM. Cardiotoxicity of anticancer drugs: the need for cardio-oncology and cardio-oncological prevention. *J Natl Cancer Inst*. 2010;102(1):14–25.
14. Liaw CC, Chen JS, Wang CH, Chang HK, Huang JS. Tumor fever in patients with nasopharyngeal carcinoma: clinical experience of 67 patients. *Am J Clin Oncol*. 1998;21(4):422–425.
15. Kinney MA, Warner ME, Nagorney DM, et al. Perianaesthetic risks and outcomes of abdominal surgery for metastatic carcinoid tumours. *Br J Anaesth*. 2001;87(3):447–452.
16. Zanella A. Noninfective complications of blood transfusions. *Tumori*. 2001;87(2):S20–S23.
17. Plouin PF, Duclos JM, Soppelsa F, Boublil G, Chatellier G. Factors associated with perioperative morbidity and mortality in patients with pheochromocytoma: analysis of 165 operations at a single center. *J Clin Endocrinol Metab*. 2001;86(4):1480–1486.
18. Lin JT, Lachmann E. Lambert-Eaton myasthenic syndrome: a case report and review of the literature. *J Womens Health (Larchmt)*. 2002;11(10):849–855.
19. Ohguro H, Nakazawa M. Pathological roles of recoverin in cancer-associated retinopathy. *Adv Exp Med Biol*. 2002;514:109–124.
20. Hurtado J, Esbrit P. Treatment of malignant hypercalcaemia. *Expert Opin Pharmacother*. 2002;3(5):521–527.
21. Mekhail N, Kapural L. Complex regional pain syndrome type I in cancer patients. *Curr Rev Pain*. 2000;4(3):227–233.
22. Ewer MS. Specialists must communicate in complex cases. *Intern Med World Rep*. 2001;16(5):17.
23. Grant MC, Yang D, Wu CL, et al. Impact of enhanced recovery after surgery and fast track surgery pathways on healthcare-associated infections: results from a systematic review and meta-analysis. *Ann Surg*. 2017(1);265(1):68–79.
24. Wessel J, Endrikat J, Buscher U. Frequency of denial of pregnancy: results and epidemiological significance of a 1-year prospective study in Berlin. *Acta Obstet Gynecol Scand*. 2002;81(11):1021–1027.

25. Wheeler M, Coté CJ. Preoperative pregnancy testing in a tertiary care children's hospital: a medico-legal conundrum. *J Clin Anesth*. 1999;11(1):56–63.

26. Manley S, de Kelaita G, Joseph NJ, Salem MR, Heyman HJ. Preoperative pregnancy testing in ambulatory surgery. Incidence and impact of positive results. *Anesthesiology*. 1995;83(4):690–693.

27. Committee on Gynecologic Practice. The American College of Obstetricians and Gynecologists. ACOG. Committee opinion: number 278, November 2002. Avoiding inappropriate clinical decisions based on false-positive human chorionic gonadotropin test results. *Obstet Gynecol*. 2002;100(5 pt 1):1057–1059.

28. Esfandiari N, Goldberg JM. Heterophile antibody blocking agent to confirm false positive serum human chorionic gonadotropin assay. *Obstet Gynecol*. 2003;101(5 pt 2): 1144–1146.

29. Bussar-Maatz R, Weissbach L, Dahlmann N, Mann K. [The "false positive" tumor marker in malignant testicular tumor]. *Urologe A*. 1993;32(3):177–182. [German]

30. Coriat P, Richer C, Douraki T, et al. Influence of chronic angiotensin-converting enzyme inhibition on anesthetic induction. *Anesthesiology*. 1994;81(2):299–307.

31. Coriat P. [Interferences between angiotensin-converting enzyme inhibitors and spinal anesthesia]. *Cah Anesthesiol*. 1994;42(6):727–733. [French]

32. Behnia R, Molteni A, Igi R. Angiotensin-converting enzyme inhibitors: mechanisms of action and implications in anesthesia practice. *Curr Pharm Des*. 2003;9(9):763–776.

33. Roshanov PS, Rochwerg B, Patel A, et al. Witholding versus continuing angiotensin-converting enzyme inhibitors or angiotensin II receptor blockers before noncardiac surgery. *Anesthesiology*. 2017;126:16–27.

34. Douketis JD, Spyropoulos AC, Spencer FA, et al. Perioperative management of antithrombotic therapy. *Chest*. 2012;141(2):e326S–e350S. doi:10.1378/chest.11–2298

35. Chen L, Bracey AW, Radovancevic R, et al. Clopidogrel and bleeding in patients undergoing elective coronary artery bypass grafting. *J Thorac Cardiovasc Surg*. 2004;128(3):425–431.

36. Keefe DL. Anthracycline-induced cardiomyopathy. *Semin Oncol*. 2001;28(4 Suppl 12):2–7.

37. Mukai Y, Yoshida T, Nakaike R, et al. Five cases of anthracycline-induced cardiomyopathy effectively treated with carvedilol. *Intern Med*. 2004;43(11):1087–1088.

38. Cardinale D, Colombo A, Lamantia G, et al. Anthracycline-induced cardiomyopathy: clinical relevance and response to pharmacologic therapy. *J Am Coll Cardiol*. 2010;55(3):213–220.

39. Moss AJ, Hall WJ, Cannom DS, et al. Cardiac-resynchronization therapy for the prevention of heart-failure events. *N Engl J Med*. 2009;361(14):1329–1338.

40. Krum H, Roecker EB, Mohacsi P, et al. Carvedilol prospective randomized cumulative survival (COPERNICUS) study group. Effects of initiating carvedilol in patients with severe chronic heart failure: results from the COPERNICUS Study. *JAMA*. 2003;289(6):712–718.

41. Feldman D, Vander Els N. Bleomycin-induced lung injury. *UpToDate*. https://www.uptodate.com/contents/bleomycin-induced-lung-injury

42. Mathes DD. Bleomycin and hyperoxia exposure in the operating room. *Anesth Analg*. 1995;81(3):624–629.

43. Donat SM, Levy DA. Bleomycin associated pulmonary toxicity: is perioperative oxygen restriction necessary? *J Urol*. 1998;160(4):1347–1352.

44. Kintzel PE. Anticancer drug-induced kidney disorders. *Drug Saf*. 2001;24(1):19–38.

45. Tassinari D, Sartori S, Drudi G, et al. Cardiac arrhythmias after cisplatin infusion: three case reports and a review of the literature. *Ann Oncol*. 1997;8(12):1263–1267.

46. Albengres E, Le Louët H, Tillement JP. Systemic antifungal agents. Drug interactions of clinical significance. *Drug Saf*. 1998;18(2):83–97.

47. Dieckmann KP, Gehrckens R. Thrombosis of abdominal aorta during cisplatin-based chemotherapy of testicular seminoma - a case report. *BMC Cancer*. 2009;9(1):459–462.

48. Cheng E, Berthold DR, Moore MJ, Duran I. Arterial thrombosis after cisplatin-based chemotherapy for metastatic germ cell tumors. *Acta Oncol*. 2009;48(3):475–477.

49. Morlese JF, Jeswani T, Beal I, Wylie P, Bell J. Acute ventricular and aortic thrombosis post chemotherapy. *Br J Radiol*. 2007;80(952):e75–e77.

50. Grenader T, Shavit L, Ospovat I, Gutfeld O, Peretz T. Aortic occlusion in patients treated with Cisplatin-based chemotherapy. *Mt Sinai J Med*. 2006;73(5):810–812.

51. Apiyasawat S, Wongpraparut N, Jacobson L, Berkowitz H, Jacobs LE, Kotler MN. Cisplatin induced localized aortic thrombus. *Echocardiography*. 2003;20(2):199–200.

52. Kaur A, Yu SS, Lee AJ, Chiao TB. Thalidomide-induced sinus bradycardia. *Ann Pharmacother*. 2003;37(7-8):1040–1043.

53. Singhal S, Mehta J. Thalidomide in cancer: potential uses and limitations. *BioDrugs*. 2001;15(3):163–172.

54. Rajkumar SV, Gertz MA, Lacy MQ, et al. Thalidomide as initial therapy for early-stage myeloma. *Leukemia*. 2003;17(4):775–779.

55. Matthews SJ, McCoy C. Thalidomide: a review of approved and investigational uses. *Clin Ther*. 2003;25(2):342–395.

56. Darby SC, Cutter DJ, Boerma M, et al. Radiation-related heart disease: current knowledge and future prospects. *Int J Radiat Oncol Biol Phys*. 2010;76(3):656–665.

57. Adams MJ, Hardenbergh PH, Constine LS, Lipshultz SE. Radiation-associated cardiovascular disease. *Crit Rev Oncol Hematol*. 2003;45(1):55–75.

58. Basavaraju SR, Easterly CE. Pathophysiological effects of radiation on atherosclerosis development and progression, and the incidence of cardiovascular complications. *Med Phys*. 2002;29(10):2391–2403.

59. Vallis KA, Pintilie M, Chong N, et al. Assessment of coronary heart disease morbidity and mortality after radiation therapy for early breast cancer. *J Clin Oncol*. 2002;20(4):1036–1042.

60. Gaya AM, Ashford RF. Cardiac complications of radiation therapy. *Clin Oncol (R Coll Radiol)*. 2005;17(3):153–159.

61. Lind PA, Pagnanelli R, Marks LB, et al. Myocardial perfusion changes in patients irradiated for left-sided breast

cancer and correlation with coronary artery distribution. *Int J Radiat Oncol Biol Phys*. 2003;55(4):914–920.

62. Pai VB, Nahata MC. Cardiotoxicity of chemotherapeutic agents: incidence, treatment and prevention. *Drug Saf*. 2000;22(4):263–302.

63. Friedman M, Landsberg R, Pryor S, Syed Z, Ibrahim H, Caldarelli DD. The occurrence of sleep-disordered breathing among patients with head and neck cancer. *Laryngoscope*. 2001;111(11 pt 1):1917–1919.

64. Sharma VK, Galli W, Haber A, et al. Unexpected risks during administration of conscious sedation: previously undiagnosed obstructive sleep apnea. *Ann Intern Med*. 2003;139(8):707–708.

65. Läubli H, Balmelli C, Bossard M, et al. Acute heart failure due to autoimmune myocarditis under pembrolizumab treatment for metastatic melanoma. *Journal for ImmunoTherapy of Cancer*. 2015;3:11.

66. Brahmer JR, Tykodi SS, Chow LQM, et al. Safety and activity of anti-PD-L1 antibody in patients with advanced cancer. *N Engl J Med*. 2012;366:2455–2465.

67. Eggermont AMM, Chiarion-Sileni V, Grob JJ, et al. Adjuvant ipilimumab versus placebo after complete resection of high-risk stage III melanoma (EORTC 18071): a randomised, double-blind, phase 3 trial. *The Lancet Oncology*. 2015;5:522–530.

68. Giza DE, Moudgil R, Lopez-Mattei, et al. Association between ibrutinib and mid-cavitary Takotsubo cardiomyopathy: a case report and a review of chemotherapy-induced Takostubo's cardiomyopathy. *European Heart Journal – Case Reports*. 2017;1(2):1–7.

69. Yun S, Vincelette ND, Mansour I, et al. Late onset ipilimumab-induced pericarditis and pericardial Effusion: a rare but life threatening complication. *Case Rep Oncol Med*. 2015;2015:1–5. doi:10.1155/2015/794842

70. Scott-Coombes D, Whawell S, Vipond MN, Thompson J. Human intraperitoneal fibrinolytic response to elective surgery. *Br J Surg*. 1995;82(3):414–417.

71. Adachi W, Koike S, Rafique M, et al. Preoperative intraperitoneal chemotherapy for gastric cancer, with special reference to delayed peritoneal complications. *Surg Today*. 1995;25(5):396–403.

72. American College of Surgeons. ACS National Surgical Quality Improvement Program. https://www.facs.org/quality-programs/acs-nsqip

73. Bilimoria KY, Liu Y, Paruch JL, et al. Development and evaluation of the universal ACS NSQIP surgical risk calculator: a decision aid and informed consent tool for patients and surgeons. *J Am Coll Surg*. 2013;217:833–842.

74. Young J, Badgery-Parker T, Dobbins T, et al. Comparison of ECOG/WHO performance status and ASA score as a measure of functional status. *J Pain Symptom Manage*. 2015;49(2):258–264. doi:10.1016/j.jpainsymman.2014.06.006

75. Adachi W, Kobayashi M, Koike S, et al. The influence of excess body weight on the surgical treatment of patients with gastric cancer. *Surg Today*. 1995;25(11):939–945.

76. Goldman L, Caldera DL, Nussbaum SR, et al. Multifactorial index of cardiac risk in noncardiac surgical procedures. *N Engl J Med*. 1977;297(16):845–850.

77. Eagle KA, Brundage BH, Chaitman BR, et al. Guidelines for perioperative cardiovascular evaluation for noncardiac surgery. Report of the American College of Cardiology/American Heart Association Task Force on Practice Guidelines. Committee on Perioperative Cardiovascular Evaluation for Noncardiac Surgery. *Circulation*. 1996;93(6):1278–1317.

78. Fleischer LA, Fleischmann KE, Auerbach AD. 2014 ACC/AHA guideline on perioperative cardiovascular evaluation and management of patients undergoing noncardiac surgery: executive summary. *J Nucl Cardiol*. 2015;22:162–215.

79. McGlynn EA, Asch SM, Adams J, et al. The quality of health care delivered to adults in the United States. *N Engl J Med*. 2003;348(26):2635–2645.

80. Justice AC, Covinsky KE, Berlin JA. Assessing the generalizability of prognostic information. *Ann Intern Med*. 1999;130(6):515–524.

81. Gibbons RJ, Balady GJ, Bricker JT, et al. ACC/AHA 2002 guideline update for exercise testing: summary article. A report of the American College of Cardiology/American Heart Association task force on practice guidelines (committee to update the 1997 exercise testing guidelines). *J Am Coll Cardiol*. 2002;40(8):1531–1540.

82. Surawicz B, Knilans T. *Chou's Electrocardiography in Clinical Practice: Adult and Pediatric*. 6th ed. Philadelphia, PA: Saunders; 2008.

83. Smith-Bindman R, Lipson J, Marcus R, et al. Radiation dose associated with common computed tomography examinations and the associated lifetime attributable risk of cancer. *Arch Intern Med*. 2009;169(22):2078–2086.

84. Cohen MC, Aretz TH. Histological analysis of coronary artery lesions in fatal postoperative myocardial infarction. *Cardiovasc Pathol*. 1999;8(3):133–139.

85. Thompson C, Bergstrome D, Parlow JL. Limitations of preoperative dobutamine stress echocardiography in identifying severe left main coronary artery stenosis: a report of two cases and a brief review. *Can J Anaesth*. 2003;50(9):933–939.

86. Silver MA, Pisano C. High incidence of elevated B-type natriuretic peptide levels and risk factors for heart failure in an unselected at-risk population (stage A): implications for heart failure screening programs. *Congest Heart Fail*. 2003;9(3):127–132.

87. Maisel A. B-type natriuretic peptide levels: a potential novel "white count" for congestive heart failure. *J Card Fail*. 2001;7(2):183–193.

88. Karthikeyan G, Moncur RA, Levine O, et al. Is a preoperative brain natriuretic peptide or N-terminal pro-B-type natriuretic peptide measurement an independent predictor of adverse cardiovascular outcomes within 30 days of noncardiac surgery? A systematic review and meta-analysis of observational studies. *J Am Coll Cardiol*. 2009;54(17):1599–1606.

89. Ryding AD, Kumar S, Worthington AM, Burgess D. Prognostic value of brain natriuretic peptide in noncardiac surgery: a meta-analysis. *Anesthesiology*. 2009;111(2):311–319.

90. Bolliger D, Seeberger MD, Lurati Buse GA, et al. A preliminary report on the prognostic significance of preoperative brain natriuretic peptide and postoperative cardiac troponin in patients undergoing major vascular surgery. *Anesth Analg.* 2009;108(4):1069–1075.

91. Rodseth RN, Padayachee L, Biccard BM. A meta-analysis of the utility of pre-operative brain natriuretic peptide in predicting early and intermediate-term mortality and major adverse cardiac events in vascular surgical patients. *Anaesthesia.* 2008;63(11):1226–1233.

92. Goei D, Schouten O, Boersma E, et al. Influence of renal function on the usefulness of N-terminal pro-B-type natriuretic peptide as a prognostic cardiac risk marker in patients undergoing noncardiac vascular surgery. *Am J Cardiol.* 2008;101(1):122–126.

93. Zustovich F, Trivello M, Ceravolo R, et al. Cardio-Toxicity during chemotherapy: feasibility of new diagnostic approaches. *Health.* 2010(2):376–380.

94. Gibson PH, Croal BL, Cuthbertson BH, et al. Use of preoperative natriuretic peptides and echocardiographic parameters in predicting new-onset atrial fibrillation after coronary artery bypass grafting: a prospective comparative study. *Am Heart J.* 2009;158(2):244–251.

95. Goei D, Hoeks SE, Boersma E, et al. Incremental value of high-sensitivity C-reactive protein and N-terminal pro-B-type natriuretic peptide for the prediction of postoperative cardiac events in noncardiac vascular surgery patients. *Coron Artery Dis.* 2009;20(3):219–224.

96. Helfand M, Buckley DI, Freeman M, et al. Emerging risk factors for coronary heart disease: a summary of systematic reviews conducted for the U.S. Preventive Services Task Force. *Ann Intern Med.* 2009;151(7):496–507.

97. Froehlich JB, Karavite D, Russman PL et al. American College of Cardiology; American Heart Association. American College of Cardiology/American Heart Association preoperative assessment guidelines reduce resource utilization before aortic surgery. *J Vasc Surg.* 2002;36(4):758–763.

98. Morgan PB, Panomitros GE, Nelson AC, Smith DF, Solanki DR, Zornow MH. Low utility of dobutamine stress echocardiograms in the preoperative evaluation of patients scheduled for noncardiac surgery. *Anesth Analg.* 2002;95(3):512–516.

99. Liu LL, Dzankic S, Leung JM. Preoperative electrocardiogram abnormalities do not predict postoperative cardiac complications in geriatric surgical patients. *J Am Geriatr Soc.* 2002;50(7):1186–1191.

100. Young EL, Karthikesalingam A, Huddart S, et al. A systematic review of the role of cardiopulmonary exercise testing in vascular surgery. *Eur J Vasc Endovasc Surg.* 2012(44):64–71.

101. Pryma DA, Ravizzini G, Amar D, Richards VL, Patel JB, Strauss HW. Cardiovascular risk assessment in cancer patients undergoing major surgery. *J Nucl Cardiol.* 2005;12(2):151–157.

102. Chopra V, Flanders SA, Froehlich JB, Lau WC, Eagle KA. Perioperative practice: time to throttle back. *Ann Intern Med.* 2010;152(1):47–51.

103. Stevens RD, Fleisher LA. Strategies in the high-risk cardiac patient undergoing non-cardiac surgery. *Best Pract Res Clin Anaesthesiol.* 2004;18(4):549–563.

104. Labib SB, Goldstein M, Kinnunen PM, Schick EC. Cardiac events in patients with negative maximal versus negative submaximal dobutamine echocardiograms undergoing noncardiac surgery: importance of resting wall motion abnormalities. *J Am Coll Cardiol.* 2004;44(1):82–87.

105. Kligfield P. ST segment analysis in exercise stress testing. In: Zareba W, Maison-Blanche P, Locati EH, eds. *Noninvasive Electrocardiology in Clinical Practice.* Armonk, NY: Futura Publishing Company; 2001:227–256.

106. Majd-Ardekani J, Clowes P, Menash-Bonsu V, Nunan TO. Time for abstention from caffeine before an adenosine myocardial perfusion scan. *Nucl Med Commun.* 2000;21(4):361–364.

107. Landesberg G, Beattie WS, Mosseri M, Jaffe AS, Alpert JS. Perioperative myocardial infarction. *Circulation.* 2009;119(22):2936–2944.

108. Pierpont GL, Moritz TE, Goldman S, et al. Disparate opinions regarding indications for coronary artery revascularization before elective vascular surgery. *Am J Cardiol.* 2004;94(9):1124–1128.

109. McFalls EO, Ward HB, Moritz TE, et al. Coronary-artery revascularization before elective major vascular surgery. *N Engl J Med.* 2004;351(27):2795–2804.

110. Kaluza GL, Joseph J, Lee JR, et al. Catastrophic outcomes of noncardiac surgery soon after coronary stenting. *J Am Coll Cardiol.* 2000;35(5):1288–1294.

111. Vicenzi MN, Ribitsch D, Luha O, et al. Coronary artery stenting before noncardiac surgery: more threat than safety? *Anesthesiology.* 2001;94(2):367–368.

112. Grines CL, Bonow RO, Casey DE Jr, et al. Prevention of premature discontinuation of dual antiplatelet therapy in patients with coronary artery stents: a science advisory from the American Heart Association, American College of Cardiology, Society for Cardiovascular Angiography and Interventions, American College of Surgeons, and American Dental Association, with representation from the American College of Physicians. *Circulation.* 2007;115(6):813–818.

113. Nuttall GA, Brown MJ, Stombaugh JW, et al. Time and cardiac risk of surgery after bare-metal stent percutaneous coronary intervention. *Anesthesiology.* 2008;109(4):588–595.

114. Rabbitts JA, Nuttall GA, Brown MJ, et al. Cardiac risk of noncardiac surgery after percutaneous coronary intervention with drug-eluting stents. *Anesthesiology.* 2008;109(4):596–604.

115. Faggioni M, Baber U, Sartori S, et al. Incidence, patterns, and associations between dual-antiplatelet therapy cessation and risk for adverse events among patients with and without diabetes mellitus receiving drug-eluting stents: results from the PARIS registry. *JACC Cardiovasc Interv.* 2017(10);7:645–654.

116. Levine GN, Bates ER, Bittl JA, et al. 2016 ACC/AHA guidelines focused update on duration of dual antiplatelet therapy in patients with coronary artery disease. *JACC.* 2016;68(10):1082–1115.

117. French KE. *Personal communication*. 2017.

118. Hayes DL. Evolving indications for permanent pacing. *Am J Cardiol*. 1999;83(5B):161D–165D.

119. Prystowsky EN, Nisam S. Prophylactic implantable cardioverter defibrillator trials: MUSTT, MADIT, and beyond Multicenter Unsustained Tachycardia Trial. Multicenter Automatic Defibrillator Implantation Trial. *Am J Cardiol*. 2000;86(11):1214–1215.

120. Bristow MR, Feldman AM, Saxon LA. Heart failure management using implantable devices for ventricular resynchronization: comparison of medical therapy, pacing, and defibrillation in chronic heart failure (COMPANION) trial. COMPANION steering committee and COMPANION clinical investigators. *J Card Fail*. 2000;6(3):276–285.

121. Pinski SL. Continuing progress in the treatment of severe congestive heart failure. *JAMA*. 2003;289(6):754–756.

122. Mazur M, Wang F, Hodge DO, et al. Burden of cardiac arrhythmias in patients with anthracycline-related cardiomyopathy. *JACC Clin Electrophysiol*. 2016;3(2):139–150. doi:10.1016/j.jacep.2016.08.009

123. Kramer DB, Tsai T, Natarajan P, et al. Frailty, physical activity, and mobility in patients with cardiac implantable electrical devices. *J Am Heart Assoc*. 2017;6(2):3004659.

124. Pili-Floury S, Farah E, Samain E, Schauvliege F, Marty J. Perioperative outcome of pacemaker patients undergoing non-cardiac surgery. *Eur J Anaesthesiol*. 2008; 25(6):514–516.

125. Trankina MF, Black S, Gibby G. Pacemakers: perioperative evaluation, management and complications. *Anesthesiology*. 2000;93:A–1193. (Meeting abstract)

126. Wilke A, Hesse H, Gorg C, Maisch B. Elevation of the pacing threshold: a side effect in a patient with pacemaker undergoing therapy with doxorubicin and vincristine. *Oncology*. 1999;56(2):110–111.

127. Crossley GH, Poole JE, Rozner MA, et al. The Heart Rhythm Society (HRS)/American Society of Anesthesiologists (ASA) Expert Consensus Statement on the perioperative management of patients with implantable defibrillators, pacemakers and arrhythmia monitors: facilities and patient management. *Heart Rhythm*. 2011;8(7):1114–1154.

128. Mahlow WJ, Craft RM, Misulia NL. A perioperative management algorithm for cardiac rhythm management devices: the PACED-OP protocol. *PACE*. 2013;36(2):238–248.

129. Gifford J, Larimer K, Thomas C, May P. ICD-ON registry for perioperative management of CIEDs: most require no change. *Pacing Clin Electrophysiol*. 2017(2);40(2): 128–134. doi:10.1111/pace.12990. Epub January 31, 2017

130. Rozner MA, Nguyen AD. Unexpected pacing threshold changes during non-implant surgery. *Anesthesiology*. 2002;96:A1070.

131. Kleinman B, Ushomirsky S, Murdoch S. Unintended discharge of an ICD in an patient undergoing total knee replacement. *APSF Newsletter*. 2017;32(1):10–11.

132. Tekin UN, Khan IA, Singh N, Nair VM, Vasavada BC, Sacchi TJ. A left atrial paraganglioma patient presenting with compressive dysphagia. *Can J Cardiol*. 2000;16(3):383–385.

133. Osranek M, Bursi F, Gura GM, Young WF Jr, Seward JB. Echocardiographic features of pheochromocytoma of the heart. *Am J Cardiol*. 2003;91(5):640–643.

134. Dluhy RG. Pheochromocytoma—death of an axiom. *N Engl J Med*. 2002;346(19):1486–1488.

135. Neumann HP, Bausch B, McWhinney SR, et al. Freiburg-Warsaw-Columbus Pheochromocytoma Study Group. Germ-line mutations in nonsyndromic pheochromocytoma. *N Engl J Med*. 2002;346(19):1459–1466.

136. Hull CJ. Phaeochromocytoma. Diagnosis, preoperative preparation and anaesthetic management. *Br J Anaesth*. 1986;58(12):1453–1468.

137. Schuiki ER, Jenni R, Amann FW, Ziegler WH. A reversible form of apical left ventricular hypertrophy associated with pheochromocytoma. *J Am Soc Echocardiogr*. 1993;6(3 pt 1):327–331.

138. Jacob JL, da Silveira LC, de Freitas CG, Cêntola CA, Nicolau JC, Lorga AM. Pheochromocytoma with echocardiographic features of obstructive hypertrophic cardiomyopathy. A case report. *Angiology*. 1994;45(11): 985–989.

139. Kocak S, Aydintug S, Canakci N. Alpha blockade in preoperative preparation of patients with pheochromocytomas. *Int Surg*. 2002;87(3):191–194.

140. Russell WJ, Metcalfe IR, Tonkin AL, Frewin DB. The preoperative management of phaeochromocytoma. *Anaesth Intensive Care*. 1998;26(2):196–200.

141. Lentschener C, Gaujoux S, Tesniere A, et al. Point of controversy: perioperative care of patients undergoing pheochromocytoma removal-time for a reappraisal? *Eur J Endocrinol*. 2011(165):365–373.

142. Lundin L, Norheim I, Landelius J, Oberg K, Theodorsson-Norheim E. Carcinoid heart disease: relationship of circulating vasoactive substances to ultrasound-detectable cardiac abnormalities. *Circulation*. 1988;77(2):264–269.

143. Kulke MH, Mayer RJ. Carcinoid tumors. *N Engl J Med*. 1999;340(11):858–868.

144. Dougherty TB, Cronau LH Jr. Anesthetic implications for surgical patients with endocrine tumors. *Int Anesthesiol Clin*. 1998;36(3):31–44.

145. Hughes EW, Hodkinson BP. Carcinoid syndrome: the combined use of ketanserin and octreotide in the management of an acute crisis during anaesthesia. *Anaesth Intensive Care*. 1989;17(3):367–370.

146. Padfield NL. Carcinoid syndrome: comparison of pretreatment regimes in the same patient. *Ann R Coll Surg Engl*. 1987;69(1);16–17.

147. Bakaeen FG, Reardon MJ, Coselli JS, et al. Surgical outcome in 85 patients with primary cardiac tumors. *Am J Surg*. 2003;186(6):641–647.

148. Lobo A, Lewis JF, Conti CR. Intracardiac masses detected by echocardiography: case presentations and review of the literature. *Clin Cardiol*. 2000;23(9): 702–708.

149. Gillam LD. Intraoperative transesophageal echocardiography. *Cardiol Rev*. 2000;8(5):269–278.

26 Advanced Heart Failure in Patients with Cancer

Sadeer G. Al-Kindi ▪ *Guilherme H. Oliveira*

INTRODUCTION

Cancer and Heart Failure (HF) have shared a similar trajectory over time. They both have transitioned from uniformly lethal diseases to chronic conditions. Therapeutical innovation has rendered both diseases more manageable, with better cure rates and longer survival for afflicted patients. Because of intensive research and major breakthroughs over the past two decades, newer antineoplastic and cardiovascular interventions have resulted in a growing population of cancer-free survivors[1] and patients with stable cardiovascular diseases. In fact, improved prevention, risk factor modification and medical and interventional advances in coronary heart disease (CHD) have transformed HF into the only cardiovascular disease with rising incidence and prevalence.[2] Therefore, it is not surprising that the sheer number patients with both HF and cancer are seen increasingly more frequently in clinical practice.

The growing overlap of these large groups of patients makes the interaction of cancer and HF a subject of pressing clinical and health policy interest. Paradoxically, this problem has been incompletely understood and more is unknown than known in the field. With vast funding availability for cancer research during the past decade, the pace of advances in cardiovascular diseases has not kept up with that of cancer.

The problem is further complicated by the fact that many of the new molecular targeted therapy for cancer has been found to be associated with cardiotoxicity and the development of HF.[3,4] Therefore, HF caused by cancer therapy has been and will likely continue to be major co-morbidity in cancer survivors. Whereas the majority of the literature has focused on anthracycline-induced cardiomyopathy, newer tyrosine kinase inhibitors (TKIs) and monoclonal antibodies have been shown to cause HF through different mechanisms and with divergent natural histories.[5] Thus, chemotherapy-related HF can no longer be lumped together as one entity, but must rather be differentiated into the various causative agents. Consequently, a classification of chemotherapy-related myocardial dysfunction that addresses that caused by the anthracyclines model (Type I) and that caused by TKI (type II)[6] model has been suggested. One similarity between both is the shared predisposing factors, such as age, pre-existing cardiac risk factors and previous cardiovascular insults.

In addition, HF caused by incidental etiologies such as hypertension, coronary artery disease, myocarditides and valvular heart disease is becoming increasingly more common to the onco-cardiology practice. Factors such as age overlap between cancer and heart disease, shared risk factors and an aging population of cancer survivors are responsible for the growing number of cancer patients with incident HF.[7] Such patients pose their own unique management challenges because pre-existing heart disease may interfere with choice of chemotherapy and magnify the complexities of surgical or radiotherapeutic interventions.

Considering the multiple etiologic factors of HF in cancer patients, their management should be as targeted and diverse as its causes. Nevertheless, because of poor mechanistic understanding and lack of molecular targeted HF therapy, all HF is treated similarly. National guidelines derived from observations in very different groups of patients have been thus far indiscriminately applied to cancer patients. Not surprisingly, the prognosis of HF in cancer remains worse than associated with other forms of ischemic and non-ischemic cardiomyopathies.[8]

Much of the activity in the research around chemotherapy-related cardiomyopathy has been spent in detection and prevention of cardiotoxicity. Multiple imaging modalities have been investigated as monitoring techniques in attempts to detect early myocardial dysfunction, with varying success. Similarly, strategies at preventing or minimizing cardiotoxicity have been explored. Unfortunately, without a clear understanding of pathogenesis, both efforts have yielded overall disappointing results.

In this chapter we will undertake an in-depth analysis of the problem concerning HF in cancer patients. We will expose the magnitude of the problem by studying the epidemiology of HF in this population. We will explore the common mechanisms that underlie myocardial dysfunction, cancer and its therapeutic targets, review pathogenesis and etiologies, and attempt to identify possible areas of future research. We will then review the methods of prevention, detection and investigation of HF in this population, and provide a framework for the systematic approach to these patients. Lastly, we will address the management of this heterogeneous and complex group of patients, emphasizing medical and device therapy for both acute decompensated and chronic HF, with special focus on myocardial recovery. In all instances, where evidence is lacking, we will dissert based on our combined acquired experience and the standard practice at our institutions.

EPIDEMIOLOGY

The prevalence and incidence of HF in the United States continues to rise with improved survival of patients with ischemic heart disease. In individuals over 80 years, the prevalence of HF reaches 12%–15%. The incidence of heart failure increases with age and by age 85 it peaks at 42 per 1000 person/years. In 2006 there were 1.2 million hospital discharges for HF and by 2030 there will be almost 6 million people in the US with HF.[2] In parallel, the yearly incidence of cancer in the United States is around 0.5% and the lifetime probability of developing cancer 50%. However, despite the fact that 1.7 million patients will be diagnosed with cancer in 2017,[9] their 5-year survival has increased to 83% from 58% in the mid-1970s.[9]

It is not surprising, therefore, that there are a significant number of people with HF who have cancer and vice-versa. In regards to this overlap, there are three epidemiological questions that are important from the clinical standpoint: 1) how many patients with heart failure also have cancer? 2) How many patients with cancer also have heart failure? 3) How many cancer survivors will develop heart failure?

The answer to the first question can be inferred from the heart failure literature. In an outcome study of 2450 HF patients with both preserved and reduced ejection fraction, the prevalence of cancer was approximately 12% amongst both groups.[10] In this population, the presence of cancer was an independent predictor of mortality, but less powerful than renal failure, cirrhosis, peripheral arterial disease, dementia and hyponatremia. Similarly, in the Candesartan in Heart Failure Assessment of Reduction in Mortality and Morbidity (CHARM) Program, among 7599 patients with HF NYHA class II-IV with both preserved and low ejection fractions (EF), the prevalence of cancer was 7%.[11] Therefore, approximately 10% of the patients with HF are also likely to have a diagnosis of cancer.

There is considerable amount of literature on the epidemiology of HF and cardiac dysfunction in cancer survivors. In over 10,000 childhood cancer survivors mean age of 26 years, followed for a mean of 17 years, the incidence of self-reported HF was 1.26%. These patients were eight times more likely to have HF than their age-matched siblings.[12] In a retrospective analysis of almost 7000 Swedish Hodgkin disease (HD) survivors, 3% had HF at a mean follow-up of 11 years.[13] In a cohort of over 4000 breast cancer patients treated with a combination of chemo and radiation therapy followed for 10 years, the incidence of heart failure or cardiomyopathy was 9.9%.[14] The likelihood of developing HF following cancer treatment is mostly dependent on the type of treatment received. The incidence of HF following adriamycin therapy in 607 children from the Netherlands after 6–15 years of follow-up was 2.8% to 5%.[15] The incidence of subclinical left ventricular dysfunction (LVD), however, may be much larger. In a series of 141 lymphoma patients treated with anthracyclines and followed for 5 years with serial echocardiographic examinations, 39 (27.6%) developed subclinical LVD while only one patient developed overt HF.[16] Thus it is possible that the problem of LVD in cancer survivors may be underappreciated.

MOLECULAR BASIS OF CARDIOTOXICITY-INTERSECTING PATHWAYS OF HF AND CANCER

From a distance, HF and cancer have nothing in common: they are the end result of two diametrically opposite cellular processes: premature demise and unnatural longevity. Within the paradox of life and death hide the molecular secrets that determine one instead of the other. Therein lies their similarity: the pathways that determine survival and death are not just intertwined, but seem to be the same. New molecular targeted cancer therapy is teaching us that the same molecular checkpoints that are switched on in cancer are switched off in HF. Signaling pathways that sustain carcinogenesis also preserve normal cardiomyocyte function and survival. Therefore, increasingly often, what kills cancer also kills the heart. Below follows a summary of selected known shared biological pathways between cardiac function and tumor genesis that help shed light on the mechanisms whereby drugs used to treat cancer cause HF.

▪ Protein p53

Known as the protector of the genome, the transcription factor p53 (TP53 in humans) is charged with maintaining gene stability.[17] It is at the core of a number of signaling pathways that are activated by multiple cellular stresses including exogenous DNA damage, hypoxia, hemodynamic load, oncogene activation and telomere erosion. Once cellular insults occur, p53 can cause transactivation-dependent and independent effects that facilitate transient cell adaptation to stressful conditions. Increased DNA repair, cell cycle arrest, induction of apoptosis, enhancement of expression of detoxifying enzymes are a few of the ways it suppresses oncogenesis and renders cells more resistant to infarction-induced hypoxia.[18] Suppression or up regulation of p53 have been shown to be associated with carcinogenesis and HF, respectively. In proliferative cells, p53 responds to DNA damage by maintaining genomic stability and preventing malignant transformation. It is therefore not surprising that most human malignancies either have loss-of-function mutations of the p53 gene or deactivate p53 by increased downstream inhibition. Failing human cardiomyocytes, subjected to hemodynamic stress, express significant up regulation of p53. In this setting p53, is an effector protein that exerts its function through nuclear gene induction and direct cytoplasmic actions resulting in myocyte hypertrophy, increased activation of caspase-3 and apoptosis.[19] Anthracyclines generate free radicals that induce cell membrane lipid peroxidation and DNA damage of all tissues, including cancer and heart cells. In cardiomyocytes, doxorubicin causes early DNA insult that lead to p53 mediated apoptosis and cell death.[20] It has been shown that inhibition of p53 can reduce doxorubicin-induced apoptosis[21] and cell death without diminishing the amount of DNA damage caused by anthracyclines.[20] This suggests that prevention of anthracycline-induced cardiotoxicity may be possible without diminishing its anti-neoplastic efficacy. The mechanism of anthracycline cardiotoxicity is discussed in greater detail in Chapter 3.

However, myocardial dysfunction and HF can occur with minimal or no apoptosis, despite activation of the same p53 mediated stress pathways. Apoptosis interruptus is a process characterized by preserved nuclei in failing human cardiomyocytes despite up regulation of caspase-3 and cytochrome—c release—i.e., activation of the apoptotic cascade without cell death.[19] This occurs through cardiomyocyte-invoked survival mechanisms, such as unregulated expression of cytosolic X-linked inhibitor of apoptosis protein (XIAP). Release of cytochrome-c into the cytoplasm causes intracellular energy depletion that impairs contractile function and may be responsible for the loss of contractility observed in failing cardiomyocytes. If the energy depletion is severe enough, necrosis can occur, otherwise the cell remains in a "zombie" state between apoptosis and necrosis. This may be the mechanism involved in myocardial hibernation or in acute reversible anthracycline cardiomyopathy. Carvedilol, reperfusion, unloading with ventricular assist devices (VADs) and other therapies with proven anti-apoptotic properties may lead to reversal of apoptosis interruptus and thus help explain the phenomenon of myocardial recovery.

■ Neuregulin-1/Erb2 Signaling

Neuregulin 1 (NGR-1) is an epidermal growth factor whose biological effects are mediated by a family of tyrosine kinase receptors of which Erb-2 (HER-2) is the most well-known. These biological effects encompass proliferation, differentiation and survival of breast epithelial cell, neurons and myocytes. ErB-2 was discovered as an oncogene product found to be overexpressed in certain breast cancers, where its presence portends aggressive biological behavior and poor prognosis. Increased Erb-2 signaling was shown to foment survival and resistance of breast cancer cells to therapy. Therefore, a monoclonal antibody, trastuzumab (Herceptin), was specifically designed to inhibit the tyrosine kinase Erb-2 and shown to have great efficacy in the treatment of Erb-2 positive breast cancer.[22] Subsequently, clinical trials have shown that 4%–7% of patients develop cardiac dysfunction with trastuzumab alone and up to 27% in those also exposed to anthracyclines.[23,24] Experimental studies with Erb-2 knockout mice have demonstrated the development of dilated hearts with poor trabeculation, impaired resistance to hemodynamic stress (aortic banding) and greater susceptibility to anthracycline toxicity.[25] Inhibition of Erb-2 signaling exposes the myocardium- and cancer cells- to unopposed effects of stress response activation by exogenous insults. However, another possible mechanism is that when trastuzumab binds to Erb-2, it may trigger downregulation of the anti-apoptotic protein BCL-X_L leading to the increased rate of apoptosis observed in cardiomyocytes that are otherwise relatively resistant to programmed cell death. Another important finding is that NRG-1/Erb-2 signaling is involved in the progression of HF. In the early stages of hemodynamic stress, myocardial NRG-1 mRNA is upregulated and parallels the onset and progression of LVH, only to start declining with progressive myocardial remodeling and neurohormonal activation.[26] Lastly, circulating levels of NRG-1may serve as a prognostic marker similar to BNP.[27] The mechanisms of trastuzumab cardiotoxicity is discussed in details in Chapter 4.

■ Vascular Endothelial Growth Factors (VEGF)

Angiogenesis is essential to both tumor progression[28] and preservation of cardiac homeostasis and function in response to pressure overload.[29] The angiogenic protein VEGF-A is overexpressed in 60% of human cancers and promotes endothelial cell activation through the tyrosine kinase receptor VEGFR-2. Several antiangiogenic small molecule kinase inhibitors have been developed and approved for the treatment of cancer. So far, three such agents, imatinib, sunitinib and sorafenib, have been associated with LVD and HF.[30-32] Imatinib was found to cause cardiotoxicity by activating endoplasmic reticulum (ER) stress response by inhibiting c-Abl, a protein overexpressed in Bcr-Abl (Philadelphia chromosome) positive CML.[30] One of the mechanisms of sunitinib cardiotoxicity was found to be inhibition AMP-activated protein kinase (AMPK), the master regulator to cardiomyocyte response to decreased energy. Finally, various degrees of VEGFR inhibition may be responsible for the differences of cardiotoxicity potency by TKI inhibitors.

■ Phosphatidylinositol 3-Kinase (PI3K) Pathway

Recent studies have shown that there are more mutations or amplifications in PI3K pathway than in any other pathway in cancer patients.[33] Inhibition of components of the PI3K pathway, such as AKT, pyruvate dehydrogenase kisase isoenzyme 1 (PDK1), mammalian target of rapamycin (mTOR), all impair both angiogenesis and cell growth and survival in cancer cells and cardiomyocytes.[34] In fact, the pathways are essentially the same in both tissues but only more extensive and persistent in neoplastic cells. The pathway is activated by tyrosine kinase receptors (RTK). The pathway ends with activation of mTORC1, which promotes cell growth, angiogenesis and inhibits apoptosis. It is likely, that suppression of any or many of the components will lead to death of cancer cells at the expense of myocyte death. This pathway epitomizes the similarities and shared mechanisms between neoplastic cell and cardiomyocyte growth and survival. Because more drug therapy are being developed targeting multiple components of this pathway, it is likely that cardiotoxicity in cancer therapy will continue to be a growing problem.

ETIOLOGY OF HF IN CANCER PATIENTS

HF occurs in patients with cancer for a variety of reasons. The etiology depends on age, type of cancer therapy, cardiovascular risk factors and clinical setting under which it occurs. Young patients previously free of cardiovascular history usually have HF directly as a result of chemotherapy or radiation therapy. In more unusual instances, they may have congenital coronary anomalies, viral myocarditides, congenital cardiomyopathies, infiltrative diseases and HF caused directly by tumor. Older patients, on the other hand, are more likely to have HF caused by the traditional cardiac risk factors, such as hypertension, valvular heart disease and coronary heart disease. In this population, it is important to always assume the presence of underlying structural heart disease, even in the setting of cardiotoxic cancer treatment. In both young and old patients, every effort should be invested in asserting the etiologic cause of HF, because of the widely different prognosis and treatment options. Lastly, HF is also common in patients of all ages in situations of acute hemodynamic and physiologic stress that lead to systemic inflammatory response syndromes, such as septic shock, but also among acutely ill patients after stem cell transplantation and with leukemia. Below is a more detailed discussion of each etiologic subtype.

■ Chemotherapy

This particular issue is addressed in more detail in other sections of this book. Nevertheless, there are certain points important to emphasize from the HF standpoint. The two types of chemotherapy agents most commonly associated with HF are anthracyclines and tyrosine kinase inhibitors (TKIs), more specifically trastuzumab. The incidence of HF associated with sunitinib therapy was reported to be 2.7%[31]; while HF associated with imatinib is a rare event, happening in less than 1% of cases.[35] Cyclophosphamide (CY) in very high doses can cause acute fulminant HF by inducing hemorrhagic myocarditis and hemorrhagic pericardial effusion from direct endothelial damage.[36] This is, however, a rare occurrence that can be facilitated by excessive doses of CY, previous or concomitant therapy with anthracycline and pre-existing LV dysfunction.[37] In clinical practice, doxorubicin and trastuzumab are the most common agents that cause LVD and heart failure.

These two classes of drugs act at the cellular level in very different ways. Doxorubicin induces cardiac damage in a dose-dependent manner,[38] and does not require any pre-existing structural heart disease to cause myocyte death, as long as the cardiotoxic doses are reached. The typical dose beyond which the risk of cardiotoxicity starts to increase is 350 mg/m². At 400 mg/m², the likelihood of cardiotoxicity is around 5%, increasing to 26% at 500 mg/m², and over 60% at doses of 700 mg/m² and above.[39] There are several studies implicating different mechanisms to explain anthracycline cardiotoxicity, including generation of free radicals, upregulation of p53, overexpression of topoisomerase IIBeta and abnormalities in calcium handling (see above discussion). The cancer population[40] most at risk of developing cardiotoxicity are those treated for lymphomas, sarcomas, leukemias and breast cancer. Breast cancer patients who are HER2/neu positive are in addition treated with trastuzumab and therefore have incremental risk of developing heart failure. Interestingly, trastuzumab on its own is not sufficient to cause heart dysfunction.[41] It is, rather, a modulator of cardiac dysfunction, acting to further disrupt a previously damaged heart. At the molecular level, inactivation of the HER2 mediated survival pathway by trastuzumab, responsible for protecting against stress-signaling pathways, leads to an irreversible loss of myocytes and heart failure. Stress pathways are activated by a number of insults,[42] such as ischemia, hypoxia, hemodynamic overload and, through mechanisms not yet fully understood, anthracyclines.

It is known that patients with pre-existing heart disease are more susceptible to the cardiotoxic effects of either one of these agents, and this group requires close monitoring of their cardiac function during and following therapy. Additionally, a thorough baseline work-up prior to initiation of the chemotherapy should be undertaken to unveil any unsuspected pre-existing structural heart disease that may render the patient more susceptible to cardiotoxicity. A baseline comprehensive echocardiographic study is ordered in every patient with planned treatment with anthracyclines and trastuzumab. Further testing is directed as indicated by a thorough history and physical examination.

Determination of the etiology of any new decrease in cardiac function in this group of patients can be challenging and requires careful attention to temporal relation to exposure to chemotherapy. As a rule, it should not be assumed that any drop in LVEF is caused by chemotherapy induced cardiotoxicity and reversible causes should be sought, especially myocardial ischemia, uncontrolled hypertensive disease, worsening valvular function and superimposed infection. See below for a more detailed discussion on this.

Radiation Therapy

Irradiation of the heart is a well-established risk factor for cardiovascular disease including pericarditis and ischemic heart disease.[43] Cardiomyopathy and heart failure are less well-recognized as serious consequences of this common type of cancer therapy. Cancer survivors treated exclusively with radiation who were followed long-term have been shown to develop heart failure characterized almost exclusively by normal systolic function and restrictive physiology.[44] Alternatively, patients may develop systolic dysfunction as a consequence of direct radiation-induced injury coupled with anthracycline therapy or myocardial infarction from radiation-induced atherosclerotic coronary disease.[45] One of the difficulties with determining the causal relationship between radiation therapy and cardiomyopathy and HF is that many of the patients were also exposed to cardiotoxic chemotherapy agents such as anthracyclines.

However, animal models have been used to study this issue. In rabbits, irradiation in progressive doses caused a stepwise pattern of injury that started with small and medium arteries inflammation, followed by a neutrophilic infiltration of the myocardium and finally a later phase characterized by endothelial capillary damage with cardiomyocyte ischemia, death and extensive fibrosis.[46] Human pathologic and autopsy studies have shown that radiation is associated with non-specific, diffuse, interstitial fibrosis and severe microvascular abnormalities.[47] This supports the clinical observation of HF with preserved systolic function and restrictive physiology common in this group of patients. In fact, restrictive physiology by echocardiography is thought to be a major reason for HF in this population.

Another reason for HF in patients treated with radiation therapy is constrictive pericarditis. Historically, up to 20%–40% of Hodgkin disease patients treated with radiation developed pericarditis. Even though modern radiotherapy techniques have reduced the irradiation of the heart, pericarditis can still occur in up 20% of patients.[48] Acutely, within days to weeks, there may be pericardial effusion from increased permeability of pericardial microvasculature but also from fibrosis of small lymphatic and venous vessels. Typically, radiation-induced pericardial effusion is exudative and can therefore be differentiated from other causes of transudative effusion. Chronically, after more than 5–10 years, patients evolve with increased pericardial inflammation and progressive thickening. Effusive-constrictive pericarditis can also result, with the co-existence of constriction and pericardial effusion; in these cases, drainage of the effusion does not alleviate HF. The diagnosis of HF caused by pericardial disease is often missed and requires a high degree of suspicion. In fact, the investigation of HF in patients with a history of radiation exposure should always include investigation of the coronaries and pericardium, irrespective of the age group.

Radiation has also been an established risk factor for valvular disease, which may be a cause of HF in this population. This manifests clinically with a latent interval of 10–20 years from radiation. It is characterized by fibrosis and calcifications following the direction of the radiation beam. In the childhood cancer survivor study, cancer survivors were 4.8-fold more likely to develop valvular disease than their unaffected siblings, with a significant increase in risk with cumulative doses of 1500 centigray or more.[49] The 30-year cumulative incidence of significant valvular disease approached 15% in patients who received 3500 centigray. Treatment of severe valvular disease due to radiation poses a dilemma, as outcomes are not favorable even in experienced centers.[50]

The dose of radiation and heart volume irradiated are important determinants in the likelihood of HF development. Doses higher than 35–40 Gy, fractionated doses of >2 Gy/day and greater heart volume exposure can result in a three-fold higher risk of cardiac death and HF. Other risk factors include younger age at irradiation, use of adjuvant chemotherapy, tumor proximity to the heart and previous heart disease.[48]

■ Cancer

HF caused by cancer is a very rare occurrence in the community but must be considered in patients with malignancies. Both primary and metastatic cardiac tumors can potentially present or cause HF. More commonly, metastatic disease to the heart can cause valvular obstruction, arrhythmias, impediment to diastolic filling, outflow obstruction, pulmonary hypertension with right ventricular failure, pericardial invasion and cardiac encasement and myocardial infiltration with a pseudo infarct physiology. The most common malignancies known to metastasize to the heart are melanoma, renal cell carcinoma, non-small cell lung cancer, and squamous cell carcinomas. These tumors can present as intracavitary lesions of varying sizes in the left or right ventricle, most commonly attached to the intraventricular septum. Lymphomas and leiomyosarcomas[51] can infiltrate the myocardium and cause regional wall abnormalities as well as substitution of cardiac myocytes that can be detected by abnormalities

in echocardiographic speckle tracking imaging and cardiac magnetic resonance. Syncope and ventricular arrhythmias can be the first clue to an intracardiac metastasis before the tumor mass progresses to cause obstructive symptoms and heart failure. Primary cardiac tumors, particularly rhabdomyosarcoma and myxomas can cause HF by valvular obstruction and pseudo mitral stenosis. The literature has abundant case reports and some case series of other tumors that evolve with cardiac involvement more rarely, including uterine cervical cancer, liposarcomas, Burkitt lymphoma, Wilm's tumor, leukemia, hepatocellular carcinomas and neuroectodermal tumors.

Treatment of intracardiac tumors depend largely on whether they are primary or metastatic, the type and chemosensitivity of the tumor, and overall status of the patient. Treatment with combination of chemotherapy and surgery is probably preferred. The advantage of attempting chemotherapy initially is that depending on the response, it may obviate the need for surgical intervention. Also, it allows assessment of the sensitivity of the tumor to the chemotherapy agent. The risks with pre-operative chemotherapy are that the patient may not respond and lose the operable window, may develop complications from chemotherapy such as sepsis and overall deterioration which may preclude surgery later on, or may develop progression of tumor related symptoms such as HF and fatal ventricular arrhythmias. Surgical excision of large intracardiac tumors has been performed using the technique of autotransplantation, where the heart is explanted, allowing tumor resection and then re-implanted.[52] One complication from this technique is post-operative HF with LV stunning and transient right ventricular dysfunction. In cases where post-autotransplantation HF develops, both the LV and RV may require inotropic support for a few days to weeks. Serial examinations with echocardiography and cardiac MR are indicated in all cases of intracardiac masses before and after treatment (Table 26-1).

TABLE 26-1 Echocardiography follow-up schedule post-treatment

ANTHRACYCLINE DOSE	1 MONTH	3 MONTHS	6 MONTHS	1 YEAR	YEARLY
200 mg/m²	–	Echo with strain	–	Echo with strain	–
>200–450 mg/m²	–	Echo with strain	Echo with strain	Echo with strain	Echo with strain At year 3,5,10
>450 mg/m²	Echo with strain	Echo with strain	Echo with strain	Echo with strain	Echo with strain yearly for life

Lastly, carcinoid heart disease has been well-described in patients with serotonin-secreting neuroendocrine tumors.[53] Patients that develop hepatic metastasis are more likely to have cardiac involvement of the heart.[54] Heart involvement is characterized by pulmonic and tricuspid valve thickening with stenosis and regurgitation and progressive right ventricular heart failure.[55] The mitral and aortic valves are involved later in the progression of the disease and less frequently, but when they are patients develop biventricular heart failure. The prognosis of patients with carcinoid heart disease is poor, but improves with valvular surgery.[56] More recently, slower progression of cardiac involvement and improved prognosis has been suggested with hepatic tumor resection.[57]

■ Ischemic Cardiomyopathy

Many of the patients first diagnosed with cancer already carry a diagnosis of ischemic heart disease (IHD) and ischemic cardiomyopathy (ICMP). Such patients pose an additional challenge to the treatment of their cancer because, not only are curative and palliative procedures such as surgery and chemotherapy riskier, but also they are more frail in general. In addition, most if not all patients with ICMP are on single or dual antiplatelet therapy. This complicates procedures such as stem cell transplantation that require bone marrow ablation with consequent severe thrombocytopenia. These patients should continue their HF treatment in parallel to their cancer treatment. In general, cardiotoxic chemotherapy should be avoided in this population.

As mentioned above, older patients that develop LVD in the setting of chemotherapy should undergo ischemic work-up. This is particularly true for those that develop severe LVD after small doses of anthracyclines and after drugs not usually associated with LVD. Also, patients who develop HF with trastuzumab therapy without a history of previous anthracyclines should be presumed to have subclinical coronary disease. Lastly, patients with cancer and co-existing CAD risk factors, in particular those with lung cancer and tobacco history, diabetes, peripheral vascular disease, who develop LVD and HF even in the setting of cardiotoxic treatment, should be presumed to have CAD. In such patients, the diagnosis of ischemic cardiomyopathy should be established or ruled out with conventional or computed tomography coronary angiography.

The new diagnosis of ICMP in a patient with cancer should trigger standard, guideline-based therapy. There are, however, some caveats to be considered in this population. Coronary revascularization with percutaneous intervention may be preferred to aorto-coronary bypass depending on the long-term prognosis from the cancer standpoint. In other words, there is no reason to bypass a patient whose prognosis is less than 5 years from the cancer standpoint. In such cases, we prefer to perform multi-vessel and left main stenting. Also, we most often use bare-metal stents because there is no need prolonged dual platelet therapy in patients that often require repeated surgical interventions. Other therapies such as implantable defibrillators (ICD) and bi-ventricular pacemakers will be discussed below.

One last point to discuss is ICMP in patients with early life exposure to radiation therapy. Radiotherapy induced coronary disease is an important contributor to early onset CAD in childhood cancer survivors. Such patients may have extensive multivessel CAD with HF by the fourth decade.

■ Non-Ischemic Cardiomyopathy

A significant proportion of cancer patients develop HF from causes other than those listed above. It is our practice to try to determine the etiologic cause of HF in all patients seen at the oncocardiology clinic. This practice has resulted in diagnoses of rare etiologies and discovery of unforeseen cardiotoxicity of novel chemotherapy agents.

A common phenomenon observed in our institution is that almost 50% of our patients with LVD improve or recover their left ventricular function within a year. This cohort includes patients with chemotherapy exposure but is mostly composed of patients who are acutely ill in the hospital.

Our experience suggests that patients undergoing stem cell transplantation may develop transient LVD with signs of severe fluid overload that not infrequently require ultrafiltration. The etiologic mechanism of this phenomenon is not yet clear but may involve a systemic inflammatory reaction similar to that of septic LVD, or be due to the high intensity anthracycline-based pre-transplant ablative therapy. When this happens acutely, most, if not all patients recover their cardiac function completely. HF that occurs months to years after stem cell transplant is most often related to high doses of anthracyclines before transplantation.

Septic cardiomyopathy is also common in the setting of cancer. Typically patients develop profound LVD and HF with neutropenic sepsis, usually in the setting of vasoactive drug therapy and multiorganism cultures. Tachyarrhythmia-related cardiomyopathy is also thought to play a role in these extremely sick neutropenic patients. Those who survive have complete recovery of their cardiac function.

Some patients with gastrointestinal malignancies that require large sections of small bowel resection may develop nutritional cardiomyopathies, more specifically thiamine and selenium deficiency. We typically measure both nutrients in patients with a history of chemotherapy or surgical induced malabsorption. We recently treated a patient with chronic platinum-induced malabsorption who was admitted to another facility where her total parenteral nutrition was interrupted for 3 weeks. She developed severe acute LVD with HF with undetectable plasma selenium levels. She was treated with selenium replacement and inotropic support and within one week recovered her left ventricular function.

Other causes of HF in our population include restrictive cardiomyopathy in patients with hemochromatosis from multiple transfusions, such as those with myelodysplastic syndromes and hemoglobinopathies. Amyloid heart disease is common in patients with multiple myeloma and can be readily diagnosed with echocardiography and right ventricular biopsies. Viral myocarditides are rare, but we recently had a breast cancer survival patient with H1N1 cardiomyopathy that required LVAD support. Recently, fulminant myocarditis has also been described in patients receiving immune checkpoint inhibitors, with an estimated incidence of 1 in 1000 patients.[4]

Lastly, valvular heart disease is not a common cause of HF in our population. Critical aortic stenosis is rare, whereas HF from endocarditis-induced aortic and mitral regurgitation are more common, but still unusual. Valvular heart disease, however, can result in significant HF in long-term survivors of cancers, as previously described.

APPROACH TO NEW LEFT VENTRICULAR DYSFUNCTION IN DURING CANCER THERAPY

The mainstay of evaluation of cardiac function during cancer treatment is echocardiography. Echocardiographic evaluation in patients undergoing chemotherapy should include a comprehensive 2D color Doppler study with tissue Doppler measurements, contrast injection unless perfect endocardial definition is obtained, 3-dimensional reconstruction for precise evaluation of ejection fraction, and speckled tracking strain analysis. At our institution (and in many institutions in the United States[58]), echocardiography is preferred to multi-gated first pass angiography (MUGA) because it allows more complete evaluation of cardiac function and earlier clues to cardiotoxicity. Therefore, echocardiograms should be performed liberally in the setting of cancer and cancer treatment. This allows for serial assessment of changes in LV systolic and diastolic changes.

The approach to patients who develop cardiac dysfunction while on cancer treatment needs to be systematic and comprehensive. It should focus on early detection, early and precise definition of etiology and early treatment. Our experience and some published data suggest that anthracycline cardiomyopathy, if detected and treated early enough, may be completely reversible. The same principle holds true to trastuzumab induced LVD. Therefore, our approach is to quickly establish the etiology of HF and treat it aggressively.

The first step when confronted with a drop in LVEF by any imaging modality without signs and symptoms of HF is to confirm it with a second modality. If an echo was done, then a repeat echo with contrast, 3D reconstruction and strain analysis is done. Alternatively, CMR or MUGA can be used. Once the diagnosis of LVD is confirmed, a thorough search for an etiologic cause is initiated. If the patient is on any known cardiotoxic treatment, that treatment is interrupted. Unless the patient is younger than 30 years, coronary anatomy is visualized by either CT angiography or conventional coronary angiography. We obtain B-type natriuretic peptide, troponin I, thyroid function tests, ferritin and viral PCR for coxackie virus, HIV, hepatitis B and C, parvovirus B19, Influenza A and H1N1. We perform plasma measurements of selenium, thiamine and zinc in selected patients. If this initial work-up is negative, a CMR with delayed gadolinium enhancement is obtained followed by endomyocardial right ventricular biopsies, if suspicion is high for a secondary etiology. Endomyocardial biopsies help rule out myocarditis, amyloidosis, hemochromatosis and when electron microscopy is used, allows for staging of anthracycline cardiotoxicity.

Once the etiology is determined, therapy with carvedilol and ACE-inhibitors or angiotensin receptor blockers, digoxin with or without spironolactone and a statin is instituted. Further details about therapy are discussed below.

If LVD is determined to be chemotherapy-induced, we recommend withholding the agent for a month and repeat echocardiographic evaluation with strain imaging after 4 weeks of HF therapy. If the LV function recovers, then chemotherapy is instituted in the presence of HF therapy. Serial echocardiograms are done at the end of each cycle and should the LV function drop in the presence of appropriate HF therapy, the decision to permanently suspend the causal agent is made on a case-by-case basis in discussion with the oncology team.

In the inpatient setting, this approach differs somewhat owing to the clinical scenario and overall condition of patients. It is often not possible to perform coronary angiography in patients that are acutely ill, with sepsis, or in the throes of stem cell transplantation. However, if there are other indications for coronary angiography, such as acute coronary syndrome or pulmonary edema, we have a low threshold to performing right and left heart catheterization in these patients.

■ Surveillance and Prevention of Cardiotoxicity

Surveillance ■ Cardiotoxicity surveillance has historically been performed invasively with right ventricular endomyocardial biopsies.[59] Staging classifications of anthracycline cardiotoxicity have been developed but are now of mostly historical interest.[60] With the advent of imaging modalities, the search for a non-invasive biopsy equivalent has become the Rosetta Stone of chemotherapy-induced cardiotoxicity. Following the biopsy era, monitoring cardiotoxicity was accomplished with the use of multigated acquisition scans (MUGA).[61] This technology has provided accurate, reproducible, relatively inexpensive and non-invasive numerical assessment of EF in patients undergoing cardiotoxic chemotherapy.[62] Based on two case series with very few patients that have suggested usefulness of MUGAs to predict overt LVD and help tailor therapy in patients receiving anthracyclines,[61,63] guidelines have been published for serial MUGAs in these patients.[64] Still today, over three decades after the publication of initial studies and the advent of multiple newer and more sophisticated imaging modalities, MUGA is still widely used by oncologists for this purpose.

Echocardiography has a number of advantages over MUGA. There is no exposure to radiation, other aspects of cardiac structure and function can be assessed at the same time, and more subtle changes in systolic and diastolic function can be detected before overt decreases in EF. In our institution, echocardiography is the preferred method for cardiac function monitoring during chemotherapy. Additional echo parameters other than EF have been explored in clinical practice as potentially useful in predicting cardiotoxicity, such as tissue Doppler velocities, left atrial volumes, Doppler transmitral E and A values and more recently, strain rate and segmental strain analysis. Unfortunately, echocardiography has important limitations. Assessment of EF can be very erratic depending on method of assessment—whether visual, M-mode or Method of disks. Additionally, problems such as poor endocardial definition, extreme obesity, hyperinflated lungs, can severely limit accurate EF assessment. Poor endocardial definition can be circumvented with the use of intravenous contrast, thus, for serial EF monitoring purposes, contrast should be used generously. Another option with echocardiography is the use of 3-D reconstruction for EF calculation, which can help with what is perhaps the greatest downfall of echocardiography: interobserver variability. Despite these issues with EF assessment, echocardiography allows the shift of focus from EF to newer and more premature changes in LV function. It is clear that a visible fall in EF is the end result of a process that started much earlier. Stress pathway activation by anthracyclines causes alterations in genetic and molecular signaling that lead to cardiomyocyte malfunction, apoptosis and drop-out, myofibrillar disarray and hypertrophy with fibrotic substitution of the myocardium, activation of the neurohormonal axis with increased hemodynamic load, changes in diastolic function and not until very late, decreases in EF. Diastolic assessment with Tissue Doppler and transmitral flow patterns may be a more sensitive way to detect cardiotoxicity in a stage immediately before a change in EF.[65] Even earlier, speckle tracking technology offers insight into the degree and quality of deformation of the myocardial fibers. Data supports its value in early detection of subclinical myocardial dysfunction before any changes in EF become apparent.[66]

Newer and as of yet clinically unproven technologies offer hope of earlier and more accurate detection of cardiotoxic changes. Cardiac magnetic resonance (CMR) has several important conceptual advantages over the current methods. It is widely considered the gold standard for EF determination and assessment of ventricular volumes and function. In cases where there are discrepancies in EF between different modalities, CMR should be used as the definitive method. In addition, delayed gadolinium enhancement (DGE) allows for visualization of myocardial edema and may serve as a surrogate for chemotherapy induced myocardial damage. In a small study of 22 patients treated with anthracyclines, the pattern and intensity of DGE at 3 days predicted a significant reduction in EF at four weeks. In another study, looking at trastuzumab cardiotoxicity in 10 patients with EF of less than 40%, subepicardial DGE by CMR was demonstrated in all patients.[67] Further studies are required to establish the utility of DGE in cardiotoxicity detection.[68]

Molecular imaging technology for detection of apoptosis and caspase 3 activity has been tested in mice with promising results. Annexin V scintigraphy has been used to image apoptotic activity occurring in acute doxorubicin cardiotoxicity in rats.[69] This and other newer modalities are subject of intense investigations.[65]

Cardiac biomarkers such as BNP and TNI have been investigated and shown to be useful in predicting cardiac dysfunction following chemotherapy. In a small series of 52 patients, persistent elevation of BNP over a period of 72h after chemotherapy with anthracyclines was strongly associated with deteriorations in EF and diastolic function at 12 months.[70] In a group of 204 patients who received high dose chemotherapy, elevations in cardiac TNI were associated with persistent decreases in LVEF in long-term follow-up. Interestingly, in this study, the degree of initial TNI elevation correlated well to the degree of left ventricular dysfunction.[71] Larger scale trials are still underway to confirm these findings.

Prevention ■ Prophylaxis of chemotherapy-related LVD and HF has been difficult to achieve. The most efficacious strategies have included decrease in dosing, formulation, and rapidity of administration of anthracyclines. Keeping the cumulative dose of doxorubicin to less than 450 mg/m2, administration over a period of 48–72h and the advent of the liposomal formulation have significantly decreased the incidence of cardiotoxicity over the last decades to less than 3%.[72,73]

Of the many cardioprotective compounds explored, dexrazoxane has met with the most success so far. When its use with anthracyclines was compared to historical controls treated with anthracyclines only, there was a significant decrease in the incidence of heart failure over 10 years.[74] It was postulated that dexrazoxane exerted its benefit through inhibition of doxorubicin-induced DNA damage and ensuing cardiomyocyte apoptosis.[75] More recently, it was shown that dexrazoxane mediated DNA protection against doxorubicin was mediated by low levels of expression of topoisomerase 2 beta in mice.[76] Other substances such as coenzyme Q, flavonoids, vitamin C, L-carnitine, N-acetylcysteine and iron chelators were used in attempts to prevent anthracycline cardiotoxicity without much convincing success.[77]

ACE-I and betablockers, both prophylactically and as rescue therapy have also been used. In a series of 112 patients with positive troponins after high-dose chemotherapy randomized to enalapril 20 mg or placebo, 43% of placebo patients developed a >10% decrease in EF as compared to no patients in the treatment arm.[78] Carvedilol, on the other hand, has a number of potential in vitro benefits that are yet to be tested in a prospective manner in the clinical setting. Some, but not all, small randomized trials have shown benefit with betablockers and ACE inhibitors to prevent cardiotoxicity. In a trial of 90 patients with hematologic malignancies receiving anthracycline therapy randomized to enalapril+-carvedilol vs placebo, LVEF decreased in the placebo arm (−3.1%, P = 0.035) but not in the intervention arm,

and rates of heart failure or LVSD were also higher in the placebo arm (6-month incidence 6.7% vs. 24.4%, P = 0.02).[79] In a recent trial 130 patients with breast cancer randomized to candesartan and metoprolol in 2×2 factorial design, candesartan, but not metoprolol, was associated with decreased incidence of cardiotoxicity (defined as 5% change in LVEF).[80]

In our institution, we routinely use both ACE inhibitors and carvedilol in patients at risk for developing cardiotoxicity. Figures 26-1 and 26-2 show the approach for risk stratification and surveillance of cardiotoxicity in patients receiving anthracycline.

THERAPY OF HEART FAILURE

Guidelines for the treatment of HF in patients with cancer and chemotherapy-induced HF are not available. Therefore, standard HF therapy is generally applied to these patients. In this section we will focus mostly on chemotherapy-induced HF and LVD.

■ Acute Decompensated Heart Failure

The treatment of acutely ill patients with heart failure decompensation is controversial and there are no universally accepted guidelines that can be applied to cancer patients. Patients with cancer often present with symptoms and signs of heart failure that can be caused by another acute illness. The most common HF impostors in patients in a cancer center are sepsis, pulmonary embolism, pericardial tamponade, pulmonary lymphangitic carcinomatosis and alveolar hemorrhage in graft-versus-host disease in patients who have undergone stem-cell transplantation. Physical examination can be notoriously unreliable in these patients, but the most sensitive and specific sign of HF is jugular venous pressure elevation and hepatojugular reflux. Pulmonary auscultatory findings are extremely unreliable and it is common to see chronic HF patients with acute exacerbations who have a pulmonary wedge pressure of over 30 mmHg and completely clear lungs. A third heart sound is very specific but notoriously insensitive because it is difficult to recognize, independent of the level of experience of the examiner. Therefore, determination of HF by invasive and non-invasive methods is the mainstay of diagnosis in our patients. Often the co-existence of low EF and sepsis warrant a pulmonary artery catheter for etiologic diagnosis and hemodynamic-guided therapy. Once the diagnosis of acute heart failure is documented, immediate treatment is instituted based on two simple but extremely important and, sometimes difficult to ascertain, questions:

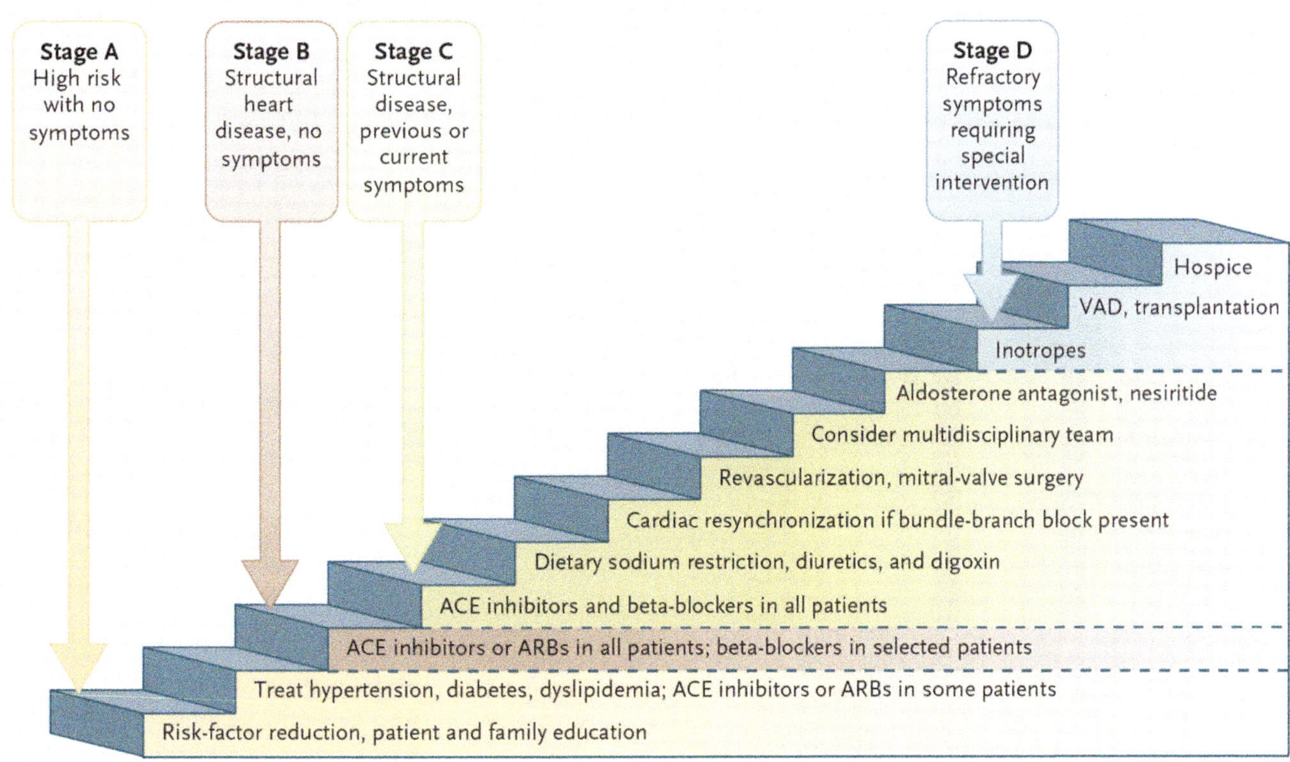

FIGURE 26-1 ACC/AHA stages of HF. (Reproduced from Jessup et al., 2003.[143])

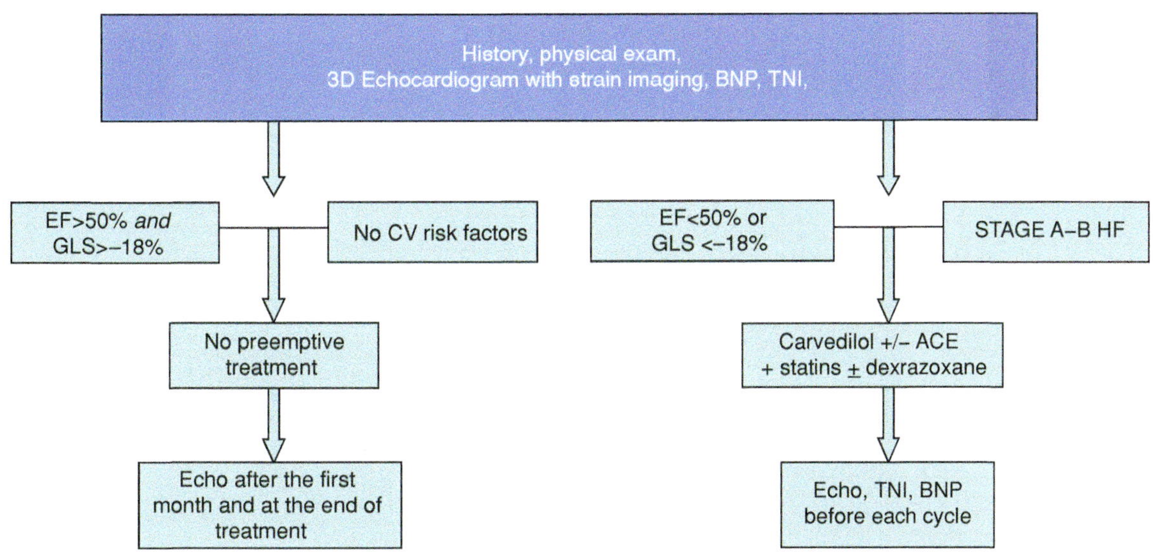

FIGURE 26-2 Approach for initial assessment of high-risk patients with planned anthracycline. (Reproduced from Al-Kindi et al., 2014.[144] Used with permission.)

1. Is the patient in a low output state? Clinical exam can offer clues to this answer with findings of cold extremities, low blood pressure and narrow pulse pressure, but the definitive answer requires invasive hemodynamic assessment. If cardiac index is below 2 L/min/m^2, it is safe to say that a low output state is present. In such cases, short-term inotropic support is warranted to rescue the patient from the inexorable downward spiral that might otherwise rapidly lead to death. In these patients, inotropic and inodilatory therapy with milrinone, dobutamine, levosimendan

or nitroprusside should be instituted. There are a few distinctions that should be borne in mind when selecting which one of these agents to use. If the patient has ischemic cardiomyopathy, dobutamine should be preferred.[81] If the patient has been on chronic beta-blocker therapy, the dose should be decreased but not discontinued,[82] and milrinone should be the drug of choice.[83] Patients not on previous beta-blocker therapy should not have these drugs initiated until they are hemodynamically stable and euvolemic (see below). Patients with HF post cardiac arrest should be treated with milrinone because it has been shown to facilitate cardiac function recovery in that setting.[84] Other considerations regarding inotropic choice are blood pressure and heart rate. An important limitation to use of milrinone and nitroprusside is hypotension with systolic blood pressure of less than 100 mmHg. Such patients benefit from the vasoconstrictive effects of higher doses of dobutamine and sometimes require concomitant use of dopamine or nor-epinephrine. Patients with atrial tachycardias, fibrillation or resting tachycardia, however, benefit from the chronotropically neutral effect of milrinone. Lastly both levosimendan and nitroprusside have been shown to be beneficial in this setting, although the former is not approved in the United States.[85,86] In some cases, however, inotropic support with drugs may not be sufficient, and intra-aortic balloon counterpulsation and other device therapy might be considered and are discussed below.

2. What is the patient's volume status? This is a crucial question to answer before initiation of therapy. In euvolemic patients, initiation of oral beta-blockade is warranted and results in better outcomes.[87] On the other hand, there is no evidence to support use of intravenous beta-blockers in this setting but rather, data demonstrating that they may be deleterious altogether. Extrapolation of data from patients with acute heart failure from myocardial infarction who received intravenous beta-blockers in a randomized fashion and had an increased incidence of cardiogenic shock and death,[88] supports the notion that intravenous beta-blockade in decompensated heart failure should be avoided. In fact, the 2007 ACC/AHA guidelines has downgraded intravenous beta-blockers to a class III indication for patients with myocardial infarction and signs of heart failure, such as resting tachycardia, low systolic blood pressure or low output state.[89]

Similarly, in patients with HF from tachyarrhythmias, the institution of intravenous calcium channel blockers for rhythm control, not only fails to achieve rhythm control, but causes worsening HF symptoms, which in turn perpetuates tachycardia. For these patients, intravenous digoxin or amiodarone are the agents of choice, with the caveat that patients with atrial fibrillation or flutter of greater than 48h duration should be fully anticoagulated before amiodarone therapy due to the potential risk of cardioversion and cerebral embolism. In cases of severe HF where the arrhythmia is thought to be the culprit, prompt cardioversion should be performed.

On the other hand, severe hypervolemia is common in newly diagnosed HF patients undergoing chemotherapy because they typically receive enormous amounts of fluids with chemotherapy. These patients do not require invasive hemodynamics because they display elevated jugular venous pressure, severe peripheral edema, symptoms of HF and extremely elevated BNPs. A documentation of depressed EF in this setting is enough to allow aggressive HF therapy. Because these patients are hypervolemic beta-blockers should be avoided initially until euvolemia is achieved, since all trials of carvedilol in class 3 and 4 HF excluded patients that were not euvolemic. Therapy with diuretics should be instituted, and for patients with cancer, torsemide and bumetamide are superior to furosemide because they have better bioavailability, are more predictably absorbed and are less dependent on albumin to be delivered to the loop of Henle. In addition, torsemide may result in better outcomes when compared to furosemide in HF patients.[90] However, aggressive diuretic treatment can sometime lead to the cardio-renal syndrome with progressive renal insufficiency and diuretic resistance. In patients that develop cardio-renal syndrome, inotropic support with dobutamine or milrinone can usually restore good diuresis, improvement in renal function and HF class. Addition of spironolactone in high doses of 100–200 mg or metolazone 5–20 mg daily can boost diuresis but also increase the need for dialysis. An intravenous drip proceeded by a loading dose of furosemide, torsemide of bumetamide is also an option in such cases. Alternatively, cardio-renal syndrome can be sometimes avoided altogether with ultrafiltration. Ultrafiltration has been shown to be superior to intravenous diuretics in activation of the neurohormonal system, decreased length of hospitalization, and total weight loss.[91] Currently, ultrafiltration is indicated for patients with gross fluid overload and that require more than 160 mg/day of furosemide with a serum creatinine of less than 3 mg/dl. Small ultrafiltration devices such as Aquadex Flex (CHF Solutions USA) can withdraw up to 500 ml/h of isotonic fluid, do not require central venous access and can be used on a regular telemetry floor.

Whatever the hemodynamic profile, the goal of therapy should be to re-establish euvolemia and hemodynamic stability. BNP can be used to assess success of therapy and help determine euvolemia in these very sick patients and are measured frequently during the course of hospitalization. Despite lack of evidence to support this practice, in our patient population, often with several concomitant disease processes, serial BNP measurement provides a compass that helps guide therapy. In our practice, we typically do not start oral beta-blocker therapy until 2 or 3 days prior to discharge if the BNP is less than 500 ng/dL.

■ Medical Therapy of Chronic Heart Failure

In patients with chemotherapy-induced HF the goal of chronic HF treatment is often to achieve recovery of LV function. Because we follow these patients so intensely, we detect early changes in systolic and diastolic function and initiate HF therapy sometimes even prophylactically when cardiotoxicity is anticipated. We have found that a high percentage of patients that develop trastuzumab cardiotoxicity with LVD recover when treated aggressively.5 This section will focus on the discussion around chemotherapy-related LVD and the available data relating specifically to this problem (Figure 26-3).

Despite a lack of strong evidence,[77] the mainstay of therapy for patients who develop chemotherapy-induced LVD and HF is carvedilol and ACE-inhibitors. In the general HF population, the benefits of carvedilol

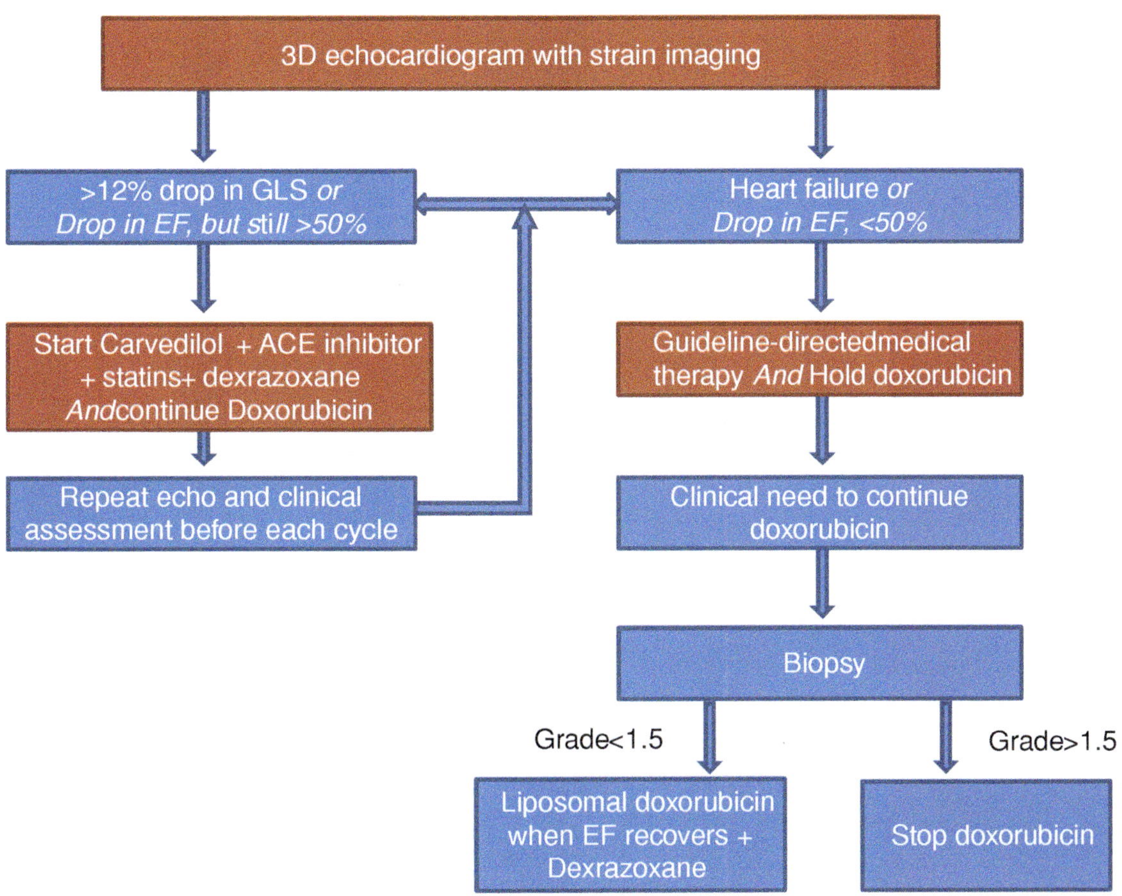

FIGURE 26-3 Approach for follow-up of patients receiving anthracyclines. (Reproduced from Al-Kindi et al., 2014.[144] Used with permission.)

are well established.[87,92] In treatment and prevention of anthracycline-induced cardiotoxicity, the use of carvedilol is supported by limited but promising data.[93,94] In addition to its multiple benefits in hemodynamic unloading and reverse remodeling, carvedilol may have specific advantages over other beta-blockers in the setting of anthracycline cardiotoxicity. Unlike other beta-blockers such as atenolol, carvedilol has been shown in vitro to prevent apoptosis by inhibiting the doxorubicin-induced activation of caspase 3.[95] This may be particular important within the concept of apoptosis interruptus (see above).

It appears that part of its beneficial effect in anthracycline-induced cardiotoxicity results from antioxidant properties rather than its beta-adrenergic antagonism.[96] Carvedilol may also conversely, potentiate the cytotoxic potential of doxorubicin against cancer cells[97] and have its own anti-proliferative effects in melanoma and leukemia cells.[98]

ACE inhibitors (ACE-I) have also been used extensively in all etiologies of HF and their impact on survival has been well established in numerous large-scale clinical trials. Angiotensin II plays an important role in carcinogenesis through its actions as a potent inducer of angiogenesis and neovascularization.[99] In humans, epidemiologic studies have associated the use of ACE-I with lower than expected incidence of cancer[100] and the antineoplastic role of ACE-I has been recently confirmed in mice injected with lung cancer cells.[101] Although the role of ACE-I in the prevention of chemotherapy-induced cardiotoxicity has been documented,[78] its usefulness in secondary treatment and rescue of cardiotoxicity has not been tested in a prospective fashion. In our own experience, 84% of patients treated with ACE-I and carvedilol who had trastuzumab-induced LVD had recovery of function.[5]

In patients with symptomatic HF as opposed to those with an asymptomatic drop in EF on screening echocardiograms, we add digoxin and in appropriate cases, spironolactone[102] to their therapy. Digoxin has been associated with symptomatic improvement and increased survival in populations of HF before the beta-blocker era.[103]

Lastly, because of the extensive body of literature supporting their use in HF and cardiovascular disease in general, we routinely treat all HF patients with statins.[104] In addition, statin therapy may have beneficial effects in doxorubicin cardiotoxicity, mediated by their antioxidant effects and inhibition of mitochondrial apoptosis in mice.[105] Interestingly, statins have been shown to have direct antineoplastic effects in tumor size reduction and chemo-sensitization.[106] They

have also been shown to induce the mammalian target of rapamycin and activate p53 deficient cells making them more susceptible to cytotoxic effects of chemotherapy agents.[107]

ADVANCED HF THERAPY IN CANCER PATIENTS

A subset of patients with HF develop progressive symptoms despite optimal medical treatment. This subset of patients has the worst prognosis in the absence of advanced therapies, such as mechanical circulatory support and heart transplantation. In this section, we discuss the epidemiology, pathophysiology and use of advanced HF therapies in chemotherapy-induced cardiomyopathy (CCMP) with advanced HF (American College of Cardiology/American Heart Association stages C-D HF). Although the majority of patients with advanced CCMP are due to anthracycline, we will also briefly discuss radiation-induced cardiomyopathy (RCMP) and implications for advanced therapies.

CCMP prevalence can be approximately extrapolated from large registries of advanced HF. For example, among hospitalized patients in the Get-with-the-Guidelines (GWTG) registry, CCMP represented 1.1% of non-ischemic cardiomyopathies and 0.46% of all patients hospitalized with heart failure.[108] However, the exact contribution of CCMP to the estimated 150,000–250,000 patients with advanced HF in the United States in 2013 is not known.[109] Analyses of the United Network of Organ Sharing (UNOS), the International Society for Heart and Lung Transplant (ISHLT) registry, and the Interagency Registry of Mechanically Assisted Circulatory Support (INTERMACS), found that CCMP patients accounted for 0.8% to 2.5% of all OHT recipients[110,111] and 0.5% of those implanted with mechanical circulatory support devices.[112] Therefore, extrapolating from large databases of highly selected patients, the prevalence of end-stage HF from CCMP is between 0.5% and 2.5%. These numbers may be an underestimation, since many CCMP patients neither have access nor are eligible for advanced therapies.

■ The Left Ventricle: Recovery of Function

The pathophysiology of CCMP has been characterized by cardiomyocyte death. Histologically, myofibrillar dropout, sarcoplasmic vacuolization, and decreased cardiomyocyte density characterize CCMP.[113] The exact mechanisms of these effects are thought to involve anthracycline-induced production of reactive oxygen species that disrupt cardiac topoisomerase 2b activity causing DNA double-strand breaks, irreversible mitochondrial dysfunction and apoptosis.[114,115] In addition, anthracyclines have been associated with depletion of progenitor stem cells responsible for restoring cardiomyocytes and promoting LV recovery.[116,117] This evidence implies that anthracycline cardiotoxicity may not be reversible. However, left ventricular dysfunction and HF seen in acute-onset anthracycline cardiotoxicity (with variable low cumulative doses of anthracyclines) may be precipitated by localized myocardial inflammation, arrhythmia, sepsis, hormonal activation, which are mistakenly attributed to anthracycline and labeled erroneously as CCMP In addition, concomitant HER2 antagonist, known to result in reversible LV dysfunction, may potentiate anthracycline-cardiotoxicity, resulting in 'reversible' pattern of CCMP.

In real-world setting, recovery of LV function has been reported in clinical studies of patients receiving anthracyclines. For example, among 104 patients receiving various chemotherapy agents and developed de novo LV dysfunction, recovery of LV function occurred in about half of the patients (55%). In another study of 226 patients who developed LV dysfunction after anthracycline, 11% had full recovery and 71% had partial recovery after receiving standard heart failure pharmacotherapy.[94]

Few cases of myocardial recovery and device explantation have been reported in CCMP-labeled patients.[118–122] In the authors' opinion, these most likely represent examples of patients with reversible cancer therapy-associated LV dysfunction rather than end-stage anthracycline-induced CCMP.

■ Right Ventricular Involvement

Pathology studies have long established right ventricular (RV) injury by anthracyclines.[59] In fact, RV biopsies have reliably diagnosed, tracked and predicted LV dysfunction in CCMP.[123,124] In CCMP, RV systolic dysfunction precedes LV dysfunction and is associated with worse outcomes. For example, breast cancer patients followed by echocardiography had significant decreases in tricuspid annular plane systolic excursion and right ventricular fractional area after only two cycles of doxorubicin.[125] Similarly, 29 of 36 (81%) breast cancer patients receiving doxorubicin and trastuzumab developed greater RV than LV impairment at 12 months by cardiac magnetic resonance imaging.[126] Among 30 patients with breast cancer undergoing anthracycline ± HER2 inhibitors compared with

age-balanced pre-treatment controls, RV fractional area change was significantly lower than controls (42 ± 7 versus 47 ± 6%, P = 0.01), while RV dysfunction (defined by global longitudinal strain < −20.3%) was seen in 40% (n = 12).[127]

RV impairment carries even more important implications in end-stage CCMP. Analyses of advanced therapies in CCMP have confirmed the prevailing clinical suspicion that these patients have increased incidence of RV failure. In fact, patients with CCMP undergoing LVAD implantation had higher risk of post-implant RV failure and death than patients with other etiologies.[128] CCMP patients were twice as likely to have required biventricular assist devices by the time of transplantation as other non-ischemic patients (5.6% vs. 2.3%, p = 0.002).[112] In INTERMACS, almost a fifth of patients with CCMP needed biventricular support, significantly more than both ischemic and other non-ischemic patients (19% vs. 6% vs. 11%, p = 0.006), Figure 26-1. Surrogate markers of RV function were also more abnormal in CCMP patients, with higher mean right atrial pressures, lower mean pulmonary artery pressure, higher central venous pressure to pulmonary capillary wedge pressure ratio and higher incidence of severe tricuspid regurgitation. These data were also observed in CCMP patients undergoing heart transplantation in the ISHLT registry, and corroborate the importance of RV impairment in CCMP, underscoring the need for careful assessment of RV function prior to LVAD.

■ Epidemiology of Advanced HF in Cancer Patients

Large databases have unveiled unique characteristics of CCMP patients (Table 26-2). They are often younger and consistently healthier, with significantly less prevalence of diabetes, hypertension, tobacco, alcohol or illicit drug use.[110,112] Additionally, there seems to be a clear female predominance. Females represented 67% of all hospitalized patients with CCMP in the GWTG registry.[108] Similarly, of the 75 CCMP patients identified in the INTERMACS registry, 54 (72%) were women, compared to ischemic and non-ischemic cardiomyopathy where men predominate at 87% and 76%, respectively.[112] Finally, two thirds of CCMP patients who received heart transplantation in the United States were women.[110,111] The reason for this gender disparity is not entirely clear although predominance of breast cancer in women has been implicated. However, factors intrinsic to female sex may play a role as is suggested by similar findings[25] among patients with hematologic malignancies that typically

TABLE 26-2   Characteristics of cancer survivors with advanced HF

CHARACTERISTICS
- Young (mean 5–10 years younger than other etiologies)
- Predominantly females (60%–70%)
- Predominantly White/Caucasian
- Lower prevalence of diabetes, hypertension, dyslipidemia, obesity
- Chest irradiation exposure, complicated by valve disease and coronary bypass

lack gender predilection as well as previous work by Lipshultz et al.[129]

Therapies

Cardiac Resynchronization Therapy and Implantable Cardiac Defibrillators ■ Cardiac resynchronization therapy (CRT) has emerged as a therapeutic option for patients with HF and mechanical dyssynchrony, increasing additive survival and quality of life to guideline-directed medical therapy.[130,131]

Small data series suggest favorable effects of resynchronization in patients with CCMP, despite its different myocardial substrate.

In a small case series, four patients with CCMP and prolonged QRS (129–171 milliseconds) were treated with CRT. All four patients experienced improved NYHA class to I or II, 6-minute walk test, quality of life and echocardiographic parameters (LVEF (21% to 46%), left ventricular end-diastolic dimension from mean of 55 mm to 47 mm) at 6-month follow-up.[132]

In a larger series, 18 patients with CCMP and prolonged QRS received CRT and were compared to 189 patients with other types of non-ischemic cardiomyopathy who received CRT. CCMP patients were more likely to be women, have narrower QRS, and less likely to have atrial fibrillation and hypertension than controls. CCMP patients were survivors of breast cancer, lymphoma and sarcoma, and the majority had received radiation. After a mean follow-up of 9.1 months, patients with CCMP patients had improvement in all echocardiographic parameters, including LVEF (from mean of $18.6 \pm 7.6\%$ to $27.2 \pm 13.5\%$), LVEDD (6.04 ± 0.63 cm to 5.56 ± 0.95 cm), mitral regurgitation severity (4.3 ± 2 to 3.1 ± 1.9) and NYHA class (2.9 ± 0.3 to 2.4 ± 0.3), comparable to patients with non-ischemic cardiomyopathy.[133]

While promising, these reports are small and the role of CRT-D in CCMP is not completely understood. The ongoing Multicenter Automatic Defibrillator Implantation Trial-Chemotherapy-Induced Cardiomyopathy (MADIT-CHIC), designed to evaluate the role of CRT-D in CCMP will likely provide further clarification on the efficacy of CRT in this population.

Whereas there are no data specifically addressing the use of implantable cardioverter defibrillator (ICD) in CCMP, significantly less CCMP patients in the INTERMACS registry had ICD compared to other etiologies (66% vs. 77%, respectively, p<0.05).[112] It is possible that CCMP patients remain undiagnosed until acute presentation and rapid progression, thus obviating ICD placement. Nevertheless, it is concerning that a high percentage of CCMP patients do not receive prophylaxis for sudden cardiac death. These observations underscore the importance of echocardiographic screening in asymptomatic or oligosymptomatic cancer survivors with a history of cardiotoxic chemotherapy to unveil subclinical left ventricular systolic dysfunction, and identify eligibility for ICD implantation.

Mechanical Circulatory Support ■ Ventricular Assist Devices (VADs) are a form of cardiac replacement therapy which allow for substitution of the heart's pumping function by that of an intracavitary electrical pump. Once initially used for short term postoperative support that required intensive care stay and very large bedside extracorporeal pumps.[134] VADs are now small intracorporeal devices that can be used for a number of years.[135]

Improved technology has culminated in the advent of short-term devices that can be percutaneously inserted via the subclavian artery and small long-term devices surgically implanted in the intraabdominal cavity. Continuous flow devices, such as the Heartmate 2 and the heartware devices have proven efficacy and safety as a bridge to transplantation or as destination therapy.[136] However, the benefits of LVADs in patients with CCMP had been unclear until recently.

The safety and efficacy of LVADs in this group was established by an INTERMACS analysis of 75 CCMP patients.[112] Despite having increased bleeding and requiring more biventricular support, CCMP patients had similar outcomes to other patients in the registry (Figures 26-4 and 26-5). It is possible that survival among CCMP patients was favorably influenced

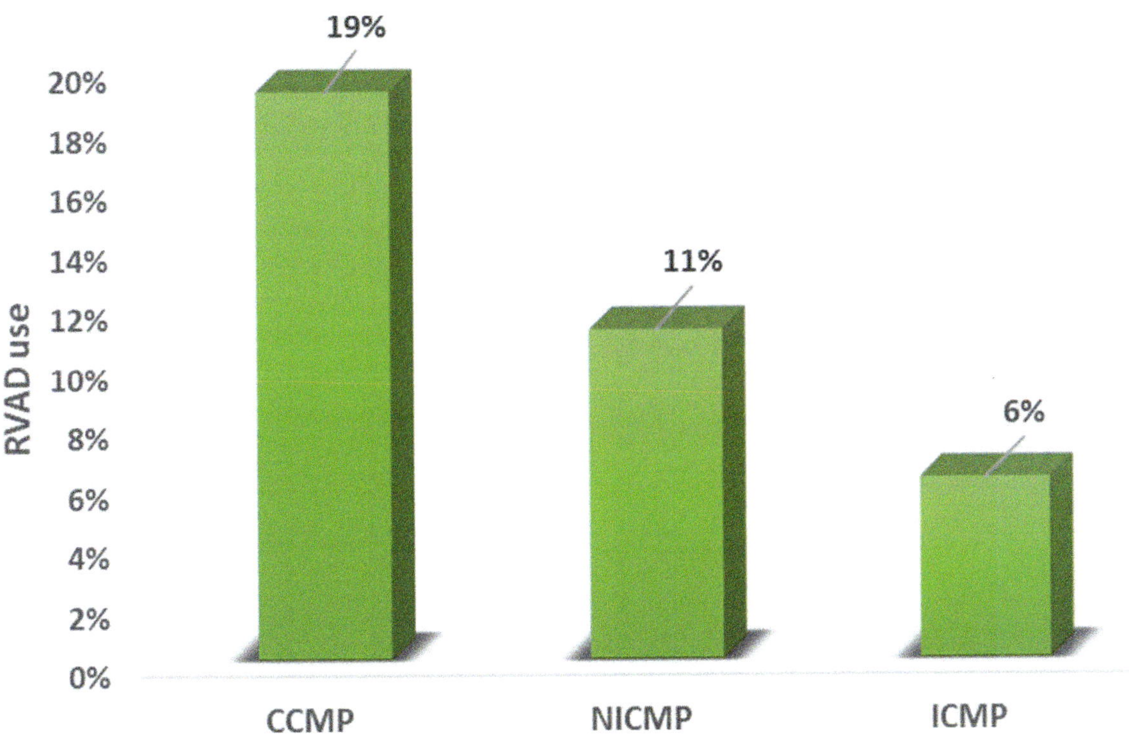

FIGURE 26-4   RVAD use according to etiology of cardiomyopathy. CCMP = chemotherapy-induced cardiomyopathy; ICMP = ischemic cardiomyopathy; NICMP = non-ischemic cardiomyopathy; RVAD = right ventricular assist device. (Adapted with permission from Oliveira, 2014.[112])

by being significantly younger, healthier and leaner than their ischemic and non-ischemic counterparts. Indeed, careful analysis of the survival curves suggests that a small survival disadvantage might be found if the sample size were larger. Because curve separates within the first 3 months, when most patients with biventricular support die (Figure 26-5F), it is possible that post-implant RV failure contributed significantly to mortality.

It was also evident that CCMP patients are more acutely ill at presentation than other groups, with a trend towards higher inotrope use, higher BNP and less use of defibrillators. Another interesting aspect of LVAD use in this population is that about a third were implanted as destination therapy, significantly higher than NICMP and ICMP (14% and 23% p<0.001). Because this occurs despite their younger age and better health, the most logical inference is that about one-third of CCMP patients present within 5 years of cancer diagnosis.

There are important considerations when implanting LVADs in patients with CCMP patients (Table 26-3). First, as mentioned earlier, careful assessment of RV function, through imaging and hemodynamic measurements, should be performed to avoid unexpected post-LVAD RV failure. Second, it is important that identify history of chest radiation, which may complicate surgery because of tpericardial

adhesions or presence of concomitant valve disease requiring valve replacement.

In conclusion, LVADs seem to be effective and safe for patients with advanced HF due to CCMP. Despite increased need for biventricular support and higher frequency of bleeding, carefully selected CCMP patients who are implanted with LVADs have survival comparable to other etiologies.

Heart Transplantation ■ Heart transplantation remains the gold standard therapy for end-stage HF with a median survival of 11 years.[137] CCMP patients are often ineligible for transplant because of current or previous history of malignancy within 5 years,[138] and their eligibility has been often mitigated by concerns for recurrent or de novo malignancies in the setting of immunosuppressive therapy. Nevertheless, there is good evidence supporting the safety of transplant in CCMP. In addition to anecdotal cases and small series, there are two large-scale reports analyzing the outcomes of CCMP patients treated with OHT.

Between 2000 and 2008, there were 232 adults with CCMP who underwent OHT in the International Society of Heart and Lung Transplantation (ISHLT) registry. The overall survival was not different between CCMP and other non-ischemic patients, with 1, 2 and 5 year survival (86% vs. 87%, 79% vs. 81%

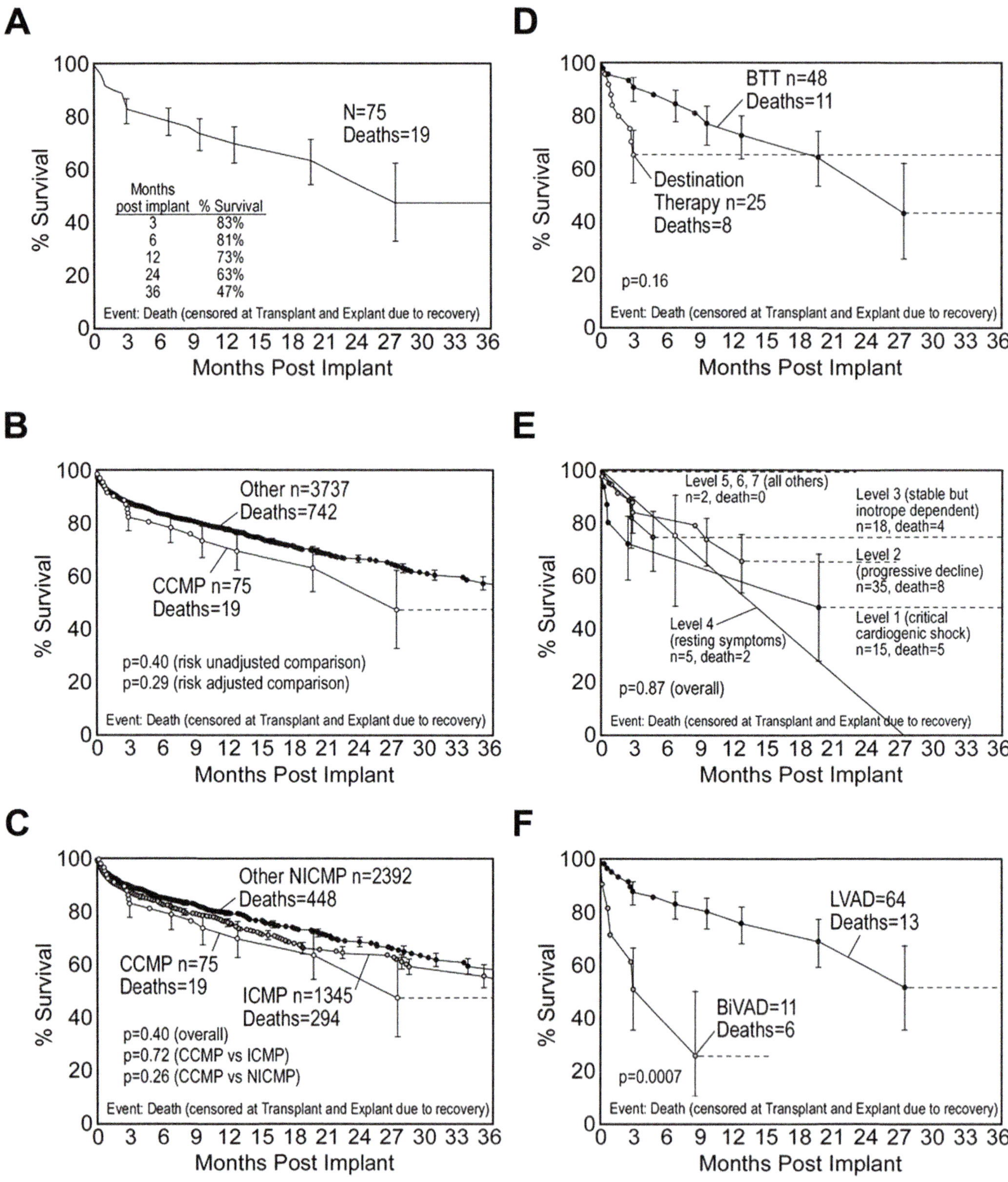

FIGURE 26-5 Survival of CCMP patients implanted with MCSD: (A) CCMP patients only; (B) CCMP versus (ICMP and NICMP) adult primary implants; (C) CCMP versus ICMP versus NICMP adult primary implants; (D) CCMP patients by device strategy; (E) CCMP by patient profile; (F) CCMP patients by device side. MCSD, mechanical circulatory support devices; BTT, bridge to transplantation; BiVAD, biventricular assist device; LVAD, left ventricular assist device; CCMP, chemotherapy-induced cardiomyopathy; ICMP, ischemic cardiomyopathy; NICMP, nonischemic cardiomyopathy. (Reproduced from Oliveira, 2014.[112])

TABLE 26-3 Special considerations for treatment of advanced HF due to CCMP

MCS	OHT
- Increased RV failure	- Difficult sternotomy (if radiation)
- Increased bleeding	- Cancer recurrence
- Increased infections	- Infections
- ? device thrombosis	- Concomitant lung disease
- Restrictive physiology if history of radiation	

and 71% vs. 74%, p = 0.19) (Figure 26-5). Interestingly, the risk of cardiac allograft rejection in the first year post-transplant was lower in CCMP than non-ischemic patients (28% vs. 38%, p = 0.03), likely reflecting immunologic down-regulation due to bone marrow suppression from cancer treatments. Consistent with this hypothesis, post-transplant infection rates were higher in the CCMP group (22% vs. 14%, p = 0.04). In line with younger age and less co-morbidities, CMMP recipients had lower incidence of post-transplant renal dysfunction (24% vs. 29%, p = 0.02), and none of the CCMP patients required renal replacement therapy or renal transplantation.[110]

Despite longstanding concerns related to cancer recurrence in this patient population, there was no increase in malignancy recurrence or death from cancer; and only skin cancer was more frequent among CCMP recipients.

In a larger study of the United Network for Organ Sharing (UNOS) registry analysis of 435 CCMP heart transplant recipients from 1987 to 2011, the 10-year survival of CCMP recipients was better than non-ischemic cardiomyopathies after multiple adjustments (hazard ratio 1.28 [1.03–1.59], p = 0.026). Overall, there was a significant increasing trend in the proportion of CCMP among non-ischemic patients from 1987 to 2011[111] (0.5% to >1.5% p<0.001), reflecting a possible increasing prevalence and/or transplant eligibility of advanced CCMP.

Not all patients with end-stage HF exposed to chemotherapy have similar outcomes with OHT. Eighty-seven patients with history of restrictive cardiomyopathy from chemotherapy and radiation listed for OHT in UNOS database (2000–2015), had worse survival compared to those with other types of restrictive cardiomyopathy and other etiologies (Figures 26-6 and 26-7). This was mainly due to early post-transplant mortality (21%). A possible explanation for this is the presence of co-existing radiation-induced restrictive lung disease in such patients, which leads to pulmonary complications reflected in increased length of stay and higher respiratory-related mortality.[139]

In conclusion, OHT is appropriate, safe and yields equivalent survival in CCMP recipients compared to those transplanted for other cardiomyopathies. Regarding the risk of cancer reactivation by immunosuppressive therapy, it should be noted that of 232 transplanted CCMP patients only one death occurred because of recurrence of the primary malignancy.[25] This implies that the arbitrary 5-year period of cancer-freedom commonly imposed before granting transplant eligibility for CCMP patients is probably too strict. Especially in patients with breast cancer and hematologic malignancies, for whom the prognosis and likelihood of recurrence can be established with reasonable certainty at presentation depending on cancer staging.[140–142] Lastly, because CCMP patients are younger, healthier and may not be as easily supported with currently approved devices, we propose that the blanket five year moratorium prior to transplant be abandoned altogether and that time to OHT eligibility be decided in consultation with an oncologist, on an individual basis, and as short as possible.

FUTURE DIRECTIONS

The therapy of cancer is likely what will direct the future of cardiovascular and HF therapeutics. Intense basic and translational research in cancer has pointed inadvertently to new mechanisms in the pathogenesis of HF and unveiled new unsuspected pathways of myocardial survival. The armamentarium of unselective small molecule tyrosine kinase targeted therapy under development will likely reveal new pathways to cardiotoxicity and thereby point towards new mechanistic hypotheses of HF development and progression. Such discoveries will hopefully result in HF therapy targeted at those same molecular pathways that are disrupted by current and future anti-cancer drugs.

In parallel, new avenues for management of HF as a result of cancer therapy will require more investments in clinical, translational and basic research, not directed at cancer, but at HF. The importance of the mechanistic intersection of HF and cancer will need to be more widely recognized by both the cardiology and oncology community, and increased cooperation must ensue.

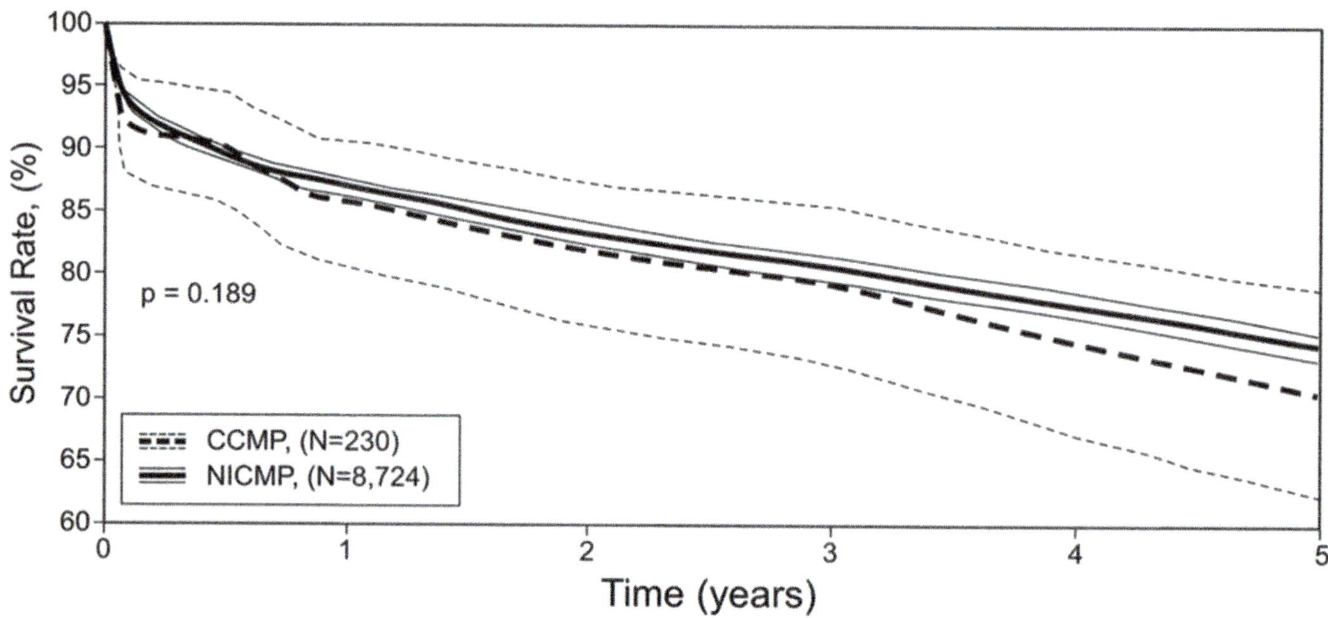

FIGURE 26-6   Post-transplant survival of anthracycline-induced cardiomyopathy (CCMP and other non-ischemic cardio-myopathy (NICMP) patients. Patients with CCMP are indicated by bold dotted lines, with the associated confident intervals as small dotted lines, and patients with NICMP are indicated by the black line, with 95% confidence intervals as faint black lines. (Reproduced from Oliveira, 2012.[110])

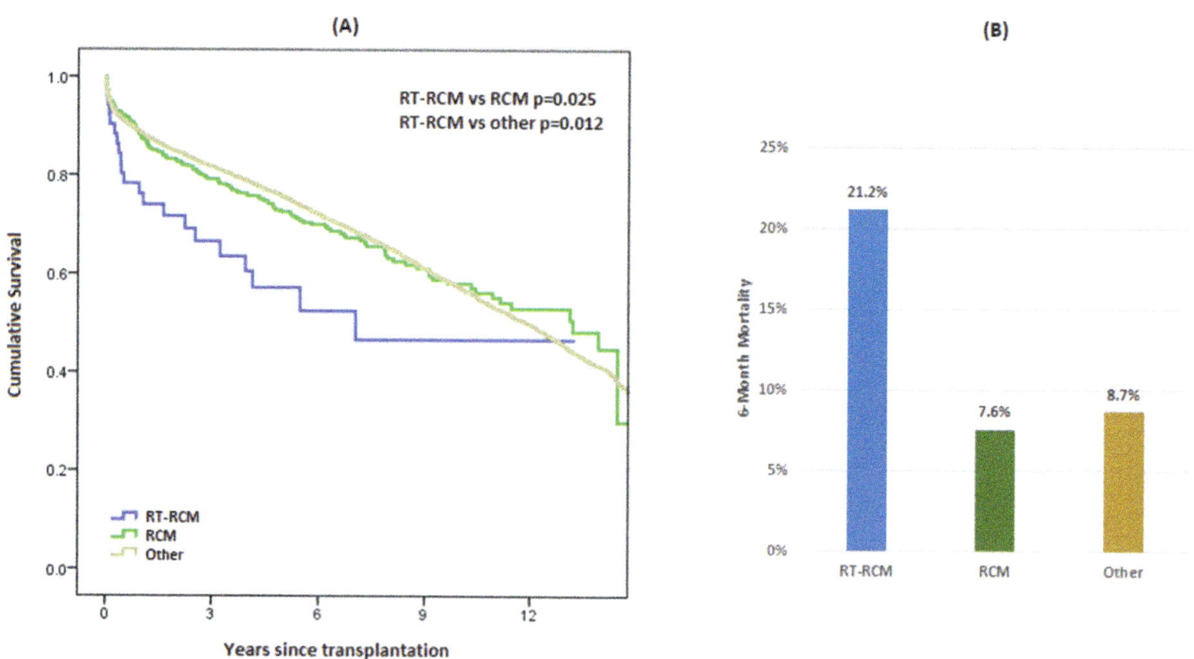

FIGURE 26-7   Post-transplantation survival by etiology in radiation-induced restrictive cardiomyopathy (RT-RCM), other restrictive cardiomyopathies (RCM) and other etiologies (A) Kaplan-Meier (B) six-month mortality. (Reproduced from Al-Kindi, 2016.[139])

In terms of diagnosis and monitoring of cardiac function during chemotherapy, new technologies involving molecular imaging, CMR with newer biological markers, may provide us with the elusive non-invasive biopsy method. Single protein testing and biomarkers specific for cardiotoxicity may become available and allow better determination of risk.

Therapeutically, in the immediate future, the hemodynamic and neurohormonal HF therapy that is now available, especially ACE-I and beta-blockers, must be tested prospectively in large-scale multicenter trials to determine their efficacy in prevention and/or rescue of chemotherapy-induced cardiomyopathy. If so, their use must be widespread; if not, a paradigm shift in HF therapy to molecular targeted therapy must occur as soon as possible. Stem cell transplantation and the mobilization of cardiac progenitor cells is an exciting prospect for anthracycline cardiotoxicity, given the recent finding that repletion of the latter may result in rescue of cardiac function.[117] Also the advent of organ cloning, total artificial hearts and improved organ replacement strategies might offer hope to patients with HF who could further benefit from additional cardiotoxic cancer therapy.

Ultimately, however, genetic profiling and gene-targeted therapy will provide the final answers to many of the most pressing problems in onco-cardiology today, and allow for truly personalized cancer and HF therapy.

REFERENCES

1. Carver JR, Shapiro CL, Ng A, et al. American Society of Clinical Oncology clinical evidence review on the ongoing care of adult cancer survivors: cardiac and pulmonary late effects. *J Clin Oncol.* 2007;25(25):3991–4008.

2. Lloyd-Jones D, Adams R, Carnethon M, et al. Heart disease and stroke statistics—2009 update: a report from the American heart association statistics committee and stroke statistics subcommittee. *Circulation.* 2009;119(3):e21–e181.

3. Yeh ET, Bickford CL. Cardiovascular complications of cancer therapy: incidence, pathogenesis, diagnosis, and management. *J Am Coll Cardiol.* 2009;53(24):2231–2247.

4. Johnson DB, Balko JM, Compton ML, et al. Fulminant myocarditis with combination immune checkpoint blockade. *N Engl J Med.* 2016;375(18):1749–1755.

5. Ewer MS, Vooletich MT, Durand JB, et al. Reversibility of trastuzumab-related cardiotoxicity: new insights based on clinical course and response to medical treatment. *J Clin Oncol.* 2005;23(31):7820–7826.

6. Ewer MS, Lippman SM. Type II chemotherapy-related cardiac dysfunction: time to recognize a new entity. *J Clin Oncol.* 2005;23(13):2900–2902.

7. Al-Kindi SG, Oliveira GH. Prevalence of preexisting cardiovascular disease in patients with different types of cancer: the unmet need for onco-cardiology. *Mayo Clin Proc.* 2016;91(1):81–83.

8. Givertz MM. Underlying causes and survival in patients with heart failure. *N Engl J Med.* 2000;342(15):1120–1122.

9. Siegel RL, Miller KD, Jemal A. Cancer statistics, 2017. *CA Cancer J Clin.* 2017;67(1):7–30.

10. Bhatia RS, Tu JV, Lee DS, et al. Outcome of heart failure with preserved ejection fraction in a population-based study. *N Engl J Med.* 2006;355(3):260–269.

11. O'Meara E, Clayton T, McEntegart MB, et al. Sex differences in clinical characteristics and prognosis in a broad spectrum of patients with heart failure: results of the Candesartan in Heart Failure: Assessment of Reduction in Mortality and Morbidity (CHARM) program. *Circulation.* 2007;115(24):3111–3120.

12. Oeffinger KC, Mertens AC, Sklar CA, et al. Chronic health conditions in adult survivors of childhood cancer. *N Engl J Med.* 2006;355(15):1572–1582.

13. Andersson A, Näslund U, Tavelin B, Enblad G, Gustavsson A, Malmer B. Long-term risk of cardiovascular disease in Hodgkin lymphoma survivors—retrospective cohort analyses and a concept for prospective intervention. *Int J Cancer.* 2009;124(8):1914–1917.

14. Hooning MJ, Botma A, Aleman BM, et al. Long-term risk of cardiovascular disease in 10-year survivors of breast cancer. *J Natl Cancer Inst.* 2007;99(5):365–375.

15. Kremer LC, van Dalen EC, Offringa M, Ottenkamp J, Voûte PA. Anthracycline-induced clinical heart failure in a cohort of 607 children: long-term follow-up study. *J Clin Oncol.* 2001;19(1):191–196.

16. Hequet O, Le QH, Moullet I, et al. Subclinical late cardiomyopathy after doxorubicin therapy for lymphoma in adults. *J Clin Oncol.* 2004;22(10):1864–1871.

17. Riley T, Sontag E, Chen P, Levine A. Transcriptional control of human p53-regulated genes. *Nat Rev Mol Cell Biol.* 2008;9(5):402–412.

18. Green DR, Kroemer G. Cytoplasmic functions of the tumour suppressor p53. *Nature.* 2009;458(7242):1127–1130.

19. Narula J, Haider N, Arbustini E, Chandrashekhar Y. Mechanisms of disease: apoptosis in heart failure—seeing hope in death. *Nat Clin Pract Cardiovasc Med.* 2006;3(12):681–688.

20. L'Ecuyer T, Sanjeev S, Thomas R, et al. DNA damage is an early event in doxorubicin-induced cardiac myocyte death. *Am J Physiol Heart Circ Physiol.* 2006;291(3):H1273–H1280.

21. Liu X, Chua CC, Gao J, et al. Pifithrin-alpha protects against doxorubicin-induced apoptosis and acute cardiotoxicity in mice. *Am J Physiol Heart Circ Physiol.* 2004;286(3):H933–H939.

22. Slamon DJ, Leyland-Jones B, Shak S, et al. Use of chemotherapy plus a monoclonal antibody against HER2 for metastatic breast cancer that overexpresses HER2. *N Engl J Med.* 2001;344(11):783–792.

23. Piccart-Gebhart MJ, Procter M, Leyland-Jones B, et al. Trastuzumab after adjuvant chemotherapy in HER2-positive breast cancer. *N Engl J Med.* 2005;353(16):1659–1672.

24. Seidman A, Hudis C, Pierri MK, et al. Cardiac dysfunction in the trastuzumab clinical trials experience. *J Clin Oncol.* 2002;20(5):1215–1221.

25. Ozcelik C, Erdmann B, Pilz B, et al. Conditional mutation of the ErbB2 (HER2) receptor in cardiomyocytes leads to dilated cardiomyopathy. *Proc Natl Acad Sci USA.* 2002;99(13):8880–8885.

26. Lemmens K, Segers VF, Demolder M, De Keulenaer GW. Role of neuregulin-1/ErbB2 signaling in endothelium-cardiomyocyte cross-talk. *J Biol Chem.* 2006;281(28):19469–19477.

27. Ky B, Kimmel SE, Safa RN, et al. Neuregulin-1 beta is associated with disease severity and adverse outcomes in chronic heart failure. *Circulation*. 2009;120(4):310–317.

28. Folkman J. Tumor angiogenesis: therapeutic implications. *N Engl J Med*. 1971;285(21):1182–1186.

29. Sano M, Minamino T, Toko H, et al. P53-induced inhibition of Hif-1 causes cardiac dysfunction during pressure overload. *Nature*. 2007;446(7134):444–448.

30. Kerkelä R, Grazette L, Yacobi R, et al. Cardiotoxicity of the cancer therapeutic agent imatinib mesylate. *Nat Med*. 2006;12(8):908–916.

31. Khakoo AY, Kassiotis CM, Tannir N, et al. Heart failure associated with sunitinib malate: a multi-targeted receptor tyrosine kinase inhibitor. *Cancer*. 2008;112(11):2500–2508.

32. Schmidinger M, Zielinski CC, Vogl UM, et al. Cardiac toxicity of sunitinib and sorafenib in patients with metastatic renal cell carcinoma. *J Clin Oncol*. 2008;26(32):5204–5212.

33. Hennessy BT, Smith DL, Ram PT, Lu Y, Mills GB. Exploiting the PI3K/AKT pathway for cancer drug discovery. *Nat Rev Drug Discov*. 2005;4(12):988–1004.

34. Cheng H, Force T. Molecular mechanisms of cardiovascular toxicity of targeted cancer therapeutics. *Circ Res*. 2010;106(1):21–34.

35. Trent JC, Patel SS, Zhang J, et al. Rare incidence of congestive heart failure in gastrointestinal stromal tumor and other sarcoma patients receiving imatinib mesylate. *Cancer*. 2010;116(1):184–192.

36. Gottdiener JS, Appelbaum FR, Ferrans VJ, Deisseroth A, Ziegler J. Cardiotoxicity associated with high-dose cyclophosphamide therapy. *Arch Intern Med*. 1981;141(6):758–763.

37. Taniguchi I. Clinical significance of cyclophosphamide-induced cardiotoxicity. *Intern Med*. 2005;44(2):89–90.

38. Carter JM, Bergin PS. Doxorubicin cardiotoxicity. *N Engl J Med*. 1986;314(17):1118–1119.

39. Yeh ET, Tong AT, Lenihan DJ, et al. Cardiovascular complications of cancer therapy: diagnosis, pathogenesis, and management. *Circulation*. 2004;109(25):3122–3131.

40. Hoshijima M, Chien KR. Mixed signals in heart failure: cancer rules. *J Clin Invest*. 2002;109(7):849–855.

41. Joensuu H, Kellokumpu-Lehtinen PL, Bono P, et al. Adjuvant docetaxel or vinorelbine with or without trastuzumab for breast cancer. *N Engl J Med*. 2006;354(8):809–820.

42. Chien KR. Stress pathways and heart failure. *Cell*. 1999;98(5):555–558.

43. Fajardo LF. Basic mechanisms and general morphology of radiation injury. *Semin Roentgenol*. 1993;28(4):297–302.

44. Tolba KA, Deliargyris EN. Cardiotoxicity of cancer therapy. *Cancer Invest*. 1999;17(6):408–422.

45. Ilhan I, Sarialioglu F, Ozbarlas N, Büyükpamukçu M, Akyüz C, Kutluk T. Late cardiac effects after treatment for childhood Hodgkin's disease with chemotherapy and low-dose radiotherapy. *Postgrad Med J*. 1995;71(833):164–167.

46. Stewart JR, Fajardo LF. Radiation-induced heart disease. Clinical and experimental aspects. *Radiol Clin North Am*. 1971;9(3):511–531.

47. Veinot JP, Edwards WD. Pathology of radiation-induced heart disease: a surgical and autopsy study of 27 cases. *Hum Pathol*. 1996;27(8):766–773.

48. Adams MJ, Hardenbergh PH, Constine LS, Lipshultz SE. Radiation-associated cardiovascular disease. *Crit Rev Oncol Hematol*. 2003;45(1):55–75.

49. Mulrooney DA, Yeazel MW, Kawashima T, et al. Cardiac outcomes in a cohort of adult survivors of childhood and adolescent cancer: retrospective analysis of the childhood cancer survivor study cohort. *BMJ*. 2009;339:b4606.

50. Donnellan E, Masri A, Johnston DR, et al. Long-term outcomes of patients with mediastinal radiation-associated severe aortic stenosis and subsequent surgical aortic valve replacement: a matched cohort study. *J Am Heart Assoc*. 2017;6(5). doi:10.1161/JAHA.116.005396.

51. Oliveira GH, Al-Kindi SG, Hoimes C, Park SJ. Characteristics and survival of malignant cardiac tumors: a 40-year analysis of >500 patients. *Circulation*. 2015;132(25):2395–2402.

52. Reardon MJ, Walkes JC, Benjamin R. Therapy insight: malignant primary cardiac tumors. *Nat Clin Pract Cardiovasc Med*. 2006;3(10):548–553.

53. Bhattacharyya S, Davar J, Dreyfus G, Caplin ME. Carcinoid heart disease. *Circulation*. 2007;116(24):2860–2865.

54. Pellikka PA, Tajik AJ, Khandheria BK, et al. Carcinoid heart disease. Clinical and echocardiographic spectrum in 74 patients. *Circulation*. 1993;87(4):1188–1196.

55. Møller JE, Connolly HM, Rubin J, Seward JB, Modesto K, Pellikka PA. Factors associated with progression of carcinoid heart disease. *N Engl J Med*. 2003;348(11):1005–1015.

56. Møller JE, Pellikka PA, Bernheim AM, Schaff HV, Rubin J, Connolly HM. Prognosis of carcinoid heart disease: analysis of 200 cases over two decades. *Circulation*. 2005;112(21):3320–3327.

57. Bernheim AM, Connolly HM, Rubin J, et al. Role of hepatic resection for patients with carcinoid heart disease. *Mayo Clin Proc*. 2008;83(2):143–150.

58. Patel T, Al-Kindi S, Oliveira G. Trends in cardiac imaging in patients receiving cardiotoxic chemotherapy. *J Am Coll Cardiol*. 2017;69:1498.

59. Billingham ME, Mason JW, Bristow MR, Daniels JR. Anthracycline cardiomyopathy monitored by morphologic changes. *Cancer Treat Rep*. 1978;62(6):865–872.

60. Mackay B, Ewer MS, Carrasco CH, Benjamin RS. Assessment of anthracycline cardiomyopathy by endomyocardial biopsy. *Ultrastruct Pathol*. 1994;18(1–2):203–211.

61. Alexander J, Dainiak N, Berger HJ, et al. Serial assessment of doxorubicin cardiotoxicity with quantitative radionuclide angiocardiography. *N Engl J Med*. 1979;300(6):278–283.

62. Strashun AM, Goldsmith SJ, Horowitz SF. Gated blood pool scintigraphic monitoring of doxorubicin cardiomyopathy: comparison of camera and computerized

probe results in 101 patients. *J Am Coll Cardiol.* 1986;8(5):1082–1087.

63. Ritchie JL, Singer JW, Thorning D, Sorensen SG, Hamilton GW. Anthracycline cardiotoxicity: clinical and pathologic outcomes assessed by radionuclide ejection fraction. *Cancer.* 1980;46(5):1109–1116.

64. Steinherz LJ, Graham T, Hurwitz R, et al. Guidelines for cardiac monitoring of children during and after anthracycline therapy: report of the cardiology committee of the childrens cancer study group. *Pediatrics.* 1992; 89(5 pt 1):942–949.

65. Jurcut R, Wildiers H, Ganame J, D'Hooge J, Paridaens R, Voigt JU. Detection and monitoring of cardiotoxicity-what does modern cardiology offer? *Support Care Cancer.* 2008;16(5):437–445.

66. Jassal DS, Han SY, Hans C, et al. Utility of tissue Doppler and strain rate imaging in the early detection of trastuzumab and anthracycline mediated cardiomyopathy. *J Am Soc Echocardiogr.* 2009;22(4):418–424.

67. Fallah-Rad N, Lytwyn M, Fang T, Kirkpatrick I, Jassal DS. Delayed contrast enhancement cardiac magnetic resonance imaging in trastuzumab induced cardiomyopathy. *J Cardiovasc Magn Reson.* 2008;10:5.

68. Yeh ET, Oliveira GH, Bickford C. Reply. *J Am Coll Cardiol.* 2010;55(2):172.

69. Bennink RJ, van den Hoff MJ, van Hemert FJ, et al. Annexin V imaging of acute doxorubicin cardiotoxicity (apoptosis) in rats. *J Nucl Med.* 2004;45(5):842–848.

70. Sandri MT, Salvatici M, Cardinale D, et al. N-terminal pro-B-type natriuretic peptide after high-dose chemotherapy: a marker predictive of cardiac dysfunction? *Clin Chem.* 2005;51(8):1405–1410.

71. Cardinale D, Sandri MT, Martinoni A, et al. Left ventricular dysfunction predicted by early troponin I release after high-dose chemotherapy. *J Am Coll Cardiol.* 2000;36(2):517–522.

72. O'Brien ME, Wigler N, Inbar M, et al. Reduced cardiotoxicity and comparable efficacy in a phase III trial of pegylated liposomal doxorubicin HCl (CAELYX/ Doxil) versus conventional doxorubicin for first-line treatment of metastatic breast cancer. *Ann Oncol.* 2004;15(3):440–449.

73. van Dalen EC, van der Pal HJ, Caron HN, Kremer LC. Different dosage schedules for reducing cardiotoxicity in cancer patients receiving anthracycline chemotherapy. *Cochrane Database Syst Rev.* 2006;(4):CD005008.

74. Testore F, Milanese S, Ceste M, et al. Cardioprotective effect of dexrazoxane in patients with breast cancer treated with anthracyclines in adjuvant setting: a 10-year single institution experience. *Am J Cardiovasc Drugs.* 2008;8(4):257–263.

75. Popelová O, Sterba M, Hasková P, et al. Dexrazoxane-afforded protection against chronic anthracycline cardiotoxicity in vivo: effective rescue of cardiomyocytes from apoptotic cell death. *Br J Cancer.* 2009;101(5):792–802.

76. Lyu YL, Kerrigan JE, Lin CP, et al. Topoisomerase IIbeta mediated DNA double-strand breaks: implications in doxorubicin cardiotoxicity and prevention by dexrazoxane. *Cancer Res.* 2007;67(18):8839–8846.

77. van Dalen EC, Caron HN, Dickinson HO, Kremer LC. Cardioprotective interventions for cancer patients receiving anthracyclines. *Cochrane Database Syst Rev.* 2008;(2):CD003917.

78. Cardinale D, Colombo A, Sandri MT, et al. Prevention of high-dose chemotherapy-induced cardiotoxicity in high-risk patients by angiotensin-converting enzyme inhibition. *Circulation.* 2006;114(23):2474–2481.

79. Bosch X, Rovira M, Sitges M, et al. Enalapril and carvedilol for preventing chemotherapy-induced left ventricular systolic dysfunction in patients with malignant hemopathies: the OVERCOME trial (preventiOn of left Ventricular dysfunction with Enalapril and caRvedilol in patients submitted to intensive ChemOtherapy for the treatment of Malignant hEmopathies). *J Am Coll Cardiol.* 2013;61(23):2355–2362.

80. Gulati G, Heck SL, Ree AH, et al. Prevention of cardiac dysfunction during adjuvant breast cancer therapy (PRADA): a 2 × 2 factorial, randomized, placebo-controlled, double-blind clinical trial of candesartan and metoprolol. *Eur Heart J.* 2016;37(21): 1671–1680.

81. Felker GM, Benza RL, Chandler AB, et al. Heart failure etiology and response to milrinone in decompensated heart failure: results from the OPTIME-CHF study. *J Am Coll Cardiol.* 2003;41(6):997–1003.

82. Fonarow GC, Abraham WT, Albert NM, et al. Influence of beta-blocker continuation or withdrawal on outcomes in patients hospitalized with heart failure: findings from the OPTIMIZE-HF program. *J Am Coll Cardiol.* 2008;52(3):190–199.

83. Lowes BD, Tsvetkova T, Eichhorn EJ, Gilbert EM, Bristow MR. Milrinone versus dobutamine in heart failure subjects treated chronically with carvedilol. *Int J Cardiol.* 2001;81(2-3):141–149.

84. Niemann JT, Garner D, Khaleeli E, Lewis RJ. Milrinone facilitates resuscitation from cardiac arrest and attenuates postresuscitation myocardial dysfunction. *Circulation.* 2003;108(24):3031–3035.

85. Mullens W, Abrahams Z, Francis GS, et al. Sodium nitroprusside for advanced low-output heart failure. *J Am Coll Cardiol.* 2008;52(3):200–207.

86. Mebazaa A, Nieminen MS, Packer M, et al. Levosimendan vs dobutamine for patients with acute decompensated heart failure: the SURVIVE randomized trial. *JAMA.* 2007;297(17):1883–1891.

87. Packer M, Coats AJ, Fowler MB, et al. Effect of carvedilol on survival in severe chronic heart failure. *N Engl J Med.* 2001;344(22):1651–1658.

88. Chen ZM, Pan HC, Chen YP, et al. Early intravenous then oral metoprolol in 45,852 patients with acute myocardial infarction: randomised placebo-controlled trial. *Lancet.* 2005;366(9497):1622–1632.

89. Antman EM, Hand M, Armstrong PW, et al. 2007 focused update of the ACC/AHA 2004 guidelines for the management of patients with ST-elevation

myocardial infarction: a report of the American College of Cardiology/American Heart Association Task Force on Practice Guidelines: developed in collaboration with the Canadian Cardiovascular Society endorsed by the American Academy of Family Physicians: 2007 Writing Group to Review New Evidence and Update the ACC/AHA 2004 Guidelines for the Management of Patients With ST-Elevation Myocardial Infarction, Writing on Behalf of the 2004 Writing Committee. *Circulation.* 2008;117(2):296–329.

90. Murray MD, Deer MM, Ferguson JA, et al. Open-label randomized trial of torsemide compared with furosemide therapy for patients with heart failure. *Am J Med.* 2001;111(7):513–520.

91. Costanzo MR, Guglin ME, Saltzberg MT, et al. Ultrafiltration versus intravenous diuretics for patients hospitalized for acute decompensated heart failure. *J Am Coll Cardiol.* 2007;49(6):675–683.

92. Packer M, Bristow MR, Cohn JN, et al. The effect of carvedilol on morbidity and mortality in patients with chronic heart failure. U.S. Carvedilol Heart Failure Study Group. *N Engl J Med.* 1996;334(21):1349–1355.

93. Kalay N, Basar E, Ozdogru I, et al. Protective effects of carvedilol against anthracycline-induced cardiomyopathy. *J Am Coll Cardiol.* 2006;48(11):2258–2262.

94. Cardinale D, Colombo A, Bacchiani G, et al. Early detection of anthracycline cardiotoxicity and improvement with heart failure therapy. *Circulation.* 2015;131(22):1981–1988.

95. Spallarossa P, Garibaldi S, Altieri P, et al. Carvedilol prevents doxorubicin-induced free radical release and apoptosis in cardiomyocytes in vitro. *J Mol Cell Cardiol.* 2004;37(4):837–846.

96. Oliveira PJ, Bjork JA, Santos MS, et al. Carvedilol-mediated antioxidant protection against doxorubicin-induced cardiac mitochondrial toxicity. *Toxicol Appl Pharmacol.* 2004;200(2):159–168.

97. Jonsson O, Behnam-Motlagh P, Persson M, Henriksson R, Grankvist K. Increase in doxorubicin cytotoxicity by carvedilol inhibition of P-glycoprotein activity. *Biochem Pharmacol.* 1999;58(11):1801–1806.

98. Stanojkovic TP, Zizak Z, Mihailovic-Stanojevic N, Petrovic T, Juranic Z. Inhibition of proliferation on some neoplastic cell lines-act of carvedilol and captopril. *J Exp Clin Cancer Res.* 2005;24(3):387–395.

99. Walther T, Menrad A, Orzechowski HD, Siemeister G, Paul M, Schirner M. Differential regulation of in vivo angiogenesis by angiotensin II receptors. *FASEB J.* 2003;17(14):2061–2067.

100. Christian JB, Lapane KL, Hume AL, Eaton CB, Weinstock MA. Association of ACE inhibitors and angiotensin receptor blockers with keratinocyte cancer prevention in the randomized VATTC trial. *J Natl Cancer Inst.* 2008;100(17):1223–1232.

101. Attoub S, Gaben AM, Al-Salam S, et al. Captopril as a potential inhibitor of lung tumor growth and metastasis. *Ann N Y Acad Sci.* 2008;1138:65–72.

102. Pitt B, Zannad F, Remme WJ, et al. The effect of spironolactone on morbidity and mortality in patients with severe heart failure. Randomized Aldactone Evaluation Study Investigators. *N Engl J Med.* 1999;341(10):709–717.

103. Digitalis Investigation Group, Ahmed A, Waagstein F, et al. Effectiveness of digoxin in reducing one-year mortality in chronic heart failure in the Digitalis Investigation Group trial. *Am J Cardiol.* 2009;103(1):82–87.

104. Ramasubbu K, Estep J, White DL, Deswal A, Mann DL. Experimental and clinical basis for the use of statins in patients with ischemic and nonischemic cardiomyopathy. *J Am Coll Cardiol.* 2008;51(4):415–426.

105. Riad A, Bien S, Westermann D, et al. Pretreatment with statin attenuates the cardiotoxicity of Doxorubicin in mice. *Cancer Res.* 2009;69(2):695–699.

106. Caner M, Sonmez B, Kurnaz O, et al. Atorvastatin has cardiac safety at intensive cholesterol-reducing protocols for long term, yet its cancer-treatment doses with chemotherapy may cause cardiomyopathy even under coenzyme-Q10 protection. *Cell Biochem Funct.* 2007;25(4):463–472.

107. Roudier E, Mistafa O, Stenius U. Statins induce mammalian target of rapamycin (mTOR)-mediated inhibition of Akt signaling and sensitize p53-deficient cells to cytostatic drugs. *Mol Cancer Ther.* 2006;5(11):2706–2715.

108. Shore S, Grau-Sepulveda MV, Bhatt DL, et al. Characteristics, treatments, and outcomes of hospitalized heart failure patients stratified by etiologies of cardiomyopathy. *JACC Heart Fail.* 2015;3(11):906–916.

109. Miller LW, Guglin M. Patient selection for ventricular assist devices: a moving target. *J Am Coll Cardiol.* 2013;61(12):1209–1221.

110. Oliveira GH, Hardaway BW, Kucheryavaya AY, Stehlik J, Edwards LB, Taylor DO. Characteristics and survival of patients with chemotherapy-induced cardiomyopathy undergoing heart transplantation. *J Heart Lung Transplant.* 2012;31(8):805–810.

111. Lenneman AJ, Wang L, Wigger M, et al. Heart transplant survival outcomes for adriamycin-dilated cardiomyopathy. *Am J Cardiol.* 2013;111(4):609–612.

112. Oliveira GH, Dupont M, Naftel D, et al. Increased need for right ventricular support in patients with chemotherapy-induced cardiomyopathy undergoing mechanical circulatory support: outcomes from the INTERMACS Registry (Interagency Registry for Mechanically Assisted Circulatory Support). *J Am Coll Cardiol.* 2014;63(3):240–248.

113. Rahman AM, Yusuf SW, Ewer MS. Anthracycline-induced cardiotoxicity and the cardiac-sparing effect of liposomal formulation. *Int J Nanomedicine.* 2007;2(4):567–583.

114. Zhou S, Starkov A, Froberg MK, Leino RL, Wallace KB. Cumulative and irreversible cardiac mitochondrial dysfunction induced by doxorubicin. *Cancer Res.* 2001;61(2):771–777.

115. Vejpongsa P, Yeh ET. Topoisomerase 2: a promising molecular target for primary prevention of anthracycline-induced cardiotoxicity. *Clin Pharmacol Ther.* 2014;95(1):45–52.

116. Jeyaseelan R, Poizat C, Baker RK, et al. A novel cardiac-restricted target for doxorubicin. CARP, a nuclear modulator of gene expression in cardiac

progenitor cells and cardiomyocytes. *J Biol Chem.* 1997;272(36):22800–22808.

117. De Angelis A, Piegari E, Cappetta D, et al. Anthracycline cardiomyopathy is mediated by depletion of the cardiac stem cell pool and is rescued by restoration of progenitor cell function. *Circulation.* 2010;121(2):276–292.

118. Pak SW, Uriel N, Song R, et al. Surgical management of chemotherapy-induced end-stage heart failure. *J Cardiac Failure.* 2010;16(8):S45–S46.

119. Castells E, Roca J, Miralles A, et al. Recovery of ventricular function with a left ventricular axial pump in a patient with end-stage toxic cardiomyopathy not a candidate for heart transplantation: first experience in Spain. *Transplant Proc.* 2009;41(6):2237–2239.

120. Freilich M, Stub D, Esmore D, et al. Recovery from anthracycline cardiomyopathy after long-term support with a continuous flow left ventricular assist device. *J Heart Lung Transplant.* 2009;28(1):101–103.

121. Khan N, Husain SA, Husain SI, et al. Remission of chronic anthracycline-induced heart failure with support from a continuous-flow left ventricular assist device. *Tex Heart Inst J.* 2012;39(4):554–556.

122. Kurihara C, Nishimura T, Nawata K, et al. Successful bridge to recovery with VAD implantation for anthracycline-induced cardiomyopathy. *J Artif Organs.* 2011;14(3):249–252.

123. Meinardi MT, van der Graaf WT, van Veldhuisen DJ, Gietema JA, de Vries EG, Sleijfer DT. Detection of anthracycline-induced cardiotoxicity. *Cancer Treat Rev.* 1999;25(4):237–247.

124. Von Hoff DD, Layard MW, Basa P, et al. Risk factors for doxorubicin-induced congestive heart failure. *Ann Intern Med.* 1979;91(5):710–717.

125. Tanindi A, Demirci U, Tacoy G, et al. Assessment of right ventricular functions during cancer chemotherapy. *Eur J Echocardiogr.* 2011;12(11):834–840.

126. Grover S, DePasquale C, Srinivasan G, et al. Contemporary breast cancer chemotherapy leads to persistent late right ventricular myocardial dysfunction: a prospective multi-centre study. *J Cardiovasc Magn Reson.* 2013;15(suppl 1):P164.

127. Calleja A, Poulin F, Khorolsky C, et al. Right ventricular dysfunction in patients experiencing cardiotoxicity during breast cancer therapy. *J Oncol.* 2015;2015:609194.

128. Baumwol J, Macdonald PS, Keogh AM, et al. Right heart failure and "failure to thrive" after left ventricular assist device: clinical predictors and outcomes. *J Heart Lung Transplant.* 2011;30(8):888–895.

129. Lipshultz SE, Lipsitz SR, Mone SM, et al. Female sex and drug dose as risk factors for late cardiotoxic effects of doxorubicin therapy for childhood cancer. *N Engl J Med.* 1995;332(26):1738–1743.

130. Russo AM, Stainback RF, Bailey SR, et al. ACCF/HRS/AHA/ASE/HFSA/SCAI/SCCT/SCMR 2013 appropriate use criteria for implantable cardioverter-defibrillators and cardiac resynchronization therapy: a report of the American College of Cardiology Foundation appropriate use criteria task force, Heart Rhythm Society, American Heart Association, American Society of Echocardiography, Heart Failure Society of America, Society for Cardiovascular Angiography and Interventions, Society of Cardiovascular Computed Tomography, and Society for Cardiovascular Magnetic Resonance. *J Am Coll Cardiol.* 2013;61(12):1318–1368.

131. Kass DA. Cardiac resynchronization therapy. *J Cardiovasc Electrophysiol.* 2005;16(suppl 1):S35–S41.

132. Ajijola OA, Nandigam KV, Chabner BA, et al. Usefulness of cardiac resynchronization therapy in the management of Doxorubicin-induced cardiomyopathy. *Am J Cardiol.* 2008;101(9):1371–1372.

133. Rickard J, Kumbhani DJ, Baranowski B, Martin DO, Tang WH, Wilkoff BL. Usefulness of cardiac resynchronization therapy in patients with Adriamycin-induced cardiomyopathy. *Am J Cardiol.* 2010;105(4):522–526.

134. Pierce WS, Parr GV, Myers JL, Pae WE Jr, Bull AP, Waldhausen JA. Ventricular-assist pumping patients with cardiogenic shock after cardiac operations. *N Engl J Med.* 1981;305(27):1606–1610.

135. Rose EA, Gelijns AC, Moskowitz AJ, et al. Randomized Evaluation of Mechanical Assistance for the Treatment of Congestive Heart Failure (REMATCH) study group. Long-term use of a left ventricular assistance for end-stage heart failure. *N Engl J Med.* 2001;345(20):1435–1443.

136. Slaughter MS, Rogers JG, Milano CA, et al. Advanced heart failure treated with continuous-flow left ventricular assist device. *N Engl J Med.* 2009;361(23):2241–2251.

137. Stehlik J, Edwards LB, Kucheryavaya AY, et al. The registry of the international society for heart and lung transplantation: twenty-eighth adult heart transplant report—2011. *J Heart Lung Transplant.* 2011;30(10):1078–1094.

138. Christiansen S. Surgical treatment of doxorubicin-induced heart failure. *Thorac Cardiovasc Surg.* 2010;58(1):8–10.

139. Al-Kindi SG, Oliveira GH. Heart transplantation outcomes in radiation-induced restrictive cardiomyopathy. *J Card Fail.* 2016;22(6):475–478.

140. Paik S, Shak S, Tang G, et al. A multigene assay to predict recurrence of tamoxifen-treated, node-negative breast cancer. *N Engl J Med.* 2004;351(27):2817–2826.

141. Paik S, Tang G, Shak S, et al. Gene expression and benefit of chemotherapy in women with node-negative, estrogen receptor-positive breast cancer. *J Clin Oncol.* 2006;24(23):3726–3734.

142. Zhou Z, Sehn LH, Rademaker AW, et al. An enhanced international prognostic index (NCCN-IPI) for patients with diffuse large B-cell lymphoma treated in the rituximab era. *Blood.* 2014;123(6):837–842.

143. Jessup M, Brozena S. Heart Failure. *N Engl J Med.* 2003;348:2007–2018.

144. Al-Kindi S, Younes A, Qattan M, Oliveira GH. Preemptive cardioprotective strategies in patients receiving chemotherapy. *Curr Cardiovasc Risk Rep.* 2014;8:406.

27 Pregnancy and the Heart in Cancer Patients and Survivors

Kara A. Thompson

INTRODUCTION

Advances in cancer therapy have resulted in remarkable improvement in survival rates among patients who are or who will be in their child-bearing years. Pregnancy in such patients may be complicated by previous or, in some cases, concomitant therapy. The goal of supportive care for these patients is to maximize the likelihood of a healthy infant and to avoid potentially serious or life-threatening sequelae for the mother.

Survival rates among children treated for cancer have increased from 58% in the 1970s to 82% in the 2000s.[1] It is estimated that there are currently 388,500 adult survivors of childhood cancer in the United States and that this number will increase to 500,000 by 2020.[2] Consequently, an increasing number of female survivors of childhood cancer will reach childbearing age and desire to become pregnant.

Cardiomyopathy is a known risk of treatment with anthracyclines. Despite this toxicity, anthracyclines are used to treat 60% of childhood cancer patients because of the effectiveness of these drugs.[1] With anthracyclines, the 5-year survival rate for patients with the most common form of childhood cancer, acute lymphoblastic leukemia (ALL), increased from 0% in 1960 to 80% in the 2000s.[3] The incidence of heart failure increases with higher cumulative doses of anthracyclines: less than 5% for doses lower than 250 mg/m^2, 10% for doses between 250 mg/m^2 and 600 mg/m^2, and more than 30% for doses higher than 600 mg/m^2.[4] Studies have also shown that no dose of anthracyclines is without cardiac risk.[1]

Radiation therapy, also widely used to treat younger patients, is associated with adverse cardiac side effects because of inflammation that can lead to premature coronary artery disease, valvular heart disease, diastolic dysfunction, pericardial disease, and dysrhythmias. Although the use of radiotherapy has decreased and techniques for reducing cardiac damage have evolved, potentially damaging radiotherapy remains an important part of treatment for some cancers, such as Hodgkin lymphoma, and many patients treated during childhood carry the burdens of clinically significant radiation exposure into their childbearing years.[1]

Other risk factors for the development of cardiac toxicity are time since cancer diagnosis and age less than 5 years at the time of diagnosis.[1] Female sex is also an independent risk factor for the development of late cardiotoxicity, especially after treatment with an anthracycline.[5] In view of the known potential cardiac effects of anthracyclines and radiation, the cardiac risk of pregnancy after childhood cancer is a crucial consideration.

PREGNANCY AND THE NORMAL HEART

Pregnancy is associated with substantial changes in cardiac physiology (Table 27-1). Blood volume begins to increase at about 6 weeks' gestation, increases rapidly until mid-pregnancy, and then continues to increase at a slower rate. Blood volume increases by an average of approximately 50% above baseline during the course of a normal pregnancy, and cardiac output increases by 30% to 50% above that of non-pregnant women.

In early pregnancy, the increase in cardiac output is predominantly caused by an increase in stroke volume. The left ventricle (LV) enlarges to accommodate this increased volume, but the shortening characteristics remain unchanged in the normal heart.[6] In late pregnancy, the increase in cardiac output is predominantly caused by an increase in heart rate.[7] With labor, cardiac output increases by 50% during contractions. Systolic and diastolic blood pressure markedly increase, and oxygen consumption increases by 3-fold. Immediately postpartum, venous return to the heart increases as compression of the inferior vena cava is relieved. This increased preload causes increased stroke volume and cardiac output immediately after delivery, and this increase normalizes during the first 24 to 72 hours of the postpartum period.

For patients with compromised cardiac reserves, these hemodynamic changes can lead to decompensation and heart failure. Often, among patients with subclinical cardiac disease, the cardiac problem will manifest itself for the first time during pregnancy.[8] Among women with clinically significant cardiac dysfunction, heart failure can develop before mid-pregnancy. Among women with moderate dysfunction, heart failure can

TABLE 27-1 Hemodynamic changes during a normal pregnancy

	TRIMESTER 1	TRIMESTER 2	TRIMESTER 3
Blood volume	Increases starting 6 weeks, rapid increase ▲	Rapid increase and then gradual ▲▲	Gradual increase and plateau (50%) ▲▲▲
SV	▲	▲▲▲	▲▼
HR	▲	▲▲	Peaks (10–20 beats) ▲▲▲
CO = HR × SV	▲	▲▲ to ▲▲▲	▲▲▲ to ▲▲
SBP	About same	Mild decrease	About same
DBP	Mild decrease	Moderate decrease	Mild decrease
Pulse pressure	Widens	Widens	About same
SVR	▼	▼▼	▼▼▼

SV, stroke volume; HR, heart rate; CO, cardiac output; SBP, systolic blood pressure; DBP, diastolic blood pressure; SVR, systemic vascular resistance

Source: Modified from Elkayam U, 1997[7]; used with permission.

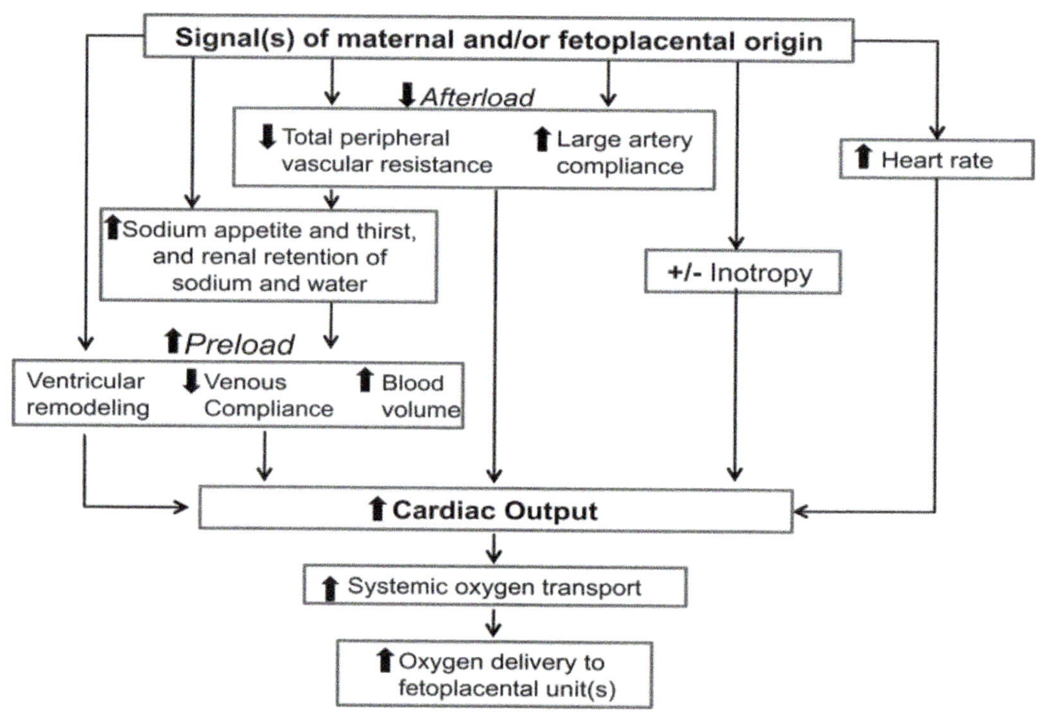

FIGURE 27-1 Regulation of cardiac output during pregnancy. (From Conrad, 2011[10]; used with permission.)

develop after 28 weeks in the setting of maximum blood volume and cardiac output. Among those with mild disease, heart failure can develop during labor and delivery and during the postpartum period.[9]

Ventricular performance during pregnancy is accommodated by a substantial decrease in systemic vascular resistance and vasodilation.[9] The mechanism of these changes involves a complex interaction between the renin-angiotensin-aldosterone system, prostaglandins, nitric oxide, and atrial and brain natriuretic factors (Figure 27-1).[10] Although cardiac output increases substantially during pregnancy to provide adequate oxygen delivery to the developing fetus, LV function remains normal; thus, pregnancy

TABLE 27-2 Pregnancy is not a continuous high-output state. COP, colloid oncotic pressure; PCWP, pulmonary capillary wedge pressure; NSC = no significant difference between the values obtained during and after pregnancy

	PREGNANT (35–38 WKS)	POSTPARTUM (11–13 WKS)	CHANGE
Mean arterial pressure (mm Hg)	90 ± 6	86 ± 8	NSC
Pulmonary capillary wedge pressure (mm Hg)	8 ± 2	6 ± 2	NSC
Central venous pressure (mm Hg)	4 ± 3	4 ± 3	NSC
Heart rate (beats/min)	83 ± 10	71 ± 10	+17%
Cardiac output (L/min)	6.2 ± 1.0	4.3 ± 0.9	+43%
Systemic vascular resistance (dyne/sec/cm^{-5})	1210 ± 266	1530 ± 520	−21%
Pulmonary vascular resistance (dyne/sec/cm^{-5})	78 ± 22	119 ± 47	−34%
Serum colloid osmotic pressure (mm Hg)	18.0 ± 1.5	20.8 ± 1.0	−14%
COP-PCWP gradient (mm Hg)	10.5 ± 2.7	14.5 ± 2.5	−28%
Left ventricular stroke work index (g/m/m^2)	48 ± 6	41 ± 8	NSC

Source: Modified from Cunningham et al., 2010[9]; used with permission.

is a eudynamic state.[9] In 1989, Clark and associates[11] studied hemodynamics in pregnancy by subjecting 10 healthy pregnant women to right heart catheterization in late pregnancy and again approximately 3 months postpartum. They found that pulmonary capillary wedge pressure did not change significantly. In addition, although cardiac output increased significantly with pregnancy, LV contractility as measured by the stroke work index did not change significantly. This finding demonstrates that pregnancy is not associated with a continuous high-output state related to hyperdynamic LV function (Table 27-2).[11]

PREGNANCY AND HEART FAILURE

Although heart disease is uncommon during pregnancy, it is the leading cause of maternal death. The incidence of pregnancy-related death has increased in the United States in recent years, and the greatest increase is in deaths attributable to cardiovascular disease during pregnancy.[9] In 1987, the pregnancy-related mortality rate was 7.2 per 100,000 live births, whereas in 2009 it was 17.8 per 100,000 live births.[12] The rate of maternal mortality due to cardiac disease increased from 1.65 per 100,000 live births in the years 1997 to 1999 to 2.31 per 100,000 live births in the years 2006–2008.[9] Possible reasons for this increase include the fact that more women are experiencing pregnancies at advanced ages, and these women exhibit risk factors and chronic conditions that increase maternal risk.[9]

The outcome of pregnancy among women with heart disease has been studied. Siu et al.[13] prospectively studied the outcomes of 562 women with heart disease. They found four predictors of maternal cardiac complications: 1) a previous cardiac event, such as heart failure, arrhythmia, transient ischemic attack, or stroke; 2) poor functional class with cyanosis or heart failure classified as New York Heart Association (NYHA) class II or higher; 3) left heart inflow or outflow obstruction with a mitral valve area of less than 2 cm^2, an aortic valve area of less than 1.5 cm^2, or an LV outflow gradient higher than 30 mm

Hg; and 4) LV systolic dysfunction with an ejection fraction of less than 40%.[13] Siu et al. developed a risk index based on these four predictors, each of which was assigned 1 point. The estimated risk of a cardiac event was 5% with 0 points, 27% with 1 point, and 75% with more than 1 point. Thus, the risk of a cardiac event for a patient with an ejection fraction of less than 40% is 27%.[13]

Another study[14] involved 32 women with idiopathic or doxorubicin-induced dilated cardiomyopathy (DCM). These women were studied prospectively during pregnancy and were compared to non-pregnant women matched for age and degree of LV dysfunction with a follow-up period of 16 months. Among women with DCM, 14 of 36 pregnancies were complicated by a maternal cardiac event, and 13 of these events occurred among the 18 women with moderate or severe LV dysfunction. In comparison, 3 of 18 non-pregnant women with moderate to severe LV dysfunction experienced cardiac events during the follow-up period. In this study, all cardiac complications during pregnancy occurred among patients with moderate or severe LV dysfunction, symptoms of NYHA class III or IV heart failure, a previous cardiac event, or some combination of these three factors. No adverse events occurred among women who exhibited none of these 3 characteristics. However, if any of these 3 factors were present, the risk of a cardiac event was 64%. Women with mild LV dysfunction generally did well during pregnancy, with the exception of those who had experienced a previous cardiac event. The cardiac events that occurred during pregnancy usually happened late in pregnancy or postpartum, at the times of maximal hemodynamic stress, and heart failure was the most common event. It is also likely that the pregnancy group, unlike the non-pregnancy group, experienced some cardiac decompensation caused by discontinuation of cardiac medications, such as angiotensin-converting enzyme (ACE) inhibitors, beta blockers, and diuretics that are contraindicated during pregnancy.

It is unknown whether pregnancy itself or the discontinuation of cardiac medications during pregnancy has a negative late effect on long-term ventricular function.[14] In normal hearts, chronic volume overloading even with multiple pregnancies does not compromise LV function.[6] One small study of women with a systemic right ventricle found that pregnancy was associated with a risk of ventricular dysfunction, which had not recovered at the last follow-up visit (mean, 31 months after pregnancy).[15]

For patients with a history of peripartum cardiomyopathy (PPCM), future pregnancies are generally not recommended. PPCM is defined as heart failure that occurs during the last month of pregnancy or during the first 5 months postpartum and is not associated with underlying heart disease or idiopathic DCM. The onset of PPCM does not coincide with the greatest hemodynamic load on the heart, which occurs during the mid-second and the third trimesters.[16] Risk factors for the development of PPCM are multiparity, advanced maternal age, multifetal pregnancy, preeclampsia, gestational hypertension, and African American race.[17]

The pathophysiology of PPCM is uncertain. One theory is that this cardiomyopathy is related to angiogenic imbalance, as is true for cardiomyopathy that develops as an adverse effect of antiangiogenic cancer therapy (Figure 27-2). Late pregnancy is associated with a strong antiangiogenic environment. The tyrosine kinase protein soluble fms-like tyrosine kinase 1 (sFLT1) is secreted by the placenta and inhibits the production of vascular endothelial growth factor (VEGF). Cardiac peroxisome proliferator-activated receptor-γ coactivator 1α (PGC-1α) is a protein that upregulates two proangiogenic pathways[18]: the production of both VEGF and manganese superoxide dismutase (MnSOD), which protects against reactive oxygen species (ROS). When ROS levels are increased, the cleavage of prolactin into a potent antiangiogenic form is also increased. Bromocriptine inhibits prolactin secretion and has shown some promise in preventing the development of PPCM. Doxorubicin toxicity, on the other hand, is worse among mice with high systemic levels of prolactin.[19]

The prognosis of patients with PPCM is variable; mortality rates range from 18% to 56%.[17] In the United States, LV function recovers in approximately half of patients with PPCM (ejection fraction [EF] > 50%), usually within 6 months.[20] The prognosis for patients with PPCM is better than that for patients with other forms of cardiomyopathy (Figure 27-3).[21] Subsequent pregnancies, however, are generally not recommended because they can be associated with a decrease in LV function or even death. A study of 44 women with 60 subsequent pregnancies found that symptoms of heart failure developed in 21% of women with recovered LV function before the subsequent pregnancy but in 44% of women with persistent LV dysfunction. The LV dysfunction persisted in 14% of the women with recovered LV function before the subsequent pregnancy and in 31% of patients without LV recovery before the subsequent pregnancy. None of the women with recovered LV function died during pregnancy, but 19% of those with persistent LV dysfunction died during pregnancy.[22] Some findings suggest that contractile reserve as documented by exercise stress echocardiography predicts a low likelihood of relapse among women with normal LV function before a subsequent pregnancy.[23,24]

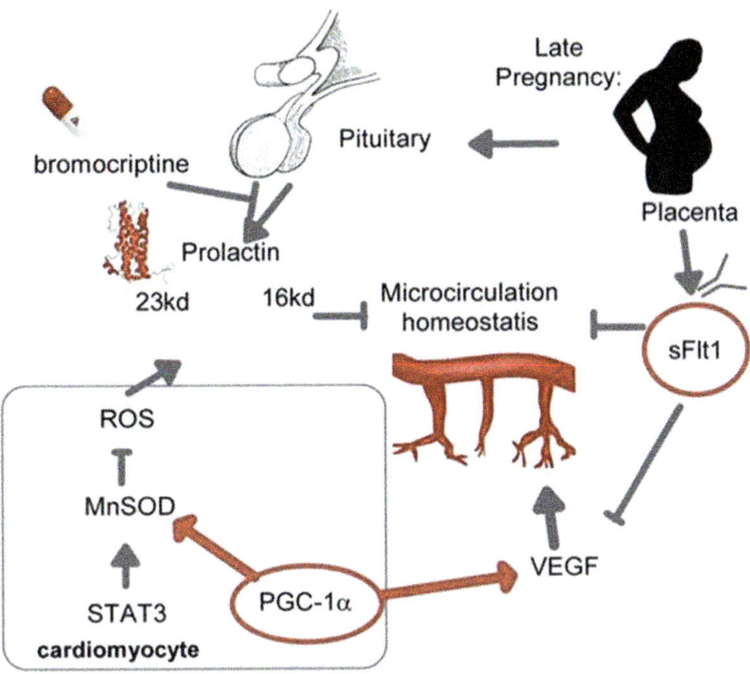

FIGURE 27-2   Angiogenic Pathways. MnSOD, manganese superoxide dismutase; PGC-1α, peroxisome proliferator-activated receptor-γ coactivator 1α; ROS, reactive oxygen species; sFlt1, soluble fms-like tyrosine kinase 1; STAT3, signal transducer and activator of transcription 3. (From Patten et al., 2012[18]; used with permission.)

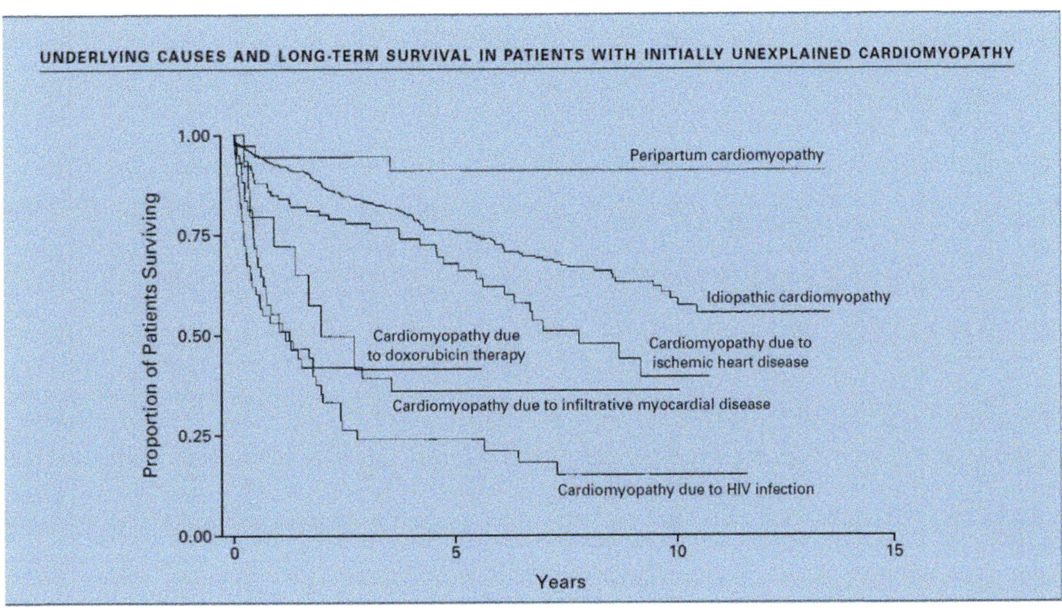

FIGURE 27-3   Adjusted Kaplan–Meier Estimates of Survival According to the Underlying Cause of Cardiomyopathy. Only idiopathic cardiomyopathy and cardiomyopathy due to causes for which survival was significantly different from that in patients with idiopathic cardiomyopathy are shown. (From Felker et al., 2000[21]; used with permission.)

Diagnosing heart failure in pregnant women can be challenging because normal pregnancy often mimics heart failure. Normal pregnancy can be associated with shortness of breath, fatigue, decreased exercise capability, lightheadedness, syncope, edema, lateral displacement of the apical impulse, and increased cardiac size as determined by chest radiography (CXR).[25] Underlying heart disease should be considered for patients with an S3 or S4 gallop, a diastolic murmur, atrial fibrillation, a loud systolic murmur, fixed split of the second heart sound, elevated levels of brain natriuretic peptide (BNP), or sinus tachycardia more than 15% higher than the normal heart rate.[25] Imaging studies with echocardiography are important and are recommended each trimester for patients with known LV dysfunction.[26]

BNP measurements are also clinically useful. One small study measured BNP levels in 78 pregnant women, 66 women with heart disease, and 12 healthy control subjects. Among the healthy control subjects, BNP levels did not increase during pregnancy. Among women with heart disease, however, BNP levels were significantly higher than among the healthy control subjects. Over the course of pregnancy, 24 (38%) women with heart disease exhibited BNP concentrations higher than 100 pg/ml, and 8 (13%) experienced adverse cardiac events. Sixteen women with heart disease had an elevated BNP level during pregnancy but did not experience an adverse cardiac event. None of the women with BNP levels lower than 100 pg/ml experienced adverse cardiac events; thus, the negative predictive value of normal BNP levels was 100%. The significance of elevated BNP levels among women who did not experience cardiac events is unknown, but these levels could be a marker of decreased cardiac reserve and could have prognostic significance.[27]

ANTHRACYCLINE EXPOSURE

Cardiac disease is the most common cause of death for childhood cancer survivors who do not experience a recurrence of the primary cancer or the development of a new cancer.[1] Often, cardiac disease among these patients is subclinical. Echocardiographic findings of cardiac dysfunction have been reported in 25% to 50% of asymptomatic patients within 20 years of exposure to treatment with anthracycline.[28] When administered to children, doxorubicin impairs myocardial growth such that the increase in LV wall thickness relative to the size of the LV cavity is inappropriately small.[29] Thus, among survivors of childhood cancer, LV dysfunction is more often related to increased afterload and heart failure with preserved EF rather than to decreased systolic function.[30]

Risk factors for the development of cardiac toxicity have been identified. A higher cumulative dose of anthracycline is known to increase the risk of cardiac dysfunction.[30] Among children with ALL, 65% of those who received a cumulative dose of 228 mg/m^2 or more of doxorubicin experienced abnormal cardiac function, as determined by echocardiography. Increased afterload was present in 59% of these children, and decreased contractility was present in 23%. Young age at time of treatment is another risk factor for anthracycline toxicity. Lipshultz et al.[29] found that, among children with ALL, treatment age less than 4 years was a significant independent predictive factor of increased afterload.[29] In addition, cardiac mortality rates are higher among patients whose cancer is diagnosed before they reach the age of 7.[31,32] The reduction in contractility is larger among female patients than among male patients, a fact possibly associated with a sex-related difference in body fat composition and the volume of distribution of doxorubicin.[5] The incidence of cardiac toxicity increases with the length of time since treatment (Figure 27-4). Lifetime follow-up is prudent because there is no time limit on the clinical expression of cardiac toxicity. Myocyte damage during therapy can gradually, over years, lead to LV dilation, LV wall thinning, and decreased contractility. With increased metabolic demand, such as that occurring during pregnancy, or sequential injury, such as that accompanying viral infection, the damaged heart is sometimes unable to compensate.[1]

STUDIES OF CARDIAC OUTCOMES OF PREGNANCY IN SURVIVORS OF CHILDHOOD CANCER

For patients with previous anthracycline exposure, the risk of symptomatic cardiac dysfunction due to excessive stress, such as pregnancy, is not well known.[28] However, case reports and small studies of cardiac outcomes of pregnancy among survivors of childhood cancer have been published. In 1988, Davis and Brown[33] described a 13-year-old patient who presented at 39 weeks' gestation with spontaneous rupture of membranes. She had a history of osteosarcoma and treatment with a cumulative dose of 525 mg/m^2 of doxorubicin at age 6. Two years before admission she had undergone echocardiography, with normal results. Acute heart failure developed 67 hours after delivery, with 4-chamber enlargement and global hypokinesis, as detected by echocardiography. Her pulmonary capillary wedge pressure was 28 mm Hg. Endomyocardial biopsy showed cardiac fibrosis consistent with doxorubicin toxicity. This was the first

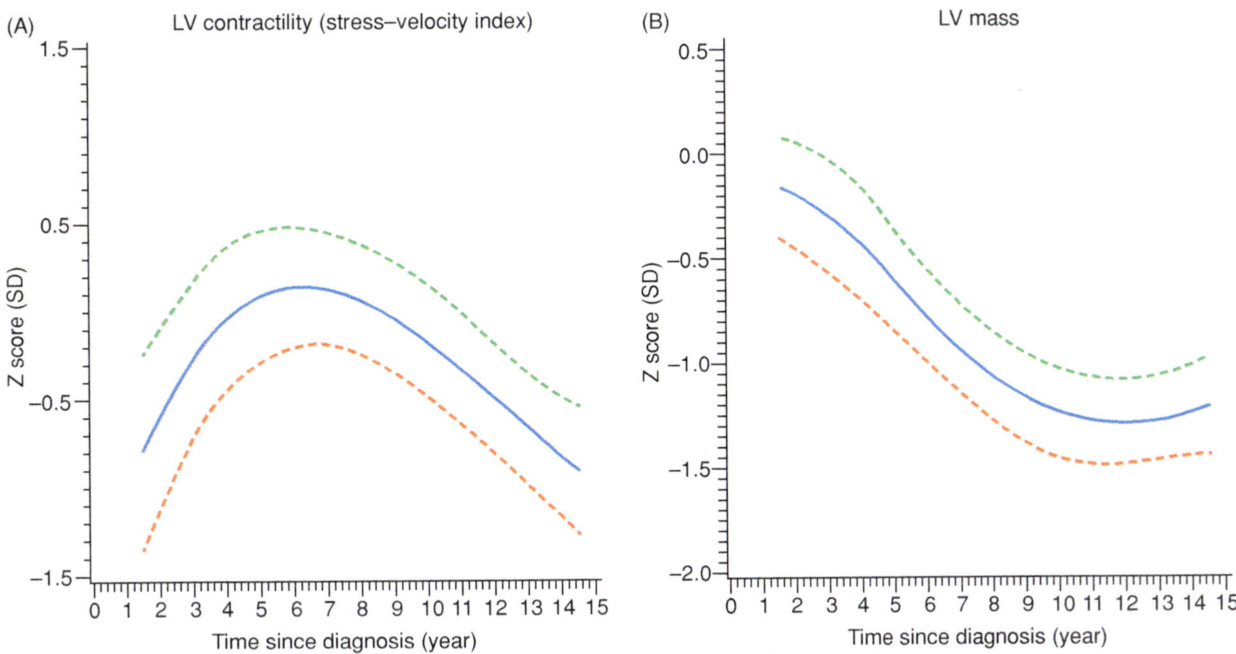

FIGURE 27-4   Z scores of left ventricular contractility (A) and left ventricular mass (B) from 115 long term survivors of acute lymphoblastic leukaemia treated with doxorubicin, by time since diagnosis. A model of follow-up data for all children is given. The solid line is the overall group mean. A Z score of zero indicates the normal population mean. The dased lines are the upper and lower 95th centile confidence bounds form the predicted mean. (From Lipschultz et al., 2008[30]; used with permission.)

report of pregnancy-associated cardiac failure related to previous doxorubicin damage; the cardiac failure was subclinical before the pregnancy.[33]

In 1997, Katz et al.[34] described a 28-year-old patient who presented with heart failure 3 months postpartum. She had a history of B-cell lymphoma treated with 270 mg/m² of doxorubicin ten years earlier. Two months after completion of chemotherapy, radionuclide scintigraphy showed an ejection fraction of 58%. When she presented to the emergency room 10 years later during the postpartum period, her EF was 20%. Despite medical therapy, one year later the patient exhibited persistent LV dysfunction with an ejection fraction of 25%.[34] Another case report[35] described a woman who presented with heart failure at 34 weeks' gestation; this patient had a history of Hodgkin disease 3 years earlier and had been treated with a low dose of doxorubicin (134 mg/m²) and radiation therapy to the chest, which is known to augment the risk of anthracycline toxicity. Her documented EF one year before presentation was 58%. At presentation, she was found to have a dilated LV, moderate mitral regurgitation, and severe LV systolic dysfunction. Her LV function improved with treatment, but she did not completely recover.[35]

Three studies have evaluated the cardiac outcome of pregnancy among survivors treated for childhood cancer.

First, Bar et al.[36] prospectively studied 37 such survivors who were pregnant. The median age at the time of cancer diagnosis was 12 years, and the median follow-up time was 17 years. Cardiac function was evaluated with fractional shortening (FS), a parameter analogous to ejection that does not assume the 3-dimensional shape of the LV; this value is more frequently used to describe LV contractility among children and is calculated with unmodified LV end-diastolic and end-systolic dimensions. The normal range for fractional shortening is 36% ± 4%. Cardiac dysfunction was defined as FS less than 30% on two sequential echocardiograms performed at least 1 month apart. The FS was higher than 30% for 29 of the 37 women and lower than 30% for 8. Cardiac failure did not develop in any of the women with FS higher than 30% but did develop in 2 of the 8 patients with FS lower than 30%. One patient experienced disease progression and was evaluated for cardiac transplantation. The other patient recovered with treatment. Although the differences between the groups were not statistically significant, FS decreased by a median of 19% among women with an initial FS lower than 30%, whereas there was no change in FS among women with an initial FS higher than 30%. This study found that pregnancy did not contribute to poorer cardiac function after the administration of anthracyclines. It is notable that all of the patients in this study received a cumulative dose of doxorubicin of less than 500 mg/m^2.[36]

Second, Van Dalen et al.[37] retrospectively reviewed the records of 53 women who became pregnant after treatment for childhood cancer. The mean age at the time of cancer diagnosis was 11.2 years, and the mean follow-up time was 20 years. Cardiac dysfunction was defined by clinical signs and symptoms. Echocardiography was not routinely performed. The mean cumulative dose of anthracycline was 267 mg/m^2. None of these patients experienced cardiomyopathy during the peripartum period (during pregnancy and within 5 months after delivery). Heart failure had been diagnosed in 2 of the patients shortly after the completion of anthracycline therapy. One had a normal fractioning shortening documented prior to pregnancy and had no signs of heart failure with pregnancy. She did not have an echocardiogram after the pregnancy. The second patient had a mildly decreased FS of 27% documented before pregnancy. She tolerated the pregnancy well, but developed heart failure 2.5 years after delivery and required treatment with medications. Her FS was 17% at her last follow-up visit. Although these findings were encouraging, this study was not adequately powered to assess cardiac risk with pregnancy.[37]

Third, a more recent retrospective study by Hines et al.[38] involved 847 female cancer survivors with 1554 subsequent pregnancies. This study gathered information by sending a questionnaire to female survivors of childhood cancer treated at St. Jude Children's Research Hospital between 1963 and 2006. Medical records, including reports of echocardiography performed at other institutions, were obtained to validate patient reports of cardiovascular disease. The median age at the time of cancer diagnosis was 10.3 years, and the median follow-up time was 26.5 years. The median cumulative anthracycline dose was 200 mg/m^2. Cardiomyopathy developed in 43 (5%) of the 847 patients; it developed before pregnancy in 26 patients, during pregnancy or during the first 5 months of the postpartum period in 3 patients, and more than 5 months after delivery in 14 patients. Cardiac function was normal in 16 patients before pregnancy, but 3 of the 16 experienced deterioration of cardiac function with pregnancy. Of the 26 patients with cardiomyopathy before pregnancy, 8 experienced worsening cardiac function with pregnancy. EF was normal before pregnancy in 3 patients, abnormal before pregnancy in 3, and unknown for 2. The results of this study suggest that cardiomyopathy associated with pregnancy is rare among survivors of childhood cancer.[38] However, the incidence is much higher among these women (approximately 1:500) than among the general population (approximately 1:3000).[20,38]

MD ANDERSON DATA ON CARDIAC OUTCOMES IN CHILDHOOD CANCER SURVIVORS

At MD Anderson, we recently evaluated the cardiac outcomes of 58 childhood cancer survivors who were treated with anthracyclines, chest irradiation, or both and subsequently had at least one pregnancy with a median follow-up time of 20 years. Characteristics of patients with adverse cardiac conditions were compared to those of patients without such cardiac conditions and to those of a control group of female survivors who did not become pregnant. Of the 58 patients, 17 experienced an adverse event defined as an EF of less than 50% on at least 2 echocardiograms or coronary artery disease. The diagnosis of cardiac disease was made before pregnancy for 3 women, during pregnancy for 9, and after pregnancy for 5. The peripartum period was defined as during pregnancy and 1 year after delivery. Of the 17 patients with adverse cardiac events, 8 (47.1%) recovered, 7 (41.2%) did not recover, and 2 (11.8%) died.[39] Although this finding was not statistically significant, the best recovery occurred among patients whose heart failure was diagnosed during pregnancy.

Certain subgroups of women had a higher risk of adverse cardiac outcomes in association with pregnancy: younger age at the time of cancer treatment, longer time from cancer treatment to first pregnancy, and higher total anthracycline dose. Pregnancy was also associated with a 2.35-fold increase in the risk of cardiotoxicity in the overall study population. Our findings suggest more concern regarding cardiac outcomes in cancer survivors with pregnancies than the results obtained by Hines et al.[38] Our study was different because the definition of cardiotoxicity was based on echocardiographic findings rather than on self-report. We also studied a higher-risk group of patients; our patients received a higher mean dose of anthracycline (272 mg/m^2) than did the patients in the Hines study (200 mg/m^2).[39]

CANCER DIAGNOSIS DURING PREGNANCY

A diagnosis of cancer during pregnancy is rare, but the incidence of such diagnoses is expected to increase as more women delay pregnancy. Breast cancer is the most common type of cancer diagnosed during pregnancy; it occurs in approximately 1 of every 3000 pregnancies.[40] Cardiotoxic chemotherapy with trastuzumab or anthracyclines may be crucial for treating patients with a cancer diagnosis during pregnancy, and the combination of both drugs can have a synergistic cardiotoxic side effect.[41] Because of its teratogenic effects, chemotherapy is generally avoided during the first trimester.[42]

Case reports have described the use of trastuzumab during pregnancy. Trastuzumab causes some decrease in LV function in approximately 14% of non-pregnant patients and symptomatic heart failure in approximately 4% of non-pregnant patients. It is unknown whether the cardiac stress of pregnancy increases the risk of drug-induced LV dysfunction.[43] One case report stated that discontinuation of trastuzumab therapy was necessary at 24 weeks' gestation because of a decrease in the EF. The patient delivered a healthy baby and resumed chemotherapy 3 weeks after delivery.[40]

One small study involving 10 pregnant women assessed the effect of anthracyclines on maternal and fetal cardiac function. The women were treated with anthracyclines during the second and third trimesters of pregnancy. Compared to a control group of 10 non-pregnant women matched for age, type of cancer, and anthracycline treatment, these women exhibited no difference in cardiac function. In addition, chemotherapy exerted no clinically significant effect on fetal cardiac function.[42] At this time, only limited amounts of data exist to guide management, but careful monitoring of the mother with echocardiography is advisable before the initiation of chemotherapy, after 3 doses of anthracyclines, and before delivery.[41]

CONCLUSIONS

Childhood cancer survivors and women with cancer who are exposed to cardiotoxic chemotherapy during pregnancy require more vigilant cardiac monitoring during pregnancy than do women in the general population. Because of insufficient data, specific guidelines for such monitoring are limited. International guidelines suggest that surveillance for cardiotoxicity is reasonable before pregnancy or during the first trimester for all women previously treated with anthracyclines, chest irradiation, or both.[44] No recommendations have been formulated for ongoing surveillance of pregnant cancer survivors who exhibited normal LV systolic function before pregnancy or during the first trimester.[4] Dutch guidelines recommend that all pregnant cancer survivors treated with any cardiotoxic treatment should undergo echocardiography during the third trimester of pregnancy.[4]

Lifelong cardiac monitoring is recommended for all survivors of childhood cancer treated with cardiotoxic therapy. Evaluation before, during, and after pregnancy is especially important. For patients who present for pre-pregnancy counselling and evaluation, performance of an exercise stress test might be reasonable. Patients who cannot achieve 70% of aerobic capability are unlikely to tolerate pregnancy.[25] And, for patients with mild LV dysfunction, myocardial contractile reserve as documented by an exercise stress echocardiogram may suggest a more favorable cardiac outcome.[23,24,45] For patients with EF less than 40% or an NYHA score higher than 2, pregnancy is not recommended.[26] During pregnancy planning, high-risk features that should be considered include younger age at the time of cancer treatment, higher doses of anthracycline, longer times from treatment to pregnancy, previous cardiac events, baseline LV dysfunction, and history of radiation therapy in addition to anthracycline therapy.

Clinical examination, echocardiography, and BNP measurements are important monitoring tools during and after pregnancy. The World Health Organization classifies women with mild LV dysfunction as risk class II or III depending on the individual and recommends cardiology evaluation each trimester for those at lower risk and monthly or bimonthly for those at higher risk.[45,46] For patients with a history of peripartum cardiomyopathy, Elkayan suggests a baseline echocardiogram, measurement of the BNP level either before pregnancy or during early pregnancy, and repeat echocardiography after the first and second trimesters, 1 month before delivery, 1 month after delivery, and upon the appearance of any symptoms.[20] With the known effects of anthracyclines and radiation on the heart, it would be ideal to develop similar guidelines or recommendations that are specific for pregnant survivors of childhood cancer. In the meantime, it is important for doctors to realize that the incidence of cardiac toxicity increases with time after treatment with anthracyclines and that the risk of heart failure with pregnancy is increased compared to the general population. Childhood cancer survivors should undergo evaluation for individual risks before pregnancy and careful monitoring before, during, and after pregnancy.

REFERENCES

1. Lipshultz SE, Adams MJ, Colan SD, et al. Long-term cardiovascular toxicity in children, adolescents, and young adults who receive cancer therapy: pathophysiology, course, monitoring, management, prevention, and research directions: a scientific statement from the American Heart Association. *Circulation.* 2013;128:1927–1995.
2. Mulrooney DA, Armstrong GT, Huang S, et al. Cardiac outcomes in adult survivors of childhood cancer exposed to cardiotoxic therapy: a cross-sectional study. *Ann Intern Med.* 2016;164:93–101.
3. Mariotto AB, Rowland JH, Yabroff KR, et al. Long-term survivors of childhood cancers in the United States. *Cancer Epidemiol Biomarkers Prev* 2009;18:1033–1040.

4. Armenian SH, Hudson MM, Mulder RL, et al. Recommendations for cardiomyopathy surveillance for survivors of childhood cancer: a report from the International Late Effects of Childhood Cancer Guideline Harmonization Group. *Lancet Oncol.* 2015;16:E123–E136.

5. Lipshultz SE, Lipsitz SR, Mone SM, et al. Female sex and higher drug dose as risk-factors for late cardiotoxic effects of doxorubicin therapy for childhood-cancer. *N Engl J Med.* 1995;332:1738–1743.

6. Katz R, Karliner JS, Resnik R. Effects of a natural volume overload state (pregnancy) on left ventricular performance in normal human subjects. *Circulation.* 1978;58:434–441.

7. Elkayam U. Pregnancy and cardiovascular disease. In: Braunwald E, ed. *Heart Disease: A Textbook of Cardiovascular Medicine.* 5nd ed. Philadelphia, PA: Saunders; 1997.

8. Warnes CA. Pregnancy and heart disease. In: Mann D, Zipes D, Libby P, Bonow R, eds. *Braunwald's Heart Disease.* 10nd ed. Philadelphia, PA: Elsevier; 2015.

9. Cunningham F, Leveno K, Bloom S, et al. Maternal physiology. In: Cunningham F, Leveno K, Bloom S, et al., eds. *Williams Obstetrics.* 23nd ed. New York, NY: McGraw Hill; 2010.

10. Conrad KP. Maternal vasodilation in pregnancy: the emerging role of relaxin. *Am J Physiol Regul Integr Comp Physiol.* 2011;301:R267–R275.

11. Clark SL, Cotton DB, Lee W, et al. Central hemodynamic assessment of normal term pregnancy. *Am J Obstet Gynecol.* 1989;161:1439–1442.

12. Centers for Disease Control and Prevention. Pregnancy Mortality Surveillance System. www.cdc.gov/reproductivehealth/maternalinfanthealth/pmss.html. Accessed April 7, 2015, 2013.

13. Siu SC, Sermer M, Colman JM, et al. Prospective multicenter study of pregnancy outcomes in women with heart disease. *Circulation.* 2001;104:515–521.

14. Grewal J, Siu SC, Ross HJ, et al. Pregnancy outcomes in women with dilated cardiomyopathy. *J Am Coll Cardiol.* 2009;55:45–52.

15. Guedes A, Mercier LA, Leduc L, Berube L, Marcotte F, Dore A. Impact of pregnancy on the systemic right ventricle after a Mustard operation for transposition of the great arteries. *J Am Coll Cardiol.* 2004;44:433–437.

16. Sliwa K, Hilfiker-Kleiner D, Petrie MC, et al. Current state of knowledge on aetiology, diagnosis, management, and therapy of peripartum cardiomyopathy: a position statement from the Heart Failure Association of the European Society of Cardiology Working Group on peripartum cardiomyopathy. *Eur J Heart Fail.* 2010;12:767–778.

17. Pearson GD, Veille JC, Rahimtoola S, et al. Peripartum cardiomyopathy: national heart, lung, and blood institute and office of rare diseases (National Institutes of Health) workshop recommendations and review. *JAMA.* 2000;283:1183–1188.

18. Patten IS, Rana S, Shahul S, et al. Cardiac angiogenic imbalance leads to peripartum cardiomyopathy. *Nature.* 2012;485:333–338.

19. Hilfiker-Kleiner D, Kaminski K, Podewski E, et al. A cathepsin D-cleaved 16 kDa form of prolactin mediates postpartum cardiomyopathy. *Cell.* 2007;128:589–600.

20. Elkayam U. Clinical characteristics of peripartum cardiomyopathy in the United States: diagnosis, prognosis, and management. *J Am Coll Cardiol.* 2011;58:659–670.

21. Felker GM, Thompson RE, Hare JM, et al. Underlying causes and long-term survival in patients with initially unexplained cardiomyopathy. *N Engl J Med.* 2000;342:1077–1084.

22. Elkayam U, Tummala PP, Rao K, et al. Maternal and fetal outcomes of subsequent pregnancies in women with peripartum cardiomyopathy. *N Engl J Med.* 2001;344:1567–1571.

23. Elkayam U. Risk of subsequent pregnancy in women with a history of peripartum cardiomyopathy. *J Am Coll Cardiol.* 2014;64:1629–1636.

24. Fett JD, Fristoe KL, Welsh SN. Risk of heart failure relapse in subsequent pregnancy among peripartum cardiomyopathy mothers. *Int J Gynecol Obstet.* 2010;109:34–36.

25. Warnes C. Pregnancy and heart disease. In *Braunwald's Heart Disease*, 9th ed. RO Bonow, DL Mann, DP Zipes, P Libby, eds. Philadelphia, PA: Elsevier; 2011.

26. Stergiopoulos K, Shiang E, Bench T. Pregnancy in patients with pre-existing cardiomyopathies. *J Am Coll Cardiol.* 2011;58:337–350.

27. Tanous D, Siu SC, Mason J, et al. B-type natriuretic peptide in pregnant women with heart disease. *J Am Coll Cardiol.* 2010;56:1247–1253.

28. Lipshultz SE, Adams MJ. Cardiotoxicity after childhood cancer: beginning with the end in mind. *J Clin Oncol.* 2010;28:1276–1281.

29. Lipshultz SE, Colan SD, Gelber RD, Perez-Atayde AR, Sallan SE, Sanders SP. Late cardiac effects of doxorubicin therapy for acute lymphoblastic leukemia in childhood. *N Engl J Med.* 1991;324:808–815.

30. Lipshultz SE, Alvarez JA, Scully RE. Anthracycline associated cardiotoxicity in survivors of childhood cancer. *Heart.* 2008;94:525–533.

31. Lipshultz SE, Lipsitz SR, Sallan SE, et al. Chronic progressive cardiac dysfunction years after doxorubicin therapy for childhood acute lymphoblastic leukemia. *J Clin Oncol.* 2005;23:2629–2636.

32. Mertens AC, Yasui Y, Neglia JP, et al. Late mortality experience in five-year survivors of childhood and adolescent cancer: the Childhood Cancer Survivor Study. *J Clin Oncol.* 2001;19:3163–3172.

33. Davis LE, Brown CEL. Peripartum heart-failure in a patient treated previously with doxorubicin. *Obstet Gynecol.* 1988;71:506–508.

34. Katz A, Goldenberg I, Maoz C, Thaler M, Grossman E, Rosenthal T. Peripartum cardiomyopathy occurring in a patient previously treated with doxorubicin. *Am J Med Sci.* 1997;314:399–400.

35. Hadar A, Sheiner E, Press F, Katz A, Katz M. Dilated cardiomyopathy in a pregnant woman after doxorubicin and radiotherapy for Hodgkin's disease: a case report. *J Reprod Med.* 2004;49:401–403.

36. Bar J, Davidi O, Goshen Y, Hod M, Yaniv I, Hirsch R. Pregnancy outcome in women treated with doxorubicin for childhood cancer. *Am J Obstet Gynecol.* 2003;189:853–857.

37. van Dalen EC, van der Pal HJH, van den Bos C, Kok WEM, Caron HN, Kremer LCM. Clinical heart failure during pregnancy and delivery in a cohort of female childhood cancer survivors treated with anthracyclines. *Eur J Cancer.* 2006;42:2549–2553.

38. Hines MR, Mulrooney DA, Hudson MM, et al. Pregnancy-associated cardiomyopathy in survivors of childhood cancer. *J Cancer Surviv.* 2016;10:113–121.

39. Thompson KA, Hildebrandt MA, Ater JL. Cardiac outcomes with pregnancy after cardiotoxic therapy for childhood cancer. *J Am Coll Cardiol.* 2017;69:594–595.

40. Shrim A, Garcia-Bournissen F, Maxwell C, Farine D, Koren G. Favorable pregnancy outcome following Trastuzumab (Herceptin®) use during pregnancy-case report and updated literature review. *Reprod Toxicol.* 2007;23:611–613.

41. Amant F, Brepoels L, Halaska MJ, Gziri MM, Calsteren KV. Gynaecologic cancer complicating pregnancy: an overview. *Best Pract Res Clin Obstet Gynaecol.* 2010;24:61–79.

42. Gziri MM, Debieve F, De Catte L, et al. Chemotherapy during pregnancy: effect of anthracyclines on fetal and maternal cardiac function. *Acta Obstet Gynecol Scand.* 2012;91:1465–1468.

43. Roberts NJ, Auld BJ. Trastuzamab (Herceptin®)-related cardiotoxicity in pregnancy. *J R Soc Med.* 2010;103:157–159.

44. Shankar SM, Marina N, Hudson MM et al. Monitoring for cardiovascular disease in survivors of childhood cancer: report from the cardiovascular disease task force of the children's oncology group. *Pediatrics.* 2008;121:e387–e396.

45. European Society of Gynecology, Association for European Paediatric Cardiology, German Society for Gender Medicine, et al. ESC Guidelines on the management of cardiovascular diseases during pregnancy: the Task Force on the Management of Cardiovascular Diseases during Pregnancy of the European Society of Cardiology (ESC). *Eur Heart J.* 2011;32:3147–3197.

46. Thorne S, MacGregor A, Nelson-Piercy C. Risks of contraception and pregnancy in heart disease. *Heart.* 2006;92:1520–1525.

28 Exercise in the Cancer Patient: Cardiovascular Considerations

Susan C. Gilchrist

CARDIOVASCULAR RISK IN CANCER PATIENTS

Cardiovascular disease (CVD) is a leading competing cause of death among patients with early-stage cancer. For example, breast cancer patients have a 30% higher risk of CVD events than the general population over an 18-year period.[1] Individuals with localized prostate cancer who are treated with radical prostatectomy and androgen-deprivation therapy (ADT) are at higher risk of death from cardiovascular causes over a median duration of 4.1 months than are patients not treated with ADT (hazard ratio [HR], 2.6; 95% confidence interval [CI], 1.4–4.7; $P = 0.002$).[2] Among patients with Hodgkin lymphoma (HL), for whom 10-year survival rates are higher than 80%, late cardiovascular complications are more common than among the general population.[3] Moreover, among women with endometrial cancer, CVD is the most frequent cause of death (36%).[4]

Direct exposures to the cardiovascular system (e.g., radiation, chemotherapy) as well as indirect exposures (e.g., weight gain, hypertension) are known to contribute to cancer patients' higher risk of CVD. For example, Darby et al. found that the risk of coronary heart events among breast cancer patients increases by 7.4% (2.9%–14.5%) per Gy of radiation exposure, and this risk is sustained for 20 years after diagnosis.[5] Treatment with cardiotoxic drugs (e.g., anthracyclines) increases the risk of a CVD event by 2-fold after the analysis has been adjusted for previous radiation exposure.[6] Importantly, the cause of the heightened risk of CVD is related both to the cardiotoxic effects of treatment and to the CVD risk factors already existing or accumulating during cancer treatment.[7,8] For example, patients undergoing chemotherapy for testicular cancer experience a worsening lipid profile and weight gain with treatment.[9] Survivors of breast, prostate, colorectal, and gynecologic cancers are more likely to be overweight or obese, to be physically inactive, and to report hypertension or diabetes than are persons with no cancer.[10] Childhood cancer survivors, even years after diagnosis and into young adulthood, exhibit poorer CVD risk profiles than do sibling control subjects.[11] Even patients with ductal carcinoma in situ (DCIS), who are not exposed to extensive chemotherapeutic agents that patients with invasive forms of breast cancer undergo, exhibit a change in CVD risk factors after diagnosis.[12]

CARDIORESPIRATORY FITNESS: A PROGNOSTIC CVD MARKER IN CANCER PATIENTS

Traditionally, treatment-related toxicities are monitored via measurements of cardiac function (e.g., left ventricular ejection fraction). However, the effects of cancer therapies can extend beyond the heart to impact the entire cardiovascular-skeletal muscle axis.[7] An assessment of the integrity of this axis can be directly measured and is manifested by the patient's attained maximal oxygen uptake (Vo_2max) or cardiorespiratory fitness (CRF).[13] CRF, assessed during an incremental exercise treadmill (or bicycle) test, reflects the integrative ability of the heart to deliver adequate oxygen to skeletal muscle and other vital organs.

Previous studies have shown that cardiorespiratory fitness (CRF) is substantially impaired among cancer patients. Breast cancer patients exhibit a 27% lower CRF than do age-matched sedentary controls.[14] For a 50-year-old woman with breast cancer, this CRF translates into a CRF equivalent to that of a sedentary 70-year-old woman. This finding was confirmed by a meta-analysis of 27 clinical trials and observational studies measuring CRF in the preadjuvant and postadjuvant treatment settings for breast cancer.[15] Alarmingly, a decline in a breast cancer patient's CRF is not transient but rather sustained, even 7 years after treatment.[16] Low CRF has also been demonstrated in other populations, such as young adult cancer survivors[17,18] and women with a history of gynecological cancers.[19]

CRF is emerging as a prognostic factor for survival after a cancer diagnosis. Jones et al. assessed the association between CRF and all-cause mortality among patients with non–small cell lung cancer (NSCLC).[20] The study used Cancer and Leukemia Group B (CALGB) protocol 9238, a multi-institutional study that assessed CRF after a lung cancer diagnosis and prior to surgical resection. The median time from CRF measurement to death was 3.7 years. Compared to the referent group with low CRF, the adjusted risk of death was 36% lower for patients with a moderate CRF level and 44% lower for those with a high CRF level. In this study, CRF corresponded to a Vo_2 peak of 12.8 ±3.3 ml kg^{-1}min^{-1} for the referent group with low CRF, a peak of 15.5 ± 3.0 ml kg^{-1}min^{-1} for patients with moderate CRF, and a peak of 19.1 ± 4.1 ml kg^{-1}min^{-1} for patients with high CRF. In a second study, the relationship between CRF and survival was assessed among patients with metastatic breast cancer.[14] The median time from CRF measurement to death was 27 months. Women with a Vo_2 peak higher than 15.4 ml kg^{-1}min^{-1} had a 68% lower adjusted risk of death than women with a Vo_2 peak lower than 15.4 ml kg^{-1}min^{-1}.

■ Postulated Mechanisms for Loss of CRF in Cancer Patients

There are several postulated mechanisms that may contribute to a decline in CRF in cancer patients. We focus on the following conditions: cardiac atrophy, diastolic dysfunction, endothelial dysfunction/impaired vascular compliance, and skeletal muscle dysfunction.[7]

Cardiac atrophy ■ Cancer patients are likely to exhibit sedentary behavior, prolonged sitting time, and bed rest during treatment. Bed rest results in chronic unloading of the heart, which has deleterious consequences on left ventricular (LV) mass and LV end-diastolic volume (the ability of blood to fill the heart), resulting in cardiac atrophy. A study by Levine et al. found that bed rest for 6 weeks decreased LV end-diastolic volume by 14% and LV mass by 8.0% ($P<0.05$ for both).[21] Cardiac atrophy leads to a reduction in cardiac work, requiring an increase in chronotropic work (e.g., heart rate) and preservation of LV contractility to maintain LVEF. Cardiac atrophy can also result in alterations in diastolic filling and orthostatic intolerance because of the reduction in standing stroke volume that is caused by a decrease in end-diastolic volume. This reduction can lead to presyncope secondary to an increased dependence on plasma volume to maintain cardiac output. These symptoms can be exaggerated among patients with attenuated baroreflex-mediated increases in sympathetic activity, such as cancer patients exposed to radiation to the neck or to anthracycline-based chemotherapy regimens.[22,23]

LV chamber compliance and diastolic dysfunction ■ A decrease in LV chamber compliance, defined as the change in pressure resulting from a given change in volume at a specific LV end-diastolic volume, is characteristic of the aging process. For cancer patients, this process can occur much earlier than would be expected on the basis of age.[24] Importantly, alterations in LV compliance can contribute to exercise intolerance, even with a normal LVEF. During exercise, the elevated heart rate shortens the duration of diastole, which reduces LV diastolic filling and forces the LV to fill more rapidly to maintain adequate stroke volume. Rapid LV filling is accomplished by accelerating LV relaxation to produce a subsequent decrease in LV end-diastolic pressure. Relaxation can be accomplished by optimizing elastic recoil, by increasing the rate of myocardial relaxation, or by increasing LV chamber compliance.[25] If LV end-diastolic volume cannot be maintained by these changes, left atrial pressure increases, and this increase is characteristic of diastolic dysfunction.

Endothelial dysfunction and impaired vascular compliance ■ Coronary endothelial function modulates vasomotor tone and is necessary for meeting the blood-flow demands of the heart under stress. The resulting downstream effect is an increase in blood pressure and subsequent hypertension resulting from several potential mechanisms, including a decrease in the bioavailability of nitric oxide (NO). Premature hypertension is a common complication of cancer therapies, with an incidence of approximately 20%.[26] Cancer patients most susceptible to hypertension are those exposed to vascular endothelial growth factor (VEGF) inhibitors, particularly inhibitors of VEGF receptor 2 (VEGFR-2), which promotes vasodilation via NO signaling pathways.[27]

Hypertension contributes not only to function but also to larger-vessel pathology, specifically arterial stiffness contributing to increased afterload or work by the heart. Increases in afterload decrease stroke volume and increase LV end-diastolic pressure by decreasing the velocity of fiber shortening and, subsequently, the rate of volume ejection, ultimately leading to a higher risk of heart failure.[28]

The heart messenger: Skeletal muscle ■ Aging of skeletal muscle can manifest itself as decreased muscle strength and function and as changes in muscle composition, as evidenced by an increase in skeletal muscle fat and the loss of lean muscle mass (sarcopenia).[29] Sarcopenia can develop among women undergoing breast cancer treatment, especially those with reduced levels of physical activity.[30] The development of this condition is concerning given the alterations in fat and lean muscle content linked to insulin resistance, a key CVD risk factor.[31] In addition, certain anticancer drugs, such as anthracyclines, can impair mitochondrial function and increase the concentration of reactive oxidative species, thereby promoting a pro-inflammatory state in the muscle.[32] Finally, the tumor itself can compete with skeletal muscle for the available energy substrate, thereby affecting skeletal muscle metabolism.[33] Each of these potential insults can impair muscle strength, muscle function, and skeletal muscle signaling to the heart (via the autonomic nervous system).[34]

■ Exercise Training in Cancer Patients to Improve CRF

An important goal of exercise training is to optimize CRF. The Table 28-1 lists the existing meta-analyses and scientific evidence regarding the effect of exercise training on CRF in cancer patients. Below, we highlight studies based on when the exercise training was performed within the cancer continuum.

Prior to cancer treatment ■ Exercise training before surgery, or prehabilitation, provides an opportunity to mitigate loss of CRF and to enhance functional capability before surgery.[35] A recent systematic review of 18 exercise training trials involving 966 cancer patients provides supportive evidence. The 6 studies that objectively measured CRF found that prehabilitation was associated with an overall improvement in CRF of 8% to 32%.[36] For lung cancer patients, for example, exercise training before resection (5 times per week at 60%–100% Vo_{2peak}) improved CRF by 14.6% or 2.4 ml kg^{-1}min^{-1}. Another study of prehabilitation involved

TABLE 28-1   Systematic reviews of the effect of exercise training on CRF among cancer patients (2005–2015)

Study	Cancer Type	Studies Reviewed (Studies measuring ΔVo_2)	Time Point of Intervention (Studies measuring ΔVo_2)	Effect of ET on CRF
Singh et al.[36]	Lung (61%), colorectal, prostate, colon, pancreatic, liver, colon, rectum, sarcoma, esophagus	Systematic review of 18 clinical trials (6)	Before surgery	↑
Loughney et al.[60]	Breast (82%), lung, mixed	Systematic review of 17 clinical trials (4)	During cancer treatment	↔
Schmitz et al.[38]	Breast (72%), colon, lung, ovarian, leukemia, lymphoma, testicular, sarcoma, stomach, prostate, other	Systematic review of 22 high-quality studies (9)	During (5) and after (4) cancer treatment	↑ (during, weak evidence) ↑(after, strong evidence)
Jones et al.[61]	Breast (67%), lymphoma, prostate, colon	Meta-analysis of 6 clinical trials (6)	During (2) and after (4) cancer treatment	↑
Wolin et al.[62]	Hematologic cancer (100%)	Review of 23 high-quality intervention studies in adult (1) and pediatric (6) populations	Receiving or not receiving hematopoietic stem cell transplant	↑ (adults, weak evidence) ↑(children, strong evidence)
Fong et al.[43]	Breast (65%), colorectal, endometrial, prostate, lung, lymphoma, gastric, colon, gynecologic	Meta-analysis of 34 randomized clinical trials (7)	After cancer treatment	↑

ET, exercise training; CRF, cardiorespiratory fitness

patients with rectal cancer who experienced a loss of CRF after neoadjuvant chemotherapy. This study, by West et al., found that patients who participated in 6 weeks of aerobic exercise training before rectal surgery exhibited significantly improved CRF (back to baseline levels) than did control subjects ($P<0.0001$).[37]

During active cancer treatment ■ A systematic review and meta-analysis by Schmitz et al. found only weak evidence to suggest that exercise interventions improve CRF during active treatment of breast cancer.[38] However, the weight of the evidence suggests that exercise mitigates the loss of CRF during active treatment. For example, a trial involving breast cancer patients found that participation in a progressive aerobic exercise training regimen 3 times per week at 70% of Vo_{2max} resulted in no change in CRF (0.2 ml kg^{-1}min^{-1}), whereas the control group experienced a significant loss in CRF (-1.6 ml kg^{-1}min^{-1}).[39] A secondary analysis of the data gathered during this study showed that a longer duration of aerobic exercise training (50–60 min per bout rather than 25–30 min per bout) at a constant intensity (70% PHR) and frequency (3 times per week) was more successful at mitigating CRF loss among breast cancer patients undergoing adjuvant chemotherapy.[40]

A combination of resistance training and aerobic exercise has been studied for prostate cancer patients undergoing radiotherapy with or without ADT. No significant change in CRF was found among patients randomly assigned to resistance exercise (Vo_{2peak}, 0.14 ml kg^{-1}min^{-1}) or aerobic exercise training (Vo_{2peak}, 0.04 ml kg^{-1}min^{-1}), while there was a loss of CRF demonstrated in the control group (Vo_{2peak}, -1.4 ml kg^{-1}min^{-1}, $P = 0.008$).[41] For children with acute lymphocytic leukemia (ALL) who were undergoing maintenance treatment (mercaptopurine daily and methotrexate weekly), an in-hospital exercise intervention improved CRF.[42] The intervention consisted of supervised moderate to vigorous aerobic exercise 3 times weekly at a minimum of 70% PHR in addition to resistance training. Significant increases in CRF were found between baseline levels and levels after 16 weeks of training (Vo_{2peak}, 24.3 ± 5.9 ml kg^{-1}min^{-1} vs 30.2 ± 6.2 ml kg^{-1}min^{-1}; $P<0.05$).

Taken together, these studies indicate that an exercise training intervention can mitigate the decline in CRF during active treatment for breast cancer and can improve CRF among patients with certain cancer types who are undergoing certain treatment regimens. This finding is important given that the loss of CRF that is experienced during active treatment can be substantial ($\sim$30%)[14]; therefore, maintaining CRF during treatment can promote quicker recovery and improvement in CRF after treatment.

After cancer treatment (Survivorship) ■ The positive effects on CRF of exercise training after treatment have been demonstrated among patients with several types of cancer. A meta-analysis of randomized controlled trials demonstrated a pooled increase in Vo_{2max} of 2.2 ml kg^{-1}min^{-1} ($P<0.01$) among survivors of breast cancer, colorectal cancer, prostate cancer, lung cancer, and lymphoma.[43] For example, postmenopausal breast cancer patients participating in aerobic exercise training 3 times per week at 70% to 75% of Vo_{2max} for 30 minutes exhibited better CRF after 15 weeks than did patients receiving standard care ($P<0.01$).[44] Jarvela et al. assessed the effect of a home-based exercise program for survivors of childhood ALL. The program instructed patients in muscular strength training and encouraged them to perform a strength exercise program 3 to 4 times per week and an aerobic exercise of choice for at least three 30-min sessions per week. After 16 weeks, CRF had increased significantly from baseline (Vo_{2peak}, 35.2 ml kg^{-1}min^{-1} ml vs 37.1 ml kg^{-1}min^{-1}; $P = 0.01$). A study by Thorsen et al. involved 111 patients treated for lymphoma, breast cancer, gynecologic cancer, or testicular cancer. Patients participated for 14 weeks in a program consisting of exercise training twice per week for 30 min at 60% to 70% of MHR, or in standard of care.[45] After the intervention, CRF was significantly better among the exercise group than among the control group ($P<0.01$). Furthermore, for patients with Stage I to Stage III colorectal cancer, a 12-week telephone-based intervention including weekly calls to monitor physical activity (PA), discuss barriers to PA, and reinforce participants' efforts resulted in significant improvements in CRF among the exercise group compared to a control group ($P = 0.002$).[46] Taken together, these findings indicate that exercise intervention protocols improve CRF after treatment for various types of cancer.

■ Integrating Exercise Training into Clinical Practice for Cancer Patients

Clinical use of cardiopulmonary exercise testing in the cancer setting ■ Measurement of CRF or Vo_{2peak} via cardiopulmonary exercise testing (CPET) is clinically feasible in the cancer setting.[47] CPET is a noninvasive test using a stationary bicycle or a treadmill for exercise and involving both cardiac (electrocardiography [ECG]) monitoring and measurements of gas exchange (requiring a facemask or mouthpiece). CPET is unique in that, unlike other imaging methods (e.g., 2D echocardiogram), it can simultaneously assess for multiple organ defects (e.g., cardiac, pulmonary, skeletal muscle) caused by cancer treatment. CPET provides an objective assessment of Vo_{2peak} even before cancer patients exhibit symptoms or overt disease. Several components of CPET can help guide decisions about cardiopulmonary readiness and can assist in developing individualized exercise prescriptions for cancer patients (Box 28-1).

Exercise prescription for cancer patients ■ Prescribing an initial exercise program involves a review of the frequency, duration, and intensity goals of exercise with a cancer patient. Exercise can be safely performed during or after cancer treatment, as demonstrated by a review of clinical studies,[48] provided that the exercise intervention is appropriate and includes emergency protocols and appropriate exclusion criteria. Contraindications to exercise for cancer patients have been previously reviewed and are summarized in the Box 28-2.[48–50] An overall guideline for prescribing exercise for cancer patients has been previously published (Table 28-2).[51]

Of note, intensity recommendations can be individualized for cancer patients based on both the resting heart rate and the maximal heart rate achieved during CPET utilizing the following formula[52]:

Exercise heart rate = ([max HR – resting HR] × % Intensity goal) + resting HR

Using this formula, for example, a patient with a resting heart rate of 90 who obtains a maximal heart rate of 160 has a target heart rate of 139, given a moderate intensity goal of 70% of Vo_{2peak}: ([160-90] × .70) + 90 = 139. This measurement may be more appropriate for cancer patients who have a higher resting HR due to cancer treatment. In addition, aerobic exercise intensity can be obtained by using the Borg scale to assess patients' feedback about their perceived exertion

---

Box 28-1 Clinically useful measurements that should be obtained from cancer patients during cardiopulmonary exercise testing

Vo_{2peak}: Peak oxygen consumption (ml kg^{-1}min^{-1}). Gold standard measure of cardiorespiratory fitness (CRF). Lower among cancer patients than among the general population.

Heart rate recovery: Heart rate (HR) at 1 min after peak exercise. Inability to reduce heart rate is a measure of autonomic dysfunction, a key metric for cancer patients.

Abnormal heart rate response: Chronotropic incompetence. Inability to increase HR commensurate to increased exercise work load. A measure of autonomic dysfunction during exercise testing.

Oxygen pulse (ml of oxygen per heart beat): Derived from Fick equation; approximates stroke volume. Measurements are abnormal among patients with cardiomyopathy, severe valvular disease, coronary artery disease, pulmonary vascular obstructive disease.

Respiratory exchange ratio (VCo_2/o_2): Ratio of exhaled carbon dioxide (Co_2) to inhaled oxygen (O_2). Measures effort among cancer patients; good effort, >1.0.

VE/VCo_2: Minute ventilation (expired volume, VE) relative to volume of Co_2 exhalation. Measure of ventilatory efficiency. Marker of lung disease, pulmonary artery hypertension, heart failure.

Ventilatory threshold (VT): Shift from aerobic to anaerobic metabolism. May be useful for debilitated cancer patients.

Box 28-2 Contraindications to and Special Considerations for Exercise by Cancer Patients

CONTRAINDICATIONS

Cardiac
  Uncontrolled symptomatic heart failure
  Acute myocarditis
  Recent myocardial infarction
  Severe symptomatic valvular disease
  Uncontrolled heart rhythm
  Acute pulmonary embolism
  Severe hypertension (>200/110 mmHg)
Findings of Laboratory Studies
  Severe anemia (<8 g/dl)
  Absolute neutrophil count <500
  Platelet count <50 k/cmm
Symptoms
  Severe shortness of breath
  Acute nausea during exercise
  Vomiting within 24 hours
  Disorientation
  Blurred vision
Other
  Acute infection
  Acute metabolic disease
  Unmanaged lymphedema
  Mental or physical impairment to exercise
Special Considerations
  Initial wound healing after surgery
  Indwelling catheter
  Bone or brain metastasis
  Recent chemotherapy or radiotherapy
(within 24 hours)

TABLE 28-2 Exercise prescription guidelines for cancer patients

PATIENT CHARACTERISTICS (EXAMPLES)	GOAL OF EXERCISE	INITIAL PRESCRIPTION	EXERCISE PROGRESSION
General (patients following the completion of adjuvant therapy for localised disease presenting with no overt underlying comorbid disease)	To improve all components of the oxygen cascade	Frequency:3–5 days/week Intensity:* light to moderate Type: aerobic endurance Time: 20–40 min/session	Frequency: 4–6 days/week Intensity:* light to vigorous Type: aerobic endurance, interval training and resistance Time: ~30–60 min/session
Cardiovascular limitation (patients presenting with chemotherapy-induced LV dysfunction and/or anaemia	Improved LV filling and relaxation, enhanced LV compliance, improvement in endothelial function, and decreased arterial stiffness	Frequency: 3 days/week Intensity:* light to moderate Type: aerobic endurance Time: ~20–30 min/session	Frequency: 3–5 days/week Intensity:* moderate Type: aerobic Time: ~20–60 min/session
Respiratory limitation (patients following pulmonary resection with concomitant COPD)	Reduced ventilatory demand and dyspnoea, with favourable skeletal muscle adaptations	Frequency: 3–4 days/week Intensity:* light to moderate Type: aerobic endurance and resistance Time: >20 min/session	Frequency: 4–5 days/week Intensity:* moderate to vigorous Type: aerobic endurance, interval and resistance Time: ~20–60 min/session
Peripheral limitation (patients presenting with tumour and/or treatment-induced cachexia or muscle atrophy)	Increased muscle mass and aerobic enzymes, and improved fibre type transition and oxidative metabolism	Frequency: 3 days/week Intensity:‡ light to moderate Type: resistance Time: 20–30 min/session	Frequency: >3 days/week Intensity:‡ moderate Type: resistance and aerobic Time: ~20–60 min/session

*Relative intensities guideline for aerobic endurance training: light (light effort, normal or slight breathing, 40%–50% of measured heart rate maximum or VO2peak); moderate (moderate effort, elevated breathing, 50%–70% of measured heart rate maximum or VO2peak); vigorous (hard effort, greater breathing, >70% of measured heart rate maximum or VO2peak). ‡Relative intensities guideline for resistance training: light (50%–60% of measured one repetition maximum), moderate (60%–80% of measured one repetition maximum), and hard (>80% of measured one repetition maximum).

COPD, chronic obstructive pulmonary disease; LV, left ventricular; VO2peak, peak oxygen consumption.

Source: Adapted from Lakoski, SG et al., 2012.[51]

during graded exercise in CPET[53] This method is used for cancer patients who do not have reliable heart rates or who desire a subjective measure of exertion in addition to a calculated exercise heart rate goal.

CONCLUSION

Cardiovascular disease is an important competing cause of death in cancer patients. As evidenced by the current review, CRF is an emerging biomarker of CVD risk in cancer patients, as it represents the overall functioning of the cardiovascular-skeletal muscle axis that may be impacted by cancer therapies. Importantly, exercise training is a key non-pharmacologic strategy to promote improvement in CRF with the goal to reduce CVD in cancer patients. Further work is now needed to formalize exercise training opportunities and programs for cancer patients. Presently, adapting cardiac rehabilitation for cancer patients is an option for broadening the accessibility of exercise to cancer patients. Most cardiac rehabilitation (CR) programs have the capacity to perform CPET as well as the infrastructure to modify existing CVD risk factors that contribute to a cancer patient's elevated risk for CVD. Utilizing CR for cancer patients has been demonstrated in a prior study and its successful results have been reviewed.[54] In addition to CR, other previously published models of exercise rehabilitation have been published.[55–58] Future studies will be necessary to test a wide range of models to identify the most cost-effective strategy that can effectively deliver exercise to improve CVD outcomes for cancer patients.[59]

REFERENCES

1. Hooning MJ, Botma A, Aleman BM, et al. Long-term risk of cardiovascular disease in 10-year survivors of breast cancer. *J Natl Cancer Inst*. 2007;99:365–375.

2. Tsai HK, D'Amico AV, Sadetsky N, Chen MH, Carroll PR. Androgen deprivation therapy for localized prostate cancer and the risk of cardiovascular mortality. *J Natl Cancer Inst*. 2007;99:1516–1524.

3. van Nimwegen FA, Schaapveld M, Janus CP, et al. Cardiovascular disease after Hodgkin lymphoma treatment: 40-year disease risk. *JAMA Intern Med*. 2015;175:1007–1017.

4. Ward KK, Shah NR, Saenz CC, McHale MT, Alvarez EA, Plaxe SC. Cardiovascular disease is the leading cause of death among endometrial cancer patients. *Gynecol Oncol*. 2012;126:176–179.

5. Darby SC, Ewertz M, Hall P. Ischemic heart disease after breast cancer radiotherapy. *N Engl J Med*. 2013;368:2527.

6. Yood MU, Wells KE, Alford SH, et al. Cardiovascular outcomes in women with advanced breast cancer exposed to chemotherapy. *Pharmacoepidemiol Drug Saf*. 2012;21:818–827.

7. Jones LW, Haykowsky MJ, Swartz JJ, Douglas PS, Mackey JR. Early breast cancer therapy and cardiovascular injury. *J Am Coll Cardiol*. 2007;50:1435–1441.

8. Jones LW, Haykowsky M, Pituskin EN, et al. Cardiovascular reserve and risk profile of postmenopausal women after chemoendocrine therapy for hormone receptor—positive operable breast cancer. *Oncologist*. 2007;12:1156–1164.

9. Gietema JA, Sleijfer DT, Willemse PH, et al. Long-term follow-up of cardiovascular risk factors in patients given chemotherapy for disseminated nonseminomatous testicular cancer. *Ann Intern Med*. 1992;116:709–715.

10. Weaver KE, Foraker RE, Alfano CM, et al. Cardiovascular risk factors among long-term survivors of breast, prostate, colorectal, and gynecologic cancers: a gap in survivorship care? *J Cancer Surviv*. 2013;7:253–261.

11. Armstrong GT, Liu Q, Yasui Y, et al. Late mortality among 5-year survivors of childhood cancer: a summary from the childhood cancer survivor study. *J Clin Oncol*. 2009;27:2328–2338.

12. Sprague BL, Trentham-Dietz A, Nichols HB, Hampton JM, Newcomb PA. Change in lifestyle behaviors and medication use after a diagnosis of ductal carcinoma in situ. *Breast Cancer Res Treat*. 2010;124:487–495.

13. McGuire DK, Levine BD, Williamson JW, et al. A 30-year follow-up of the Dallas Bedrest and Training Study: I. Effect of age on the cardiovascular response to exercise. *Circulation*. 2001;104:1350–1357.

14. Jones LW, Courneya KS, Mackey JR, et al. Cardiopulmonary function and age-related decline across the breast cancer survivorship continuum. *J Clin Oncol*. 2012;30:2530–2537.

15. Peel AB, Thomas SM, Dittus K, Jones LW, Lakoski SG. Cardiorespiratory fitness in breast cancer patients: a call for normative values. *J Am Heart Assoc*. 2014;3:e000432.

16. Lakoski SG, Barlow CE, Koelwyn GJ, et al. The influence of adjuvant therapy on cardiorespiratory fitness in early-stage breast cancer seven years after diagnosis: the Cooper Center Longitudinal Study. *Breast Cancer Res Treat*. 2013;138:909–916.

17. Miller AM, Lopez-Mitnik G, Somarriba G, et al. Exercise capacity in long-term survivors of pediatric cancer: an analysis from the cardiac risk factors in childhood cancer survivors study. *Pediatr Blood Cancer*. 2013;60:663–668.

18. De Caro E, Smeraldi A, Trocchio G, Calevo M, Hanau G, Pongiglione G. Subclinical cardiac dysfunction and exercise performance in childhood cancer survivors. *Pediatr Blood Cancer*. 2011;56:122–126.

19. Peel AB, Barlow CE, Leonard D, DeFina LF, Jones LW, Lakoski SG. Cardiorespiratory fitness in survivors of cervical, endometrial, and ovarian cancers: the Cooper Center Longitudinal Study. *Gynecol Oncol*. 2015;138:394–397.

20. Jones LW, Watson D, Herndon JE 2nd, et al. Peak oxygen consumption and long-term all-cause mortality in nonsmall cell lung cancer. *Cancer*. 2010;116:4825–4832.

21. Perhonen MA, Franco F, Lane LD, et al. Cardiac atrophy after bed rest and spaceflight. *J Appl Physiol (1985)*. 2001;91:645–653.

22. Sharabi Y, Dendi R, Holmes C, Goldstein DS. Baroreflex failure as a late sequela of neck irradiation. *Hypertension*. 2003;42:110–116.

23. Lakoski SG, Jones LW, Krone RJ, Stein PK, Scott JM. Autonomic dysfunction in early breast cancer: incidence, clinical importance, and underlying mechanisms. *Am Heart J*. 2015;170:231–241.

24. Brouwer CA, Postma A, Vonk JM, et al. Systolic and diastolic dysfunction in long-term adult survivors of childhood cancer. *Eur J Cancer*. 2011;47:2453–2462.

25. Little WC, Kitzman DW, Cheng CP. Diastolic dysfunction as a cause of exercise intolerance. *Heart Fail Rev*. 2000;5:301–306.

26. Wu S, Chen JJ, Kudelka A, Lu J, Zhu X. Incidence and risk of hypertension with sorafenib in patients with cancer: a systematic review and meta-analysis. *Lancet Oncol*. 2008;9:117–123.

27. Nazer B, Humphreys BD, Moslehi J. Effects of novel angiogenesis inhibitors for the treatment of cancer on the cardiovascular system: focus on hypertension. *Circulation*. 2011;124:1687–1691.

28. Zile MR, Bennett TD, St John Sutton M, et al. Transition from chronic compensated to acute decompensated heart failure: pathophysiological insights obtained from continuous monitoring of intracardiac pressures. *Circulation*. 2008;118:1433–1441.

29. Stenholm S, Harris TB, Rantanen T, Visser M, Kritchevsky SB, Ferrucci L. Sarcopenic obesity: definition, cause and consequences. *Curr Opin Clin Nutr Metab Care*. 2008;11:693–700.

30. Demark-Wahnefried W, Peterson BL, Winer EP, et al. Changes in weight, body composition, and factors influencing energy balance among premenopausal breast cancer patients receiving adjuvant chemotherapy. *J Clin Oncol*. 2001;19:2381–2389.

31. Goodpaster BH, Theriault R, Watkins SC, Kelley DE. Intramuscular lipid content is increased in obesity and decreased by weight loss. *Metabolism*. 2000;49:467–472.

32. Gouspillou G, Scheede-Bergdahl C, Spendiff S, et al. Anthracycline-containing chemotherapy causes long-term impairment of mitochondrial respiration and increased reactive oxygen species release in skeletal muscle. *Sci Rep*. 2015;5:8717.

33. Fearon KC. Cancer cachexia and fat-muscle physiology. *N Engl J Med*. 2011;365:565–567.

34. Christensen JF, Jones LW, Andersen JL, Daugaard G, Rorth M, Hojman P. Muscle dysfunction in cancer patients. *Ann Oncol*. 2014;25:947–958.

35. Silver JK. Cancer prehabilitation and its role in improving health outcomes and reducing health care costs. *Semin Oncol Nurs*. 2015;31:13–30.

36. Singh F, Newton RU, Galvao DA, Spry N, Baker MK. A systematic review of pre-surgical exercise intervention studies with cancer patients. *Surg Oncol*. 2013;22:92–104.

37. West MA, Loughney L, Lythgoe D, et al. Effect of prehabilitation on objectively measured physical fitness after neoadjuvant treatment in preoperative rectal cancer patients: a blinded interventional pilot study. *Br J Anaesth*. 2015;114:244–251.

38. Schmitz KH, Holtzman J, Courneya KS, Masse LC, Duval S, Kane R. Controlled physical activity trials in cancer survivors: a systematic review and meta-analysis. *Cancer Epidemiol Biomarkers Prev*. 2005;14:1588–1595.

39. Courneya KS, Segal RJ, Mackey JR, et al. Effects of aerobic and resistance exercise in breast cancer patients receiving adjuvant chemotherapy: a multicenter randomized controlled trial. *J Clin Oncol*. 2007;25:4396–4404.

40. Courneya KS, McKenzie DC, Mackey JR, et al. Effects of exercise dose and type during breast cancer chemotherapy: multicenter randomized trial. *J Natl Cancer Inst*. 2013;105:1821–1832.

41. Segal RJ, Reid RD, Courneya KS, et al. Randomized controlled trial of resistance or aerobic exercise in men receiving radiation therapy for prostate cancer. *J Clin Oncol*. 2009;27:344–351.

42. San Juan AF, Fleck SJ, Chamorro-Vina C, et al. Effects of an intrahospital exercise program intervention for children with leukemia. *Med Sci Sports Exerc*. 2007;39 13–21.

43. Fong DY, Ho JW, Hui BP, et al. Physical activity for cancer survivors: meta-analysis of randomised controlled trials. *BMJ*. 2012;344:e70.

44. Courneya KS, Mackey JR, Bell GJ, Jones LW, Field CJ, Fairey AS. Randomized controlled trial of exercise training in postmenopausal breast cancer survivors: cardiopulmonary and quality of life outcomes. *J Clin Oncol*. 2003;21:1660–1668.

45. Thorsen L, Skovlund E, Stromme SB, Hornslien K, Dahl AA, Fossa SD. Effectiveness of physical activity on cardiorespiratory fitness and health-related quality of life in young and middle-aged cancer patients shortly after chemotherapy. *J Clin Oncol*. 2005;23:2378–2388.

46. Pinto BM, Papandonatos GD, Goldstein MG, Marcus BH, Farrell N. Home-based physical activity intervention for colorectal cancer survivors. *Psychooncology*. 2013;22:54–64.

47. Jones LW, Eves ND, Haykowsky M, Joy AA, Douglas PS. Cardiorespiratory exercise testing in clinical oncology research: systematic review and practice recommendations. *Lancet Oncol*. 2008;9:757–765.

48. Rajarajeswaran P, Vishnupriya R. Exercise in cancer. *Indian J Med Paediatr Oncol*. 2009;30:61–70.

49. American College of Sports Medicine. *ACSM's Guide to Exercise and Cancer Survivorship*. Indianapolis, IN: American College of Sports Medicine; 2012.

50. American College of Sports Medicine. *ACSM's Guidelines for Exercise Testing and Prescription*. 9th ed. Philadelphia, PA: Lippincott Williams and Wilkin; 2013.

51. Lakoski SG, Eves ND, Douglas PS, Jones LW. Exercise rehabilitation in patients with cancer. *Nat Rev Clin Oncol*. 2012;9:288–296.

52. Karvonen MJ, Kentala E, Mustala O. The effects of training on heart rate; a longitudinal study. *Ann Med Exp Biol Fenn*. 1957;35:307–315.

53. Wilson RC, Jones PW. A comparison of the visual analogue scale and modified Borg scale for the measurement of dyspnoea during exercise. *Clin Sci (Lond)*. 1989;76:277–282.

54. Dittus KL, Lakoski SG, Savage PD, et al. Exercise-based oncology rehabilitation: leveraging the cardiac rehabilitation model. *J Cardiopulm Rehabil Prev*. 2015;35:130–139.

55. Segal R, Evans W, Johnson D, et al. Oncology rehabilitation program at the Ottawa Regional Cancer Centre: program description. *CMAJ*. 1999;161:282–285.

56. Grabois M. Integrating cancer rehabilitation into medical care at a cancer hospital. *Cancer*. 2001;92:1055–1057.

57. Chasen MR, Feldstain A, Gravelle D, Macdonald N, Pereira J. An interprofessional palliative care oncology rehabilitation program: effects on function and predictors of program completion. *Curr Oncol*. 2013;20:301–309.

58. Canestraro A, Nakhle A, Stack M, et al. Oncology rehabilitation provision and practice patterns across Canada. *Physiother Can*. 2013;65:94–102.

59. Alfano CM, Ganz PA, Rowland JH, Hahn EE. Cancer survivorship and cancer rehabilitation: revitalizing the link. *J Clin Oncol*. 2012;30:904–906.

60. Loughney L, West MA, Kemp GJ, Grocott MP, Jack S. Exercise intervention in people with cancer undergoing neoadjuvant cancer treatment and surgery: a systematic review. *Eur J Surg Oncol*. 2016 Jan;42(1):28–38.

61. Jones LW, Liang Y, Pituskin EN, et al. Effect of exercise training on peak oxygen consumption in patients with cancer: a meta-analysis. *Oncologist*. 2011;16:112–120.

62. Wolin KY, Ruiz JR, Tuchman H, Lucia A. Exercise in adult and pediatric hematological cancer survivors: an intervention review. *Leukemia*. 2010;24:1113–1120.

Index

A

Abscopal effects, 132
ACEI. *See* Angiotensin-converting enzyme
Acute arterial ischemic events, 270–271
Acute cardiac ischemia, 206
Acute coronary syndrome
    causes, 426–427
    risk factors, 426–427
    treatment, 427–429, 430t
Acute decompensated heart failure, 570–573
Acute heart failure, 438
Acute leukemia, 266
Acute lymphoblastic leukemia (ALL), 450
Acute pericarditis, 252–253
Acute pulmonary embolism, 359–360, 362–364
Acute respiratory distress syndrome (ARDS), 375
ADCC. *See* Antibody-dependent cell-mediated cytotoxicity
Adjuvant therapy, 302
Advanced echocardiographic techniques, 188
Advanced therapy, heart failure (HF)
    cardiac resynchronization therapy, 576
    epidemiology, 575–576
    heart transplantation, 577–579
    implantable cardiac defibrillators, 576
    left ventricle, recovery of function, 574–575
    mechanical circulatory support, 576–577
    right ventricular involvement, 575
Afatinib, 97
Aflibercept, 331
Airway disease, 390–393
AL amyloidosis, 185, 191
Alemtuzumab (campath), 7
Alkylating agents, 2
ALL. *See* Acute lymphoblastic leukemia
All-*trans* retinoic acid, 251
Altered vascular tone, 128
Alveolar lung disease, 388–389
American Society of Clinical Oncology (ASCO), 317
American Society of Echocardiography (ASE), 507
Amifostine, 467–468
Amyloid amyloidosis (AA), 185
Amyloid protein, 186
Anaphylaxis, 390–393
Angina
    pectoris, 186
    treatment of, 190
Angiosarcomas, 246, 281, 300
Angiotensin-converting enzyme (ACEI), 27
    inhibitors, 64
Angiotensin II receptor blocker (ARB), 27
ANP. *See* Atrial natriuretic peptide

Anthracenediones, 71–72
Anthracycline-associated cardiac dysfunction, 64–66
Anthracycline-associated cardiotoxicity, 461–462
Anthracycline-associated myopathy, 58
Anthracycline cardiotoxicity, 23–25, 25f, 27, 28t, 64
    anthracycline toxicity. *See* anthracycline toxicity
    introduction and general considerations, 47–50
    primary prevention of, 22–27
Anthracyclines, 5, 12, 47, 62t, 251, 448–453
    conversion, 27
    effect, 51
    pregnancy, 592
Anthracycline toxicity
    anthracycline-associated cardiac dysfunction, 64–66
    cardiac monitoring during anthracycline treatment, 62–63
    cardioprotection, 66–71
    clinical recognition of cardiac damage, 54–61
    cumulative dose of doxorubicin *vs.* congestive heart failure relationship, 52–54
    doxorubicin and anthracenediones, 71–72
    early and late doxorubicin cardiotoxocity, 50–51
    risk factors for doxorubicin cardiotoxicity, 61–62
Antiangiogenic therapy
    cardiovascular adverse events, 333
    classes, 330–331, 332t
    fibroblast growth factor, 329
    G-protein-coupled receptors, 330
    monoclonal antibodies, 331, 332t
    placental growth factor, 329
    small-molecule tyrosine kinase inhibitors, 333
    tumor angiogenesis factor, 329
Antiarrhythmic medications, 203
Antibody-dependent cell-mediated cytotoxicity (ADCC), 95
Anti-cancer therapies, 199
Anticoagulation, 281
Anti-ErbB2 drugs, 98
Anti-ErbB2 signaling, 98
Antigen-presenting cells (APCs), 103
Anti-HER2 cardiotoxicity
    cardiotoxicity of anti-ERBB2 signaling, 98
    ERBB signaling, 98–99
    ERBB2 signaling in cancer, 89–91
    ERBB2 signaling in heart, 91–93
    next-generation ERBB2 antagonists differ from trastuzumab, 95–98
    trastuzumab, ERBB2-targeted drug, 94–95
Anti-HER2 therapies, 87
Antimetabolites, 4
Antiplatelet agents, 36
Antitumor antibiotics, 5

Antitumor drugs and heart, 11–12
Antitumor immunity, 103
Anxiety
    causes, 528t
    clinical consequences, 528
    mechanisms, 528
    prevalence, 528
ARB. *See* Angiotensin II receptor blocker
ARDS. *See* Acute respiratory distress syndrome
Arrhythmias, 197, 281, 282, 358–359
Arsenic trioxide (ATO), 31–32
Arterial thrombosis, 21
    disease-related, 33–34
ASCO. *See* American Society of Clinical Oncology
ASE. *See* American Society of Echocardiography
Atezolizumab, 106
ATO. *See* Arsenic trioxide
Atrial flutter and fibrillation, 202–204
Atrial natriuretic peptide (ANP), 167
Atrial premature complex (APC), 199–200
Atrioventricular (AV) block, 210–211
Atrioventricular nodal reentrant tachycardia
    (AVNRT), 200
Atrioventricular reentry tachycardia
    (AVRT), 200
Avelumab, 106

B

Ballon aortic valvuloplasty, 518–519
Balloon pericardiotomy, 517
Bayes' law, 54, 55f
Benign pericardial tumors, 245
Beta-adrenergic blocking drugs, 64
Beta blockers, 462
Bevacizumab, 7, 331
Biopsy specimens, 58
Bivalent NRG-1, 92, 99t
Bleeding, 343
Bleomycin, 5, 387
Blood and blood component transfusion, 268
Blood biomarkers
    natriuretic peptides, 167
    troponins, 163–167
Blood cultures, 482
BNP. *See* Brain natriuretic peptide
Bortezomib, 8, 191
Bradyarrhythmias, 210–212
Brain natriuretic peptide (BNP), 167
Breast cancer, 250
Breast cancer radiotherapy
    cardiac mortality after, 136–137
    heart disease after, 137
    injury to cardiac structures after, 139
    trends in cardiac exposure from, 138–139
Bronchospasm, 390–393
Bruton's tyrosine kinase (BTK) inhibitor, 8, 205
B-type natriuretic peptide (BNP), 58, 438

C

CAD, 358
Calcium channel blockers, 190
Camptothecin analogs, 6
Cancer, 359
    role of checkpoints in, 105
Cancer patient, cardiac arrhythmias in, 197
    bradyarrhythmias, 210–212
    cardiac implantable electronic devices
        (CIEDs), 212–213
    characterization of arrhythmia, 197
    supraventricular arrhythmias, 198–204
    ventricular arrhythmias, 204–210
Capecitabine, 5, 267
Carbonyl reductase (CBR), 27
Carboplatin, 2
Carcinoembryonic antigen (CEA) levels, 249
Carcinoid heart disease
    cardiac physical examination, 309
    cardiac ultrasonography, 310
    characteristic finding, 309
    clinical presentation, 309–313, 310f–312f
    echocardiography, 310
    etiology, 309
    magnetic resonance imaging, 310
    management, 313
    pathophysiology, 309
    prognosis of patients, 313–314
    valve surgery, 313
Cardiac adverse events, 107–110
Cardiac amyloidosis, 186, 191, 221, 266–267
    classification of, 185
    clinical conditions associated with AL and AA
        amyloidosis, 185–186
    diagnostic approach, 187
    incidence and prevalance, 185
    investigations, 187–190
    prognosis, 191–192
    treatment, 190–191
    types of amyloid protein, 186–187
Cardiac arrhythmias in cancer patient, 197
    bradyarrhythmias, 210–212
    cardiac implantable electronic devices, 212–213
    characterization of arrhythmia, 197
    supraventricular arrhythmias, 198–204
    ventricular arrhythmias, 204–210
Cardiac atrophy, 600
Cardiac autotransplantation, 288–294, 293f–294f
Cardiac biopsies, 50, 58, 67, 71
Cardiac blood biomarkers after radiation therapy (RT), 163,
    164t–166t
Cardiac catheterization, 284
Cardiac computed tomography (CCT), 241, 279
Cardiac damage, 54–61
Cardiac development and myocardial stress, 79–80
Cardiac disease, preexisting, 112–113
Cardiac disorders, 318

Cardiac dose, variation in risk with, 137–138
Cardiac emergencies
    acute coronary syndrome, 426–429, 430t
    acute heart failure, 438
    approaches, 423, 424t
    dysrhythmia, 429–432
    pericardial tamponade, 438–439
    sudden cardiopulmonary arrest. *See* Sudden
        cardiopulmonary arrest
Cardiac endothelial cells, 13
Cardiac examination, 187
Cardiac glycosides, 201
Cardiac implantable electronic devices (CIEDs), 212–213
    MRI, 491–492
    neoplasms, 554
    non-conditional devices, 493–495
    photon therapy, 495–496
    preoperative evaluation, 552–553
    proton therapy, 496
    radiation therapy management, 496–498
Cardiac irAEs, 115t, 116
Cardiac magnetic resonance imaging (CMRI), 224, 239–240,
    279
Cardiac manifestations, treatment of, 190
Cardiac monitoring, 455
    during anthracycline treatment, 62–63
    common terminology criteria for adverse events, 315,
        316
    common toxicity criteria, 315
    congestive heart failure, 323
    doxorubicin, 323–324
    FDA approval process, 319–321
    left ventricular ejection fraction, 317, 323
    National Cancer Institute, 315
    National Heart, Lung, and Blood Institute, 315
    phase I clinical trials, 321
    phase II clinical trials, 321–322
    phase III clinical trials, 322
    phase IV clinical trials, 322–323
    trastuzumab, 324–326, 325t
    tyrosine kinase inhibitors, 317
Cardiac magnetic resonance imaging (CMRI)
    delayed enhancement, 241
    first-pass perfusion, 241
    T1 and T2 tissue characterization, 240–241
Cardiac neoplasms, 279
Cardiac output, 221
Cardiac perfusion scans, 57
Cardiac physical examination, 309
Cardiac radionuclide imaging, 56
Cardiac resynchronization therapy, 576
Cardiac Review and Evaluation Committee (CREC), 317, 322
Cardiac stem cells, 13
Cardiac tamponade, 227, 256, 281
Cardiac thrombi, echocardiographic assessment of, 232–233
Cardiac transplant patients, immune checkpoint inhibitors
    for, 113
Cardiac troponin T (cTnT), 163
Cardiac tumors, 230–232

adjuvant therapy, 302
aggressive biologic nature, 302
anatomic approaches, 285
cardiac autotransplantation, 288–294, 293f–294f
cardiac neoplasms, 279
clinical presentation, 281–284
diagnosis, 237–241
infradiaphragmatic tumors, 295–296
left atrial tumor resection, 286
left ventricular tumor resection, 286–288, 289f
management, 279
minimally invasive approaches, 296
primary benign tumors, 297–299, 298f, 299f
primary malignant tumors, 300–301f
pulmonary artery tumor resection, 295
recurrence, 301
research, 303
right atrial tumor resection, 285–286, 285f
right ventricular outflow tract, 295
sarcoma therapy, 302
secondary cardiac tumors, 301
surgical approach, pathologic features affecting,
    296–297
surgical historical perspective, 280–281
surgical treatment, 284–285
Cardiac ultrasonography, 310
Cardiac/vascular toxicity, 16t–20t
Cardiomyopathy, 121–122
    in pregnancy, 587
Cardio-oncology
    antitumor drugs and heart, 11–12
    cardiotoxicity and role of non-cardiomyocyte cells, 13
    emerging paradigms, 29–36
    new drugs and scenarios, 39
    pharmacological approaches to clinical, 15–22
    pharmacologic principles of primary prevention, 22–29
    pharmacologic principles of secondary prevention,
        36–39
    preclinical mechanisms and clinical facts, 12–13
    predictiveness of preclinical models, 13–15
Cardioprotection, 66–71
    before irradiation, 509–510
Cardiorespiratory fitness (CRF)
    cardiac atrophy, 600
    diastolic dysfunction, 600
    endothelial dysfunction, 600
    exercise training, 601–602, 601t
    impaired vascular compliance, 600
    integrating exercise training, 602–604, 604t
    LV chamber compliance, 600
    skeletal muscle, 600–601
Cardiotoxicity, 13, 113
    from any agent, 27–29
    detection of, 222–223
    late, 36
    outcome of, 85–86
    potential mechanisms of, 110–111
    prevention, 570
    surveillance, 569–570

Cardiotoxicity-intersecting pathways, 562–564
Cardiotoxic therapies, childhood cancer
    amifostine, 467–468
    anthracycline-associated cardiotoxicity, 461–462
    anthracyclines, 448–453
    beta blockers, 462
    cardiac monitoring, 455
    continuous anthracycline infusion, 464–465
    derivatives, 464
    dexrazoxane, 465–467
    dyslipidemia, 459–460
    echocardiography, 455–456
    growth hormone, 462–463
    insulin resistance, 459–460
    liposomal formulations, 463–464
    mechanical support, 463
    metabolic supplements, 468
    obesity, 459
    physical inactivity, 460–461
    prevention, 463
    radiotherapy, 453–454
    serum cardiac troponin concentrations, 456
    serum NT-PROBNP concentrations, 457
    tobacco use, 459
    traditional risk factors, 457–459
    tyrosine kinase inhibitors, 454–455
Cardiovascular adverse events, antiangiogenic therapy
    bleeding, 343
    congestive heart failure, 338–340
    hypertension, 333–337
    left ventricular dysfunction, 338–340
    proteinuria, 341–343
    QTc prolongation, 340–341
    thromboembolism, 337–338
Cardiovascular interventions
    ballon aortic valvuloplasty, 518–519
    balloon pericardiotomy, 517
    cardioprotection before irradiation, 509–510
    chemotherapy cardioprotection, 508–509
    coronary artery bypass grafting, 517
    endomyocardial biopsy, 518
    fractional flow reserve, 514
    intravascular ultrasonography, 514–515
    malignancy and coronary disease, 501–503
    optical coherence tomography, 516
    percutaneous coronary intervention, 516–517
    pericardiocentesis, 517, 518f
    radiation therapy, 503–504
    stable angina, 510–511
    thrombocytopenia, 511–513
    transcatheter aortic valve implantation, 518–519
    University of Texas MD Anderson Cancer Center,
      515–516
    vascular access considerations, 513–514, 514t
Cardiovascular magnetic resonance imaging, 189
Cardiovascular mortality, 148t
Cardiovascular system, radiation therapy on, 119
    radiation-related cardiovascular disease, 120–133
    radiation-related heart disease. *See* Radiation-related
      heart disease

Carfilzomib, 8
Carotid sinus hypersensitivity, 211–212
Catheter-based pericardiotomy, 256
CBR. *See* Carbonyl reductase
CCT. *See* Cardiac computed tomography
CDER. *See* Center for Drug Evaluation and Research
    (CDER)
Cell cycle, 1
Cell cycling drugs, 1
Center for Drug Evaluation and Research (CDER), 320
Cerebrovascular disease, 124–125
Cetuximab (erbitux), 7
Checkpoint inhibitors
    administration, 106
    of CTLA-4, 105
    immune checkpoint cardiotoxicity, 113–114
    immune-related adverse events, 106–110
    monitoring for cardiotoxicity, 114–115
    of PD-1, 105
    of PD-L1, 106
    potential mechanisms of cardiotoxicity, 110–111
    preexisitng immune/cardiac disease and rechallenge,
      111–113
    role of checkpoints in cancer, 105
    role of immune checkpoints in normal immunity, 103,
      104f
    T cells, 103
    therapy, 115, 115f
Chemical cardioprotectors, 68–70
Chemoradiation, 250
Chemotherapeutic medications, 205
Chemotherapeutic related cardiac dysfunction (CTRCD),
    317
Chemotherapeutics, 321
Chemotherapy, 267, 564–565
Chemotherapy agents
    alkylating agents, 2
    anthracyclines, 5
    antimetabolites, 4
    antitumor antibiotics, 5
    camptothecin analogs, 6
    epipodophyllotoxins, 5–6
    5-fluorouracil (5FU), 4–5
    folate analogs, 4
    natural products, 5
    new antifolates, 4
    nitrosoureas, 2
    platinum agents, 2–4
    taxanes, 6
    vinca alkaloids, 6
Chemotherapy cardioprotection, 508–509
Chemotherapy-related pericardial disease, 250–251
Chest roentgenograms, 57
Childhood cancer survivors studies, 592–594
Childhood cancer treatment, 146–149
Chronic cardiomyopathy, 50
Chronic heart failure (CHF), 323
    medical therapy for, 573–574
Chronic obstructive pulmonary disease
    (COPD), 375

Chronic thromboembolic pulmonary hypertension (CTEPH), 376
CIEDs. *See* Cardiac implantable electronic devices
Circumferential pericardial effusion, 227, 228f
Cisplatin, 2, 267
Clinical cardio-oncology, 15–22
Clinical practice guidelines (CPG), 317
CMRI. *See* Cardiac magnetic resonance imaging
Coagulation, abnormal, 128
Coenzyme Q, 468
Common adverse events, 106–107
Common terminology criteria for adverse events (CTCAE), 315, 316
Common toxicity criteria (CTC), 315
Compensatory proliferation and repair, 131
Complex signaling system, 79
Comprehensive in vitro Proarrhythmia Assay (CiPA), 30
Computed tomography (CT), 283
Conduction abnormalities, 57
Conduction system abnormalities, 124
Conduction system disease, 109
Congestive heart failure (CHF), 11, 81f, 186, 281, 321, 338–340
    treatment of, 190
Constrictive pericarditis, 227–228
Continuous anthracycline infusion, 464–465
Continuous positive airway pressure (CPAP), 359
Conventional echocardiography, 162
Coronary arteriography, 113
Coronary artery bypass grafting (CABG), 517
Coronary artery disease (CAD), 120–121
Corticosteroids, 212
CTC. *See* Common toxicity criteria
CTEPH. *See* Chronic thromboembolic pulmonary hypertension
Culture-negative infectious endocarditis, 485
Cumulative dose of doxorubicin *vs.* congestive heart failure relationship, 52–54
Cyclophosphamide, 61
CYP3A4, 272
Cytarabine (1β-D-arabinofuranosyl cytosine; Ara C), 5
Cytokines, 501
    activation, 126–128
Cytotoxic T lymphocyte–associated antigen 4 (CTLA-4), 105

D

Dasatinib, 7, 8, 12
DCM. *See* Dilated cardiomyopathy
2D echocardiography signal, 221
Deep venous thrombosis (DVT), 263
Defibrillators, 190
    devices, 495
Definitive chemoradiotherapy (dCRT), 149, 152–153
Delayed enhancement, cardiac MRI, 241
Depression
    biological and behavioral mechanisms, 530–531
    clinical symptoms, 529–530, 530t, 532f
    definition, 528–529
    management, 533–534
    medications, 530, 530t
    prevalence, 529
    screening, 531–533, 531t
Depsipeptide, 8
Dermatologic toxicity, 107
Dexrazoxane, 25, 26, 26f, 36, 69–70, 69t, 465–467
DHFR. *See* Dihydrofolate reductase
Diabetes mellitus, 460
Diastolic dysfunction, 38, 57, 600
Diastolic function, 221–223
Digoxin, 203
Dihydrofolate reductase (DHFR), 4
Dihydropyrimidine dehydrogenase (DPD), 2
Dilated cardiomyopathy (DCM), 590
DILI. *See* Drug-induced lung injury
3-Dimensional echocardiography, LV assessment with, 223
DNA damage, 132
Doppler echocardiography, left ventricular assessment with, 221–223
Doppler tissue imaging (DTI), 221
Dose limitation, 67
Doxetacel, 6
Doxorubicin, 47, 47t, 53, 54, 61f, 68, 71–72, 323–324
    cardiotoxicity of, 50–51, 61–62
Doxorubicin-iron, 50
Dronedarone, 199
Drug-induced lung disease (DILD), 380–386
Drug-induced lung injury (DILI)
    clinical manifestations, 381
    conventional chemotherapy, 382t–383t
    diagnosis, 381
    focal nodular consolidations, 381
    immune checkpoint inhibitors, 384t–385t
    molecular targeted therapies, 384t–385t
    risk factors, 381
    treatment, 386
Durvalumab, 106
DVT. *See* Deep venous thrombosis
Dyslipidemia, 459–460
Dysrhythmia, 57, 429–432, 433t–437t
    causes, 432
    primary dysrhythmia, 432
    secondary dysrhythmia, 432
    treatment, 432

E

EACI. *See* European Association of Cardiovascular Imaging
Early asymptomatic cardiotoxicity, 36–37
Early cardioprotection, 66
Echocardiography (Echo), 188, 229, 233, 252, 279, 455–456
    2D-based strain analysis, 225, 225f
    2D LV assessment with, 219–221
    2D strain (2DS) imaging, 224
    3D, LV assessment with, 223
    heart, general location within, 238
    superior vena cava, indwelling catheters, 238
    vascularization, 238–239
    wall motion abnormalities, 239
Echo imaging quality, 56

Ectopic atrial tachycardia, 202
Effusive-constrictive disease, 257
EGF. *See* Epidermal growth factor
Ejection fraction, 219
  accurate estimate of, 223–224
  three-dimensional, 224–225
EKG-gated cardiac magnetic resonance imaging, 482
EKG-gated multi-slice computed tomography, 482
Electrocardiogram (ECG), 57, 188
Electrocardiography, 168, 187–188, 197
Electron microscopic evaluation, 49
Embolic symptoms, 281
Endocardial biopsies, 111
Endocardial tracing, 219, 220f
Endomyocardial biopsy, 113, 189–190, 518
  assessments, 67
Endothelial cells (ECs), 126
  damage and dysfunction of, 126, 600
  death of, 131
End-stage heart failure, 191
Enhanced permeability, 23
Enterococci, 484
Eosinophilic lung disease, 388
Epidermal growth factor (EGF)
  in heart, 79
  signaling system, 79–80
Epidermal growth factor receptor (EGFR), 2
Epipodophyllotoxins, 5–6
Epirubicin, 5, 24, 47, 47f, 72
ErbB receptors, 90f
ErbB signaling, 90f, 98–99
ErbB2 antagonists, 95–98
ErbB2 signaling, 89
  in cancer, 89–91
  in heart, 91–93
ErbB2-targeted drug, 94–95
Erlotinib hydrochloride, 8
Erythropoetin (EPO), 268
Esophageal cancer radiotherapy, 151
Esophageal cancer treatment, 151
Etoposide, 5
European Association of Cardiovascular Imaging (EACI), 507
European Heart Rhythm Association, 204
European Society of Medical Oncology (ESMO), 317
Everolimus, 8
Exercises/fitness
  cardiorespiratory fitness, 599–600
  cardiovascular risk, 599
Exercise training, 601–602, 601t
Exertional dyspnea, 186

F

Fat pad biopsy, 190
FDG PET-CT. *See* F18 fluorodeoxyglucose positron emission tomography-computed tomography
F18 fluorodeoxyglucose positron emission tomography (FDG-PET), 158, 482

F18 fluorodeoxyglucose positron emission tomography-computed tomography (FDG PET-CT), 241
Fibroblast growth factor (FGF), 329
Fibromas, 298
Fibrosis, 129–130
First-pass perfusion, cardiac MRI, 241
Fludarabine, 5
Fluid analysis, 249
5-Fluoro-2-deoxyuridine monophosphate (FdUMP), 4
5-Fluorouracil (5FU), 4–5
5-Fluorouracil, 267
Folate analogs, 4
Fractional flow reserve, 514
Fungal infectious endocarditis, 485

G

Gated myocardial perfusion imaging (GMPI), 150, 151
Gefitinib, 8
Gemcitabine, 5, 267
Gene therapy, 302
Genetic susceptibility, 168
GMPI. *See* Gated myocardial perfusion imaging
G-protein-coupled receptors, 330
Growth hormone, 462–463

H

HAART. *See* Highly active antiretroviral therapy
Hacek microorganisms, 484
Heart failure (HF), 358
  acute decompensated heart failure, 570–573
  advanced therapy for, 574–579, 577f, 578f
  cardiotoxicity-intersecting pathways, 562–564
  chemotherapy, 564–565
  chronic heart failure, medical therapy of, 573–574
  epidemiology, 562
  etiology, 564–568
  new left ventricular dysfunction, 568–570
  phosphatidylinositol 3-kinase pathway, 564
  pregnancy, 589–592
  radiation therapy, 565–566
  therapy for, 570–574
  treatment of, future directions, 564–568
  tyrosine kinase inhibitors (TKIs), 561
Heart failure with reduced ejection fraction (HFrEF), 323
Heart-lung interactions
  critically ill patients, 403–406
  drug-induced lung injury. *See* Drug-induced lung injury
  lung infections, 395–401, 397t, 398f
  physiological basis, 351–352
  pulmonary disease. *See* Pulmonary disease, cardiac consequences of
  ventilatory control disorders, 401–403
Heart Success Program model, 535
Heart transplantation, 577–579
Hematopoietic stem cell transplantation (HSCT), 375
Hemodynamic assessment, cardiac catheterization with, 188–189

Heparin-induced thrombocytopenia (HIT), 364
Hereditary amyloidosis, 185–186
Highly active antiretroviral therapy (HAART), 251
Histone deacetylation inhibitors, 8
HIV. *See* Human immunodeficiency virus
Hodgkin lymphoma, 159t–161t, 250
    evolution of radiotherapy techniques for, 146
Hodgkin lymphoma survivors
    cardiac morbidity of, 140, 144t–145t
    cardiac mortality in, 140, 141t–143t
Hormonal therapy, 268
Human immunodeficiency virus (HIV), 251
5-hydroxyindoleacetic acid (5-HIAA), 310
Hypereosinophilic syndrome, 233
Hypersensitivity-like reactions, 388
Hypertension
    association with antitumor efficacy, 334–335
    management, 336–337
    monitoring, 336
    pretreatment assessment, 335
    VSPi-induced hypertension, 335
Hypoxia, 128–129

I

Ibrutinib, 199, 205
Idarubicin, 5, 71–72
Idarubicin (IDA)-based therapy, 464
Imaging techniques
    cardiovascular magnetic resonance imaging, 163
    CT angiography and CT calcium scores, 162–163
    echocardiography, 158–162
    nuclear medicine imaging, 155–158
Imatinib, 333, 455
IMID, 9
Immune-checkpoint blocking antibodies, 9
Immune checkpoint cardiotoxicity, 113–114
Immune checkpoint inhibitors (ICI), 206, 211, 323,
    384t–385t
    myocarditis, 111, 111f
    therapy, 107f
Immune disease, 111
Immune-related adverse events (IRAEs), 106–110, 108t, 109,
    323
Immunotherapy, 6–7
Impaired vascular compliance, 600
Implantable cardiac defibrillators, 576
Implantable cardiac defibrillators (ICDs), 213
Implanted pacemaker, 495
Infection-related pericardial disease, 251
Infectious endocarditis (IE)
    blood cultures, 482
    complications, 485, 487
    culture-negative, 485
    diagnosis, 480–483
    echocardiography, 480–482
    EKG-gated cardiac magnetic resonance imaging, 482
    EKG-gated multi-slice computed tomography, 482
    enterococci, 484

    18F-fluorodeoxyglucose positron emission
        tomography, 482
    fungal, 485
    hacek microorganisms, 484
    histopathology, 482
    microorganisms, 477–480, 478f–479f
    modified Duke criteria, 480t
    molecular methods, 483
    non-hacek gram-negative organisms, 485
    radiolabeled white blood cell single-photon emission
        CT, 482
    risk factors, 487–488
    serology, 482
    staphylococci, 484
    streptococci, 483–484
    surgery indications, 485, 486t–487t
    treatment, 483
Infra-diaphragmatic radiotherapy, 154
Infradiaphragmatic tumors, 295–296
Innovative delivery systems, 50, 70–71
Insulin resistance, 459–460
Integrating exercise training, 602–604, 604t
Intensity modulated proton therapy (IMPT), 153
Interstitial lung disease (ILD), 386–387
Intracardiac masses, echocardiographic assessment of,
    228–229
Intraoperative transesophageal echocardiography (TEE),
    285, 286
Intravascular ultrasonography, 514–515
Ipilimumab, 105
IRAEs. *See* Immune-related adverse events
Irinotecan, 2
Ischemic cardiomyopathy, 567
Isolated atrial amyloidosis (IAA), 186
I131 tositumomab (Bexxar), 7
I131 Tositumomab Rituximab, 6

J

JNKs. *See* Jun N-terminal kinases
Jun N-terminal kinases (JNKs), 12

L

Lapatinib, 97
    ditosylate, 8
Late cardiotoxicity, 36
L-carnitine, 468
Left atrial tumor resection, 286
Left atrium, evaluation of, 232
Left ventricle
    evaluation of, 232–233
    recovery of function, 574–575
Left ventricular assessment
    with 3-dimensional echocardiography, 223
    with doppler echocardiography, 221–223
    with strain imaging, 224–226
    with two-dimensional echocardiography,
        219–221

Left ventricular chamber
  compliance, 600
  measurement, 223–224
Left ventricular dimensions, 219
Left ventricular dysfunction, 321, 338–340
Left ventricular ejection fraction (LVEF), 56–57, 219, 317, 323
Left ventricular mass, 219–221
Left ventricular tumor resection, 286–288, 289f
Lenalidomide, 9
Lipomas, 298
Liposomal anthracycline, 71
Liposomal doxorubicin, 70, 71
Liposomal formulations, 23f, 463–464
Liver metabolism, 1
Low molecular weight heparins (LMWH), 34–36
Lung cancer radiotherapy, 153
Lung infections, 395–401, 397t, 398f
5-Luorouracil (5-FU), 2

M

Macrophage-monocyte tissue factor, 267
Magnesium therapy, 209
Magnetic resonance conditional cardiac implantable
  electronic devices, 492–493
Magnetic resonance imaging (MRI), 283
  carcinoid heart disease, 310
  CIED. *See* Cardiac implantable electronic devices
  defibrillator devices, 495
  implanted pacemaker and, 495
  magnetic resonance conditional cardiac implantable
    electronic devices, 492–493
  magnetic resonance non-conditional cardiac
    implantable electronic devices, 493–495
  radiation effects, 495–496
Magnetic resonance non-conditional cardiac implantable
  electronic devices, 493–495
Major adverse cardiac events (MACE), 206
Malignancy and coronary disease, 501–503
Malignant effusions, 255
Malignant mesothelioma, 300
Massive pulmonary embolism (MPE), 360, 364–366
Maximum tolerated dose (MTD), 39, 321
Measured matrix metalloproteinase 3 (MMP-3), 167
Mechanical circulatory support, 576–577
Mediastinal tumors, 199
Mesothelioma, 245–246, 298
Metabolic supplements, 468
Metastatic cardiac tumors, 301
Metastatic disease, 246–249
Methotrexate (MTX), 4
Metoprolol, 29
Microvascular damage, 150–151
Mitocondrial DNA (mtDNA), 12
Mitochondrial dysfunction, 50
Mitoxantrone, 72
MM-111, 97–98
Modern radiotherapy modalities, 153
Molecular targeted therapies, 384t–385t

Monitoring for cardiotoxicity, 114–115
Monoclonal antibodies, 6–7, 331, 332t
  against VEGF, 331
Monovalent NRG-1, 98, 99t
Morphologic grading scale, 58, 59t
MPE. *See* Massive pulmonary embolism
mtDNA. *See* Mitocondrial DNA
Multifocal atrial tachycardia (MAT), 201
Multi-gated acquisition (MUGA), 323
Multiple-hit hypothesis, 37
Myeloproliferative disorders, 265
Myelosuppression, 6
Myocardial damage, 150–151
Myocardial ErbB2 signaling, 91
Myocardial infarction (MI), 504
Myocardiocytes, direct radiation damage to, 132
Myocarditis outcome, 112
Myocbacterium tuberculosis, 251

N

National Cancer Institute (NCI), 315
National Comprehensive Cancer Network (NCCN), 272
National Heart, Lung, and Blood Institute (NHLBI), 315
Natural products, 5
NCCN. *See* National Comprehensive Cancer Network
NCPE. *See* Noncardiogenic pulmonary edema
Necitumumab, 331
Neratinib, 97
Neuregulin 1 (NGR-1), 563
Neutrophil extracellular traps (NETs), 501
New antifolates, 4
New drugs and scenarios, 39
New left ventricular dysfunction, 568–570
New oral anticoagulants (NOACs), 34–36
New York Heart Association (NYHA), 534
Nilotinib, 7, 8
Nitrosoureas, 2
Nivolumab, 105
Nonanthracycline chemotherapeutics, 39
Noncardiogenic pulmonary edema (NCPE), 388–389
Non-cardiomyocyte cells, 13
Non-conditional devices, 493–495
Non-HACEK gram-negative organisms, 485
Non-Hodgkin lymphomas, 2, 4
Non–immune-mediated myocarditis, 113
Noninvasive cardiac testing, 49
Noninvasive studies, 57–58
  of systolic dysfunction, 59
Noninvasive tests, 54–56, 62
Non-Ischemic cardiomyopathy, 567–568
Nonmalignant pericardial disease, 249–251
  chemotherapy-related pericardial disease,
    250–251
  infection-related pericardial disease, 251
  radiation-induced pericardial disease, 249–250
Non-small-cell lung carcinoma (NSCLC), 2
Non-sustained VT, 206

Non-vitamin K antagonist oral anticoagulants (NOACs), 204
Normal immunity, role of immune checkpoints in, 103, 104f
NRG-1/ErbB signaling, 91f, 92
Nuclear scintigraphy, 189

O

Obesity, 459
Observational data, 133–137
Obstructive sleep apnea (OSA)
    arrhythmias, 358–359
    CAD, 358
    cancer, 359
    heart failure, 358
    hypertension, 358
    pulmonary hypertension, 358
Obstructive symptoms, 281
Oncogene addiction, 89
Optical coherence tomography (OCT), 516
Organ toxicity, 107
OSA. *See* Obstructive sleep apnea
Oxaliplatin, 4
Oxidative phosphorylation (OXPHOS), 12
Oxidative stress, 128–129
Oxygen radical formation, 5

P

Pacemakers, 190
Paclitaxel (Taxol), 6
Panitumumab (vectibix), 7
Papillary fibroelastomas, 298
Parasympathetic tone, 211
Parietal pericardium, 244
Paroxysmal arrhythmias, 202
Paroxysmal supraventricular tachycardia (PSVT), 200–202
Patient health questionnaire (PHQ-9), 532f
PCWP. *See* Pulmonary capillary wedge pressers
Pembrolizumab, 105
Percutaneous coronary intervention, 516–517
Pericardial constriction, 257–259
Pericardial cyst, 245, 245f
Pericardial disease, 123–124, 227–228
    acute pericarditis, 252–253
    cardiac tamponade, 256
    etiology, 243
    function, 244
    malignancy, 243
    metastatic disease, 246–249
    non-malignant pericardial disease, 249–251
    pericardial constriction, 257–259
    pericardial effusion, 253–256
    primary tumors, 244–245, 244t
    structure, 244
    symptoms, 243
Pericardial effusions, 150, 227, 253–256
Pericardial innervation, 244
Pericardial lipomas, 246

Pericardial space, 244
Pericardial tamponade, 438–439
    diagnosis, 439
    symptoms and signs, 439
    syncope, 439–441, 440t
    treatment, 439
Pericardiocentesis, 227, 284, 517, 518f
Pericarditis, 109, 150
Peripartum cardiomyopathy (PPCM), 590
Peripheral artery disease (PAD), 112, 505
Peripheral vascular disease, 125
Pertuzumab, 97
Pharmacodynamic variability, 1–2
Pharmacogenomic variability, 2
Pharmacokinetic variability, 1–2
Pharmacologic cardioprotectors, 50, 68–70
Pharmacologic principles
    of primary prevention, 22–29
    of secondary prevention, 36–39
Pheochromocytomas, 210, 299
Phosphatidylinositol 3-kinase (PI3K) pathway, 564
Photon therapy, 495–496
Physical inactivity, 460–461
Pixantrone, 24, 72
Placental growth factor (PlGF), 329
Platinum agents, 2–4
Platinum-derived drugs, 1
Pleural disease, 388
Podophyllum peltatum, 5
Pomalidomide, 9
Ponatinib, 14, 15, 36
PORT. *See* post-operative radiotherapy
Post-chemotherapy chronic health conditions, 37–38
Post-operative radiotherapy (PORT), 152
Posttransplant lymphoproliferative disorder (PTLD), 113
Potential therapeutic modalities, 64
Pralatrexate, 4
Preclinical mechanisms and clinical facts, 12–13
Preclinical models, predictiveness of, 13–15
Preexisitng immune/cardiac disease and rechallenge, 111–113
Pregnancy
    anthracycline exposure, 592
    cancer diagnosis, 594–595
    cardiomyopathy, 587
    childhood cancer survivors studies, 592–594
    heart failure, 589–592
    MD Anderson data, 594
    normal heart, 587–589
    radiation therapy, 587
Preoperative evaluation
    background, 543–544
    cardiac evaluation, 548–549
    cardiac implantable electronic devices (CIEDs), 552–553
    chemotherapy, 546–547
    echocardiographic evaluation, 549
    goals, 544–546
    immunotherapy, 548
    preoperative cardiac stress testing, 550–552

Preoperative evaluation (*Continued*)
    preoperative revascularization, 552
    radiation therapy, 547–548
    serum biomarkers, 549–550
    testing guidelines, MD Anderson Cancer Center, 545t,
      546t
Primary arrhythmias, 197
Primary benign tumors, 297–299, 298f–299f
Primary cardiac lymphoma, 246
Primary malignant tumors, 300–301f
Primary tumors, pericardial disease, 244–245, 244t
    angiosarcoma, 246
    mesothelioma, 245–246
    pericardial cyst, 245, 245f
    pericardial lipomas, 246
    primary cardiac lymphoma, 246
    teratoma, 245
Programmed cell-death 1 (PD-1), 105
Programmed cell-death ligand 1 (PD-L1), 106
Protein p53, 562–563
Proteinuria, 341–343
Proton beam therapy (PBT), 146, 151
Proton therapy, 496
PSVT. *See* Paroxysmal supraventricular tachycardia
Psychosocial considerations
    anxiety, 527–528
    depression, 528–534, 530t, 532f
    disease-management programs, 534–538, 534f,
      536f–537f
    strategies for improving symptom, 538
Pulmonary arterial hypertension (PAH)
    histopathologic changes, 373
    HIV, 372
    nitric oxide, 372
    pathogenesis, 372–373
    portopulmonary hypertension, 371–372
    vasoconstriction, 372
Pulmonary artery tumor resection, 295
Pulmonary capillary hemangiomatosis (PCH). *See*
    Pulmonary veno-occlusive disease
Pulmonary capillary wedge pressers (PCWP), 390
Pulmonary disease, cardiac consequences of
    chronic obstructive pulmonary disease, 352–355, 352t
    sleep-related breathing disorders, 355–359, 356f, 357f
Pulmonary hypertension
    algorithm for evaluation, 371f
    classification, 366, 366t
    definition, 366
    future screening tests, 370–371
    hypoxia, 375–376
    invasive therapies, 380
    patients studies, 369–370
    PH owing to left heart disease, 374–375
    pulmonary arterial hypertension, 371–372
    pulmonary hypertension, 380
    screening studies, 367–369
    signs and symptoms, 366–367, 367t
    treatment, 378–380, 379f
    unclear/multifactorial mechanisms, 376–378

Pulmonary thromboembolism
    clinical presentation, 360–362
    etiology, 359–360
    management, 362–366
    pathophysiology, 360
Pulmonary vascular disease
    pulmonary hypertension. *See* Pulmonary hypertension
    pulmonary thromboembolism, 359–366, 362f–363f
Pulmonary vascular disorders (PVD)
    pulmonary veno-occlusive disease, 389–390
    thromboembolic disease, 389–390
Pulmonary veno-occlusive disease (PVOD)
    chronic deposition, 374
    histologic hallmark, 374
    physical examination, 373
    pleural effusions, 374
    pulmonary vasodilator therapy, 374
    radiation and chemotherapy, 373
    treatment, 373
PVD. *See* Pulmonary vascular disorders

Q

QTc prolongation, 340–341
QT prolongation, 29–33

R

Radiation dose-response relationships for cardiac
    morbidity, 146
Radiation effects, magnetic resonance imaging (MRI),
    495–496
    cardiac implantable electronic devices, 496–498, 497f,
      498f
    proton therapy, 496
Radiation-induced cardiovascular disease (RICD), 168
Radiation-induced heart disease, 168, 169t
Radiation-induced lung injury, 393–395
Radiation-induced pericardial disease, 249–250
Radiation-induced skin telangiectasia, 168
Radiation-related atherosclerosis, 131–132
Radiation-related heart disease (RRHD), 150
    breast cancer treatment, 133–139
    detection and monitoring of, 155–168
    esophageal cancer treatment, 149–151
    Hodgkin lymphoma treatment, 140–149
    lung cancer treatment, 151–153
    testicular cancer treatment, 153–154
    treatment for other cancers, 154–155
Radiation sensitizing agents, 395t
Radiation therapy, 213, 269, 269f, 503–504, 565–566
    cardiovascular interventions, 503–504
    heart failure, 565–566
    management, 496–498
    pregnancy, 587
    screening cancer patients, 505–508
    vascular effects, 504–505
Radiolabeled white blood cell single-photon emission CT,
    482

Radiotherapy, 453–454
Ramucirumab, 331
Randomized data, 133
R-CEOP. *See* Rituximab-CHOP
Reactive oxygen species (ROS), 24
Real-time 3-dimensional echocardiography (RT3DE), 223
Real-time three-dimensional echocardiography, 230–231
Real-time three-dimensional transesophageal
    echocardiography, 231–232
Recombinant human neuregulin 1 (rhNRG-1)
    in animal models, 92, 92t
    as treatment for heart failure, 92, 93t
Recombinant monoclonal antibodies, 331
Reflex-mediated bradycardia, 211–212
Regional function, assessment of, 219
Regional systolic function, 219
Renin-angiotensin-aldosterone (RAA) system, 130–131
Retention Effect, 23
Revised Cardiac Risk Index (RCRI), 509
Right atrial tumor resection, 285–286, 285f
Right ventricular involvement, 575
Right ventricular outflow tract, 295
Rituximab-CHOP (R-CEOP), 6
ROS. *See* Reactive oxygen species (ROS)

S

Sarcoma therapy, 302
SBD. *See* Sleep-related breathing disorders
Schedule modification, 67
Secondary arrhythmias, 197
Secondary cardiac tumors, 301
Senile systemic amyloidosis, 186, 191
Serum biomarkers, 187
Serum cardiac troponin concentrations, 456
Serum NT-PROBNP concentrations, 457
Serum troponins, 187
SHR. *See* Spontaneously hypertensive rats
Sinus bradycardia, 210
Sinus node dysfunction, 210
Sinus tachycardia, 199
Sirtuin-3, 50
Skeletal muscle, 600–601
Sleep-related breathing disorders (SBD)
    cancer, 355–356
    cardiovascular disease, 356
    central sleep apnea, 356–357
    definition, 355
    obstructive sleep apnea, 357–358
Small-molecule tyrosine kinase inhibitors, 333
Society for Cardiovascular Angiography and Interventions
    (SCAI), 508
Somatostatin analogs, 313
Sorafenib, 333
    administration, 503
    tosylate, 8
Sorafenib Tosylate Sunitinib, 8
Spironolactone, 64
Spontaneously hypertensive rats (SHR), 13

Stable angina, 510–511
Staphylococci, 484
Stem cell transplantation (SCT), 167
Strain imaging, LV assessment with, 224–226
Streptococci, 483–484
Stroke volume, 221
Structural cardiovascular toxicity, 14
Subxiphoid pericardiotomy, 255
Sudden cardiopulmonary arrest
    causes, 423
    resuscitation, 425–426
    treatment-related causes, 425
    tumor-related causes, 424–425
Sunitinib, 333
Sunitinib Malate, 8
Superior vena cava (SVC), indwelling catheters, 238
Supraventricular arrhythmias, 198
    atrial flutter and fibrillation, 202–204
    atrial premature complex, 199–200
    ectopic atrial tachycardia, 202
    multifocal atrial tachycardia, 201
    paroxysmal supraventricular tachycardia, 200–201
    sinus tachycardia, 199
Supraventricular tachycardias, 198, 198t
Syncope, 439–441, 440t

T

Tachycardia-bradycardia syndrome, 210
Tamponade, 256
T1 and T2 tissue characterization, cardiac MRI, 240–241
Targeted therapies, 7–8
Taxanes, 6
T-cells, 103
    inactivation, 103, 104f
Temsirolimus, 8
Teratoma, 245
Testicular cancer, 153
Thalidomide, 9
Thiopurine methyltransferase (TPMT), 2
Thiotepa, 227
Thrombocytopenia, 511–513
Thromboembolic sequelae, 203
Thromboembolism, 33–36, 337–338
Thrombosis, 33–36, 128
Thyrotoxicosis, 203
Tissue Doppler imaging, 162
TKIs. *See* Tyrosine kinase inhibitors (TKIs)
Tobacco use, 459
Topotecan, 6
Torsades de pointes, 206–210
Total body irradiation (TBI), 154, 155
TPMT. *See* Thiopurine methyltransferase
Traditional risk factors, 457–459
Transcatheter aortic valve implantation, 518–519
Translocations disrupt genes, 303
Transthoracic echocardiogram, 248
Transthoracic echocardiography, 158
Transthyretin amyloid cardiomyopathy, 192

Transthyretin cardiac amyloidosis, 191
Trans-vascular cardiac biopsy, 58
Trastuzumab, 7, 81, 94–95, 94f, 95f, 324–326, 325t
    ERBB2 antagonists differ from, 95–98
Trastuzumab-anthracycline interaction, 80–82
Trastuzumab-associated cardiotoxicity, 80, 80f
    basic science considerations, 79–80
    in clinical trials, 82–87
        trastuzumab-anthracycline interaction,
          80–82
Trastuzumab-emtansine, 96–97
Tricuspid valve replacement, 313
Troponins, 51
Tuberculous pericarditis, 251
Tumor angiogenesis factor (TAF), 329
Tumor growth pattern, 1
Type I cardiotoxicity, 48, 48t
Type II cardiotoxicity, 48, 48t
Tyrosine kinase inhibitors (TKIs), 317, 454–455, 561

U

UDP-glucoronosyltransferase (UGT)1A1 enzyme, 2
Ultrasonography, cardiac, 310

V

Valve surgery, 313
Valvular heart disease, 122–123
Vascular access considerations, 513–514, 514t
Vascular disorders, 318
Vascular endothelial growth factors, 502, 563–564
    inhibitor, 268
Vascularization, 238–239
Vascular permeability, 126–128
VEGF. *See* Vascular endothelial growth factors
Venous thromboembolism (VTE), 21, 33, 34, 204
    cancer therapies, 267–269
    chemotherapy, 267–269

duration of therapy, 273
hypercoagulability, 263–264
incidental venous thromboembolism, 273
malignancies, 265–267
management, 269, 271–272
mechanisms, 263
paraneoplastic syndrome, 264–265
pathophysiology, 263
prevalence, 263
prophylaxis, 269–270
pulmonary embolism, 273–274
thrombocytopenia and VTEs, 273
upper extremity DVT, 273
Venous thrombosis, 33
Ventilatory control disorders, 401–403
Ventricular arrhythmias, 204–205
    torsades de pointes, 206–210
    ventricular fibrillation, 206
    ventricular premature complexes, 205
    ventricular tachycardia, 205–206
Ventricular fibrillation, 206
Ventricular premature complexes, 205
Ventricular tachycardia (VT), 200, 205–206
Vinca alkaloids, 6
Visceral pericardium, 244
Vitamin K antagonists (VKA), 34–36
Vorinostat, 8
VSPi-induced hypertension, 335
VT. *See* Ventricular tachycardia

W

Wall motion abnormalities, 239
Weaning patients from mechanical ventilation, 406
Wolff–Parkinson–White syndrome, 200–201

Y

Y90 ibritumomab tiuxetan (Zevalin), 6, 7